FREE Study Skills Videos/L

Dear Customer,

Thank you for your purchase from Mometrix! We consider it an honor and a privilege that you have purchased our product and we want to ensure your satisfaction.

As part of our ongoing effort to meet the needs of test takers, we have developed a set of Study Skills Videos that we would like to give you for <u>FREE</u>. These videos cover our *best practices* for getting ready for your exam, from how to use our study materials to how to best prepare for the day of the test.

All that we ask is that you email us with feedback that would describe your experience so far with our product. Good, bad, or indifferent, we want to know what you think!

To get your FREE Study Skills Videos, you can use the **QR code** below, or send us an **email** at <u>studyvideos@mometrix.com</u> with *FREE VIDEOS* in the subject line and the following information in the body of the email:

- The name of the product you purchased.
- Your product rating on a scale of 1-5, with 5 being the highest rating.
- Your feedback. It can be long, short, or anything in between. We just want to know your impressions and experience so far with our product. (Good feedback might include how our study material met your needs and ways we might be able to make it even better. You could highlight features that you found helpful or features that you think we should add.)

If you have any questions or concerns, please don't hesitate to contact me directly.

Thanks again!

Sincerely,

Jay Willis
Vice President
<u>jay.willis@mometrix.com</u>
1-800-673-8175

SCAN HERE

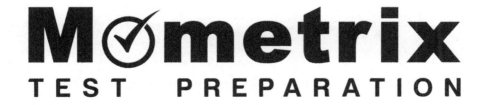

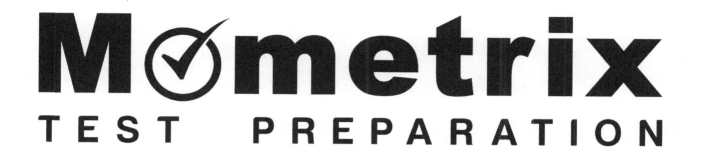

Advanced EMT

Exam Secrets
Study Guide

Exam Review and Practice Test for
the NREMT Advanced EMT Test

Written and edited by Mometrix Test Prep

Printed in the United States of America

This paper meets the requirements of ANSI/NISO Z39.48-1992 (Permanence of Paper).

Mometrix offers volume discount pricing to institutions. For more information or a price quote, please contact our sales department at sales@mometrix.com or 888-248-1219.

Mometrix Media LLC is not affiliated with or endorsed by any official testing organization. All organizational and test names are trademarks of their respective owners.

Paperback
ISBN 13: 978-1-5167-1433-9
ISBN 10: 1-5167-1433-4

DEAR FUTURE EXAM SUCCESS STORY

First of all, **THANK YOU** for purchasing Mometrix study materials!

Second, congratulations! You are one of the few determined test-takers who are committed to doing whatever it takes to excel on your exam. **You have come to the right place.** We developed these study materials with one goal in mind: to deliver you the information you need in a format that's concise and easy to use.

In addition to optimizing your guide for the content of the test, we've outlined our recommended steps for breaking down the preparation process into small, attainable goals so you can make sure you stay on track.

We've also analyzed the entire test-taking process, identifying the most common pitfalls and showing how you can overcome them and be ready for any curveball the test throws you.

Standardized testing is one of the biggest obstacles on your road to success, which only increases the importance of doing well in the high-pressure, high-stakes environment of test day. Your results on this test could have a significant impact on your future, and this guide provides the information and practical advice to help you achieve your full potential on test day.

Your success is our success

We would love to hear from you! If you would like to share the story of your exam success or if you have any questions or comments in regard to our products, please contact us at **800-673-8175** or **support@mometrix.com**.

Thanks again for your business and we wish you continued success!

Sincerely,
The Mometrix Test Preparation Team

Need more help? Check out our flashcards at:
http://MometrixFlashcards.com/EMT

TABLE OF CONTENTS

Introduction

Thank you for purchasing this resource! You have made the choice to prepare yourself for a test that could have a huge impact on your future, and this guide is designed to help you be fully ready for test day. Obviously, it's important to have a solid understanding of the test material, but you also need to be prepared for the unique environment and stressors of the test, so that you can perform to the best of your abilities.

For this purpose, the first section that appears in this guide is the **Secret Keys**. We've devoted countless hours to meticulously researching what works and what doesn't, and we've boiled down our findings to the five most impactful steps you can take to improve your performance on the test. We start at the beginning with study planning and move through the preparation process, all the way to the testing strategies that will help you get the most out of what you know when you're finally sitting in front of the test.

We recommend that you start preparing for your test as far in advance as possible. However, if you've bought this guide as a last-minute study resource and only have a few days before your test, we recommend that you skip over the first two Secret Keys since they address a long-term study plan.

If you struggle with **test anxiety**, we strongly encourage you to check out our recommendations for how you can overcome it. Test anxiety is a formidable foe, but it can be beaten, and we want to make sure you have the tools you need to defeat it.

1

Secret Key #1 – Plan Big, Study Small

There's a lot riding on your performance. If you want to ace this test, you're going to need to keep your skills sharp and the material fresh in your mind. You need a plan that lets you review everything you need to know while still fitting in your schedule. We'll break this strategy down into three categories.

Information Organization

Start with the information you already have: the official test outline. From this, you can make a complete list of all the concepts you need to cover before the test. Organize these concepts into groups that can be studied together, and create a list of any related vocabulary you need to learn so you can brush up on any difficult terms. You'll want to keep this vocabulary list handy once you actually start studying since you may need to add to it along the way.

Time Management

Once you have your set of study concepts, decide how to spread them out over the time you have left before the test. Break your study plan into small, clear goals so you have a manageable task for each day and know exactly what you're doing. Then just focus on one small step at a time. When you manage your time this way, you don't need to spend hours at a time studying. Studying a small block of content for a short period each day helps you retain information better and avoid stressing over how much you have left to do. You can relax knowing that you have a plan to cover everything in time. In order for this strategy to be effective though, you have to start studying early and stick to your schedule. Avoid the exhaustion and futility that comes from last-minute cramming!

Study Environment

The environment you study in has a big impact on your learning. Studying in a coffee shop, while probably more enjoyable, is not likely to be as fruitful as studying in a quiet room. It's important to keep distractions to a minimum. You're only planning to study for a short block of time, so make the most of it. Don't pause to check your phone or get up to find a snack. It's also important to **avoid multitasking**. Research has consistently shown that multitasking will make your studying dramatically less effective. Your study area should also be comfortable and well-lit so you don't have the distraction of straining your eyes or sitting on an uncomfortable chair.

 The time of day you study is also important. You want to be rested and alert. Don't wait until just before bedtime. Study when you'll be most likely to comprehend and remember. Even better, if you know what time of day your test will be, set that time aside for study. That way your brain will be used to working on that subject at that specific time and you'll have a better chance of recalling information.

Finally, it can be helpful to team up with others who are studying for the same test. Your actual studying should be done in as isolated an environment as possible, but the work of organizing the information and setting up the study plan can be divided up. In between study sessions, you can discuss with your teammates the concepts that you're all studying and quiz each other on the details. Just be sure that your teammates are as serious about the test as you are. If you find that your study time is being replaced with social time, you might need to find a new team.

2

Secret Key #2 – Make Your Studying Count

You're devoting a lot of time and effort to preparing for this test, so you want to be absolutely certain it will pay off. This means doing more than just reading the content and hoping you can remember it on test day. It's important to make every minute of study count. There are two main areas you can focus on to make your studying count.

Retention

It doesn't matter how much time you study if you can't remember the material. You need to make sure you are retaining the concepts. To check your retention of the information you're learning, try recalling it at later times with minimal prompting. Try carrying around flashcards and glance at one or two from time to time or ask a friend who's also studying for the test to quiz you.

To enhance your retention, look for ways to put the information into practice so that you can apply it rather than simply recalling it. If you're using the information in practical ways, it will be much easier to remember. Similarly, it helps to solidify a concept in your mind if you're not only reading it to yourself but also explaining it to someone else. Ask a friend to let you teach them about a concept you're a little shaky on (or speak aloud to an imaginary audience if necessary). As you try to summarize, define, give examples, and answer your friend's questions, you'll understand the concepts better and they will stay with you longer. Finally, step back for a big picture view and ask yourself how each piece of information fits with the whole subject. When you link the different concepts together and see them working together as a whole, it's easier to remember the individual components.

Finally, practice showing your work on any multi-step problems, even if you're just studying. Writing out each step you take to solve a problem will help solidify the process in your mind, and you'll be more likely to remember it during the test.

Modality

Modality simply refers to the means or method by which you study. Choosing a study modality that fits your own individual learning style is crucial. No two people learn best in exactly the same way, so it's important to know your strengths and use them to your advantage.

For example, if you learn best by visualization, focus on visualizing a concept in your mind and draw an image or a diagram. Try color-coding your notes, illustrating them, or creating symbols that will trigger your mind to recall a learned concept. If you learn best by hearing or discussing information, find a study partner who learns the same way or read aloud to yourself. Think about how to put the information in your own words. Imagine that you are giving a lecture on the topic and record yourself so you can listen to it later.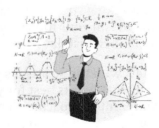

For any learning style, flashcards can be helpful. Organize the information so you can take advantage of spare moments to review. Underline key words or phrases. Use different colors for different categories. Mnemonic devices (such as creating a short list in which every item starts with the same letter) can also help with retention. Find what works best for you and use it to store the information in your mind most effectively and easily.

3

Secret Key #3 – Practice the Right Way

Your success on test day depends not only on how many hours you put into preparing, but also on whether you prepared the right way. It's good to check along the way to see if your studying is paying off. One of the most effective ways to do this is by taking practice tests to evaluate your progress. Practice tests are useful because they show exactly where you need to improve. Every time you take a practice test, pay special attention to these three groups of questions:

- The questions you got wrong
- The questions you had to guess on, even if you guessed right
- The questions you found difficult or slow to work through

This will show you exactly what your weak areas are, and where you need to devote more study time. Ask yourself why each of these questions gave you trouble. Was it because you didn't understand the material? Was it because you didn't remember the vocabulary? Do you need more repetitions on this type of question to build speed and confidence? Dig into those questions and figure out how you can strengthen your weak areas as you go back to review the material.

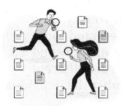 Additionally, many practice tests have a section explaining the answer choices. It can be tempting to read the explanation and think that you now have a good understanding of the concept. However, an explanation likely only covers part of the question's broader context. Even if the explanation makes perfect sense, **go back and investigate** every concept related to the question until you're positive you have a thorough understanding.

As you go along, keep in mind that the practice test is just that: practice. Memorizing these questions and answers will not be very helpful on the actual test because it is unlikely to have any of the same exact questions. If you only know the right answers to the sample questions, you won't be prepared for the real thing. **Study the concepts** until you understand them fully, and then you'll be able to answer any question that shows up on the test.

It's important to wait on the practice tests until you're ready. If you take a test on your first day of study, you may be overwhelmed by the amount of material covered and how much you need to learn. Work up to it gradually.

On test day, you'll need to be prepared for answering questions, managing your time, and using the test-taking strategies you've learned. It's a lot to balance, like a mental marathon that will have a big impact on your future. Like training for a marathon, you'll need to start slowly and work your way up. When test day arrives, you'll be ready.

Start with the strategies you've read in the first two Secret Keys—plan your course and study in the way that works best for you. If you have time, consider using multiple study resources to get different approaches to the same concepts. It can be helpful to see difficult concepts from more than one angle. Then find a good source for practice tests. Many times, the test website will suggest potential study resources or provide sample tests.

Practice Test Strategy

If you're able to find at least three practice tests, we recommend this strategy:

UNTIMED AND OPEN-BOOK PRACTICE

Take the first test with no time constraints and with your notes and study guide handy. Take your time and focus on applying the strategies you've learned.

TIMED AND OPEN-BOOK PRACTICE

Take the second practice test open-book as well, but set a timer and practice pacing yourself to finish in time.

TIMED AND CLOSED-BOOK PRACTICE

Take any other practice tests as if it were test day. Set a timer and put away your study materials. Sit at a table or desk in a quiet room, imagine yourself at the testing center, and answer questions as quickly and accurately as possible.

Keep repeating timed and closed-book tests on a regular basis until you run out of practice tests or it's time for the actual test. Your mind will be ready for the schedule and stress of test day, and you'll be able to focus on recalling the material you've learned.

Secret Key #4 – Pace Yourself

Once you're fully prepared for the material on the test, your biggest challenge on test day will be managing your time. Just knowing that the clock is ticking can make you panic even if you have plenty of time left. Work on pacing yourself so you can build confidence against the time constraints of the exam. Pacing is a difficult skill to master, especially in a high-pressure environment, so **practice is vital**.

Set time expectations for your pace based on how much time is available. For example, if a section has 60 questions and the time limit is 30 minutes, you know you have to average 30 seconds or less per question in order to answer them all. Although 30 seconds is the hard limit, set 25 seconds per question as your goal, so you reserve extra time to spend on harder questions. When you budget extra time for the harder questions, you no longer have any reason to stress when those questions take longer to answer.

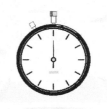

Don't let this time expectation distract you from working through the test at a calm, steady pace, but keep it in mind so you don't spend too much time on any one question. Recognize that taking extra time on one question you don't understand may keep you from answering two that you do understand later in the test. If your time limit for a question is up and you're still not sure of the answer, mark it and move on, and come back to it later if the time and the test format allow. If the testing format doesn't allow you to return to earlier questions, just make an educated guess; then put it out of your mind and move on.

On the easier questions, be careful not to rush. It may seem wise to hurry through them so you have more time for the challenging ones, but it's not worth missing one if you know the concept and just didn't take the time to read the question fully. Work efficiently but make sure you understand the question and have looked at all of the answer choices, since more than one may seem right at first.

Even if you're paying attention to the time, you may find yourself a little behind at some point. You should speed up to get back on track, but do so wisely. Don't panic; just take a few seconds less on each question until you're caught up. Don't guess without thinking, but do look through the answer choices and eliminate any you know are wrong. If you can get down to two choices, it is often worthwhile to guess from those. Once you've chosen an answer, move on and don't dwell on any that you skipped or had to hurry through. If a question was taking too long, chances are it was one of the harder ones, so you weren't as likely to get it right anyway.

On the other hand, if you find yourself getting ahead of schedule, it may be beneficial to slow down a little. The more quickly you work, the more likely you are to make a careless mistake that will affect your score. You've budgeted time for each question, so don't be afraid to spend that time. Practice an efficient but careful pace to get the most out of the time you have.

Secret Key #5 – Have a Plan for Guessing

When you're taking the test, you may find yourself stuck on a question. Some of the answer choices seem better than others, but you don't see the one answer choice that is obviously correct. What do you do?

The scenario described above is very common, yet most test takers have not effectively prepared for it. Developing and practicing a plan for guessing may be one of the single most effective uses of your time as you get ready for the exam.

In developing your plan for guessing, there are three questions to address:

- When should you start the guessing process?
- How should you narrow down the choices?
- Which answer should you choose?

When to Start the Guessing Process

Unless your plan for guessing is to select C every time (which, despite its merits, is not what we recommend), you need to leave yourself enough time to apply your answer elimination strategies. Since you have a limited amount of time for each question, that means that if you're going to give yourself the best shot at guessing correctly, you have to decide quickly whether or not you will guess.

Of course, the best-case scenario is that you don't have to guess at all, so first, see if you can answer the question based on your knowledge of the subject and basic reasoning skills. Focus on the key words in the question and try to jog your memory of related topics. Give yourself a chance to bring the knowledge to mind, but once you realize that you don't have (or you can't access) the knowledge you need to answer the question, it's time to start the guessing process.

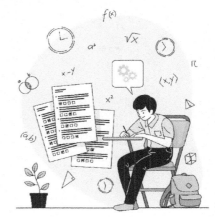

It's almost always better to start the guessing process too early than too late. It only takes a few seconds to remember something and answer the question from knowledge. Carefully eliminating wrong answer choices takes longer. Plus, going through the process of eliminating answer choices can actually help jog your memory.

Summary: Start the guessing process as soon as you decide that you can't answer the question based on your knowledge.

How to Narrow Down the Choices

The next chapter in this book (**Test-Taking Strategies**) includes a wide range of strategies for how to approach questions and how to look for answer choices to eliminate. You will definitely want to read those carefully, practice them, and figure out which ones work best for you. Here though, we're going to address a mindset rather than a particular strategy.

Your odds of guessing an answer correctly depend on how many options you are choosing from.

Number of options left	5	4	3	2	1
Odds of guessing correctly	20%	25%	33%	50%	100%

You can see from this chart just how valuable it is to be able to eliminate incorrect answers and make an educated guess, but there are two things that many test takers do that cause them to miss out on the benefits of guessing:

- Accidentally eliminating the correct answer
- Selecting an answer based on an impression

We'll look at the first one here, and the second one in the next section.

To avoid accidentally eliminating the correct answer, we recommend a thought exercise called **the $5 challenge**. In this challenge, you only eliminate an answer choice from contention if you are willing to bet $5 on it being wrong. Why $5? Five dollars is a small but not insignificant amount of money. It's an amount you could afford to lose but wouldn't want to throw away. And while losing

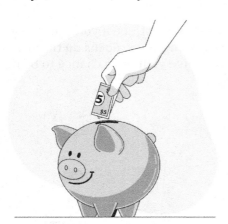

$5 once might not hurt too much, doing it twenty times will set you back $100. In the same way, each small decision you make—eliminating a choice here, guessing on a question there—won't by itself impact your score very much, but when you put them all together, they can make a big difference. By holding each answer choice elimination decision to a higher standard, you can reduce the risk of accidentally eliminating the correct answer.

The $5 challenge can also be applied in a positive sense: If you are willing to bet $5 that an answer choice *is* correct, go ahead and mark it as correct.

Summary: Only eliminate an answer choice if you are willing to bet $5 that it is wrong.

Which Answer to Choose

You're taking the test. You've run into a hard question and decided you'll have to guess. You've eliminated all the answer choices you're willing to bet $5 on. Now you have to pick an answer. Why do we even need to talk about this? Why can't you just pick whichever one you feel like when the time comes?

The answer to these questions is that if you don't come into the test with a plan, you'll rely on your impression to select an answer choice, and if you do that, you risk falling into a trap. The test writers know that everyone who takes their test will be guessing on some of the questions, so they intentionally write wrong answer choices to seem plausible. You still have to pick an answer though, and if the wrong answer choices are designed to look right, how can you ever be sure that you're not falling for their trap? The best solution we've found to this dilemma is to take the decision out of your hands entirely. Here is the process we recommend:

Once you've eliminated any choices that you are confident (willing to bet $5) are wrong, select the first remaining choice as your answer.

Whether you choose to select the first remaining choice, the second, or the last, the important thing is that you use some preselected standard. Using this approach guarantees that you will not be enticed into selecting an answer choice that looks right, because you are not basing your decision on how the answer choices look.

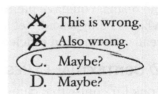

This is not meant to make you question your knowledge. Instead, it is to help you recognize the difference between your knowledge and your impressions. There's a huge difference between thinking an answer is right because of what you know, and thinking an answer is right because it looks or sounds like it should be right.

Summary: To ensure that your selection is appropriately random, make a predetermined selection from among all answer choices you have not eliminated.

Test-Taking Strategies

This section contains a list of test-taking strategies that you may find helpful as you work through the test. By taking what you know and applying logical thought, you can maximize your chances of answering any question correctly!

It is very important to realize that every question is different and every person is different: no single strategy will work on every question, and no single strategy will work for every person. That's why we've included all of them here, so you can try them out and determine which ones work best for different types of questions and which ones work best for you.

Question Strategies

☑ READ CAREFULLY

Read the question and the answer choices carefully. Don't miss the question because you misread the terms. You have plenty of time to read each question thoroughly and make sure you understand what is being asked. Yet a happy medium must be attained, so don't waste too much time. You must read carefully and efficiently.

☑ CONTEXTUAL CLUES

Look for contextual clues. If the question includes a word you are not familiar with, look at the immediate context for some indication of what the word might mean. Contextual clues can often give you all the information you need to decipher the meaning of an unfamiliar word. Even if you can't determine the meaning, you may be able to narrow down the possibilities enough to make a solid guess at the answer to the question.

☑ PREFIXES

If you're having trouble with a word in the question or answer choices, try dissecting it. Take advantage of every clue that the word might include. Prefixes can be a huge help. Usually, they allow you to determine a basic meaning. *Pre-* means before, *post-* means after, *pro-* is positive, *de-* is negative. From prefixes, you can get an idea of the general meaning of the word and try to put it into context.

☑ HEDGE WORDS

Watch out for critical hedge words, such as *likely, may, can, sometimes, often, almost, mostly, usually, generally, rarely,* and *sometimes.* Question writers insert these hedge phrases to cover every possibility. Often an answer choice will be wrong simply because it leaves no room for exception. Be on guard for answer choices that have definitive words such as *exactly* and *always.*

☑ SWITCHBACK WORDS

Stay alert for *switchbacks.* These are the words and phrases frequently used to alert you to shifts in thought. The most common switchback words are *but, although,* and *however.* Others include *nevertheless, on the other hand, even though, while, in spite of, despite,* and *regardless of.* Switchback words are important to catch because they can change the direction of the question or an answer choice.

⊘ Face Value

When in doubt, use common sense. Accept the situation in the problem at face value. Don't read too much into it. These problems will not require you to make wild assumptions. If you have to go beyond creativity and warp time or space in order to have an answer choice fit the question, then you should move on and consider the other answer choices. These are normal problems rooted in reality. The applicable relationship or explanation may not be readily apparent, but it is there for you to figure out. Use your common sense to interpret anything that isn't clear.

Answer Choice Strategies

⊘ Answer Selection

The most thorough way to pick an answer choice is to identify and eliminate wrong answers until only one is left, then confirm it is the correct answer. Sometimes an answer choice may immediately seem right, but be careful. The test writers will usually put more than one reasonable answer choice on each question, so take a second to read all of them and make sure that the other choices are not equally obvious. As long as you have time left, it is better to read every answer choice than to pick the first one that looks right without checking the others.

⊘ Answer Choice Families

An answer choice family consists of two (in rare cases, three) answer choices that are very similar in construction and cannot all be true at the same time. If you see two answer choices that are direct opposites or parallels, one of them is usually the correct answer. For instance, if one answer choice says that quantity x increases and another either says that quantity x decreases (opposite) or says that quantity y increases (parallel), then those answer choices would fall into the same family. An answer choice that doesn't match the construction of the answer choice family is more likely to be incorrect. Most questions will not have answer choice families, but when they do appear, you should be prepared to recognize them.

⊘ Eliminate Answers

Eliminate answer choices as soon as you realize they are wrong, but make sure you consider all possibilities. If you are eliminating answer choices and realize that the last one you are left with is also wrong, don't panic. Start over and consider each choice again. There may be something you missed the first time that you will realize on the second pass.

⊘ Avoid Fact Traps

Don't be distracted by an answer choice that is factually true but doesn't answer the question. You are looking for the choice that answers the question. Stay focused on what the question is asking for so you don't accidentally pick an answer that is true but incorrect. Always go back to the question and make sure the answer choice you've selected actually answers the question and is not merely a true statement.

⊘ Extreme Statements

In general, you should avoid answers that put forth extreme actions as standard practice or proclaim controversial ideas as established fact. An answer choice that states the "process should be used in certain situations, if…" is much more likely to be correct than one that states the "process should be discontinued completely." The first is a calm rational statement and doesn't even make a definitive, uncompromising stance, using a hedge word *if* to provide wiggle room, whereas the second choice is far more extreme.

⊘ BENCHMARK

As you read through the answer choices and you come across one that seems to answer the question well, mentally select that answer choice. This is not your final answer, but it's the one that will help you evaluate the other answer choices. The one that you selected is your benchmark or standard for judging each of the other answer choices. Every other answer choice must be compared to your benchmark. That choice is correct until proven otherwise by another answer choice beating it. If you find a better answer, then that one becomes your new benchmark. Once you've decided that no other choice answers the question as well as your benchmark, you have your final answer.

⊘ PREDICT THE ANSWER

Before you even start looking at the answer choices, it is often best to try to predict the answer. When you come up with the answer on your own, it is easier to avoid distractions and traps because you will know exactly what to look for. The right answer choice is unlikely to be word-for-word what you came up with, but it should be a close match. Even if you are confident that you have the right answer, you should still take the time to read each option before moving on.

General Strategies

⊘ TOUGH QUESTIONS

If you are stumped on a problem or it appears too hard or too difficult, don't waste time. Move on! Remember though, if you can quickly check for obviously incorrect answer choices, your chances of guessing correctly are greatly improved. Before you completely give up, at least try to knock out a couple of possible answers. Eliminate what you can and then guess at the remaining answer choices before moving on.

⊘ CHECK YOUR WORK

Since you will probably not know every term listed and the answer to every question, it is important that you get credit for the ones that you do know. Don't miss any questions through careless mistakes. If at all possible, try to take a second to look back over your answer selection and make sure you've selected the correct answer choice and haven't made a costly careless mistake (such as marking an answer choice that you didn't mean to mark). This quick double check should more than pay for itself in caught mistakes for the time it costs.

⊘ PACE YOURSELF

It's easy to be overwhelmed when you're looking at a page full of questions; your mind is confused and full of random thoughts, and the clock is ticking down faster than you would like. Calm down and maintain the pace that you have set for yourself. Especially as you get down to the last few minutes of the test, don't let the small numbers on the clock make you panic. As long as you are on track by monitoring your pace, you are guaranteed to have time for each question.

⊘ DON'T RUSH

It is very easy to make errors when you are in a hurry. Maintaining a fast pace in answering questions is pointless if it makes you miss questions that you would have gotten right otherwise. Test writers like to include distracting information and wrong answers that seem right. Taking a little extra time to avoid careless mistakes can make all the difference in your test score. Find a pace that allows you to be confident in the answers that you select.

⊘ Keep Moving

Panicking will not help you pass the test, so do your best to stay calm and keep moving. Taking deep breaths and going through the answer elimination steps you practiced can help to break through a stress barrier and keep your pace.

Final Notes

The combination of a solid foundation of content knowledge and the confidence that comes from practicing your plan for applying that knowledge is the key to maximizing your performance on test day. As your foundation of content knowledge is built up and strengthened, you'll find that the strategies included in this chapter become more and more effective in helping you quickly sift through the distractions and traps of the test to isolate the correct answer.

Now that you're preparing to move forward into the test content chapters of this book, be sure to keep your goal in mind. As you read, think about how you will be able to apply this information on the test. If you've already seen sample questions for the test and you have an idea of the question format and style, try to come up with questions of your own that you can answer based on what you're reading. This will give you valuable practice applying your knowledge in the same ways you can expect to on test day.

Good luck and good studying!

A Note About EMT Interventions

Each EMS certification level has a specific scope of practice that dictates which interventions a certification holder may perform in the course of their job. An individual with an EMR certification is not permitted to perform all of the same interventions that an individual with an EMT certification may. Similarly, an Advanced EMT certification authorizes an individual to perform interventions that neither an EMT nor an EMR certification would allow.

As you read through this study guide, you will notice that we frequently provide information about all of the interventions that may be performed for a given emergency, not just those that are appropriate for this level of certification. Even though you may not be authorized to perform all of these interventions, we believe it will be helpful for you to be aware that they exist, as you may find yourself working with others in the EMS community with a higher level of certification, and knowing about what they are permitted to do may help you respond more effectively in a given situation. **You should never attempt to perform any intervention that is outside the scope of practice for your certification.**

As you continue your journey toward certification, we at Mometrix applaud you for your desire to serve your community in this way. Best of luck in your studying!

Foundational Knowledge and Skills

Medical Terminology

BODY PLANES AND ANATOMIC TERMS

Body planes include the following:

- **Sagittal/Lateral**: Vertical plane separating right from left
- **Median/Midsagittal**: Sagittal plane at the midline (middle) separating the body into equal halves
- **Coronal/Frontal**: Vertical plane separating anterior (front) from posterior (back)
- **Axial/Transverse**: Horizontal plane that separates the body into superior (upper) and inferior (lower) parts

A **cross section** is an axial/transverse (horizontal) cut through a tissue specimen or body structure, whereas a **longitudinal section** is a sagittal or coronal (vertical) cut. **Medial** is toward the midline, whereas **lateral** is away from the midline and to the side. **Distal** is farther from the point of reference, and **proximal** is closer. When describing an area of the patient's body, the description should be patient oriented, using phrases such as "patient's left" and "patient's right" to ensure accurate interpretation.

Body planes and anatomic terms

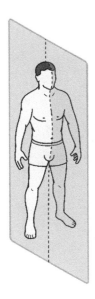 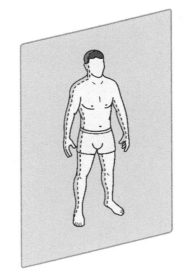 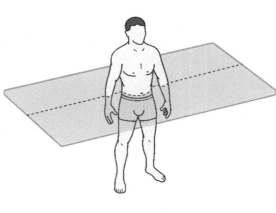

Sagittal/Lateral   Coronal/Frontal   Axial/Transverse

15

COMMON MEDICAL PREFIXES

Term	Meaning	Examples
Cardio-	Heart	Cardiovascular (heart and vessels), cardiology (study of the heart)
Neuro-	Nerves	Neurology (study of the nerves), neuron (nerve cell)
Hyper-	Enlarged, excessive, high	Hypertrophy (enlarged tissue), hyperemesis (excessive vomiting), hyperactive (overactive), hypertension (high BP)
Hypo-	Under, beneath, low	Hypoglycemia (low blood sugar), hypotension (low BP), hypoxia (low oxygen)
Naso-	Nose	Nasopharyngeal (nose and throat), nasal (referring to the nose)
Oro-	Mouth	Oropharyngeal (mouth and throat), oral (referring to the mouth)
Arterio-	Artery	Arteriovenous (artery and vein), arterial (referring to arteries)
Hemo- Hemato-	Blood	Hemolysis (breakdown of blood), hemoglobin (blood component), hematology (study of blood)
Therm-	Temperature	Thermoregulation (temperature regulation), thermometer (temperature measurement)
Vaso-	Vessels	Vasoconstriction (narrowing of vessels), vasodilation (widening of vessels)
Tachy-	Rapid	Tachycardia (rapid heart rate), tachypnea (rapid respirations)
Brady-	Slow	Bradycardia (slow heart rate), bradypnea (slow respirations)

Pharmacology

FIVE RIGHTS OF MEDICATION ADMINISTRATION

The EMS provider may assist patients to self-administer medications or administer them directly depending on the scope of practice and protocols. Medical direction may be offline, which means standing orders are available to treat specific conditions or written protocols have been established that must be followed. Online medical direction requires verbal contact with a medical director. When receiving an online medication order, the EMS provider should use the echo (read-back) technique (repeating back the orders to ensure that they were understood correctly) and clarify any orders that are confusing or unclear.

The **five rights of medication administration** include the following:

1. **Right patient**: Prescribed specifically for that patient
2. **Right medication**: Correct choice for the patient's condition and matches the prescription
3. **Right route**: Appropriate for the patient's condition, enteral or parenteral
4. **Right dose**: As prescribed and appropriate for the patient's age, weight, and condition
5. **Right time**: Medication not expired, is administered at the time ordered (e.g., "stat" (immediately) or "every 5 minutes × 3")

> **Review Video: Top 5 Pharmacology Review Mnemonics**
> Visit mometrix.com/academy and enter code: 119193

PRINCIPLES OF PHARMACOKINETICS

Pharmacokinetics relates to the route of administration, the absorption, the dosage, the frequency of administration, the distribution, and the serum levels achieved over time.

- The **drug's rate of clearance (elimination)** and **doses needed** to ensure therapeutic benefit are considered. Most drugs are cleared through the kidneys, with water-soluble compounds excreted more readily than protein-soluble compounds.
- **Volume of distribution** (IV drug dose divided by plasma concentration) determines the rate at which the drug passes into tissue. Drug distribution depends on the degree of protein binding and ion trapping that takes place.
- **Elimination half-life** is the time needed for the concentration of a particular drug to decrease to half of its starting dose in the body. Approximately five half-lives are needed to achieve steady-state plasma concentrations if giving doses intermittently.
- **Context-sensitive half-life** is the time needed to reach 50% concentration after withdrawal of a continuously-administered drug.
- **Recovery time** is the length of time it takes for plasma levels to decrease to the point that the effect is eliminated. This is affected by plasma concentration.
- **Effect-site equilibrium** is the time between administration of a drug and clinical effect (the point at which the drug reaches the appropriate receptors) and must be considered when determining dose, time, and frequency of medications.
- The **bioavailability** of drugs may vary, depending upon the degree of metabolism that takes place before the drug reaches its site of action.

FIRST PASS METABOLISM AND DRUG CLEARANCE

First pass metabolism is the phenomenon that occurs to ingested drugs that are absorbed through the gastrointestinal tract and enter the hepatic portal system. Drugs metabolized on the first pass travel to the liver, where they are broken down, some to the extent that only a small fraction of the active drug circulates to the rest of the body. This first pass through the liver greatly reduces the bioavailability of some drugs. Routes of administration that avoid first pass metabolism include intravenous, intramuscular, and sublingual.

Drug clearance refers to the ability to remove a drug from the body. The two main organs responsible for clearance are the liver and the kidneys. The liver eliminates drugs by metabolizing, or biotransforming the substance, or excreting the drug in the bile. The kidneys eliminate drugs by filtration or active excretion in the urine. Drugs use either renal or hepatic methods of clearance. Kidney and liver dysfunction inhibit the clearance of drugs that rely on that organ for removal. Toxicity results from poor clearance.

ENTEROHEPATICALLY RECIRCULATED DRUGS AND RENALLY-EXCRETED DRUGS

Enterohepatically recirculated drugs are effectively removed from circulation and then reabsorbed. These drugs are secreted in bile, which is collected in the gall bladder and emptied into the small intestine, from which part of it is reabsorbed and part is excreted in the feces. This reabsorption reduces the clearance of these drugs and increases their duration of action. Generally, drugs susceptible to enterohepatic recirculation are those with a molecular weight greater than 300g/mole and those that are amphipathic (have both a lipophilic portion and a polar portion).

Renally-excreted drugs are metabolized (biotransformed) by the liver to a form that can be excreted by the kidneys. Others are excreted by the kidneys unchanged. Infants with decreased renal function demonstrate decreased urine output or elevated levels of BUN and creatinine. The EMT should avoid using drugs that depend on the kidneys for clearance if the infant has renal impairment as overdose may result.

ABSORPTION IN RELATION TO ROUTES OF MEDICATION ADMINISTRATION

The absorption rate of a drug depends on its transfer from its site of administration to the circulatory system. Different **routes of administration** have different absorption characteristics:

- **Oral**: Ingested medications pass from the gastrointestinal tract into the blood stream. Most absorption occurs in the small intestine and is affected by gastric motility and emptying rate, drug solubility in gastrointestinal fluids, and food presence. Orally administered drugs are susceptible to first pass metabolism by the liver.
- **Intravenous**: Medications directly administered to the blood stream have 100% absorption. Peak serum levels are rapidly achieved. Some drugs are not tolerated intravenously, due to vein irritation or toxicity, and others must be given as an infusion.
- **Intramuscular**: Medications injected into a muscle are fairly rapidly absorbed because muscle tissue is highly vascularized. Drugs in lipid vehicles absorb more slowly than those in aqueous vehicles.
- **Subcutaneous**: Medications injected beneath the skin absorb more slowly because the dermis is less vascularized than muscle. Hypoperfusion and edema decrease absorption further.

DRUG CLASSIFICATION

The following are different ways to classify drugs:

- **Therapeutic classification**: The common uses for the drug will place it in a certain therapeutic classification.
- **Pharmacological classification**: The action of the drug determines which pharmacological category a drug will be in.

All drugs have a **chemical name** and a simpler **generic name**. A company making the drug can give it a trade or **brand name**. The generic form of a drug is generally cheaper but may differ in efficacy from a brand name drug due to a difference in the amount of drug that is absorbed for use in the body. The Controlled Substances Act restricts usage of certain drugs and classifies them according to schedules that include:

- **Schedule I**: Ecstasy, LSD, marijuana, peyote, mescaline, psilocybin, heroin, and others.
- **Schedule II**: Amphetamine, cocaine, codeine, fentanyl, Dilaudid, Demerol, Ritalin, morphine, opium, and others.
- **Schedule III**: Anabolic steroids, barbiturates, codeine, Vicodin, pentothal.
- **Schedule IV**: Xanax, Librium, Klonopin, Tranxene, Redux, Darvocet, Valium, Ativan, Versed, phenobarbital, Restoril, Sonata, Ambien.
- **Schedule V**: Lomotil and others.

BLOOD DRUG LEVELS

Plasma drug levels are used for **therapeutic drug monitoring** because, although plasma is often not the site of action, plasma levels correlate well with therapeutic (effective) and toxic (dose-related adverse effects) responses to most drugs. The therapeutic range of a drug is that between the minimum effective concentration (level at which there is no therapeutic benefit) and the toxic concentration (level at which toxic effects occur). To achieve drug plateau (steady state), the drug half-life (time needed to decrease drug concentration by 50%) must be considered. Most drugs reach plateau with administration equal to four half-lives and completely eliminate a drug in 5 half-lives. Because drug levels fluctuate, peak (highest drug concentration) and trough (lowest drug concentration) levels may be monitored. Samples for trough levels are taken immediately prior to administration of another dose while peak samples are taken at various times, depending on the average peak time of the specific drug, which may vary from 30 minutes to 2 hours or so after administration.

SIDE EFFECTS OF MEDICATIONS

All drugs can have **side effects** and some are toxic at certain levels or in combination with other drugs. Some side effects will be minor and may go away after a week or two. Others can be severe or life threatening, such as anaphylaxis. Common side effects include nausea, vomiting, diarrhea, and rashes. Side effects may vary with individuals according to age, gender, and condition and may be related to non-compliance with treatment, incorrect dosage, poly-pharmacy, or drug interactions. Drug compendiums will list all possible side effects according to system or incidence. Pharmacologically similar medications usually have some common side effects among the drugs in that class. EMT actions include:

- Always question the patient about allergies or previous drug reactions before administering medication if possible.
- Educate the patient about possible side effects of all medications.
- Watch out for drug-drug or food-drug combinations that are dangerous.

DRUG INTERACTIONS

Drug interactions occur when one drug interferes with the activity of another in either the pharmacodynamics or pharmacokinetics:

- With **pharmacodynamic interaction**, both drugs may interact at receptor sites causing a change that results in an adverse effect or that interferes with a positive effect.
- With **pharmacokinetic interaction**, the ability of the drug to be absorbed and cleared is altered, so there may be delayed effects, changes in effects, or toxicity. Interactions may include problems in a number of areas:
  - **Absorption** may be increased or (more commonly) decreased, usually related to the effects within the gastrointestinal system.
  - **Distribution** of drugs may be affected, often because of changes in protein binding.
  - **Metabolism** may be altered, often causing changes in drug concentration.
  - **Biotransformation** of the drug must take place, usually in the liver and gastrointestinal system, but drug interactions can impair this process.
  - **Clearance interactions** may interfere with the body's ability to eliminate a drug, usually resulting in an increased concentration of the drug.

SPECIFIC INTERACTIONS

Some drugs will either increase or inhibit the actions of other drugs. They may interfere with receptor-site binding or the way in which the drug is metabolized or excreted. Certain drugs may cause drowsiness when taken together or with alcohol. Some foods will inhibit drug action, such as the inhibition of warfarin by vitamin K-containing foods. Other foods may cause toxic levels of a drug to accumulate. Grapefruit juice, for example, is metabolized by the same enzyme that metabolizes about 50 drugs, including digoxin and statins. This can prevent the liver from breaking down drugs and lead to severe reactions. One should always obtain a complete medication list from the patient, including prescription and over-the-counter medications, herbals, vitamins, minerals, and dietary supplements that are taken regularly and occasionally. All medications taken should be checked for potential interactions with drugs or foods.

MEDICATION LEGISLATION

Legislation relevant to medications and medication administration include:

- **Pure Food and Drug Act (1906)**: Consumer protection act intended to prevent the manufacture, sale, and transportation of adulterated foods, drugs, and alcoholic beverages.
- **Federal Food, Drug, and Cosmetic Act (1938)**: Provides authority to the FDA to oversee food, drug, and cosmetic safety.
- **Harrison Narcotics Tax Act (1914)**: Provides authority for regulation and taxation of production, importation, and distribution of cocaine/opium products, such as narcotics.
- **Controlled Substances Act (1970)**: Establishes U.S. drug policy and five schedules under which drugs are classified. It is implemented by the DEA and the FDA.
- **Food and Drug Administration (FDA)**: Consumer protection agency that protects public health through the control and supervision of drugs, vaccines, blood transfusions, medical devices, cosmetics, foods, tobacco, and dietary supplements.
- **Drug Enforcement Agency (DEA)**: Law enforcement agency, part of the Department of Justice, enforces the Controlled Substances Act and combats drug smuggling and use.

NALOXONE FOR OPIOID OVERDOSE

Naloxone (Narcan) autoinjector contains a single dose of 2 mg naloxone in 0.4 mL solution and is delivered IM or SQ only. Naloxone autoinjector is used to treat suspected opioid overdose in adult and pediatric patients. Opioid overdose is characterized by lethargy, respiratory depression, sleepiness, pinpoint pupils, confusion, and non-responsiveness. The label contains printed directions, and the electronic voice instruction system guides the user as well. Procedure:

1. Remove red safety guard.
2. Administer into the anterolateral aspect of the thigh. May be administered through clothing if necessary. For infants under one year, pinch the thigh muscle before administering the medication.
3. Injections may be repeated every 2-3 minutes as needed with new devices.

Naloxone (Narcan) 4 mg nasal spray is used to treat opioid overdose in adults and pediatric patients. Procedure:

1. Open container and remove the device.
2. Place thumb on the plunger and 2 fingers on the nozzle.
3. Place the tip of the nozzle into one of the patient's nostrils until the fingers contact the patient's nose.
4. Depress the plunger. Additional doses may be given every 2-3 minutes using a new device each time.

AUTOINJECTORS FOR NERVE AGENT EXPOSURE

Autoinjectors are spring-loaded syringe/needle devices that contain preloaded doses of medication and can be easily administered by following the directions on the devices. Autoinjectors are available for nerve agent treatment for emergency medical personnel—Mark I and DuoDote.

- **Atropine autoinjector**: For symptoms of nerve damage (increases heart rate, dries secretions, dilates pupils, and reduces GI upset)
- **Pralidoxime (2-PAM chloride) autoinjector**: For symptoms of nerve damage, twitching, and difficulty breathing
- **Diazepam autoinjector**: For convulsions associated with nerve agents

Wear appropriate PPE, remove the safety cap, cleanse the skin with alcohol, and (holding the device perpendicular to the skin) apply firm pressure with the tip of the injector against the skin in the outer thigh until the device fires the needle into the muscle tissue (avoid jabbing). Then, hold the autoinjector in place for at least 10 seconds to ensure that the medication is completely injected. Carefully remove the needle from the skin. Avoid touching the needle, and do not attempt to recap it. Dispose of the intact device in a sharps container.

NEBULIZED, INHALED AND SUBLINGUAL ROUTES OF MEDICATION ADMINISTRATION

Nebulized medications are delivered with compressed air or high flow oxygen (6-8 L/min) to aerosolize the small volume of liquid into a mist. The patient breathes the aerosolized medication through a mouthpiece or a securely fitted mask. Nebulized medications, such as albuterol and steroids, are often given to patients with respiratory diseases, such as asthma and COPD. Nebulizers are often easier for patients to use than **inhaled medications** per a metered-dose-inhalers, especially if they are at all confused. Inhaled medications are provided per a metered-dose inhaler (MDI) that delivers a specific dose of aerosolized medication, but the patient must be able to coordinate breathing with the dose (puff) and to hold her breath for 10 seconds after delivery of the drug. For both nebulized and inhaled medications, patients should sit upright.

Mucosal/sublingual/buccal medications are usually provided in thin wafers that dissolve on contact with saliva. Sublingual medications are placed under the tongue and mucosal/buccal medications between the gums and the cheek. The medications are absorbed quickly into the bloodstream so dosage is often lower than other routes. Eating, drinking fluids, and smoking can affect absorption of the drugs.

METERED-DOSE INHALER (MIDI/MDI) AND THE SMALL-VOLUME NEBULIZER

The EMT may administer or assist the patient with use of a metered-dose inhaler (MIDI/MDI) or a small-volume nebulizer for medications such as albuterol, according to protocol, as follows:

- The **MIDI/MDI** is a pressurized cartridge that is used for the administration of a specific dose of an aerosolized medication. Shake the medication vigorously before use, prime if it is the initial use, position 4 cm (two finger widths) away from the patient's mouth or between the lips, have the patient exhale and breathe in slowly and completely while the MIDI is activated, and then have the patient hold his breath for 10 seconds, waiting 1 minute between puffs. Stop the treatment if the patient becomes shaky, dizzy, coughs uncontrollably, has palpitations, or has a pulse increase of ≥20 bpm. Resume slowly after 5-10 minutes.
- A **small-volume nebulizer** includes a nebulizer cup that holds 2-4 mL of medication, air tubing, a compressor to aerosolize the medication, and a T-piece and mouthpiece or face mask for delivery. Dilute the medication with sterile water or NS, not tap water, if necessary. Have the patient sit upright for treatment, breathing normally through the mouth, using the mouthpiece or face mask.

COMMONLY ADMINISTERED MEDICATIONS BY THE EMT

Medication	Dose/Route/Use	Side effects/Interactions
Aspirin	Orally, 325 mg, chew and swallow for fast action when having a heart attack.	Avoid with signs of stroke or gastrointestinal (GI) bleeding. Decreases clotting time and may increase the risk of bleeding.
Glucose	Orally for hypoglycemia. May be in liquid or tablet form, or a glass of orange juice may be given.	Minimal unless hyperglycemic.
Oxygen	Inhaled; usually 2-6 L, but it varies according to protocol.	Minimal, although oxygen toxicity can occur with high doses for prolonged periods of time.
Bronchodilators (albuterol, levalbuterol)	Inhaled; usually two puffs of a handheld inhaler. Dosage varies according to the medication. Used for bronchospasm, wheezing.	Adverse effects: tachycardia, dizziness, nervousness, tremor, headache, rhinitis, increased cough.
Epinephrine (EpiPen)	Autoinjector; 0.3 mg at 1:1000 for ≥66 lb, 0.15 mg at 1:2000 for 33-66 lb for severe allergic reaction/anaphylaxis.	Avoid using with antihistamines, thyroid hormones, and alpha blockers. Adverse effects: drowsiness, headache, palpitations, nervousness, tremors.
Nitroglycerin	Sublingually for angina (chest pain); 0.3-0.6 mg, repeated every 5 minutes up to 3 times.	Avoid with myocardial infarction. Adverse effects: headache, flushing, dizziness, orthostatic hypotension, palpitations. Interactions: Avoid with erectile dysfunction drugs (sildenafil, tadalafil, vardenafil).

ROUTES OF DRUG ADMINISTRATION FOR THE EMT

The route of administration is the manner by which a drug is introduced into the body. The most **common routes of administration** utilized by the EMT are:

- Enteral (oral, rectal, or by feeding tube)
- Topical (on the skin, in the eyes or nose, vaginal, or inhaled)
- Parenteral (IV, subcutaneous, intramuscular, intracardiac, intraosseous, intradermal, intrathecal, intraperitoneal, transdermal, transmucosal, intravitreal, and epidural)

There are many variations on these three basic routes of administration. The FDA acknowledges 111 different routes of administration. When deciding on the route of administration, the ordering provider must consider:

- How fast the patient requires the drug
- How effective it will be by a given route
- The likelihood of toxicity
- The discomfort it will cause
- How likely the patient is to comply with the route
- How likely the route is to play into the patient's addictive habits

TYPES OF INJECTIONS

The three most common types of injections and the preferred injection sites are as follows:

- **Subcutaneous injection**: Deliver the drug under the skin with a ½ inch, 24- or 25-gauge needle held at a 45° angle to reach the fat. Choose the upper arm, abdomen, thigh, or lower back as the site. The maximum amount of subcutaneous medication is 0.5 mL. An example is insulin for a patient with diabetes.
- **Intramuscular injection**: Deliver the drug into the muscle at a 90° angle to reach the deep tissue. Standard needle length is 1 to 1.5 inches depending on the weight of the individual. CDC guidelines recommend the use of a 22- to 25-gauge needle for adult intramuscular injections. Recommended sites for injection on the adult include deltoid (most recommended), vastus lateralis (thigh), ventrogluteal (hip), or dorsogluteal (buttocks). The maximum recommended amount of IM medication is 3 mL. An example is Vitamin B12 for a patient with pernicious anemia.
- **Intravenous Injection**: Deliver the drug into a vein of the arm, hand, leg, foot, scalp, or neck with an Angiocath, butterfly, or Insyte Autoguard needle. Use a size from 14 gauge to 26 gauge, depending on the fluid and the patient. The nurse sets the drip rate per minute by adjusting the clamp and monitoring the drip chamber. An example of a drug requiring intravenous injection is Zoledronate, which is given yearly to prevent bone fractures for individuals with osteoporosis.

> **Review Video: Calculating IV Drip Rates**
> Visit mometrix.com/academy and enter code: 396112

Two less frequently used forms of injection are: Intradermal (into the skin; Paramedics only), and intraosseous access (IO) into the bone, which is used in emergency situations when other access sites are not available.

ADMINISTRATION OF IMMUNIZATIONS

Emergency medications that may be administered by EMS personnel include **immunizations.**

EMS personnel may be called upon by local health departments to assist with immunizations, especially with outbreaks such as H1N1 or COVID-19. State regulations regarding EMS personnel may vary somewhat. EMS personnel must follow all public health safety guidelines, including the use of appropriate PPE to protect the EMS personnel and the patients. EMS personnel should complete training regarding immunizations and should be familiar with the pharmacology of the immunizations, mode of administration, adverse effects (including allergic reactions), and vaccination follow-up (if indicated). The EMS personnel should question patients about prior allergic reactions to immunizations and any history of Guillain-Barré syndrome before administration of an immunization.

ADMINISTRATION OF INHALED NITROUS OXIDE (NITROX)

Inhaled nitrous oxide (Nitrox) may be administered by EMS personnel at the AEMT level and higher to control moderate to severe pain. Nitrox is provided by a 2-cylinder device that mixes nitrous oxide and oxygen (1:1) per a face mask with a demand valve. An airtight seal must be maintained with the face mask and the patient must be able to hold the mask and self-administer. The effects of nitrous oxide dissipate within 2-5 minutes of discontinuation. Nitrox is a mild intoxicant so patients may talk and laugh during administration. Nitrox is contraindicated for those with altered level of consciousness, head injury, confusion, respiratory distress (COPD, pneumothorax, air embolism, pulmonary edema, decompression sickness), pre-delivery pregnancy, and Abdominal distension.

Nitrox should only be administered with good ventilation in the transport because it may accumulate on the floor of the transport and affect EMS personnel, especially if administration exceeds 15 minutes.

MEDICATIONS ADMINISTERED INTRAVENOUSLY

The following **emergency medications** may be administered intravenously although state regulations regarding which medications the EMT can administer IV may vary:

- **Analgesics**: Utilize a standard pain assessment tool, such as the 1-10 numeric rating scale when determining the appropriate analgesic, which may include morphine, hydromorphone, ketorolac, IV acetaminophen, and ketamine. Analgesics are often diluted with 10 mL NS and administered over 3-5 minutes to avoid phlebitis. Common adverse effects include nausea, vomiting, hypotension, respiratory depression, diaphoresis, and dizziness.
- **Dextrose/Glucose**: 50 mL of 50% solution IV for adults; 2-4 mg of 25% solution for those under age 8; 4 mg/kg of 12.5% solution for neonates. IV administration for pediatric patients must be administered slowly. Indicated to combat hypoglycemia and unconsciousness of unknown origin. Contraindicated with delirium tremens with dehydration, and intracranial/intraspinal hemorrhage or with BS of greater than 60 mg/dL. Glucose level should be checked prior to administration.
- **Antiemetics**: Antinausea agents are usually restricted to adult patients only with EMS personnel. Commonly used drugs include:
  - **Prochlorperazine**, 5-10 mg. Adverse effects include hypotension, sedation, tremors, slurring of speech, dystonia, restlessness, and cardiac dysrhythmias. Tissue necrosis may occur with extravasation, so IM is often preferred. Contraindicated with narrow angle glaucoma, hepatic or cardiac disease, and altered level of consciousness.
  - **Metoclopramide**, 5-10 mg IV, adverse effects may include diarrhea, neuroleptic malignant syndrome (rare), with hyperthermia and rigidity. Contraindicated with MAO inhibitors, seizure disorders, and intestinal obstruction.
  - **Ondansetron**, 4-8 mg IV. (Dosages over 16 mg may cause prolongation of QT interval.) Drug must be diluted in 50 mL of D5W or NS and infused over 15 minutes. Adverse effects are rare but may include blurred vision, headache, sedation, hypoxia, rash, and chills. Contraindicated with use of apomorphine and used cautiously with liver disease.
- **Epinephrine**: Onset of action IV is immediate and can cause cardiac arrest at 1:1000 dosage, so IM is preferred for anaphylaxis although IV may be given at 1:10,000 solution over 5-10 minutes for anaphylaxis and resultant respiratory distress associated with bronchospasm. For cardiac arrest, 10 mL of 1:10,000 solution can be administered every 3-5 minutes (equal to 1 mg every 3-5 minutes). Mix with D5W, lactated Ringer, or NS immediately prior to use and monitor VS and ECG continuously. Autoinjector cannot be used intravenously.
- **Naloxone**: 2-4 mg administered initially to adults and 0.1 mg/kg to pediatric patients. This may be repeated in 2-3 minutes to 10 mg for adults to reverse the effects of opioid overdose and associated respiratory depression. Adverse effects include tremor, agitation, seizures, and withdrawal symptoms.

EMT Assessment

PRIMARY ASSESSMENT

After surveying the environment for safety issues, the EMS provider should quickly conduct a **primary assessment** to identify conditions that are life-threatening, as follows:

- **Level of consciousness**: Alert, responsive to verbal stimuli, responsive to painful stimuli, nonresponsive
- **Breathing status**: Normal, abnormal, rate abnormalities (>24 or <8), apnea, choking, normal or abnormal chest movement, chest rise and fall, noisy respirations, use of accessory muscles, tripod position, nasal flaring
- **Circulatory status**: Radial, carotid pulse, pulse abnormalities, major bleeding, skin color (pink, blue [cyanotic], pale), skin temperature, skin moisture, capillary refill, signs of shock

Life-threatening conditions must be treated immediately, as follows:

- Carotid pulse present with no radial pulse: Lay the patient flat and elevate his or her feet 8-12 inches.
- No pulse: Begin CPR.
- Shock: Lay the patient flat, elevate his or her feet 8-12 inches, and administer oxygen at 15 L/min.
- Bleeding: Apply pressure to control any bleeding.
- Abnormal breathing: Provide oxygen with a nonrebreather mask. If the patient is unresponsive, cyanotic, or in respiratory distress, use a BVM with supplemental oxygen.
- Unresponsive: Ensure a patent airway.

Based on the assessment, the patient is classified as stable, potentially unstable, or unstable.

HISTORY TAKING ON ARRIVAL AT A SCENE

History taking should include the following:

- **Chief complaint**: If the patient is unable to explain, information may be gathered from his or her family, friends, or others who are present. Look for a medical alert bracelet or other such jewelry.
- **Nature of the illness or mechanism of injury**: Reason for calling EMS, cause of injury, type of illness. Look for environmental clues (fire, drug paraphernalia, motor vehicle accident).
- **Signs and symptoms observed or reported by the patient**: Skin temperature, open wounds, BP abnormalities, pain, or difficulty breathing.
- **Precipitating events**: Falls, accidents, violence, eating, exercising, walking, driving.
- **Pediatric considerations**: Check capillary refill to assess blood flow in infants and children younger than 6. Assess the pulse at the brachial artery (inside of the upper arm) for infants up to 1 year of age and the carotid artery in the neck for children older than 1 year. May need to use distraction to gain trust and alleviate fear. Encourage the parents/caregivers to hold the child if possible and assist in calming the child.
- **Geriatric (older adult) considerations**: Determine if the patient needs assistive devices, such as hearing aids, eyeglasses, cane, walker, or dentures.

OPQRST METHOD OF HISTORY TAKING

O	Onset	The time that the symptoms associated with this event started.
P	Provocative; palliative.	That which makes it better; that which makes it worse.
	Positioning	The position that the patient is in on arrival and the need to remain in this position or to move him or her.
Q	Quality of discomfort	Burning, stabbing, nagging, crushing, sharp, or dull.
R	Radiation of pain	Area to which the pain moves from the original site.
S	Severity of pain	Based on a 1-to-10 or other appropriate scale.
T	Time	Historical onset, such as earlier, similar events.

SAMPLE METHOD OF HISTORY TAKING

S	Signs and symptoms	Pain, bleeding, shortness of breath, injuries, fever, rash.
A	Allergies	Medications, environmental (foods, insects, plants, animals).
M	Medications	Prescribed, over-the-counter (OTC) vitamins/minerals, birth control and erectile dysfunction medications, herbal preparations, recreational drugs, other people's medications.
P	Past pertinent history	Especially related to the current event.
L	Last oral intake	Foods, fluids, other substances.
E	Events (precipitating)	Occurrence just prior to event.

TAKING A HISTORY OF SENSITIVE TOPICS

When asking a patient about **sensitive topics,** the EMS provider should try to provide as much privacy as possible in an emergent situation in order to maintain confidentiality and protect the patient from reprisals. The EMS provider should ask questions directly in a straightforward and nonjudgmental manner, stressing the need for information in order to help the patient, especially if the patient is reluctant to answer. Sensitive topics include the following:

- **Sexual history**: People who engage in unusual or unhealthy sexual practices, such as sadomasochism, autoerotic asphyxiation, swinging, and prostitution, are often reluctant to admit to those practices. Adolescents may be especially reluctant to admit they are pregnant or have engaged in sexual activity or have had an abortion. Males (especially those older than age 40) should be asked about the use of erectile dysfunction drugs (such as Viagra) because they are a contraindication to some medical treatments.
- **Physical/Sexual abuse and/or violence**: Victims often lie about abuse to defend the abuser or out of shame or fear of further violence.
- **Alcohol/Drug use and abuse**: Patients often underreport the extent of their drinking or drug taking or deny it altogether. Patients may be concerned about legal actions, such as if they have been driving drunk and gotten into an accident.

SPECIAL HISTORY-TAKING CHALLENGES

Special history-taking challenges include the following:

- **Silent patient**: Be patient, sensitive, and alert for nonverbal clues.
- **Talkative patient**: Allow the patient to speak freely for a few minutes and then periodically summarize.
- **Anxious patient**: Be patient, provide reassurance, and explain all procedures.
- **Patient with multiple complaints**: Ask the patient to help prioritize his or her issues.
- **Hostile/angry patient**: Remain calm; respond as appropriate.
- **Intoxicated patient**: Avoid cornering, belittling, or challenging the patient or asking the patient to lower his or her voice or stop swearing. Remain calm and treat the patient with respect.
- **Depressed, crying patient**: Question the severity of the patient's depression; listen and remain supportive and nonjudgmental.
- **Patient with a language barrier**: Use a translator if possible. Use hand gestures. Show the equipment before using it; point to the part of the body where the equipment will be used.
- **Patient with a visual impairment**: Announce one's presence and explain all procedures verbally. Tell the patient before touching him or her.
- **Patient with a hearing impairment**: Determine if the patient has a hearing aid, and obtain it if possible. Speak slowly and clearly, facing the patient for any hearing deficit. If the patient has no hearing, use writing, hand gestures, and demonstrations to communicate.

SECONDARY ASSESSMENT

Following completion of the primary assessment and after attending to any life-threatening problems that are identified, carry out a **secondary assessment** as follows:

- **Measure vital signs**: Pulse (radial to carotid for adults and brachial for infants and small children), respiration rate, and BP. Using the correct BP cuff size is essential for accuracy. The length of the bladder in the cuff should be equal to 80% of the arm's circumference, and the lower edge of the cuff when positioned should end about one inch above the antecubital fossa (inner elbow). Inflate the cuff to 160-180 initially, and increase the pressure if pulse sounds are heard at that level.
- **Ask further questions as indicated**: These may focus on the primary complaint or others, depending on the situation.
- **Conduct a physical examination**: Examine the body; palpate for areas of tenderness or swelling; auscultate heart, lung, and abdominal sounds; and note any injuries. Do a brief head-to-toe assessment, and compare one side of the body with the other, noting any asymmetry.
- **Treat any life-threatening injuries or conditions** noted immediately.

REASSESSMENT

Reassessment involves ongoing monitoring of the patient at regular intervals to determine changes in his or her condition or trends such as decreasing BP or increasing agitation. **Reassessment** is done after a secondary assessment. Unstable patients should be reassessed at least every 5 minutes and stable patients every 15 minutes. Reassessment should include reviewing the primary assessment, taking vital signs, repeating the physical examination (including evaluation of mental status), and monitoring the chief complaint and response to interventions. Reassessment findings should be compared to baseline findings. The patient's airway, ventilation, and circulation should be reassessed as well as the patient's degree of pain—stable, better, or worse. Each intervention should be reassessed for effectiveness and the need for modifications of treatment or if new interventions should be determined. If the patient is receiving oxygen, the tank and all of the equipment should be checked to ensure that they are functioning properly.

NORMAL VITAL SIGNS FROM NEONATE TO LATE ADULTHOOD

Age	Heart rate	Respirations	BP (mmHg)
Neonate (0-12 mo.)	100–220 (average 140–160); slows after ~3 months	40–60 for a few minutes, then 30–40	Systolic 70–90
Toddler (12–36 mo.)	80–130	20–30	Systolic 70–100
Preschooler (3-5)	80–120	20–30	Systolic 80–110
School aged (6–12)	70–110	20–30	80–120/60–80
Adolescent (13–18)	55–100	12–20	110–131/64–84
Early adult (19–40)	60–100 (average 80)	12–20	100–119/60–79 to 140/90 (high)
Middle adult (41–60)	60–100 (average 80)	12–20	100–119/60–79 to 140/90 (high)
Late adult (61+)	60–100 (average 70)	12–20	100–119/60–79 to 140/90 (high)

ASSESSMENT OF FUNCTIONAL ABILITIES

Functional abilities should ideally be assessed in an active manner, with the person demonstrating the ability to sit; stand; get on and off of the toilet; walk; bend down; remove shoes, shirt, or jacket and then put them on again; listen; read; and answer questions. However, in an emergent situation, this type of assessment is often not possible. Careful questioning about the home environment can help with approximating the type of activities required and physical limitations that the patient experiences. A careful history of functional ability can pinpoint when and if changes occurred. Again, specific questioning guides patients: "When did you begin to use a cane?" "How old were you when you stopped using the tub?" "What is the biggest problem with caring for yourself?" or "When did you have a hip replacement, and how has that changed your life?"

INSTRUMENTAL ACTIVITIES OF DAILY LIVING (IADL) ASSESSMENT TOOL

Instrumental Activities of Daily Living (IADL) assessment tool measures eight activities necessary for an adult to function independently. This tool helps to determine the need for supportive services. Eight activities are each assigned as 0 (cannot do independently) or 1 (minimal or adequate degree of ability), so the total score ranges from 0 to 8, with a higher score indicating more independence in care. Abilities that are measured include the following:

- Telephone use (ability to look up numbers and/or call numbers)
- Shopping for food, clothes, or needed items
- Food preparation (plans diet and prepares food)
- Housekeeping (ability to perform all or part of household duties)
- Laundry (can wash all or some of personal clothes and linen)
- Transportation availability (ability to drive or use public transportation)
- Medication (ability to be responsible for managing prescriptions and taking medications)
- Financial responsibility (ability to keep track of finances, pay bills, and budget correctly)

Labs and Point of Care Testing

BLOOD GLUCOSE MONITORING

Blood glucose monitoring is done with a glucometer. Testing is indicated with a decreased level of consciousness or confusion in a diabetic patient or a decreased level of consciousness with the cause being unknown. The glucometer must be calibrated and tested regularly. Test results from capillary blood tend to be lower than test results on venous blood. The **testing procedure** is as follows:

- Wipe the site with an alcohol swab. The alcohol must be thoroughly dried before puncture, or it may interfere with the test results.
- Prick the side of the finger pad with a lancet or lancing device rather than the fingertip because the fingertip is more sensitive.
- Express a drop of blood onto the test strip.
- Insert the test strip into the glucometer according to the manufacturer's recommendations.
- Read the test results.
- Dispose of the lancet in a sharps container.

Warming the hand or lowering it may help to ensure adequate blood for the test. Hypoglycemia (low blood sugar/insulin reaction) is a reading of ≤70 mg/dL. Hyperglycemia (high blood sugar) is a reading of ≥160 mg/dL.

COMPLETE BLOOD COUNT (CBC)
Total erythrocytes (RBCs) normal values:

- Males >18 years: 4.5–5.5 million per mm^3
- Females >18 years: 4–5 million per mm^3

Hemoglobin: Carries oxygen; it is decreased in anemia and increased in polycythemia. Normal values:

- Males >18 years: 14–18 g/dL
- Females >18 years: 12–16 g/dL

Hematocrit: Indicates the proportion of RBCs in a liter of blood (usually about 3× the hemoglobin number). Normal values:

- Males >18 years: 45-52%
- Females >18 years: 36-48%

Reticulocyte count (immature RBCs): Measures marrow production and should rise with anemia. Normal values:

- 0.5-1.5% of total RBCs

Leukocytes (WBCs) normal values:

- Normal WBC for adults: 4800–10,000
- Acute infection: 10,000+
- Severe infection: 30,000+
- Viral infection: ≤4000

The differential provides the percentage of each different type of leukocyte. An increase in the WBC count is usually related to an increase in one type and often an increase in immature neutrophils, known as bands, referred to as a "shift to the left," an indication of an infectious process.

I-STAT CHEM 8+

There are many point-of-care testing devices available; the one most commonly used for comprehensive blood analysis is the **i-STAT CHEM 8+,** which includes the following tests plus hemoglobin and hematocrit:

Blood urea nitrogen (BUN)

- Normal values: 7–20 mg/dL
- Measures kidney function
- Increases with kidney disease

Carbon dioxide (CO_2)

- Normal values: 20–29 mmol/L
- Measures acid/base balance
- Measures bicarbonate

Anion gap

- Normal values: 8–16 mEq/L
- Measures sodium (chloride + bicarbonate)
- Helps identify metabolic acidosis

Creatinine

- Normal values: 0.8–1.4 mg/dL
- Measures kidney function
- Increases with kidney disease

Glucose

- Normal values: 70–128 mg/dL
- Measures blood sugar level
- Increase can indicate diabetic ketoacidosis; decrease can indicate an insulin reaction

Serum chloride

- Normal values: 101–111 mmol/L
- Measures electrolyte level
- Increase can indicate metabolic acidosis and respiratory alkalosis; decrease can indicate respiratory acidosis and metabolic alkalosis

Serum sodium

- Normal values: 136–144 mEq/L
- Measures electrolyte level
- Increase can indicate excess sweating, diarrhea, burns, or the use of diuretics; decrease can indicate dehydration, vomiting, and diarrhea

Calcium (ionized)

- Normal values: 4.4–5.4 mg/dL (1.1–1.35 mmol/L)
- Critical values:
  - <2 mg/dL (<0.5 mmol/L) may result in tetany
  - >7 mg/dL (>1.75 mmol/L) may result in coma
- Measures electrolyte level

Review Video: Lab Values
Visit mometrix.com/academy and enter code: 120244

CARDIAC BIOMARKERS

When the heart is damaged, it releases **cardiac biomarkers**, substances that aid in diagnosis. Biomarkers include the following:

- **Creatine kinase (CK) and isoenzyme (MB),** also known as CK-MB, is specific to the heart muscle, and the level increases within 4–8 hours after a heart attack; it peaks at about 24 hours after the heart attach (earlier with thrombolytic therapy), and it remains elevated for 72 hours.
- **Myoglobin (heme protein that transports oxygen)** is found in skeletal and cardiac muscles. The level increases 1–3 hours after a heart attack and peaks within 12 hours. Although an increase is not specific to a heart attack, a failure to increase can be used to rule out an MI.
- **Troponin I** is found only in the heart muscle. Levels increase 3–6 hours after a heart attack, peak in 14–20 hours, and return to normal within 5–7 days.
- **Troponin T** is found in heart and skeletal muscle. Levels increase 3–6 hours after a heart attack, peak in 12–24 hours, and return to normal in 10–15 days.
- **Brain natriuretic peptide (BNP)** is secreted by the ventricular muscle with increased volume and pressure. An increased level indicates heart failure.

Airway, Respiration, and Ventilation

Airway, Respiration, and Ventilation Management

UPPER RESPIRATORY SYSTEM

Air enters the upper respiratory system through the **nasal cavity** and/or mouth, where it is warmed and moistened by **nasal and oral mucosa**. The four pairs of **paranasal sinuses** aid in warming and moistening the air (see graphic below). The air passes through the **pharynx**: **nasopharynx**, **oropharynx**, and **laryngopharynx/hypopharynx** (below and behind the larynx and epiglottis). Air passes behind or past the **soft palate** (the soft tissue at the back of the mouth) and the **uvula**, which hangs from the soft palate and into the lower respiratory system. The **hyoid bone** is above the Adam's apple and helps support the larynx. The **vallecula** ("spit trap") is at the root of the tongue. The **adenoids** (pharyngeal tonsils) are located on the posterior wall of the nasopharynx, and the **palatine tonsils** are on the back of the mouth on either side of the tongue. The adenoids and tonsils may become infected and swollen, obstructing the airway. The jawbones include the maxilla (upper) and mandible (lower). The jugular notch is the visible depression between the neck and clavicles (collarbones).

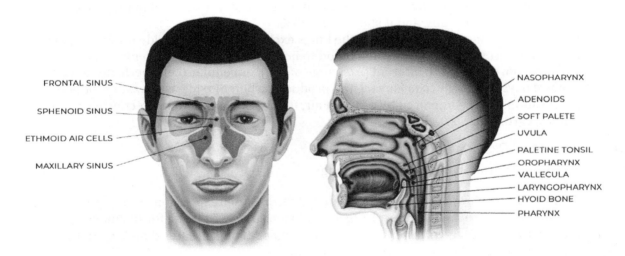

FRONTAL SINUS

SPHENOID SINUS

ETHMOID AIR CELLS

MAXILLARY SINUS

NASOPHARYNX

ADENOIDS

SOFT PALETE

UVULA

PALETINE TONSIL

OROPHARYNX

VALLECULA

LARYNGOPHARYNX

HYOID BONE

PHARYNX

> **Review Video: Respiratory System**
> Visit mometrix.com/academy and enter code: 783075

LOWER RESPIRATORY SYSTEM

Air passes from the upper respiratory system and the pharynx to the lower respiratory system and the **larynx** (voice box) into the **trachea** (windpipe). The **epiglottis** is a cartilage flap attached to the **thyroid cartilage** (above the cricoid cartilage), and it closes over the larynx and **glottis** (vocal cords) when swallowing, so food enters the esophagus. The trachea branches into two (right and left) **bronchi** that carry the air into the **lungs**. Each bronchus branches into smaller **bronchioles** and **alveoli** (small air sacs), which are connected to the ends of the bronchioles. The alveoli are covered with webs of tiny venous capillaries that deliver carbon dioxide and arterial capillaries that pick up oxygen. Muscles of respiration are the **diaphragm**, which is enervated by the **phrenic nerve**, and the **intercostal muscles**, but **accessory muscles** in the neck and collarbone area may help during respiratory distress.

PHYSIOLOGY OF RESPIRATION

The physiology of respiration includes the following:

1. **Ventilation**: Movement of air in and out of the lungs during inhalation and exhalation. Breathing may be impaired by disease (muscular dystrophy), drugs, trauma, bronchoconstriction, allergic reactions, foreign body obstructions, and infection.
2. **Oxygenation**: The process by which oxygen molecules bind to hemoglobin in the blood. The blood saturation level reflects the amount of oxygen that is dissolved in the blood and available to body tissues, and it should be ≥95%.
3. **Respiration**: The process by which the lungs exchange carbon dioxide for oxygen in the alveoli and provide this oxygenated blood to body tissues. Respiration may be external (inspiration, expiration), internal (exchange of gas), or cellular (cells perform tasks that require oxygen and glucose [sugar] and produce carbon dioxide as a waste product). Respiration may be impaired by a lack of air, toxins/poisons, and ineffective circulation (shock, cardiac arrest).

KEY ELEMENTS OF RESPIRATION

Key elements of respiration include the following:

- **Tidal volume**: Normal volume of gas inhaled during one respiration cycle (approximately 500 mL in a healthy adult, 6–8 mL/kg for children, and 5–7 mL/kg for neonates)
- **Inspiratory reserve volume**: Volume of air inhaled that is greater than the tidal volume during forced deep inhalation (up to 3000 mL)
- **Dead space**: Volume of inhaled gas that does not take part in gas exchange
- **Alveolar dead space**: Volume of alveoli that are ventilated but not perfused
- **Vital capacity**: Maximum volume of gas that can be forcefully exhaled from the lungs following a full inhalation
- **Minute volume**: Volume of gas expelled from the lungs in one minute (the respiratory rate × the tidal volume)
- **Residual volume**: Volume of gas remaining in the lungs after one full, forced exhalation
- **Total lung capacity**: Vital capacity plus residual volume; the total volume that the lungs can contain (usually about 6000 mL for adults)
- **Cellular respiration**: Use of oxygen and glucose to produce energy at the cellular level and the creation of water and carbon dioxide as by-products of metabolism

THE ROLE OF THE LUNGS IN EXTERNAL AND INTERNAL RESPIRATION

The lungs, located in the thoracic cavity and surrounded by pleural membranes, facilitate breathing through changes in pressure. When inhaling, the lungs and thoracic cavity expand, decreasing air pressure inside and forcing air from outside to enter. When exhaling, the pressure increases as the lungs and thoracic cavity contract, forcing air out of the lungs. The phrenic and intercostal nerves cause the diaphragm and intercostal muscles to contract and relax.

- **External respiration** occurs with gas exchange (oxygen for carbon dioxide) at the alveoli. The respiratory center in the brain (medulla oblongata) controls the breathing rate in response to chemoreceptors in the arteries that monitor levels of oxygen and carbon dioxide.
- **Internal respiration** occurs with gas exchange in the tissue cells. Physiologic dead spaces are those areas of the lung (including impaired alveoli) where gas exchange does not occur.

OXYGENATION AND PERFUSION IN THE LIFE SUPPORT CHAIN

Critical to the life support chain are oxygenation and perfusion. **Oxygenation** involves gas exchange of carbon dioxide for oxygen at the alveolar/capillary level and the cell/capillary level. **Perfusion** involves the transport of blood, which carries oxygen, glucose, and other nutrients as well as waste products throughout the body. Oxygen and glucose are essential for cell functioning. Glucose is produced by the digestion of carbohydrates (starches). Glucose is the primary energy source for the body, and its use is controlled by insulin, which is produced by the pancreas. Excess glucose is stored in the liver as glycogen for later use or is converted to fat. These fundamental elements are affected by the composition of ambient air (usually 21% oxygen), airway patency, ventilation, regulation of respiration, blood volume and transport, heart action, and blood vessel size and resistance.

PEDIATRIC AND OLDER ADULT AIRWAYS

Special **considerations** should be given to both pediatric and older adult airways:

- **Pediatric airways**: Infants are obligate nasal breathers for the first two to four months and usually only breathe through the nose, although they can generally breathe through the mouth if necessary. However, if nasal passages are blocked, they may quickly develop respiratory distress. Chest wall compliance is greater in infants and small children, so they must work harder than an adult to move the same amount of air. Additionally, proportionally the airway is smaller, the tongue is larger, and the cartilage is softer, increasing the risk of obstruction.
- **Older adult airways**: Breathing capacity tends to decline after age 40 because the number of alveoli decreases and the size of alveoli increases, resulting in less surface for, and less efficient, gas exchange. Lung elasticity also decreases, resulting in decreased vital capacity. The chest muscles tend to weaken and stiffen with age, and older adults have a lowered ability to cough and clear the airways.

AIRWAY ASSESSMENT AND MANUAL MEASURES TO CLEAR THE AIRWAY

Indications of an adequate airway include a normal voice and speaking ability and audible and visible air exchange. Indications of inadequate airway include unusual breathing sounds (wheezing, stridor), hoarse voice/inability to speak, and no audible or visible air exchange. Airway obstruction may result from the tongue falling back, food, a foreign body, vomit, blood, teeth, and edema (swelling). **Maneuvers** include the following:

- **Head tilt/chin lift**: Hyperextend the neck by tilting the patient's head back with one hand on his or her forehead to straighten the airway and lift the tongue. Then lift the chin and pull forward with the fingers of the other hand under the chin with the thumb on top. The chin lift pulls the mandible (jaw) forward. This prevents the tongue from blocking the pharynx. Contraindications to the head tilt/chin lift include suspected cervical spine and neck injuries.
- **Jaw thrust**: This technique is used with a suspected spinal cord or neck injury in which extending the neck must be avoided. From behind, place the fingers behind the angles of the patient's lower jaw and place your thumbs on the chin; move the jaw upward until it is extended while using the thumbs to slightly open the patient's mouth. Contraindications include severe facial injuries.
- **Modified chin lift/jaw thrust**: This technique is used with a suspected spinal cord/neck injury with an unstable cervical spine. From the head of the patient, place the thumbs on his or her cheekbones, place the fingers under the patient's mandible, and then pull the mandible upward with the fingers while applying pressure with the thumbs. If using a mask for ventilation, place the mask in position and secure it with the thumbs while the fingers thrust the patient's jaw forward.

ASSESSMENT OF OXYGENATION

Assessment of oxygenation includes the following:

1. **Evaluate respirations**: Note the signs of respiratory distress—rapid breathing, slow breathing, use of accessory muscles, nasal flaring, and sternal retraction—because they may indicate inadequate oxygenation.
2. **Assess mental status**: Confusion may be associated with hypo-oxygenation (low oxygen), but it's important to determine a baseline mental status if possible because the patient may have dementia or may be confused because of medications.
3. **Assess skin**: Note cyanosis (blue tinge) especially around the mouth, fingertips, and oral mucous membranes because this indicates a lack of oxygen. Another sign is pallor. Mottling of the skin, purplish or reddish discoloration especially on the knees and feet, indicates hypo-oxygenation and is a common indication that death is near.
4. **Monitor pulse oximetry**: Oxygen saturation should be 95%–100%. If a patient has mild respiratory disease, the pulse oximetry level may be as low as 90% and still be within the normal range for the patient. Readings of less than 90%–92% indicate hypoxemia (low oxygen in the blood).

ASSESSMENT OF RESPIRATIONS AND SUPPLEMENTAL OXYGEN ADMINISTRATION

When assessing respirations, the EMS provider should note the patient's gag reflex and rate of respirations (whether it is normal for the patient's age or too fast, too slow, or absent). The provider should also evaluate the rise and fall of the chest and any abnormal movements (such as sternal retraction, nasal flaring) noisy breathing (gurgling, wheezing), the use of accessory muscles, or the tripod position (sitting, leaning forward, and supporting the body with the hands).

If breathing is abnormal or the pulse oximetry is less than 95%, the EMS provider should take precautions against bloodstream infection (BSI) and administer **supplemental oxygen** with a **nonrebreather mask** with the oxygen set at 12–15 L. The reservoir bag of the mask must be completely filled before applying the mask to the patient, securing it with an elastic band about the head. If the patient cannot tolerate the nonrebreather mask, then a **nasal cannula** may be used with the oxygen flow set at 4–6 L, the prongs inserted into the nostrils, and tubing secured by looping over the ears and tightening under the chin.

ASSESSMENT OF VENTILATION

Ventilation is adequate if the respiratory rate, depth of respiration, and effort of breathing are normal. **Signs of inadequate ventilation** include the following:

1. **Increased effort of breathing**: Nasal flaring, sternal retraction (infants), use of abdominal or intercostal (between the ribs) muscles, sweating, sitting in the tripod position (upright, leaning forward, hands on knees).
2. **Abnormal breath sounds**: Wheezes, rales (crackles), and/or rhonchi (snoring/whistling sounds).
3. **Abnormal depth of breathing**: Hypoventilation (too shallow) or hyperventilation (too deep).
4. **Abnormal rate of breathing**: Tachypnea (too fast) or bradypnea (too slow).
5. **Abnormal chest wall movement**: Splinting, asymmetric, paradoxical (chest wall/diaphragm move in during inhalation and out during exhalation—opposite of normal).
6. **Irregular breathing pattern**: May include periods of apnea (no breathing).

Patients with inadequate ventilation or apnea in which there is no breathing or only occasional gasping require ventilation assistance, such as with a pocket mask or bag-valve mask (BVM).

NEGATIVE-PRESSURE BREATHING VS. POSITIVE-PRESSURE BREATHING

Negative-pressure (normal) breathing:

- The movement downward of the diaphragm (triggered by the phrenic nerves) creates a negative pressure in the lungs, drawing air into them.
- Blood flows from the lungs to the heart and back and to the body at a steady rate in normal breathing.
- The epiglottis closes the esophagus during inhalation, preventing air from entering the stomach.

Positive-pressure breathing:

- Ventilation forces air into the lungs, and this can result in dysfunction of the diaphragm because it is responding to a change in pressure rather than stimulation by the phrenic nerve.
- Blood flow from the lungs is reduced, resulting in decreased cardiac (heart) output.
- The epiglottis may stay open during ventilation, allowing air into the stomach and increasing the risk of vomiting.

BAG-VALVE MASK (BVM)

Bag-valve mask (BVM) ventilation equipment used for positive-pressure ventilation (PPV) includes a mask, a ventilator bag, an oxygen reservoir bag, and an attachment for oxygen delivery. The correct mask size is important: The mask should not cover the chin. BVM is contraindicated if the airway is not patent, but it is used for abnormal breathing and for respiratory distress/failure. BVM requires two EMS personnel—one to control the mask and the other to control the bag. Steps are as follows:

1. Position oneself behind the patient's head, place the mask over the patient's nose and mouth, and make a tight seal by holding it in place with the thumbs and index fingers while the other fingers slide under the patient's jaw to lift the chin.
2. Squeeze the bag with inhalations initially for 5 to 10 breaths and then adjust the rate to at least 12 breaths per minute, slowly adjusting the rate and tidal volume delivered.

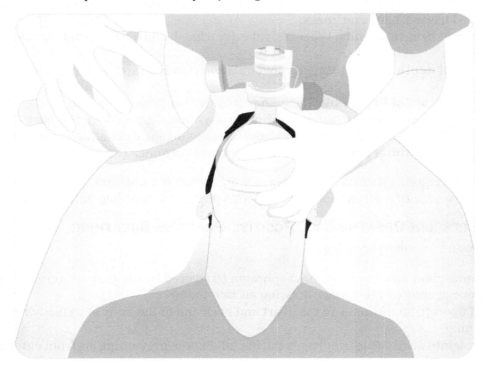

Assessment of lung compliance (the ability to expand and contract) includes observation of chest movement, rate of respirations, and the feel of BVM. Difficult ventilation suggests impaired compliance. Note: The BVM can be used with or without oxygen.

POCKET-MASK VENTILATION

Pocket-mask ventilation is used when administering cardiopulmonary resuscitation (CPR) to a patient who is in cardiac arrest and apneic (not breathing). If two EMS personnel are available, one should be positioned at the patient's head to administer pocket-mask ventilation while the other does compressions. If there is only one EMS personnel, then that person should be positioned at the patient's side. Administration is as follows:

1. Remove the mask from the container and push the flattened mask to open it.
2. Wipe the patient's face clean with alcohol swab if necessary to remove secretions, vomitus.
3. Do a chin tilt or jaw thrust and place the mask over the patient's nose and mouth, holding it in place with both hands to seal it tightly.

38

4. Take a deep breath and blow in through the one-way valve, watching the chest rise to ensure that ventilation has occurred.
5. Continue to ventilate the patient at a rate of 30 compressions to 2 ventilations for CPR.
6. Attach supplemental oxygen if available to improve oxygenation.
7. Upon patient recovery or completion of CPR, remove the mask, discard the valve, and disinfect the mask.

Pocket Mask

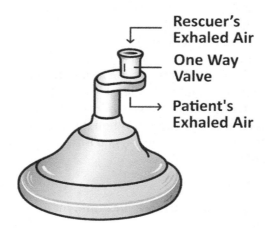

Rescuer's Exhaled Air

One Way Valve

Patient's Exhaled Air

SELLICK'S MANEUVER (CRICOID PRESSURE)

Sellick's maneuver (cricoid pressure) may be used with PPV to prevent air from flowing down the esophagus and into the stomach rather than down the trachea and into the lungs because stomach distension increases the risk of vomiting. This maneuver may also be used with intubation to prevent regurgitation of stomach contents and aspiration. **Sellick's maneuver** may be used on unconscious patients receiving a mask or BVM. The procedure consists of applying pressure downward to the cricoid cartilage of the neck (which is at the bottom of the larynx and blocks the upper esophagus) with the thumb and index finger. Pressure is usually applied at 30 to 40 newtons but no greater than 40 newtons because too great of force may block the airway. The maneuver may also cause nausea and vomiting and, with severe pressure, may result in rupture of the esophagus. Vomiting is a contraindication.

UPPER AIRWAY SUCTIONING

Suctioning devices may be vehicle mounted or portable and should be checked to ensure that the tubing is intact and the canister has an airtight seal. Patients at risk for aspiration include those with an altered level of consciousness, those having difficulty swallowing or breathing, trauma patients, obese patients, and those with recurrent vomiting. **Oral suctioning** is used to remove secretions, vomitus, and blood. Suctioning may be done with a rigid-tip catheter (Yankauer) or a soft-tip catheter. Steps include the following:

1. Don a mask and gloves.
2. Measure the patient from the tip of the ear to the corner of the mouth to determine how far to insert the catheter.
3. Turn on the suction.
4. Use the cross-finger technique to open the mouth.
5. Insert the tube and apply suction. The rigid catheter has a finger control to start and stop suction.

6. Move the catheter around the gum line and over the tongue to the back of the mouth, but avoid stimulating the gag reflex.
7. Suction for no longer than 15 seconds at a time.

Note: Clear a small infant's airway by suctioning the nose with a bulb syringe.

PORTABLE OXYGEN CYLINDERS

Two commonly used sizes of **portable oxygen cylinders** are D tanks (M15; 350 L) and E tanks (M24; 625 L). The EMS provider should use protective equipment (goggles, gloves). The cylinder should be placed upright. A label over the holes on the top of the cylinder indicates that the cylinder is full. Remove the label, leaving the washers in place unless the washers are built into the regulator. Face the opening of the tank away and use the key to crack the cylinder by letting out a small amount of oxygen. Apply the regulator and slide it into place. Tighten and then open the cylinder to check for pressure (there should be at least 200 psi). Close the cylinder, attach the oxygen tubing to the regulator, set the oxygen flow to the correct number of liters, and then open the cylinder and administer oxygen to the patient. When discontinuing use of the cylinder, turn off the cylinder, remove the oxygen tubing, turn the oxygen flow setting up to bleed air from the regulator, and remove the regulator.

OXYGEN DELIVERY DEVICES

Oxygen delivery devices provide oxygen-enriched air. Ambient air is about 21% oxygen, so the fraction of inspired air (FiO_2) is 21%.

- **Nasal cannula (prongs)**: FiO_2 of 24–40% with flows of ≤6 liters per minute (LPM). Humidification should be used for prolonged flow rates of >4 LPM.
- **Partial rebreather face mask**: This mask covers the nose and mouth, delivering FiO_2 of 30–60%, but the flow of oxygen should be maintained at 6–12 LPM to decrease the risk of rebreathing. Because of the higher flow rate, humidification should be used.
- **Venturi mask**: Oxygen entrainment masks come with different-sized color-coded nozzles to more accurately control FiO_2, with different sizes providing different FiO_2 levels, usually ranging from 24–50%, although an FiO_2 reading of >35% is not always reliable. The flow rate is 12–15 LPM. Humidifiers may be used.
- **Non-rebreather mask**: This mask covers the mouth and nose with a reservoir bag of oxygen. A one-way valve prevents the patient from rebreathing exhaled air. FiO_2 is about 60–80% or greater at a flow rate of 15 LPM.

RECOVERY POSITION

The recovery position is used for patients who are unconscious but breathing (such as those with a drug overdose or after a seizure) and have no life-threatening injuries. This position helps to maintain a patent airway and reduces the risk of aspiration from vomitus.

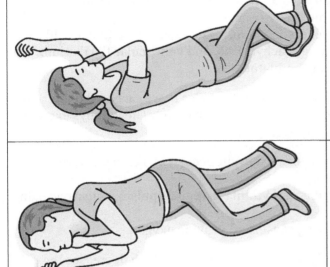	Kneeling beside the patient, lift his or her chin to ensure that the airway is open and place his or her closest arm at a right angle to the body with hand up. Place the patient's farthest arm around his or her neck with the hand touching the opposite cheek. Flex the patient's knee to 90° until the foot is flat on the floor/surface.
	Using the patient's knee as a fulcrum and supporting the farthest arm and shoulder, roll the patient onto his or her side by pulling on the farthest knee. Make sure that the top knee contacts the floor/surface to support the patient's body and that the top hand is under his or her head/neck to keep the neck in a neutral position.

ARTERIAL BLOOD GASES

Arterial blood gases are monitored to assess the effectiveness of oxygenation, ventilation, and acid-base status and to determine oxygen flow rates. The partial pressure of a gas is the pressure that is exerted by each gas in a mixture of gases, proportional to its concentration, based on total atmospheric pressure of 760 mmHg at sea level. Normal values include the following:

1. Acidity/alkalinity (pH): 7.35–7.45
2. Partial pressure of carbon dioxide ($PaCO_2$): 35–45 mmHg
3. Partial pressure of oxygen (PaO_2): 80 mmHg
4. Bicarbonate concentration (HCO_3): 22–26 mEq/L (a lower level is a base deficit, and a higher level is a base excess)
5. Oxygen saturation (SaO_2): ≥95%

The relationship between these elements, particularly the $PaCO_2$ and the PaO_2, indicates the respiratory status. For example, $PaCO_2$ >55 and PaO_2 <60 in a patient previously in good health indicates respiratory failure. There are many issues to consider. Ventilator management may require a higher $PaCO_2$ to prevent barotrauma and a lower PaO_2 to reduce oxygen toxicity.

ACID/BASE BALANCE

Respiratory acidosis: Hypoventilation (decreased breathing or inadequate mechanical ventilation) retains carbon dioxide and increases acid, which decreases the pH (acidity) to less than 7.35 (more acidic). The kidneys retain bicarbonate to compensate.

- **Causes**: COPD, pneumonia, muscle weakness, sedative/barbiturate overdose, obesity, muscle weakness (Guillain-Barré syndrome).
- **Symptoms**: Drowsiness, dizziness, headache, confusion, seizures, flushing, and low BP, tachypnea (tachy- = rapid; -pnea = breathing), tachycardia, and ventricular fibrillation.
- **Treatment**: Improved ventilation and bronchodilators.

Respiratory alkalosis: Hyperventilation (increased breathing) exhales more carbon dioxide and decreases acid, which increases the pH to greater than 7.45 (more alkalotic). The kidneys excrete increased bicarbonate to compensate.

- **Causes**: Hypoxia (low oxygen), brain injury, acetylsalicylic acid (ASA, i.e., aspirin) overdose, pulmonary embolism (clot), and septicemia.
- **Symptoms**: Confusion, lethargy, tachycardia, arrhythmia (irregular pulse), epigastric pain, nausea, and vomiting.
- **Treatment**: Identify and treat the underlying cause, and provide oxygen.

Metabolic acidosis: The kidneys excrete less acid, causing acid retention which decreases the pH, or the body excretes excess bicarbonate (through diarrhea), also decreasing the pH. Hyperventilation occurs in order to exhale additional carbon dioxide and acid to compensate.

- **Causes**: Diarrhea (it causes a loss of sodium bicarbonate), starvation, kidney disease, liver failure, excessive alcohol, shock, severe dehydration, and diabetic ketoacidosis (it causes acidic ketone bodies to build up).
- **Symptoms**: Headache, confusion, abnormal pulse, nausea, vomiting, diarrhea, and low BP.
- **Treatment**: Identify and treat the underlying cause. Bicarbonate is rarely administered, but it may be indicated in severe cases.

Metabolic alkalosis: Vomiting excretes excessive acid and/or the kidneys retain salt and potassium to compensate for vomiting, but in doing so, excrete more hydrogen ions (acid). This increases the body's pH, and hypoventilation occurs to retain carbon dioxide and acid.

- **Causes**: Excessive prolonged vomiting, low potassium level, advanced kidney failure.
- **Symptoms**: Confusion, anxiety, tremors, muscle cramping, seizures, tachycardia (rapid pulse), nausea, and vomiting.
- **Treatment**: Patient may respond to 0.9% IV saline (50-100 mL/hr.), but the underlying cause must be identified and treated. Some patients may require hemodialysis.

> **Review Video: Blood Gases**
> Visit mometrix.com/academy and enter code: 611909

OXYGEN VIA FACEMASK

Ensuring that a **facemask** (Ambu bag) is the correct fit and type is important for adequate ventilation, oxygenation, and prevention of aspiration. Difficulties in management of facemask ventilation relate to risk factors: >55 years, obesity, beard, edentulous, and history of snoring. In some cases, if dentures are adhered well, they may be left in place during induction. The facemask is applied by lifting the mandible (jaw thrust) to the mask and avoiding pressure on soft tissue. Oral or nasal airways may be used, ensuring that the distal end is at the angle of the mandible. There are a number of steps to prevent mask airway leaks:

- Increasing or decreasing the amount of air to the mask to allow better seal.
- Securing the mask with both hands while another person ventilates.
- Accommodating a large nose by using the mask upside down.
- Utilizing a laryngeal mask airway if excessive beard prevents seal.

VENTURI FACEMASK VENTILATION AND HUMIDIFIERS

The **Venturi facemask** is a high flow air-entrainment mask that mixes air and oxygen and provides a fixed flow of oxygen to the patient, usually ranging from FiO_2 of 24-50%, although FiO_2 above 35% is not always reliable. The mask comes with a set of different color-coded jets that control the mixture of air and oxygen in order to provide the desired oxygen concentration. The Venturi mask is used primarily with patients, such as those with COPD, who require oxygen supplementation but have a hypoxic drive to breathe and may be used if the EMS is concerned that the patient will retain carbon dioxide. The oxygen flow rate is set between 12 and 15 L/min.

The Venturi mask does not require the use of a **humidifier** because of the large amount of air mixed with the oxygen. However, a humidifier may be used if the patient has an artificial airway, such as a tracheostomy, as the humidification helps to loosen secretions, but the risk of infection increases. The oxygen flow rate must be between 10 and 15 L/min. Humidifiers are no longer routinely used with oxygen administration because studies show they have little effect on upper respiratory dryness.

NASOPHARYNGEAL AIRWAY (NPA)

The nasopharyngeal airway (NPA), a blind-insertion airway device, is indicated for unconscious or semiconscious patients who still have a gag reflex or those who cannot tolerate an oropharyngeal airway (OPA), but it should be avoided with severe head injury, risk of basal skull fracture, nasal bleeding, and history of deviated septum or nasal fracture. It's important to use the appropriate size. To insert the NPA, perform the following steps:

1. Choose a size that is slightly smaller in diameter than the patient's nostril.
2. Measure from the tip of the earlobe to the tip of the nose.
3. Lubricate the NPA with water-soluble lubricant and insert it in the larger and most patent (open) nostril. If inserting into the right nostril, insert with the bevel (tip) angled toward the nasal septum (the bony cartilage division between the nostrils). If inserting it into the left nostril, invert the NPA to angle the bevel toward the septum.
4. When the NPA reaches the throat, rotate it 180° into the proper position.

Nasopharyngeal Airway Placement

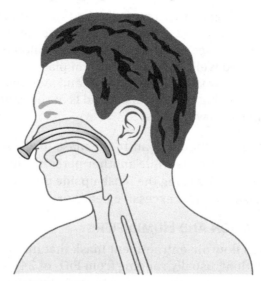

POSITIVE AIRWAY PRESSURE (PAP) DEVICES

All positive airway pressure (PAP) devices, such as **continuous positive airway pressure** (CPAP), have an air blower that delivers pressurized room air to an interface/mask. Pressure can be increased or decreased by adjusting the speed or the amount of airflow, with most machines generating from 2-20 cm of water pressure. Carbon dioxide is expelled through a vent or a nonrebreather valve on expiration. **Bilevel PAP** (**BiPAP**, **BPAP**) devices deliver two levels of pressure, which can be preset. Inspiratory PAP (IPAP) is set at a higher level (10 cmH$_2$O) than is expiratory PAP (EPAP) (5 cmH$_2$O) to allow a higher pressure needed to open the airway during inspiration but reduce the pressure to facilitate expiration. PAP is indicated for pulmonary edema, CHF, COPD, asthma, and near drowning.

The procedure includes the following:

1. Fill the humidifier with distilled water.
2. Program the settings.
3. Fit the mask and headgear/straps.
4. Begin with the pressure at the lowest setting, usually 5 cmH$_2$O (CPAP), and increase it slowly at 1 cmH$_2$O every few minutes until the optimal level is reached.
5. Monitor the oxygen saturation and respirations.

PULSE OXIMETRY

Pulse oximetry uses an external oximeter that attaches to the patient's finger or earlobe to measure arterial oxygen saturation (SPO$_2$), the percentage of hemoglobin that is saturated with oxygen. The oximeter uses light waves to determine SPO$_2$. Oxygen saturation should be maintained >95%, although some patients with chronic respiratory disorders, such as COPD, may have lower SPO$_2$ readings (generally > 88% is acceptable). Results may be compromised by impaired circulation, excessive light, poor positioning, and nail polish. If the SPO$_2$ reading falls, the oximeter should be repositioned because incorrect positioning is a common cause of inaccurate readings. Oximetry is used for monitoring when patients are on supplemental oxygen or mechanical ventilation. Oximeters do not provide information about carbon dioxide levels, so they cannot monitor carbon dioxide retention. Oximeters also cannot differentiate between different forms of hemoglobin, so if the hemoglobin has picked up carbon monoxide, the oximeter will not recognize that.

CAPNOGRAPHY, END-TIDAL CO₂ (ETCO₂), AND PEAK FLOW METER

Capnography provides a visual display of end-tidal carbon dioxide ($ETCO_2$/$PETCO_2$) levels in inhalation and exhalation. **Capnography** is recommended to establish the correct placement of an endotracheal tube, to assess the effectiveness of CPR, to evaluate respiratory distress (asthma, COPD, overdose), and to assess the patient's response to treatment. Normal **ETCO₂** is 35–45 mmHg. Hypercarbia (a measurement of >45 mmHg) occurs with hypoventilation (overdose, sedation, post-seizure, head trauma, stroke), and hypocarbia (a measurement of <35 mmHg) with hyperventilation (anxiety, bronchospasm, pulmonary edema, decreased cardiac output). $ETCO_2$ levels are less accurate with sidestream measurement used for the nasal cannula and face mask than with the mainstream sensor used with an endotracheal tube, so it's important to keep the sensor close to the mouth and secured.

The normal capnogram is a waveform that represents the varying CO_2 level throughout the breath cycle.

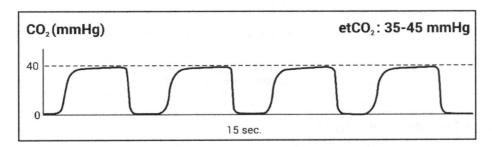

The **peak flow meter** is a handheld device that is used to determine the maximum flow rate of air on a forceful exhalation. Peak flows are used to monitor asthma and COPD. Peak flow measures are taken three times, and the highest flow rate is recorded. Optimal levels are individualized for all patients.

OROPHARYNGEAL AIRWAY (OPA)

The oropharyngeal airway (OPA), a blind-insertion airway device, may be inserted to provide better ventilation, but the OPA requires the head tilt/chin lift or modified jaw thrust as well because the device alone does not ensure a patent airway. The OPA is indicated for unconscious patients, patients with no gag reflex, and patients who are apneic (not breathing) and require ventilatory aid. The OPA is often inserted if a patient stops breathing, such as with a cardiac arrest. The OPA is contraindicated in conscious patients and those with a gag reflex. To insert the OPA, perform the following steps:

1. Estimate the length of the OPA by measuring the patient from the angle of the jaw or the tip of the earlobe to the corner of the mouth.
2. Select the correct size.
3. Open the patient's mouth using the cross-finger technique. Suction any secretions.
4. Tilt the head back (if possible). Insert the device with the tip of the OPA pointing upward for adults and downward for children.
5. Rotate the OPA into position for adults.
6. Ensure that the phalanges of the mouthpiece are securely against the patient's mouth.
7. Check to make sure the OPA is patent (open).

Oropharyngeal Airway

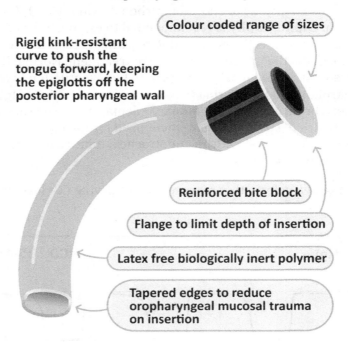

Rigid kink-resistant curve to push the tongue forward, keeping the epiglottis off the posterior pharyngeal wall

Colour coded range of sizes

Reinforced bite block

Flange to limit depth of insertion

Latex free biologically inert polymer

Tapered edges to reduce oropharyngeal mucosal trauma on insertion

LARYNGEAL-MASK AIRWAY (LMA)

The laryngeal-mask airway (LMA), a blind-insertion airway device, is an intermediate airway allowing ventilation but not complete respiratory control. The LMA consists of an inflatable cuff (mask) with a connecting tube. It may be used when tracheal intubation can't be done or as a conduit for later blind insertion of an endotracheal tube. The head and neck must be in a neutral position for insertion. If the patient has a gag reflex, then conscious sedation or topical anesthesia (deep oropharyngeal) is required. The LMA is inserted by sliding the airway along the hard palate, using the finger as a guide, into the pharynx, and the ring is inflated to create a seal around the opening to the larynx, allowing ventilation with mild positive pressure. The LMA ProSeal has a modified cuff that extends onto the back of the mask to improve the seal. The CobraPLA (perilaryngeal airway) has a larger pharyngeal cuff and provides a better seal. The LMA is contraindicated in morbid obesity, with obstructions or abnormalities of the oropharynx, and in non-fasting patients because some aspiration is still possible.

Laryngeal Mask Airway

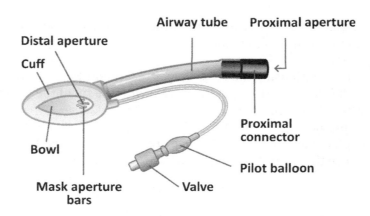

Distal aperture

Cuff

Airway tube   Proximal aperture

Bowl

Mask aperture bars

Valve

Proximal connector

Pilot balloon

TRACHEOBRONCHIAL SUCTIONING

Tracheobronchial suctioning may be done after intubating a patient so that secretions will not be forced into the lungs during artificial ventilation. A flexible "whistle-tip" catheter is used for suctioning. The patient should be on a cardiac monitor because hypoxia may produce cardiac arrhythmias (abnormal pulse). A pulse oximeter should be in place to monitor oxygen saturation.

The procedure is as follows:

1. Preoxygenate the patient for at least 5 minutes with 100% oxygen to prevent suction-related hypoxia.
2. Lubricate the catheter with a water-soluble lubricant.
3. Detach the ventilation equipment and inject 3–5 mL sterile water/saline into the endotracheal tube (ETT) to loosen up any secretions.
4. Gently insert the catheter into the ETT until resistance (the carina) is met.
5. Then, apply suction while slowly withdrawing and rotating the catheter. Suction for no more than 15 seconds.
6. If arrhythmias occur or if the oxygen saturation falls, discontinue suctioning immediately.
7. Reattach the ventilation equipment.
8. Preoxygenate again for at least 30 seconds if suctioning must be repeated.

Respiratory Emergencies

ASSESSMENT OF LUNG SOUNDS

The lungs should be auscultated for normal and abnormal **breath sounds.**

- **Vesicular**: Normal low-pitched sound over lung bases and most lung fields.
- **Bronchovesicular**: Medium-pitched sound heard over the main bronchi. Duration is the same in expiration and inspiration.
- **Bronchial**: Normal high-pitched loud sound heard over the trachea. The expiratory sound is as long or longer than the inspiratory sound. It is abnormal if it is heard over the lung bases.
- **Rales (crackles)**: High-pitched crackles usually heard at the end of expiration in the lung bases, indicating fluid in the alveoli. May be fine or coarse.
- **Rhonchi**: Deep rumbling sound that may be high-pitched and sibilant (whistling) or low-pitched and sonorous (snoring) caused by constricted airways or large amounts of secretions in the airways. It is more pronounced on expiration.
- **Wheezes**: High- or low-pitched whistling or musical sounds most pronounced on expiration. They often indicate asthma or foreign-body obstruction.
- **Stridor**: Crowing sound caused by inflammation and swelling of the larynx and trachea. Common finding in croup (associated with cough).
- **Grunts**: Indicates respiratory distress in a newborn.
- **Friction rub**: Grating sound heard over the area of the lungs where the pleura is inflamed.

> **Review Video: Lung Sounds**
> Visit mometrix.com/academy and enter code: 765616

COMMON RESPIRATORY CONDITIONS

ASTHMA

Asthma is the result of an immune response that causes constriction of bronchi and inflammation and increased secretions in the lower airways. Symptoms include cough, wheezing, diminished breath sounds, dyspnea, and difficulty speaking. Children's symptoms are often intermittent, whereas adults' symptoms tend to be persistent. Death from asthma is most common in those older than 65. Geriatric patients are most at risk from influenza, pneumonia, and pneumococcal pneumonia.

Prehospital Interventions: Administer albuterol (nebulized/metered dose) per protocol and oxygen (6-8 L per minute), and provide airway management and ventilation. Provide CPAP for moderate/severe cases. If severe, provide rapid transport.

PERTUSSIS (WHOOPING COUGH)

Pertussis consists of a severe persistent whooping cough, thick sputum, post-cough emesis, petechiae on the upper body, and sclera from exertion. Infants may develop CNS damage, apnea, or pneumonia; children may develop hernia or muscle damage; and adults may develop hernia or a fractured rib.

Prehospital Interventions: Use standard and droplet precautions, provide the patient a position of comfort, and manage the patient's airway, ventilation, and oxygen supplementation as needed.

CYSTIC FIBROSIS (CF)

CF is a progressive congenital disease that particularly affects the pancreas and lungs, causing the production of thick mucus that clogs the lungs and causes recurrent bacterial infections of the lower respiratory tract. Symptoms include severe cough, sputum, fever, and dyspnea.

Prehospital Interventions: Use standard and droplet precautions, and provide the patient a position of comfort. Manage the patient's airway, ventilation, and oxygen supplementation. Start an IV access line. If severe, provide rapid transport.

CHRONIC PULMONARY OBSTRUCTIVE DISEASE (COPD)

COPD is a disease with limitations of airflow, narrowing airways, exertional dyspnea, chronic cough, right-sided heart failure (cor pulmonale), damaged and distended alveoli, barrel chest, and clubbed fingers. Symptoms include severe dyspnea, cough, sputum, cyanosis, and the tripod position. Specific types of COPD include:

- Chronic Bronchitis: Chronic inflammation of bronchial passages with cough and sputum production, resulting in narrowed airway passages and dyspnea. Symptoms usually persist for more than 3 months per year.
- Emphysema: Chronic inflammation of the alveoli of the lungs results in ruptures and large, distended air sacs that trap air. Symptoms include dyspnea, cyanosis, difficulty exhaling, barrel chest, altered mental status, and pursed-lip breathing.

Prehospital Interventions: Manage the patient's airway and ventilation and provide oxygen per nasal cannula or Venturi mask to maintain oxygen saturation >90%, provide the patient with a position of comfort or capnography near 35-45 mmHg, peak flow, and consider CPAP. Administer a beta-agonist bronchodilator (albuterol) according to protocol. Severe: Provide rapid transport.

PNEUMONIA

Pneumonia is inflammation of the lung, filling the alveoli with exudate and interfering with ventilation. It is common throughout childhood and adulthood. **Pneumonia** may be a primary disease, or it may occur secondary to another infection or disease, such as lung cancer. Pneumonia may be caused by bacteria, viruses, parasites, fungi, or toxins. Pneumonia is characterized by location (lobar, bronchial/lobular, interstitial). Symptoms include fever, chills, cough, purulent sputum, and difficulty breathing, chest pain on cough or deep inhalation, and headache. Bacterial pneumonia is treated with antibiotics, and viral pneumonia is treated with antivirals. Geriatric patients may exhibit confusion. Pediatric patients with undeveloped or poor immune systems, or chronic illnesses such as cystic fibrosis and asthma, have an increased risk.

Prehospital Interventions: Use standard and droplet precautions, including wearing a protective face mask. Place the patient in a position of comfort (usually with his or her head elevated), manage the airway and ventilation, provide supplemental oxygen, and provide IV access line if indicated.

> **Review Video: Pneumonia**
> Visit mometrix.com/academy and enter code: 628264

SPONTANEOUS PNEUMOTHORAX

Spontaneous pneumothorax is air in the pleural space that causes the lung to collapse but without an obvious cause. Symptoms include an abrupt onset of sharp chest pain on the affected side, dyspnea, difficulty breathing, and decreased or absent respirations on the affected side.

- **Primary** (no underlying lung disease): It is most common in tall, thin adolescents and young adults and is associated with cigarette smoking. It often resolves without treatment and rarely progresses to tension pneumothorax.
- **Secondary** (underlying lung disease): It is most common in those with chronic obstructive pulmonary disease (COPD), cystic fibrosis, and severe asthma, and it poses a risk of death because of respiratory compromise. Patients may develop hypoxemia, altered mental status, coma, and tension pneumothorax.

Prehospital Interventions: Manage the patient's airway, ventilation, and oxygen supplementation. Place the patient in a position of comfort and transport. A large spontaneous pneumothorax will require catheter aspiration of air or insertion of a chest tube.

PULMONARY EDEMA

Pulmonary edema occurs when the alveoli in the lungs fill with fluid.

- **Cardiogenic**: The left ventricle weakens, so the heart cannot pump adequate amounts of blood, resulting in back pressure in the left atrium and the vessels in the lungs, forcing fluid into the alveoli. Left ventricular damage can result from coronary artery disease, cardiomyopathy, myocardial infarction, defective heart valves, and uncontrolled hypertension.
- **Non-cardiogenic**: Damage to the capillaries in the lungs causes them to leak fluid into the alveoli. Conditions causing noncardiogenic pulmonary edema include acute respiratory distress syndrome (ARDS), adverse drug reactions, pulmonary embolism, lung injury, viral infections, nervous system conditions, toxin exposure, smoke inhalation, near drowning, and high-altitude pulmonary edema (HAPE).

Symptoms include severe dyspnea, orthopnea, tachycardia, cough, and chest pain.

Prehospital Interventions: Manage airway, ventilation, and supplemental oxygen/CPAP or intubation with PEEP, and start an IV access line. Medications may include dopamine, dobutamine, nitroglycerin, and furosemide (per protocol). Severe cases require rapid transport. For HAPE, immediately descend to a lower altitude (500-1000 m), provide supplemental oxygen and a portable hyperbaric chamber, and administer acetazolamide or dexamethasone (per protocol).

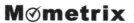

EPIGLOTTITIS

Acute epiglottitis (supraglottitis) occurs in children (primarily 1-8 years old) and in young adults. Acute epiglottitis requires immediate medical attention because it can rapidly become obstructive. The onset is usually very sudden and often occurs during the night. The patient may awaken suddenly with a fever, but he or she usually does not have a cough.

Symptoms include the following:

- **Tripod position**: Sits upright, leaning forward with the chin out, mouth open, and tongue protruding.
- **Agitation**: Appears restless, tense, and agitated.
- **Drooling**: Excess secretions combined with pain or dysphagia and a mouth-open position cause drooling.
- **Voice**: No hoarseness, but the voice sounds thick and "froglike."
- **Cyanosis**: Color is usually pale and sallow initially but may progress to frank cyanosis.
- **Throat**: On examination, the epiglottis appears bright red and swollen. Note: The patient's throat should not be examined with a tongue blade unless intubation and tracheostomy equipment are immediately available because the examination can trigger an obstruction.

Prehospital Interventions: Provide rapid transport, administer high-flow oxygen with a blow-by mask, or provide slow ventilation with a BVM.

ACUTE PULMONARY EMBOLISM

Acute pulmonary embolism occurs when a pulmonary artery or arteriole is blocked by a blood clot originating in the venous system or the right heart. While most **pulmonary emboli** are from thrombus formation, other causes may be air, fat, or septic embolus. Common originating sites for thrombus formation are the deep veins in the legs, the pelvic veins, and the right atrium. Causes include atrial fibrillation and stasis related to damage to the endothelial wall and changes in blood coagulation factors. Symptoms include dyspnea, tachypnea, tachycardia, anxiety, restlessness, chest pain, fever, rales, cough (sometimes with hemoptysis), and hemodynamic instability.

Prehospital Interventions: Assess vital signs, oxygen saturation, lung sounds, signs of jugular vein distention, signs of DVT, and signs of shock. Provide the patient with high-flow oxygen per nasal cannula (C-PAP or BIPAP if hypoxia persists), insert a large bore IV line in the antecubital fossa (to facilitate CT scan with dye), administer NS if the patient is hypotensive but limit to 500-1000 mL to avoid pulmonary edema. Monitor ECG, typical pattern is S1Q3T3—elevated S wave (lead 1) and Q wave and inverted T wave (lead III). Provide analgesia per protocol (avoid morphine). Administer norepinephrine for persistent hypotension. Provide immediate anticoagulation, such as IV heparin, if available.

Cardiology and Resuscitation

Cardiovascular Emergencies

CIRCULATORY SYSTEM

The circulatory system controls blood flow throughout the body and to the tissues, controls gas exchange (carbon dioxide and oxygen), serves as a reservoir for blood, maintains blood pH through a buffer system, responds to infections, and facilitates coagulation (blood clotting). The circulatory system includes the cardiovascular system (heart and blood vessels) and the blood.

- **Heart**: The heart has four chambers, upper (right atrium and left atrium) and lower (right ventricle and left ventricle). The heart muscle receives blood from two major coronary arteries and their branches. The myocardium (heart muscle) receives blood from two major coronary arteries and their branches. The inner lining of the heart is the endocardium, and the lining that surrounds the heart is the pericardium, which has an inner double-layered serous membrane (visceral pericardium) and a fibrous outer layer (parietal pericardium).
- **Vessels**: The venous system includes veins, venules, and venous capillaries and brings blood back to the heart via the inferior and superior vena cava. The arterial system, including the coronary arteries, branches from the aorta after it leaves the heart and includes arteries, arterioles, and arterial capillaries.
- **Blood**: Blood consists of red blood cells (erythrocytes); white blood cells (leukocytes including monocytes, lymphocytes, basophils, neutrophils, and eosinophils); platelets (thrombocytes); and plasma, the liquid portion of the blood (which contains clotting factors).

> **Review Video: Functions of the Circulatory System**
> Visit mometrix.com/academy and enter code: 376581

CONDUCTION SYSTEM OF THE HEART

Normal conduction of the heart has the following four stages:

1. **Generation of an impulse at the sinoatrial (SA) node** (primary pacemaker) located at the junction of the right atrium and superior vena cava: The electrical impulse travels the cells of the atria along internodal pathways, causing electrical stimulation and contraction of the atria, including Bachmann's bundle, which stimulates the left atrium.
2. **Atrioventricular node conduction of impulse**: This occurs when the impulses from the SA node reach the AV node in the right atrial wall near the tricuspid valve. There is a slight delay (about one-tenth of a second), allowing the atria to empty.
3. **Atrioventricular bundle (bundle of His) conduction**: The AV node relays the impulse to the ventricles through the atrioventricular bundle—specialized conduction cells in the ventricular septum that branch to the right and left ventricles, carrying the electrical impulse.
4. **Purkinje fiber conduction**: Impulses are conducted down the AV bundles to the base of the heart where they divide into the Purkinje fibers, which stimulate the myocardial cells to contract the ventricles.

CARDIAC CYCLE AND BLOOD FLOW THROUGH THE HEART

The cardiac cycle involves one complete heartbeat with systole (ventricular contraction) and diastole (relaxation) phases. **Stroke volume** is the volume of blood ejected from the left ventricle in one cardiac cycle (about 60–70 mL), and **cardiac output** is the heart rate times the stroke volume.

The **blood flows** as follows:

- Deoxygenated venous blood returns to the heart per the inferior vena cava, superior vena cava, and coronary sinus (bringing blood from the coronary arteries) into the right atrium, and then it flows through the tricuspid valve into the right ventricle.
- From the right ventricle, blood flows through the pulmonic (semilunar) valve into the pulmonary artery and to the lungs to exchange carbon dioxide for oxygen.
- Oxygenated blood flows from the lungs through the pulmonary veins into the left atrium and through the mitral (bicuspid) valve into the left ventricle.
- From the left ventricle, blood flows through the aortic valve and into the aorta, the coronary arteries, and the general circulation through the thoracic and abdominal aorta.
- After blood flows through the valves, they close to prevent backflow. Both atria and both ventricles contract simultaneously.

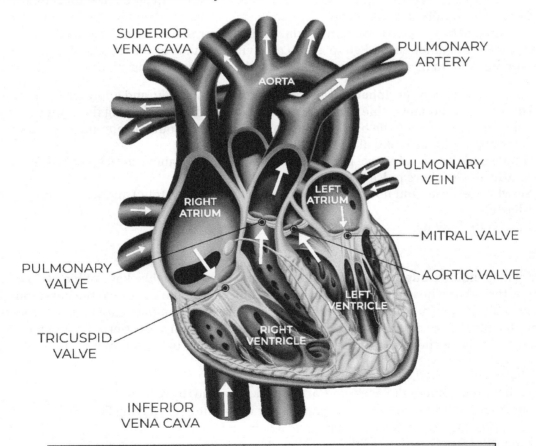

Review Video: Heart Blood Flow
Visit mometrix.com/academy and enter code: 783139

Review Video: Diastolic vs Systolic
Visit mometrix.com/academy and enter code: 898934

PERFUSION, OXYGENATION OF TISSUES, AND CARDIAC COMPROMISE

Perfusion depends on an adequate supply of red blood cells, which carry oxygen. Perfusion may be impaired if the heart does not pump adequately, if the rate of heart contractions is too low or too rapid to be effective, and if the volume of blood and/or red blood cells pumped is not adequate to provide oxygenation to the tissues. With adequate perfusion, **oxygenation of tissues** occurs when blood flows throughout the body, and gas exchange of carbon dioxide and waste products for oxygen occurs at the capillaries. **Cardiac compromise** results in inadequate circulation and/or perfusion of vital organs. Cardiac compromise may result from atherosclerosis (plaques/fatty deposits) in the arterial lumens, resulting in obstructed blood flow and inadequate dilation and constriction of arteries. Ischemia (low oxygenation) occurs with decreased blood flow and can damage tissues, but occlusion (obstruction) can result in the death of tissue. Cardiac compromise may result from heart damage causing an inadequate heart rate and/or pumping. Cardiac compromise may also result from an inadequate volume of circulating blood.

OBTAINING A MANUAL BLOOD PRESSURE

When obtaining **a** manual blood pressure, a correctly sized cuff is essential. The cuff width should be 40% of the circumference (or 20% wider than the diameter) of the middle of the limb to which the blood pressure cuff will be applied. The bladder (which fills with air as the cuff is inflated) should circle at least 80% of the limb and the cuff width (when used on the upper arm) should cover two-thirds of the length of the upper arm. Small or extra-large blood pressure cuffs may be indicated. Cuffs should not be applied to a limb receiving IV fluids or one that is traumatized. The forearm (or leg) should be at heart level and the hand turned up if using an arm. Procedure:

1. Palpate brachial or peripheral artery, deflate cuff completely, and apply snugly to the site (two fingers should be able to fit between the cuff and arm), aligning the centering arrows correctly or centering the bladder over the artery. Cuff should be one-inch above site of arterial pulsation (popliteal or antecubital).
2. Inflate bladder and increase pressure to about 30 mmHg above anticipated base or 30 mmHg above where pulse is no longer palpable.
3. Slowly release air and note when heart sound appears (systolic) and when it disappears (diastolic).
4. Record BP reading.

ANGINA

Chest pain may indicate **angina** (pain from temporary constriction/blockage of blood flow in the coronary arteries) or a heart attack (pain caused by blockage of blood flow to the heart muscle because of a blood clot (most common) or hemorrhage, resulting in the death of heart tissue). Heart problems in children are often associated with congenital heart disease. Geriatric and female patients may not have chest pain with a heart attack. Make note of the following:

- Character, location, and severity of the pain.
- Radiation of pain to the neck, jaw, arms, back, jaw, and/or stomach.
- Shortness of breath at rest, with exertion, or worsening when lying flat.
- Cold, clammy skin is common with a heart attack.
- Note BP, pulse (rapid, irregular, slow), and respirations.
- Note nausea and/or vomiting and dizziness/lightheadedness.

ANGINA PECTORIS (STABLE)

Impairment of blood flow through the coronary arteries leads to ischemia of the cardiac muscle and **angina pectoris**—pain that may occur in the sternum, chest, neck, arms (especially the left arm), or back. The pain frequently occurs with crushing pain substernally, radiating down the left arm or both arms, although this type of pain is more common in males than females, whose symptoms may appear less acute and may include nausea, shortness of breath, and fatigue. Elderly or diabetic patients may also have pain in their arms, no pain at all (silent ischemia), or weakness and numbness in both arms.

Stable angina episodes usually last for <5 minutes and are fairly predictable, exercise-induced episodes caused by atherosclerotic lesions blocking >75% of the lumen of the affected coronary artery. Precipitating events include exercise, a decrease in the environmental temperature, heavy eating, strong emotions (such as fright or anger), or exertion, including coitus. Stable angina episodes usually resolve in less than 5 minutes by decreasing the activity level and administering sublingual nitroglycerin. Provide supportive care, oxygen, and assist the patient to take nitroglycerin if available.

ANGINA PECTORIS (UNSTABLE, VARIANT/PRINZMETAL'S)

Unstable angina (also known as preinfarction or crescendo angina) is a progression of coronary artery disease, and it occurs when there is a change in the pattern of stable angina. The pain may increase, may not respond to a single nitroglycerin dose, and may persist for >5 minutes. Usually pain is more frequent, lasts longer, and may occur at rest when sitting or lying down. Unstable angina may indicate a rupture of an atherosclerotic plaque and the beginning of thrombus formation, so it should always be treated as a medical emergency with rapid transport because it may indicate a myocardial infarction.

Variant angina (also known as **Prinzmetal's angina**) results from spasms of the coronary arteries. It can be associated with or without atherosclerotic plaques and is often related to smoking, alcohol, or illicit stimulants. Variant angina frequently occurs cyclically at the same time each day and often while the person is at rest. Nitroglycerin or calcium channel blockers are used for treatment.

MANAGEMENT OF A PATIENT WITH ANGINA

Management of a patient with angina begins with a thorough assessment, primary and secondary survey, and use of the OPQRST and SAMPLE methods of history taking. Patients are often very frightened, so the EMS provider should provide clear feedback and reassurance. The patient should be placed in the semi-Fowler's position, especially if he or she is experiencing shortness of breath, and the oxygen saturation should be monitored. Respiratory compromise may require supplemental oxygen, bag-mask ventilation (BVM) assistance, PEEP, CPAP/BiPAP, manually triggered ventilators (MTVs), or automatic transport ventilators (ATVs). If an EMT is the first to arrive at the scene, the EMT should determine the need for the assistance of an advanced emergency medical technician (AEMT) or a paramedic.

Pharmacological interventions (assist the patient with medication administration, or administer the medication according to protocol) may include the following:

- **Aspirin** (for suspected heart attack; Bayer, Heartline, ZORprin, Empirin): Provide 162 to 325 mg chewable (preferred). Contraindicated with GI bleeding, stroke.
- **Nitroglycerin** (for suspected angina; Nitro-Dur, Nitrolingual, NitroMist): Provide 0.4 mg sublingually repeated every 3–5 minutes up to three doses. Contraindicated if the patient has recently taken Viagra, had a stroke, or has excessive bleeding.
- **Oral glucose** (for suspected hypoglycemia/insulin reaction): Glucose tablets, solution.

All patients with chest pain should be transported because even mild chest discomfort may indicate that the patient is having a heart attack, especially in older patients and female patients, who often have atypical symptoms.

MYOCARDIAL INFARCTION

Myocardial infarction (also referred to as an MI or heart attack) may occur after an episode of unstable angina caused by a rupture of an atherosclerotic plaque and thrombosis associated with coronary artery spasm, but it may also result from vasoconstriction, acute blood loss, decreased oxygen, and ingestion of cocaine. Symptoms may vary considerably, with males having the more "classic" symptom of a sudden onset of crushing chest pain. Elderly and diabetic patients may complain primarily of weakness. Symptoms include the following:

- Angina with pain in the chest that may radiate to the neck or arms, crushing pain, tightness (often more than 30 minutes and unrelieved by rest or nitroglycerin).
- Hypertension or hypotension.
- Palpitations, tachycardia, bradycardia, and dysrhythmias.
- Dyspnea.
- ECG changes (ST segment and T-wave changes), tachycardia, bradycardia, and dysrhythmias.
- Pulmonary edema, peripheral edema, weak/absent peripheral pulses.
- Nausea and vomiting.
- Pallor, cold and clammy skin, diaphoresis.
- Neurological/psychological disturbances: Anxiety, light-headedness, headache, visual abnormalities, slurred speech, and fear.

Prehospital Interventions: Manage the patient's airway/ventilation/oxygen supplementation, provide supportive care, perform CPR/defibrillation if needed, and provide rapid transport.

> **Review Video: Myocardial Infarction**
> Visit mometrix.com/academy and enter code: 148923

ECG ANALYSIS OF MYOCARDIAL INFARCTION

Myocardial ischemia results in ST-segment depression and T-wave inversion. **Myocardial injury** results in ST-segment elevation and T-wave inversion. **Myocardial infarction** results in hyperacute T waves (initial stage), ST-segment elevation, T-wave inversion, and pathologic Q waves. Arrhythmias common to MI include sinus tachycardia (rapid heart rate), sinus bradycardia (slow heart rate), heart blocks, ventricular fibrillation, pulseless electrical activity (PEA), and asystole. Rapid transport is indicated for patients having no relief from medication, hypotension, hypoperfusion, and/or significant ECG changes/abnormalities. No transport is indicated only for patient refusal.

Q wave MI:

- Characterized by a series of abnormal Q waves (wider and deeper) on ECG, especially in the early morning (related to adrenergic activity)
- Infarction is usually prolonged and results in necrosis (This may indicate extensive transient ischemia)
- Usually transmural

Non-Q wave MI:

- Characterized by changes in the ST-T wave with ST depression (usually reversible within a few days)
- Usually reperfusion occurs spontaneously, so the infarct size is smaller; contraction necrosis related to reperfusion is common
- Usually nontransmural

ELECTROCARDIOGRAM (ECG)

The electrocardiogram (ECG) records and shows a graphic display of the electrical activity of the heart through a number of different waveforms, complexes, and intervals as follows:

- **P wave**: Start of the electrical impulse in the sinus node and spreading through the atria, muscle depolarization
- **QRS complex**: Ventricular muscle depolarization and atrial repolarization
- **T wave**: Ventricular muscle repolarization (resting state) as cells regain a negative charge
- **U wave**: Repolarization of the Purkinje fibers

A modified lead II ECG is often used to monitor basic heart rhythms and dysrhythmias. Typical placement of leads for a two-lead ECG is 3 to 5 cm inferior to the right clavicle and left lower rib cage. Typical placement for a three-lead ECG is the right arm (RA) near the shoulder, the V_5 position over the fifth intercostal space (LA), and the left upper leg (LL) near the groin.

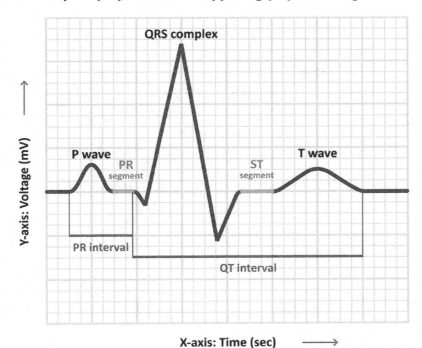

57

12-Lead Electrocardiography

The most common electrocardiography setup is the **12-lead ECG**, which assesses 12 different views of the heart. The 12-lead ECG actually comprises 10 electrodes and 12 sources of measurement as follows:

- Four limb electrodes: right and left arm and right and left leg (RA, LA, RL, LL). Put in place, avoiding heavily muscled areas.
- Six precordial (in front of the heart/pericardium) electrodes:
  - V1—Right sternum, fourth intercostal space
  - V2—Left sternum, fourth intercostal space
  - V3—Halfway between V2 and V4
  - V4—Midclavicular line, fifth intercostal space
  - V5—In line with V4 at the anterior axillary line
  - V6—In line with V4 and V5 at the midaxillary line

The patient should be placed in the flat supine position for the ECG, although he or she can sit in the semi-Fowler's position if unable to tolerate a flat position. The skin should be dry and the hair clipped or shaved to improve the electrode contact, and conductive gel is applied to the electrode. The skin can be wiped with an alcohol pad to remove oils or other residue before applying the electrodes. Electrodes should not be placed directly over a bone.

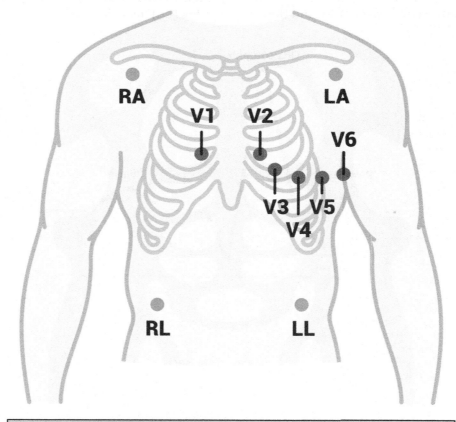

Review Video: Cardiovascular Assessment
Visit mometrix.com/academy and enter code: 323076

HEART SOUNDS

Normal and abnormal heart sounds include the following:

- **First and second sounds**: The first heart sound (S1—"lub") is closure of the mitral and tricuspid valves (heard at the apex/left ventricular area of the heart). The second heart sound (S2—"dub") is closure of the aortic and pulmonic valves (heard at the base of the heart). There may be a slight splitting of the S2.
- **Gallop rhythms**:
  - S3 occurs after S2 in children and young adults, but it may indicate heart failure or left ventricular failure in older adults (heard with the patient lying on the left side).
  - S4 occurs before S1 and occurs with ventricular hypertrophy, such as from coronary artery disease, hypertension, or aortic valve stenosis.
- **Opening snap**: Unusual, high-pitched sound occurring after S2 with stenosis of mitral valve from rheumatic heart disease
- **Ejection click**: Brief, high-pitched sound occurring immediately after S1 with stenosis of the aortic valve
- **Friction rub**: Harsh, grating sound heard in systole and diastole with pericarditis
- **Murmur**: Sound caused by turbulent blood flow from stenotic or malfunctioning valves, congenital defects, or increased blood flow

HEART FAILURE

Heart failure (HF, aka congestive HF) includes disorders of contractions (systolic "left-sided" dysfunction) or filling (diastolic dysfunction) or both, which result in hypertrophy (thickening, enlarging, and stiffening) of the myocardium (heart muscle). The most common causes are coronary artery disease, myocardial infarction, systemic or pulmonary hypertension, cardiomyopathy, and valvular disorders. The incidence of HF correlates with age. Left-sided HF may cause pulmonary edema that impairs ventilation, leading to hypoxia, especially when the patient is lying in a supine position, and right-sided HF may cause abdominal and peripheral edema of the feet and legs. The circulatory time with HF decreases overall, so changes in oximetry to show hypoxia may be delayed. The autonomic nervous system's regulation of breathing to control oxygen levels may be impaired, resulting in periodic breathing patterns, Cheyne-Stokes breathing, or central sleep apnea. Medications used to treat HF include ACE inhibitors (captopril, lisinopril), angiotensin receptor blockers (ARBs) (losartan, valsartan), beta-blockers (metoprolol, carvedilol), aldosterone agonists (spironolactone), and diuretics (hydrochlorothiazide, furosemide).

CHRONIC VS ACUTE HEART FAILURE

Chronic heart failure develops insidiously over time as the heart muscles weaken and enlarge, so initially patients may only note fatigue, weight gain, and swelling in their feet and ankles. **Acute heart failure** is characterized by impairment of gas exchange and decreased cardiac output because of changes in preload, contractibility, and heart rhythm; symptoms are more acute and may include irregular heartbeat, chest pain, cough, and rapid breathing, wheezing, and cyanosis from lack of adequate oxygen. Patients may also suffer from anxiety, decreased activity tolerance, and disturbances in sleep patterns. Medical management is aimed at increasing cardiac function, providing support, and monitoring treatment. Patients often are acutely short of breath and sitting upright, with rales evident in their lungs. Assessment includes conducting primary and secondary surveys, taking a complete medical history including medication use and home oxygen use, and assessing the patient's level of consciousness, airway status (cough, sputum, labored breathing, tripod position), heart rate/rhythm, peripheral pulses, edema (pitting/nonpitting, ascites, sacral), and complications.

Prehospital Interventions: Manage the patient's airway/ventilation/oxygen supplementation with a nonrebreather mask or BVM with high-flow oxygen. Position the mask for comfort and suction if necessary.

HYPERTENSIVE CRISIS

Hypertensive crisis (aka malignant hypertension) is a marked elevation in BP that can cause severe organ damage if left untreated. Causes include encephalopathy, intracranial hemorrhage, aortic dissection, eclampsia, and heart failure. Classifications are as follows:

- **Hypertensive emergency**: Acute hypertension, usually >120 mmHg diastolic, must be treated immediately to lower the BP in order to prevent damage to vital organs, such as the heart, brain, or kidneys.
- **Hypertensive urgency**: Acute hypertension must be treated within a few hours, but the vital organs are not in immediate danger. The blood pressure is lowered more slowly to avoid hypotension, ischemia of vital organs, or failure of autoregulation with a one-third reduction in 6 hours.

Symptoms include headache, dizziness, dyspnea, weakness, visual disturbances, anxiety, chest pain (atypical), heart failure, acute coronary syndrome, and stroke.

Prehospital Interventions: Asymptomatic hypertension requires referral to a physician, whereas severe symptoms require rapid transport. Interventions include airway support/ventilation with oxygen supplementation and advanced life support as needed. Patients with severe dyspnea and pulmonary edema may need CPAP.

THROMBOEMBOLISM AND PULMONARY EMBOLISM

Thromboembolism includes the formation of a thrombus (such as in the heart with atrial fibrillation and in the deep veins with immobilization) and an embolism in which a clot breaks off and travels through the circulatory system. Although thromboembolism may cause a heart attack or stroke, the most common presentation is a **pulmonary embolism (PE)** resulting from deep vein thrombosis. The patient may or may not complain of pain at the thrombus site, which may be swollen and erythematous (red), typically in a lower extremity. When the patient develops PE, the usual presentation is acute onset of dyspnea and tachycardia and sitting in the tripod position. Some patients may have ECG abnormalities, frothy sputum, cough, fever, hemoptysis, and jugular vein distension.

Prehospital Interventions: Provide supportive care, manage the patient's airway/ventilation/intubation as needed with oxygen to maintain oxygen saturation >94%, establish an IV access line, administer up to 1 L of NS, and give norepinephrine if indicated. If protocol permits, administer heparin for PE.

Shock and Resuscitation

SYMPTOMS AND INTERVENTIONS FOR SHOCK

Shock is a life-threatening condition that occurs when the tissues do not receive adequate oxygen, such as with severe bleeding or fluid loss, severe infection, heart failure, or abnormal dilation of the blood vessels. Indications of shock include extreme thirst; anxiety and restlessness; weak, rapid pulse; altered mental status progressing to loss of consciousness; rapid, shallow respirations; hypotension (low BP—often a late sign); and cool, clammy, pale skin with mottling sometimes on the extremities from inadequate perfusion. If left untreated, shock may lead to cardiac arrest. Note that geriatric patients may have a higher baseline respiration and heart rate and an irregular pulse.

Prehospital Interventions: Apply pressure to control the bleeding, perform spinal stabilization if needed, place the patient in the shock position (flat with feet elevated above the level of the heart, 8-12 inches), manage the patient's airway and ventilation and administer high-concentration oxygen, provide warming blankets to maintain the body temperature, provide reassurance, apply a pneumatic anti-shock garment (PASG), insert an IV access line, and administer fluids for hemorrhage/severe hypotension. Provide rapid transport if needed.

STAGES AND TYPES OF SHOCK

Shock generally occurs in stages as the body tries to compensate. **Compensated shock** occurs in the early stage while the body speeds up the heart rate and respirations and diverts blood to the vital organs (resulting in pale, cool skin) to maintain adequate perfusion and BP. **Decompensated shock** occurs when the body can no longer compensate and the BP falls and symptoms worsen. With irreversible shock, recovery is no longer possible because of cell damage caused by inadequate oxygenation and perfusion. **Types of shock** include the following:

- **Cardiogenic**: Heart failure, myocardial infarction, drug overdose, dysrhythmia, congenital heart disease
- **Distributive**: Anaphylaxis, drug overdose
- **Hypovolemic**: Hemorrhage, severe vomiting and/or diarrhea, severe burns, dehydration
- **Obstructive**: Pneumothorax, pericardial tamponade
- **Neurogenic**: Spinal cord injury (a form of distributive shock because of decreased vascular tone)
- **Septic**: Sepsis, severe infections (also a form of distributive shock)

Signs and symptoms are similar for all types of shock even though the mechanisms are different (excluding neurogenic shock which can present with bradycardia instead of tachycardia).

HYPOVOLEMIC SHOCK

Hypovolemic shock occurs when the total circulating volume of fluid decreases, leading to a fall in venous return that in turn causes a decrease in ventricular filling and preload. This results in a decrease in stroke volume and cardiac output. This in turn causes generalized arterial vasoconstriction, increasing afterload (increased systemic vascular resistance), and causing decreased tissue perfusion.

Hypovolemic shock is **classified** according to the degree of fluid loss as follows:

- **Class I**: <750 mL or ≤15% of total circulating volume (TCV) (usually well tolerated)
- **Class II**: 750-1500 mL or 15-30% of TCV (tachycardia, anxiety, narrow pulse pressure, and increased respirations)
- **Class III**: 1500-2000 mL or 30-40% of TCV (hypotension, pallor, cold, clammy skin, delayed capillary refill, severe tachycardia, and altered mental status)
- **Class IV**: >2000 mL or >40% of TCV (severe shock, a weak thready pulse, cyanosis, and death without aggressive resuscitation)

Prehospital Interventions: Control the patient's bleeding upon arrival to the scene. The EMS provider should insert two large-bore, short IV catheters, give 250-500 cc of warm isotonic boluses (20-30 mL/kg), keep the patient warm, maintain the patient's airway/ventilation/oxygen supplementation to maintain oxygen saturation at 90-92%, maintain the systolic BP at 70-90 mmHg, place him or her in the shock position, and provide rapid transport.

RESPIRATORY FAILURE/ARREST

Respiratory failure occurs when ventilation is insufficient for adequate gas exchange so that levels of carbon dioxide in the blood increase and levels of oxygen decrease. **Respiratory failure** may result from respiratory infection (pneumonia, tuberculosis), heart failure, chronic respiratory illness (asthma, chronic bronchitis, COPD), trauma, and depression of the CNS (usually from medications or trauma). Respiratory failure may be acute with sudden onset or chronic, developing over time. If untreated, respiratory failure can lead to **respiratory arrest**, which in turn leads to cardiac arrest. Indications of respiratory failure include altered mental status, cyanosis, labored breathing (dyspnea and orthopnea), coughing, fatigue, diminished breath sounds, and the presence of rales (crackles) and rhonchi (snoring/whistling sound). Patients may have hemoptysis (bloody sputum). The patient's oxygen saturation level is lower than 90% per pulse oximeter.

Prehospital Interventions: Manage the patient's airway/ventilation/oxygen supplementation; positive-pressure ventilation may be needed. Place the patient in a position of comfort (usually high Fowler's).

HEIMLICH MANEUVER FOR CHOKING

INFANTS

Indications of choking in **infants younger than 1 year old** include lack of breathing, gasping, cyanosis, and the inability to cry. The procedure for **Heimlich chest thrusts** includes the following:

- Position the infant in the prone position along your forearm with the infant's head lower than the trunk, being sure to support the head so the airway is not blocked.
- Using the heel of the hand, deliver five forceful upward blows between the shoulder blades.
- Sandwich the child between your two arms, and turn the infant into the supine position and drape over your thigh with his or her head lower than the trunk and the head supported.
- Using two fingers (as for CPR compressions), give up to five thrusts (about 1.5 inches deep) to the lower third of the sternum.
- Only do a finger sweep and remove a foreign object if the object is visible. Repeat five back blows, five chest thrusts until the foreign body is ejected.
- If the infant loses consciousness, begin CPR. If a pulse is noted but spontaneous respirations are absent, continue with ventilation only.

CHILDREN AND ADULTS

The universal sign of choking is when a person clutches his or her throat and appears to be choking or gasping for breath. If the person can speak ("Can you speak?") or cough, the Heimlich maneuver is not usually necessary. The Heimlich maneuver can be done with the victim sitting, standing, or supine. The Heimlich maneuver for **children (≥1 year) and adults** is as follows:

- Wrap both arms around the victim's waist from the back if sitting or standing. Make a fist and place the thumb side against the victim's abdomen slightly above the umbilicus. Grasp this hand with the other and thrust sharply upward to force air out of the lungs.
- Repeat as needed.
- If the victim loses consciousness, ease him or her into a supine position on the floor, and initiate chest compressions (CPR). Assess the airway and remove any visible obstruction. The blind finger sweep is no longer recommended. Repeat compressions and ventilations until recovery or emergency personnel arrive.

CARDIOPULMONARY RESUSCITATION (CPR) FOR CARDIAC ARREST

Cardiac arrest of unknown cause in adults or children is usually treated as though it were ventricular fibrillation or pulseless ventricular tachycardia, but the protocol varies. **Cardiopulmonary resuscitation (CPR)** involves the following components:

- Immediate defibrillation is performed according to protocol with an AED/manual defibrillator (preferred) followed by CPR, beginning with compressions (30:2 compression to ventilation at the rate of 100-120 per minute at least 2 inches deep; two-finger compressions, to one-third of the chest depth for infants and children) for 2 minutes or 5 cycles and repeat defibrillation.
- Repeat cycles of 2 minutes of CPR and defibrillation. (Laypeople may use compression-only CPR.)
- If a defibrillator is not readily available, CPR may begin first. Note that if a BVM is used, the break in compressions should not exceed 10 seconds. If an advanced airway/intubation is in place, ventilation should be at the rate of 8-10 per minute, maintaining oxygen saturation ≥94% but <100% with ventilation between compressions.
- The $ETCO_2$ value should be 10-20 mmHg if chest compressions are adequate, increasing to 35-45 mmHg with the return of spontaneous circulation (ROSC).

DEFIBRILLATION USING AN AUTOMATED/SEMI-AUTOMATED DEFIBRILLATOR

Emergency defibrillation is indicated for acute ventricular fibrillation or ventricular tachycardia with no audible or palpable pulse; it is ineffective for asystole or pulseless electrical activity. Defibrillation delivers an electrical discharge through paddles or pads applied to both sides of the chest. Automated external defibrillators (AEDs) are frequently used by first responders although manual defibrillators require less downtime from CPR. Procedure:

- Turn on the AED.
- Apply pads to chest (position may vary according to manufacturer). For infants and small children, if pads touch when applied in the directed positions for an adult, apply one to chest and one to back.
- Plug in the connector if necessary.
- Do not touch the patient while the AED analyzes heart rhythm.

- Follow directions for shocking (or resuming CPR if rhythm is not shockable) and warn others to stand clear.
- Continue CPR beginning with compressions immediately after shock is delivered for 2 minutes or 5 cycles between defibrillations.

If the patient is wet, wipe off the chest before applying pads. Remove any transdermal patches on the chest, and shave excessive hair before applying pads. If the patient has an implanted device, the pads should be placed at least 1 in (2.5 cm) away.

SPECIAL ARRESTS AND PERI-ARREST SITUATIONS

Special arrests and peri-arrest situations include:

- **Drowning**: For water rescue, start with ventilation because compressions are ineffective. On land, open the patient's airway and check for breathing (respiratory arrest may occur before cardiac arrest). If there are no respirations, ventilate twice and check his or her pulse. If there is no pulse, begin CPR at a 30:2 ratio and defibrillate as soon as possible for VT/VF or follow asystole protocol, depending on the situation. If the patient vomits (common), turn him or her to one side, clear the mouth/suction, and resume CPR.
- **Electrical shock or lightning**: Begin CPR following standard protocol. Early intubation may be necessary if face, mouth, or neck burns are present. Maintain spinal stabilization because of the risk of back/neck injury. Provide an IV access line and fluids for extensive tissue injury after resuscitation.
- **Pregnancy**: Begin CPR following standard protocol. If the fundus height is at or above the umbilicus, use lateral uterine displacement (LUD) during CPR to relieve aortocaval compression. Alert resources for immediate peri-mortem C-section (in the second half of a pregnancy) if ROSC is not achievable or resuscitation is futile.
- **Hypothermia**: If no pulse or respiration is detectable, begin immediate CPR (30:20) and defibrillate as soon as possible. Remove any wet clothing (during resuscitation if possible) and begin with warming protocols. Manage the patient's airway/ventilation/oxygen supplementation with warm, humidified oxygen. After ROSC, warm the patient to 32-34 °C. Treat the underlying cause, such as drug overdose. Do not consider terminating efforts until the patient is rewarmed.
- **Electrolyte imbalance**: Sodium, magnesium (except for extreme hypermagnesemia), and calcium abnormalities rarely lead to cardiac arrest. However, hyperkalemia (high potassium) (>6.5 mEq/L/mmol/L) may be lethal. Stabilize the heart cells with 5-10 mL of 10% calcium chloride or 10-20 mL of 10% calcium gluconate; shift potassium to the cells with 1 mEq/kg sodium bicarbonate and 25 g 50% glucose (unless he or she is hyperglycemic) with 10 U regular insulin (if available, to prevent hyperglycemia) and 2.5 mg albuterol (per nebulizer); and provide diuresis with 20-40 mg furosemide (per protocol).
- **Trauma**: Follow standard protocol, but the patient may require cervical spine stabilization and advanced airway/ventilation or cricothyrotomy, depending on the injuries. Use barriers to protect yourself from blood. Note: A chest blow may cause VF, requiring rapid defibrillation.

POST-RESUSCITATION RETURN OF SPONTANEOUS CIRCULATION (ROSC)

If a patient undergoing resuscitation has **return of spontaneous circulation (ROSC)**, his or her ventilation and oxygenation must be supported to maintain the oxygen saturation ≥94% but less than 100% to avoid hyperoxia. Ventilation should be maintained at 10-12 breaths per minute with an ETCO$_2$ value at 35-40 mmHg. Hyperventilation must be avoided. Hypotension (systolic BP <90 mmHg) should be treated with an IV bolus (1-2 L saline) and vasopressor infusion. Treatable causes (the five H's and five T's) should be addressed, and a 12-lead ECG should be used to monitor the patient's condition. If the patient is nonresponsive, therapeutic hypothermia (to 32-34 °C) for 12-24 hours may be considered as a neuroprotective measure. If the patient is responsive and able to follow commands, he or she should be immediately transported to the appropriate receiving facility: the ICU or cardiac cath lab for acute myocardial infarction (AMI) or ST-elevated myocardial infarction (STEMI) for percutaneous coronary intervention (PCI). Note: Brain damage begins within 4-6 minutes of cardiac arrest, and it is irreversible after 8-10 minutes.

TERMINATION OF RESUSCITATION EFFORTS

Criteria for termination of resuscitation efforts include the following considerations:

- ≥18 years
- Arrest is cardiac-related and not a condition that may respond to hospital treatment
- Endotracheal intubation was successful and maintained throughout resuscitation efforts
- Standard advanced cardiac life support efforts were used
- Resuscitation efforts maintained for 25 minutes or asystole through four rounds of drugs
- At the time of the decision to terminate, the patient exhibits asystole or an agonal rhythm (the bizarre, ineffective, wide ventricular rhythm associated with dying)
- Official DNR order
- Newborn: No heartbeat detected after 10 minutes of CPR

Note: Older age, quality of life, and time of collapse prior to EMS arrival are not criteria for termination. Generally, resuscitation efforts are continued until arrival at the receiving facility on those patients younger than 18 unless the child has a terminal disease and an advance directive that limits resuscitation efforts. Prior to termination, the EMS provider should have direct communication with medical oversight and consult/advise the family members that are present. Family resistance must be noted and reported. Criteria for withholding resuscitation include DNR status, obvious signs of death (such as rigor mortis/lividity), or conditions that are unsafe for the rescuer.

WITHHOLDING RESUSCITATION ATTEMPTS

Although the goal of EMS is to save lives, it is not always possible or ethical to carry out resuscitation efforts. **Withholding resuscitation** is justified under the following conditions:

- The patient's condition is not compatible with life (massive injuries, decapitation, crushed chest, severe open head injury with loss of brain tissue), and the patient is not breathing and has no pulse.
- The patient exhibits obvious signs of death, such as rigor mortis or livor mortis, indicating that he or she can no longer be resuscitated.
- The patient has a do-not-resuscitate (DNR) form available, and it is properly signed. Note: The EMS provider cannot accept the word of family or friends that the patient does not want to be resuscitated without a DNR order.
- Conditions are unsafe to approach the patient and/or administer resuscitation efforts. This may occur, for example, if there are gunshots heard in the area, if the patient is pinned under a motor vehicle, or if the patient cannot safely be reached in time because of difficult terrain.

65

CPR ASSISTIVE DEVICES

IMPEDANCE THRESHOLD DEVICE (ITD)

The impedance threshold device (such as the ResQPOD ITD) is a small, single-use device that fits into the airway circuit (face mask or advanced airway) with CPR. During CPR, compressions generate both positive pressure that promotes cardiac output and, when released completely, negative pressure (a vacuum) within the thorax that refills the heart, so adequate negative pressure ensures better filling. During compressions with an ITD, a valve in the device allows air to escape, but, when the compressions are released, the valve closes to prevent the intake of air, increasing negative pressure and improving circulation on subsequent compressions; however, the device allows the EMS provider to ventilate the patient, and it has flashing timing lights every 6 seconds (so 1 ventilation with every flash equals 10 per minute). The ITD may double the blood flow to the heart and double the systolic BP as well as increase cerebral perfusion.

AUTOMATED CHEST COMPRESSION DEVICES

With automated chest compression devices for CPR, manual CPR should be started while the equipment is obtained and readied. These devices are only intended for adults and nontraumatic arrests, and they must be removed for defibrillation.

- **Piston-driven device (Thumper)**: Uses pneumatic (air) power on a piston device set at a prescribed compression depth. The backboard must first be secured with straps, the device is slid into a slot in the backboard, the massager pad is placed over the sternum, the device is turned on, and the compression depth is then set. The device can also control ventilations and tidal volume.
- **LUCAS device**: It is also piston driven and is similar to the Thumper, but it applies decompression suction on recoil to increase negative pressure, and it does not provide for ventilations.
- **Load-distributing band/Vest CPR (AutoPulse)**: A device that contains a backboard and fits like a vest around the patient's chest and applies compression to the chest and around the thorax, increasing perfusion pressure. It can be set for continuous compressions or 30:2, and it automatically adjusts to the patient's size.

SPECIAL CONSIDERATIONS FOR FLUID RESUSCITATION

Special considerations for fluid resuscitation include the following:

- **Geriatric patients**: Underlying hypertension may result in shock with systolic BP >100 mmHg. Even small amounts of bleeding may lead to shock, especially if the patient has anemia and is less able to tolerate excessive fluids because of underlying anemia or electrolyte imbalances.
- **Pediatric patients**: Infuse up to 20 mL/kg of warmed isotonic solution, and start a second or third infusion if he or she is nonresponsive to the first infusion. Use continuous infusion for uncontrolled hemorrhage to maintain perfusion en route. It is important to manage temperature control to maintain perfusion. Use an age-specific vital sign chart to monitor vital signs.
- **Pregnant patients**: Shock results in the shunting of maternal blood away from the fetus to the mother's vital organs, so it is critical to maintain the patient's BP as close as possible to normal.

Trauma

Trauma Overview

BLUNT TRAUMA

Blunt trauma can be the result of a variety of accidents/injuries:

- **Motor vehicle crashes**: Result in 30–40% of accidental deaths and half of closed-head and spinal cord injuries with injuries usually more serious with ejection, lateral (T-bone) impacts, and unrestrained patients, although lap belts increase the risk of abdominal injury (bowel injury in children). Shoulder belts may cause vascular injuries. Injuries include crush (compression), shear (tearing), and burst (rupture from sudden increase in pressure). The risk of death increases if another vehicle occupant dies. Most frontal collisions result in injuries from impact with the steering wheel, dashboard, windshield, or floorboards. More severe injuries occur at speeds of >25 mph.
- **Motorcycle crashes**: Approximately 75% of deaths are from head injuries, but injuries to the spine, pelvis, and extremities, including limb loss, are common.
- **Pedestrian and motor vehicle impacts**: Often results in Waddell's triad (tibiofibular or femur fracture, trunk injury, and head/face injury). Small children are often run over, and adults are thrown over the car by the impact. Intra-abdominal injury and pelvic fractures may occur from fender contact with the hips.
- **Falls**: The most common cause of accidental death in geriatric patients is by falling. Anticoagulants increase the risk of injury with falls. The degree of injury depends on the patient's weight and the fall distance. Injuries are most severe with a fall distance of >20 feet for adults and >10 feet for children. A three-story fall results in 50% mortality; the mortality is almost 100% for five-story falls. Horizontal landings cause fewer injuries (hand, wrist, head/face, and abdominal) than feet-first landings, which often result in fractures of the heel, leg, pelvis, and/or vertebrae.
- **Sports injuries/play**: Injuries vary depending on the type of injury but can include head injuries, musculoskeletal injuries, and abdominal injuries. Helmet or knee contact to the flank area may cause kidney injury. The most common injuries are strains, sprains, and knee injuries.
- **Assaults**: Assaults are most common in young males and include facial and head injuries. Severe torso injuries may occur with kicking/stomping. If the patient is intoxicated and has altered consciousness, then he or she is treated as having a head injury. Assaults include domestic violence and child abuse, with distinctive patterns of injury.

PENETRATING TRAUMA

Penetrating traumas are most often the result of violence, such as gunshot wounds and puncture wounds.

- **Gunshot wounds**: Solid organs (brain, liver, spleen) often suffer more damage than more elastic tissues (fat, lungs). If a bullet is not deformed after entering the tissue, it tends to tumble (180°), creating a tunnel of injury (permanent cavity) and damage to the surrounding tissue (temporary cavity). If the bullet is deformed, it causes more severe localized tissue damage. Bullets usually have a straight trajectory, but they may be deflected if they strike bone. Shotgun blasts within 15 feet cause more damage than other gunshot wounds, but they are usually less severe at a distance.
- **Puncture wounds**:
  - *Stab:* Includes hand-driven objects (knives, glass shards, ice picks, or pieces of metal/wood). Surface puncture wounds are often small, but their depth varies according to the instrument used, which should be removed surgically.
  - *Slash:* These are usually long but not deep lacerations.
  - *Impalement:* This usually results from objects larger than a knife, often from a fall onto an object, but it can include arrows and nails from pneumatic tools.

BLEEDING

IDENTIFYING TYPE AND SOURCE OF BLEEDING

Any type of trauma can induce bleeding, internal or external. Identifying the **type and source of bleeding** is critical in managing the bleed.

- **Arterial**: Bright-red spurting blood that is difficult to control; lessens as the BP falls
- **Venous**: Dark-red blood flowing in a steady stream; may be copious, but is easier to control than an arterial bleed
- **Capillary**: Oozing; usually clots spontaneously
- **Internal**: Usually evidenced by increasing signs of shock or discolored swollen, painful tissue, guarding, coughing up blood, or rectal bleeding. Long-bone fractures (femur) and pelvic fractures may result in severe blood loss.

Prehospital Interventions: Using standard precautions and PPE as indicated, apply sterile gauze dressing and pressure with the fingertips if it is a small bleed or apply direct hand pressure if it is more copious. As dressings saturate, add new dressings but don't remove the old ones. A tourniquet may be needed if the bleeding is uncontrolled. Maintain the patient in the shock position, especially with an arterial bleed or severe blood loss, and keep him or her warm. Avoid giving food or fluids, and transport immediately for severe bleeding. Severity relates to the rate of blood loss volume and the age and health of patient. The blood volume is less with pediatric patients. Moving the injured area, a change in body temperature, medications, and the removal of bandages may impair clotting.

CONTROLLING VISIBLE HEMORRHAGE

Many types of hemorrhage exist, but hemorrhage in the general sense means severe bleeding or significant loss of blood. When the source of a patient's blood loss can be visualized, there are ways to control the hemorrhage. First and foremost, the patient's airway, breathing, and circulation should be assessed. Once those have been evaluated, the hemorrhage site should be freed from constrictive clothing or attire of any kind so that the site is exposed. In cases of minor bleeding, direct pressure should be applied to the injury site to stop the bleeding, the site should be cleansed with soap and water, and a sterile dressing should be applied. In cases of serious hemorrhage, the risks of causing further damage to an injured site should be considered against the possible benefits of applying direct pressure to the area.

TOURNIQUETS

Tourniquets are recommended as life-saving devices for uncontrolled arterial hemorrhage of the extremities that cannot be controlled with pressure or other means. The types of trauma tourniquets that are recommended were developed by the military but are now in common use for emergency care. The Combat Application Tourniquet (CAT) and the SOF Tactical Tourniquet (SOF-T) are adjustable bands with a windlass stick to tighten and a windlass clip and strap. The tourniquet is applied about 2 inches above the wound or above the knee for lower leg wounds and above the elbow for lower arm wounds. After the tourniquet is applied, the windlass is twisted to tighten until the distal pulse disappears and bleeding slows considerably or stops. Once bleeding is controlled, the windlass is secured. The tourniquet should be kept open to the field of vision so it is constantly monitored. If no tourniquet is available, a BP cuff can be applied and inflated.

REVISED TRAUMA SCORE (RTS) AND PRIMARY ASSESSMENT OF TRAUMA PATIENTS

The revised trauma score (RTS) uses the Glasgow Coma Scale (GCS) score, systolic BP, and respiration rate to establish a score for triage. A score of 0-4 is assigned for each category:

	GCS Score	Systolic BP	Respirations
4	13-15	90+	10-29
3	9-12	76-89	30+
2	6-8	50-75	6-9
1	4-5	1-49	1-5
0	3	0	0

For triage purposes, an RTS of 12 indicates delayed treatment; 11 indicates urgent, and a score of 3-10 indicates that immediate treatment is required. A score of less than 3 indicates death or an unsurvivable condition.

In the hospital setting, the RTS is further interpreted using a weighted scale for more accuracy in predicting survival. The scores (0-4) are combined using a weighting formula: RTS = (0.9368 × GCS score) + (0.7326 × BP score) + (0.2908 × RR score). Thus, an RTS can range from 0 to 7.84.

Primary assessment of trauma patients should include evaluation of the airway, breathing, and circulation (including observing for deviated septum, changes in chest wall motion, fractures, sucking chest wounds, and crepitation [of the neck and chest] from air), as well as an assessment of disability with a brief neurological exam (pupils, limb movement) and GSC/RTS. Removing the patient's clothing for examination and logrolling him or her are part of the assessment.

ISSUES OF TRANSPORT MODE AND DESTINATION

Issues that arise surrounding transport modes and destination when handling trauma include:

- Patient's triage status and duration of time needed for transport
- Distance from receiving institution
- Patient's need for specialized equipment or medical specialists and availability in ambulance and at receiving institution
- Airlift vs ambulance transport for critically ill
- Low acuity patient's insistence on transport to hospital when transport is deemed unnecessary
- Patient refusal to be transported to hospital
- Patient incompetent to make decisions about transport or unconscious and unable to make decisions
- Use of lights or sirens continuously, intermittently, or not at all (Lights-only may be used to minimize patient's anxiety and to reduce distractions for EMS. Sirens may be used intermittently at intersections and when traffic congestion is slowing progress.)
- Patient dies prior to transportation
- Patient dies en route (Regulations may vary by state and jurisdiction but may require the ambulance to wait for the medical examiner.)

Chest Trauma

CHEST WOUNDS

Chest wounds can be characterized as sucking wounds or impalements.

- **Sucking**: This is an open pneumothorax in which air is sucked into the thoracic cavity, deflating the lung, usually through a penny-size or larger wound. Patients will exhibit respiratory distress, absent breath sounds on the affected side, wound gurgling on inspiration, and bubbling of blood around the wound. Prehospital Interventions: Apply an occlusive dressing with an Asherman Chest Seal dressing or with Vaseline gauze covered with secured (taped on three sides) plastic wrap or aluminum foil and place the patient in a position of comfort.
- **Impalement**: This is a penetrating wound with an object impaled into the chest. Symptoms may be similar to those listed above, depending on the site of impalement and the depth. Impalement may cause hemothorax, tension pneumothorax, or pericardial tamponade. Prehospital Interventions: Expose the wound area, and secure the object manually with a bulky dressing. Do not remove the object unless it is necessary for performing chest compressions (CPR). Control any bleeding.

FRACTURED RIBS AND FLAIL CHEST

Fractured ribs usually result from severe blunt trauma (motor vehicle accident, physical abuse). Underlying injuries should be expected according to the area of fractures as follows:

- Upper two ribs: Injuries to the trachea, bronchi, or great vessels
- Right-sided ≥ rib 8: Liver trauma
- Left-sided ≥ rib 8: Spleen trauma

Pain may be the primary symptom of rib fractures, resulting in shallow breathing.

Flail chest (more common in adults and adolescents than children) occurs when at least three adjacent ribs are fractured, anteriorly and posteriorly, so that they float free of the rib cage. Variations include the sternum floating with ribs fractured on both sides. With flail chest, the chest wall cannot support changes in intrathoracic pressure, so paradoxical respirations occur with the flail area contracting on inspiration and expanding on expiration. Ventilation decreases.

Prehospital Interventions: Manage the patient's airway/ventilation/oxygen supplementation (PPV with BVM or intubation). Provide cardiac monitoring, an IV access line, and supportive care. Observe for signs of tension pneumothorax or hemothorax.

TENSION PNEUMOTHORAX

If not treated promptly, a sucking chest wound (open pneumothorax) may progress to a **tension pneumothorax,** especially if mechanical ventilation is used. A tension pneumothorax occurs when pressure in the pleural space exceeds that of the atmosphere, causing a mediastinal shift (which is usually difficult to assess visually) with displacement of the trachea away from the affected site, putting pressure against the great vessels (decreasing cardiac output), and putting pressure against the heart (resulting in tachycardia). Patients are usually in severe respiratory distress with jugular vein distension, absent breath sounds on the affected side, narrow pulse pressure, pulsus paradoxus, and unequal chest rise.

Prehospital Interventions: Place an airtight seal or Asherman Chest Seal over the open wound, manage the patient's airway/ventilation/oxygen supplementation to an oxygen saturation level of

≥94%, provide cardiac monitoring, start an IV access line, and provide rapid transport. Tension pneumothorax will require needle decompression or insertion of a chest tube (according to protocol).

HEMOTHORAX

Hemothorax occurs with bleeding into the pleural space, usually from major vascular injury such as tears in the intercostal vessels, lacerations of the great vessels, or trauma to the lung tissue. Hemothorax is most common with penetrating wounds. A small bleed may be self-limiting and seal, but a tear in a large vessel can result in massive bleeding, followed quickly by hypovolemic shock from decreased circulating blood. The pressure from the blood may result in the inability of the lung to ventilate and a mediastinal shift. Clots in the chest area may trigger fibrinolysis, which breaks down clots and increases bleeding. Often a hemothorax occurs with a pneumothorax, especially in severe chest trauma. Further symptoms include severe respiratory distress, decreased breath sounds, unequal breath sounds, dullness on auscultation, jugular venous distension, and shock.

Prehospital Interventions: Manage the patient's airway/ventilation/oxygen supplementation, provide an IV access line and fluid bolus for shock but avoid aggressive fluids because of the risk of hemodilution, provide the patient a position of comfort (the shock position if necessary), and provide rapid transport.

CARDIAC TAMPONADE

Cardiac tamponade occurs when fluid, usually blood, accumulates in the pericardial sac. If the fluid accumulates rapidly, the walls of the pericardial sac do not have time to stretch to accommodate the fluid, so the patient may quickly develop pulseless electrical activity (PEA) with fluid accumulation of 50-250 mL. If fluid accumulates slowly, such as with pericardial effusions associated with cancer, patients may tolerate up to 2 L of fluid before symptoms become acute. Cardiac tamponade compresses the heart and limits the venous return to the heart and blood flow into the ventricles, thereby reducing cardiac output. Symptoms: Beck's triad includes decreased arterial BP, increased jugular venous distension, and muffled heart sounds. Patients may be anxious, dyspneic, dizzy, and have angina-like pain.

Prehospital Interventions: Manage airway/high concentration oxygen, monitor the ECG, provide an IV access line and fluids as indicated, and provide rapid transport for pericardiocentesis.

BLUNT CARDIAC TRAUMA

Blunt cardiac trauma most often occurs as the result of motor vehicle accidents, falls, or other blows to the chest, which can result in respiratory distress as well as hypovolemia from rupture of the great vessels of the heart and/or cardiac failure from cardiac tamponade or increasing intrathoracic pressure. The heart is particularly vulnerable to chest trauma, with the right atrium and right ventricle being the most commonly injured because they are anterior to the rest of the heart. **Commotio cordis,** an often-lethal dysrhythmia from a blow to the pericardial area, may occur (most common in young males with sports injuries). Cardiac trauma may be difficult to identify because of other injuries, but if it is suspected, an ECG should be done and any abnormalities (dysrhythmias, ST changes, sinus tachycardia, or heart block) should be noted.

Decreased cardiac output and cerebral oxygenation may result in severe agitation with combative behavior.

Prehospital Interventions: Provide CPR and defibrillation if indicated; manage the patient's airway/ventilation/oxygen supplementation; provide an IV access line with severe injury; and monitor changes in the patient's level of consciousness.

MYOCARDIAL AND PULMONARY CONTUSION

A **myocardial contusion** occurs when the heart muscle is bruised. Patients often sustain myocardial contusion from motor vehicle accidents, aggressive chest compressions during cardiopulmonary resuscitation (CPR) efforts, and/or blunt chest trauma resulting from a fall. Symptoms of the condition are typically mild. Many patients with myocardial contusion feel as though their heart is racing, and they also frequently experience pain in their breastbone.

A **pulmonary contusion** occurs when the lung becomes bruised. High-velocity motor vehicle accidents are a common cause of pulmonary contusion. Symptoms of the condition may include the presence of rales during inhalation, an increased rate of respiration, and/or breathing difficulties.

TRAUMATIC ASPHYXIA

Traumatic asphyxia occurs when severe crushing pressure on the chest pushes against the heart, forcing blood from the right side of the heart back into the venous system (superior vena cava), including the neck and head veins, resulting in inadequate oxygenation to the upper extremities, face, and brain. Symptoms include altered mental status, seizures, swollen tongue, subconjunctival hemorrhages in the eyes, and cyanosis of the arms.

Prehospital Interventions: Manage the patient's airway/ventilation/oxygen supplementation, provide supportive care, provide cardiac monitoring, and start an IV access line with fluid bolus for shock.

TRAUMATIC AORTIC DISRUPTION

Traumatic aortic disruption occurs when the aorta is torn or ruptures as the result of trauma, usually blunt injury, such as in a motor vehicle accident. Massive bleeding may occur and the trauma is often fatal unless the tear is partial-thickness and the blood is contained in a pseudo aneurysm (sac). Patients may complain of chest, back, or abdominal pain and may exhibit signs of shock (dyspnea, pallor, hypotension, tachycardia, cool/clammy skin). A harsh systolic murmur may be evident, and circulation to the lower extremities may be impaired, with faint or absent palpable pulses and decreased blood pressure.

Prehospital Interventions: Continually assess vital signs, oxygen saturation, and ECG. Assess level of pain (1-10 numeric scale), provide 100% oxygen with non-rebreather mask, administer analgesia per protocol and antiemetic if nauseated to prevent vomiting, insert large bore IV and provide NS infusion and transfusions if indicated and available. Rapid transit to ED is essential.

Abdominal and Genitourinary Trauma

ABDOMINAL AND GENITOURINARY ORGANS

The **peritoneum** lines the abdominal cavity. The anterior (front) area is the **intraperitoneal space**, which contains the stomach, the first part of the duodenum, the small intestines, and part of the large intestines and rectum as well as the liver, bile ducts, spleen, ovaries, part of the pancreas and ureters, and bladder. The posterior (back) **retroperitoneal space** contains part of the duodenum, the ascending and descending colon, and part of the rectum as well as part of the pancreas and ureters, the kidneys, the adrenal glands, the uterus, and the fallopian tubes. The ovaries, uterus, and fallopian tubes comprise the female reproductive system. **Solid organs** include the liver, spleen, ovaries, uterus, pancreas, kidneys, and adrenals. **Hollow organs** include the bile ducts, stomach, large and small intestines, fallopian tubes, ureters, and bladder.

EVISCERATIONS AND IMPALED OBJECTS

Eviscerations occur with open abdominal wounds, such as opening incisions or traumatic injuries, which allow the internal organs (often the intestines) to protrude externally. Surgical repair is required to reinsert the organs into the abdomen. The patient may go into shock, especially if the evisceration is part of other major injuries (common in trauma cases).

Prehospital Interventions: Provide supportive care; cover the eviscerated organs with thick, sterile gauze dressings moistened with NS, but do not attempt to reinsert them, manage the patient's airway/ventilation/oxygen supplementation as needed, and provide rapid transport.

Impalements occur when an object penetrates the abdomen and remains in place and may be associated with multiple internal injuries and bleeding.

Prehospital Interventions: Do not remove the object, but do expose the abdomen and manually secure the object with bulky dressings and control any bleeding. Provide supportive care, manage the patient's airway/ventilation/oxygen supplementation as needed, and provide rapid transport.

BLUNT ABDOMINAL WOUNDS

Abdominal trauma may result in **blunt wounds**, which may occur as the result of motor vehicle accidents, motorcycle accidents, pedestrian injuries, sports injuries, falls, blast injuries, and assaults. Blunt injuries comprise crush (compression), shear (tearing), and burst (sudden increased pressure) injuries. Motor vehicle accidents often result in liver injury in the passenger with impact on that side of the vehicle and spleen injury in the driver with impact on the driver's side. Other injuries from blunt trauma include damage to the diaphragm, retroperitoneal hematomas, and intestinal injuries, including perforation. Symptoms of internal injuries include pain, guarding, abdominal distension, discoloration, tenderness on movement, and evidence of lower rib fractures. Some patients may exhibit rectal bleeding and/or vomiting of blood.

Prehospital Interventions: Provide airway/ventilation/oxygen supplementation as needed, place in a position of comfort, treat for shock if indicated (especially with suspected internal bleeding), and provide rapid transport for patients in an unstable condition.

PENETRATING ABDOMINAL WOUNDS

Abdominal trauma may result in **penetrating wounds**, which are almost always related to gunshot wounds (high energy), shotgun wounds (medium energy), or knife wounds (low energy). Gunshot and shotgun wounds tend to cause more extensive damage than stab wounds, especially to the colon, liver, spleen, and diaphragm, and they may have an exit wound. Interior injuries may be extensive because the bullet damages tissues and may ricochet off of bone. Hemorrhage and peritonitis (especially with perforation of the intestines) are common complications. Pain is often more acute with injury to hollow organs than to solid organs, although blood loss may be severe with injury to the liver, spleen, or kidneys, and blood collecting in the retroperitoneal space may not be evident on inspection, palpation, or auscultation.

Prehospital Interventions: Control external bleeding, manage the patient's airway/ventilation/oxygen supplementation, mobilize the spine if indicated, and apply a pneumatic antishock garment (PASG) if indicated for shock or pelvic fracture (contraindicated with difficulty breathing, pregnancy [second and third trimesters], evisceration, an impaled object, and open fractures).

HEPATIC (LIVER) INJURY

Hepatic (liver) injury is the most common cause of death (mortality rates of 8–25%) from abdominal trauma and is often associated with multiple organ damage, so symptoms may be nonspecific. **Liver injuries** are classified according to the degree of injury, as follows:

I. Tears in the capsule with hematoma
II. Laceration(s) of the parenchyma (<3 cm)
III. Laceration(s) of the parenchyma (>3 cm)
IV. Destruction of 25–75% of a lobe from burst injury
V. Destruction of >75% of a lobe from burst injury
VI. Avulsion (tearing away)

Hemorrhage is a common complication of hepatic injury. Treatment often includes intravenous fluids for fluid volume deficit as well as blood products (plasma, platelets) for coagulopathies.

Prehospital Interventions: Manage the patient's airway/ventilation/oxygen supplementation, control external bleeding, treat signs of shock, start an IV access line with fluid bolus if indicated (but beware of hemodilution), provide rapid transport for an unstable patient.

SPLENIC INJURY

The spleen is the most frequently injured solid organ in blunt trauma because it's not well protected by the rib cage and it is very vascular. Symptoms may be very nonspecific. Kehr's sign (radiating pain in the left shoulder) indicates intra-abdominal bleeding, and Cullen's sign (ecchymosis around the umbilicus) indicates hemorrhage from a ruptured spleen. Some may have right upper abdominal pain, although diffuse abdominal pain often occurs with blood loss, associated with hypotension. **Splenic injuries** are classified according to the degree of injury, as follows:

- Tear in splenic capsules or hematoma
- Laceration of parenchyma (<3 cm)
- Laceration of parenchyma (>3cm)
- Multiple lacerations of parenchyma or burst-type injury

Treatment may be supportive if the injury is not severe; otherwise, suturing or removal of the spleen may be needed.

Prehospital Interventions: Control external bleeding, manage the patient's airway/ventilation/oxygen supplementation, treat signs of shock, start an IV access line with fluid bolus if indicated (but beware of hemodilution), and provide rapid transport for an unstable patient.

TRAUMATIC INJURIES TO GENITALIA
PENIS
- Blunt, penetrating, crushing, or amputating injuries as well as urethral penetration. Pain and bleeding may be severe.
- **Prehospital Interventions**: Control external bleeding, do not removed the impaled object. Provide pain management, an ice pack to reduce swelling, and emotional support.

SCROTUM
- Blunt, penetrating, or crushing injury may result in severe pain and swelling.
- **Prehospital Interventions**: As above but do not attempt to relieve scrotal pressure except with ice packs.

VAGINA
- May have external bruising and tearing (especially with sexual assault) at the vaginal opening. There may be pain, swelling, and bleeding.
- **Prehospital Interventions**: Control external bleeding, and provide emotional support, but do not remove impaled objects.

VULVA
- May include blunt, penetrating, or crushing injury as well as bite marks (with sexual assault) with pain, swelling, and bleeding.
- **Prehospital Interventions**: As above. Report sexual assaults according to protocol.

ABDOMINAL VASCULAR INJURIES
Vascular injuries usually result from penetrating injuries, which may partially or completely transect a vessel, or blunt injuries, which may damage the wall or dissect the vessels. Acceleration/deceleration may result in shearing injuries. Indications of **vascular injuries** include pulsatile bleeding, enlarging hematoma, and ischemia distal to the vascular injury, as noted by the six P's (pain, pallor, pulseless, paresthesia, poikilothermia [unstable core body temperature], and paralysis) as well as audible bruit or palpable thrill and signs of increasing shock or compartment syndrome. Abdominal vessel injuries are most common in the aorta and inferior vena cava (45% mortality), but additional injuries, such as to the hepatic veins and portal vein, increase mortality rates (90%). Internal venous hemorrhage may be more severe than arterial.

Prehospital Interventions: Control external bleeding, manage the patient's airway/ventilation/oxygen supplementation, start an IV access line with fluid bolus if needed for shock (but beware of hemodilution with bleeding), and provide rapid transport (surgical repair within 1 hour is critical).

Orthopedic Trauma

MUSCULOSKELETAL SYSTEM

The musculoskeletal system includes 206 bones including long bones (e.g., the femur in the thigh), short bones (e.g., the carpal bones in the fingers), and flat bones (e.g., the sternum). The outer hard shell of the bone is the cortex, and the inner porous area is the trabecular bone. The vertebrae lack the cortex layer. Long bones have three parts: The middle section is the diaphysis, followed by the metaphyses, and then the epiphyses (the bone ends). In growing children, an epiphyseal plate of cartilage separates the metaphyses and epiphyses, allowing bone growth. This closes in adults, but damage to this area in a child may impair bone growth. The middle part of the short bones contains yellow bone marrow (fatty tissue). Red bone marrow, which produces blood cells, is found in the middle of the flat bones (pelvis, sternum, ribs, and scapula) and at the ends (epiphyses) of long bones. The skeletal system is connected by cartilage and tendons, and it is protected, supported, and allowed movement by about 700 soft-tissue muscles.

> **Review Video: Muscular System**
> Visit mometrix.com/academy and enter code: 967216
>
> **Review Video: Skeletal System**
> Visit mometrix.com/academy and enter code: 256447

ASSESSMENT OF MUSCULOSKELETAL INJURIES

Assessment of musculoskeletal injuries should include the following:

- Palpation/inspection for tissue damage, swelling, deformity, and tenderness
- Comparison with the opposite side if a limb is involved
- Assessment of neurovascular status (pulse, color, sensation, and function) distal to (below) the fracture
- Assessment of the six P's:
  - **Pain** (site of pain, degree, character)
  - **Pallor** (below the fracture or generalized)
  - **Paresthesia** (impaired sensation below fracture)
  - Distal **pulses** (intact, weak, absent)
  - **Paralysis** (with or without impaired sensation)
  - **Pressure** (often associated with swelling and pain)
- Assessment of age and general condition (geriatric patients are more likely to have fractures from relatively minor injuries because of osteoporosis)

If a fracture or dislocation is suspected, then the area should be splinted or immobilized for transport. Types of splints include rigid (should be padded), nonrigid (moldable), traction, air (pneumatic devices), pillow/blanket, short spine board, and long spine board. Splinting procedures are similar for adults, pediatric patients, and geriatric patients.

FRACTURES

Fractures usually result from trauma (falls, auto accidents), but **pathologic (nontraumatic) fractures** can result from minor force to diseased bones (osteoporosis or cancerous lesions). **Stress fractures** are caused by repetitive trauma (forced marching). **Salter-Harris fractures** involve the cartilaginous epiphyseal plate near the ends of long bones in children who are growing, and this can impair bone growth. Fractures can be classified as open or closed:

- **Open fractures** have soft-tissue injury and a break in the skin overlying the fracture, including puncture wounds from external forces or bone fragments; these can result in osteomyelitis (bone infection).
- **Closed fractures** involve a broken bone but no break in the skin.

Symptoms include pain, deformity or angulation, swelling, bruising, inability to move the joint or bear weight, grating on movement, and impaired function or circulation. Isolated fractures are usually not life threatening, but pelvic and femur fractures may involve severe blood loss.

Prehospital Interventions: Cover open wounds with sterile dressings, manually stabilize and immobilize the fracture area, but do not replace protruding bones, apply a cold pack, and place the patient in a position of comfort.

NONTRAUMATIC FRACTURES

Nontraumatic fractures occur when the bone weakens and can no longer support the body, such as may occur with a cancerous tumor of the bone or osteoporosis. Common fractures associated with osteoporosis include fractures of the vertebrae and hip. Osteoporotic fractures are most common in older adults, but they may also occur in adolescents with eating disorders. Infants and young children with multiple nontraumatic, non-abusive fractures may have a genetic disorder, such as osteogenesis imperfecta. Assessment of suspected fractures includes evaluating pain/tenderness, swelling around the fracture site, loss of sensation or movement, circulatory impairment (note the color of the skin, pallor or cyanosis), and deformity (especially noticeable in limb fractures).

Prehospital Interventions: Splint extremity fractures; manage the patient's airway/ventilation/oxygen supplementation as needed; and provide transport for treatment.

TYPES OF FRACTURES

Fractures can be classified by the location and style of the break.

Spiral: Common in toddlers who fall on an extended leg, breaking the tibia, but it may also occur with abuse in small children as a result of jerking on or twisting an extremity (usually the arm).

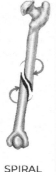

SPIRAL

Greenstick: Most common in children whose bones are less hard. It is usually quite painful but without deformity.

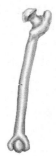

GREENSTICK

Displaced: Poses a risk of damage to surrounding tissues, including nerves and blood vessels and may lead to an open fracture if not properly splinted. The deformity is usually evident.

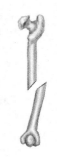

DISPLACED

Transverse: Usually occurs in long bones and is at risk of displacement unless it is splinted to prevent movement. Most often occurs from direct impact, such as sports injuries. May suggest abuse if occurring in small children.

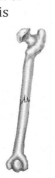

TRANSVERSE

Comminuted: Usually result from high-impact trauma, such as with motor vehicle accidents, and it is more common in older adults or those with weakened bones. This fracture is very painful and is often accompanied by swelling and muscle spasms.

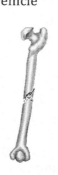

COMMINUTED

The femur is the long bone in the thigh. Although any part of the femur may fracture, fractures in the upper femur are common and are generally referred to as hip fractures. **Femur fractures** in young patients usually result from high-impact trauma, such as motor vehicle or pedestrian/motor vehicle accidents, whereas femur fractures in geriatric patients are most often from falls and are associated with osteoporosis. Patients may have many comorbidities and may present with dehydration and blood loss. Mortality rates for **hip fractures** are high, with 10% during the initial treatment and 25% over the next year. Symptoms of femur fractures include pain and deformity at the fracture site and an inability to walk or bear weight. A hematoma may be present.

Prehospital Interventions: Splint the leg in the position it was found in with a traction splint (Hare Traction Splint/Sager Emergency Traction Splint), flush open fractures with NS to remove debris, and apply an NS-moistened sterile gauze dressing, monitor vital signs and neurovascular status, and assess soft tissue for damage. Provide an IV access and fluids if indicated.

PREHOSPITAL MANAGEMENT OF FRACTURES

Prehospital management of fractures depends on the location and severity of the fracture:

- **Tibia/Fibula (lower leg)**: Manually immobilize during splinting. Splint the joint above and below the fracture(s) (upper thigh to ankle) with a padded rigid long-leg splint or a pneumatic splint, and then secure it to the other leg for additional support.
- **Shoulder**: Apply a sling to the affected side and secure the patient's arm against the body with a swathe to limit movement.
- **Knee**: If the pulse below the fracture is adequate and there is no deformity, splint with the knee straight. If there is deformity, splint the leg in the position it was found. If there is no pulse below the fracture, consult with medical assistance immediately. Never use a traction splint.
- **Clavicle (upper chest)**: Apply a sling to the affected side. (Common in young children who fall with an arm outstretched.)
- **Humerus (upper arm)**: Apply a sling to the affected side and swathe the arm to the body to limit movement.
- **Radius/Ulna (forearm)**: Splint from the elbow to the wrist and secure above and below the fracture. Elevate the arm.
- **Elbow**: Apply a sling to the affected side (often results from a fall).

AMPUTATIONS

Amputations may be partial or complete and result from crush, guillotine (cutting), or avulsion (twisting) injuries. A **simple amputation** requires no extrication and other injuries or shock are absent, but a **complex amputation** may involve multiple injuries, shock, and delayed treatment because of extrication. The amputated limb should be treated initially as though it could be reattached, although single digits (except the thumb) and lower limbs are not usually reattached. The part should be irrigated with normal saline (NS) to remove debris; wrapped in NS-moistened gauze; and placed in a sealed plastic bag, which should be immersed in ice water. The body part should not freeze and should not be placed directly on ice.

Prehospital Interventions: Manage the patient's airway/ventilation/oxygen supplementation; control bleeding by direct pressure or, if there is severe hemorrhage, by applying a BP cuff proximal to (above) the injury 70 mmHg greater than the systolic BP for <30 minutes. Irrigate the stump with NS if it is dirty, cover the open area with NS-moistened gauze, and elevate the stump.

PELVIC FRACTURES

Pelvic fractures represent about 3% of total fractures, but they pose a greater risk than most other types of fractures. **Pelvic fractures** most often result from a motor vehicle accident (50-60%) in adults and a pedestrian/motor vehicle impact (60-80%) in children. Pelvic fractures may be accompanied by major injuries to soft tissue and internal organs, especially the bladder, urethra (especially in children and women), and colon. A fracture on one side often results in a fracture on the other side as well. The primary cause of death after a pelvic fracture is hemorrhage with 50-70% of patients with unstable fractures requiring multiple transfusions. Geriatric patients have higher mortality rates than do younger patients. Symptoms include pain and tenderness, bloody urine, rectal bleeding, vaginal bleeding, retroperitoneal bleeding, hematoma over the fracture site, pain on hip motion, and signs of shock (with blood loss).

Prehospital Interventions: Monitor vital signs for indications of shock, position supine, apply PASG or a pelvic wrap device (per protocol) to stabilize and prevent excessive movement, and monitor the patient's airway, ventilation, and oxygen supplementation. Provide an IV access (large bore) and fluid as indicated.

PNEUMATIC ANTISHOCK GARMENT (PASG)

The pneumatic antishock garment (PASG) is indicated for hypovolemic shock and hypotension associated with and stabilization of pelvic and bilateral femur fractures. PASG is contraindicated with respiratory distress, pulmonary edema, pregnancy (second and third trimesters), heart failure, myocardial infarction, stroke, evisceration, abdominal or leg impalement, head injuries, and uncontrolled bleeding above the garment.

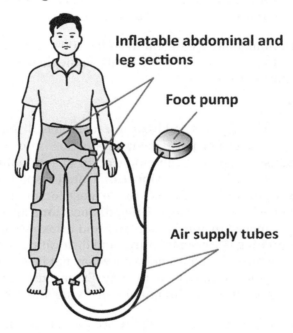

Inflatable abdominal and leg sections

Foot pump

Air supply tubes

The **procedure** for PASG use is as follows:

1. Place the garment flat on the patient-transport device/stretcher and transfer the patient onto the garment.
2. If the patient is already on the stretcher, place the garment under his or her legs first and then lift the patient's buttocks and slide the garment upward until the upper garment edge is 1 inch below the bottom ribs.
3. Secure the legs first and then the abdominal section with the Velcro straps. Attach the pump hoses to each leg and the abdominal section at the valves and close the stopcocks.
4. Open the stopcock for each leg and abdominal section one at a time, and inflate them one at a time.

After inflating each section, close the stopcock and check the vital signs. Stop inflating if the systolic BP ≥90 mmHg. If the systolic BP is still <90 mmHg, then proceed to filling the next section or sections until all three are filled.

FAT EMBOLISM

Fat embolism, a life-threatening complication of fractures, can occur when fat enters the venous circulatory system, typically lodging in the pulmonary microvasculature, causing increased pulmonary vascular resistance. Patients most at risk are the young with multiple injuries, the elderly, and those with preexisting disease (pulmonary hypertension, right ventricular disorder, or metastatic cancer). Preventive methods include stabilizing fractures of long bones or the pelvis within 24 hours of injury. Signs of fat embolism include abrupt bradycardia, hypertension, jugular venous distension, hypoxemia, decreased $ETCO_2$ concentration, chest and upper extremity petechiae, fat globules in the retina, and various cardiac irregularities such as dysrhythmias. As the pulmonary artery pressure increases, cardiac output decreases.

Prehospital Interventions: Immediate treatment includes 100% oxygen with mechanical ventilation per endotracheal tube with adequate IV fluids. Epinephrine or related drugs may be used for hemodynamic support per protocol.

JOINT DISLOCATIONS

Subluxation (partial dislocation of a joint) and **luxation** (complete dislocation of a joint) can cause neurovascular compromise, which can be permanent if reduction is delayed. This is especially a problem with **hip dislocations**, which most commonly occur in automobile accidents when the person's knees impact the dashboard. **Elbow dislocations** often result from athletic injuries and may cause nerve damage. **Shoulder dislocations** are the most common type and also often result from athletic injuries. They may become chronic. **Knee dislocations** may result in severe injury to the popliteal artery, and this can lead to amputation, so rapid transport and emergent surgical repair are indicated. Differentiating between fractures and dislocations can be difficult because the symptoms and appearance are often similar. A deformity may not be evident or may be obscured by edema, or edema may give the appearance of a deformity. Extensive bruising may occur with all types of injuries, and pain may occur even with minor soft-tissue injuries.

Prehospital Interventions: Splint and immobilize the area, and place the patient in a position of comfort.

SHOULDER INJURIES

A **sternoclavicular sprain** results from tearing of the ligaments that connect the sternum to the clavicle, usually resulting from a direct blow or twisting of an arm extended backward. Symptoms include pain near the top of the chest (below the neck). The pain increases on activity (such as lifting) and when lying on the affected side.

The **rotator cuff** comprises the muscle and ligaments of the shoulder joint. The bones in the joint include the scapula and humerus. Muscles (subscapularis, supraspinatus, infraspinatus, spines minor) and tendons anchor to the head of the humerus so that the arm can move in all directions, and ligaments connect the bones. Part of the rotator cuff is under the scapula. The most common injury to the rotator cuff is a tear in the supraspinatus tendon, so that the tendon is separated from its attachment, resulting from a violent pull on the arm, an abnormal rotation, or fall on an outstretched hand.

Prehospital Interventions: Provide a protective sling.

STRAINS AND SPRAINS

A **strain** is an overstretching of a part of the musculature ("pulled muscle") that causes microscopic tears in the muscle, usually resulting from excess stress or overuse of the muscle. The onset of pain is usually sudden with local tenderness on use of the muscle. A **sprain** is damage to a joint, with a partial rupture of the supporting ligaments and/or tendons, usually caused by wrenching or twisting that may occur with a fall. The rupture can damage blood vessels, resulting in edema, tenderness at the joint, and pain on movement with pain increasing over 2–3 hours after the injury. An avulsion fracture (the bone fragment is pulled away by a ligament) may occur with strain.

Prehospital Interventions: Immobilize the area for transport, use rest, ice, compression, and elevation (the RICE protocol), and monitor the patient's neurovascular status (especially for sprains) by checking the pulse, capillary refill, color, and sensation distal to (below) the injury.

SPLINTING AND SPINAL MOTION RESTRICTION

LONG SPINAL BOARD AND SPLINTING BY TRACTION

Various methods of splinting and spinal motion restriction should be considered by the emergency medical responder, based on the patient's method of injury and symptoms:

- **Long spinal board**: If spinal injury is suspected, place a cervical collar on the patient before placing the patient on the long board. With one person stabilizing the head and neck, the patient is logrolled onto one side and the board is positioned against the patient so that the patient can be logrolled back onto the board. Once the patient is positioned on the board, padding such as rolled towels should be placed about the head, neck, and shoulders to provide further support and to ensure the head remains in a neutral position. The patient is secured by straps.
- **Splinting by traction**: Assess patient for signs/symptoms of mid-shaft femur fracture without lower leg or hip injury. Ask partner to apply the ankle hitch and apply manual traction and then to elevate the leg. Slide the long-leg device under the leg and secure with the ischial strap by the hip. Fasten the ankle hitch to the device and apply traction according to manufacturer's guidelines until the patient feels some relief of discomfort. Secure the rest of the leg with straps. Reassess circulation, sensation, and motor function. Place patient on a long spinal board and secure the patient and the device to the long board.

SEATED SPINAL MOTION RESTRICTION USING THE KENDRICK EXTRICATION DEVICE

Seated spinal motion restriction (SMR) using the Kendrick Extrication Device (KED) is indicated for a seated patient who is unable to self-extricate, is conscious and stable, and complains of head, neck, or back pain. Ask another person to continually stabilize the patient's head from behind and then check the patient's hands and feet for sensation and movement:

1. Apply cervical collar. Support the chest and lean the patient forward ≤45 degrees and place the KED in position behind the patient.
2. Move the patient back to upright position and fasten the straps (usually color coded) across the abdomen first and then the chest. Before fastening the chest strap, ask the patient to take a deep breath to ensure the strap doesn't restrict breathing.
3. Then fasten leg straps by bringing each strap under the buttocks and up between the legs and then to the side to fasten. Male patients may need to adjust their genitals.
4. Last make sure the head contacts the padding of the device, bring the flaps about the sides of the face, and then apply the chin strap and the forehead strap.

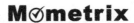

5. Check sensations and movement in the hands and feet again and then move the patient onto a long board and then onto a stretcher.
6. Remove KED but leave the cervical collar in place.

COMPARTMENT SYNDROME

Compartment syndrome occurs when muscle perfusion is inadequate because of constriction caused by a cast or tight dressing or because of an increase in the contents of the enclosed compartment of a muscle sheath resulting from edema or hemorrhage. This increases pressure and compression, often related to fractures, crush injuries, burns, rhabdomyolysis, and snakebites. **Compartment syndrome** most often affects the forearm and leg muscles. Symptoms include severe throbbing pain unrelieved by opiates, numbness and tingling as pressure on the nerves increases, cyanosis and decreased or absent pulse distal to injury, limb paralysis, and edema (with tissue often being rigid). Necrosis and permanent damage may occur within 4 hours if treatment is inadequate or delayed.

Prehospital Interventions: Remove the constriction (cast, splint, or dressing), elevate the limb, apply an ice compress, provide pain management, and provide rapid transport because the patient may need surgical fasciotomy to relieve the pressure.

Soft Tissue Trauma

OPEN SOFT-TISSUE INJURIES

Injury	Characteristics	Prehospital Interventions
Abrasion	Painful superficial scraping of the outermost layer of skin. There is little or no bleeding.	Irrigate with water or NS to remove debris and cover with nonadherent dressing.
Laceration	A cut or break in the skin from impact with a sharp object. Bleeding may vary from mild to severe.	Apply pressure to control the bleeding, irrigate to remove debris if necessary, and cover with a dry sterile gauze dressing.
Puncture	Wound from impact with a sharp pointed object (knife, bullet); it may exhibit little external bleeding but major internal bleeding and soft-tissue damage. An exit wound may be present.	Apply pressure to control any bleeding, manage the patient's airway/ventilation/oxygen supplementation, and provide rapid transport if the patient's condition is unstable.
Impaled object	Penetrating object remains in wound.	Leave the object in place and pad with bulky dressings.
Foreign body in eye(s)	Patient has pain, tearing, redness, and blurred or impaired vision from dirt, dust, chemicals, or other materials in the eye(s).	Cover both eyes loosely (avoiding pressure) to prevent movement. If it is chemical contamination, flush the eye(s) with copious amounts of NS or water.
Avulsions	The skin and underlying soft tissue are torn away, such as with a degloving injury, from any part of the body, although lower extremity injury is the most common. Bleeding may be severe, especially if vessels are torn or exposed.	Flush with sterile water or NS to remove debris if necessary, apply pressure and dressings to control bleeding and protect tissue, apply an ice pack, seal the avulsed skin and tissue in a plastic bag, and place in ice water for possible reimplantation or skin grafts. Return loose flaps to their anatomic positions.
Blast injury	Involves varying degrees of soft-tissue injury and sometimes amputations, fractures, impalements, traumatic brain injuries, ruptured eardrum, pulmonary injury, perforated bowel, and burns.	Manage the patient's airway/ventilation/oxygen supplementation, control bleeding and shock, provide CPR if necessary, supportive care, and rapid transport.

CLOSED SOFT TISSUE INJURIES

Injury	Characteristics	Prehospital Interventions
Contusion	Results from blunt or compressive pressure to a muscle and is a common sports injury. These may include other injuries, such as sprains, strains, fractures, and damage to internal organs. Symptoms include tenderness, pain on movement, and bruising. If bruising is in the shape of an instrument, it usually indicates abuse.	Provide RICE therapy and supportive care.
Hematoma	Collection of blood within the tissue because of damaged blood vessels from injury, underlying fracture, or medications (such as warfarin). These may be small or very large, and patients may lose ≥1 L of blood. Symptoms may include pain and swelling.	Provide supportive care for small contusions (which often resolve spontaneously), RICE therapy, and monitor for signs of continued bleeding.
Crush injury	External pressure may cause severe internal injuries, such as fractures and organ rupture.	Manage the patient's airway, ventilation, oxygen supplementation, and shock as needed, control bleeding, and provide supportive care.

CLASSIFICATION OF BURNS AND RULE OF NINES

Burn injuries may be chemical, electrical, or thermal and are assessed by the area affected, percentage of the body burned, and the depth of the burn, as follows:

- **First-degree burns** are superficial and affect the epidermis, causing erythema and pain.
- **Second-degree burns** extend through the dermis (partial thickness), resulting in blistering and sloughing of the epidermis and severe pain.
- **Third-degree burns** affect the underlying tissue, including the vasculature, muscles, and nerves (full thickness). Depending on the extent of the nerve damage, third-degree burns may present with less pain.

Burns are **classified** according to the American Burn Association's criteria as follows:

- **Minor**: <10% body surface area (BSA) or 2% BSA with third-degree burns without serious risk to the face, hands, feet, or perineum
- **Moderate**: 10–20% BSA combined second-degree and third-degree burns in adults; age <10 years or ≤10% third-degree without serious risk to the face, hands, feet, or perineum
- **Major**: ≥20% BSA; ≥10% third-degree burns; all burns are to the face, hands, feet, or perineum and will result in functional/cosmetic defect; or burns with inhalation or other major trauma

The **rule of nines** estimates the BSA burned:

- **Adults**: Head 9%, trunk (front) 18%, trunk (back) 18%, arm 9%, leg 18%, perineum 1%
- **Infants/Children**: Head 18%, trunk (front) 18%, trunk (back) 18%, arm 9%, leg 13.5%, perineum 1%

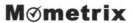

ELECTRICAL BURNS

Low-voltage **electrical contact** most often causes a localized burn (first to third degree) to the hand or mouth (toddlers) with various degrees of tissue damage, although mouth contact may also result in cardiac or respiratory arrest. High-voltage electrical contact results in an entry and an exit wound with internal damage occurring between these wounds. Electrical current takes the shortest route to leave the body (flowing along blood vessels and nerves), so if the current passes from hand to hand, damage is usually more severe than if it passes from a hand to a foot. Severe injury may result in damage to bones, compartment syndrome, organ failure, and cardiac arrest from asystole or ventricular fibrillation. Vessels may be mildly or severely damaged. Abdominal organs may be damaged. Neurological damage with unconsciousness is common, especially if the current passes through the head. Peripheral nerve damage is also common, and damage to the spinal cord may occur.

Prehospital Interventions: Manage the patient's airway, ventilation, and oxygen supplementation, provide CPR/defibrillation as needed, provide rapid transport (with the head elevated if it was involved), start an IV access line, and give fluid resuscitation if needed.

LIGHTNING BURNS AND INJURIES

Lightning injuries may occur with a direct strike (≤5%), side splash from a strike nearby, contact voltage when touching an item that has been struck, ground current (from a more distant strike), and blunt trauma from being too close to a strike (which often results in the patient being thrown). Symptoms may vary, but they can include external burns (Lichtenberg figures) in a fernlike pattern, acute pain, fixed and dilated pupils (temporary), eye injuries, confusion, headache, hearing loss, perforated eardrum, hypotension, paralysis/paresis, spinal cord injury, altered mental status, brain injury, fractures, and cardiac arrest. Patients may be responsive initially but lapse into unconsciousness as cerebral edema increases, resulting in secondary respiratory and/or cardiac arrest. Burns are usually mild because of the brief contact.

Prehospital Interventions: Manage the patient's airway, ventilation, and oxygen supplementation, provide CPR/defibrillation as needed, provide rapid transport (with the head elevated), start an IV access line, and give fluid resuscitation.

GENERAL MANAGEMENT OF CHEMICAL AND ELECTRICAL BURNS

Patients with severe burns may develop shock and impairment of all major body systems. If the burning process is ongoing, room-temperature water or NS should be applied to stop the burning and any smoldering clothes or jewelry should be removed, although if the clothing is adhered to the skin, it should be left in place. With facial or airway burns, the airway must be monitored constantly with interventions as necessary, and an IV access line should be provided for fluid replacement, based on the patient's weight and the extent of the burn (Parkland formula: 4 mL/kg/wt × BSA per 24 hours). The burned area should be covered with nonadherent dry clean dressings, and the patient should be kept warm for transport. Children experience greater fluid and heat loss because of their greater body surface relative to their size, and the EMS provider should be alert to the possibility of child abuse. With **chemical burns**, any dry powder should be brushed off, and wet chemicals should be flushed with copious amounts of water (by a provider wearing gloves and eye protection). With **electrical burns**, internal burns may be more severe than external burns, and the patient is at risk of cardiac arrest.

DRESSINGS AND BANDAGES

Dressings and bandages may be appropriate when handling specific wounds or burns. Each type of dressing has specific characteristics meant to be used for specific purposes.

- **Sterile gauze**: 4×4 (sponge) or roller/wrapping gauze (Kerlix) used to protect skin or pack wounds to control bleeding. Roller gauze may be used to secure other dressings.
- **Nonadherent dressings**: Designed not to stick to open wounds because of their special coating (Teflon, foam, petrolatum, hydrogel). Used on abrasions, burns, and lightly draining wounds.
- **Occlusive dressings**: These have a waxy coating to make an air- and water-tight seal, but they are not as absorbent as gauze. Used for sucking chest wounds, abdominal eviscerations, and lacerations of the external jugular vein or carotid.
- **Trauma dressings**: Dressings that often include a nonadherent pad, a clotting agent embedded in the dressing, and an elastic wrap in one piece so that they can be rapidly applied (e.g., an ACE bandage), include QuikClot Combat Gauze and Celox Rapid hemostatic gauze. Especially useful to control bleeding and to apply pressure to a wound.
- **Adhesive, roller bandages**: May be elastic or nonelastic, and they are used to secure other dressings and/or apply compression.

CRUSH SYNDROME

Crush syndrome results from injury associated with crushing pressure to skeletal muscle from heavy weight, such as when trapped under falling debris for extended periods, especially more than four hours. Injuries include:

- Direct damage to cells
- Decreased circulation and impaired oxygenation of tissue, which cause leakage of cells and buildup of lactic acid
- Dying cells leak substances, such as toxins, proteins, and electrolytes, into surrounding tissue but remain localized because of pressure
- With release of pressure, these substances enter general circulation:
  - *Potassium*: Causes cardiac dysrhythmias
  - *Myoglobin*: Damages kidneys
  - *Purines*: Damages lungs and liver

Symptoms vary depending on severity.

Prehospital Interventions: Assess airway, breathing, circulation, oxygen saturation, and VS. Provide oxygen at high concentration, establish IV access with NS infusion, monitor ECG for changes consistent with hyperkalemia. If hyperkalemia is evident, administer calcium chloride 500 mg IV over 2 minutes or administer aerosolized albuterol. Provide analgesia as indicated.

HIGH-PRESSURE INJECTION

With high-pressure injection of substances, such as water, air, paint, kerosene, solvents, or oil, the substance travels until it meets resistance, such as from muscle or bone, and then spreads through the tissues. Injuries to the hand are most common. Damage may include dissection, damage to nerves, impaired oxygenation, tissue necrosis, bleeding into the tissues, and clot formation. Some substances may be toxic to cells, and the substance may be contaminated with bacteria. The injection site may be quite small and initial symptoms may be mild (pain, numbness) but pain and swelling tend to increase over time and can lead to compartment syndrome. Some substances may cause systemic symptoms (fever, elevated white blood cell count, and kidney damage).

Prehospital Interventions: Inspect, clean, and cover injection site. Provide analgesia as appropriate and elevate affected body part, assessing for signs of compartment syndrome (edema, tautness, severe pain and/or numbness, impaired circulation and sensation).

TRAUMATIC BITES

ANIMAL AND HUMAN BITE WOUNDS

Animal bites: Dog bites may cause any type of soft-tissue injury (lacerations, punctures, crush injury, avulsions) depending on the extent of the bite. Cat bites are often puncture bites with a high risk of infection. Pediatric and geriatric patients are most at risk of infection. Children are the most common victims of animal bites.

Prehospital Interventions: Check that the scene is safe and the animal is secured, control any bleeding, flush the wound with sterile NS or water, apply dressings, manage the patient's airway/ventilation/oxygen supplementation (especially with bites to the face/throat), and treat shock if needed. Check the rabies status of the animal involved if known. Report the bite according to legal requirements.

Human bites: If the bite is on the genitals, it indicates abuse. Most commonly bites are on the fingers from fist contact with someone's mouth. Human bites are prone to infection, especially if treatment is delayed.

Prehospital Interventions: Flush the wound with NS or water, apply a sterile dressing, and provide emotional support for victims of abuse. Document the patient's statement accurately in the event the bite becomes a legal matter.

SPIDER BITES

Certain spider bites can be lethal if not treated in a timely fashion:

BLACK WIDOW

Initially there are two faint fang marks with a pale area surrounded by a red-blue ring. Muscle cramps, pain radiating to the upper chest (arm bites) or abdomen (leg bites) and weakness within 2 hours increasing to generalized pain, headache, itching chills, nausea, vomiting, dyspnea, hypertension, cardiac abnormalities, shock, and coma.

Prehospital Interventions: Provide supportive care and analgesia and benzodiazepine to relieve muscle spasms (per protocol). Take the spider in a sealed plastic bag to the receiving facility.

BROWN RECLUSE

Red, swollen bite site with severe pain and itching; "red, white, and blue" sign (a pale center with a central blister and reddish-blue peripheral discoloration with the blister becoming ischemic and necrotic) leaving an open ulcerated area that covers with black eschar and may expand in size. The following systemic reactions may occur within 6–12 hours in some patients: fever, vomiting, jaundice, hypotension, change in mental status, hemolytic anemia, disseminated intravascular coagulation, renal failure, seizures, coma, and death.

Prehospital Interventions: Provide supportive care and analgesia. If symptoms are severe, provide an IV access line and fluids.

INSECT BITES AND STINGS

Insect bites should be treated by first identifying the insect (through the recognition of bite characteristics), and then treating as appropriate.

FIRE ANTS

Fire ant bites cause hives and blistering with severe itching, redness, pain, and burning. Some patients may develop systemic reactions and anaphylaxis.

Prehospital Interventions: Provide supportive care and cold compresses. Use the anaphylaxis protocol if necessary.

WASPS/BEES

Wasp and bee stings cause pain, itching, redness, and swelling (most common), but they may also cause severe allergic (hives) and/or anaphylactic (life-threatening) reactions.

Prehospital Interventions: Wipe the area with gauze or scrape it with a sharp instrument to remove the stinger, wash with soap and water, apply ice, and elevate. Give antihistamines for an allergic response. Use the anaphylaxis protocol if necessary.

TICKS

With tick bites, pain may occur at the bite site. Ticks carry numerous infections, including Lyme disease, so follow-up is essential.

Prehospital Interventions: Grasp the tick near the skin with tweezers and pull with steady upward pressure, disinfect the site, and save the tick in a plastic bag.

SCORPION STINGS

Scorpion stings typically cause local burning, itching, pain, and redness, and may cause severe neurologic or other systemic reactions, such as paresthesia, stroke, hypertension, tachycardia, respiratory distress, priapism, hemorrhage, nausea, and vomiting. Pregnant women may miscarry.

Prehospital Interventions: Immobilize the affected part below the level of the heart, apply cool compresses (the first 2 hours), monitor the patient's airway, ventilation, and oxygen supplementation, start an IV access and give fluids if needed, and administer norepinephrine for severe hypotension.

SNAKE BITES

Pit vipers include rattlesnakes, copperheads, and cottonmouths. They have erectile fangs that fold until they are aroused; their venom is primarily hemotoxic and cytotoxic, but it may also have neurotoxic properties (affecting the blood, cells, and nerves at the bite site and systemically). Symptoms vary depending on the amount of venom that is injected (many bites are dry).

- Wounds usually show one or two fang marks.
- Swelling may begin immediately, or it may be delayed for up to 6 hours.
- Pain may be severe.
- There may be a wide range of symptoms, including hypotension and impairment of blood clotting that can lead to excessive blood loss, depending upon the type and amount of venom.
- Progressive weakness, vision problems, nausea, vomiting, altered consciousness, and seizures are expected.

Prehospital Interventions: Note the time elapsed from the time of the bite to the time of transport, reassure the patient, immobilize the extremity, cleanse the wound with soap and water, apply an ice pack to slow venous return and reduce swelling, transport immediately for further treatment such as with antivenom, and mark the extent of the swelling on the skin every 15 minutes.

COMPLICATIONS ASSOCIATED WITH BURN INJURIES

Burn injuries begin with the skin but can affect all organs and body systems, especially with a major burn. Complications include the following:

- **Cardiovascular***: Cardiac output may fall by 50% as capillary permeability increases with vasodilation and fluid leaks from the tissues, resulting in hypovolemia and hypothermia. Vasoconstriction occurs as a compensatory mechanism, but it may impair circulation and result in further hypoxia.
- **Pulmonary***: Injury may result from smoke inhalation or (rarely) aspiration of hot liquid. Pulmonary injury is a leading cause of death from burns and is classified according to the degree of damage as follows:
    o **First**: Singed eyebrows and nasal hairs with possible soot in airways and slight edema, increasing hypoxia.
    o **Second**: Stridor, dyspnea, and tachypnea with edema and erythema of the upper airway, including the area of the vocal cords and epiglottis, resulting in severe hypoxia, sometimes with rapid onset.
- **Infection**: Open wounds are vulnerable to infection.
- **Circumferential burns**: Swelling beneath eschar can create a tourniquet effect, impairing distal circulation.

SKIN DAMAGE CAUSED BY RADIATION TREATMENT

Skin damage/burns caused by radiation treatment vary widely depending upon the dose, duration, fraction-size, treatment area, type of equipment, and condition of the patient. Acute radiation dermatitis usually occurs when radiation is higher than 10 Gy. Patients vary in the progression of symptoms. There may be an initial inflammatory response in the tissue, with increased perfusion and WBCs to the area.

STAGING OF SKIN DAMAGE

Acute skin damage begins within 2-3 weeks of exposure to radiation with changes that are reversible. Because the cells in the skin are constantly going through mitotic division, they are vulnerable to the effects of irradiation. Most reactions subside 1-3 months after therapy ends. Damage is staged according to the type and degree of reaction, and staging determines treatment:

- **Stage I**: Slight edema and inflammation with erythema that may result in burning, itching and discomfort, caused by dilation and increased permeability of capillaries
- **Stage II**: Dry, itching, scaly skin with partial sloughing of epidermis, caused by inability of basal epidermal cells to adequately replace surface cells and decreased functioning of skin glands.
- **Stage III**: Moist blistering skin with loss of epidermal tissue, serous drainage, and increased pain with exposure of nerves, caused by continued deterioration of skin.
- **Stage IV**: Loss of body hair and sweat gland suppression resulting in permanent hair loss, atrophy, pigment changes, and ulcerations, caused by accumulation of radiation in the tissues.

Head, Face, Neck, and Spine Trauma

ANATOMY OF THE BRAIN AND SPINAL CORD

The **brain** is protected by the skull and the meninges, the three layers of lining: the dura mater, arachnoid mater, and the pia mater. Brain tissue is comprised of gray matter (neurons [nerve cells]) and white matter (covered nerve pathways that conduct messages). The main part of the brain is the cerebrum, which is comprised of two hemispheres that contain the frontal parietal, temporal, and occipital lobes. The cerebrum controls higher brain functions, including thought, speech, vision, hearing, and action. The cerebellum lies in the back of the brain below the cerebrum and controls the equilibrium and coordination. The brain stem controls involuntary functions, such as respirations, heart rate, temperature control, and nerve transmission. The brain stem is continuous with the **spinal cord**, which is also protected by the meninges and the vertebrae (cervical, thoracic, and lumbar). Cerebrospinal fluid circulates within the subarachnoid space of the brain and the spinal cord.

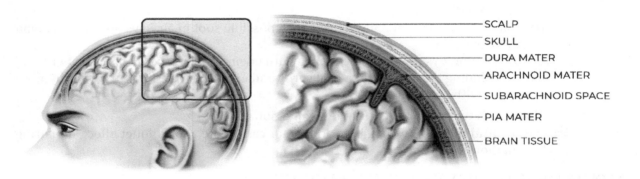

SCALP
SKULL
DURA MATER
ARACHNOID MATER
SUBARACHNOID SPACE
PIA MATER
BRAIN TISSUE

BRAIN AND CERVICAL SPINE INJURIES

Direct injury to **brain** tissue or damage from bleeding inside of the skull may occur with head injury. Altered mental status is likely. Cerebrospinal fluid may leak from the nose/ears. Symptoms include the pupils being unequal, nausea, vomiting, bradycardia (slow heart rate), elevated BP, and irregular breathing.

Prehospital Interventions: Immobilize spine, manage the patient's airway, ventilation, and oxygen supplementation, provide shock prevention, control bleeding, and provide rapid transport.

Suspect injury to the **spine** with motor vehicle/pedestrian accidents, falls, hanging, blunt or penetrating trauma to the head, neck, or torso, diving accidents, and unresponsive trauma patients. Patients may have tenderness in the area, pain on moving, numbness, tingling, or weakness, inability to feel or move below the injury, difficulty breathing, and incontinence (bowel or bladder).

Prehospital Interventions: If patient is responsive, manually stabilize the head and neck in the position found until a cervical collar and backboard are in place. Evaluate the patient's pain, sensations, and ability to move. If patient is unresponsive, stabilize the head and neck as above, manage the airway, ventilation, and oxygenation, question witnesses, and provide rapid transport.

BRAIN INJURIES, THE COUP/CONTRECOUP PATTERN, AND POSTURING

Primary brain injuries are those that result from the original trauma and include direct damage to brain tissue, such as may occur with a gunshot wound. **Secondary brain injuries** result from the effects of the primary injury, such as increasing intracranial pressure, ischemia (most common), hemorrhage, edema, and brain herniation.

Coup/Contrecoup injuries are common in motor vehicle accidents and shaken baby syndrome. With acceleration/deceleration and contact injuries where the head hits a fixed object (such as a windshield) and snaps back from the impact, coup (on the side of impact) and contrecoup (on the opposite side) contusions may both occur.

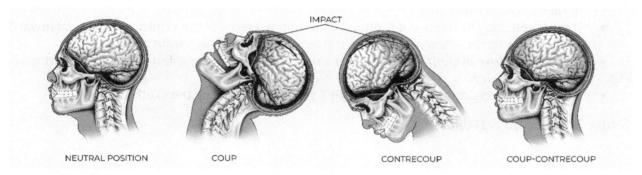

NEUTRAL POSITION   COUP   CONTRECOUP   COUP-CONTRECOUP

Decerebrate (extension) posturing (with the body stiff, legs straight, feet extended, arms straight, and the head/neck arched back) is associated with severe midbrain damage. **Decorticate (flexion) posturing** (with the body stiff, legs straight, and hands clenched on the chest) is associated with damage to the pathway connecting the brain and spinal cord and may include damage to the cerebral cortex, white matter, or basal ganglia.

DECEREBRATE POSTURING

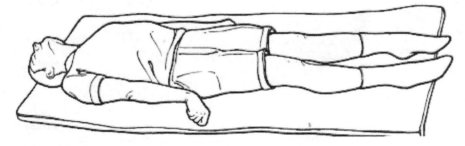

DECORTICATE POSTURING

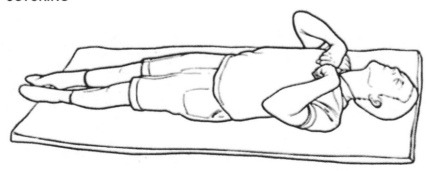

SKULL FRACTURES

The skull is divided into eight cranial bones: one frontal bone (over the frontal lobe), two parietal bones (over the parietal lobes), two temporal bones (over the temporal lobes), one occipital bone (over the occipital lobe and cerebellum), one sphenoid bone (it forms part of the eye orbit), and one ethmoid bone (it separates the nasal cavity from the brain). **Skull fractures** include the following:

- **Basilar**: Occurs in the bones at the base of the brain and can cause severe brain stem damage.
- **Comminuted**: The skull fractures into small pieces.
- **Compound**: A surface laceration extends to a skull fracture, which may be overlooked because of heavy bleeding.
- **Depressed**: May be open and is often comminuted. Pieces of the skull are depressed inward on the brain tissue, often producing dural tears and underlying brain trauma.
- **Linear/hairline**: A skull fracture forms a thin line without any splintering, usually without underlying injury.
- **Diastatic**: Affects children younger than 3 years old, widening the skull sutures.

SKULL BONES AND SUTURES

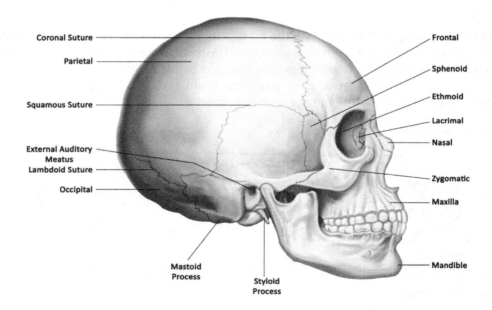

94

HEAD, SCALP, AND FACIAL INJURIES

Injury	Characteristics	Prehospital
Head	Open: Bleeding. Closed: Swelling and bruising, may have depression of the skull and underlying injury. Battle's sign (bruising over the mastoid process) and/or raccoon eyes (bruising about eyes) may indicate a basal skull fracture.	Apply direct pressure to control the bleeding; apply dry, sterile dressings. Monitor the patient's mental status. Be alert for signs of skull fracture.
Scalp	Copious bleeding may occur. May cause shock in infants and young children. Injuries above the ears increase the risk of brain injury.	As above. Manage the patient's airway, ventilation, and oxygen supplementation if needed. Rapid transport is required with shock. Avoid closing the patient's mouth with bandages.
Facial	May include soft-tissue damage, facial bone fractures (nasal, orbital), eye injuries, and oral/dental injuries (tooth avulsions, mandibular/maxillary fractures). May have severe swelling, airway compromise, impaired vision, and bloody nose.	Maintain a patent airway, but avoid nasopharyngeal airways; suction as needed; take broken teeth to the hospital; examine the eyes; and control bleeding. Patch both eyes if one or both eyes are injured. Stabilize impaled objects in the eye(s), but remove impaled objects from the cheeks if any bleeding obstructs the patient's airway.

NON-SPINAL NECK INJURIES AND NASAL FRACTURES

Non-spinal neck injuries may result from blunt trauma or penetrating trauma, and they must be carefully assessed for underlying spinal cord injury. Open wounds may bleed profusely, especially if the carotid artery is breached, resulting in rapid exsanguination and death. The airway may be compromised. Difficulty swallowing indicates esophageal injury, whereas voice changes indicate laryngeal injury. Crackling on palpation indicates air in the tissues.

Prehospital Interventions: Apply single-digit (gloved) pressure to control bleeding of the carotid artery or jugular veins; apply an occlusive dressing for an injury to the large vessels after the bleeding is controlled to prevent air from entering the bloodstream, which is life-threatening; and manage the patient's airway/ventilation/oxygen supplementation (advanced life support may be needed). Rapid or air medical transport may be needed.

Nasal fractures (40% of facial fractures) may cause persistent bleeding and should be assessed for drainage of the cerebrospinal fluid and injury of the surrounding structures, including brain injury, skull fracture, and neck and cervical spine injury.

Prehospital Interventions: Control any bleeding, elevate the patient's head, and manage the airway, but do not use a nasopharyngeal airway.

MANDIBULAR FRACTURES, LARYNGOTRACHEAL INJURIES, AND NON-CNS-ASSOCIATED SPINAL TRAUMA

Additional non-CNS fractures of the face, neck and spine include:

- **Mandibular fractures** are most common in males 21 to 30 and result from a blow to the jaw from an assault, motor vehicle accident, or gunshot wound and are often associated with other injuries, such as head injury or midface fractures. Symptoms include malocclusion of teeth, pain, point tenderness, and ecchymosis of the floor of the mouth.
  Prehospital Interventions: Manage the patient's airway/ventilation/oxygen supplementation (avoid the nasal airway), use an ice pack to reduce edema, elevate the patient's head, and monitor him or her closely.
- **Laryngotracheal injuries** result from direct trauma and may result in swelling and hemorrhage. Symptoms include swelling, changes in voice, hemoptysis, subcutaneous emphysema (from open wounds), and structural irregularities. The patient must be assessed for associated injuries.
  Prehospital Interventions: Manage the patient's airway/ventilation/oxygen supplementation because airway obstruction is common, elevate the patient's head, and provide supportive care. May require a surgical airway.
- With **non-CNS-associated spinal trauma**, patients complain of pain and point tenderness, but neurological findings are intact.
  Prehospital Interventions: Provide sitting or standing spinal mobilization and supportive care and manage the patient's airway, ventilation, and oxygen supplementation as needed.

DENTAL INJURIES

Dental fractures, most commonly of the maxillary teeth, may occur in association with other oral and facial injuries and may be overlooked unless a careful dental examination is carried out. Fractures may range from chipping of the enamel to fracture of the tooth root.

Dental avulsions are complete displacement of a tooth from its socket. The tooth may be reimplanted if done within 1-2 hours after displacement, although only permanent teeth are reimplanted, not primary teeth, so question the parents of children to determine if an avulsed tooth is permanent.

Prehospital Interventions: Manage the patient's airway, ventilation, and oxygen supplementation as needed, elevate the patient's head, and place the avulsed tooth in NS for transport.

Nervous System Trauma

CONCUSSIONS

A concussion is a brain injury in which structural damage is not apparent but neurological functioning is impaired. Patients may experience a brief loss of consciousness after a head injury and may experience confusion and even bizarre behavior (if the frontal lobe is affected). Other symptoms include severe headache, somnolence, dizziness, lack of coordination, confusion, disorientation, inappropriate emotional response, nausea, and vomiting. Symptoms are usually transient (lasting from minutes to hours), but up to 50% may have recurrent symptoms (such as difficulty concentrating, headaches, and dizziness) for months. The **American Academy of Neurology classifies concussions** as follows:

- **Grade 1**: Transient confusion without loss of consciousness, with symptoms resolving in <15 minutes
- **Grade 2**: Transient confusion without loss of consciousness, with symptoms resolving in >15 minutes
- **Grade 3**: Any loss of consciousness of any duration

Prehospital Interventions: Provide supportive care and reassurance, monitor vital signs and neurological status for signs of increasing intracranial pressure that may indicate more severe injury, and elevate the patient's head.

SIGNS OF INCREASING INTRACRANIAL PRESSURE

Head trauma may result in **increased intracranial pressure** and cerebral edema. Patients often suffer initial hypertension, which increases intracranial pressure and decreases perfusion, and significant swelling, which also interferes with perfusion, causing hypoxia and hypercapnia (increased carbon dioxide), which trigger increased blood flow. This increased volume at a time when injury impairs autoregulation further increases cerebral edema, which, in turn, increases intracranial pressure and results in a further decrease in perfusion with resultant ischemia (impaired circulation). If the pressure continues to rise, the brain may herniate. The mean arterial pressure must remain between 65 and 150 mmHg for the brain to autoregulate intracranial pressure (the normal pressure is 2–12 mmHg). Symptoms include Cushing's triad: wide pulse pressure, bradycardia, and irregular respirations.

Initially: Decreased levels of consciousness, increased BP, and decreased pulse, Cheyne-Stokes (irregular) respirations, and reactive pupils. Middle brain stem involvement: Wide pulse pressure, bradycardia, pupils sluggish or nonreactive, and hyperventilation. Lower brain stem: Pupil blown on the side of injury, irregular respirations, flaccid response to painful stimulation, and the BP and pulse decrease.

Prehospital Interventions: Elevate the patient's head, manage the patient's airway/ventilation/oxygen supplementation, provide rapid transport, and start an IV access line.

INTRACRANIAL HEMATOMAS

Type	Characteristics	Prehospital
Epidural	Bleeding between the dura and the skull, pushing the brain downward and inward. The hemorrhage is usually caused by arterial tears, so bleeding is often rapid, leading to severe neurological deficits and respiratory arrest. The patient may be lucid and without symptoms for 2–6 hours after the injury.	Provide supportive care, keep the patient's head elevated to reduce intracranial pressure, note neurological status (movement, strength, mental status, pupils equal and reactive or unequal/fixed), and provide rapid transport. Provide an IV access line and fluids.
Subdural	Bleeding between the dura and the arachnoid mater, usually from tears in the cortical veins of the subdural space. It tends to develop more slowly than an epidural hemorrhage. If the bleeding is acute and develops within minutes or hours of injury, then the prognosis is poor. Subacute hematomas that develop more slowly cause varying degrees of injury.	
Intracerebral	Bleeding into the substance of the brain from an artery. Sudden onset; it results in a hemorrhagic stroke with a lack of nutrients and oxygen to parts of the brain. May result from degenerative changes, hypertension, brain tumors, medications, or illicit drugs (crack, cocaine). Symptoms vary depending on the site, but they may include one-sided weakness, paralysis, difficulty speaking, severe headache, and altered mental status.	Provide supportive care, keep the patient's head elevated to reduce intracranial pressure, note neurological status (movement, strength, mental status, pupils equal and reactive or unequal/fixed), provide rapid transport, start an IV access line, and give fluids.
Subarachnoid	Bleeding in the space between the meninges and brain and into the cerebrospinal fluid, usually resulting from aneurysm, arteriovenous malformation (AVM), or trauma. This type of hemorrhage compresses the brain tissue. The first presenting symptoms are severe headache, nausea and vomiting, nuchal rigidity, palsy related to cranial nerve compression, retinal hemorrhages, and papilledema.	

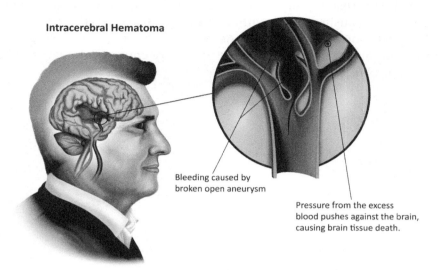

Intracerebral Hematoma

Bleeding caused by broken open aneurysm

Pressure from the excess blood pushes against the brain, causing brain tissue death.

SPINAL INJURIES AND SPINAL CORD INJURIES (SCIs)

Spinal injuries of the vertebrae include fractures, dislocations, open wounds, and flexion and extension injuries. Because the spinal cord lies within the vertebral column, injury to the vertebrae may cause **spinal cord injuries (SCIs)** and disrupt transmissions in nerves that connect the body and the brain. SCI may affect only a few nerves, or they may completely transect the spinal cord, resulting in permanent paralysis below the site of injury. SCIs should be suspected with head trauma, penetrating trauma, direct blunt trauma, falls, diving injuries, motor vehicle accidents, rapid deceleration accidents, and multisystem trauma. Assessment includes evaluating extremity movement, respiration control, sensation, reflexes, pain/tenderness, and vital signs.

Prehospital Interventions: Logroll the patient to examine his or her back, immobilize the patient (seated or standing), apply a rigid cervical collar, lift and move him or her with care, and provide rapid transport. Elevate the torso of children 2–3 cm with padding so that the head is in a neutral position if using an adult immobilization device. Immobilize infants in their car seats, padding all the voids.

Spinal cord injuries (SCIs) may result from blunt trauma (such as automobile accidents), falls from a height, sports injuries, and penetrating trauma (such as a gunshot or knife wound). Damage results from mechanical injury and secondary responses resulting from hemorrhage, edema, and ischemia. The types of symptoms relate to the area and degree of injury, as below:

- **Anterior cord**: This results from pressure/damage to the anterior spinal cord. The posterior column functions remain, so there are sensations of touch, vibration, and position remaining below the injury but with complete paralysis and loss of the sensations of pain and temperature. The prognosis is poor.
- **Brown-Séquard**: The cord is hemisected from penetrating trauma, resulting in spastic paresis, loss of sense of position and vibration on the injured side, and loss of pain and temperature sensation on the other side. The prognosis is good.
- **Posterior cord**: Motor function is preserved but without sensation.
- **Conus medullaris**: Injury to the lower spine (lower lumbar and sacral nerves).

99

- **Central cord**: This results from hyperextension or hyperflexion and ischemia or stenosis of the cervical spine, causing spinal contusion and quadriparesis (more severe in the upper extremities) with some loss of sensations of pain and temperature. Prognosis is good, but fine motor skills are often impaired in the upper extremities with paresis being more acute distally than proximally in the arms.

Trauma in Special Populations

PREGNANCY AND PEDIATRIC TRAUMA

Pregnancy trauma: The mother and fetus are each considered to be patients. Pregnant patients are susceptible to falls and domestic abuse. Pregnant women have an increased blood volume and heart rate, impaired venous return if in the supine (flat) position in the third trimester, and an increased risk of vomiting and aspiration. Hypovolemia/shock lowers oxygen to the fetus, resulting in fetal stress. Vaginal bleeding may occur.

Prehospital Interventions: Have suction available, monitor the patient's airway, ventilation, and oxygen supplementation with 100% oxygen per nonrebreather mask and ventilation assistance if needed, transport on the left side (tilt the immobilization board if necessary), provide an IV access line and fluids if indicated and rapid transport.

Pediatric trauma: Assess the pediatric triangle (appearance, work of breathing, and circulation). The respiration rate varies with age, but the use of accessory muscles and sternal retraction indicate respiratory distress. Assess the brachial pulse in infants—a slow pulse indicates hypoxia.

Prehospital Interventions: Manage hypovolemia/shock, prevent hypothermia, and manage the patient's airway, ventilation, and oxygen supplementation as needed. Ventilate if he or she is bradycardic (BVM is preferred for children).

TRAUMA IN GERIATRIC PATIENTS

Geriatric patients are more susceptible to trauma because of aging processes, and they may be less able to maintain normal vital signs during hemorrhage. Polypharmacy is common, and medications may affect vital signs and blood clotting. The risk of cerebral bleeding is increased because of brain shrinkage. The cough reflex may be lessened. Fractures are common because of osteoporosis, especially hip fractures.

Prehospital Interventions: Splint fractures, monitor the patient's airway, ventilation, and oxygen supplementation, monitor oxygenation with pulse oximetry, suction if necessary, and check the mouth for dentures (which may obstruct the airway). Spinal curvature may require padding of the spinal board.

TRAUMA IN THE COGNITIVELY IMPAIRED PATIENT

Disorders that result in cognitive impairment may include Alzheimer's or other forms of dementia, traumatic brain injuries, strokes, Down syndrome, and autistic spectrum disorders. Patients may be more at risk of trauma, and assessment and history taking may be difficult. Perceptions of pain may be altered, and psychological reactions may vary.

Prehospital Interventions: Remain supportive, reassure the patient, obtain information from the caregiver if necessary, and treat as indicated by the patient's condition.

Environmental Emergencies

TEMPERATURE-RELATED TRAUMA
GENERALIZED HYPOTHERMIA
Generalized hypothermia occurs when the body temperature falls to below-normal levels:

- Mild: 34–36 °C (93.2–96.8 °F)
- Moderate: 30–34 °C (86.0–93.2 °F)
- Severe: <30 °C (<86.0 °F)

Contributing factors include wet and cold environments, wind, age (geriatric/pediatric), medical conditions, substance abuse (alcohol, drugs), and poison. Up to 50% of trauma patients with severe injuries become hypothermic because of exposure, blood loss, shock, and standard procedures (such as administration of cold fluids and clothing removal). Indications of hypothermia include cold skin, shivering, decreased mental status (confusion, memory loss, lethargy, dizziness, mood changes, impaired judgment, difficulty speaking), decreased sensation of touch, decreased motor function (muscle rigidity, stiff posture, muscle/joint stiffness), and bradycardia.

Prehospital Interventions: Remove the patient from the cold environment, remove any wet clothing, wrap in warm blankets, begin CPR if no pulse is obtained after 30–45 seconds of assessment, and use an AED if it indicates the need to defibrillate.

FROSTBITE/FREEZING
Frostbite is tissue damage from freezing, most often affecting the nose, ears, and distal extremities (hands/feet). The affected part feels numb and aches or throbs, becoming hard and insensate as the tissue freezes, resulting in circulatory impairment, necrosis of tissue, and gangrene. **Degrees of frostbite/freezing** are as follows:

1. Partial freezing with erythema and mild edema, stinging, burning, and throbbing pain.
2. Full-thickness freezing with increased edema in 3–4 hours and clear blisters in 6–24 hours; sloughing of skin with eschar formation, numbness, and then aching and throbbing pain.
3. Full-thickness freezing into the subdermal tissue with cyanosis, hemorrhagic blisters, skin necrosis, a "wooden" feeling, severe burning, throbbing, and shooting pains.
4. Freezing extends into the subcutaneous tissue (muscles, tendons, and bones) with a mottled appearance, non-blanching cyanosis, and eventually deep black eschar.

Prehospital Interventions: Remove the patient from the cold environment with care, remove wet clothing, cover the patient with a blanket, remove jewelry, manually stabilize the affected area, and transport rapidly. Do NOT break blisters, rub or massage the area, apply heat, rewarm if the area may refreeze, allow the patient to walk, or give him or her anything by mouth.

HEAT-RELATED ILLNESSES

Heat-related illnesses include:

- **Heat Stress**: Increased temperature causes dehydration. Symptoms may include swelling of the hands and feet, flushing, itching, sunburn, dizziness, muscle cramps, and hyperventilation. The patient's temperature is normal.
  Prehospital Interventions: Remove the patient from heat, give fluids to rehydrate, and give oxygen with a nonrebreather mask.
- **Heat Exhaustion**: Dehydration results in sodium depletion. Symptoms may include flu-like symptoms, headache, dizziness, fainting, nausea, vomiting, weakness, muscle cramping, rapid pulse, diaphoresis, and cold clammy skin. The patient's temperature is usually <41 °C (105.8 °F), and it may be normal.
  Prehospital Interventions: Remove the patient from heat; use evaporative cooling techniques such as ice packs to the axilla, groin, and neck; rehydrate (half glass of water every 15-20 minutes). Give oxygen as above.
- **Heat Stroke**: There are two types, which may progress to multiorgan dysfunction syndrome with liver and kidney failure, and death. **Exertional**: Sudden onset after exertion. The patient's temperature varies because he or she is still sweating; there is diaphoresis, syncope, and loss of consciousness. **Non-exertional**: Sudden onset after heat exposure. The temperature is usually >41 °C (105.8 °F) rectally or >39.4 °C (102.9 °F) orally. There can be mild irritability, decorticate posturing, seizures, coma, and tachycardia.
  Prehospital Interventions: Remove the patient from heat, apply evaporative cooling and ice packs as above; provide airway/ventilation/oxygenation support as needed, IV access line and fluids, and rapid transport.

SUBMERSION/DROWNING

Submersion may cause aspiration (wet drowning) or trigger severe laryngospasm (dry drowning), although some people will be pulled from the water still breathing. **Drowning** is the leading cause of death in children younger than age 5, and it is the second leading cause of death in children younger than age 15. Most infant submersions are in bathtubs and result from intentional injury or lack of supervision. Adolescent and adult submersions are often related to drugs, alcohol, or risk-taking behaviors. Submersion asphyxiation can cause profound damage to multiple organ systems, including the brain, heart, and lungs, from a lack of oxygen and aspiration. Hypothermia related to near drowning has some protective effect because blood is shunted to the brain and heart. Indications of submersion include coughing, vomiting, difficulty breathing, and respiratory and cardiac arrest.

Prehospital Interventions: Initiate CPR if the patient is in arrest, manage the patient's airway/ventilation/oxygen supplementation with 100% oxygen (may need intubation), place him or her in the recovery position if he or she is unconscious or vomiting, provide suction as needed, start an IV access line, and provide rapid transport.

Multisystem Trauma

MULTI-SYSTEM TRAUMA

Multi-system trauma involves injury to more than one major system, which is quite common. Care includes the following points:

- Ensure the safety of the patient and all rescue personnel and determine the need for additional resources.
- Consider the mechanism of injury and identify and manage life-threatening conditions.
- Manage the patient's airway, ventilation, and oxygen supplementation (high concentration) as well as necessary spinal immobilization with him or her in a lying/sitting position, and make positioning decisions.
- Control hemorrhage, provide shock therapy, and maintain body temperature.
- Splint musculoskeletal injuries.
- Suspect additional injuries.
- Prioritize interventions and continue care en route rather than delaying transport.
- Evaluate the patient's condition by the injuries sustained (bleeding, difficulty breathing, lack of pulse) rather than by the patient's response (screaming, yelling).
- Complete the primary and secondary assessments, and obtain a medical history.
- Platinum ten—the first 10 minutes on the scene in which the patient should be extricated and stabilization efforts should be started.
- Golden hour—the first 60 minutes during which the patient should be stabilized and transported to the receiving facility.
- Notify the receiving facility so that resources are prepared.

BLAST INJURIES

Blast injuries may result from high-order explosives (TNT, nitroglycerin) or low-order explosives (pipe bombs, Molotov cocktails). Enclosed explosions usually cause more injury than do open-air blasts. Blast waves occur only with high-order explosives and result from high-pressure impulses. Blast wind may occur with either type of explosive and involves superheated air. Ground shock may cause further injury. Immediate death may occur.

Injuries may include the following:

- **Primary**: Blast wave injury affects gas-filled organs/structures including the lungs, eardrum, abdomen, eyes, and brain (20% of victims).
- **Secondary**: Penetrating injuries from flying shrapnel affecting any part of the body along with abrasions, contusions, and lacerations. (Secondary injury is the most common cause of death.)
- **Tertiary**: Injuries from being thrown by blast wind, such as fractures, spinal and brain injuries, and traumatic amputations.
- **Quaternary**: Other injuries and complications, such as difficulty breathing because of smoke inhalation, burns, and crush injuries.

Prehospital Interventions:

- Be alert for a second explosive device or a device on a victim (who may be a perpetrator).
- Carry out rapid triage.
- Control any bleeding and manage shock.
- Manage the patient's airway, ventilation, and oxygen supplementation. Provide CPR if necessary.
- Splint musculoskeletal injuries.
- Start an IV access and give fluid resuscitation.
- Provide rapid transport.

Medical/Obstetrics/Gynecology

Neurological Emergencies

NEUROLOGICAL SYSTEM

The neurological (nervous) system consists of the **central nervous system (CNS)**, which contains the brain, spinal cord and nerves, and the **peripheral nervous system (PNS)**, which contains the sensory neurons, ganglia (nerve clusters), and nerves connecting to the CNS. The brain consists of the **cerebrum** (frontal, temporal, parietal, and occipital lobes); the **cerebellum**; and the **brain stem**, which is continuous with the spinal cord. The PNS is divided into the **autonomic nervous system (ANS)** and the **somatic nervous system (SoNS)**. The autonomic nervous system controls the body's organs and maintains homeostasis (balance). Functions of the ANS include control of the heart rate and function, respiration, digestion, sexual arousal, and other systems. The SoNS comprises cranial and spinal nerves that connect the CNS to the skeletal muscles and skin. The SoNS is the voluntarily controlled component of the PNS, and it receives and responds to external sensory stimuli from the skin and sensory organs.

> **Review Video: Brain Anatomy**
> Visit mometrix.com/academy and enter code: 222476

GLASGOW COMA SCALE (GCS)

The Glasgow coma scale (GCS) measures the depth and duration of coma or impaired level of consciousness; it is a critical part of the neurological assessment and, when trended, can mark progress/recovery or neurological decline. The GCS measures three parameters: best eye response, best verbal response, and best motor response, with a total possible score that ranges from 3 to 15. The same scale is used with slight modifications for infants.

Eye opening	4: Spontaneous 3: To verbal stimuli 2: To pain (not of face) 1: No response
Verbal	5: Oriented 4: Conversation confused, but can answer questions 3: Uses inappropriate words 2: Speech incomprehensible 1: No response
Motor	6: Moves on command 5: Moves purposefully respond pain 4: Withdraws in response to pain 3: Decorticate posturing (flexion) in response to pain 2: Decerebrate posturing (extension) in response to pain 1: No response

Injuries/conditions are classified according to the total score: 3-8 Coma; ≤8 Severe head injury likely requiring intubation; 9-12 Moderate head injury; 13-15 Mild head injury.

> **Review Video: Glasgow Coma Scale**
> Visit mometrix.com/academy and enter code: 133399

STROKES

Strokes result from interruption of blood flow to an area of the brain.

- **Ischemic strokes** (80%) are caused by blockage of an artery supplying the brain, usually from a thrombus (blood clot) or embolus (traveling clot).
- **Hemorrhagic strokes** (20%) result from a ruptured cerebral artery, causing not only a lack of oxygen and nutrients but also edema (swelling) that causes widespread pressure and damage. With both types, patients may experience weakness, paralysis, and loss of sensation in one or more extremities; difficulty speaking or loss of speech; vision impairment; difficulty swallowing; headache; an altered state of consciousness (confusion, disorientation); or coma.
- **Transient ischemic attacks** (TIAs) from small clots cause similar but short-lived (minutes to hours) symptoms. Emergent treatment includes placing the patient in the semi-Fowlers or Fowler's position and administering oxygen. The patient may require oral suctioning if the secretions pool. The patient's airway, breathing, and circulation should be assessed. Patients should be transported immediately to the receiving facility because thrombolytic therapy to dissolve blood clots should be administered within 1-3 hours.

CINCINNATI PREHOSPITAL STROKE SCALE

The Cincinnati Prehospital Stroke Scale should be administered to any patient who is suspected of having a stroke. The patient may be experiencing a stroke if he tests positive for any of the three signs and should be transported to the receiving facility as soon as possible.

Signs	Directions to patient	Abnormal results
Facial drooping	Smile. Show your teeth.	One side of the face is weak or paralyzed and doesn't move as well as the other.
Arm drifting	Close your eyes and hold your arms out straight and hold them there for 10 seconds.	One arm doesn't move at all or drifts downward.
Speaking abnormality	Repeat after me: "Don't count your chickens before they are hatched."	Patient slurs words, uses inappropriate words, or is unable to respond.

LOS ANGELES PREHOSPITAL STROKE SCREEN

The Los Angeles Prehospital Stroke Screen is used to assess patients in a prehospital setting who have symptoms that suggest a stroke (such as altered state of consciousness, difficulty speaking, one-sided weakness, or paralysis). The results are positive for stroke if all criteria are met or are unable to be measured and the physical exam shows an unequal response. Note: A patient may still be having a stroke even if all the criteria are not met.

General criteria	Yes	No	Unknown
Age >45			
No history of epilepsy or seizures			
Onset of symptoms <24 hours			
Patient was able to walk before the onset of symptoms			
Blood glucose between 60 and 400 mg/dL			

Physical criteria	Equal	Right	Left
Facial smile	Normal	Droop	Droop
Grip strength	Normal	Weak or no grip	Weak or no grip
Arm strength	Normal	Drifts or falls down	Drifts or falls down

SEIZURES

GRAND MAL SEIZURES

Seizures are sudden, involuntary, abnormal electrical disturbances in the brain that can manifest as alterations of consciousness, spastic tonic and clonic movements, convulsions, and loss of consciousness.

- **Tonic-clonic (grand mal)**: Occurs without warning.
  - *Tonic period* (10–30 seconds): The eyes roll upward with loss of consciousness, the arms flex, and the body stiffens in symmetric contractions with cyanosis and salivating.
  - *Clonic period* (usually 30 seconds or longer): Violent rhythmic jerking with contraction and relaxation and sometimes incontinence of urine and feces.

During the seizure, the patient's head and body should be protected from injury but no attempt should be made to insert anything into the mouth or restrain the patient. If possible, the patient should be screened from spectators and turned onto his or her side (the recovery position) to prevent aspiration. Following seizures, there may be confusion, disorientation, and impairment of motor activity and speech and vision for several hours. Headache, nausea, and vomiting may occur.

> **Review Video: Seizures**
> Visit mometrix.com/academy and enter code: 977061

Prehospital Interventions: Monitor the airway, breathing, and circulation and suction. Administer oxygen as needed. Insert a nasopharyngeal airway for assisted ventilation if the patient is cyanotic.

PARTIAL SEIZURES

Partial seizures are caused by an electrical discharge to a localized area of the cerebral cortex, such as the frontal, temporal, or parietal lobes with seizure characteristics related to the area of involvement. They may begin in a focal area and become generalized, often preceded by an aura.

- **Simple partial**: Unilateral motor symptoms including somatosensory, psychic, and autonomic.
  - *Aversive*: Eyes and head are turned away from the focal side.
  - *Sylvan* (usually during sleep): Tonic-clonic movements of the face, salivation, and arrested speech.
- **Special sensory**: Various sensations (numbness, tingling, prickling, or pain) spreading from one area. May include visual sensations, posturing, or hypertonia. These are rare in patients <8 years old.
- **Complex (psychomotor)**: There is no loss of consciousness, but there may be altered levels of consciousness, and patients may be nonresponsive with amnesia. May involve complex sensorium with bad tastes, auditory or visual hallucinations, and a feeling of déjà vu or strong fear. Patients may carry out repetitive activities, such as walking, running, smacking lips, chewing, or drawling. Patients are rarely aggressive. The seizure is usually followed by prolonged drowsiness and confusion. Occurs from age 3 through adolescence.

NEUROLOGICAL ASSESSMENT
ASSESSING THE PATIENT'S LEVEL OF CONSCIOUSNESS

The **AVPU** is a quick assessment done to determine the **patient's level of consciousness**. This may be one of the first assessments done when initially attending to a patient.

Alert, voice, pain, unresponsive (AVPU)			
A	Alert and awake; aware of person, place, time, and condition. Follows commands. Pediatric: Active and responds to external stimuli and to caregiver.	Yes	No
V	Responds to verbal stimuli, but the eyes do not open spontaneously. Pediatric: Responds only when the caregiver calls the child's name.	Yes	No
P	Responds to painful stimuli, such as pinching the skin/earlobe, but not to verbal stimuli. Pediatric: Responds only to painful stimuli, such as pinching the nailbed.	Yes	No
U	Unresponsive; does not respond to painful or verbal stimuli. Pediatric: Unresponsive.	Yes	No

ASSESSMENT OF A PATIENT'S MENTAL STATUS

When assessing a patient's mental status, make note of the following:

- **Level of consciousness**: Using the AVPU assessment.
- **Posture and behavior**: Abnormal findings include restlessness, agitation, bizarre posturing, catatonia (immobility), and tics or other abnormal movements.
- **Dress, grooming, and hygiene**: Kempt or unkempt, clean or dirty.
- **Facial expressions**: May vary widely (anxious, depressed, angry, sad, elated, or fearful). Note whether the patient's expressions seem appropriate to the situation/words.
- **Speech/Language**: Quantity, rate, fluency, appropriate/inappropriate. Note aphasia (inability to speak and/or understand words), dysphonia (abnormal voice/difficulty speaking), or dysarthria (difficulty speaking words).
- **Mood**: Nature and duration of the patient's current mood. Note suicidal ideation.
- **Thoughts/Perceptions**: Note logic, relevance, and organization of thoughts and abnormal findings, such as thought blocking (sudden period of silence in the middle of a sentence while speaking), flight of ideas (racing thoughts), incoherence, confabulation (producing distorted memories), loose association (responses not connected to questions or one sentence not connected to the next), or transference (redirecting emotions to a substitute). Note homicidal or suicidal thoughts, obsessions, compulsions, delusions, illusions, and hallucinations.
- **Judgment**: Note the patient's insight, ability to make decisions, and ability to plan.

CAUSES OF ALTERED MENTAL STATUS

Altered mental status occurs because brain functioning is disrupted. Signs of altered mental status may be subtle (such as slight agitation, lethargy, sleepiness, or forgetfulness) or more obvious (such as disorientation, confusion, personality changes, violent behavior, somnolence, seizures, and coma). An **altered mental status** may occur abruptly or may have a slower onset, depending on the cause:

- **Inadequate oxygenation**: Brain cells can only survive about 6 minutes without oxygen, but damage begins to occur after about 60 seconds.
- **Inadequate ventilation**: Even if oxygen is plentiful, gas exchange is inadequate with impaired ventilation.
- **Overdose of medication**: May occur with numerous drugs, including opioids/narcotics (such as heroin and oxycodone), antipsychotics, hallucinogens, inhalants, cocaine, methamphetamines, and benzodiazepines.
- **Poisoning**: Includes arsenic; lead; cyanide; and overdose of medications such as acetaminophen, clonidine, salicylates, calcium channel blockers, and beta blockers.
- **Infection**: Systemic infections (sepsis), brain abscesses, chronic infections (human immunodeficiency virus/acquired immune deficiency syndrome [HIV/AIDS]).
- **Psychological/psychiatric condition**: Includes bipolar disorder, schizophrenia, post-traumatic stress disorder (PTSD), and depression.
- **Diabetes**: Hyperglycemia and hypoglycemia (especially insulin reaction).

AEIOU TIPS MNEMONIC TO OUTLINE THE POTENTIAL CAUSES FOR ALTERED MENTAL STATUS

Many different conditions can lead to altered mental status, and the EMS provider should consider all possibilities because emergent treatment may vary depending on the cause. Always check for medical alert jewelry. The following **AEIOU TIPS mnemonic** is a helpful guide to recalling potential causes:

A	Alcohol/Acidosis	Note the smell of alcohol, empty alcohol containers.
E	Endocrine/Epilepsy	Consider electrolyte imbalance, encephalopathy; note oral trauma, urinary incontinence.
I	Infection	Consider urinary infection in older adults, meningitis, encephalitis, sepsis.
O	Opiates/Overdose	Note if the pupils are constricted, drug paraphernalia, history of drug taking, empty medicine containers.
U	Uremia/Underdose	Note generalized edema, history of kidney failure, failure to take prescribed medicines.
T	Trauma	Consider head injury, excessive bleeding, assault.
I	Insulin	Check refrigerator/medicine cabinet for diabetes medications; check the blood glucose level.
P	Poisoning/Psychosis	Note any history of psychiatric illness; observe the environment for poisons.
S	Stroke/Seizures	Note one-sided weakness, incontinence, difficulty speaking, somnolence.

MENTAL STATUS EXAM (MSE)

Mental status is usually assessed through normal interactions, and the **mental status exam** (MSE) can be used as a guide when assessing patients. Some components require only observation, whereas others require questioning. Components include the following:

- **Appearance**: Kempt, unkempt
- **Behavior/attitude**: Appropriate, inappropriate
- **Consciousness/alertness**: Conscious, arousable, able to focus
- **Orientation**: Person, place, time, event
- **Speech/language**: Normal, abnormal, bizarre, tone, volume
- **Thought processes/content**: Logical/Illogical thinking, delusions, hallucinations, paranoia, fixations, suicidal ideation
- **Affect**: Flat (no expression), blunted (little expression), broad (a wide range of expressions), inappropriate (inconsistent), and restricted (one expression at all times)
- **Mood**: Happy, sad, depressed, elated, withdrawn
- **Attention span**: Appropriate, short, scattered
- **Memory**: Intact, short- or long-term memory loss
- **Judgment/reasoning**: Ability to make reasonable decisions and ability to understand and reason
- **Suicidal or homicidal ideation**: Present, absent

ASSESSMENT OF MEMORY AND ATTENTION

Techniques for the assessment of memory and attention include the following:

- **Orientation**: Ask patient questions to determine if he or she knows person (their name), place (where they are), time (date and hour), and event (what's happening). If a patient knows all of that information, then he or she is oriented ×4.
- **Digit span test**: Tell or show the patient a sequence of six or seven numbers and ask him or her to recall and repeat them.
- **Word recall**: Name three unrelated items and ask the patient to remember them. Wait a few minutes, and then ask the patient to name the items.
- **Serial 7s test**: Ask the patient to count backward from 100 by 7s (100, 93, 86. . .).
- **Spell backward test**: Ask the patient to spell "world" backward (D-L-R-O-W).
- **Remote memory**: Ask the patient to tell her birthdate or that of a close family member.
- **Recent memory**: Ask the patient to describe events earlier in the day.
- **Current memory**: Ask the patient to recall your name or the name of someone else present and to whom the patient was recently introduced.

HEADACHES AND MIGRAINES

Types of headaches/migraines include the following:

- **Tension**: Steady, constant pressure-like pain usually starting in the forehead, temples, or the back of the neck.
- **Cluster**: Unilateral, occurring one to eight times daily, often for several weeks and associated with severe pain in the eye and orbit and radiating to the face and temporal area.
- **Migraine**: Severe recurring headaches often characterized by a prodrome phase, aura phase, headache phase, and recovery phase.
- **Head/neck trauma-related headaches**: Vary but may start at neck or shoulders and radiate to the top of the head.
- **Bleeding/stroke-related headaches**:
  - *Epidural*: Sudden severe, intense
  - *Subdural*: Progressive headache worsening over time
  - *Subarachnoid*: "Thunderclap" severe headache with abrupt onset; may be worse at the back of the head
  - *Stroke*: Tension-type headache with the site of pain relating to the area of injury, often associated with alterations in mental status and other symptoms, such as weakness, paralysis, nausea and vomiting, and photophobia.

STATUS EPILEPTICUS

Status epilepticus (SE) is usually generalized tonic-clonic seizures that are characterized by a series of seizures with the intervening time being too short for the regaining of consciousness. The constant seizures and periods of apnea can lead to exhaustion, respiratory failure with hypoxemia and hypercapnia, hyperthermia, cardiac failure, and death. SE may result from uncontrolled epilepsy, noncompliance with anticonvulsive treatment, stroke, encephalopathy, drug toxicity, brain trauma, brain tumors (neoplasms), and metabolic disorders. SE is life threatening, so treatment should begin as soon as possible.

Prehospital Interventions:

- Place an intravenous (IV) line.
- If opioid drug intoxication is the suspected cause, administer naloxone.
- Administer midazolam (intramuscular [IM]) (5 to 10 mg), lorazepam (IV), or diazepam (IV) to control seizures.
- Intubate and ventilate if in respiratory distress.
- Provide supportive care for seizures to prevent injury.
- Control hyperthermia with room-temperature water to skin and an IV normal saline (NS) bolus of 500 mL.

Gastrointestinal Emergencies

GASTROINTESTINAL (GI) TRACT

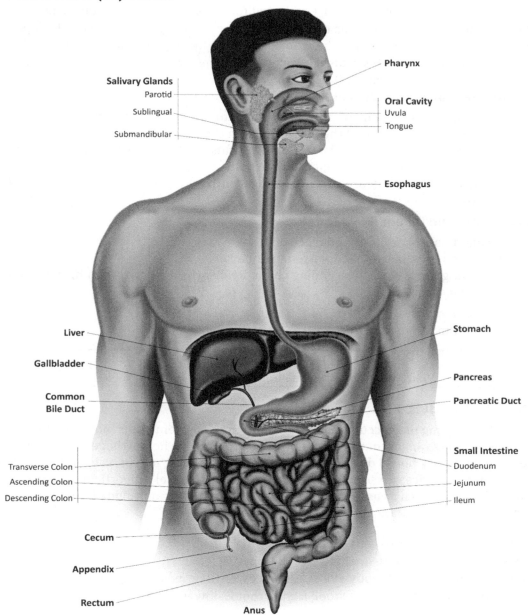

Elements of the **gastrointestinal tract**:

- **Mouth**: Chews, moistens, begins carbohydrate hydrolysis (the breakdown of food by enzymes), creates a bolus of food. Connected to the esophagus by the pharynx.
- **Esophagus**: Transports a bolus through the lower esophageal sphincter (which prevents backflow up the esophagus) to the stomach by peristalsis (wavelike contractions)
- **Stomach**: Churns, secretes acids and enzymes, begins hydrolysis of proteins, and creates chyme (a more fluid substance)
- **Small intestine (about 20 feet long)**:
  - Duodenum: Accepts chyme and digests food to prepare for absorption
  - Jejunum: Absorbs most of the nutrients from the food, including vitamin B_{12}; accepts bile from the liver and gallbladder to digest fats and pancreatic enzymes from the pancreas to digest proteins, fats, and carbohydrates
  - Ileum: Contains the ileocecal valve, which controls the flow of chyme into the large intestine
- **Large intestine (about 5 feet long)**:
  - Cecum: Reabsorbs fluids and electrolytes
  - Appendix: Is believed to store useful gut bacteria
  - Ascending, transverse, descending colon: Reabsorbs water, vitamin K, and electrolytes to form feces
- **Rectum**: Stores feces
- **Anus**: Contains sphincters that control the expelling of feces

---

Review Video: Gastrointestinal System
Visit mometrix.com/academy and enter code: 378740

GASTROINTESTINAL BLEEDING

Gastrointestinal bleeding may occur anywhere within the GI system but is most common from the upper GI. Bleeding may range from slow and insidious to massive hemorrhage. Causes include esophageal inflammatory bowel disease (IBD), HIV/CMV infection, polyps, cancer, hemorrhoids, diverticulosis, ulcers, varices (associated with liver disease), Meckel's diverticulum, anticoagulation, and overuse of NSAIDS, such as aspirin and ibuprofen, so history can provide important clues. Output may help to differentiate upper GI bleeding from lower:

- Hematemesis/Coffee ground emesis: Upper GI
- Melena (dark, tarry, foul-smelling stool): Upper GI
- Hematochezia (bright bloody stool)/Clots: Lower GI or massive upper GI
- Bright blood about outside of stool: Hemorrhoids, lower GI

Prehospital Interventions: Assess vital signs and oxygen saturation, abdominal tenderness, and signs of hypovolemic shock (pallor, hypotension, tachycardia, cool/clammy skin, loss of consciousness). With rectal bleeding, place absorbent pads on stretcher. Start two large-bore IVs and begin resuscitation with 1-2 L of crystalloid (NS/Lactated Ringer's) with signs of hypovolemia. Provide supplemental oxygen as needed to maintain oxygen saturation above 94%. Monitor ECG readings. With upper GI bleeding, vomiting, and abdominal distention, insertion of an NG tube may be indicated. Provide blood transfusions if indicated and available.

PERITONITIS

Peritonitis is a bacterial infection of the peritoneum (lining of the abdominal cavity) that can lead to septicemia and death. Patients with kidney failure (especially those patients on peritoneal dialysis), liver disease, or infection of the GI tract are especially at risk. Other causes include an abdominal wound, ruptured appendix, perforated colon, diverticulitis, abdominal surgery, and inflammatory bowel disease. Symptoms include signs of acute abdomen: abdominal pain and distension, rigid abdomen, nausea and vomiting, diarrhea, fever, and chills. Other symptoms may include decreased urine output, excessive thirst, and tachycardia (rapid pulse). Peritonitis may be associated with ulcerative diseases, such as Crohn's disease (open sores through all layers of the walls of any part of the GI tract, most commonly in the ileum) and ulcerative colitis (open sores in the inner lining of the colon).

Prehospital Interventions: Obtain an accurate medical history, note the condition of the abdomen with gentle palpation, provide supplemental oxygen/ventilation as needed, and position the patient for comfort because he or she may be experiencing severe pain.

ULCERATIVE COLITIS AND CROHN'S DISEASE

Ulcerative colitis is superficial inflammation of the mucosa of the colon and rectum, causing ulcerations ranging from pinpoint to extensive. Ulcerations may bleed and produce purulent material. The mucosa of the bowel becomes swollen, erythematous (red), and granular. Onset is usually between ages 15 and 30. Ulcerative colitis may affect only the rectum, the entire colon, or only the left colon. Indications include abdominal pain (usually absent or mild unless disease is severe), bloody diarrhea, rectal bleeding, fecal urgency, and tenesmus (a constant feeling of having to defecate).

> **Review Video: Ulcerative Colitis**
> Visit mometrix.com/academy and enter code: 584881

Crohn's disease is chronic inflammation of any area of the GI system but most commonly the small intestine and the beginning of the large intestine, resulting in ulcers that may involve the full thickness of the intestinal wall. An acute flare-up may mimic appendicitis. Indications include diarrhea (watery), rectal bleeding, abdominal cramping and pain (usually in the right lower quadrant), nausea, vomiting, fever, and night sweats.

Prehospital Interventions: Provide supportive care, manage the patient's airway/ventilation/oxygen supplementation (to maintain oxygen saturation of ≥94%), and provide shock treatment per protocol if necessary.

Immunological Emergencies

ALLERGIC REACTIONS AND ANAPHYLAXIS

Allergic reactions are the response of the body's immune system to an antigen (substance), such as peanuts or shellfish. The body produces antibodies (immunoglobulins, such as IgE or non-IgE) that can identify and attempt to neutralize or destroy antigens. Allergic responses may be mild (local rash, redness, itching, swelling, congestion), moderate (generalized itching, difficulty breathing), or severe (life-threatening anaphylaxis).

With **anaphylaxis,** an antigen triggers the release of substances that affect the skin, cardiopulmonary system, and GI tract. Histamine causes initial redness and swelling by inducing vasodilation. In some cases, initial reactions may be mild, but subsequent contact can cause a severe, life-threatening response. Symptoms include a sudden onset of weakness, dizziness, and confusion; tachycardia; generalized swelling; itching; severe low BP leading to shock; airway obstruction; nausea and vomiting; hives; diarrhea; seizures; coma; and death.

Prehospital Interventions: Inject epinephrine to the lateral thigh and repeat every 5-10 minutes as needed; provide an antihistamine (diphenhydramine) for itching, a vasopressor for hypotension, a bronchodilator (salbutamol/magnesium sulfate) for respiratory distress, supplemental oxygen/ventilation, intubation if necessary, an IV access line, and immediate transport.

> **Review Video: Immune System**
> Visit mometrix.com/academy and enter code: 622899

Infectious Disease

INFECTIOUS AND CONTAGIOUS DISEASES

Infectious diseases, which may be communicable or noncommunicable, are those that are caused when microorganisms (such as bacteria, viruses, retroviruses, protozoa, helminths [worms], and fungi) invade the body and cause disease.

- **Noncommunicable diseases** may spread from an environmental source, such as contaminated water or food (such as with food poisoning), or from insects that carry the disease (such as with Lyme disease). However, they do not spread from person to person, so only standard precautions are needed when caring for these patients.
- **Contagious (communicable) diseases** are infections that are spreadable from person to person. They may be transmitted through direct physical contact and sneezing or coughing as well as through contact with blood or other body fluids (feces, urine, semen, or sweat). With contagious diseases, the type of precautions needed depends on the mode of infection, and they may range from contact to droplet to airborne precautions. The type of PPE needed also varies.

PROCEDURES FOR EXPOSURE/CONTAMINATION

Any exposure/contamination should be reported at hand-off and to the appropriate infection control person following protocols, and follow-up care should be sought if necessary. **Decontamination procedures** are as follows:

- **Skin**: Cleanse the area thoroughly with soap and water.
- **Eyes**: Flush with water for 20 minutes.
- **Needlestick**: Wash the area with soap and water and report immediately.
- **Clothing**: Remove the clothing as soon as possible, and wash visible soiling of skin with soap and water if a shower is not immediately available, but shower as soon as possible. Clothes should be washed separately in a washing machine at the workplace.
- **Equipment/Vehicle**: Clean thoroughly with disinfectant. Dispose of equipment if unable to adequately decontaminate it.

When reporting exposures/contamination, note the type of exposure, the date and time of exposure, circumstances, actions taken to decontaminate, and any other required information.

DECONTAMINATING AN AMBULANCE

Decontaminating an ambulance begins with the removal of any debris with sharps being deposited in a sharps container and soiled linen being red-bagged. Then, the equipment and surfaces that have had contact with a patient or with contaminated materials must be cleaned, disinfected, or sterilized, depending on the type of equipment/surface and the type of contamination. Between patients, surfaces and equipment should be wiped down with a disinfectant, such as a 1:100 chlorine bleach solution or premixed wipes. Alcohol-based products are effective for many organisms, but not for *Clostridium difficile* (which is spread through fecal contamination). If equipment is left with a patient at a receiving facility, that facility must clean the equipment or place it in a red bag before returning it. At the end of the day, the entire ambulance should be cleaned. Various methods of sterilization, including the use of fogging agents and UV lights, are available. All cleaning procedures must be recorded for compliance purposes.

INFECTIOUS VIRAL DISEASES

Disease	Vaccine	Characteristics/Considerations
Chickenpox (varicella)	Varicella or MMRV	Fever, flu-like symptoms, headache, and generalized vesicular rash. Complications: Viral encephalitis, meningitis, pneumonia, Reye's syndrome. Use contact and airborne precautions until lesions are crusted over in 1–3 weeks.
Mumps	MMR or MMRV	Fever, earache, swelling of parotid gland(s), pain, stiff neck (15%). Complications: Spreads to testicles or other parts of the body (heart, kidneys, ovaries, pancreas, brain). There may be hearing impairment. Use standard and droplet precautions.
German measles (rubella)	MMR or MMRV	Low-grade fever, headache, sore throat, anorexia for 1–5 days and then a pink maculopapular rash on the face progressing to the neck, trunk, and legs. Complications: Encephalitis, arthritis (in adolescents). The disease is usually mild, but it poses a risk for the fetus if the mother is infected. Use standard and droplet precautions.
Measles (rubeola)	MMR or MMRV	High fever, conjunctivitis, cough, photophobia, Koplik spots in the mouth, and then a generalized dark-red maculopapular rash, subsiding in 4–7 days. Complications: Diarrhea, otitis media, bronchitis, pneumonia, encephalitis, death. Use airborne precautions while the patient is contagious.
Whooping cough (pertussis)	Dtap or tDap	**Catarrhal stage** (2 weeks): Nasal congestion, runny nose, low-grade fever, nonproductive cough. **Paroxysmal stage** (1–6 weeks): Severe "whooping" coughing spasms with thick sputum, especially at night. Infants may have apnea rather than whooping. **Convalescent stage** (up to 6 weeks): Gradual decrease in coughing. Treated with antibiotics. Use droplet precautions until 5 days after initiating antibiotics.
Influenza	Annual influenza	Abrupt fever, chills, aching, cough, runny nose, sore throat, and headache. Infants and young children: May have croup, conjunctivitis, nausea, vomiting, diarrhea, abdominal pain. Complications (most common in pediatric and geriatric patients): Otitis media, worsening of chronic lung conditions, pneumonia, myocarditis, encephalitis, Guillain-Barré syndrome, Reye's syndrome. Use droplet and contact precautions.
Mononucleosis	N/A	Fever (2–3 days), sore throat, swollen tonsils, lymphadenopathy, enlarged spleen and liver, fatigue, malaise. Infants and young children may be asymptomatic. Symptoms usually last 2–3 weeks, although weakness may persist for months. Complications (rare): Encephalitis, meningitis, Guillain-Barré syndrome, ruptured spleen, low platelet count. Use standard precautions.

Disease	Vaccine	Characteristics/Considerations
Herpes simplex 1	N/A	A blistering oral lesion or lesions on any other area of the skin. Cold sores typically occur at the border of the lip. Herpetic whitlow (infected finger) is from an infected child sucking a finger. Neonatal infection may be disseminated and may affect the liver, lungs, and brain. Herpetic gingivostomatitis syndrome includes fever, bilateral lymphadenopathy, and lesions in the mouth and tongue, progressing to open painful ulcers making swallowing difficult, so the patient drools. Symptoms usually last 1–2 weeks. Treatment is with acyclovir. Use standard precautions.
Hantavirus pulmonary syndrome	N/A	Hantavirus is transmitted through contact with the nesting material, feces, or urine of infected rodents or contaminated food. Initial symptoms are flu-like with fatigue, fever, and muscle aches. Half of those patients who are infected also experience headaches, chills, nausea and vomiting, diarrhea, and abdominal pain. Late symptoms occur within 4–10 days and include cough, shortness of breath, and a feeling of smothering progressing to pulmonary edema and respiratory failure. **Prehospital Interventions**: Use standard precautions, manage the airway/ventilation/intubation and supplemental oxygen as needed, provide an IV access line.
Rabies	Rabies vaccine (CDC recommends this vaccine only to those at high risk of exposure)	Viral disease with an incubation period of 30–90 days. It is transmitted through contact with the saliva of an infected animal (dog, cat, fox, skunk, raccoon, bat). The virus enters through open skin and travels along the nerves to the brain. Initial symptoms: Fever, chills, malaise, and pain at the bite site. Late: Anxiety, agitation, hallucinations, weakness, paralysis, hydrophobia, coma, respiratory failure, and death. **Prehospital Interventions**: Wash animal bites with soap and water and irrigate with povidone iodine. Notify the receiving facility of the possible need for rabies prophylaxis. Use standard and droplet precautions, provide supportive care, manage airway/ventilation/intubation/supplemental oxygen as needed, and provide an IV access line.

HUMAN IMMUNODEFICIENCY VIRUS/ACQUIRED IMMUNE DEFICIENCY SYNDROME

Human immunodeficiency virus infection (HIV) is the retrovirus that causes acquired immune deficiency syndrome (AIDS). Diagnosis is determined by the CD4+ T-cell count with AIDS currently being diagnosed with a CD4+ count of <200 cells per mm³. HIV is transmitted in bodily fluids (blood, semen, vaginal secretions, and breast milk) that contain free virions and infected CD4+ T-cells. The categories are as follows:

- **Category A** (CD4+ count <500): Asymptomatic or lymphadenopathy, sore throat, and fatigue.
- **Category B** (CD4+ count 200 to 499): Conditions include candidiasis, pelvic inflammatory disease, bacillary angiomatosis, fever, diarrhea, herpes zoster, low platelet count, weight loss, and peripheral neuropathy.
- **Category C** (AIDS) (CD4+ count <200): Invasive diseases are common. Conditions include cervical cancer, candidiasis, cytomegalovirus, encephalopathy, TB, *Pneumocystis jirovecii* pneumonia (formerly known as *P. carinii* pneumonia), Kaposi's sarcoma, toxoplasmosis, and wasting syndrome.

About 1.2 million people in the United States have HIV infection, but 13% are unaware of it. Risk factors include unprotected sex, especially males having sex with other males, and needle sharing.

Prehospital Interventions: Provide supportive care, manage the airway, support ventilation, and provide IV access if necessary. Use droplet precautions for cough.

HEPATITIS B

Hepatitis B virus (HBV) is a virus transmitted through contact with blood either directly, through sexual contact, or sharing needles. The DNA enters the host cell nucleus, copies, and replicates. The cell-mediated immune response that destroys the virus also causes damage to liver cells, resulting in acute hepatitis. Symptoms include jaundice, anorexia, arthralgia, nausea, vomiting, and abdominal pain. Most people recover completely from hepatitis B. Adults are more likely to experience symptoms than children, although children are more at risk of developing chronic infection. Acute infections persist for <6 months. Ninety percent of chronic HBV infections occur in infants and young children, but only 6% of those are more than 5 years old (including adults). Chronic infections are often undetected until marked liver damage has occurred.

Prehospital Interventions: Use of standard precautions, including face shield with danger of blood splashing, is essential. Any accidental contact with blood or needlestick should be reported so that prophylaxis may be provided. Needlesticks and blood contamination should be washed with soap and water, and blood splashes to the face should be flushed with water. Eyes should be irrigated with water or NS. Prophylaxis (within 24 hours of contact) is with hepatitis B immune globulin.

COVID-19

COVID-19 is caused by an extremely virulent coronavirus strain that can be spread through droplet and airborne transmission. The incubation period appears to extend up to 14 days with many showing symptoms on days 4-5. Symptoms range from mild to severe and life-threatening. Common signs/symptoms include fever/chills, cough, shortness of breath, severe dyspnea, congestion, muscle aches, headache, acute loss of sense of smell and/or taste, and sore throat. Some have chest pain and may appear to be having a heart attack. Some have primarily GI symptoms with nausea, vomiting, and diarrhea. Bilateral interstitial pneumonia and respiratory failure are common complications with severe disease. Oxygen saturation may be quite low before patients that feel short of breath. Children and adults may develop a severe multisystem inflammatory syndrome with toxic shock syndrome and cardiac dysfunction.

Prehospital Interventions: Treatment depends on symptoms. With severe disease, administer high flow oxygen at 100% or if respiratory failure, ketamine for induction and oxygen per BVM/non-invasive ventilation. Some require emergent intubation and ventilation. Insert an IV and administer NS, monitor temperature, VS, oxygen saturation, and ECG. EMS personnel must wear protective PPE including N95 respirator and face shield.

DRUG-RESISTANT BACTERIAL CONDITIONS

Drug-resistant bacterial conditions are an increasing problem because of the widespread use of antibiotics. **Reasons for resistance** to develop include the following:

- Failure to complete a course of antibiotics as prescribed, allowing for development of superinfections or resistant bacteria, or mismanaged or inappropriate antibiotic therapy, such as treating viral infections with antibiotics to placate patients
- Prophylactic antibiotic use in livestock, poultry
- Use of antibiotic soaps and lotions

Patients who are hospitalized, have undergone surgery, have medical devices in place (such as urinary catheters or intravenous lines), are under the care of healthcare providers, have been previously treated with antibiotics (particularly for long periods of time), or are immunocompromised are especially susceptible to developing drug resistance.

Common drug-resistant infections include the following:

- Multidrug-resistant tuberculosis (MDR-TB)
- Extensive drug-resistant tuberculosis (XDR-TB)
- Methicillin-resistant *Staphylococcus aureus* (MRSA): Often seen in skin infections, wound infections, and pneumonia
- Vancomycin-resistant *S. aureus* (VRSA): Infections nonresponsive to methicillin or vancomycin, leaving few drugs to treat patients
- Vancomycin-resistant enterococcus (VRE)

Endocrine Emergencies

ENDOCRINE SYSTEM ORGANS AND GLANDS

The endocrine system consists of the following organs and glands:

- **Hypothalamus**: Links the endocrine and nervous systems; produces hormones that are stored in the posterior lobe of the pituitary gland; stimulates the pituitary to release hormones
- **Pineal gland**: Secretes melatonin and dimethyltryptamine, which control sleep cycles and dreaming
- **Pituitary gland**: The posterior lobe secretes oxytocin (it stimulates uterine contractions/lactation) and vasopressin (aka antidiuretic hormone, which raises BP and promotes water reabsorption); the anterior lobe secretes hormones that control cell growth (somatotropin), body growth (growth hormone), release of hormones by the thyroid (thyrotropin), release of steroids from the adrenal glands (corticotropin), and reproductive functions (follicle-stimulating hormone and luteinizing hormone)
- **Thyroid gland**: Secretes hormones that control protein production, basal metabolic rate, and oxygen consumption (T3, T4, and calcitonin)
- **Parathyroid glands**: Secretes parathyroid hormone, which controls the use of calcium
- **Adrenal glands**: Produce cortisol (roles in metabolism), aldosterone (water and sodium levels), and androgens (male hormones)
- **Ovaries**: Secrete female hormones (estrogen and progesterone)
- **Testes**: Secrete androgens (testosterone)

> **Review Video: Endocrine System**
> Visit mometrix.com/academy and enter code: 678939

DIABETIC CONDITIONS

Diabetes mellitus is a group of metabolic disorders that involve hyperglycemia (increased blood glucose [sugar]) because of defective production and/or action of insulin. Insulin metabolizes glucose to produce energy as fuel for body cells.

- **Type 1**: Autoimmune destruction of beta cells in the pancreas results in no or deficient insulin production. Treatment is with insulin. Symptoms include rapid onset, increased thirst, frequent urination, increased hunger, delayed healing, weight loss, frequent infections, and blurred vision.
- **Type 2**: Insulin baseline may be normal or deficient, but there is no or an inadequate increase in response to a meal, so the glucose level rises but there is decreased uptake by the tissues. Insulin resistance occurs because there is decreased sensitivity to insulin by the tissues. Type 2 diabetes is often related to older age and obesity. Treatment is with oral diabetic agents. Symptoms include slow onset, increased thirst, increased urination, candidal (fungal) infections, delayed healing, and weight gain.
- **Gestational**: Beta cells in the pancreas are unable to produce adequate insulin during pregnancy, but normal production resumes after delivery. Treatment varies. Symptoms include increased thirst, urinary frequency, or sometimes no symptoms at all.

> **Review Video: Diabetes Mellitus**
> Visit mometrix.com/academy and enter code: 501396

HYPERGLYCEMIA AND DIABETIC KETOACIDOSIS

Hyperglycemia is high blood glucose (sugar) with a level >126 mg/dL after fasting for 8 hours or >180 mg/dL 2 hours after eating. Hyperglycemia may occur in undiagnosed diabetic patients, diabetic patients who have taken inadequate insulin, those who have eaten a diet too high in carbohydrates (sugars), or those who are ill, such as with an infection. It can also be induced by certain medications, such as steroids, statins, thiazide diuretics, and some antipsychotics. Initial signs include polyuria (increased urine), polyphagia (hunger), polydipsia (increased thirst), headaches, lethargy, fatigue, and blurred vision, but if the blood sugar is very high (>250 mg/dL), then patients may become increasingly somnolent, and he or she may develop **diabetic ketoacidosis** from the buildup of ketones as fat is broken down by the body for energy because sugar/glucose cannot be used. The patient may exhibit Kussmaul's breathing (fruity-smelling breath from ketones), lapse into a coma, and die if left untreated.

Prehospital Interventions: Question the patient about diabetes and the use of diabetes medications. Check the patient's blood sugar level, and monitor the vital signs and oxygen saturation. Manage the airway and assisted ventilation as needed, and provide an IV access line and crystalloid fluids and regular insulin if indicated. Rapid transport is required with altered levels of consciousness.

HYPERGLYCEMIC HYPEROSMOLAR NONKETOTIC SYNDROME (HHNS) OR COMA (HHNK)

Hyperglycemic hyperosmolar nonketotic syndrome (HHNS) or coma (HHNK) occurs in people without a history of diabetes or in people with mild type 2 diabetes but with insulin resistance resulting in persistent hyperglycemia, which causes osmotic diuresis. Fluid shifts from intracellular to extracellular spaces to maintain osmotic equilibrium, but the increased glycosuria and dehydration result in hypernatremia and increased osmolality (concentration). This condition is most common in persons 50–70 years old, and it often is precipitated by an acute illness such as a stroke, medications such as thiazides, or dialysis treatments. HHNS differs from ketoacidosis because although the insulin level is not adequate, it is high enough to prevent the breakdown of fat. Symptoms include polyuria, dehydration, hypotension, tachycardia, blood glucose >500 mg/dL, changes in mental status, hallucinations, seizures, and hemiparesis.

Prehospital Interventions: Question the patient about his or her history of diabetes and use of diabetes medications. Check the patient's blood sugar level, monitor the vital signs and oxygen saturation, and provide supportive care and an IV access line as needed. Rapid transport is needed for altered levels of consciousness.

HYPOGLYCEMIA

Hypoglycemia (low blood sugar/glucose) is most often caused by an insulin reaction (too much insulin for the amount of glucose/sugar intake) or an overdose of oral diabetes medications, which stimulate the overproduction of insulin. Hypoglycemia may occur if patients took insulin but skipped a meal, vomited, or exercised too strenuously, depleting the body of sugar/glucose while insulin levels remain high. Increased insulin levels cause glucose levels to fall to ≤70 mg/dL, initially resulting in tremors, headache, blurred vision, dizziness, and pallor leading to confusion, bizarre behavior, lack of coordination, combative behavior, personality changes, tachycardia, and irregular heartbeat. Severe hypoglycemia may lead to seizures, coma, and death. Hypoglycemia is life threatening if untreated. Infants may have dehydration and seizures; geriatric patients may have dehydration and stroke.

Prehospital Interventions: Ask the patient about his or her diabetes status and use of diabetes medications. Check the patient's glucose level, and administer oral glucose tablets, one tablespoon of sugar, or a glass of orange juice if the patient is able to swallow. Provide rapid transport for altered levels of consciousness.

Psychiatric Conditions

BEHAVIORAL ALTERATIONS

Behavioral alterations may include agitation, anger, throwing temper tantrums (children), acting aggressively (adolescents/adult), exhibiting poor judgment, and acting inappropriately. **Behavioral alterations** may result from psychiatric disorders (e.g., depression, schizophrenia, bipolar disorder) and psychiatric medications as well as numerous other causes, including the following:

- Hypoglycemia/low blood sugar (insulin reaction)
- Lack of adequate oxygen interfering with brain function
- Shock (low BP; a rapid pulse results in inadequate blood supply to the brain)
- Mind-altering substances (cocaine, methamphetamine, LSD, Rohypnol [date-rape drug])
- Brain infection (meningitis, encephalitis, brain abscess)
- Seizure disorders (epilepsy, other causes of seizures)
- Poisoning/Overdose (lead poisoning, drug overdose)
- Malnutrition resulting in inadequate nourishment of brain tissue
- Substance abuse (drug or alcohol abuse/withdrawal)
- Heat extremes (hypothermia/hyperthermia)

Indications of being a danger to self or others include severe agitation, hallucinations, delusional thinking, paranoia, self-destructive behavior (e.g., cutting, drug/alcohol abuse, promiscuity, risk-taking activities), depression, and suicide attempts. A patient may pose a risk to others if he or she is behaving in a threatening or violent manner and has a weapon (e.g., gun, knife, baseball bat).

ASSESSMENT OF PSYCHIATRIC PATIENTS

Assessment of patients with psychological/psychiatric symptoms should begin with a history that includes the patient's age and cultural/spiritual background and whether the patient has experienced similar symptoms previously or has a history of a psychiatric disorder as well as any history of substance abuse. **Assessment** includes the following:

- **General appearance:** Note hygiene, grooming, appropriate dress, eye contact, unusual movements (twitching, posturing, repetitive movements), and the appearance and condition of the skin.
- **Speech**: Note speech cadence and abnormal word use, such as neologisms (invented words), clang associations (rhyming), word salad (string of random words), and associative looseness (ideas shifting from one to another).
- **Posture/Gait:** Note automatisms (purposeless behaviors, such as drumming fingers), slowed motions, waxy flexibility (maintaining an awkward position for extended periods of time), ability to walk, and abnormalities of gait.
- **Mental status**: Note the patient's state of being alert versus non-alert, responsive versus unresponsive, and coherent versus incoherent; clarity of ideas; suicidal ideation; and desire for self-harm.
- **Mood and affect**: Note facial expressions, expressed emotions, and affect (blunted, broad, flat, inappropriate, restricted).
- **Memory/Intellectual processes**: Note if memory and intellectual processes are intact or impaired. Is the patient disoriented and confused or alert and responsive?
- **Attention**: Note if the patient's attention is focused or unfocused.

Assessing For Risk of Suicide

Suicidal ideation occurs frequently in those with mood disorders or depression (common in geriatric patients). Although females are more likely to attempt suicide, males actually successfully commit suicide three times more often, primarily because females tend to take overdoses from which they can be revived, whereas males choose more violent means (jumping from a high place, shooting, or hanging). This holds true for adolescents and adults. Risk factors include psychiatric disorders (schizophrenia, bipolar disorder, post-traumatic stress disorder [PTSD], and substance abuse), physical disorders (HIV/AIDS, diabetes, traumatic brain injury, spinal cord injury), and social problems (bullying). Passive suicidal ideation involves wishing to be dead or thinking about dying without making plans, whereas active suicidal ideation involves making plans. Patients at risk should be questioned about their feelings, problems, plans for suicide, and access to weapons. High-risk findings include the following:

- Violent suicide attempt (knives, gunshots) or access to a weapon
- History of a suicide attempt and a suicide attempt with a low chance of rescue
- Ongoing psychosis or disordered thinking
- Ongoing severe depression and feelings of helplessness
- Lack of a social support system

Schizophrenia and Psychosis

Schizophrenia, a thought disorder, causes psychotic episodes and distortion of reality and the inability to determine the line between fantasy and reality. The onset may be acute or more insidious. Symptoms are positive (delusions, hallucinations, disorganized or catatonic behavior, disorganized speech) or negative (flat affect/decreased emotional range, social isolation, poverty of speech, lack of interest and drive). Patients may have bizarre delusions (thought broadcasting) or hear voices (which they may try to drown out by turning the TV, radio, or music volume up loud). Patients may isolate themselves socially, exhibit poor hygiene, exhibit catatonia (a stiff, unmoving position), and have odd speech. Treatment is with typical and atypical antipsychotics and antidepressants (such as selective serotonin reuptake inhibitors [SSRIs]).

Psychosis is not a disease but a description of a condition and may apply to various diagnoses (such as schizophrenia and bipolar disease). Psychosis is characterized by marked derangement of the personality and a distorted view of reality. Patients may experience hallucinations (seeing/hearing something not present), delusions (false or distorted beliefs), and illusions (false impressions).

Prehospital Interventions: Provide supportive care.

Delirium

Delirium is an acute sudden change in consciousness, characterized by reduced ability to focus or sustain attention, language and memory disturbance, disorientation, confusion, audiovisual hallucinations, sleep disturbance, and psychomotor activity disorder. **Delirium** differs from disorders with similar symptoms in that delirium is fluctuating. Delirium occurs in 10%–40% of hospitalized older adults and about 80% of patients who are terminally ill. Delirium may result from drugs such as anticholinergics and numerous conditions including infection, hypoxia, trauma, dementia, depression, vision and hearing loss, surgery, alcoholism, untreated pain, fluid/electrolyte imbalance, and malnutrition. Delirium increases the risks of morbidity and death, especially if untreated. Asking the patient to count backward from 20 to 1 and spell his or her first name backward can identify an attention deficit.

Prehospital Interventions: Ensure the patient's safety, manage the patient's airway, ventilation, and oxygen supplementation, and reorient the patient frequently.

AGITATED/EXCITED DELIRIUM

Patients with agitated/excited delirium are often very combative, aggressive, violent, and uncooperative, and they may exhibit shouting, threaten violence, and behave bizarrely. The patient may experience hallucinations, disorientation, paranoia, and panic. Patients may be exceptionally strong and seem insensitive to pain. They are often hyperthermic (high temperature). Agitated or excited delirium may be associated with hypoglycemia, brain damage, chemical imbalance, and substance abuse (methamphetamine, cocaine, phencyclidine [PCP, angel dust], and LSD). Patients often require restraints for their own or for others' safety, but they are at risk of death by asphyxiation or restraint (positional) because they fight desperately against the restraints.

Prehospital Interventions: The EMS provider should use active listening and try to establish rapport while assessing the patient's intellectual functioning, orientation, judgment and thought processes, language, mood, and appearance to determine if law enforcement or other assistance is needed. The patient may refuse care, but implied consent is legal for patients with abnormal behavior. The patient must be transported safely for treatment. The EMS provider should look for medications or drugs on site and take them to the receiving facility.

CALMING PATIENTS WITH BEHAVIORAL EMERGENCIES

Patients with **behavioral emergencies** are often agitated and may be confused, fearful, and/or aggressive, so the paramedic must remain calm and approach the patient slowly; remain at a safe distance; and avoid fast movements, threatening postures, or attempts at physical contact, acknowledging the patient's agitation and offering assistance ("I can see that you're upset, and I want to help") and maintaining eye contact (unless the person is violent and reacts aggressively). The EMT should encourage the patient to talk about what is causing the behavior and should answer questions honestly while avoiding threatening, arguing, or challenging the patient. If the patient is suffering hallucinations or delusional thinking, the EMT should avoid playing along ("I don't see what you do") but should also avoid contradicting the patient directly when responding. Family or friends may assist with intervention. The EMT should not leave the patient unattended and should try to lower distressing stimuli (such as lights and noise) and consider contacting law enforcement. Restraints should be avoided if possible.

RESTRAINTS

If a combative patient poses a risk to him- or herself or EMS personnel, **restraints** may be necessary to safely assess, treat, and transport the patient, keeping in mind that the altered state of consciousness may result from drug or alcohol use; traumatic injury; or from a mental or physical disorder, such as schizophrenia, dementia, or hypoglycemia (insulin reaction). Protocols for use of restraints must be followed, and restraints should be applied under medical direction. If possible, the police should be present and there should be one EMS personnel for each limb, staying beyond the limb's range of motion until ready to secure the limb, with one EMT talking to the patient and explaining the procedure. The EMT should avoid unnecessary force, which may result in increased combativeness and injury to the patient or others. Patients should not be restrained in the prone (face-down) position. Documentation must include the reason for restraining the patient, the time, and the method of restraint.

TYPES OF RESTRAINTS

Patients needing restraints are often agitated, confused, and refuse care, but implied consent is legal for patients with abnormal behavior. **Types of restraints** include the following:

- **Verbal:** Try to calm the patient while being firm.
- **Nonverbal:** Use body language and a show of force (with a number of EMS personnel being present) to convince the patient.
- **Physical:** Use standard precautions; one person is assigned to each limb, while a fifth person reassures and tries to calm the patient. Apply multiple restraints as necessary, including across the trunk, being careful not to restrict the patient's breathing.
- **Chemical:** Use as a last resort (usually after physical restraints). Includes benzodiazepines (lorazepam) and neuroleptics (haloperidol).
- **Tasers/electrical stun guns:** These may be used by law enforcement to subdue a severely agitated patient. They may cause burns, dart injuries, fall injuries, or cardiac arrest. Stun guns require direct contact, but Tasers may be shot from 20 feet away.

Document the reason for restraint, the types of restraints, the restraint technique, and the time the patient is restrained. Monitor the patient's condition continuously, including the heart rate, airway, ventilation, oxygen supplementation, and circulation.

TYPES OF PHYSICAL RESTRAINTS

Common types of physical restraints include the following:

- **Soft:** Padded cuffs (often leather) that fasten about the wrists and ankles and are attached to a long board. These are the most commonly used restraints.
- **Stretcher/Spinal board straps:** These may be strapped across the chest (not too tight), abdomen, or legs to help restrict movement.
- **Long board/Spinal board:** Patient should be restrained to the long board and then placed on a wheeled stretcher and never tied to or fastened to the stretcher.
- **Spit sock:** This is a hood that fits over the patient's head to prevent him or her from biting or spitting.
- **Cervical collar:** This is used to protect the patient's cervical spine and to prevent him or her from biting.

The EMT should not place the patient in handcuffs or hard plastic ties. If these were placed on a patient by a law enforcement officer and must stay in place, such as with a criminal suspect or an extremely violent patient, then a law enforcement officer must stay with the patient at all times.

Toxicology

ROUTES OF POISONING

Routes of poisoning include:

- **Ingestion**: Drugs, overdose, toxic/caustic liquids (bleach, cleaning solution, antifreeze, gasoline), mouse/rat poison, pesticides, some plants, and alcohol. There is a wide range of symptoms, depending on the substance: anaphylaxis, lethargy, constricted pupils, mouth burns, nausea and vomiting, pain, diarrhea, difficulty breathing, confusion, seizures, and coma. (Toddlers are particularly at risk.)
- **Inhalation**: Toxic gases, smoke, hair spray, carbon monoxide, chlorine, halogens. Symptoms include difficulty breathing, lethargy, confusion, nausea, vomiting, headache, cyanosis, seizures, slurred speech, and coma.
- **Injection**: Heroin, morphine, drug overdose. Symptoms include local irritation, lethargy, confusion, slurred speech, nausea, vomiting, difficulty breathing, seizures, and coma. (Adolescents are prone to experimentation with drugs.)
- **Absorption**: Cleaning products, various chemicals. Symptoms include local irritation, anaphylaxis, burns, tissue damage, rash, nausea, vomiting, shortness of breath, and confusion.

Prehospital Interventions: Treatment varies according to the severity. Contact a poison control center if necessary, provide supportive care, remove the substance residue from the patient's mouth, place the patient in the recovery position, manage the patient's airway/ventilation/oxygen supplementation, provide CPR as necessary, induce vomiting or administer activated charcoal only if advised by the poison control center or another expert, and provide rapid transport. If the contamination is by inhalation, remove the patient from the source as soon as possible. If the contamination is by absorption, remove the contaminated clothes, wash the patient's skin with large amounts of soap and water, and flush the affected eyes with water or NS.

NERVE AGENTS/CHOLINERGICS

Nerve agents/cholinergics are toxic chemicals (organophosphates) that damage the nervous system and bodily functions, leading to death in a short time. Nerve agents include tabun (GA), sarin (GB), soman (GD), and VX, and they are used in terrorist attacks. GA, BG, and GD persist in the environment for 10 minutes to 24 hours during the summer and 2 hours to 3 days during the winter (cold weather), and they have very fast action. VX persists longer in the environment and is more lethal. Symptoms of exposure (gas/aerosol) include salivation, lacrimation, urination, defecation, GI upset, and emesis; runny nose; pupil contraction; vision impairment; slurred speech; chest pain; hallucinations; respiratory distress; and coma. High doses may cause immediate seizures and death.

Prehospital Interventions: Move away from the area quickly or shelter in place, remove the patient's clothing, and wash the patient's body with large amounts of soap and water. Use an autoinjector for atropine and pralidoxime (separate injections [Mark I] or combined dose [DuoDote]), unless there is only mild tearing or a runny nose, and use diazepam for seizures. Provide airway/ventilation/oxygen supplementation and circulation support.

CARBON MONOXIDE POISONING

Carbon monoxide poisoning occurs when people breathe in carbon monoxide, usually related to industrial or household accidents or suicide attempts. Carbon monoxide binds to hemoglobin 200 times more readily than oxygen, and once the carbon monoxide binds to hemoglobin (creating carboxyhemoglobin), the hemoglobin can no longer bind to or transport oxygen, resulting in hypoxemia. Symptoms vary depending on the percentage of saturation with carbon monoxide. At 10%, patients may complain of headache and nausea. At >20%, a patient becomes increasingly weak and confused with alterations in mental status. At >30%, a patient may have dyspnea, chest pain, and increased confusion. When the level continues to increase, a patient may experience seizures, coma, and death. The patient's skin color may be cyanotic, pink, or bright cherry red (but this is not a reliable sign).

It is critical to note that pulse oximetry is not an accurate measure of oxygen saturation in patients with carbon monoxide poisoning because the technology cannot differentiate between oxygen and carbon monoxide binding to the blood.

Prehospital Interventions: Administer 100% oxygen with a nonrebreather mask and transport.

POISON CONTROL RESOURCES

The **National Capital Poison Center** provides a website with an online tool (called webPOISONCONTROL) and a telephone number (800-222-1222) for people who swallow or come into contact (absorbed, inhaled, or injected) with toxic substances.

- **webPOISONCONTROL** can be used for patients (ages 6 months to 79 years and nonpregnant women) who are asymptomatic and unintentionally came into contact with a single drug or medication, household product, or berries over a short period of time (minutes to a few hours) but are otherwise healthy.
- **Telephone contact** is used for all other situations, including a patient with symptoms, pregnant women, non-swallowing contact, those aged <6 months or >79, or those who swallowed materials or substances other than those listed for online assistance. Telephone contact can be made for any poisoning if it is preferred to online assistance.

This service is free and usually requires about 3 minutes for a response. When calling, be prepared to describe the substance (include the product name and dosage for medications), amount swallowed, age of patient, weight of patient, time since exposure, and the patient's ZIP Code and email address. If unsure of the amount of poison or the weight of the victim, estimates are acceptable.

AGE-RELATED CONCERNS RELATED TO TOXICOLOGY

Age-related concerns related to toxicology include the following:

- **Toddlers** are at risk of ingestion of toxic substances because their taste buds are not yet fully developed and this allows them to drink foul-tasting substances, such as cleaning supplies, which may be kept under a sink where a child has easy access if the cabinet is not secured. Household substances that pose a substantial risk include perfumes, cosmetics, and alcohol. Toddlers may also ingest unsecured medications.
- **Adolescents**, who often experiment with drugs and alcohol, are at risk from alcohol poisoning and overdose or severe reaction to illicit drugs. Additionally, adolescents often attempt suicide with acetaminophen (Tylenol), sometimes to gain attention, without realizing that it can cause liver failure and death even after resuscitation.
- **Geriatric patients** are most at risk from medication errors, such as taking the wrong medication, taking medications belonging to friends or family, or taking the wrong dose of a medication.

SUBSTANCE ABUSE

Many people with substance abuse (alcohol or drugs) are reluctant to disclose this information. Common agents include:

- Cannabis (marijuana)
- Hallucinogens (LSD)
- Stimulants (cocaine, methamphetamine)
- Barbiturates (secobarbital [Seconal] amobarbital [Amytal])
- Sedatives (zolpidem [Ambien], eszopiclone [Lunesta])
- Hypnotics/benzodiazepines (alprazolam [Xanax], diazepam [Valium]
- Lorazepam [Ativan])
- Opiates (heroin, morphine, fentanyl, oxycodone, hydrocodone)

A number of indicators are suggestive of **substance abuse**.

Physical Signs

- Needle tracks on arms or legs
- Burns on fingers or lips
- Pupils abnormally dilated or constricted, eyes watery
- Slurring of speech, slow speech
- Lack of coordination, instability of gait
- Tremors
- Sniffing repeatedly, nasal irritation
- Persistent cough
- Weight loss
- Dysrhythmias (abnormal pulse)
- Pallor, puffiness of face

Other Signs

- Odor of alcohol/marijuana on clothing or breath
- Labile emotions, including mood swings, agitation, and anger
- Inappropriate, impulsive, and/or risky behavior
- Lying
- Missing appointments
- Difficulty concentrating/short-term memory loss, disoriented/confused
- Blackouts
- Insomnia or excessive sleeping
- Lack of personal hygiene

ETHANOL (ALCOHOL) ABUSE AND WITHDRAWAL

Ethanol (the alcohol that is found in alcoholic beverages, flavorings, and some medications) is a multisystem toxin and CNS depressant. It is often the drug of choice of teenagers, young adults, and those >60 years old. **Ethanol overdose** affects the CNS and other organs. If patients are easily aroused, they can usually safely sleep off the effects, but if a patient is semiconscious or unconscious, emergency medical treatment is needed. Young children frequently ingest alcohol in products such as perfumes and cleaning solutions, which are often more toxic than alcoholic beverages.

Infants/Young Children

- Seizures, coma, death
- Respiratory depression and hypoxia
- Hypoglycemia (especially infants and toddlers)
- Hypothermia

Teenagers/Adults

- Altered mental status, coma, circulatory collapse, death
- Hypotension, bradycardia with arrhythmias
- Respiratory depression and hypoxia
- Cold, clammy skin or flushed skin
- Acute pancreatitis/abdominal pain

Chronic abuse of ethanol (alcoholism) is associated with **alcohol withdrawal syndrome** (delirium tremens) with abrupt cessation of alcohol intake, resulting in hallucinations, tachycardia, diaphoresis, sometimes psychotic behavior, and a high mortality rate.

Prehospital Interventions: Manage the patient's airway, ventilation, and oxygen supplementation and provide CPR if necessary, maintain body temperature, and reduce noise/light.

NARCOTIC OVERDOSE

Narcotics include opiates (drugs derived from opium) and opioids (synthetic narcotics). Drugs frequently abused include heroin and many prescription drugs such as morphine, meperidine, fentanyl (pills and patches), oxycodone, hydrocodone, buprenorphine, and methadone. Patients often crush pills and snort or inject them to increase the effects. As their tolerance increases, patients tend to take higher and higher doses, resulting in addiction and an increasing risk of overdose. Narcotics reduce pain and provide a feeling of euphoria or well-being as well as drowsiness. Symptoms of **overdose** may include slurred speech, pupil (pinpoint) constriction, nausea, hypotension, vomiting, lack of coordination, alterations of consciousness, coma, respiratory depression, cyanosis, and cardiac arrest (death). Patients may have a runny, irritated nose from snorting drugs or may have needle marks from injecting.

Prehospital Interventions: Manage the patient's airway, ventilation, and oxygen supplementation and provide CPR if necessary. Administer naloxone (an opioid reversal agent) per autoinjector or nasal spray if protocol allows.

TREATMENTS FOR TOXIC INGESTIONS

Treatment for toxic ingestions includes the following:

- **Administration of a reversal agent** (antidote) if the toxic substance is known and an antidote exists. Antidotes for common toxins include the following:
    - **Opiates**: Naloxone (Narcan)
    - **Acetaminophen**: N-acetylcysteine
    - **Calcium channel blockers, beta-blockers**: Calcium chloride, glucagon
    - **Tricyclic antidepressants**: Sodium bicarbonate, physostigmine
    - **Ethylene glycol and toxic alcohols**: Fomepizole and ethanol infusion (and, later, dialysis)
    - **Iron**: Deferoxamine
    - **Digitalis/Digoxin**: Digibind
    - **Cyanide**: Methylene blue, glyceryl trinitrate
    - **Benzodiazepines**: Flumazenil
    - **Warfarin (Coumadin)**: Phytomenadione (vitamin K)
- **GI decontamination** at one time was standard procedure (syrup of ipecac and gastric lavage followed by activated charcoal). It is no longer advised for routine use, although selective gastric lavage may be appropriate if done within 1 hour of ingestion.
- **Activated charcoal** (1 g/kg) orally or per NG tube binds to many toxins if given within 1 hour of ingestion. It may also be used in multiple doses (every 4–6 hours) to enhance elimination.

Hematologic Emergencies

COMPONENTS OF THE BLOOD

Blood cells are produced in the bone marrow. Blood is a viscous, dark-red fluid comprised of cells, gases, and plasma. Blood components include the following:

- **Erythrocytes** (red blood cells [RBCs]): RBCs carry hemoglobin, which transports oxygen. If the RBC count is low (such as from blood loss) or the oxygen-carrying capacity is impaired (such as with anemia), the patient may experience hypoxemia (low oxygen). The life cycle of RBCs is normally 120 days.
- **Leukocytes** (white blood cells [WBCs]): WBCs defend the body against invading organisms (viruses, bacteria, fungi, and parasites), and in the bloodstream and tissues they respond to allergies. WBCs include lymphocytes (B, T, natural killer, and null cells), monocytes, eosinophils, basophils, and neutrophils.
- **Thrombocytes** (platelets): Platelets release clotting factors and have an active role in forming blood clots.
- **Plasma** (55% of blood): Plasma carries water, proteins, electrolytes, lipids (fats), blood cells, and glucose as well as clotting factors.

The primary blood types are A, B, AB, and O. Blood is either Rh– or RH+, and patients must receive transfusions of blood that are type and Rh compatible.

HEMATOLOGICAL CONDITIONS

Hematological conditions include:

- **Anemia**: Anemia occurs when there are deficient numbers of RBCs or the hemoglobin doesn't bind to sufficient oxygen to meet body demands. Anemia results in a decrease in oxygen transportation and decreased perfusion throughout the body, causing the heart to compensate by increasing cardiac output. The types include iron-deficiency (inadequate iron), blood-loss, hemolytic (red cells destroyed), aplastic (bone marrow damaged), and pernicious (vitamin B_{12} deficiency) anemia.
- **Leukopenia**: A low WBC count (<4000) makes the patient vulnerable to infection. Causes include chemotherapy, autoimmune disorders, cancer, viral infections, medications (such as antibiotics), radiation, HIV/AIDS, and TB.
- **Lymphomas**: Cancer of the lymphocytes (the WBCs involved in the immune response). Two main types are Hodgkin's and non-Hodgkin's lymphoma.
- **Polycythemia**: Excessive RBC count, resulting in viscous (thick) blood and an increased risk of clots.
- **Multiple myeloma**: Cancer of the plasma cells, resulting in tumor in the bone marrow, bone pain, anemia, kidney failure, and infection.
- **Thrombocytopenia**: Low platelet count, increasing the risk of bruising and bleeding.

SICKLE CELL DISEASE

Sickle cell disease is a recessive genetic disorder of chromosome 11, causing hemoglobin to be defective so that the red blood cells (RBCs) are sickle-shaped and inflexible, resulting in their accumulating in small vessels and causing painful blockages. Although normal RBCs survive for 120 days, sickled blood cells may survive only 10–20 days, stressing the bone marrow that can't produce RBCs fast enough and resulting in anemia. Different types of **crises** occur (aplastic, hemolytic, vaso-occlusive, and sequestering), which can cause infarctions in organs, severe pain, damage to organs, and rapid enlargement of the liver and spleen. Vaso-occlusive crisis is common in adolescents and adults, and it can be triggered by sickness, stress, dehydration, temperature changes, and high altitude. Young children are prone to splenic sequestration (RBCs trapped in the spleen, causing it to enlarge and sometimes rupture), which is characterized by pain in the left abdomen.

Prehospital Interventions: Manage the patient's airway, ventilation, and oxygen supplementation and circulation, provide emotional support, and provide rapid transport for severe symptoms.

CLOTTING DISORDERS

Clotting disorders include the following:

- **Hemophilia** is an inherited disorder in which the person lacks adequate clotting factors, which results in bleeding with trauma, bruising, spontaneous hemorrhage (often in the joints), and epistaxis. There are three primary types: A (80–90%), B, and C.
- **Disseminated intravascular coagulation (DIC)** (consumption coagulopathy) is a secondary disorder that is triggered by another event, such as trauma, congenital heart disease, necrotizing enterocolitis, sepsis, and severe viral infections. DIC triggers coagulation (clotting) and hemorrhage through a complex series of events, with clotting and hemorrhage occurring simultaneously, putting the patient at risk of death.
- **Von Willebrand's disease** is a group of congenital bleeding disorders (inherited from either parent) affecting 1-2% of the population, associated with deficiency or lack of von Willebrand factor (vWF), a glycoprotein.

Prehospital Interventions: Monitor for signs of bleeding, and manage the patient's airway/ventilation/oxygen supplementation. Provide rapid transport for hemorrhage or acute blood loss resulting in hypotension.

Genitourinary Emergencies

COMPONENTS OF THE GENITOURINARY SYSTEM

The **genitourinary system** encompasses the organs of the urinary system and the organs of the reproductive system. The **urinary system** is comprised of two kidneys (which are located in the right and left flank areas) that filter the blood of toxins and excess fluid, creating urine. The ureters carry the urine to the bladder where urine is stored, and the urethra carries the urine from the bladder to the external meatus (opening) during urination. The male urethra is about 18-20 cm long, while the female urethra is only 3-4 cm long, placing females at more at risk for ascending infections.

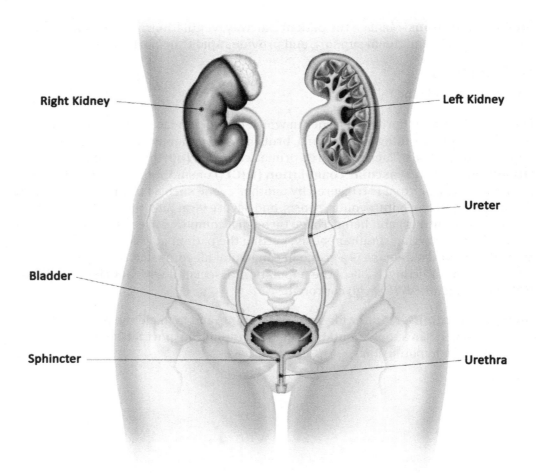

Review Video: Urinary System
Visit mometrix.com/academy and enter code: 601053

The **male reproductive system** includes the scrotum, two testes, the epididymis, spermatic cords and vas deferens, seminal vesicles, ejaculatory duct, prostate, urethra, Cowper's glands, and penis. The **female reproductive system** includes the ovaries, fallopian tubes, uterus, and vagina as well as the breasts.

> **Review Video: Reproductive Systems**
> Visit mometrix.com/academy and enter code: 505450

RENAL AND URINARY CALCULI

Renal (kidney) and urinary calculi (stones) occur frequently, more commonly in males, and they can be related to diseases (hyperparathyroidism, renal tubular acidosis, and gout) and lifestyle factors, such as sedentary work. Their incidence is highest between ages 35 and 45. Additionally, some medications can precipitate calculi. Calculi can form at any age, most are composed of calcium, and can range in size from very tiny to >6 mm. Stones of <4 mm can usually pass in the urine easily.

Symptoms occur with obstruction and are usually of sudden onset and acute.

- Severe flank pain radiating to the abdomen and labia or testicle on the same side as the stone (adolescents and adults), abdominal or pelvic pain (young children)
- Nausea and vomiting
- Diaphoresis
- Hematuria (blood in urine)

Prehospital Interventions:

- Analgesia: Opiates and NSAIDs as needed (per protocol)
- Provide supplemental oxygen if needed
- Start an IV access line and give fluids if indicated
- Transport

RENAL FAILURE

Acute renal failure is an abrupt and almost complete failure of kidney function, occurring over a period of hours or days. It most commonly occurs in hospitalized patients, but it may occur in others as well. Causes include MI, heart failure, sepsis, anaphylaxis, burns, trauma, infections, transfusion reactions, medications (NSAIDs and ACE inhibitors), and obstruction. Symptoms include reduced or absent urinary output, increased nocturia (nighttime urination), altered mental status, tinnitus, a metallic taste in the mouth, tremors, seizures, flank pain, abdominal pain, hypertension, increased bruising.

Chronic renal failure occurs after years of disease that damages the kidneys, often being essentially asymptomatic until the damage is severe. Early symptoms may include anorexia, general malaise, headaches, itching, and weight loss. Later symptoms include fluid retention (pulmonary edema, peripheral edema, ascites), headache, bruising, dry skin, muscle cramping, bone pain, weakness, breath odor, excessive thirst, frequent hiccups, dyspnea, vomiting (especially in the morning), and hypertension.

Prehospital Interventions: Manage the patient's airway/ventilation/oxygen, provide an IV access line (if the patient is hypotensive or if there is evidence of pulmonary edema), and transport.

END-STAGE RENAL DISEASE (ESRD)

Acute and chronic renal failure may progress to **end-stage renal disease (ESRD)** when the kidneys are no longer able to function and the patient needs dialysis or a kidney transplant. The patient may develop uremic syndrome, which results in decreased production of red blood cells and platelets, electrolyte imbalances, bone disease, multiple endocrine disorders, cardiac problems (especially congestive heart failure), anorexia, and malnutrition. Symptoms include altered mental status, hallucinations, and confusion from the accumulation of waste products in the blood; increasing edema and shortness of breath from accumulated fluids; chest and bone pain; severe pruritus; nausea, vomiting, and diarrhea; tremors, muscle twitching, and seizures; and increased bruising and discoloration of the skin.

> **Review Video: End Stage Renal Disease**
> Visit mometrix.com/academy and enter code: 869617

Prehospital Interventions: Manage the patient's airway/ventilation/oxygen, start an IV access line (if the patient is hypotensive or if there is evidence of pulmonary edema), and transport.

MANAGEMENT

HEMODIALYSIS

Hemodialysis is used primarily for those who have progressed from renal insufficiency to uremia with end-stage renal (kidney) disease (ESRD). With hemodialysis, blood is circulated outside of the body through a dialyzer (a synthetic semipermeable membrane), which filters the blood and removes waste products and excess fluids. A vascular access device, such as a catheter, fistula, or graft, must be established for hemodialysis, with fistulas and grafts usually placed in an arm and a catheter placed in the upper chest (into the superior vena cava). Tubing from the dialysis machine attaches to the access device for treatments, which are usually done for 4 hours three times weekly. Emergent conditions include low BP, nausea/vomiting, irregular pulse, cardiac arrest, bleeding from the access site, and difficulty breathing. Missed treatments may result in electrolyte excess, weakness, and pulmonary edema.

Prehospital Interventions: Manage the patient's airway/ventilation/oxygen supplementation, apply pressure to stop any bleeding, position the patient flat if he or she is in shock, and position upright if there is difficulty breathing. Provide an IV access, but avoid placing the IV and measuring the BP on the arm with the access site.

PERITONEAL DIALYSIS

Peritoneal dialysis is used to remove waste products and excess fluids from those with ESRD. A catheter is placed into the peritoneal cavity of the abdomen. The peritoneum comprises the visceral peritoneum (the lining of the gut and other viscera), which makes up about 80% of the total peritoneal surface area, and the parietal perineum (lining the abdominal cavity), which is the most important for peritoneal dialysis. A dialysate solution is instilled (usually about 2 L for adults but less for children, taking about 10 minutes) through the catheter, the catheter is clamped, and the solution is left in place for 3–6 hours (dwell time). The solution is then drained (usually for about 20 minutes), and the process is repeated with new dialysate. Peritoneal dialysis increases the risk of obesity, peritonitis, hernia, malnutrition, hypertriglyceridemia, and back pain. Obesity, older adulthood, and lack of social support are contraindications for peritoneal dialysis.

Prehospital Interventions: Manage the patient's airway/ventilation/oxygen supplementation, use contact precautions if there is purulent drainage from the catheter site, and position the patient for comfort.

URINARY CATHETER MANAGEMENT

A **urinary catheter** is inserted through the urethra and into the bladder to drain urine. Straight catheterizations are done with sterile catheters periodically to empty the bladder or to relieve urinary retention, whereas retention catheters (Foley) have a balloon that inflates to keep the catheter in place for continuous drainage. Foley catheters may be indicated for patients with neuromuscular disorders, incontinence, urinary retention, dementia, or urinary disorders. Catheters may also be inserted suprapubically (above the pubis bone) directly into the bladder, especially for males with long-term catheterization. Urinary collection bags should be kept below the level of the bladder, and the tubing is secured so that the catheter is not inadvertently pulled out, causing trauma to the urethra, especially in males. Thick, cloudy urine may indicate infection. Scant urine and lower abdominal pain/distension may indicate blockage of the catheter. Milking the catheter may help relieve a blockage. When removing a Foley catheter, the balloon must first be deflated.

Prehospital Interventions: Provide supportive care, start an IV access line, and give fluids to keep the vein open if there is severe abdominal pain.

Eyes

MANUAL EYE IRRIGATION

Manual eye irrigation is indicated to remove foreign bodies, exudate, and chemicals from the eye. With chemicals, continuous irrigation with copious amounts of fluids (NS or lactated ringers ideally, though tap water may be used in emergent situations) should be carried out for at least 15 minutes. Procedure:

1. If possible, remove contact lenses, but with chemical burns, leave lenses in place to avoid delay unless the eye is swelling rapidly. Change gloves after removing contact lenses.
2. Place absorbent pads under the face and place a curved kidney-shaped basin below cheek on affected side.
3. Wipe secretions or visible reside (inner canthus to outer) from eyelids with gauze moistened with NS.
4. Retract upper and lower eyelids to expose conjunctival sacs.
5. Irrigate from inner canthus (using a dropper, IV tubing, or irrigation syringe), toward the outer canthus, ensuring that the tip remains 1 inch from inner canthus.
6. Ask the patient to look upward and continue irrigation.
7. Allow the patient to periodically blink.
8. When completed, blot moisture and assess eye for reactivity, visual acuity, and comfort.

Nose

NOSEBLEED (EPISTAXIS)

Recurrent nosebleed (epistaxis) is common in young children (ages 2–10), especially boys, and it is often related to nose picking, dry climate, trauma, or central heating. Its incidence also increases between 50 and 80 years of age and may be associated with NSAIDs, hypertension, and anticoagulants. Patients abusing cocaine may suffer nosebleeds because of damage to the mucosa. The anterior nares have plentiful blood vessels and may bleed easily, usually from one nostril. Bleeding in the posterior nares is more dangerous and can result in considerable blood loss. Blood may flow through both nostrils or backward into the throat, and the person may swallow and vomit blood. The blood may block the airway in unconscious patients

Prehospital Interventions: Have the patient sit in an upright position, leaning forward so blood doesn't flow down the throat. Have the patient pinch the nostrils together firmly for at least 10 minutes. Advise the patient to avoid sniffing or blowing the nose.

Obstetric Emergencies

PREMONITORY SIGNS OF LABOR

Premonitory signs of labor include:

- **Lightening**: As the fetal head engages and moves toward the birth canal, the fundal pressure on the diaphragm lessens, so the mother can breathe more easily, but pressure in the pelvic area increases, causing urinary frequency. The lower abdomen may protrude more than previously. Increased circulatory impairment may cause venous stasis and ankle edema as well as increased vaginal secretions as the vaginal mucous membranes become congested. Pressure on the nerves may result in leg cramps or increased pelvic, back and leg pain.
- **Braxton Hicks (BH)**: BH contractions are short in duration, occur at irregular intervals in the lower abdomen, and do not change the cervix. They are often relieved by activity or mild analgesia. The intensity and frequency of BH contractions often increase immediately prior to the onset of true labor.
- **Cervical changes**: The cervix ripens (softens) to allow for effacement (thinning) and dilation.
- **Bloody show**: A mucous plug from pooled secretions forms at the opening of the cervical canal during pregnancy; when the cervix begins to efface, this mucous plug is expelled, exposing capillary vessels that bleed. Bloody show typically appears as pink mucus and usually occurs within 24 to 48 hours of the onset of labor.
- **Ruptured membranes**: Rupture of the membranes occurs in about 12% of women prior to the onset of labor, which usually then occurs within 24 hours. Before rupture, the membranes typically bulge through the dilating cervix; fluid comes in a gush, although it may come in smaller spurts in some cases. If the membranes rupture before engagement of the fetal head, the umbilical cord may prolapse with the fluid, increasing the risk to the fetus, so mothers should always seek medical attention after rupture. If the mother is at term and labor does not start within 24 hours of rupture, labor may be induced.

STAGES OF LABOR

The stages of labor proceed as follows:

- **First stage (dilation stage)**: Consists of three phases
  - **Latent phase**: The cervix begins to dilate from 0-3 cm; contractions are mild to moderate and occur every 3-30 minutes and are of short duration.
  - **Active phase**: The cervix dilates from 4-7 cm; contractions are every 1-5 minutes, lasting 20-40 seconds. Pain is increased.
  - **Transitional phase**: The cervix dilates from 8-10 cm; contractions come every 1.5-2.0 minutes, lasting 60-90 seconds. There is increased pain, hyperventilation, crying, moaning, vomiting, and rectal pressure.
- **Second stage (expulsion stage)**: Starts when the cervix is fully dilated and ends with delivery of the baby. The patient feels an uncontrollable urge to push, the perineum begins to bulge, and the fetal head crowns as the mother begins to bear down and birth is imminent. Pressure on the rectum and anus may cause stool to be expelled. Birth occurs head first if it is a normal delivery, feet first if it is a breech delivery.
- **Third stage (placental stage)**: Delivery of the placenta should occur 5-30 minutes after birth. There are two phases: placental separation and placental expulsion. Normal blood loss as a result of placental separation is 300-500 mL. Retained placenta may occur if more than 30 minutes elapse.
- **Fourth stage**: The period of 1-4 hours after birth, which involves 250-400 mL blood loss, moderate hypotension (low BP), and tachycardia (rapid pulse).

ANATOMICAL STRUCTURES OF PREGNANCY

The anatomical structures involved with pregnancy and fetal development are contained within the female **uterus** (womb). The **placenta** is attached to the walls of the uterus; it includes the **umbilical cord**, which provides blood, nutrients, and oxygen to the fetus. The fetus is inside an **amniotic sac**, which contains amniotic fluid that cushions the fetus. The opening to the uterus is the **cervix**, which thins and dilates for delivery. The cervix opens into the **vagina**, which acts as the birth canal.

VAGINAL BLEEDING DURING PREGNANCY

Vaginal bleeding may occur during any part of a pregnancy and may be related to any of the structures within the uterus. Vaginal bleeding during the **first trimester** of pregnancy may indicate spontaneous abortion, ectopic pregnancy, or infection, although light occasional spotting may be normal. All vaginal bleeding during pregnancy should be assessed by a physician, and a large amount of bleeding may indicate a medical emergency. Bloody show near term may indicate that delivery is near.

Prehospital Interventions: Use standard precautions and position the patient on her left side. Place a sanitary pad over the vaginal opening and save any soaked pads in a plastic bag so the physician can estimate the amount of blood loss. Manage the patient's airway, ventilation, and oxygen supplementation and provide emotional support. Provide an IV access line and fluids if indicated.

DELIVERY OF A NEWBORN

If the fetal head is obvious at the vaginal opening (crowning), delivery is imminent. Steps to delivery include the following:

1. Wash hands and don PPE for standard precautions and obtain an OB kit and supplies.
2. Position the patient on her back with hips and knees flexed, feet flat on the stretcher, and legs apart.
3. Position one person at the mother's head to support and care for the mother, while the other person delivers the baby.
4. Provide oxygen to the mother, and if time allows, provide an IV access line and NS, cardiac monitoring, and analgesia as needed.
5. As the infant's head is crowning, support the perineum with the palm of your hand, also supporting the baby's head as it delivers.
6. Palpate the neck to determine if the umbilical cord has wrapped around the neck. If there is a nuchal cord, carefully attempt to slip it over the infant's head.
7. Once the body delivers, make note of the time of birth.
8. If the infant is not vigorous, stimulate by drying with a towel, and possibly suctioning the mouth and nose with a bulb syringe. Blow-by oxygen or bag-mask ventilation is utilized if the infant is not breathing.
9. If the infant is stable, place the baby skin to skin on mom's chest.
10. After about 2 minutes, place a cord clamp about 4 cm from the neonate's abdomen, and another cord clamp or hemostat a few centimeters down, then cut the cord in between the clamps.
11. Monitor the baby and assign an Apgar score at one and five minutes after birth.
12. Placental separation and delivery usually occur within 10-20 minutes after birth. Never pull on the umbilical cord as it may cause uterine inversion or placental tearing.
13. Place a sanitary pad over the vaginal opening to contain any bleeding. Observe for hemorrhage.
14. The uterus should be massaged to promote contractions and control excessive bleeding.

INITIAL ASSESSMENT OF THE PREGNANT PATIENT

Initial assessment of a pregnant patient should determine if the patient's emergency is related to the pregnancy (bleeding, cramping, pain, contractions), to an accident (fall or other injury), or to an unrelated illness:

- Assess patient's vital signs, including oxygen saturation. Monitor ECG.
- Assess pain using the 1-10 numeric scale.
- Determine the patient's week of gestation, singleton vs multiples, gravida, and parity.
- Determine if the patient has had prenatal care.
- If the patient is having contractions, determine the onset, frequency, and duration.
- If the patient is bleeding, determine if it is associated with trauma and estimate the amount, observe the character (dark, bright, scant, flowing, massive), and ask patient about onset and number of pads used in an hour.
- If BP is elevated, ask the patient about headaches, weight gain, seizures, and visual disturbances as these may indicate preeclampsia.
- If patient has supine hypotension, position patient on the left side with a blanket or roll under the left hip.
- Ask about medications including illegal drugs and history of substance abuse.

SPONTANEOUS AND ELECTIVE ABORTION

Spontaneous abortion: The unplanned loss of pregnancy at or before 20 weeks may result from trauma, fetal abnormality, or another cause. Indications include vaginal bleeding (mild to severe) and contractions. The patient may be very emotionally upset.

Prehospital Interventions: Use the term *miscarriage* rather than *abortion*, which has negative connotations for many. Gather any products of conception in a plastic bag to take to the hospital. Provide supportive care. Place a sanitary pad over the vagina. Provide reassurance and emotional support.

Elective abortion: Planned loss of pregnancy at or before 20 weeks per surgical procedure or abortion pills (during the first 10 weeks). Patients may develop bleeding after surgery or as the fetus is expelled.

Prehospital Interventions: Gather any products of conception in a plastic bag to take to the hospital, provide supportive care, place a sanitary pad over the vagina, and provide reassurance and emotional support.

ECTOPIC PREGNANCY

Ectopic pregnancy: Pregnancy in which the egg fertilizes and attaches outside of the uterus (usually in the fallopian tubes), resulting in abdominal pain, absent menstrual periods, and vaginal bleeding. There is a risk of the fallopian tube rupturing, resulting in internal hemorrhage, which is a life-threatening emergency.

Prehospital Interventions: As above. In the case of a rupture, start an IV and provide fluids. Monitor vital signs and level of consciousness. This patient will be rushed in for immediate surgery.

DELIVERY OF THE PRETERM INFANT

A **preterm** infant is one born prior to 37 weeks gestational age. In the United States, preterm birth is the most important factor influencing infant mortality, accounting for 75-80% of all neonatal morbidity and mortality. Preterm birth is often associated with comorbidities. The original cause of the preterm birth (such as maternal infection) may also play an integral role in the likely health problems associated with the infant's prematurity. Findings may include the following:

- Respiratory distress syndrome because of inadequate surfactant production (hyaline membrane disease)
- Hypothermia because of inadequate subcutaneous fat, small amounts of brown fat, and large skin surface area to mass ratio
- Hypoglycemia secondary to poor nutritional intake, poor nutritional stores, and increased glucose consumption associated with sepsis
- Skin trauma or infection secondary to fragile, transparent, immature skin with less subcutaneous fat
- Periods of apnea because of an immature respiratory center in the brain
- Intraventricular hemorrhage
- Large trunk and short extremities

Prehospital Interventions: Attempt resuscitation with signs of life, suction, ventilate/oxygenate, give compressions if indicated, administer epinephrine for bradycardia, and maintain body temperature.

COMPLICATIONS OF PREGNANCY AND LABOR

Complication	Characteristic	Prehospital Interventions
Preterm labor	Labor between weeks 20 and 37 weeks; presents a risk to the fetus.	Provide supportive care in the left lateral position. Manage the patient's airway, ventilation, and oxygen supplementation (100%). Transport rapidly if there is severe bleeding or a risk of imminent preterm delivery. Start an IV access line and give NS for placental abruption.
Premature rupture of membranes	Membranes rupture before the onset of labor; this may lead to preterm labor and risk to the fetus.	
Substance abuse	May result in damage to the fetus and preterm labor. Many drugs restrict blood flow to the fetus, resulting in growth restriction and low oxygen. Some drugs, such as cocaine, affect the fetal nervous system. Sudden withdrawal of opiates may trigger preterm labor. Alcohol may result in fetal alcohol syndrome, characterized by facial abnormalities, growth restriction, and neurological defects.	
Placental abruption	The placenta prematurely detaches, partially or completely, from the uterus. Risk factors: maternal hypertension, traumatic injury, cigarette smoking, and cocaine use. Partial detachment interferes with the functioning of the placenta, causing intrauterine growth restriction. Severe bleeding occurs with total detachment.	Provide supportive care in the left lateral position. Manage the patient's airway, ventilation, and oxygen supplementation (100%). Transport rapidly if there is severe bleeding or a risk of imminent preterm delivery. Start an IV access line and give NS for placental abruption.
Placenta previa	The placenta implants over or near the internal cervical opening. Implantation may be complete (covering the entire opening), partial, or marginal (to the edge of the cervical opening). Results in increased incidences of hemorrhage in the third trimester. Symptoms include painless bleeding after the 20th week of gestation.	Provide supportive care in the left lateral position. Manage the patient's airway, ventilation, and oxygen supplementation (100%). IV access line and NS. Transport rapidly if there is severe bleeding, high BP ≥160/110, seizures, or altered mental status. Provide ECG monitoring. Administer magnesium sulfate for preeclampsia/ eclampsia.
Pregnancy-induced hypertension/ Preeclampsia/ Eclampsia	Hypertension >140/90 associated with increased protein in the urine and edema (peripheral or generalized) or increase of ≥ 5 pounds of weight in one week after the 20th week of gestation. Severe preeclampsia is BP ≥ 160/110. Symptoms include headache, abdominal pain, and visual disturbances. May progress to eclampsia (seizures) and death.	

Complication	Characteristic	Prehospital Interventions
Cephalic (vertex) presentation	**Military**: Head straight, neck not flexed. **Brow**: Neck extended, brow presents first, can cause birth trauma, so episiotomy or cesarean section (C-section) is usually required. **Face**: Severely extended neck with face presentation, may prolong labor, increase swelling of the fetus, and cause neck trauma.	Provide supportive care. Manage the patient's airway, ventilation, and oxygen supplementation (100%). Transport rapidly.
Breech presentation	**Frank breech** (buttocks presentation with legs extended upward) is the most common, but **single- or double-footling breech** (incomplete breech) or **buttocks** presentation with legs flexed (complete breech) can also occur. Breech presentation is most common with placenta previa, hydramnios, fetal anomalies, and multiple gestations. Cord prolapse is more likely. Head trauma may occur because molding does not occur, and the head can become entrapped.	

PROLAPSE OF THE UMBILICAL CORD

A prolapse of the umbilical cord occurs when the umbilical cord precedes the fetus in the birth canal and becomes entrapped by the descending fetus. With an **occult cord prolapse**, the umbilical cord is beside or just ahead of the fetal head. With a **nuchal cord prolapse**, the cord tightly wraps about the fetal neck. About half of the time, prolapses occur in the second stage of labor and relate to premature delivery, multiple gestations, or other complications. As contractions occur and the head descends, pressure to the umbilical cord occludes the blood flow, causing hypoxia and bradycardia. The decrease in blood flow through the umbilical vessels can cause impaired gas exchange, and if pressure on the cord is not relieved, the fetus can suffer severe neurological damage or death.

Prehospital Interventions: Elevate the presenting part off the cord, pull the cord off of the fetus's neck if possible, elevate the mother's knees to the chest to relieve pressure on the cord, provide 100% oxygen, and transport rapidly.

HYPEREMESIS GRAVIDARUM (HG) AND RH INCOMPATIBILITY

About 60–80% of pregnant woman suffer from nausea and vomiting (N/V), especially during the first trimester, but only about 2% suffer **hyperemesis gravidarum** (HG). Symptoms of HG include severe (sometimes intractable) N/V, weight loss, and dehydration.

Prehospital Interventions: Provide intravenous fluids with 5% glucose in NS or Ringer's lactate; administer antiemetic drugs, including promethazine (Phenergan), prochlorperazine (Compazine), or chlorpromazine (Thorazine).

Rh incompatibility occurs if the mother is Rh-negative and the father is Rh-positive, putting their infant at risk for hemolytic disease of the newborn (HDN). The blood from an Rh-positive baby can mix with the Rh-negative blood of the mother, causing the mother's immune system to make antibodies to destroy the Rh factor. This immune response is called Rh sensitization and can occur during C-section or vaginal delivery, miscarriage, abortion, placental abruption, amniocentesis, chorionic villus sampling, ectopic pregnancy, toxemia, and trauma during pregnancy. Women who are Rh-negative with an Rh-positive mate receive the serum RhoGAM, containing anti-Rh (anti-D) immunoglobulin in order to agglutinate any fetal red blood cells that pass over into the mother's circulatory system and thus prevent the mother from forming antibodies against them that will attack the infant and sensitize her for future pregnancies.

MULTIPLE GESTATIONS

In vitro fertilization and ovulation-inducing drugs have increased the incidence of high-order **multiple gestations** over the past 30 years. The trend of delayed childbearing has led to an increase in twin/multiple gestations. Infants born from multiple gestations are more likely to be born prematurely and with low birth weights. The incidence of premature birth and low birth weight is proportional to the number of fetuses. There may be growth restriction/growth discordance, oligohydramnios, and restriction of movement of one or more fetuses. Approximately 50% of twins and 90% of triplets are born premature, compared to 10% of singletons. With this increase in prematurity and proportion of infants born with low birth weight, there are increased morbidities, such as cerebral palsy and intellectual disabilities. The risk for genetic disorders, such as neural tube defects and GI and cardiac abnormalities, is twice that of single gestations.

Gynecological Emergencies

FEMALE REPRODUCTIVE SYSTEM

The female reproductive system includes the ovaries, fallopian tubes, uterus, cervix, vagina, vulva, labia minora, labia majora, clitoris, and breasts. Functions include ovulation, fertilization, menstruation, pregnancy, and lactation. **Menarche** (onset of menses) is usually between 9 and 15, but it may occur in younger girls and should be considered as a possibility with younger girls. **Menopause** occurs at approximately age 50, usually following a period of about 10 years of irregular periods during which time the person may become pregnant. The normal menstrual cycle is 28 days, but it may be up to 45 days in adolescents. Assessment should include abdominal or vaginal pain, vaginal bleeding or discharge, fever, nausea and vomiting, and dizziness. Patients should have their privacy protected during an examination, and the EMS provider should communicate openly, asking for permission to touch the patient. The provider should consider the possibility of pregnancy or sexually transmitted infection (STI) with any abnormal condition.

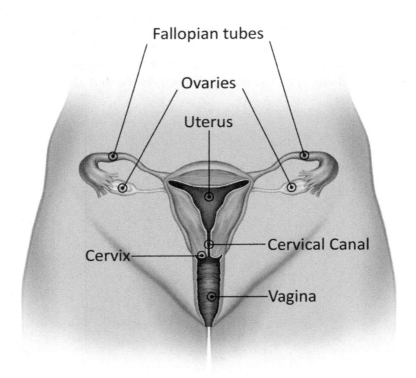

148

VAGINAL BLEEDING

Vaginal bleeding may indicate heavy menstrual bleeding (**menorrhagia**) or abnormal bleeding between cycles (**metrorrhagia**). Vaginal bleeding may also be an indication of an ectopic pregnancy or spontaneous abortion; in postmenopausal women, it may be a sign of endometrial cancer. Menorrhagia may result from hormonal imbalance, clotting disorders, uterine fibroids, and endometrial polyps. Metrorrhagia may result from infection, cancer, and cervical/endometrial polyps. Symptoms may include cramping and abdominal pain, depending on the cause. It's important to determine when the bleeding started and about how much blood has been lost (the number of sanitary pads that are saturated per hour, for example) as well as the presence or absence of pain. If the blood loss is excessive, the patient may exhibit signs of shock.

Prehospital Interventions: Use standard precautions, manage the patient's airway, ventilation, and oxygen as needed. Monitor vital signs. Position the patient flat for shock and provide IV access and fluids.

SEXUAL ASSAULT AND LEGAL ISSUES

The **crime scenes** associated with a **sexual assault** include the patient (body, injuries, clothing, and emotional response) and the place the assault occurred. A victim of sexual assault has the right to consent to or refuse each element of a sexual assault evaluation, although some states may mandate reporting of sexual assault to the authorities. The EMS provider should wear disposable gloves when handling clothing, and clothing should be handled gently so that evidence, such as strands of hair or other materials, is not lost in transfer. Documenting the assault should be done in detail with direct quotations. If the patient refuses transport, the best approach is to point out services that could benefit the patient, such as prophylaxis to prevent STIs and pregnancy. Patients are often frightened and confused, so pressuring them to protect others or trying to frighten them more by suggesting that they might be pregnant or develop an STI is a negative approach that may backfire.

Special Populations

INITIAL CARE OF THE NEWBORN

Dr. Virginia Apgar developed the **APGAR assessment** in 1952. APGAR stands for **a**ppearance, **p**ulse, **g**rimace, **a**ctivity, and **r**espiration. The APGAR is the first test given to a newborn. It is used as a quick evaluation of a newborn's physical condition to determine if any emergency medical care is needed, and it is administered 1 minute and 5 minutes after birth. The test is administered more than once because the baby's condition may change rapidly. It may be administered for a third time 10 minutes after birth if needed. The baby is rated on the five subscales, and scores are added together. A total score of ≥7 is a sign of good health.

Sign	0	1	2
Appearance (skin color)	Cyanotic or pallor over entire body	Acrocyanosis	Pink
Pulse (heart rate)	Absent	<100 bpm	>100 bpm
Grimace (reflex irritability)	Unresponsive	Grimace	Infant sneezes, coughs, and recoils
Activity (muscle tone)	Absent	Flexed limbs	Infant moves freely
Respiration (breathing rate and effort)	Absent	Slow, irregular; weak cry	Vigorous cry

> **Review Video: Newborn APGAR Score**
> Visit mometrix.com/academy and enter code: 253451

ROUTINE CARE OF THE NEWBORN

Infants have poor temperature regulation ability, particularly preterm infants who lack brown fat, which is one of the body's tools to regulate body temperature, so **providing warmth** is critical as a component of resuscitation. An infant who is just seconds old and wet will need aggressive measures to keep him or her warm while any resuscitation efforts are being initiated. Infants lose heat through their heads, so one of the first steps should be to place a hat on the head or cover the head in some way. The infant should be vigorously dried with warmed blankets. Often, this stimulation, drying and warming, is all that is needed to establish a regular respiration pattern in the neonate. Preterm infants weighing <1500 grams should be placed in a plastic bag (made specifically for this purpose), if available, up to the height of the shoulders to prevent cold shock. A term infant with no distress can be placed on the mother's chest and covered with a warm blanket.

ABCs of Resuscitation of the Neonate

The **ABCs of resuscitation** should begin immediately after delivery with assisted ventilation begun within 60 seconds if required.

- **Airway:** An airway should be established as the very first thing tended to; if there is no airway, air cannot be moved during resuscitation attempts. This step includes using a bulb syringe to clear the mouth, then the nose of secretions and properly positioning the infant's head in the sniffing position.
- **Breathing**: This step involves initiating breathing after the airway has been established; this can be done with stimulation, supplemental oxygen, or through artificial ventilation if there is apnea, gasping, or heart rate below 100 bpm. Attach pulse oximeter, consider cardiac monitor, and give PPV at 40-60 breaths per minute.
- **Circulation**: Start compressions if heart rate is <60 bpm after 30 seconds of PPV with chest movement. Check HR every 60 seconds. Compress one-third of the anterior-posterior diameter of the chest, using two thumbs or two fingers. Give 3 compressions to 1 breath every 2 seconds (90 compressions to 30 ventilations per minute). Increase oxygen to 100% during compressions. If the HR remains <60 bpm after 60 seconds of CPR, administer epinephrine by IV or ET. Volume expanders (isotonic crystalloid at 10 mL/kg) can be given IV if the neonate is hypovolemic.

Establishing an Airway

To establish an airway, the infant is placed supine with the head slightly extended in the sniffing position. A small neck roll may be placed under the shoulders to maintain this position in a very small premature infant. Once the proper position is established, the mouth and nose are suctioned (suction the mouth first to prevent reflex inspiration of secretions when the nose is suctioned) with a bulb syringe or catheter if necessary. The infant's head can be turned momentarily to the side to allow secretions to pool in the cheek where they can be more easily suctioned and removed to establish the airway. Stimulating the newborn is often all that is needed to initiate spontaneous respirations. This tactile stimulation can be accomplished by gently rubbing the back or trunk of the infant. Another technique that is used to provide stimulation is flicking or rubbing the soles of the feet. Slapping neonates as stimulation is no longer practiced and should NOT be used.

Managing Airway and Ventilation

Airway management is based on the severity of respiratory distress:

- **Blow-by oxygen**: Provide if the newborn is cyanotic and heart rate is >100 bpm and respiratory effort is adequate. Provide warm oxygen at 5 L/min. with a direct flow on the face. Avoid oral airways.
- **Bag-valve mask (BVM)**: Provide if the newborn is apneic, the heart rate <100, and/or there is inadequate respiratory effort. Use an appropriate size and avoid excess pressure, which may cause pneumothorax, although initial ventilation requires higher pressure to expand the lungs. Disable the pop-off valve.
- **Intubation**: Provide if other measures are ineffective and the heart rate is <60. Use a straight-blade laryngoscope size #1 for full term and size #0 for preterm with ETT 2.5-4.0 mm, depending on the weight of newborn. Confirm placement through visualization, auscultation (lateral, superior chest wall, epigastric region), improvement in respirations, $ETCO_2$ detector, and pulse oximetry. Secure the ETT. Provide PEEP as indicated at 5 cmH_2O. Gastric decompression may be necessary if the abdomen is distended. Provide CPR as needed.

GROWTH AND DEVELOPMENT OF PEDIATRIC PATIENTS

Normal growth and development by age, in the first two years of life, is as follows:

- **0–2 months**: Sleeps up to 16 hours per day but should rouse easily. Cries for a reason; persistent crying may indicate illness. Limited head control. Gazes at faces.
- **2–6 months**: Smiles voluntarily and makes eye contact, uses both hands, begins to hold his or her head up, rolls over, and sleeps through the night.
- **6–12 months**: Sits, crawls, has pincer grasp, mouths objects (increasing risk of poisoning and aspiration), babbles, and speaks first words by 12 months. Exhibits separation anxiety from parents.
- **12–18 months**: Begins to walk; imitates others; knows body parts and 4-6 words; lacks molars for grinding food, increasing the risk of aspiration; and has increased mobility.
- **18–24 months**: Begins to run and climb, knows 100 words (24 months), clings to parents, attaches to special objects, labels objects, and begins to understand cause and effect.
- **2–5 years**: Walks, runs, throws, catches, is toilet trained, has magical thinking and irrational fears, learns acceptable behavior, has temper tantrums, and develops modesty.
- **6–12 years**: Loses baby teeth; thinks logically; becomes self-conscious; understands the finality of death; attaches importance to school, popularity, and peers.
- **12–20 years**: Puberty begins, reasons (imperfectly), is self-conscious, seeks independence and peer approval, and takes risks.

PEDIATRIC CONSIDERATIONS

Pediatric patients have the following physiologic considerations:

- Proportionately greater body surface area to body mass ratio, so they are at greater risk of fluid and heat loss, burns, and absorption of toxins
- Higher respiratory rates and heart rates than adults, resulting in higher oxygen demand
- Immature blood/brain barrier, resulting in more neurological symptoms
- Immature immune system, resulting in a higher risk of infection
- Narrower and shorter airway and smaller jaw, so the tongue may easily obstruct the airway
- Soft tracheal cartilage that increases the risk of airway collapse, and a large epiglottis
- More pliable ribs, which provide less protection for abdominal organs, which are more forward
- Liver and spleen that are proportionately larger and at risk of injury
- Bones that are softer with open growth plates (an open growth plate injury can impair growth)
- Less protection for the brain and spinal cord (increasing the risk of injury) and less subarachnoid space
- Cerebral blood flow needs twice that of adults, increasing the risk of hypoxia
- Limited glucose stores and risk of hypothermia (especially in the first month)
- Anterior fontanel that closes by 12 months and posterior fontanel that closes by 3-4 months

PEDIATRIC ASSESSMENT

The pediatric assessment should include the following:

- **Pediatric assessment triangle**:
  - *Appearance* (abnormal tone, decreased interactivity, decreased consolability, abnormal look/gaze, and abnormal speech or cry)
  - *Work of breathing* (abnormal sounds [wheezing, stridor], position, retractions [sternum], flaring [nostrils], and apnea/gasping)
  - *Circulation* (pallor, mottling, and cyanosis)
- **Assess airway, breathing, and circulation (heart rate/pulse)**: Place in the shock position and provide a warming blanket for signs of shock.
- **Ventilation/oxygenation**: Administer oxygen and assist with ventilation if it is abnormal.
- **Determine the patient's level of consciousness**: Use the alert, voice, pain, unresponsive (AVPU) assessment. Note movement of the extremities and whether the pupils are normal, dilated, constricted, reactive, or fixed.
- **Prevent hypothermia**: Cover with a warming blanket, cover the head, and avoid unnecessary exposure of the skin.
- **Obtain the medical history from the caregiver/parent**: Include the type and duration of symptoms, fever, level of activity, recent foods/fluids, medications, medication allergies, past or chronic illnesses, and events leading to the current problem.
- **Head-to-toe physical examination**: Note any bruising, swelling, drainage, loose teeth, unusual odors, bleeding, rashes, deformities, and pain on movement.

PEDIATRIC SEIZURES

Febrile seizure is a generalized seizure associated with fever, usually >38.8 °C (101.8 °F) from any type of infection (upper respiratory, urinary tract) but without intracranial infection or other cause, occurring between 6 months and 5 years of age. Seizures usually last <15 minutes and are without subsequent neurological deficit.

Prehospital Interventions: Provide fever control (acetaminophen OR ibuprofen) and a tepid-water bath.

Other types of seizures may result from pathology, such as meningitis, cerebral edema, brain trauma, or brain tumors, but most seizures in children >3 are related to idiopathic epilepsy, which predisposes the child to recurrent seizures, usually of the same type. Seizures are characterized as focal (localized), focal with rapid generalization (spreading), and generalized (widespread). In most children, seizures become generalized with loss of consciousness. Seizure disorders with onset younger than 4 years of age usually cause more neurological damage than those with onset at older than 4 years of age.

Prehospital Interventions: Place the patient on the floor or on a safe surface, loosen clothes, and protect him or her from injury during seizure. Afterward, place the patient in the recovery position, monitor the airway/ventilation, and provide oxygen supplementation (the patient may need assisted ventilation if he or she is cyanotic), and suction if needed.

BRIEF, RESOLVED, UNEXPLAINED EVENT AND SUDDEN INFANT DEATH SYNDROME

Brief, resolved, unexplained event (BRUE) refers to a group of alarming symptoms that can occur in infants. They involve a sudden appearance of apnea, altered responsiveness, and change in color or muscle tone. The event lasts <1 minute in an infant <1 year of age, in which there is no underlying cause, and there is a quick spontaneous return to their baseline state of health. With **sudden infant death syndrome (SIDS)**, which is almost always related to respiratory arrest, the child cannot be resuscitated. There are numerous proposed causes for SIDS, so a careful history, including familial history of SIDS, and physical examination or postmortem examination can provide important information, such as indications of child abuse or metabolic/infectious disorders.

Prehospital Interventions: Continue resuscitative efforts (airway, ventilation, oxygen supplementation, and compressions as indicated) and stabilize the infant if possible. The child with BRUE should be hospitalized for observation, further studies, and apnea monitoring because these children are at increased risk for SIDS. For SIDS patients, the EMS provider should provide support and information to the family. The protocol for reporting SIDS varies by state, but it usually involves notifying the coroner's office.

GERIATRIC CONSIDERATIONS

Geriatric patients have the following special considerations and characteristics:

- Decreased sensory input (hearing, vision, touch, pain), impaired depth perception and night vision, and decreased ability to differentiate colors
- Hypertension, increasing the risk of heart attack and stroke
- Decreased breathing capacity and decreased cough, increasing the risk of infection
- Difficulty chewing and swallowing, digestive problems, and reflux when lying flat, which increases the risk of aspiration
- Short-term memory deficit and slower reflexes
- Decreased bone density, increasing the risk of breaks; loss of muscle tone
- Increased risk of infection and less obvious symptoms of infection
- Arthritis in the neck, interfering with airway assessment
- Dentures that can obstruct the airway (leave them in place if possible, during ventilation)
- Skin that is fragile and tears easily
- Irregular pulse from underlying heart problems
- Dementia (incidence increases with age), making history taking and treatment difficult
- Atypical symptoms for illnesses, even if severely ill
- Multiple comorbidities and multiple medications
- Shock with BP greater than 100

ADDITIONAL PATIENT POPULATIONS WITH SPECIAL CHALLENGES

HOMELESS/INDIGENT

These patients often are without medical care, increasing the risk of disease, and they may lack insurance. They are more likely to have mental health and substance abuse problems.

Prehospital considerations: Know who will treat indigent patients and what resources are available in the community.

BARIATRIC

These patients have increased risk of chronic disease. Patients pose handling/moving problems and require special bariatric equipment and multiple personnel to assist. Patients often have trouble breathing and must have their head elevated.

Prehospital considerations: Recognize the need for bariatric equipment and know how/where to obtain it. Notify the receiving facility. Use properly sized equipment, such as BP cuffs.

TECHNOLOGY/DEVICE-ASSISTED

These patients may have a wide range of issues including ventilators, apnea monitors, vascular devices, dialysis shunts, colostomies, ileostomies, and feeding tubes. Patients may have special needs regarding care and transport.

Prehospital considerations: Ask about the patient's equipment and needs. Avoid disturbing/damaging the devices if possible.

EMS Operations

Overview of EMS Operations

APPARATUS AND EQUIPMENT READINESS

The EMS provider should ensure that the ambulance is ready for use at all times and that the tires are properly inflated, the gas tank is full, warning devices are working, and engine fluid levels are appropriate. All necessary safety equipment, such as PPE (masks, gowns, gloves, and goggles or face guards) and safety devices (safety vests, road flares, and signs) as well as seat belts and harnesses, should be available and in proper working condition. All equipment in the cab, the compartments, and the rear of the ambulance should be in the proper place, labeled, and secured to prevent shifting during transportation. High-risk situations include going through intersections, inclement weather (especially with poor visibility), careless drivers, highway access, unpaved roads, and driver distractions (conversation, eating, drinking, mobile devices, music, GPS devices, and fatigue). During transportation, all personnel as well as patients should be properly secured with safety equipment.

SCENE-OF-INCIDENT SAFETY CONSIDERATIONS

The EMS provider must do a 360° **assessment of the scene of incident** on arrival and determine safety considerations. The provider should make note of any gunshots heard, downed power lines, buildings in a state of collapse, leaking fuels/fluids, fire, smoke, broken glass, and other hazards. EMS personnel may need to wait until the site is safe to proceed. The EMS provider should assess the mechanism of injury (accidents) and the need for appropriate PPE (gloves, gown, mask, face guard) and must keep the patient informed of all actions and prevent harm or further injury. The ambulance should be parked off of the roadway if possible or parked at a 45° angle (front wheels out) to shield the work area, making sure not to block access for other emergency vehicles. Parking uphill is safer than downhill, and upwind is safer than downwind. If flares are used to warn other drivers, they should extend at least 300 feet from a collision. Yellow warning lights at the scene are the safest, but excessive lighting may blind other drivers at night.

ENVIRONMENTAL RISK FACTORS

When assessing a patient, it's important to consider that **environmental factors** may place the patient at an increased risk for harm or may be a factor in disease. There are a number of different types of environmental factors to consider.

Factors	Examples	Effects
Toxic chemicals	Lead, arsenic, muriatic acid, sulfuric acid, ammonia, lime	May result in poisoning (lead, arsenic) or burns (acids, ammonia, lime) through direct exposure or inhalation
Physical objects	Guns, cars, knives, equipment	Accidents, gunshot wounds, stabbings, various injuries (blunt and penetrating)
Biological organisms	Bacteria, fungi, viruses	Infections
Temperature variations	Heat, cold	Burns, dehydration, heat stroke, hyperthermia, hypothermia, frostbite
Ambient noise	Sirens, loud music, traffic noise, work-related noise	Hearing loss/deafness, increased anxiety
Psychosocial	Increased stress	Anxiety, hypertension, suicidal ideation

156

RESCUES IN CONFINED SPACES

A confined space is one in which access is limited and the space is surrounded by walls or structures that are not suitable for habitation. A **confined space** may occur in a building (such as with a collapse), a silo, a motor vehicle (such as a large vehicle involved in a crash), a cistern or septic tank, or a well. A confined space may pose a risk to the patient and EMS personnel because of difficulty moving about and accessing the patient as well as decreased ventilation that may result in the buildup of toxic gases and/or a lack of oxygen. Before entering a confined space, the EMS provider should test the atmosphere and use the correct breathing equipment. This is especially important if the patient is nonresponsive, which is often an indication of poor air quality. The provider should also carefully assess his or her ability to access the patient and the best means of doing so.

TRANSFERRING A PATIENT FROM THE SCENE TO AN AMBULANCE

Different types of **stretchers** and **transfer equipment** may be used for prehospital transfer, including the following:

- **Wheeled**: Stretcher that can be lowered and raised with a wheeled base allowing it to slide into the ambulance.
- **Scoop**: Two- to four-piece stretcher that can be connected and placed under a patient.
- **Transfer sheet**: A heavy plastic sheet can be used with patients up to 800 lb to facilitate transfer.
- **Flexible stretcher**: Lightweight flexible (plastic, rubberized canvas) stretcher with webbing handles on both sides. Can be used to transfer patients around corners and up and down stairs where a wheeled stretcher cannot be used.
- **Stair chair**: Safety chair that can be used to transfer patients in tight spaces and up and down stairs.
- **Folding stretcher**: A stretcher made of lightweight materials that allows folding for compact storage in an ambulance.
- **Basket stretcher** (Stokes basket): Used primarily for rescues in the wilderness or from cliffs.

PATIENT POSITIONING

Patient positioning should be according to the possible or probable injury, with safety restraints always securing the patient to the gurney and the gurney to the vehicle.

- **Left-side-lying:** Pregnant patients should be placed in this position to increase circulation to the placenta, and unconscious patients should be placed in this position to prevent aspiration and choking if there is no indication of a spinal injury.
- **Supine** (flat on the back): Patient has a suspected pelvic fracture or neck injury (also requires a cervical collar).
- **Supine** (feet elevated above the heart): This is the position for patients in shock to increase circulation to the heart and brain as the BP falls.
- **Trendelenburg** (the entire stretcher is tilted so that the head is below the feet): Position for patients with a suspected spinal cord injury.
- **Semi-Fowler's** (30-45° position): For patients with chest pain, stroke, and/or shortness of breath and no indication of a spinal cord injury.
- **Fowler's** (upright, 90° position): For patients with severe shortness of breath.

BACKBOARDS AND CERVICAL COLLARS

Backboards were originally designed to transfer patients. However, **backboards and cervical collars** have been routinely used for EMS rescues for many years without evidence-based studies supporting their use. The premise was that stabilizing the spine and neck would prevent further injury in case a spinal injury had occurred, but spinal injuries are relatively rare, and some studies indicate that these devices do not provide any protection and, in fact, may cause damage. Additionally, cervical collars restrict the airway by 20% or more and may worsen injuries if not properly sized for the patient. Because of these findings, some EMS no longer routinely use backboards but use a vacuum mattress in a scoop basket instead. The American Association of Neurological Surgeons/Congress of Neurological Surgeons (AANS/CNS) 2013 guidelines advise that spinal immobilization using a backboard be reserved for known or suspected spinal cord injury without penetrating injury, although the use of the cervical collar is still recommended until the cervical spine is assessed for injury. Short backboards may be used to support a patient's back in a sitting position.

EMERGENCY MOVES

Emergency moves may be needed if the patient and/or EMS provider is in immediate danger from fire, explosives, or other hazards; if the patient requires life-saving treatment, such as cardiopulmonary resuscitation (CPR); or if the patient is in water, such as a pond or lake. **Emergency moves** include the following:

- **Blanket drag**: Logroll the patient onto a blanket, wrap the patient in the blanket, grasp the blanket near the patient's head while in a squatting position with your back straight, and drag. If there are two rescuers, the other should be positioned at the patient's feet and should be pushing.
- **Clothing drag**: Squat down by the patient's head, securely grasp the clothing near the patient's neck or shoulders (avoid grasping by a T-shirt), and drag the patient.
- **Arm drag**: Squat down by the patient's head. Fold the patient's arms across his or her chest. Grasp the patient under the arms, wrapping your arms about the torso and grasping the patient's wrists to stabilize his or her arms. Drag the patient.

Urgent moves, such as with altered mental status, shock, or breathing difficulties, should also be done as quickly as possible.

Emergency moves can be carried out by one rescuer if no other assistance is available, as follows:

- **Firefighter's drag**: Tie the patient's wrists together with any available material. Straddle the patient and pull the patient's arms over your neck and then crawl forward, dragging him or her beneath you.

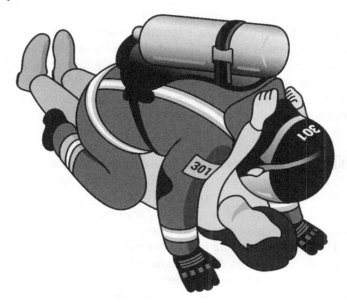

- **Firefighter's carry**: Grasp the patient's knees and pull them together and up. Stand on the patient's feet and reach out and grab one of the patient's arms with one hand. Pull the patient upright, and, as the patient elevates, place your other hand between the patient's legs. Place the patient's arm behind your neck and continue to pull the patient and lift until he or she is draped across your upper back with the arm hanging free. Then grasp the patient's arm that is hanging with the hand that is between the legs to secure the patient.

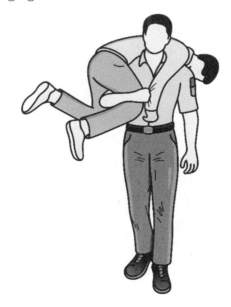

DRIVING SAFETY

The **ambulance driver** should stop briefly or slow significantly at intersections because other drivers may not hear or may ignore sirens. The driver should keep the brake covered with the left foot for fast braking and avoid excessive speeds because of the increased risk of accidents, especially on curves. The speed should be adjusted for road and weather conditions and should not be influenced by use of the siren (siren syndrome). Snow and ice should be cleared from the ambulance before driving it. At least one vehicle length should separate the ambulance from other vehicles for every 10 mph of speed. A spotter should always be used when backing up the ambulance because of poor visibility. All personnel in the ambulance should be seated and secured with seat belts or safety harnesses before the ambulance moves. Studies have shown that CPR is most effective if done from a sitting position in an ambulance rather than standing, despite common practice. Patients and gurneys should also be secured.

LIGHTS AND SIRENS

Lights and sirens should be used together, and they are indicated when going to a scene and when transporting a patient in a serious emergent situation. There are four types of warning lights used on emergency vehicles such as ambulances: rotating lights (resulting in a flashing sensation), fixed flashes (usually red or blue), strobe lights, and LED lights. Red (the most common) and blue lights are generally used to indicate emergency vehicles and can be used to obtain the right-of-way or to block the right-of-way. These colors may be interchangeable, although in some states the color blue is restricted to law enforcement vehicles. Amber lights are warning lights and can be used by all vehicles, but they do not require others to stop. Some emergency vehicle lights change to amber when the vehicle is parked. Green lights are sometimes used to indicate a mobile incident command post, but in some states, green lights may also indicate private security vehicles or volunteer firefighters.

Incident Management

FEMA IS-700.A NIMS

FEMA IS-700.A outlines the **National Incident Management System (NIMS)**, which, under the direction of the **Federal Emergency Management Agency (FEMA)**, an agency of the U.S. Department of Homeland Security, provides the foundation for collaboration among different governmental and nongovernmental agencies, jurisdictions, and specialties/disciplines in handling large-scale incidents that threaten life, property, and/or the environment. Components of FEMA IS-700.A include the following:

- **Preparedness**: Focuses on planning, procedures and protocols, training and exercises, personnel qualifications/certification, and equipment certification, and it includes the National Response Framework, which establishes protocols and ensures that local jurisdictions retain control while still using a unified approach.
- **Communications and information management**: Systems must be interoperable, reliable, portable, scalable, resilient, and redundant.
- **Resource management**: This includes personnel, equipment, supplies, and facilities, which must be inventoried and categorized using a standardized approach.
- **Command and management**: This includes the Incident Command System (this standardized approach outlines the responsibilities of the incident commander, area command, command staff, and general staff), multiagency coordination systems, and public information.
- **Management and maintenance**: The National Integration Center (NIC) is responsible for NIMS management.
- **Flexibility**: Components are scalable and adaptable to all types of incidents.
- **Standardization**: The NIC develops standards in cooperation with standards development organizations.

ICS-100.B

ICS-100.B, the **Incident Command System** course, meets NIMS requirements for operational personnel and outlines a standardized approach to incident management. ICS is used for any type of major event, planned or otherwise, and large- or small-scale incidents, including natural (disasters), technological (hazmat release), and human-caused (civil disturbance) hazards. ICS outlines the chain of command; the incident commander is in control and orders go through supervisors. Every incident requires an incident action plan, resource management, and processes for reimbursement. The incident commander establishes an incident command post and staging areas (gathering places) as well a base (coordination area for logistic and administrative functions), camps (for sleeping, eating, and sanitary services), helibases, and helispots. Primary features of ICS include common terminology, establishment/transfer of command, chain of command/unity of command, management of objects, incident action planning, modular organization, manageable span of control, comprehensive resource management, incident facilities and locations, integrated communications, information and intelligence management, accountability, and dispatch/deployment.

CHAIN OF COMMAND, UNITY OF COMMAND AND UNIFIED COMMAND

Each organization must establish the **chain of command** for its incident command system. Although these may vary somewhat, an incident commander is ultimately in charge with individuals assigned as incident managers in different areas, such as triage, treatment, transport, security, and liaison.

Unity of command means that each incident commander should have control over personnel assigned to his or her area, and each individual within the chain of command should have a clear understanding of whom to report to at the scene so that communication is efficient and timely.

Unified command means that when multiple agencies are involved from multiple jurisdictions, the chain of command that has been established is recognized and respected even though each agency retains its own authority and accountability and is responsible for carrying out its own duties. A unified command system prevents duplication of effort as well as neglect of important functions.

INCIDENT ACTION PLAN

The purpose of the **incident action plan** is to outline control objectives, resources, and strategies for dealing with an incident. Incident action plans should be updated frequently. Incident action plans may be designed for various types of incidents (terrorist attack, disease outbreak, hurricane) and modified as needed and should include the following:

- Goals and objectives, including expected outcomes
- Strategies and tactics for responding and accomplishing the goals and objectives
- An outline of the chain of command for the incident command system, including the span of control (the number of people reporting to an individual)
- Tasks assigned to each level in the chain of command
- Safety/Health plan for responders to prevent injury/illness and to treat victims as needed
- Communications plan outlining how information will be exchanged, including alternative methods of command if, for example, cell phone towers are out of commission
- Logistics plan regarding the acquisition and use of resources, such as supplies, personnel, and equipment
- Maps and demographic information

INCIDENT COMMANDER

When a multiple-casualty or mass-casualty event occurs, the first lead emergency medical responder on the scene generally assumes the role of **incident commander**, carries out a rapid assessment of the scene, and calls for additional resources as indicated while another medical responder begins triage. The incident commander should begin to establish a command center in an area that is safe and out of the way of emergency vehicles while awaiting assistance. This first incident commander will relinquish the role when the staffed and/or assigned incident commander arrives to take command and should then report to the person who is assuming the role of staging officer. The incident commander's duties include establishing command, assessing needs, developing a plan, coordinating all activities, delegating responsibilities, ensuring the safety of all personnel and patients, liaising with other agencies, and communicating information.

TRIAGE

PRIMARY TRIAGE AND RESOURCE MANAGEMENT

Primary triage is a rapid method (30–60 seconds) of prioritizing patients based on the severity of their condition, and it is carried out at the scene of multiple-casualty incidents. All patients are triaged and tagged according to the following international color-coding priority (P) guidelines on the foot or wrist (not on the clothing):

- **P1—Red**: Immediate care is needed for urgent systemic life-threatening conditions, such as airway/breathing problems, severe bleeding, severe burns (especially with breathing problems), decreased mental status, shock, and severe medical problems, or a Glasgow Coma Scale score of ≤13.
- **P2—Yellow**: Delayed care, patient is able to wait 45–60 minutes for treatment. Conditions include burns (without breathing problems), multiple bone/joint injuries, back and/or spinal cord injuries (unless the patient is in respiratory distress).
- **P3—Green**: Hold, patient is able to wait hours for treatment of minor injuries.
- **P4—Black**: Patient is deceased.

Resource management involves identifying a triage officer, who remains at the scene during the event and identifying the need for additional personnel and equipment and providing those to the patients with the highest priority.

SECONDARY TRIAGE/RE-TRIAGE

During a mass-casualty incident, triage is done quickly, and patients may be scattered over a wide area with many patients being red-tagged for emergency care. Patients coded black are left in place, but those with other-color tags should be moved and segregated in separate sections of a holding area to await treatment and/or transport. The patients should be **re-triaged** as they are moved into the holding area to determine if the tagging color is still appropriate. Additionally, **secondary triage** may be carried out in the separate sections, especially if some must be airlifted, to determine which patients have the best chance of survival and should receive priority for transfer and treatment. Secondary triage may also help to determine which trauma center (based on location or level of care) or hospital is most appropriate for the patient considering the patient's condition, transport time, and the surge capacity of the healthcare institutions.

CDC GUIDELINES FOR FIELD TRIAGE OF INJURED PATIENTS

The CDC's guidelines for field triage of injured patients is a four-step algorithm that is used to identify the most seriously ill patients and transport them to an appropriate treatment center.

Step	Assess	Findings requiring priority treatment	Plan
1	Vital signs/ Level of consciousness	Glasgow Coma Scale score of ≤13, systolic BP <90 mm Hg, respiratory rate <10 or >29 per minute (<20 in an infant <1 year), or need of ventilatory support.	Highest level trauma center
2	Anatomy of injury	Penetrating injuries, flail chest, two or more long-bone fractures, crushed/mangled/pulseless extremity, amputations, pelvic fractures, open/depressed skull fracture, or paralysis.	Highest level trauma center
3	Mechanism of injury/High-energy impact	Falls—adults >20 feet and children >10 feet or 2–3 times their height. High-risk auto crash with intrusions, partial or complete ejection, or there is a death in the same passenger compartment. Auto vs. pedestrian/bicycle with victim thrown, run over, or sustaining a significant impact. Motorcycle crash >20 mph.	Trauma center
4	Special patient/ system considerations	Older adults, children, pregnancy >30 weeks, burns, patients on anticoagulants or with bleeding disorders (based on the EMS provider's best judgment).	Trauma center/ hospital

START METHOD OF TRIAGE

With the START method of triage, the EMS provider starts triage with the first victim encountered, tags the patient, and then moves to the next patient, assessing in order: (1) respirations, (2) perfusion, and (3) mental status (RPM) and using the standard red-yellow-green-black color-coding system. Walking wounded are tagged as green.

Respirations	Present	Red tag if >30 Continue to perfusion assessment if <30
	Not present—position the airway	Red tag if respirations recur or black tag (death) if none
Perfusion	Radial pulse absent or capillary refill of greater than 2 seconds	Control bleeding and red tag
	Radial pulse present and capillary refill time of less than 2 seconds	Continue to mental status assessment
Mental status	Cannot follow simple directions	Red tag
	Can follow simple directions	Yellow tag

JumpSTART Method of Triage for Pediatric Patients

JumpSTART is a pediatric triage method developed only for use in multiple-casualty incidents.

Able to walk	No	Continue to breathing assessment.
	Yes	Green tag. Carry out secondary triage.
Breathing	No	Step 1: Position upper airway and red tag if breathing. Step 2: Give five rescue breaths and red tag if breathing. Black tag if breathing does not recur.
	Yes	Respiratory rate <15 or >45, red tag. Respiratory rate 15 to 45, continue to pulse assessment.
Palpable pulse	No	Red tag.
	Yes	Continue to AVPU assessment.
Alert, voice, pain, unresponsive (AVPU) assessment	Inappropriate pain, posturing, or unresponsive	Red tag.
	A, V, or P is appropriate	Yellow tag.

Air Medical Transport

Air medical transport is indicated when the patient is in need of a high level of care that may be available on an aircraft but not an ambulance, when the patient's condition and need for treatment are time critical, when the patient is located in a remote area where access by ambulance is difficult or would be delayed (helicopter), or when local medical services have exceeded their capacity. Helipads are often available at large hospitals, so the patient can be treated immediately after arrival. Some disadvantages include inclement weather (which may interfere with flight plans) as well as altitude and airspeed limitations. Depending on the aircraft, the cabin size may be inadequate for the patient, personnel, and equipment. Difficult terrain, such as forested or hilly areas may not provide an adequate landing site. Cost is the biggest difference between ground and air transport with air transport often costing tens of thousands of dollars with only part, or in some cases none, of the costs being covered by insurance.

Helicopters

Helicopters have the advantage over fixed-wing aircraft of being able to load a patient at or near the scene rather than having to transport the patient by ambulance to an airport. A paved surface is not necessary for a helicopter landing site, but level grassy or paved sites are preferred, ideally with 100 × 100 feet of clear space, but a minimum area of 60 × 60 feet may be used. Additionally, the area should be free of debris that may be disrupted by the rotor blades and should be clear of structures that may interfere with the aircraft, such as power poles, tall trees, power lines, cables, and antennas. A rotor aircraft does not require that people approach in a crouching position, but people should avoid holding anything over their heads and should generally approach from the front of the aircraft and avoid the rear of the aircraft and the rear rotors.

SAFETY ISSUES DURING AIR TRANSPORT

The pilot in command (PIC) of rotorcraft and fixed-wing aircraft is responsible for the **safety** of the aircraft, crew, emergency medical personnel, and the patient. As with all takeoffs and landings, medical staff and crew must be seated and secured by seat belts. Helmets should be in place and secure. Patients who are violent, confused, or combative should be physically restrained for transport and may also require chemical restraints to ensure their own personal safety as well as the safety of the medical and flight crew. Patients should be offloaded ONLY when a crew member signals the receiving medical personnel to approach the aircraft. With high-altitude fixed-wing air transports, cabins are pressurized but only to the equivalent of 6000–8000 feet, not to sea level. Rotorcraft are usually used to transfer a patient from the scene of an incident to a primary care facility or from the primary care facility to another type of facility, whereas a fixed-wing aircraft is usually used from one facility to another over longer distances.

COMMUNICATION ISSUES

A **communication specialist** should coordinate all air medical services, including communications within an agency and between agencies regarding all aspects of transport. The communication specialist should have radio communication skills and knowledge of medical terminology, including knowledge of how to obtain information about a patient, navigation, map usage, customer service, weather, aircraft emergencies, as well as **Federal Aviation Administration (FAA)** and **Federal Communications Commission (FCC)** regulations that relate to air medical transport. The communication specialist should be familiar with radio frequencies used by EMS. The dispatcher determines whether an aircraft should take off. The communication center may be located in a medical facility, airport, or other space, but it should be free of distractions and have emergency backup electrical power. All air medical transport team members should have knowledge of the radio communication system. Some systems include radio or radio-phone communication, and some systems require the team members to carry pagers, such as two-way satellite pagers. All incoming and outgoing communication should be recorded.

STATE AND FEDERAL REGULATIONS

State **statutes** require that aircraft used for air ambulance service must be licensed to provide that service, and the service must ensure that all required medical equipment is available. Although statutes may vary slightly from one state to another, most require that the service be able to provide basic and advanced life support and should provide patients with a description of services and costs. Additionally, the aircraft and crew must comply with FAA regulations and carry insurance to cover injuries that may occur in transport. The FAA carries out periodic inspections of aircraft and issues resource documents regarding safety and operations. Federal regulations establish weather guidelines for safe flying. The **U.S. Department of Transportation** provides guidelines regarding standards of care. The **Commission on Accreditation of Medical Transport Systems** establishes voluntary accreditation standards, but air medical services associated with hospitals must meet hospital accreditation standards, typically those of the Joint Commission.

SAFE EXTRICATION FROM A MOTOR VEHICLE (CAR, TRUCK)
SCENE MANAGEMENT

Scene management at the site of an accident that requires vehicle extrication incudes initial evaluation of any hazards at the site (360° evaluation), such as oncoming traffic, fallen wires, spilled fuel, and fire/explosion risk or presence. The scene must be secured (45° parking, police security, flares, and cones) and the EMS provider should don protective equipment as necessary and access the patient to provide life-saving care. The patient must be disentangled from the motor vehicle as much as can be done safely. The patient is prepared for extrication (such as by applying pressure to bleeding sites and placing a cervical collar), removed from the vehicle, and then prepared for ground or air transport and provided emergent treatment. For extrications in difficult terrain, assess the following:

- **Terrain**: Forests, desert, cliff, water, snow
- **Obstacles**: Trees, rocks, light, unavailability of landing sites
- **Methods to be used**: Helicopter extrication, overland carry, or other type of extrication
- **Alternative solutions**: Abort, contact search and rescue
- **Safety issues**: Review all safety concerns

INITIAL ACTIONS

For **vehicle extrication**, the vehicle must be stabilized before the EMS personnel attempt to enter the vehicle or administer aid to the patient, especially if the vehicle may slide or is on its side and the personnel must access the vehicle from the top because the vehicle may shift and further endanger the patient as well as EMS personnel. EMS personnel can access the vehicle through a window, breaking it if necessary, or a door if one is operable (the patient may be able to assist in opening a window or door). EMS personnel should carry an airway (in case the patient requires ventilation), dressings (to apply pressure if the patient is bleeding), and a rigid cervical collar (to protect against spinal injury or further spinal damage) and should do rapid triage on access to the patient. Oxygen is usually not administered until after the patient is extracted because of the danger of fire, especially if the patient is saturated with fuel, and CPR is not done until the patient is in the supine position on a solid surface. If patients are apneic and pulseless, they must be removed as quickly as possible even with only manual protection of the spine being provided.

EXTRICATION PROCESS

For vehicle extrication, once EMS personnel have gained access to the motor vehicle, they should unlock its doors, if possible, to allow others to more easily gain access. The EMS personnel should ensure that the engine is turned off, the parking brake is set, and the transmission is set to park. If possible, an emergency response person should disconnect the battery to decrease the risk of fire and explosion. If the patient can be removed, a short backboard should be applied before moving the patient. If the patient is wedged between the seat and the steering wheel, the seat may be slid back manually while rescuers support the patient. If the seat has become dislodged from the track, then the patient should be completely immobilized because this type of mechanical damage can result in severe physical injury. If the patient's legs are trapped, lifting the steering wheel away may also lift the dashboard and help to release the patient.

CUTTING A VEHICLE

If a patient must be **cut from a vehicle** (such as when the vehicle is on its side and access must be through a U-shaped flap in the roof), he or she should be warned of the noise and should be covered with a safety blanket (heavy aluminized). In some accidents, **air bags** may deploy with the movement of the patient or vehicle, resulting in danger to the patient and EMS personnel. If the air bags have not deployed, then the battery cables should be disconnected or cut (negative side first) to prevent deployment and personnel should avoid being in front of the path of deployment. EMS personnel should check for side air bags as well as front. The air bags should be deactivated before the steering column is moved (keeping in mind that deactivation can take up to 30 minutes), and care should be taken to avoid cutting or drilling into an air bag.

SEAT BELT PRETENSIONERS

Since the 1990s, vehicles have been equipped with **seat belt pretensioners** on three-point (shoulder harness) systems in the front and often also in the back. The purpose of seat belt pretensioners is to tighten any slack in the belts in an accident, pulling the person back into the seat and in the proper position for deployment of the air bag. Evidence of pretensioners is not always visible, although an accordion sleeve near the buckle end may be an indication. This sleeve compresses if the pretensioner fires. Although an undeployed pretensioner poses less threat to EMS personnel than an undeployed air bag, it can increase the risk of injury to the patient or EMS personnel, so the seat belt should be disconnected or cut immediately on access to the patient. If the patient was not wearing the seat belt on impact and the pretensioner fired, the seat belt will be tightly vertical along pillar B. If the seat belt pretensioner fired while being worn, it will be extended and will not be retractable.

TOOL KIT

Although large and heavy pieces of equipment, such as hydraulic rescue tools (including the Jaws of Life, cutters, spreaders, truck jacks, and rams), pneumatic tools, and come-along tools, are often used in vehicle extrication, a **tool kit** with simple hand tools should also be readily available. They may also be needed to access and safely remove a patient from a vehicle. Tools that may be needed for disassembly include adjustable wrenches, screwdrivers (flat and Phillips), flashlight, penlight, medical scissors, headlamp, pliers, bolt cutters, hammers, axes, crowbars, rescue knives (specially designed to cut through seat belts and clothing), and tin snips. Combination rescue tools are available that can be used for a variety of purposes, such as shutting off gas valves, prying open windows, and cutting through battery cables. Tool belt pouches are available to hold small tools that may be needed during an extrication.

CRIBBING AND CHOCKING

Cribbing and chocking are used to raise a vehicle and prevent it from rolling, such as when a patient is caught beneath a vehicle. **Cribbing** consists of 2×4 blocks and wedges and 4×4 blocks and wedges that are used to create crib boxes to hold an air bag. Cribs are usually made of Douglas fir or southern yellow pine, which can hold 500 psi and crush slowly. The cribbing is stacked with a 4-inch overhang (to allow for compression), and it should not exceed 48 inches in height. The crib box is put in place with the air bag on top. **Chocks** are large stepped wedges that are placed in front of or behind wheels to keep them from rolling when the air bag is inflated. As the air bag is slowly inflated, capture cribbing stacks are placed on both sides behind it to hold the vehicle when the air bag is deflated. Once the vehicle is elevated and secured, the air bag is deflated and the crib box is removed to allow room for the extrication of the patient.

VEHICLES POWERED BY ALTERNATIVE FUELS

Some vehicles are powered by **alternative fuels**, such as compressed natural gas (CNG) or liquefied natural gas (LNG), so EMS personnel should look for CNG/LNG logos, often on the right rear or near the refueling port or the right rear of the cab (semitruck). A "natural gas vehicle" warning may be located near the bottom of the rear doors. CNG tanks may be located behind the cabs in semi-trucks, and some may have additional saddle tanks. The power should be turned off, and the 12-volt battery positive and negative cables should be cut. The emergency shut-off valve should be located and turned off, although each tank can also be turned off manually. Electric vehicles pose the risk of stranded energy. Batteries should always be considered energized with a potential for high-voltage injury. Damaged lithium ion batteries that are leaking or sparking are at risk for thermal runaway (fire). The car battery should be shut down immediately. If the battery is damaged, the vehicle must be relocated at least 50 feet from any combustible material.

BUS EXTRICATION

Before accessing patients involved in a **bus crash,** the bus must be stabilized, especially if it is on its side or if it is upside down. If the engine is still running, a stop button is often located on the left side of the front panel. Access to the bus may be through the front door if possible. Access may also be through the front windshield (which can be removed through removal of the rubber locking strip that surrounds the window), side windows, the emergency exit door or window, the bathroom window, or an opening cut into the top of the vehicle. Removal of injured patients, usually on stretchers, from inside the vehicle often requires rapid triage and the assistance of multiple EMS personnel. If the vehicle remains upright but patients are completely or partially beneath the vehicle, they should be removed quickly because they may be crushed if the air suspension system deflates.

AIRCRAFT EXTRICATION

Communication is essential if EMS personnel are responding to an **aircraft crash site** because they need to know when the crash occurred, the type and size of the aircraft, the number of passengers and crew, reports of fire or explosion, and whether the aircraft is private, commercial, or military, as well as the status (fire, collapse) of any structure(s) that the aircraft may have impacted. For a small plane with the cabin still reasonably intact, extrication may be similar to a motor vehicle, but severe crashes in which the cabin is destroyed and large airplane crashes pose significantly different problems because passengers may have been thrown about inside or outside of the aircraft and seats and belongings and body parts may block access. Victims may lie in the roadway, so emergency vehicles must proceed with caution. Fire and explosions may be a severe risk, and rescuers may need to wait for fire suppression. Triage may begin outside of the aircraft while the aircraft (or the remains of the aircraft) is secured.

ADDITIONAL EXTRICATION CONSIDERATIONS
CONTROL ZONES

Part of the stabilization of the scene is ensuring that it is secure. An outer perimeter is established to block public and media access, and an inner perimeter is established immediately about the scene of the rescue and the working crew. Three **control zones** are established as follows:

- **Hot (coded red)**: This encompasses the inner perimeter and the crew as well as any area that is dangerous, such as an area contaminated by hazardous material or one in danger of a release of toxins.
- **Warm (coded orange)**: Area for trained personnel in support of those in the hot zone. Decontamination of patients, crew, and equipment is carried out in this zone.
- **Cold (coded yellow)**: This is the staging area and the command post (if necessary, for the emergent situation). No members of the public or media should be allowed in the cold zone.

Zones are usually established by placement of police cars and fire-line tape.

PATH OF LEAST RESISTANCE

The path of least resistance is an important concept to understand for rescues, especially if they involve fire and any products of combustion (smoke, heat, gas). Fire's path of least resistance is usually vertical and upward, although fire also spreads horizontally, especially if a vertical path is not available. It's for this reason that if there is a fire on the top floor of a building, the roof is breached to prevent horizontal spread. External factors, such as gusts of wind, can affect the path of least resistance. Water, on the other hand, also flows vertically, but downward and then horizontally if the downward flow is blocked. If the EMS provider is rescuing patients from a building, they will often be found near the path of least resistance, such as near a door or window. Patients should also be transported according to the path of least resistance, that is, the route that is the easiest and safest.

MULTISTEP RESCUE PROCESS

The multistep rescue process includes the following 10 steps:

1. **Preparation**: Training, readying equipment, and preparing for different types of rescues
2. **Response**: Using protocols for dispatch; contacting others, such as utility companies, which may have the necessary knowledge or equipment
3. **Situation size-up**: 360° site survey to identify hazards and determine the need for additional personnel or equipment (Determine if the situation is rescuer/equipment intensive.)
4. **Stabilization**: Establishing perimeters and control zones, monitoring hazardous atmosphere, carrying out lockout/tagout of industrial equipment
5. **Access**: Gaining access to the patient and providing emergent care
6. **Disentanglement**: Freeing the patient
7. **Removal**: Continuing critical and life support while assisting the patient to move or carrying the immobilized patient (Rapid extraction if his or her condition is life threatening.)
8. **Transport**: Transporting by various means with decontamination done as needed
9. **Scene security**: Police or others providing protection of the scene, crew, and patients
10. **Post-event analysis**: Reviewing the procedures performed and the problems encountered

CRITICAL INCIDENT STRESS MANAGEMENT (CISM)

Critical incident stress management (CISM) is a procedure to help people cope with stressful events, such as disasters, in order to reduce the incidence of **post-traumatic stress syndrome (PTSS)**.

- **Defusing sessions** usually occur very early, sometimes during or immediately after a stressful event, and they are used to educate personnel who are actively involved about what to expect over the next few days and to provide guidance in handling their feelings and stress levels.
- **Debriefing sessions** usually follow in one to three days and may be repeated periodically as needed. These sessions may include people who were directly involved as well as those who were indirectly involved. People are encouraged to express their emotions about the event. Critiquing the event or attempting to place blame is not productive as part of the CISM process.
- **Follow-up** is done at the end of the process, usually after about a week, but this time frame can vary.

Mass Casualty and Terrorism

MULTIPLE-CASUALTY INCIDENTS VERSUS MASS-CASUALTY INCIDENTS

Multiple-casualty incidents involve more than one person, but different jurisdictions may quantify the total number of persons differently. It usually refers to the following:

- An incident involving at least three patients
- An incident involving only one jurisdiction and only one to three agencies (ambulance, fire department, and police)
- An incident requiring triage, but generally only primary triage
- Standards of care are maintained, and all patients not coded black (deceased) are transported for care

Mass-casualty incidents also involve more than one person, but may involve much larger numbers—dozens, hundreds, or thousands.

- Often involves multiple jurisdictions and agencies
- Requires triage but may also involve separate waiting areas for color-coded individuals and secondary triage
- Standards of care may be modified, and patients coded black (expectant) and not expected to live may be left in the field and/or receive delayed care if they are still living after the red- and yellow-coded individuals are transported

ROLE OF THE TRANSPORTATION OFFICER IN A MASS-CASUALTY INCIDENT

During a mass-casualty event, the **transportation officer** must maintain constant communication with hospitals and trauma centers, triage officers, police, ground ambulance services, and air medical transport services. The transportation officer controls the flow of patients for treatment and must determine where to route patients in order to prevent a backlog at the receiving facility. They must also coordinate incoming and outgoing ambulances in the transportation staging area. The transportation officer must obtain information about each facility's surge capacity and the number and types of patients the facility is prepared to care for. The transportation officer must also coordinate air medical transport flights and determine, with the triage officer, which patients to transport by air according to their severity of injuries, availability of treatment options, and appropriate levels of care. Speed of transportation and care is often critical in a mass-casualty incident because delays often result in increased death rates.

ROLE OF TRIAGE

In a mass-casualty incident related to terrorism or a disaster, **rapid triage** and tagging must occur and patients must be sorted according to priority for transportation or field treatment. Because of the large numbers of casualties, triage should begin with the first patient encountered, proceeding from one to another. According to some plans, patients who are alive but expected to die are coded red, but this can result in overtriage, with too many red-coded individuals having to be transported and/or treated, resulting in patients dying during the wait. With other plans, patients expected to die are black-coded as "expectant" and left in the field or left aside until red- and yellow-coded individuals are transported and/or treated. If patients are undertriaged (such as patients who should be coded red being coded yellow instead) this can also result in increased deaths while other patients are waiting for transport or treatment.

GUIDANCE FOR INCREASING SURVIVAL RATES IN MASS-CASUALTY EVENTS

Terrorist or other attacks that involve active shooters or improvised explosive devices (IEDs) often result in injuries similar to those encountered in combat situations in which the most common causes of death are extremity hemorrhage, tension pneumothorax, and airway obstruction. The **THREAT acronym** provides guidance for dealing with these situations in the following ways:

- **Threat suppression**: Use of police protection, ballistic vests, concealment, cover, and situational awareness. One concern is that most of the protective gear available to emergency medical personnel is for ballistics rather than explosive devices.
- **Hemorrhage control**: Use of tourniquets (military style) and hemostatic dressings (QuikClot) to control bleeding.
- **Rapid Extrication to safety**: Move patients and personnel out of the danger zone to prevent further injuries.
- **Assessment by medical providers**: Includes provision of a nasopharyngeal airway or upright seating and leaning forward for airway compromise and spinal precautions.
- **Transport to definitive care**: Medical treatment should continue during transport.

SAFETY CONSIDERATIONS ASSOCIATED WITH ACTIVE SHOOTERS AND TERRORIST BOMB ATTACKS

With **active shooters**, standard protocol has been for emergency response services to wait until the police have removed the threat and secured the area before moving in to care for victims; however, this delay in treatment may result in death, so some authorities are now recommending that emergency response personnel enter the scene with police while wearing appropriate protective equipment, although this does pose some risk, especially with additional shooters or a secondary attack.

With a **terrorist bombing** and improvised explosive devices (IEDs), situational awareness is critical because multiple explosive devices (some undetonated) may be at the scene. IEDs may be inside backpacks, suitcases, and packages left unattended, and in emergency situations innocent people often drop backpacks and packages and run away, making it difficult to tell identify a threat. Additionally, attackers wearing suicide vests or belts may mix in with other victims or people escaping the blast area.

BOMB THREAT STANDOFF RECOMMENDATIONS

Threat	Explosive capacity (lb)	Mandatory evacuation distance (ft)	Preferred evacuation distance (ft)	Shelter-in-place zone (ft)
Pipe bomb	5	70	1200+	71–1199
Suicide bomber	20	110	1700+	111–1699
Suitcase/Briefcase	50	150	1850+	151–1849
Automobile	500	320	1900+	321–1899
SUV/Van	1000	400	2400+	401–2399
Small truck	4000	640	3800+	641–3799
Container truck	10,000	860	5100+	861–5099
Semitrailer	60,000	1570	9300+	1571–9299

Source: U.S. Department of Homeland Security.

B-NICE Hazardous Material (Hazmat) Incidents Associated with Terrorist Attacks

Category	Response
B—Biological (bacteria, viruses, fungi, toxins)	Inhalation type—evacuate for 80 feet, shut down air-handling systems, wear appropriate PPE and SCBA, and avoid contamination. Visible agent—decontaminate with soap and water. Symptoms may vary but are usually delayed.
N—Nuclear/ Radiological	Inhalation type (most common)—Isolate/Secure the area, avoid smoke/fumes, stay upwind, and use PPE and SCBA. Isolate victims and decontaminate as appropriate. Symptoms are usually delayed.
I—Incendiary	Be on alert for multiple devices and sabotaged fire suppression equipment. Symptoms include burns, pain, and trauma.
C—Chemical	Isolate/Secure the area, decontaminate victims with soap and water, and be on alert for chemical dispersal devices. Approach toward uphill and upwind. Isolate symptomatic patients from others. Symptoms vary but may include burns, blistering, vomiting, breathing difficulty, and neurological damage.
E—Explosives	Be alert for secondary devices, undetonated devices, and secondary hazards (unstable buildings and debris). Remove victims from the area, secure the perimeter, and stage away from the incident area. Decontaminate as necessary. Symptoms include burns, amputations, cuts, and penetrating and blunt trauma.

"All-Hazards" Safety Approach to Mass-Casualty Incidents

The "all-hazards" safety approach to mass-casualty incidents aims to provide plans that can be used to deal with all types of hazards (natural disasters, terrorist attacks, and mass-casualty incidents) as well as encompassing the four components of emergency management: mitigation, preparedness, response, and recovery. Organizations in an area coordinate to develop joint action plans that can be activated in response to incidents, with the chain of command clearly outlined. This approach lowers costs to individual organizations and provides for a faster and more effective response. However, although the basic structure may be the same for responding to all hazards, there are inevitable differences between (for example) a terrorist attack with active shooters and a natural disaster, such as a hurricane, which can be anticipated and mitigated to some degree. For this reason, modifying existing incident action plans to meet the needs of a situation is essential.

Treating Terrorists and Criminals

In mass-casualty incidents, **terrorists and criminals** involved in the incident may be injured and require treatment, and EMS personnel may feel conflicted about providing treatment when others have been injured or killed, but it's important to provide treatment to terrorists and criminals the same as any other individuals both because they are in need of help and because their survival may be critical to identifying co-conspirators and to providing reasons for the attack.

However, these individuals may pose risks to emergency medical personnel, so they should be examined while under police guard. The individual's hands should be examined first to check for weapons and detonators and secured (with handcuffs, if possible). Clothes should be examined and removed very carefully in case the person is wearing a suicide device of some type. Emergency medical personnel should also be aware that the individual may be feigning injury or unconsciousness.

EMS Regulations

EMS HISTORY

Historically, the **first use of an ambulance** was in the Siege of Málaga in Spain in 1487, when horse-drawn wagons were used to carry the wounded to safety. Military ambulances became more common in Europe throughout the following centuries. Napoleon Bonaparte assigned battlefield vehicles and attendants in 1793. The first ambulance service in the United States was instituted by the US army in 1865 in Cincinnati, followed by an ambulance service in New York just four years later. Hospital-based ambulance services increased in the 1900s, but many hospital ambulance services shut down during World War II, so fire and police departments filled the roles. At this time, there were no laws regarding minimum training for ambulance personnel. Following World War II, the use of ambulance services increased, but the quality was often poor until basic training standards were developed in 1968 along with the 911 emergency system. The **first paramedic program** was developed in 1969. The EMS Systems Act was passed in 1973, the EMS for Children Act in 1983, and the Trauma Care Systems Planning and Development Act in 1990. In 1991, standards and benchmarks for ambulance services were established by the Commission on Accreditation of Ambulance Services.

EMS SYSTEMS

The **National Highway Traffic Safety Administration (NHTSA)** is the lead agency for coordinating and promoting evidence-based emergency medical services (EMS) (fire based, third service, and hospital based) and the 911 system. The **public safety answering point (PSAP)** is the designated call-receiving site that directs calls to the appropriate emergency services. Each state defines the scope of practice, licensure, and credentialing for prehospital personnel and sets education standards based on national EMS standards. The EMS provider of any level is expected to maintain certification through maintenance of skills and continuing education and should exhibit professional behavior, including working with integrity and empathy, being an effective member of a team, showing respect and tact, maintaining a professional appearance, communicating effectively, and advocating for patients. The provider must be alert to patient safety and recognize that most errors result from skills-based, rules-based, and knowledge-based failures. Error reduction requires the use of decision aids and protocols, asking for assistance when appropriate, questioning assumptions, and making debriefing calls.

ROLES AND RESPONSIBILITIES OF EMS PERSONNEL

Roles and responsibilities of EMS personnel include the following:

- Maintain the readiness of all equipment, including disinfecting, packaging, and storing.
- Monitor personal safety, patient safety, and the safety of others on the scene.
- Evaluate the scene for additional resources when indicated.
- Gain access to the patient only when it is safe to do so.
- Perform an assessment of the patient's condition and needs.
- Provide emergency medical care as needed (or until additional resources arrive).
- Provide emotional support to the patient, family, and other providers.
- Maintain the continuity of care.
- Ensure that medical and legal standards are upheld and that patient privacy is protected.
- Communicate with others and maintain community relations.
- Practice professional behavior (integrity, self-motivation, self-confidence, tact, respect, and professional appearance).
- Maintain certification and meet continuing education requirements.

NATIONAL EMS EDUCATION AGENDA FOR THE FUTURE: A SYSTEMS APPROACH

The National EMS Education Agenda for the Future: A Systems Approach proposed an education system for EMS with five primary components, establishing the following goals for 2020:

- **Core content**: Core content to be developed by the EMS medical community, educators, and providers under leadership of the National Highway Traffic Safety Administration (NHTSA) to ensure consistency of content and reciprocity of certification. The core content should be tied to licensure and accreditation.
- **Scope-of-practice model**: National models to be used by states for all levels of EMS certification/licensure.
- **Education standards**: Standards that are developed by EMS educators with input from the medical community and regulators and that are peer reviewed.
- **Education program accreditation**: A single national accreditation agency will develop standards and guidelines.
- **EMS certification:** Four levels of national certification with different educational requirements, standards, scopes of practice, and certification:
  - (1) Entry-level emergency medical responder (EMR)
  - (2) Emergency medical technician (EMT)
  - (3) Advanced EMT (AEMT)
  - (4) Paramedic

Patient Safety and Quality Improvement

PATIENT SAFETY AND HIGH-RISK SITUATIONS

Up to 250,000 patients die each year because of medical errors. Patients are especially at risk of further injury or death in **high-risk situations** and activities such as the following:

- **Hand-off**: A standard procedure, such as **SBAR**, should be used.
  - S = Situation: Overview of current situation and important issues
  - B = Background: Important history and issues leading to current situation
  - A = Assessment: Summary of important facts and condition
  - R = Recommendation: Actions needed
- **Communications**: Problems may result in delayed or inadequate care, wrong address, or wrong destination.
- **Dropping**: Patients can be easily dropped if the gurney isn't positioned properly or if too few personnel are involved in transport.
- **Ambulance crashes**: Unnecessary speeding and failing to stop at intersections are the most common causes of ambulance crashes.
- **Inadequate spinal immobilization**: If unsure, it's always best to immobilize.
- **Medication errors**: Administration of wrong medication, wrong mode of administration, and wrong dosage.

QUALITY IMPROVEMENT

Quality improvement requires that an organization or system continually evaluates processes and outcomes and takes measures to improve the quality of care. The focus of quality improvement is on patient safety in access, provision of care, transport, and hand-off. Errors are often related to these different types of failures:

- **Skills-based**: Includes slips and mistakes. Slips occur when the EMS provider has the correct intent but does not carry out an action as intended, such as mistakenly using the wrong piece of equipment. Mistakes occur when the EMS provider has an incorrect intention that leads to incorrect action.
- **Rules-based**: The EMS provider incorrectly applies a rule, applies a bad or wrong rule, or fails to apply the correct rules. For example, an EMS provider is injured because of failing to assess safety before approaching a patient.
- **Knowledge-based**: The EMS provider's knowledge is not adequate for the situation.

EMS personnel can help reduce errors by debriefing, constantly reevaluating and questioning assumptions, using established protocols and decision aids, and asking for assistance when needed.

CONTINUOUS QUALITY IMPROVEMENT (CQI)

Continuous quality improvement (CQI) emphasizes the organization and systems and processes within that organization rather than emphasizing individuals. It recognizes internal customers (staff) and external customers (patients) and uses data to improve processes. CQI represents the concept that most processes can be improved. CQI uses the scientific method of experimentation to meet needs and improve services and uses various tools, such as brainstorming, multivoting, storyboarding, and meetings. **Core concepts** include the following:

- Quality and success are meeting or exceeding internal and external customers' needs and expectations.
- Problems relate to processes, and variations in processes lead to variations in results.
- Change can be made in small steps.

Steps to CQI include the following:

1. Forming a knowledgeable team
2. Identifying and defining measures used to determine success
3. Brainstorming strategies for change
4. Planning, collecting, and using data as part of making decisions
5. Testing changes and revising or refining as needed

Research and Evidence-Based Practice

DATA COLLECTION AND RESEARCH

Research is especially important in identifying the need for changes in procedures and protocols in order to improve patient outcomes. Research depends on the gathering of data. **Data collection** may include direct observations, surveys, interviews, and various other sources of information, such as documents and audiovisual materials. **Literature research** requires a comprehensive evaluation of current (≤5 years) and/or historical information. Most literature research begins with an internet search of databases, which provides listings of books, journals, and other materials on specific topics. Databases vary in content, and many contain only a reference listing with or without an abstract, so once the listing is obtained, the researcher must do a further search (publisher, library, etc.) to locate the material. Some databases require a subscription, but access is often available through educational or healthcare institutions. In order to search effectively, the researcher should begin by writing a brief explanation of the research to help identify possible keywords and synonyms to use as search words.

METHODS OF DATA COLLECTION

When developing **data collection procedures** to determine needs, the following must be considered: the purpose of the data collection, the audience for which the data are intended, the types of questions to be answered, the scope of the research, and the resources available to carry out data collection. Methods of collection and subsequent issues regarding those procedures are discussed below:

- **Direct observation**: Observers must be selected and trained on how to observe and when and how to record observations.
- **Interviews**: Interview questions must be developed and validated, and the interviewers must be given practice time.
- **Questionnaires**: The type of questionnaire, the questions, and the Likert scale must be determined as well as the method of distribution (one-on-one, group, email, internet).
- **Record review**: A form or checklist should be developed to guide record review, and the records should be selected based on criteria established for the research.
- **Secondary analysis**: The databases to be mined should be selected, and the criteria for the research should be established, including keywords, time frames, and populations.

EVIDENCE-BASED DECISION-MAKING

Although traditional medical practice has been based on knowledge, intuition, and judgment, these practices have not always been supported by evidence. **Evidence-based decision-making** results in best practices based on best evidence. Steps include the following:

1. Formulating a question regarding treatment and/or procedures
2. Conducting a search of the appropriate medical literature, often beginning with the search of an online database to find research that is related to the question
3. Determining the validity (measure of accuracy) and reliability (consistency) of the evidence
4. Evaluating the level of evidence (1-5, 1 being the most reliable)
5. Assessing data (information) to determine if they apply to current needs
6. Drawing up a plan for change with input from all staff members
7. Implementing changes
8. Monitoring changes and outcomes

Workplace Safety and Wellness

STRESS MANAGEMENT

The EMS provider must often deal with **stressful incidents**, such as dangerous situations (storm conditions, gunshots, falling debris); critically ill patients; unpleasant sights, sounds, and odors; multi-patient incidents; and angry/upset patients, family members, and bystanders. The EMS provider should not argue or become defensive but should remain calm and supportive, allowing the patient to express his or her feelings and trying to defuse the situation while administering medical care and cooperating with other first responders. If a patient has no pulse or respirations and does not have a valid do-not-resuscitate (DNR) order, the EMS provider should attempt resuscitation unless doing so puts the provider at risk; the injuries are not compatible with life; or obvious signs of death are present, such as tissue decay, livor mortis, which is discoloration in the lowermost blood vessels from pooled blood shortly after death, or rigor mortis, which is stiffening of the joints that occurs within 2-6 hours of death (verified by checking two or more joints). After 24-48 hours of rigor mortis, the muscles become flaccid.

WARNING SIGNS OF STRESS

Warning signs of stress often begin with difficulty sleeping and nightmares about work, loss of appetite, and lack of interest in usual activities, including work and intimacy. The individual may feel increasingly sad and depressed and may have difficulty concentrating, making decisions, and carrying out tasks. The individual may also begin to isolate from others and exhibit irritability with coworkers, family, and friends. Some individuals develop physical symptoms related to stress, such as stomach upset, headaches, nausea, and high blood pressure (BP), whereas others may experience panic attacks. Some individuals may try to self-medicate with alcohol or drugs. When experiencing the warning signs of stress, the individual should talk about the problems with someone trusted, such as a physician, coworker, supervisor, or family member, and he or she may need to seek assistance from a professional counselor. Lifestyle changes, such as decreasing the use of alcohol or drugs, exercising regularly, and practicing relaxation exercises, may help to relieve stress.

STRESS REACTIONS

Stress reactions include the following:

- **Acute stress reaction**: This reaction usually occurs quickly (minutes to hours) in response to an event that is stressful (such as the death of a child or a multiple-casualty incident). The individual may experience physical symptoms (with the release of adrenaline) such as rapid pulse, nausea, chest tightness, headache, fast respirations, and increased perspiration. An acute stress reaction usually recedes quickly, but it may persist for weeks in some individuals.
- **Delayed stress reaction**: Although the individual may cope well with a stressful event initially, months later, the person may begin to have nightmares, anxiety, and other indications of post-traumatic stress.
- **Cumulative stress reaction**: This type of stress reaction occurs when the individual has repeated stressors (either in the workplace or in his or her personal life) that cause repeated acute stress reactions, resulting in various physical and psychological problems. This is especially common in EMS personnel.

PREVENTION OF RESPONSE-RELATED INJURIES

Prevention of response-related injuries includes the following:

- **Infectious diseases**: Use PPE and understand the spread of infectious diseases—air (coughing), direct contact (blood, vomitus, other body fluids), needlestick, contaminated food/equipment, and sexual transmission. Maintain current immunizations.
- **Personal habits**: Obtain adequate sleep, nutrition, and exercise. Avoid excessive alcohol and tobacco.
- **Environmental hazards**: Conduct a 360° assessment. Note traffic hazards, the vehicle's condition, fire, leaking fluids, downed power lines, hazardous materials (look for placards and warning symbols; avoid the area until it is cleared). Use PPE and respirators as indicated.
- **Violence**: Defuse situations, make a safe response (with the assistance of law enforcement), and use restraints if necessary, for dangerous or violent individuals.
- **Collisions**: Drive safely; avoid speeding and driving through stop signs and red lights when possible. Wear seat belts and/or safety harnesses.

PRINCIPLES OF BODY MECHANICS

Basic principles of body mechanics include the following:

- Avoid reaching overhead or for prolonged periods of time or more than 20 inches away.
- Avoid pulling—push, roll, or slide instead.
- Avoid lifting—push, roll, or slide instead.
- Lift with leg muscles, not with the back.
- Hold weight close to the body rather than at arm's length.
- Flex at the hips and knees, not the waist.
- Carry patients head first upstairs and feet first downstairs.
- Maintain a straight back and avoid twisting.
- Assess weight and recognize limitations in lifting/carrying.
- Get help when necessary, and communicate every step with your partner ("Lift on the count of three").
- Maintain a firm base of support with feet apart (shoulder width) to stabilize your stance.
- Maintain the line of gravity (the imaginary line between your center of gravity and the ground) within the base of support.
- Position yourself close to an object that is to be lifted or carried.
- Lift patients from stable ground.

MOVING AND LIFTING PATIENTS

Techniques for moving patients include the following:

- **Direct ground lift**: Use only for lightweight individuals with no suspected spinal injuries. Three EMS providers line up on one side of the patient, and each kneels on the same knee. The EMS provider at the head places one arm under the patient's neck and shoulder and the other arm under the patient's lower back. The middle provider places his or her arms above and below the patient's waist, and the provider at the patient's feet places his or her arms under the knees and lower legs. On the count of three, they roll the patient onto their knees and toward their chests. On the count of three, they stand and move the patient.
- **Power lift**: Place feet shoulder width apart and pointing slightly outward; tighten the back and abdominal muscles. Squat down as though sitting. Place hands 10 inches apart with the palms upward (power grip) while grasping the stretcher and lift with the upper body becoming vertical before the hips rise.
- **Extremity lift**: Requires two EMS providers. One provider squats at the patient's head and another is at one side by the patient's knees. The provider at the head folds the patient's arms across the chest and grasps the patient by wrapping both arms around the torso under the patient's arms and grasping the patient's wrists. The second provider slides his or her hands beneath the patient's knees and lower legs, and together they stand and lift the patient.
- **Squat lift**: Requires two EMS providers. One provider squats with the back straight and the weak foot slightly forward at the head of patient, and the other provider is in the same position at the patient's feet. Grasp the patient's upper body as for the extremity lift and grasp the patient's feet. Both EMS providers push up with the stronger foot and lift with the upper body becoming vertical before the hips rise.
- **Logroll**: Used to position carrying devices under the patient and for some transfers; it requires two EMS providers positioned on the same side of the patient. Place the patient's arm on the side that he or she is being turned to above his or her head or over the chest. Place the patient's other arm across his or her chest. If on the ground, squat close to the patient. The provider at the patient's head reaches across the patient and grasps his or her shoulders and trunk while the second provider grasps his or her trunk and legs. On the count of three, they turn the patient in one smooth move.
- **Draw-sheet transfer**: Requires four EMS providers with two positioned on one side of the patient and two positioned on the other side but on the opposite side of the bed or stretcher to which the patient will be transferred. The logroll technique is used to place a draw sheet under the patient. Providers on both sides roll the edges of the draw sheet until the edges are close to the patient. On the count of three, they lift the patient slightly and move the patient across to the bed.

Occupational Safety

Occupational Safety and Health Administration (OSHA)

The Occupational Safety and Health Administration (OSHA) is part of the U.S. Department of Labor, and it is charged with ensuring safe, healthful working conditions and setting and enforcing workplace standards. OSHA covers most employers in the private sector, but state and federal safety regulations also generally conform to OSHA standards. Employers must provide safety training, inform workers of chemical hazards, and provide required PPE. OSHA must be notified of a workplace-related death within 8 hours and a workplace-related injury that results in hospitalization, the loss of an eye, or amputation within 24 hours. Workers may file a complaint about workplace conditions with OSHA and request an inspection. OSHA's Whistleblower Protection Program prohibits retaliation by the employer. OSHA provides Hazardous Waste Operations and Emergency Response Standard (HAZWOPER) training courses (8-hour, 24-hour, 40-hour, and refresher) for first responders. OSHA has established regulations and guidelines that are industry specific. For example, OSHA has regulations regarding EMS. OSHA requires that hazardous material be color coded, with red indicating danger; yellow, caution; orange, warning; and fluorescent orange/orange-red, biological hazard.

> **Review Video: Intro to OSHA**
> Visit mometrix.com/academy and enter code: 913559

Safety Data Sheets (SDSs)

Safety data sheets (SDSs), formerly known as material safety data sheets (MSDSs), explain how to handle caustic substances in the event of an accident or injury and provide pertinent information on the composition and toxic effects of chemicals in a lab. SDSs outline the proper storage of chemicals, procedures for the cleanup and dumping of caustic substances, procedures in the event of a chemical spill or injury, and the proper locations in the facility for cleanup. SDSs should also contain information indicating which substances may cause allergic effects or asthma from contact or inhalation. Emergency rescue services should obtain SDSs for common chemicals and products. Manufacturers and suppliers should have SDSs on file and can be contacted for copies. The OSHA/Environmental Protection Agency (EPA) Occupational Chemical Database provides links for SDSs for some products. SDSs are available from various other sources, including the Toxicology Data Network (TOXNET) and poison control centers. There are also pathogen safety data sheets for biological hazards.

Hazardous Materials, Exposure, and Absorption

Hazardous materials are any materials that may cause harm to humans or animals by themselves or through interaction with something else. **Hazardous materials** may be any of the following:

- **Chemical**: Blister agents, blood agents, choking agents, nerve agents, asphyxiants, or irritants that can enter the body through inhalation, absorption, ingestion, or injection
- **Radiological**: Nuclear material and radioactive substances (alpha/beta particles)
- **Physical/Biological**: Infectious wastes, blood and other body fluids, and biotoxins

Almost any material or substance can be classified as hazardous depending on various factors such as its location, amount, and interactions. **Exposure** occurs when a person/animal comes in contact with the hazardous material, and contamination is the residue resulting from exposure. **Absorption** is the method by which hazardous material enters the bloodstream. Exposure and contamination may result in an immediate response (blistering, itching, and pain) or a delayed response (nausea, vomiting, cancer, and lung disease).

CLASSIFICATION OF HAZARDOUS WASTE

The Environmental Protection Agency (EPA) **classifies hazardous wastes** according to the following characteristics:

- **Ignitable**: Liquids and nonliquids that can ignite and cause fires with flash points of <60 °C (140 °F)
- **Corrosive**: Based on pH (<2 or >12.5) or its ability to corrode steel
- **Reactive**: Wastes that are unstable, may react with water, may result in toxic gases, or may explode
- **Toxic**: Heavy metal compounds that are harmful if ingested or absorbed

Wastes may also be classified as **listed wastes**. These include wastes from manufacturing and industrial processes. Hazardous wastes are often produced in manufacturing, nuclear power plants (nuclear wastes), and healthcare facilities (needles and materials contaminated with body fluids). Nuclear wastes are classified as mixed waste because they contain a radioactive component as well as a hazardous component. Hazardous wastes can result in disease (such as from needle punctures), injury (from fire and explosions), and death (from toxic exposure and disease).

HAZARDOUS WASTE SITE CHARACTERIZATION

The purpose of hazardous waste site characterization is to identify hazards and select the appropriate PPE. The team leader is responsible for the assessment, but he or she may request assistance from outside experts, such as chemists. The three **steps to hazardous waste site characterization** include the following:

1. **Off-site characterization**: Gather information/data before personnel enter the site, including the location, a description of the activities, the duration of the event, terrain information (photographs, maps), habitation/population data, accessibility, paths of least resistance, and properties of any hazardous materials/substances. Conduct the needed interviews and review of records. Perimeter reconnaissance is done with observations, air sampling, and development of a preliminary site map.
2. **On-site survey**: Verify the information gathered from perimeter reconnaissance, survey the area and situation, note potential exposure to hazardous materials (dust, liquid, dead animals, gas) and safety hazards (obstacles, terrain, poisonous plants), and develop a site safety plan. The entry team should have at least four members: two to enter and two for outside support who can enter the site in an emergency.
3. **Ongoing monitoring**: Monitoring should be continuous.

CHEMICAL HAZARDOUS WASTE MATERIALS

Types of chemical hazardous waste materials include the following:

- **Blister agents**: Include sulfur mustard (mustard gas) and nitrogen mustard, which are both highly toxic. Exposure by inhalation, contact, or ingestion results in skin (erythema and blistering) and eye irritation and injury to the respiratory system as well as bone marrow suppression and gastrointestinal and neurological damage. The patient should be decontaminated within 1 to 2 minutes by flushing the eyes with water for up to 20 minutes and removing clothing and showering with soap (if available) and water for 20 minutes. Rescuers should use a self-contained breathing apparatus (SCBA), PPE (including eye protection), and chemical-protective gloves.
- **Asphyxiants**: Gas exposure (such as by butane, helium, and propane) lowers oxygen levels and results in suffocation. Patients require oxygen administration and may need CPR. This is especially a risk in confined spaces. Rescuers should use an SCBA.
- **Blood agents**: These include cyanide chloride, hydrogen cyanide, and arsine. Exposure by inhalation or ingestion. They prevent oxygen transfer from blood to cells. The patient may need oxygen and the antidote. Rescuers should use an SCBA.
- **Carcinogens**: Agents such as asbestos, nickel compounds, and ionizing radiation that result in genetic mutation and cancer. There are various types of exposure. Patients must be removed from exposure. The rescuer must wear adequate PPE, and in some cases, he or she should use a mask or SCBA.
- **Choking agents**: Often, a chemical weapon is used (ammonia, chlorine) that is designed to inhibit breathing and incapacitate the person. Exposure is by inhalation, contact, or ingestion (rare). They may be corrosive to the skin and result in fluid in the lungs, leading to suffocation. Patients require supportive treatment and oxygen. Rescuers should use PPE and SCBA for most agents.
- **Convulsants/Nerve agents**: These include hydrazine and strychnine. Exposure may be by inhalation, contact, and ingestion. The severity of convulsions and nervous system impairment is dose related. Patients require supportive treatment. Rescuers need SCBA and protective suits (according to the exposure level of the agent).

HAZARD SIGNS AND SYMBOLS

Sign/Symbol	Interpretation
	Flame: Includes flammable, self-heating, or self-reactive materials and gases.
	Corrosion: Includes substances that can cause skin burns, metal corrosion, and eye damage.
	Health hazard: Includes carcinogens, toxic substances, and respiratory irritants.
	Poison: Includes materials, gases, or substances that are extremely toxic and may result in death or severe illness.
	Irritant: Includes materials, gases, or substances that are irritants to the skin, eyes, and/or respiratory tract, are acutely toxic, or have a narcotic effect.
	Biohazard: Includes biological substances, such as body fluids, that pose a threat to humans. Appears on sharps containers that hold contaminated needles.

Infection Control

DISEASE PREVENTION

CDC ISOLATION GUIDELINES

The **2007 CDC Guideline for Isolation Precautions** includes the standard precautions that apply to all patients and transmission-based precautions for those with known or suspected infections.

Standard precautions should be used for all patients because all body fluids (sweat, urine, feces, blood, and sputum) and non-intact skin and mucous membranes may be infected. Standard precautions include the following:

- **Hand hygiene**: Use an alcohol-based hand rub or wash with soap and water before and after each patient contact and after any contact with body fluids and contaminated items. Always use soap and water when hands are visibly soiled.
- **Protective equipment**: Use personal protective equipment (PPE), such as gloves, gowns, and masks, eye protection, and/or face shields, when anticipating contact with body fluids or contaminated skin.
- **Respiratory hygiene/Cough etiquette**: Use source-control measures, such as covering cough, disposing of tissues, using a surgical mask on the person coughing or on staff to prevent inhalation of droplets, and properly disposing of dressings and used equipment. Wash hands after contacting respiratory secretions. Maintain a distance of >3 feet from a coughing person when possible.
- **Sharps**: Dispose of sharps, such as needles, carefully in sharps containers. Do not recap needles.

Transmission-based precautions should be used for those with known or suspected infections as well as those with excessive wound drainage, other discharge, or fecal incontinence. Transmission-based precautions include the following:

- **Contact**: Use PPE, including gown and gloves, for all contacts with the patient or the patient's immediate environment.
- **Droplet**: Appropriate for influenza, streptococcus infection, pertussis, rhinovirus, and adenovirus and pathogens that remain viable and infectious for only short distances. Use a mask while caring for the patient. Maintain the patient at a distance of >3 feet away from other patients (with a curtain separating them in an emergency department). Use a patient mask if transporting a patient.
- **Airborne**: Appropriate for measles, chickenpox, tuberculosis, severe acute respiratory syndrome [SARS] and COVID-19 because pathogens remain viable and infectious for long distances. Use ≥N95 respirators (or masks) while caring for the patient. The patient should be placed in an airborne infection isolation room (with negative air pressure if possible) in an emergency department.

PERSONAL PROTECTIVE EQUIPMENT (PPE)

Personal protective equipment (PPE) should be readily available in the appropriate sizes for each EMS individual.

- **Gowns**: Should be worn for risk of splash or spray with body fluids (severe bleeding, childbirth) and should be fluid resistant.
- **Eye protectors**: Should be worn for risk of splash or spray with body fluids or contact with debris, such as at a worksite or in a collapsing building. Goggles should fit snugly and have antifog features. (Prescription eyeglasses do not take the place of goggles.)
- **Face shields**: Provide protection for face, eyes, nose, and mouth. These are preferred to goggles when there is risk of spray or splash of body fluids. They should wrap around and cover the forehead and extend to below the chin.
- **Masks**: Protect the nose and mouth from fluids and particles and should be fluid resistant, fit snugly, and have a flexible nosepiece.
- **Respirators** (such as N95, N99, and N100): Protect the nose, mouth, and airway passages exposed to hazardous or infectious aerosols, including bacteria and viruses (tuberculosis [TB], measles, COVID-19).

HAND HYGIENE AND GLOVES

Hand hygiene should be done before eating, before and after direct contact with a patient's skin, after contact with any body fluids, after contact with inanimate objects in the patient's immediate vicinity, when moving hands from a dirty to a clean area, after removing gloves, and after using the restroom.

Hand hygiene is carried out in the following two manners:

- **Antiseptic soaps/detergents**: For visible soiling, after exposure to diarrhea stool or a patient with diarrhea, before eating, and after using the restroom. Wet hands, apply product, rub hands together vigorously for 15 seconds, covering all surfaces, rinse hands with water, and use a disposable towel to dry them.
- **Alcohol-based hand sanitizers** (the most effective way to kill bacteria): For all other situations. Apply product and rub hands together, including between the fingers, for about 20 seconds until the skin surfaces are dry.

Gloves must be worn when touching any body fluids, nonintact skin, open wounds, or mucous membranes (eyes, mouth, nose); gloves should be changed when moving from a dirty area to a clean one or from one patient to another.

IMMUNIZATIONS FOR EMS PERSONNEL

The Centers for Disease Control and Prevention (CDC) recommends the following **immunizations** for all healthcare workers, including EMS personnel:

- **Hepatitis B**: Three-dose series (now, in one month, and five months later) followed by an anti-HBs serologic test 30-60 days after the third immunization
- **Measles, mumps, rubella (MMR)**: Two-dose series with the second immunization at least 28 days after the first for those born during or after 1957 and those born before 1957 without proof of immunity
- **Varicella (chickenpox)**: Two doses, four weeks apart (A combined MMRV immunization is available.)
- **Influenza**: Annually
- **Tetanus, diphtheria, and pertussis (Tdap)**: One time, with a tetanus (TD) booster every 10 years (The TD injection does not protect against pertussis (whooping cough).)
- **Meningococcal**: One dose

Screening for **tuberculosis** with a chest x-ray or skin test is also recommended.

Documentation

MINIMUM DATA SETS

Minimum data sets are the minimum data specifically required for EMS services. These consist of the following:

- **Patient information**: This derives from the assessment including the patient's primary complaint and the findings during the initial assessment—the patient's name and address; vital signs (blood pressure [BP], pulse [P], and respiration rate [R]); and descriptions of any wounds, injuries, pain, or other symptoms. The patient's demographics (age, gender, ethnic background) should be noted as well as any other identifying or essential information.
- **Administrative information**: This includes the time of the initial report, time the EMS unit was notified, time of arrival at the incident, time of leaving the scene, time of arrival at the destination (hospital, trauma center), and time of hand-off.
- **Accurate/Synchronous clocks**: All members of the EMS system should use accurate and synchronous clocks so that they all are set to the same time to ensure there is no disparity in time reporting.

PREHOSPITAL CARE REPORT

The prehospital care report serves as a legal document to show that emergent care was provided. It describes the condition of the patient upon EMS arrival at the scene, interventions provided, and changes in the patient's condition; it is essential to ensure continuity of care. The documenting EMS provider may be called in to legal proceedings. The **prehospital care report** may also be used for educational purposes, such as through debriefing and case review. Additionally, the report is used administratively as the basis for billing as well as for the collection of data for research and evaluation of continuous quality improvement. Required elements of documentation include the time of events (receipt of call, arrival at incident, time of transport, arrival at destination), assessment findings (vital signs, injuries, bleeding, mental status), emergent care, changes in the patient's condition, response to the treatment provided, scene observations (specific place/area), hazards, and disposition of patient (care refusal, transportation, hand-off). Documentation may be on paper or may be done electronically and may combine checkboxes and narrative reports. **Run data** (or ambulance run report data) are those data elements that are required for reporting each run.

NARRATIVE DOCUMENTATION IN THE PREHOSPITAL CARE REPORT

With **narrative documentation**, the EMS provider should take care not to repeat the same information already provided in checkboxes. The provider should describe what was observed directly rather than the conclusions based on those observations and should record all pertinent information and observations, avoiding non-standardized abbreviations and radio codes, which may be misunderstood or misinterpreted. Any pertinent negatives, such as patient or family complaints, must be documented. If the incident has legal implications, such as in the case of assault, any pertinent comments or sensitive information ("I was raped") should be quoted directly and the source should be noted. Care should be taken to write clearly and spell correctly. Time should be documented for every intervention and reassessment. Any state or local reporting requirements must be met in documentation, and the contents of the prehospital report should remain confidential and be distributed only to appropriate healthcare providers. No data may be falsified, and any errors and steps taken to correct those errors must be documented.

DOCUMENTING PATIENT REFUSAL OF MEDICAL CARE

According to the Patient Self-Determination Act (1990), competent patients have the **right to refuse** any medical treatment, and parents have the right to make this decision for minor children. If a patient refuses care, then the EMS provider should inform the patient of the reasons to get medical care and possible consequences of refusal. The patient should be asked to sign the refusal form, and a family member, police officer, or bystander should sign as a witness to the patient's signing or witness the patient's refusal to sign. The EMS provider should complete documentation of any assessment carried out and any refusal of the patient to assessment. The provider should carefully document the conversation between the provider and patient regarding refusal of care and consequences and should document the proposed care as well as the information the provider gave the patient about alternate care (such as a visit to the personal physician) and the willingness to return if the patient has a change of mind.

SPECIAL DOCUMENTATION SITUATIONS

Additional documentation situations that should be handled according to protocol include:

- **Documentation errors**: In handwritten documents, draw one line through the error, initial, and write the correct information beside the error. If information was omitted, add a note with the date and initials. If documentation was electronic, follow the method prescribed for corrections.
- **Multiple-casualty incidents**: Record information temporarily for later complete documentation, if necessary, following the procedures in place for such an incident.
- **Incident reports**: Fill out forms as soon as possible, document any witnesses to the incident, and file forms according to protocol. Incident reports are often maintained separately from prehospital reports.
- **Special-situation reports**: Used for events/incidents that must be reported to an outside authority or as a supplement to the prehospital report. Fill out the report as soon as possible and include the names of all parties involved; use objective descriptions, and avoid stating conclusions. Maintain a personal copy.
- **Transfer reports**: Ensure that they contain minimum data sets and provide a transfer signature. These are used during hand-off.

EMS Communication

DYNAMICS OF THE COMMUNICATION PROCESS

The communication process, which includes the sender-receiver feedback loop, is based on Claude Shannon's article, "A Mathematical Theory of Communication" (1948), in which he provided the basis for information theory and described three necessary steps of successful communication: encoding a message, transmitting it through a channel, and decoding it. The resultant communication process begins with the sender, who serves as the encoder and determines the content of the message. The medium is the form the message takes (digital, written, audiovisual), and the channel is the method of delivery (mail, radio, TV, phone, email, text message). The recipient (receiver), who acts as the decoder, determines the meaning from the message. Feedback helps to determine whether or not the communication is successful and whether the message is understood as intended. This process is referred to as the sender-receiver feedback loop. Context is the environment (physical and psychological) in which the communication occurs, and interference is any factor that impacts the communication process. Interference may be external (such as environmental noise) or internal (such as emotional distress or anxiety).

EMS SYSTEM COMMUNICATION

With the **EMS personnel arrival** at the scene of an incident, he or she should assess the situation and the need for added resources, such as additional EMS personnel or police, and contact the appropriate authorities to request assistance. When additional EMS personnel arrive or contact is made with medical control or the receiving facility, the EMS provider should self-identify and provide a verbal report of the patient's current condition, including demographic information such as age and gender. The provider should report the patient's chief complaint and provide any history that is pertinent as well as the condition of the patient on arrival and any history of major illnesses. The EMS provider should also report the results of the patient assessment, including the vital signs and any physical/psychological findings, as well as any treatment provided and the patient's response to the treatment. The provider should communicate with law enforcement officers and other responders, such as firefighters, especially regarding safety concerns.

COMPONENTS

Components of an **EMS communication system** include the base station of a two-way radio system, which is in a fixed location, such as a dispatch center. The base station facilitates communication among a number of hand-held/mobile radios. There is often only one channel per base station, so additional base stations may be installed to add more channels. Radio transmitters/receivers may be vehicular mounted or mobile, although mobile transmitters/receivers may have limited range because they tend to have lower power (1–5 watts) than do base stations (20–50 watts). Typically, the mobile device has a range of 10–15 miles over average terrain, but it is shorter in rugged terrain. The Federal Communications Commission (FCC) controls radio frequencies, and those used for EMS are in the public safety pool.

COMMUNICATION WITH MEDICAL CONTROL

The EMS provider may be in communication with **medical control** regarding a patient's condition and need for medication. Medical control may be at the receiving facility or at a separate site. Upon receiving an order by phone or radio, the EMS provider should repeat back the order and dosage to ensure that the message was received correctly. When using the radio, the radio must be turned on and the press-to-talk (PTT) button must be pressed before beginning transmission. The provider should address the medical control person by name and give the name of their EMS unit. Transmissions should be brief and to the point, avoiding unnecessary pleasantries, codes, agency-specific terms, profanity, and meaningless phrases, keeping in mind that the airways are public. The EMS provider should give individual digits for long numbers, use "affirmative" and "negative" in place of "yes" and "no," and say "over" when the transmission is finished. Reports should be objective rather than opinion based and should avoid offering a diagnosis. The dispatcher must be notified when the unit leaves the scene.

Phone/cellular communication is similar to radio communication, but EMS personnel should be familiar with important phone numbers (such as medical control, hospitals, trauma centers) or have the numbers prominently posted for access. They should also be aware of dead spots that may prevent communication and should have a backup plan (radio) for when cellular transmission fails.

EFFECTIVE COMMUNICATION AND INTERVIEW TECHNIQUES

Effective communication begins with a self-introduction and an introduction of other team members to the patient and family and includes respecting the patient's privacy by shielding the patient from passersby if possible and avoiding loudly repeating any patient information. If possible, the EMS provider should adjust lighting and limit outside distractions such as noise.

If possible, the patient should be **interviewed** alone or should be asked if he or she wants family members present. Verbal and nonverbal responses should be observed during an interview. Information should include not only the patient's facts but also the patient's attitude and concerns. The EMS provider should ask one question at a time in language that the patient understands and avoid providing false reassurances and advice or interrupting. Strategies include the following:

- Ask **open-ended informational questions** (as opposed to yes/no) with "who," "what," "where," "when," and "how," but avoid questions with "why" if possible.
  - Instead of "Why do you continue to use heroin?" ask "Have you tried to quit drug use?"
- Ask brief **clarifying questions**: "How long have you had weakness in your left side?"
- Provide a **list of options**: "Is your headache throbbing, stabbing, or dull?"
- **Rephrase/reflect** to encourage clarification.
  - Patient: "My husband had the same type of fall and died a month later."
  - EMS Provider: "You're afraid you might die from this fall."

SPECIAL INTERVIEW SITUATIONS

HOSTILE, AGGRESSIVE, OR IMPAIRED PATIENTS

Interviewing **hostile patients** requires a calm response, avoiding negative responses and using reflective statements, such as "I can understand your feelings." The EMS provider should maintain eye contact (50–60% of the time) and try to defuse the situation, but he or she should avoid staring or standing too close and having crossed arms because this may be misinterpreted as threatening behavior. If patients are **sexually aggressive**, it's important to tell them that the behavior is inappropriate and to ask them to stop. When interviewing patients under the **influence of drugs or alcohol**, try to ask essential questions such as the type and amount of drug/alcohol ingested. Obtain information from family or friends if necessary. When patients are **hearing impaired**, the EMS provider should face the person directly, speak slowly and distinctly (but avoid shouting), provide information in writing if possible, use pantomime, and try to reduce environmental noise. Knowledge of the alphabet in sign language can be very useful to communicate with the deaf, especially if a sign-language translator is unavailable.

ELDERLY PATIENTS

When interviewing **elderly patients**, EMS personnel should be alert to possible cognitive, hearing, or vision impairments, especially if the patient appears confused upon questioning or his or her answers are inappropriate. They should ask if the patient has eyeglasses or a hearing aid and should obtain them if possible. The patient's family may be able to assist with the interview. If the patient's speech is unclear, he or she may need to put in dentures. When communicating with a **pediatric patient**, the EMS provider should have the parent or caregiver comfort the child and answer questions, especially if the child is an infant or is very young. The provider should use simple sentences and age-appropriate language and explain to the child what he or she is doing to help alleviate the child's fear. Adolescents should be addressed directly even if a parent or caregiver is providing some information, and, in some cases, the adolescent will provide more information if the parent/caregiver is not present.

NON-ENGLISH OR LIMITED ENGLISH-SPEAKING PATIENTS

The EMS provider should begin an interview with a **non-English or limited English-speaking patient** first in English. If a patient does not respond verbally and appears confused and/or frightened when questioned, and it is suspected that the patient doesn't speak English, the provider should ask directly if he or she can understand English. When a patient is a non-English speaking or a limited English speaker, the important thing is to communicate. Although children, friends, bystanders, and family are not usually used as translators, in emergent or life-threatening situations, an exception is made. The EMS provider may use signs, gestures, and pantomime to communicate and use simple words or phrases, such as "Pain?" and "OK?" because even non-English speakers may understand a few words. The provider may use a language line if available and the situation permits, and he or she should alert the receiving hospital of the need for a translator as well as providing information about the patient's language. The EMS provider should point to a body part before touching it.

THERAPEUTIC COMMUNICATION TECHNIQUES

Therapeutic communication begins with respect for the individual/family and the assumption that all communication, verbal and nonverbal, has meaning. Listening must be done empathetically. Techniques that facilitate communication include the following:

Introduction	Make a personal introduction and use the individual's name: "Mrs. Brown, I am Toby Williams, your EMS provider."
Encouragement	Use an open-ended opening question: "Is there anything you'd like to discuss?" Acknowledge comments: Say "yes" and "I understand." Allow silence and observe nonverbal behavior rather than trying to force a conversation. Ask for clarification if the patient's statements are unclear. Reflect the patient's statements back (use sparingly): • Individual: "I hate this hospital." • EMS Provider: "You hate this hospital?"
Empathy	Make observations: "You are shaking," and "You seem worried." Recognize feelings: • Individual: "I want to get well." • EMS Provider: "It must be hard for you to deal with this illness." Provide information as honestly and completely as possible about the patient's condition, treatment, and procedures and respond to the individual's questions and concerns.
Exploration	Verbally express implied messages: • Individual: "This treatment is too much trouble." • EMS Provider: "Do you think the treatment isn't helping you?" Explore a topic, but allow the individual to terminate the discussion without further probing: "I'd like to hear how you feel about that."
Orientation	Indicate reality: • Individual: "Someone is screaming." • EMS Provider: "That sound was a police siren." Comment on distortions without directly agreeing or disagreeing: • Individual: "That policeman promised I could go to St. John's Hospital." • EMS Provider: "Really? That's surprising because this ambulance is based at County Hospital."
Collaboration	Work together to achieve better results: "Maybe if we talk about this, we can figure out a way to make the treatment easier for you."
Validation	Seek validation: "Do you feel better now?" or "Did the medication help you breathe better?"

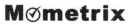

NONTHERAPEUTIC COMMUNICATION

Although using therapeutic communication is important, it is equally important to avoid interjecting **nontherapeutic communication**, which can effectively block effective communication. **Avoid the following**:

Stating meaningless clichés	"Don't worry. Everything will be fine." "Isn't it a nice day?"
Providing advice	"You should…" or "The best thing to do is…." It's better when individuals ask for advice to provide facts and encourage individuals to make their own decisions.
Providing inappropriate approval	This can prevent the individual from expressing true feelings or concerns. Individual: "I shouldn't cry about this." EMS Provider: "That's right. You're an adult."
Asking for explanations of behavior not directly related to individual care	Asking for explanations such as "Why are you upset?" may require analysis and an explanation of feelings on the individual's part.
Agreeing rather than accepting and responding	Agreeing with individual's statements "I agree with you" or "You are right" can make it difficult for the individual to change his/her statement or opinion later.
Making negative judgments	"You should stop arguing with the paramedics."
Devaluing an individual's feelings	"Everyone gets upset at times."
Disagreeing directly	"That can't be true" or "I think you are wrong."
Defending against criticism	"The doctor was not being rude; he's just very busy today."
Changing the subject	This avoids dealing with uncomfortable subjects: Individual: "I'm never going to get well." EMS Provider: "We'll contact your family in a few minutes."
Making inappropriate literal responses	Even as a joke, this is not appropriate, especially if the individual is confused or having difficulty expressing ideas: Individual: "There are bugs crawling under my skin." EMS Provider: "I'll get some bug spray."
Challenging to establish reality	This often increases confusion and frustration: Individual: "I'm dying!" EMS Provider: If you were dying, you wouldn't be able to yell and kick."
Filling silence with words	Some cultures and individuals allow more silent time in communication.

CULTURAL COMPETENCE

There are a number of issues related to cultural competence in communicating with others.

- **Eye contact:** Many cultures use eye contact differently than what is common in the United States. Some patients and families, such as Asians, Native Americans, and Arabs, may avoid direct eye contact, considering it rude, or they may look away to signal disapproval or may look down to signal respect. Careful observation of the way family members use eye contact can help to determine what will be most comfortable for the patient/family.
- **Distance**: Some cultures stand close to others (<4 feet) when speaking (Middle Easterners, Hispanics), and others stand at a greater distance (>4 feet) (Northern Europeans, many Americans). There is a considerable difference relating to concepts of personal space among cultures. Allowing the family to approach or observing whether they tend to move closer, lean forward, or move back can help to determine a comfortable distance for communication.
- **Time**: Americans tend to be time oriented, and they expect people to be on time, but time is viewed more flexibly in many other cultures.

CULTURAL CONSIDERATIONS

Cultural considerations when communicating with patients include the following:

Mexican

- Mexican culture perceives time with more flexibility than does American culture, so if patients/family need to be present at a particular time, the EMS provider should specify the exact time ("be here at 1:30 PM") and explain the reason rather than saying something that is more vague, such as "be here after lunch."
- People may appear to be unassertive or unable to make decisions when they are simply showing respect to the EMS provider by being deferent.
- In traditional families, the males make decisions, so a woman may wait for the husband or other males in the family to make decisions about her treatment or care.

Middle Eastern

- In Middle Eastern countries, males make the decisions, so issues for discussion or decision should be directed to males, such as the patient's spouse or son, and males may be direct in stating what they want, sometimes appearing demanding.
- Middle Easterners often require less personal space and may stand very close.
- If a male EMS provider must care for a female patient, then the family should be advised that *only* medical treatments, not personal care, will be done by the male provider.

Asian

- Asian families may expect EMS personnel to remain authoritative and to give directions and may not question their authority.
- Disagreeing is considered impolite. "Yes" may only mean that the person is heard, not that they agree with the person. When asked if they understand, they may indicate that they do even when they clearly do not so as not to offend the EMS provider.
- Asians may avoid eye contact as an indication of respect.

Legal and Ethical Issues

NEGLIGENCE

Negligence indicates that proper care has not been provided, based on established standards. Reasonable care uses a rationale for decision-making in relation to providing care. State regulations regarding negligence may vary, but they all have some statutes of limitation, governmental immunity, and Good Samaritan laws that may provide a defense. **Types of negligence** include:

- **Negligent conduct**: Failure to provide reasonable care or to protect/assist another, based on existing standards and expertise.
- **Gross negligence**: Willfully providing inadequate care while disregarding safety/security.
- **Contributory negligence**: The injured party contributes to his or her own harm.
- **Comparative negligence**: The amount of negligence attributed to each individual involved.

If the charge of negligence is supported, the patient may collect physical (lost earnings due to injury), psychological (pain and suffering), and punitive damages. The four necessary elements of negligence (failure to follow the standards of care) are as follows:

1. **Duty of care**: The defendant (healthcare provider) had a duty to provide adequate care and/or protect the plaintiff's (patient's) safety.
2. **Breach of duty**: The defendant failed to carry out the duty to care, resulting in danger, injury, or harm to the plaintiff.
3. **Damages**: The plaintiff experienced illness or injury as a result of the breach of duty.
4. **Causation**: The plaintiff's illness or injury is directly caused by the defendant's negligent breach of duty.

ADDITIONAL CIVIL AND CRIMINAL OFFENSES

Abandonment occurs if the EMS provider withdraws from providing care contrary to a patient's desire or knowledge and fails to arrange for appropriate care by others, resulting in harm to the patient. **Assault** occurs if an EMS provider threatens a patient in such a way that the patient becomes fearful of harm, whereas **battery** occurs when the EMS provider intentionally injures a patient, such as by hitting or shoving the person. Assault and battery often occur together.

STATUTORY RESPONSIBILITIES AND MANDATORY REPORTING

The EMS provider must practice within the **scope of responsibility**, which is outlined by each state's medical practice act. The EMS provider must be certified/licensed according to state requirements and meet appropriate educational standards regarding preparation and continuing education. The provider has a duty to the patients, the medical director, and the public and functions under government and medical oversight.

Although laws about **mandatory reporting** vary from state to state, healthcare providers, including EMS personnel, are considered mandatory reporters in all states and must report suspected cases of child and elder abuse and neglect. The EMS provider must follow state guidelines for reporting because simply notifying the receiving facility of suspected abuse or neglect is not adequate. The EMS provider should be familiar with the signs of abuse and neglect (certain types of fractures; unexplained or multiple bruises; suspicious bruise patterns; burns; hair loss; and inadequate food, clothing, and shelter).

EVIDENCE PRESERVATION

When an incident may involve **court cases**, such as with gunshot wounds, knife wounds, and rape, the EMS provider should take steps to **preserve evidence**, although providing emergent medical care takes priority. The provider should try to avoid disturbing items at the scene of the incident and should assess the environment and document any unusual findings, remembering that the environment and the patient are both considered to be part of the crime scene. The EMS provider should collaborate with law enforcement officers at the scene. If the patient has had a gunshot wound or a knife wound, the provider should not cut through the holes in the clothing but should cut along seams or away from the injuries. Any clothing or belongings removed during treatment should be secured separately in a paper bag (or plastic if paper is not available) and delivered with the patient to the receiving facility or to law enforcement officers. When the patient is describing the event, the EMS provider should document using quotations rather than summarizing.

ETHICS

ETHICAL PRINCIPLES AND MORAL OBLIGATIONS

Ethics is a branch of philosophy that studies morality—concepts of right and wrong. Applied ethics is the use of ethical principles, such as autonomy (right to self-determination), beneficence (acting to benefit another), nonmaleficence (doing no harm), verity (being truthful), and justice (equally distributing resources/care). Ethical conflicts may occur because of differences in cultural and ethical values, but they may also result from decisions that must be made regarding care, such as whether to provide CPR in a wilderness situation when the treatment is likely futile. They can also involve situations involving triage in which some patients are given priority over others, situations that involve professional misconduct (such as EMS personnel being abusive toward patients), and incidents of patient dumping because the patient has inadequate insurance or an inability to pay. EMS personnel have a moral obligation to make decisions about care in good faith and in the patient's best interest.

DECISION-MAKING MODELS

Decision-making models help guide the decision-making process on the basis of ethical principles:

- **Do no harm**: This model is based on nonmaleficence, the requirement that a treatment provided do no harm; however, by their nature, some treatments can and often do harm patients, so the underlying intent and goal of treatment must be considered when making decisions. For example, CPR may be carried out to save a patient's life and may be done with correct technique but still may result in rib fractures.
- **In good faith**: The motive for a decision should be honest and fair, and decisions should be made with a sincere intention to do good even though the outcome may be negative. For example, EMS personnel may provide a treatment for a patient in good faith although the treatment proves to be ineffective for that particular patient.
- **Patient's best interest**: Making a decision in the patient's best interest includes considering the patient's or parents' (in the case of children) wishes, the best clinical judgment, the best choice of various options, the chances for improvement/decline, and religious/cultural preferences.

Patient Rights

HEALTH INSURANCE PORTABILITY AND ACCOUNTABILITY ACT OF 1996 (HIPAA)

Sensitive information is classified under the **Health Insurance Portability and Accountability Act of 1996** (HIPAA) as protected health information (PHI) and includes the following:

- Any information about an individual's past, present, or future health or condition (mental or physical)
- Provision of health care
- Any identifying information related to payment for healthcare services, including name, address, Social Security number, or birth date, and any document or material that contains the identifying information

Personal information can be shared with a spouse, legal guardians, those with durable power of attorney for the patient, and those involved in the care of the patient, such as physicians, without a specific release. HIPAA mandates the following privacy and security rules to ensure that health information and individual privacy are protected:

- **Privacy rule**: Protected information includes any information included in the medical record (electronic or paper), conversations between the doctor and other healthcare providers, billing information, and any other form of health information.
- **Security rule**: Any electronic health information must be secure and protected against threats, hazards, or nonpermitted disclosure.

> **Review Video: HIPAA**
> Visit mometrix.com/academy and enter code: 412009

INFORMED CONSENT

Patients or their families must provide informed consent for all treatments that they receive. This includes a thorough explanation of all procedures, treatments, and associated risks. Patients/families should be apprised of all options and allowed input on the type of treatments. Patients/families should be apprised of all reasonable risks and any complications that might be life threatening or increase morbidity.

The American Medical Association has established **guidelines for informed consent**. Informed consent includes all of the following components:

- Explanation of the diagnosis
- Nature of and reason for the treatment or procedure
- Risks and benefits
- Alternative options (regardless of cost or insurance coverage)
- Risks and benefits of alternative options
- Risks and benefits of not having a treatment or procedure

Obtaining informed consent is a requirement in all states. The requirement for informed consent may be waived in life-threatening situations and if the EMS provider cannot obtain informed consent because the patient cannot communicate and legal consent cannot be obtained.

CONDITIONS FOR CONSENT

The conditions for consent for care and decision-making capacity include the following:

- **18 years or older OR court-emancipated minors**: Patients who are younger (and not court-emancipated) may have the right to give consent for all or some medical treatment in some states. State laws vary; for example, the age of consent for medical treatment in Alabama is 14.
- **Mentally competent to make decisions**: Impairment by mental disability, injury, illness, or substance abuse (intoxication) may impede an adult's ability to provide consent.

Consent may be expressed if the patient is able to give informed consent, or it may be implied, such as when care is provided in an emergent situation in which the patient is unable to give consent. Parents or caregivers give consent for minors younger than the age of 18 unless they have been emancipated. If parents or caregivers are unavailable to give consent, life-saving emergent care, general medical assessment, and medical care to prevent further injury or harm can be provided without consent.

ADVANCE DIRECTIVES, DURABLE POWER OF ATTORNEY, AND DO-NOT-RESUSCITATE (DNR) ORDER

In accordance with federal and state laws, individuals have the **right to self-determination** in health care, including decisions about end-of-life care through **advance directives** such as living wills and the right to assign a surrogate person to make decisions through a **durable power of attorney**. Patients should routinely be questioned about an advanced directive because they may present at a healthcare organization without the document. Patients who have indicated that they desire a **do-not-resuscitate (DNR) order** should not receive resuscitative treatments for terminal illness or conditions in which meaningful recovery cannot occur. Patients and families of those with terminal illnesses should be questioned as to whether the patients are hospice patients. For those with DNR requests or those withdrawing life support, staff should provide the patient palliative rather than curative measures, such as pain control and/or oxygen, and emotional support to the patient and family. Religious traditions and beliefs about death should be treated with respect.

HUMAN RESEARCH SUBJECT PROTECTION

Protection of human subjects is covered in the Health and Human Services, Title 45 Code of Federal Regulations, part 46. This regulation provides guidance for institutional review boards (IRBs) for those involved in research and outlines requirements. Institutions engaged in nonexempt research must submit an assurance of compliance (document) to the **Office for Human Research Protections** (OHRP), agreeing to comply with all requirements for research projects. Subjects cannot be used solely as a means to an end, but research should hold the possibility of benefit to the subject. Risks should be minimal, and selection of subjects should be equitable. Some research populations are granted additional protections because of their vulnerability and susceptibility to coercion; these populations include children, prisoners, pregnant women, human fetuses and neonates, mentally disabled people, and people who are economically or educationally disadvantaged. When cooperative research projects are conducted involving more than one institution, then each must safeguard the rights of subjects, ensuring informed consent and privacy.

Abuse and Neglect

ELDER ABUSE

Types of elder abuse include the following:

- **Physical**: Various types of assault related to hitting, kicking, pulling hair, shoving, and pushing. Patients may be forcibly confined, forced into seclusion, and/or force-fed to the point that they choke on food.
- **Psychological**: Caregivers may threaten to hit the patient, brandish a weapon, and/or tell the person to commit suicide. Ongoing intimidation may make the patient terrified and anxious. Sometimes, caregivers threaten to injure pets or family members, increasing the patient's fear.
- **Sexual**: Types of sexual abuse include the following:
  - Physical: Fondling, kissing, and rape
  - Emotional: Exhibitionism
  - Verbal: Sexual harassment, using obscene language, and threatening
- **Financial**: Financial abuse includes the following:
  - Outright stealing of property or persuading patients to give away possessions
  - Forcing patients to sign away property
  - Emptying bank and savings accounts and using stolen credit cards
  - Convincing the person to invest money in fraudulent schemes
  - Taking money for home renovations that are not done

CHILD ABUSE

Children rarely admit to abuse (physical, sexual, or emotional) and often attempt to protect the abusing parent. Therefore, suspicion of abuse depends on other indicators such as the following:

- **Behavioral**: The child may be overly compliant or fearful with obvious changes in demeanor when a parent/caregiver is present. Some children act out with aggression toward other children or animals. Children may become depressed, suicidal, or present with sleeping or eating disorders. Behaviors may become increasingly self-destructive as the child ages, including inappropriate sexualized behavior.
- **Physical/Sexual**: The type, location, and extent of injuries can raise the suspicion of abuse. Head and facial injuries and bruising are common signs of physical abuse, as are bite or burn marks and spiral fractures. There may be handprints or grab marks and unusual bruising, such as across the buttocks. Any bruising, swelling, or tearing of the genital area and the identification of sexually transmitted infections are also causes for concern.

Suspected abuse must be reported to the appropriate authorities, according to protocol, with careful documentation of findings and statements by the child or caregivers.

INJURIES CONSISTENT WITH DOMESTIC VIOLENCE/ABUSE

Injuries consistent with domestic violence/abuse include the following:

- Characteristic injuries:
  - Ruptured eardrum
  - Rectal/genital injury—burns, bites, trauma
  - Scrapes and bruises about the neck, face, head, trunk, arms
  - Cuts, bruises, and fractures of the face
- Patterns of injuries:
  - "Bathing suit" pattern—injuries on parts of body that are usually covered with clothing because the perpetrator wants to hide the evidence of abuse
  - Head and neck injuries (50%)
- Abusive injuries (rarely attributable to accidents):
  - Bites, bruises, rope and cigarette burns, and welts in the outline of weapons (belt marks)
  - Bilateral injuries of the arms/legs
- Defensive injuries:
  - Back-of-the-body injury from being attacked while crouched on the floor facedown
  - Located on the soles of the feet from kicking at a perpetrator
  - Located on the ulnar aspect of the hands or palm from blocking blows

NEGLECT AND LACK OF SUPERVISED CARE

Children and older or impaired adults may suffer from profound **neglect or a lack of supervision** that places them at risk. Indicators include the following:

- Appearing dirty and unkempt, sometimes with infestations of lice, and wearing ill-fitting, torn clothing and shoes.
- Being tired and sleepy during the daytime.
- Having excessive medical or dental problems, such as extensive dental caries.
- Missing doctor appointments and not receiving proper immunizations.
- Being underweight for their current stage of development.
- Lacking assistive devices or misplaced hearing aids/eyeglasses.
- Left in soiled or urine-/feces-soiled clothing.
- Clothing is inadequate (such as lack of a coat/sweater during winter or dirty, torn, ill-fitting clothes).

Neglect can be difficult to assess, especially if the EMS provider is serving a homeless or very disadvantaged population. Home visits may be needed to ascertain if there is adequate food, clothing, or supervision, and this is beyond the scope of care provided by the EMS provider. Thus, suspicions should be reported to the appropriate authorities who can arrange a follow-up assessment of the home environment.

Public Health

PUBLIC HEALTH SYSTEM

EMS are part of the **public health system**, a network of private, nonprofit, and government agencies and healthcare providers providing public health services in a wide range of areas. The primary services provided by the public health system include the following:

- Monitoring community health
- Identifying hazards to health in the environment and the community
- Educating people about health issues
- Mobilizing various agencies and individuals to take action
- Enforcing public safety laws and regulations
- Ensuring that healthcare providers are qualified, licensed, and certified as required
- Ensuring that health care is available
- Assessing the effectiveness of health care
- Researching health problems and finding solutions

Public health laws and regulations may be federal, state, or tribal and may cover issues such as immunization requirements, drinking water and sewage system standards, air quality, water fluoridation, restrictions on tobacco use (age and place), restrictions on drinking (age, driving), speed limits, prenatal care, abuse (child, older adult, sexual, and domestic), safety equipment, and safe lifting. Healthy People 2030, from the U.S. Department of Health and Human Services, provides goals and objectives for health-related public policies.

PUBLIC EDUCATION REGARDING SAFETY MEASURES

EMS personnel are often involved in **public education** regarding the following safety measures:

- **Car seats**: Car seats should be properly secured in the backseat of a motor vehicle. They should be rear facing for infants and toddlers up to 2 years of age (or the maximum recommended height and weight) and forward-facing with a harness for toddlers and preschoolers. School-aged children should use booster seats with a belt and harness until they are at least 4 feet 9 inches tall. Children younger than age 13 should not ride in a front seat.
- **Seat belts**: All people in a motor vehicle should be secured with seat belts and shoulder harnesses.
- **Helmets**: Helmets should fit properly and snugly, cover the top of the forehead, and have a securing chinstrap. They should be worn when riding a bicycle or motorcycle and engaging in sports activities such as rollerblading but not on playground equipment or when climbing trees.

Additional safety equipment that EMS personnel should be familiar with includes home alarms (smoke alarms and carbon monoxide alarms) and mobility aids for fall prevention such as safety rails, grab bars, canes, and walkers.

LEVELS OF DISEASE PREVENTION

Levels of disease prevention include the following:

- **Primary**: The goal is to prevent the initial occurrence of a health problem, such as a disease or injury, through activities such as immunizations, smoking cessation, fluoride supplementation of water, promotion of seat belt and helmet use, and use of child car seat restraints. Interventions are often aimed at the general public or large groups of people.
- **Secondary**: The goal is to identify diseases or conditions quickly and provide prompt intervention to provide treatment and prevent further disability through activities such as BP screenings, breast and testicular self-examinations, hearing and vision screenings, mammography, and pregnancy testing.
- **Tertiary**: The goal is to assist those who already have disease or disability to prevent further progress of the disease and to allow people to achieve the maximum quality of life through activities such as support groups, counseling, diet and exercise, stress management, and supportive services.

Advanced EMT Practice Test

Want to take this practice test in an online interactive format?
Check out the bonus page, which includes interactive practice questions and
much more: **mometrix.com/bonus948/advancedemt**

SCAN HERE

1. All of the following can produce an Antabuse-like reaction except

   a. Antibiotics
   b. Metronidazole
   c. Cocaine
   d. Diabetic medications

2. Lead II on the ECG indicates

   a. Presence of an MI
   b. Regularity of the heartbeat
   c. Pumping capability of the heart
   d. Location of an MI

3. Regular PVCs at intervals greater than every fourth beat are known as

   a. Frequent PVCs
   b. Multifocal PVCs
   c. Ventricular quadrigeminy
   d. Trigeminal PVCs

4. Which of the following statements regarding VT is FALSE?

   a. VT may be associated with cardiac arrest.
   b. P waves are usually not discernible.
   c. If the rhythm results in a pulse, VT is not significant.
   d. Pulseless VT should be treated the same as VF.

5. The absence of any electrical activity in the heart is known as

   a. PEA
   b. Asystole
   c. Pericardial tamponade
   d. VF

6. The first step in caring for a patient with cardiac arrest should be to

   a. Set up oxygen and IV lines
   b. Immediately apply the AED
   c. Interpret the patient's cardiac rhythm
   d. Begin CPR

7. All of the following steps in the defibrillation process are valid except

    a. Double-checking the rhythm before delivering a countershock

    b. Turning on the synchronized mode when defibrillating VF

    c. Removing NTG patches before defibrillation

    d. Checking the carotid pulse if the rhythm changes

8. The best line of care for a patient who is hyperventilating is to

    a. Plug the portals of the oxygen mask to induce rebreathing

    b. Ask the patient to breathe into a paper bag

    c. Administer oxygen

    d. Administer a nebulized bronchodilator

9. Spontaneous pneumothorax may be caused by

    a. Menstruation

    b. Anxiety

    c. Carbon monoxide

    d. Oral contraceptives

10. Which of the following may be useful in a patient with carbon monoxide poisoning?

    a. Pulse oximetry

    b. Oxygen saturation

    c. Hyperbaric oxygen

    d. Blood glucose

11. All of the following may cause coma except

    a. Vitamin deficiency

    b. Hypercalcemia

    c. Hyperglycemia

    d. Fever

12. A common cause of seizures in adults is

    a. Fever

    b. Infection

    c. Vitamin deficiency

    d. Catatonia

13. Which of the following statements regarding seizure is FALSE?

    a. Seizure patients may bite their tongue.

    b. Seizure may result in a neurological condition similar to stroke.

    c. Restraining muscle movement may stop a seizure.

    d. A patient may become violent after a seizure.

14. The roommate of a 21-year-old woman calls you to their apartment. The young woman has severe abdominal pain and vaginal bleeding and has gone into shock. This patient is most likely suffering from

    a. Appendicitis

    b. PID

    c. Bowel obstruction

    d. Ectopic pregnancy

15. The best course of treatment for a patient with hypoglycemia is to give the patient

 a. Saccharine
 b. Aspartame
 c. Oral glucose
 d. Insulin

16. Which of the following conditions is associated with an acetone-like breath odor?

 a. Hypoglycemia
 b. Hyperglycemia
 c. Diabetes
 d. DKA

17. Signs and symptoms of HHNC include

 a. Kussmaul respirations
 b. Fruity breath odor
 c. Altered mental status
 d. Rapid pulse

18. When treating a poisoning victim, which of the following takes LOWEST priority?

 a. Determining the exact substance the patient has taken
 b. Placing the patient on a cardiac monitor
 c. Proper positioning of the patient
 d. Pulse oximetry

19. Proper care for a patient with heat stroke includes

 a. Salt pills
 b. Diuretics
 c. Air conditioning
 d. Cold drinks

20. Which of the following statements regarding hypothermia is FALSE?

 a. Hypothermia may resemble cardiac arrest
 b. Rewarming the extremities may increase body temperature
 c. Hypothermia may mimic death
 d. Rewarming the extremities may decrease body temperature

21. Asthma in children is associated with

 a. Age 6 to 18 months
 b. Viral infection
 c. Family history
 d. Pneumonia

22. In pediatric patients, bronchiolitis is

 a. Seasonal
 b. Caused by a virus
 c. Associated with asthma
 d. Responsive to medication

23. The most important intervention in a child with head trauma is

  a. Immobilization
  b. Ventilation
  c. Resuscitation
  d. Transport

24. The first line of treatment for a child with severe hypothermia should include

  a. Performing CPR
  b. Rubbing the affected extremities
  c. Endotracheal intubation
  d. High-concentration oxygen

25. All of the following may be used in patients with shock except

  a. Lactated Ringer's solution
  b. 5% Dextrose in water
  c. Normal saline
  d. Plasma

26. All of the following are symptoms of cholinergic crisis except

  a. Salivation
  b. Incontinence
  c. Cardiac arrest
  d. Emesis

27. In patient triage, which of the following conditions would be considered high-priority?

  a. Respiratory arrest
  b. Burns
  c. Shock
  d. Spinal cord damage

28. An Apgar score of 10 in a newly born infant indicates

  a. Moderate distress
  b. No distress
  c. Severe distress
  d. Cyanosis

29. The first step in treatment of cardiopulmonary arrest in a newly born infant is

  a. Intubation
  b. IV fluids
  c. Ventilation
  d. Atropine

30. The Apgar score should be obtained

  a. One to five minutes after birth
  b. Before beginning resuscitation
  c. Immediately at birth
  d. Only if resuscitation is needed

31. The "G" component of the Apgar score stands for

 a. Grimace
 b. Grasp
 c. Good respiratory effort
 d. Growth

32. Which of the following may be administered to a newborn with hypoglycemia and altered consciousness?

 a. 25% dextrose and water
 b. 10% dextrose and water
 c. 50% dextrose and water
 d. Ringer's lactate

33. After an infant's head is delivered, the first line of action should be to

 a. Suction the nose
 b. Suction the mouth
 c. Cover the head
 d. Dry the head

34. Secondary apnea in a newborn is treated by

 a. Touching the infant
 b. Suctioning the mouth
 c. Suctioning the nose
 d. Assisted ventilation

35. Drug withdrawal or overdose may be treated by

 a. Antabuse
 b. Oxygen
 c. Ice immersion
 d. Ipecac

36. All of the following may mimic alcohol intoxication EXCEPT

 a. Hypoglycemia
 b. Head trauma
 c. Antabuse
 d. Drug abuse

37. In elderly patients, symptoms of which of the following can mimic those of cardiac or respiratory conditions?

 a. Alcohol abuse
 b. Drug abuse
 c. Depression
 d. Psychosis

38. The drug cocaine is classified as a

 a. Hallucinogen
 b. Stimulant
 c. Narcotic
 d. Depressant

39. The suffix "phasia" refers to

a. Speech
b. Fear
c. Order
d. Eating

40. The prefix "endo" refers to

a. On
b. Swelling
c. Within
d. Outer

41. Cardiac tamponade typically results from

a. Head trauma
b. Bleeding
c. Cardiac arrest
d. Chest trauma

42. COPD and respiratory failure may result in

a. Respiratory alkalosis
b. Respiratory acidosis
c. Stroke
d. Pneumothorax

43. Which of the following drugs is used for patients with acute MI?

a. Adenosine
b. Aspirin
c. Amiodarone
d. Dexamethasone

44. Vasopressin may be given in all of the following cases EXCEPT

a. As an alternative to epinephrine
b. To treat PEA
c. To pediatric patients with VF
d. To treat asystole

45. Epinephrine is contraindicated in

a. Hypotension
b. Hypertension
c. Cardiac arrest
d. Asthma

46. An area of potential threat in law enforcement operations is known as the

a. Hot zone
b. Warm zone
c. Cold zone
d. HAZMAT zone

47. A common cause of asymmetric pupils in an elderly patient is

   a.   COPD
   b.   Skull fracture
   c.   CHF
   d.   Glaucoma

48. Treatment of a child with hypothermia with a discernible heart rate should include

   a.   Tracheal intubation
   b.   CPR
   c.   Resuscitation
   d.   Starting an IV

49. Which of the following statements regarding chest and abdominal trauma in a child is FALSE?

   a.   Treatment of chest and abdominal trauma should be the same as that for an adult.
   b.   Respiratory distress may be a sign of abdominal trauma.
   c.   The ideal treatment for a child with chest trauma is rapid transport to a hospital.
   d.   Abdominal trauma should ideally be treated in the field.

50. Which of the following is recommended for cervical spine immobilization in a small child?

   a.   Using a KED
   b.   Using cravats
   c.   Strapping the child under the axillae
   d.   Pulling the child's head from the safety seat

51. All of the following may be used to treat seizures in a child EXCEPT

   a.   Rectal diazepam
   b.   IV glucose
   c.   IV lorazepam
   d.   IV lactated Ringer's solution

52. Stiffness of the neck and Kernig's sign are symptoms of

   a.   Epilepsy
   b.   Head trauma
   c.   Meningitis
   d.   Shock

53. Rales are indicative of which pediatric condition?

   a.   Shock
   b.   Pneumonia
   c.   Bronchiolitis
   d.   Croup

54. In a child, shock may be indicated by

   a.   Mottling of the skin
   b.   Hypertension
   c.   Rales
   d.   Respiratory distress

55. Which of the following may be used during intraosseous infusion in a child?

a. Hypodermic needles
b. Spinal needles
c. Normal saline
d. Nasal cannula

56. Compared with adults, which of the following is less likely to be injured in children?

a. Head
b. Ribs
c. Liver
d. Nerves

57. Which of the following statements regarding a pregnant trauma victim is FALSE?

a. The heart rate is increased.
b. The BP is lower.
c. The patient should be supine.
d. The patient should be placed on her left side.

58. A condition in pregnant women marked by hypertension and fluid retention is known as

a. Ectopic pregnancy
b. Gestational diabetes
c. Preeclampsia
d. Uterine rupture

59. A typical sign of placenta previa during pregnancy is

a. Severe abdominal pain
b. Painless bright red bleeding
c. Minimal vaginal bleeding
d. Palpable fetus in abdomen

60. In the case of a prolapsed cord presentation, the Advanced EMT should

a. Place the mother in a knee-to-chest position
b. Push the cord back inside
c. Form a "V" with the fingers on either side of the infant's nose and mouth
d. Cut the umbilical cord

61. Which of the following should NOT be used for resuscitation of the newly born?

a. Atropine
b. Epinephrine
c. Dextrose in water
d. Naloxone

62. Postpartum hemorrhage may be treated by all of the following EXCEPT

a. Uterine massage
b. Fluid bolus
c. IV line
d. Trendelenburg positioning

63. Right lower quadrant abdominal pain is usually indicative of

a. Cirrhosis
b. Appendicitis
c. Bowel obstruction
d. Diverticulitis

64. Epigastric pain is associated with

a. Appendicitis
b. Ectopic pregnancy
c. Myocardial ischemia
d. Hernia

65. In which of the following cases is NTG contraindicated?

a. BP greater than 100 mmHg
b. NTG prescription
c. BP below 100 mmHg
d. Headache

66. Which of the following statements regarding use of NTG is FALSE?

a. NTG may be associated with hypotension
b. NTG tablets may retain potency for months or years
c. NTG may be associated with headache
d. NTG tablets may become inactivated by exposure to air or light

67. Patients with chest pain should be assumed to have

a. Angina
b. Cardiac arrest
c. Congestive heart failure
d. MI

68. Acute MI often presents as

a. Indigestion
b. Nephrolithiasis
c. Peptic ulcer
d. Cholecystitis

69. All of the following are indicative of cardiogenic shock except

a. Altered mental status
b. Hypotension
c. Peripheral vein collapse
d. Respiratory distress

70. Which of the following drugs is contraindicated in pulmonary edema?

a. NTG
b. Morphine
c. Furosemide
d. Epinephrine

71. The signs and symptoms of pulmonary embolism may mimic those of all of the following except

  a. Pneumonia
  b. MI
  c. CHF
  d. Pneumothorax

72. A barrel-shaped chest is a sign of

  a. Asthma
  b. COPD
  c. Pulmonary embolism
  d. Spontaneous pneumothorax

73. Plasma is also known as

  a. Intracellular fluid
  b. Extracellular fluid
  c. Interstitial fluid
  d. Intravascular fluid

74. Lactated Ringer's solution is a type of

  a. Hypertonic solution
  b. Isotonic solution
  c. Hypotonic solution
  d. Electrolyte

75. Which of the following is an example of a cation?

  a. ATP
  b. Chloride
  c. Sodium
  d. Phosphate

76. The delivery of oxygenated blood to the tissues is known as

  a. Perfusion
  b. Aerobic metabolism
  c. Anaerobic metabolism
  d. Oxygenation

77. Kussmaul breathing is indicative of

  a. Metabolic alkalosis
  b. Metabolic acidosis
  c. Respiratory acidosis
  d. Respiratory alkalosis

78. Shock is typically caused by all of the following EXCEPT

  a. Fluid loss
  b. Vasodilation
  c. Hypertension
  d. Pump failure

79. Sites in the body where two bones converge are known as

a. Cartilage
b. Joints
c. Tendons
d. Ligaments

80. An abnormal accumulation of fluid in the pleural cavity is known as

a. Pneumothorax
b. Pleural effusion
c. Respiratory alkalosis
d. Cardiac tamponade

81. Which of the following components of the APVU mnemonic is incorrect?

a. A = awake and alert
b. U = unresponsive
c. V = vision impaired
d. P = responsive to painful stimuli

82. The carotid pulse is used to assess the circulation when

a. The patient is responsive.
b. The patient is unresponsive.
c. The patient is less than 1 year old.
d. The patient is pulseless.

83. Which of the following statements regarding baseline vital signs is FALSE?

a. Vital signs may vary by age.
b. Vital signs should be assessed constantly.
c. Vital signs should be assessed as a set.
d. Vital signs should be assessed individually.

84. A normal respiratory rate for an adult would be

a. 60 times per minute
b. 40 times per minute
c. 30 times per minute
d. 20 times per minute

85. Melena is characterized by

a. Vomiting of blood
b. Bright red blood in stool
c. Black, tarry stool
d. Acute MI

86. Acute abdomen is caused by all of the following EXCEPT

a. Black widow spider bite
b. Diabetic ketoacidosis
c. Myocardial infarction
d. Dog bite

87. Which of the following is a sign of increased heat production?

a. Sweating
b. Shivering
c. Decreased appetite
d. Decreased voluntary activity

88. All of the following are signs and symptoms of heat stroke EXCEPT

a. Altered level of consciousness
b. Shortness of breath
c. Profuse sweating
d. Minimal or no sweating

89. Which of the following is NOT a sign of heat exhaustion?

a. Profuse sweating
b. Altered mental status
c. Pallor
d. Hypotension

90. In treating a patient with hypothermia, the Advanced EMT should

a. Start an IV line with lactated Ringer's solution
b. Rewarm the extremities
c. Immerse the patient in warm water
d. Cover the patient with a blanket

91. Which of the following is associated with the best prognosis?

a. Dry drowning
b. Wet drowning
c. Secondary drowning
d. Seawater drowning

92. All of the following are used to assess successful ET tube placement in an infant except

a. Passage of the tube through the vocal cords
b. Breath sounds
c. Improvement in color
d. Rise and fall of the chest

93. Which of the following statements regarding PPE is FALSE?

a. Prescription glasses with side shields are acceptable eye protection.
b. Surgical masks protect against TB.
c. Coveralls are preferable to gowns as protection against body fluid exposure.
d. Vinyl gloves should never be reused.

94. An effective alternative to commercial disinfectants would be

a. Soap and water
b. Antiseptics
c. Bleach and water
d. Antibacterials

95. Treatment of a severely injured patient who is under arrest would be permissible according to

  a. Implied consent
  b. Involuntary consent
  c. Informed consent
  d. Expressed consent

96. Which of the following statements regarding refusal of care is FALSE?

  a. Mentally incompetent patients cannot give consent.
  b. Unemancipated minors cannot refuse care.
  c. Emancipated minors can refuse care.
  d. Mentally incompetent patients can refuse care.

97. All of the following types of patients can be treated under implied consent EXCEPT

  a. Mentally incompetent adult
  b. Intoxicated adult
  c. Emotionally disturbed minor
  d. Minor when a guardian is unavailable

98. The most common neurotransmitter in the sympathetic nervous system is

  a. Acetylcholine
  b. Norepinephrine
  c. Adrenaline
  d. Epinephrine

99. An example of a parasympathetic response is

  a. Tachycardia
  b. Nervousness
  c. Abdominal distress
  d. Elevated blood pressure

100. Which of the following is almost always indicative of an abnormality?

  a. S_3
  b. S_4
  c. Murmur
  d. SA node

101. Guaifenesin is classified as a _____ drug.

  a. Schedule I
  b. Schedule V
  c. Schedule IV
  d. Schedule II

102. Morphine is an example of a _____ drug.

  a. Schedule II
  b. Schedule I
  c. Schedule IV
  d. Schedule V

103. A drug classified as Pregnancy Category A is considered

    a. Contraindicated in pregnant women
    b. At remote risk of fetal harm
    c. At risk of fetal harm in animals but not humans
    d. Acceptable for use in life-threatening conditions when benefits outweigh risks

104. Acetaminophen concentrations would appear significantly higher in

    a. A 75-year-old obese patient
    b. A 25-year-old obese patient
    c. A 21-year-old normal-weight patient
    d. A 45-year-old slim patient

105. All of the following can be administered in drug form except

    a. Edrophonium
    b. Pilocarpine
    c. Acetylcholine
    d. Atropine

106. An example of a sympathetic agonist drug is

    a. Propranolol
    b. Atropine
    c. Albuterol
    d. Acetylcholine

107. Drugs given by the sublingual route are

    a. Applied directly to the skin
    b. Placed under the tongue
    c. Dissolved between the cheek and gum
    d. Injected into the dermis

108. All of the following drugs can be administered through the endotracheal tube EXCEPT

    a. Epinephrine
    b. Naloxone
    c. Metaproterenol
    d. Lidocaine

109. The fastest route of drug administration is the _____ route.

    a. Oral
    b. Intravenous
    c. Topical
    d. Endotracheal

110. An acute systemic reaction to a drug on subsequent exposure is known as

    a. Drug toxicity
    b. Tachyphylaxis
    c. Drug dependence
    d. Anaphylaxis

111. An example of drug synergism is

a. Antacids taken with tetracycline
b. Sedatives taken with barbiturates
c. Cimetidine taken with imipramine
d. Morphine taken with meperidine

112. All of the following produce a drug interaction except

a. Epinephrine taken with digoxin
b. Phenergan taken with meperidine
c. Amiodarone taken with digoxin
d. Methyldopa taken with MAO inhibitors

113. In a critically injured patient, an IV line should be placed

a. En route to the hospital
b. At the scene before transport
c. In sclerotic veins
d. After circulatory collapse

114. Lactated Ringer's solution contains

a. Free water
b. HCO_3
c. Calcium
d. Calories

115. Which of the following can be administered with blood products?

a. Lactated Ringer's solution
b. Sodium chloride 0.9%
c. Five percent dextrose in water
d. Glucose

116. No restriction of fluid flow from the IV bag to the patient is known as the

a. TKO rate
b. KVO rate
c. Wide-open rate
d. Macrodrip

117. Large-bore catheters should be used for all of the following except

a. Administration of 50% dextrose
b. Administration of blood
c. Shock patients
d. Elderly patients

118. For patient in cardiac arrest, the preferred site for IV cannulation is the

a. Jugular vein
b. Saphenous vein of the leg
c. Peripheral veins of the antecubital fossa
d. Peripheral veins of the distal extremities

119. Use of an armboard may be required in all of the following situations EXCEPT

 a. When the antecubital fossa is the venipuncture site
 b. When the wrist is the venipuncture site
 c. In a disoriented or confused patient
 d. In elderly patients

120. Which of the following statements regarding documentation of IV cannulation is FALSE?

 a. Unsuccessful attempts to start the IV must be documented.
 b. Tape should be applied over the dressing and then labeled.
 c. Tape should be labeled and then applied over the dressing.
 d. Type and gauge of the needle should be documented.

121. A pyrogenic reaction may result from

 a. Bacteria in the venipuncture site
 b. Air entering the vein
 c. Foreign proteins in the IV solution
 d. Injury to the blood vessel

122. All of the following may be helpful in placing an IV line in a moving patient EXCEPT

 a. Using an armboard to immobilize extremities
 b. Choosing smaller veins
 c. Choosing the largest vein available
 d. Using a crossover taping technique

123. Which of the following drugs can only be administered by IV push?

 a. Atropine
 b. Epinephrine 1:1000
 c. 1 g/5 mL lidocaine
 d. Adenosine

124. Two syringes are required for preparation of

 a. Ampules
 b. Reconstituted medications
 c. Piggyback infusions
 d. Intradermal TB tests

125. The subcutaneous route is used for administration of all of the following EXCEPT

 a. Vaccines
 b. Insulin
 c. Lidocaine
 d. Epinephrine

126. Which of the following IM injection sites is not recommended for young children?

 a. Dorsogluteal muscle
 b. Vastus lateralis muscle
 c. Ventrogluteal muscle
 d. Deltoid muscle

127. The needle is injected at a 90-degree angle to the skin in which type of injection?

a. Intradermal
b. Intramuscular
c. Subcutaneous
d. Endotracheal

128. Medications may be delivered via the pulmonary route through all of the following EXCEPT

a. Nebulizer
b. ET tube
c. IO infusion
d. MDI

129. Which of the following statements regarding ET administration is FALSE?

a. Drug dosages should be 2 to 2.5 times those used for IV or IO administration.
b. Medications must be diluted with normal saline.
c. The needle should be injected through the side of the ET tube.
d. CPR should be stopped during ET administration.

130. The space between the lungs is known as the

a. Thoracic cavity
b. Mediastinum
c. Abdominal cavity
d. Pelvic cavity

131. The number of cervical vertebrae in the neck is

a. 5
b. 33
c. 7
d. 12

132. How many ribs form the rib cage?

a. 10 pairs
b. 12 pairs
c. 2 pairs
d. 4 pairs

133. The forearm is composed of which of the following?

a. Carpals
b. Metacarpals
c. Phalanges
d. Radius

134. Which of the following statements regarding the lymphatic system is FALSE?

a. Lymph originates from excess cellular fluid.
b. Lymph nodes trap bacteria.
c. Swelling of the lymph nodes indicates dysfunction of the lymphatic system.
d. Swelling of the lymph nodes indicates proper functioning of the lymphatic system.

135. In assessing a patient, the resuscitation phase may be performed concurrently with the

    a. Focused history
    b. Initial survey
    c. Physical examination
    d. Rapid trauma assessment

136. During rapid trauma assessment, the Advanced EMT should assess which part of the body first?

    a. Abdomen
    b. Chest
    c. Lungs
    d. Head

137. All of the following may be used to obtain a more accurate respiratory rate EXCEPT

    a. Continuing to take the pulse but counting respirations instead
    b. Placing the patient's arm across his or her chest but counting respirations instead
    c. Keeping your hands on the patient but counting respirations instead
    d. Assessing the rise and fall of the patient's chest

138. Absence of breathing is known as

    a. Eupnea
    b. Bradypnea
    c. Apnea
    d. Tachypnea

139. Pulse oximetry is reliable in monitoring arterial oxygen saturation in

    a. Patients in stable condition
    b. Patients in cardiac arrest
    c. Patients with anemia
    d. Patients with hypotension

140. Which of the following statements regarding the detailed assessment is FALSE?

    a. Detailed assessment of a priority patient should be done during transport.
    b. A head-to-toe examination is required before transport.
    c. An elderly patient should be addressed by his or her formal name.
    d. Patient history may be obtained from bystanders.

141. All of the following may be indicative of drug use EXCEPT

    a. Unequal pupils
    b. Dilated pupils
    c. Constricted pupils
    d. Unresponsive pupils

142. Which of the following is symptomatic of subcutaneous emphysema?

    a. Neck vein distention
    b. Battle's sign
    c. Crackling below the skin
    d. Ecchymosis

143. The maximum score on the Glasgow coma scale is

a. 6
b. 9
c. 3
d. 15

144. Elastic connective tissue covered by mucous membranes that prevents foreign materials from entering the airway is known as the

a. Glottis
b. False vocal cords
c. True vocal cords
d. Adam's apple

145. Carbon dioxide is carried to the lungs by all of the following means except

a. In plasma
b. With hemoglobin
c. With oxygen
d. With water

146. With 50% oxygen saturation, the PO_2 falls to

a. 27 mmHg
b. 20 mmHg
c. 40 mmHg
d. 60 mmHg

147. Upper airway obstruction may be caused by all of the following except

a. Teeth
b. Cricoid pressure
c. Vomiting
d. Smoke inhalation

148. The whistle-top suctioning catheter is useful in

a. Removing large volumes of secretions
b. Removing large food particles
c. Laryngoscopy
d. Removing fluids from the lower respiratory tract

149. All of the following are useful in providing assisted breathing except

a. Demand-valve resuscitator
b. Whistle-top suctioning catheter
c. Mouth-to-mouth breathing
d. Mouth-to-mask breathing

150. The esophageal-tracheal Combitube should be used in

a. Semiresponsive patients
b. Patients with esophageal disease
c. Unconscious patients
d. Patients with a gag reflex

Answer Key and Explanations

1. C: Some commonly prescribed drugs can produce a reaction similar to that of the drug disulfiram (Antabuse), used in patients with chronic alcohol abuse, following alcohol ingestion; these drugs include metronidazole, antibiotics, and oral diabetic medications.

2. B: Lead II on the ECG is most commonly used for continuous patient monitoring in the prehospital setting and indicates the rate and regularity of the patient's heartbeat; however, it does not indicate the presence or location of a myocardial infarction (MI) or the pumping capability of the heart.

3. A: Regular premature ventricular complexes (PVCs) occurring at intervals greater than every fourth beat are simply called frequent PVCs; a PVC at every fourth beat is known as ventricular quadrigeminy and at every third beat, ventricular trigeminy or a trigeminal PVC. PVCs arising in several areas of the ventricles that differ from each other are known as multifocal PVCs.

4. C: Ventricular tachycardia (VT) is a condition in which three or more PVCs occur in a row, P waves are usually not discernible, and T waves may or may not be present. VT should always be considered significant, even if the rhythm results in a pulse as it may lead to cardiac arrest. Patients with pulseless VT should be treated the same as those with ventricular fibrillation (VF).

5. B: The absence of any electrical activity in the heart is known as asystole. Pulseless electrical activity (PEA) is a condition in which electrical activity in the heart is not properly converted to effective cardiac contraction; pericardial tamponade is a reversible cause of PEA. Ventricular fibrillation (VF) is the erratic firing of multiple sites in the ventricle.

6. D: The first step in caring for a patient with cardiac arrest is to immediately begin CPR. If only one Advanced EMT is present, he or she should perform CPR according to local protocols and then apply the automated external defibrillator (AED); if two or more Advanced EMTs are present, one should perform CPR and the other operate the AED. Defibrillation should not be delayed to set up oxygen or IV lines. Because the AED automatically analyzes heart rhythm, it is not necessary for an Advanced EMT to interpret cardiac rhythms to use an AED.

7. B: When defibrillating a patient with ventricular fibrillation (VF), the Advanced EMT should ensure that the synchronized mode is turned off. NTG patches should be removed before defibrillation to prevent the patch from exploding and burning the patient. Before delivering a countershock, the Advanced EMT should double-check the rhythm to ensure that the patient has not reverted to another rhythm. Upon changes in the rhythm or following three sequential shocks, the carotid pulse should be checked.

8. C: When treating hyperventilation, oxygen should be given by nasal cannula. Having the patient breathe into a paper bag or blocking off the portals of an oxygen mask to induce rebreathing is no longer considered acceptable practice as it may lead to hypoxia. Nebulized bronchodilators are used to treat acute chronic obstructive pulmonary disease (COPD).

9. A: Spontaneous pneumothorax is frequently caused by rupture of a congenital defect on the surface of the lung and may be secondary to the swelling and rupture of endometrial tissue in the lung during the menstrual cycle. Anxiety is a cause of pulmonary embolism, which is associated with obesity, thrombophlebitis, and use of oral contraceptives. Carbon monoxide poisoning is not associated with spontaneous pneumothorax.

10. C: In the case of carbon monoxide poisoning, pulse oximetry and oxygen saturation readings may be inaccurate. Hyperbaric oxygen may be useful if the patient is unresponsive, combative, or hallucinating. Measuring the blood glucose level may be useful in stroke patients.

11. D: Coma may result from intracranial causes, such as intracranial bleeding, stroke, and infection or from causes outside of the nervous system, such as vitamin deficiency, hyper- or hyponatremia, hypercalcemia, and hyper- or hypoglycemia. Fever may induce seizures in children, and rarely, in adults.

12. B: In adults, seizures may be caused by infections (such as meningitis or encephalitis), trauma, metabolic abnormalities (such as hypercalcemia and hypoglycemia), and liver or kidney failure. Febrile convulsions may cause seizures in children; however, fever is rarely the cause of seizures in adults. Psychiatric conditions such as catatonia may result in coma.

13. C: Restraining a patient during a seizure is not effective in stopping the seizure; placing a pillow or rolled blanket under the patient's head may help prevent injury. During a seizure, patients may bite their mouth or tongue. Following a seizure, patients may become violent. In some patients, a condition may develop that resembles the paralysis experienced by stroke victims; however, the paralysis only lasts for one to two hours.

14. D: Vaginal bleeding and severe abdominal pain in a woman of child-bearing age is most probably due to a ruptured ectopic pregnancy. Appendicitis is associated with right lower quadrant abdominal pain and bowel obstruction with Abdominal distension; pelvic inflammatory disease (PID) is inflammation of the female internal genitalia due to sexually transmitted disease and is marked by lower abdominal pain, vaginal discharge, fever, and chills.

15. C: For a patient with hypoglycemia, the best course of treatment is to give the patient oral glucose or sugar. Sugar substitutes such as saccharine or aspartame are not effective because they do not contain sugar. Insulin should never be given to a patient who may be diabetic.

16. D: Diabetic ketoacidosis (DKA) is associated with a fruity, acetone-like odor of the breath; however, this does not occur in all patients with DKA.

17. C: Hyperosmolar hyperglycemic nonketotic coma (HHNC) typically occurs in patients older than 60 years living in a nursing home or institutional setting and may result from infection, extreme cold, or dehydration. HHNC is usually associated with gradual deterioration of mental status. Kussmaul respirations and fruity breath odor are associated with DKA and are absent in patients with HHNC.

18. A: In treating a patient who has ingested poison, it is not necessary for the Advanced EMT to determine the exact substance the patient has taken. The airway should be maintained and pulse oximetry monitored; the patient should be placed on a cardiac monitor and positioned in the left lateral recumbent position to prevent aspiration.

19. C: In caring for a patient with heat stroke, placing the patient in a cool environment, such as an air-conditioned ambulance, as soon as possible is vital to prevent brain damage. Salt pills or cold, salty, or sweet drinks should not be given to prevent nausea and vomiting. Heat exhaustion commonly occurs in patients taking diuretics.

20. B: Severe hypothermia may mimic cardiac arrest or clinical death. In treating a patient with hypothermia, rewarming of the extremities may actually decrease body temperature and lead to shock.

21. C: In pediatric patients, asthma can occur at any age and may be a response to allergy or exercise; most pediatric asthma patients have a family history of asthma. Viral infection is associated with bronchiolitis. Pneumonia is an infection of the lower airway or lung caused by a bacteria or virus.

22. B: In pediatric patients, bronchiolitis is an infection of the lower respiratory tract caused by a virus; it may occur at any time and is not associated with a history of asthma. Bronchiolitis is often unresponsive to medication.

23. B: The most important intervention in a child with head trauma is ventilation by either bag-valve-mask device or endotracheal intubation to prevent further injury and sustain neurologic function.

24. D: The first priority in treating a child with severe hypothermia is to maintain the airway by providing high-concentration oxygen. Stimulation, including endotracheal intubation, CPR, or suctioning, should be avoided to prevent ventricular fibrillation; rubbing the affected extremities can cause further tissue damage.

25. B: Normal saline and lactated Ringer's solution may be used in patients with shock; however, 5% dextrose in water is not recommended. Plasma may be given in the hospital setting.

26. C: The acronym SLUDGE may be used as a mnemonic device for the symptoms of cholinergic crisis: Salivation, Lacrimation, Urinary incontinence, Defecation (or fecal incontinence), Generalized weakness, and Emesis.

27. C: According to proper triage methods, a patient with signs and symptoms of shock would be considered highest priority; those with burns but without airway compromise or with back injuries with or without spinal cord damage would be considered second priority. A patient in respiratory or cardiopulmonary arrest would be considered lowest priority.

28. B: An Apgar score of 7 to 10 in a newly born infant indicates mild or no distress; a score of 4 to 6 indicates moderate distress, such as cyanosis, and a score of 0 to 3 indicates severe distress.

29. C: The first step in treatment of cardiopulmonary arrest in a newly born infant is to provide ventilation and oxygenation. If the problem does not resolve, intubation, IV fluids, and medications such as atropine, epinephrine, lidocaine, or naloxone should be administered.

30. A: The Apgar score should be obtained in a newly born infant 1 to 5 minutes after birth; waiting to obtain the Apgar score before beginning resuscitation may have disastrous consequences.

31. A: The components of the Apgar score are as follows: A indicates appearance or color; P, pulse or heart rate; G, grimace or irritability; A, activity or muscle tone; and R, respirations.

32. B: Only 10% dextrose and water can be safely given to a newborn infant with hypoglycemia and altered consciousness. Hyperosmotic agents such as 25% dextrose and water or 50% dextrose and water may cause hemorrhage. Ringer's lactate is used in the treatment of hypovolemia.

33. B: Immediately after the infant's head is delivered, suction the mouth and then the nose to stimulate breathing. The infant's head, face, and body should then be dried; after this, the head should be covered with a blanket, towel, or hat to prevent heat loss.

34. D: Primary apnea occurs when a newborn is not visibly breathing and may be reversed by touching and stimulating the infant and/or suctioning. Secondary apnea occurs if oxygen deprivation continues. Secondary apnea cannot be reversed by stimulation or suctioning and may require assisted ventilation, including bag-mask ventilation with high-concentration oxygen.

35. B: In the case of drug withdrawal or overdose, maintain the airway and monitor the patient's respiratory status; oxygen may be given by nasal cannula or non-rebreather mask as per local protocol. Ipecac is seldom prescribed for use in the field and has largely been replaced by activated charcoal and gastric lavage, usually in the hospital. Ice immersion is a form of street treatment and is ineffective. Antabuse, or disulfiram, is a medication taken by patients with chronic alcohol abuse.

36. C: Drug abuse, head trauma, and medical conditions such as hypoglycemia and diabetic ketoacidosis may mimic alcohol intoxication; Antabuse, or disulfiram, is a medication prescribed for patients with chronic alcohol abuse.

37. C: In elderly patients, depression can present as organic illness, such as cardiac or respiratory disease.

38. B: Cocaine is the most widely abused stimulant drug; heroin, morphine, and hydrocodone (Vicodin) are classified as narcotics. LSD, PCP, and mescaline are common hallucinogens; marijuana and barbiturates are common depressants.

39. A: The suffix "phasia" refers to speech; thus, the term aphasia means inability to speak.

40. C: The prefix "endo" refers to within or inner; thus, the term endometrium means within the uterus.

41. D: Cardiac tamponade is associated with penetrating chest trauma in which the pericardial sac fills with fluid, resulting in the signs and symptoms of shock.

42. B: COPD and respiratory failure may block the ability of the lungs to blow off carbon dioxide, causing a build-up of acid in the blood; this condition is referred to as respiratory acidosis. Respiratory alkalosis results from a deficit of carbon dioxide due to hyperventilation, making the blood more alkaline or basic.

43. B: Aspirin is indicated for patients with acute myocardial infarction. Adenosine is indicated for supraventricular tachycardia (SVT) and paroxysmal SVT (PSVT). Amiodarone is indicated for ventricular fibrillation (VF) and ventricular tachycardia (VT) and dexamethasone is indicated for shock and various inflammatory and allergic disorders.

44. C: Children and geriatric patients have an increased sensitivity to vasopressin; thus, vasopressin is contraindicated in these patients. Vasopressin is indicated as an alternative to the first or second dose of epinephrine for the treatment of shock-refractory ventricular fibrillation (VF), asystole, or pulseless electrical activity (PEA).

45. B: Epinephrine is contraindicated in patients with hypertension, hypothermia, and pulmonary edema; it is indicated in cardiac arrest and asthma.

46. B: During law enforcement operations, the area of immediate or direct threat is known as the hot zone or kill zone; an area of potential threat is known as the warm zone, and an area posing no threat is known as the cold zone.

47. D: Asymmetric pupils in an elderly patient may result from glaucoma, other ocular diseases, or cataract surgery.

48. C: In treating a child with hypothermia, if a heart rate is present, any form of stimulation, including tracheal intubation, CPR, or suctioning, should be avoided to prevent ventricular fibrillation. Resuscitation should continue until the child's temperature returns to normal.

49. D: A child with chest or abdominal trauma should ideally be treated in the same manner as an adult; that is, by rapid transport to a hospital. In the case of a child with suspected abdominal trauma, treatment in the field may result in decompensation. Respiratory distress may be a sign of abdominal trauma.

50. B: An adult vest device such as the Kendrick extrication device (KED) is not recommended for cervical spine immobilization in a small child; placing large, wide straps under the axillae can inhibit brachial circulation. If it is necessary to remove the child from a child safety seat, the child should be moved as a unit; pulling on the head or neck can cause additional injury. Because abdominal excursion is a necessary part of ventilation in a child less than 7 years of age, cravats are preferable to straps.

51. D: Treatment of seizures in a child may include IV diazepam or lorazepam; rectal diazepam is available in a gel and may be easier to use than the IV form. IV glucose may be needed to correct hypoglycemia due to prolonged seizure activity. IV lactated Ringer's solution is used to treat shock in a child with meningitis.

52. C: The presence of neck stiffness and Kernig's sign, or pain on leg extension, is symptomatic of meningitis.

53. B: Rales are indicative of pneumonia in children older than 1 year.

54. A: Because a child's skin is thinner than that of an adult, changes in color or temperature such as mottling may indicate shock. The presence of two different skin colors is common in children in shock.

55. C: Intraosseous infusion is performed in children in severe shock or cardiac arrest; during the procedure, IV fluids such as lactated Ringer's solution or normal saline should be given. Hypodermic needles or spinal needles are not recommended.

56. B: Compared with those of adults, a child's ribs are more pliable and can withstand more force; however, in children, the head is larger and heavier and is more likely to be injured. In children, the internal organs are larger in proportion to body size and the skeletal structure is smaller; thus, children are more prone to internal injuries. The organ most likely to be injured is the liver. Children have immature nervous systems and the nerves are not well insulated.

57. C: In pregnant women, the heart rate is increased, and the blood pressure (BP) is lower. A pregnant patient should be positioned on her left side rather than in the supine position.

58. C: Preeclampsia is a condition occurring in pregnant women marked by hypertension and fluid retention. Ectopic pregnancy refers to pregnancy outside the uterus and is characterized by significant vaginal bleeding, abdominal pain, hypotension, and shock. Gestational diabetes may occur in women with preexisting diabetes but may also occur in women who are not diabetic; this condition results in high blood sugar levels and may be treated with diet and exercise. Uterine rupture most commonly occurs after the onset of labor and is marked by severe abdominal pain and a tearing sensation in the abdomen.

59. B: Placenta previa is the abnormal positioning of the placenta within the uterus and is characterized by painless bright red bleeding. Abruptio placentae, also called placenta abruptio, is the premature detachment of the placenta and is characterized by severe abdominal pain, minimal vaginal bleeding, and a palpable fetus in the abdomen.

60. A: In the case of a prolapsed umbilical cord in which the cord presents first during delivery, the mother should be placed in a knee-to-chest or head-and-torso-down position; the cord should never be pushed back inside or cut. In the case of a breech presentation, the Advanced EMT should form a "V" with his or her fingers on either side of the infant's nose and mouth, and gently guide the head out by lifting the body in a slight anterior position.

61. C: When ventilation and oxygenation are not sufficient in resuscitating a newly born infant, IV fluids and medications such as atropine, epinephrine, naloxone, or lidocaine may be given; dextrose in water is not indicated in resuscitation of the newborn.

62. D: Postpartum hemorrhage may result from vaginal or cervical tearing, bleeding or clotting disorders, or a retained placenta and should be treated with uterine massage. A second IV line may also be started and a fluid bolus administered. Positioning the mother in the knee-to-chest or Trendelenburg position is useful for a prolapsed cord presentation.

63. B: Right lower quadrant abdominal pain is usually indicative of appendicitis unless proven otherwise. Symptoms of bowel obstruction include Abdominal distension and tenderness. Diverticulitis is characterized by left lower quadrant pain. In cirrhosis, severe abdominal pain may be associated with infected peritoneal fluid.

64. C: Epigastric pain is associated with gastritis, esophagitis, pancreatitis, cholecystitis, abdominal aortic aneurysm, and myocardial ischemia; appendicitis is associated with right lower quadrant pain and hernia with right or left lower quadrant pain. A ruptured ectopic pregnancy is associated with left lower quadrant pain.

65. C: Nitroglycerin (NTG) is contraindicated in patients with systolic BP less than 100 mmHg, in patients with head injury, and in infants and children. Typically, the Advanced EMT can assist a patient with a prescription for NTG and a systolic BP greater than 100 mmHg in administering a sublingual tablet or spray. NTG administration may be associated with headache; however, headache is not a contraindication for use of NTG.

66. B: Nitroglycerin (NTG) tablets or spray have an expiration date and may lose potency after exposure to air or light. NTG use may be associated with headache or hypotension.

67. D: Because it is difficult to distinguish acute myocardial infarction (MI) from angina, a patient with chest pain should be assumed to have MI. Cardiac arrest and congestive heart failure are complications of MI.

68. A: Acute MI often presents as epigastric pain; some patients, particularly the elderly, complain of indigestion rather than chest pain.

69. B: Hypotension is not necessarily indicative of cardiogenic shock. Patients with preexisting hypertension may have nearly normal blood pressure. Signs and symptoms of cardiogenic shock include altered mental status, collapse of peripheral veins, and respiratory distress.

70. D: Nitroglycerin (NTG), furosemide, and morphine sulfate are indicated for use in patients with pulmonary edema; however, epinephrine is contraindicated.

71. C: Pulmonary embolism may be associated with pleuritic chest pain, respiratory distress, and shortness of breath. Signs and symptoms are similar to those of pneumonia, myocardial infarction (MI), and spontaneous pneumothorax.

72. B: A barrel-shaped chest is a sign of chronic obstructive pulmonary disease (COPD).

73. D: Plasma is also known as intravascular fluid; this component of the blood is noncellular and is found within the blood vessels. Intracellular fluid is found within individual cells, and extravascular fluid is outside of cell membranes. Interstitial fluid is located outside of the blood vessels in the spaces between the cells.

74. B: Isotonic solutions have an osmotic pressure equal to normal body fluid; lactated Ringer's solution and 0.9% normal saline are examples of isotonic solutions. Hypotonic solutions have an osmotic pressure less than that of normal body fluids, and hypertonic solutions have an osmotic pressure greater than that of normal fluids. Electrolytes are salts that break into ions when dissolved in a solvent.

75. C: Anions and cations are two types of electrolytes. Anions have a negative charge and cations a positive charge. Examples of cations include sodium, potassium, calcium, and magnesium, and examples of anions include chloride, phosphate, and bicarbonate. Adenosine triphosphate (ATP) is a chemical substance produced in the mitochondria.

76. A: The delivery of oxygenated blood to the tissues is known as perfusion. Aerobic metabolism allows the body to use food for energy and involves a combination of oxygen and glucose. Anaerobic metabolism is metabolism without oxygen and is experienced by patients in shock.

77. B: Kussmaul breathing, or deep, rapid respirations, is indicative of metabolic acidosis, a condition in which bicarbonate levels are low in relation to carbonic acid levels. In metabolic alkalosis, bicarbonate levels are higher than carbonic acid levels; symptoms include slow, shallow respirations. Respiratory acidosis occurs when exhalation of carbon dioxide is inhibited, and respiratory alkalosis occurs when carbon dioxide exhalation is excessive.

78. C: The primary mechanisms of shock are fluid loss, significant vasodilation, and pump failure.

79. B: A joint is a site in the body where two or more bones converge. Cartilage is connective tissue that enables bones to move freely. Fibrous tissues that attach muscles to bones are known as tendons. Ligaments are a type of fibrous tissue that connects bones or cartilage.

80. B: An abnormal accumulation of fluid in the pleural cavity is known as pleural effusion; a collection of air in the pleural cavity is known as pneumothorax. Respiratory alkalosis is a condition in which a deficit of carbon dioxide causes the blood to become more alkaline. Cardiac tamponade is associated with chest trauma and results when the pericardial sac fills too rapidly with blood, preventing the heart from filling adequately and inducing shock.

81. C: The APVU mnemonic is used to determine the level of the patient's responsiveness to stimuli. A = awake and alert, P = responsive to painful stimuli, V = responsive to verbal stimuli, and U = unresponsive.

82. B: If the patient is responsive, the radial pulse should be checked; however, in unresponsive patients, the carotid pulse should be checked first. In children less than 1 year of age, the brachial or femoral pulse should be palpated.

83. D: No one vital sign can provide adequate information about a patient's condition; thus, vital signs should be assessed as a set. Vital signs can vary widely among individuals and may vary by age. Vital signs should be assessed constantly to evaluate changes in the patient's condition.

84. D: The normal respiratory rate for an adult is 12 to 20 times per minute. Newborns breathe at a rate of 40 to 60 times per minute; children 1 year of age breathe 30 to 40 times per minute, and children 3 years of age breathe 25 to 30 times per minute.

85. C: Melena is the presence of black, tarry stool caused by the passing of digested blood through the gastrointestinal tract. Hematochezia is the presence of bright red blood in the stool. Hematemesis is the vomiting of blood and is characterized by vomitus with a coffee ground-like appearance due to the digestion of blood by the stomach acid.

86. D: Acute abdomen is the presence of acute abdominal pain not caused by injury and may result from a variety of illnesses not necessarily originating within the abdominal cavity, such as myocardial infarction and diabetic ketoacidosis. Acute abdomen may also be caused by a black widow spider bite; however, it is not associated with a dog bite.

87. B: Shivering is a sign of increased heat production. Sweating is a sign of increased heat loss associated with hyperthermic compensation. Decreased appetite and decreased voluntary activity are signs of decreased heat production.

88. C: Signs and symptoms of heat stroke include altered level of consciousness, shortness of breath, and minimal or no sweating.

89. B: Altered mental status is associated with heat stroke and is rarely seen in patients with heat exhaustion. Signs and symptoms of heat exhaustion include profuse sweating, pallor, and hypotension.

90. D: The first step in treating a patient with hypothermia is to remove the patient from the cold environment; if wet, the patient should be dried as much as possible and covered with a blanket, insulating material, and moisture barriers and transported to a warm environment. The Advanced EMT should not attempt to rewarm the extremities as this may lead to vasodilation of the arms and legs. Warmed IV fluids may be helpful; however, lactated Ringer's solution should not be given because the liver may not be able to metabolize the lactate. Warm water immersion is not useful in the pre-hospital setting.

91. A: In victims of dry drowning, anoxia results from laryngeal spasm, which prevents the entrance of both water and air into the lungs. Dry drowning may result in cerebral anoxia, edema, and unconsciousness; however, victims of dry drowning have the best chance of survival. In wet drowning, the victim exerts a violent respiratory effort, filling the lungs with water. Secondary drowning is the recurrence of respiratory distress after recovery from the initial drowning episode. In victims of seawater drowning, the presence of seawater in the lungs results in an influx of hypotonic serum, leading to profound hypoxemia.

92. B: The definitive method for assessing successful endotracheal (ET) tube placement in an infant is watching the passage of the tube through the vocal cords. Breath sounds alone may not indicate successful placement, as sounds are easily transmitted due to the small size of the infant's chest. Improvement in color and heart rate and the rise and fall of the chest indicate successful placement.

93. B: Surgical masks do not provide adequate protection against some airborne pathogens, such as those causing tuberculosis (TB). Although goggles provide the best protection against bloodborne pathogens, prescription glasses with side shields are acceptable. Because coveralls are closer-fitting than gowns, overall-type coveralls with approved barrier shielding are preferable to gowns as protection against exposure to body fluids. Latex, vinyl, and rubber gloves should never be reused.

94. C: Bleach solution diluted in water is an effective alternative to commercial disinfectants. Antiseptics destroy germs on living tissue rather than on nonliving objects. Soap and water and antibacterials are not effective alternatives to disinfectants.

95. B: Involuntary consent involves treatment of a patient granted under authority of law whether or not the patient agrees to treatment. This may apply to a patient held for mental health evaluation or a patient who is under arrest. Implied consent involves treatment of a patient who is severely ill or injured under the assumption that the patient would want care if able to respond. In the case of expressed consent, the patient gives verbal or written permission to be treated. In the case of informed consent, the patient gives consent to be treated only after receiving all information needed to understand his or her condition.

96. D: An adult who has been legally determined mentally incompetent cannot consent to or refuse care. In this case, consent is usually given by a legal guardian; however, if the guardian is not available, the patient may receive care under implied consent. Unemancipated minors, or patients younger than 18 years of age, are not able to give or withhold consent; however, emancipated minors who have been legally absolved from the need for parental consent, such as those who are married, parents, or in the armed forces, can give their own consent.

97. C: In most states, minors, or patients under the age of 18 years, cannot legally consent to or refuse care; however, if a parent or guardian is not available, minors can be treated under implied consent. Adults who have been legally declared mentally incompetent can also receive care if a legal guardian is not available. Adults experiencing alcohol or substance intoxication, emotional or psychiatric problems, or other medical conditions that may temporarily impair the ability to make rational decisions may also be treated under implied consent.

98. B: Norepinephrine is the most common neurotransmitter in the sympathetic nervous system. Norepinephrine is related to epinephrine or adrenaline, which also functions as a sympathetic neurotransmitter. Acetylcholine is the most common neurotransmitter in the parasympathetic nervous system.

99. C: The parasympathetic nervous system controls intestinal activity, respiratory rate, and pupillary response. Examples of a parasympathetic response include abdominal distress and nausea and vomiting. The sympathetic nervous system controls the fight or flight response and causes constriction of blood vessels and elevation of heart rate and blood pressure; sympathetic responses include nervousness and tachycardia.

100. B: The third (S_3) and fourth (S_4) heart sounds are not typically heard in normal individuals; however, while S_3 is sometimes heard in healthy young people, S_4 is almost always indicative of an abnormality. A murmur is an abnormal whooshing sound indicating turbulent blood flow. Many heart murmurs are benign and disappear over time. The SA, or sinoatrial, node is a normal component of the circulatory system.

101. B: Guaifenesin, an ingredient in many cough medicines, is classified as a Schedule V drug, with the lowest potential for abuse; Schedule I drugs have the highest potential for abuse and include heroin, LSD, and mescaline.

102. A: Morphine, codeine, cocaine, and amphetamines are examples of Schedule II drugs with a high potential for abuse; Schedule I drugs, such as heroin, LSD, peyote, and mescaline, have the highest potential for abuse and no accepted medical use in the United States. Schedule V drugs, including guaifenesin and difenoxin/atropine sulfate, have the lowest potential for abuse.

103. B: A drug classified as a Pregnancy Category A drug carries only a remote risk of fetal harm. Drugs in Pregnancy Category X are contraindicated in pregnant women. Drugs in Category C have shown evidence of fetal harm in animal studies and have not undergone adequate human studies. Drugs designated Pregnancy Category D may be used to treat life-threatening conditions when the potential benefits of the drug outweigh the risks.

104. A: Certain drugs, such as acetaminophen, morphine, or meperidine, are affected by body weight and appear in significantly higher concentrations in elderly and obese patients than in younger or slim patients. Thus, dosage modifications are necessary in elderly or obese patients to prevent overdose.

105. C: Acetylcholine cannot be administered as a drug because it is broken down by cholinesterase in the blood and synapses before it can occupy receptors; however, some drugs, such as pilocarpine, which is used to treat glaucoma, mimic the action of acetylcholine. Edrophonium is a cholinesterase inhibitor. Atropine is used to treat cardiovascular conditions.

106. C: Sympathetic agonists affect the alpha- and beta-adrenergic receptors. The asthma drugs albuterol and metaproterenol are known as beta-2 agonists. Propranolol is a common beta blocker. Acetylcholine affects the parasympathetic division but cannot be given as a drug because it is broken down by cholinesterase in the blood and synapses before it can reach the receptors. Atropine is an acetylcholine antagonist.

107. B: A drug given by the sublingual route is placed under the tongue. Drugs given via the buccal route are dissolved between the cheek and gum. Topical or transdermal medications are applied directly to the skin. Intradermal administration is injection of the drug into the dermis.

108. C: Five drugs can be administered through the endotracheal tube: atropine, epinephrine, lidocaine, naloxone, and vasopressin. Metaproterenol is a bronchodilator and is administered via a nebulizer or metered dose inhaler.

109. B: The intravenous route is the fastest route of drug administration while the oral route is the slowest. Drugs administered via the endotracheal route are absorbed rapidly but not immediately. The topical route has a moderate rate of absorption.

110. D: An acute systemic reaction to a drug on subsequent exposure is known as anaphylaxis; anaphylaxis occurs when an individual becomes sensitized to the drug and experiences a sudden, severe whole-body allergic reaction. Tachyphylaxis is the rapid development of tolerance to a drug. Drug dependence is the development of a physical or psychological need to use a drug; drug toxicity results from overdosage, ingestion of a drug meant for external use, or the buildup of a drug concentration in the blood resulting from impaired metabolism or excretion.

111. B: Synergism occurs when two drugs work together to produce an effect neither drug can produce alone; for example, sedatives taken with barbiturates can cause central nervous system depression. Antagonism occurs when one drug prevents the absorption of another drug; for example, antacids taken with tetracycline block the absorption of tetracycline. Potentiation occurs when one drug multiplies the effect of another; for example, cimetidine taken with imipramine increases the blood levels of imipramine. Meperidine and morphine are both members of the opiate class of drugs.

112. B: Phenergan, a nonnarcotic emetic, and meperidine, a synthetic narcotic analgesic, have a synergistic effect when taken together; that is, both drugs taken together are more effective for pain relief than either drug alone. Epinephrine taken with digoxin produces a drug interaction that increases the risk of cardiac dysrhythmias. When amiodarone is taken with digoxin, it increases serum digoxin levels, resulting in drug toxicity. Methyldopa taken with monoamine oxidase (MAO) inhibitors may lead to hypertension.

113. A: In a critically injured patient, the Advanced EMT should not delay transport to the hospital by attempting to start an IV line on the scene; rather, the IV should be started en route to the hospital. An IV line should not be started in sclerotic veins or after the patient experiences circulatory collapse.

114. C: Lactated Ringer's solution contains sodium, potassium, calcium, chloride, and lactate but not HCO_3; it does not provide free water or calories.

115. B: Sodium chloride 0.9% is the only IV solution that can be given with blood products.

116. C: No restriction of fluid flow from the IV bag to the patient is known as the wide-open rate. The TKO, or "to keep open" rate, is equal to approximately 8 to 15 drops of fluid per minute; it is also known as the KVO, or "keep vein open" rate. The macrodrip is a drip chamber used when a large amount of fluid is needed.

117. D: Large-bore, or 14- to 16-guage catheters, may be used for administration of viscous fluids, such as blood or blood components, or viscous medications, such as 50% dextrose. Large-bore catheters should be used for patients in shock, cardiac arrest, or other life-threatening conditions; however, they are not indicated for patients with small or fragile veins, such as infants and children or the elderly.

118. C: In patients in cardiac arrest, the preferred site for IV cannulation is the peripheral veins of the antecubital fossa (the area anterior to and below the elbow); distal peripheral veins are the least preferred site because blood flow from distal extremities is diminished during circulatory collapse. Use of the jugular vein is sometimes contraindicated by local protocols because the catheter and tubing are difficult to tape down and may be easily displaced. The saphenous vein of the leg should only be used as a last resort because of the risk of thrombus formation.

119. D: Use of an armboard may be necessary when the venipuncture device is inserted near a joint, such as in the antecubital fossa or in the dorsum of the hand or wrist. It may also be used with restraints in disoriented or confused patients. Use of the armboard is usually not necessary in noncritical patients.

120. B: In documenting IV placement, the Advanced EMT should place a piece of tape on a flat surface, write the information on the tape, and then place it directly over the dressing; the tape should not be labeled after it has been applied over the dressing as this may irritate the venipuncture site. Information that should be documented includes the initials of the individual who placed the IV, the date and time of insertion, and the type and gauge of the needle as well as all unsuccessful attempts to start the IV.

121. C: A pyrogenic reaction occurs when foreign proteins capable of producing a fever are present in the administration set or the IV solution. A hematoma may result from injury to a blood vessel; a local infection may occur when appropriate cleansing techniques have not been used and bacteria enter the venipuncture site. An air embolism occurs when air enters the vein.

122. B: In placing an IV line in a patient who is moving or having a seizure, the extremity should be held as still as possible. An armboard may be useful to immobilize the extremity and prevent accidental displacement of the cannula. Choose the largest vein available; using smaller veins increases the risk of the needle passing through the vein in the event of sudden movement. Using a crossover taping technique is acceptable to prevent the catheter from being dislodged from the vein.

123. D: Adenosine, an atrial antidysrhythmic, can only be given by IV push, whereas atropine, a parasympatholytic, can be given endotracheally, intramuscularly, or by IV push. Epinephrine in a 1:1000 concentration can be given subcutaneously, whereas epinephrine in a 1:10,000 concentration may be administered either endotracheally or by IV push. Administration of 1g/5 mL lidocaine by IV push may result in severe adverse events.

124. B: Two syringes are required for preparation of reconstituted medications. The first syringe is used to add the sterile liquid, and the second is used to inject the medication after it has been mixed. Ampules are breakable glass containers from which drugs are drawn with a syringe. Attaching a continuous infusion to a primary IV line is known as a piggyback infusion. Intradermal tuberculin (TB) skin tests are administered using a TB syringe.

125. C: The subcutaneous route is used for the administration of epinephrine, insulin, heparin, and some vaccines. Lidocaine is administered by the IV route.

126. A: The dorsogluteal injection site is not recommended for children under the age of 3 years because the muscle is not yet developed, and injection at this site may result in penetration of the sciatic nerve. The vastus lateralis muscle is the preferred site for injection in children less than 3 years of age; the ventrogluteal and deltoid muscles may be used for young children.

127. B: When administering an intramuscular injection, the needle is injected at a 90-degree angle to the skin. With an intradermal injection, the angle of the needle is 15 degrees and with a subcutaneous injection, 45 degrees. In endotracheal administration, drugs are introduced directly through the endotracheal tube in an intubated patient.

128. C: Medications may be administered as an aerosol via the pulmonary route using a nebulizer, metered dose inhaler (MDI), or endotracheal (ET) tube. Intraosseous (IO) infusion is the infusion of fluid or medication directly into the bone marrow.

129. C: Drug levels achieved through endotracheal (ET) administration are less than those achieved through the IV or intraosseous (IO) routes; thus, drug dosages should be 2 to 2.5 times the recommended dose for IV or IO administration. Medications must be diluted with normal saline before ET administration. The needle should not be injected through the side of the ET tube for medication delivery. If CPR is being delivered at the same time as ET drug injection, chest compressions should be stopped temporarily until several ventilations are given.

130. B: The space between the lungs is known as the mediastinum; the thoracic cavity is located between the base of the neck and the diaphragm and is formed by the boundary of the rib cage. The abdominal cavity extends from the diaphragm to the pelvic bones and comprises the gastrointestinal and urinary systems. The pelvic cavity comprises the lower portion of the abdominal cavity and is bordered by the pelvic bones.

131. C: The spine consists of 33 bones called vertebrae and is divided into 5 sections; there are 7 cervical vertebrae in the neck. There are 12 thoracic vertebrae in the posterior chest.

132. B: A total of 12 pairs of ribs form the rib cage; the upper 10 attach directly to the sternum and the remaining 2 pairs are held together by cartilage. Four vertebrae are fused into the coccyx or tailbone.

133. D: The forearm is composed of two bones: the radius and the ulna. The carpals comprise the wrist and the metacarpals form the hand. The phalanges are the small bones that comprise the fingers.

134. C: Lymph originates from excess cellular fluid and circulates throughout the body in lymph vessels. Lymphatic fluid is filtered in the lymph nodes and travels back to the circulatory system via the thoracic duct. Bacteria and viruses are trapped in the lymph nodes until they are destroyed by the immune system; thus, swelling of the lymph nodes during an infection indicates that the lymphatic system is functioning properly.

135. B: In the resuscitation phase, life-saving procedures such as relief of airway obstruction, CPR, and control of hemorrhage should be performed. The resuscitation phase may be performed concurrently with the initial survey. If a life-threatening condition is detected during the initial survey, the survey should be stopped and the condition treated before continuing the survey. The Advanced EMT should reconsider the mechanism of injury before beginning the focused history and physical examination. Rapid trauma assessment is a hands-on examination of the patient to evaluate his or her condition and should be performed after the focused history and physical examination.

136. D: During rapid trauma assessment, the head and neck should be assessed first, followed by the chest. Chest inspection should be followed by auscultation of the lungs, then palpation of the abdomen.

137. D: Because some patients attempt to control their respiratory rate during assessment, it may be necessary to count respirations to obtain a more accurate reading. After assessing the pulse, the Advanced EMT should keep his or her hands in place but count respirations instead. When obtaining a radial pulse, place the patient's arm across the chest, finish taking the pulse, and count respirations instead. Because some patients are abdominal breathers, chest movement is not adequate in assessing breathing.

138. C: Apnea is the absence of breathing; normal breathing is known as eupnea. Bradypnea is characterized by slow respirations and tachypnea by rapid and shallow respirations.

139. A: Pulse oximetry is unreliable in unstable patients, such as those with hypotension or hypothermia, anemia, or severe vascular disease, and in patients in cardiac arrest.

140. B: The detailed assessment is a subjective and objective examination of a patient to obtain more detailed patient information than that provided by the initial and focused assessments. In the case of priority patients, detailed assessment should be performed en route to the hospital. In the case of a patient with a life-threatening condition, immediate transport may be necessary and there may not be sufficient time to complete the detailed assessment. If a patient is not able to provide a patient history, the history may be obtained from bystanders. Elderly patients should be addressed by their formal names, such as "Mr." or "Mrs.," unless the patient asks otherwise.

141. A: Unequal pupils normally occur in 2% to 4% of the population. Unequal pupils may be caused by head injury, bleeding in the brain, eye trauma, or cataract surgery; however, this condition is not indicative of drug use.

142. C: Subcutaneous emphysema is caused by air entering the subcutaneous tissue through a hole in the trachea; patients often complain of a crackling or crunching sensation below the skin. Neck vein distention may be indicative of congestive heart failure or cardiac tamponade; ecchymosis may signify neck trauma and subsequent airway obstruction. Battle's sign is a discoloration of the area behind the ear and may indicate skull fracture.

143. D: The Glasgow coma scale is used for neurologic assessment of a patient in critical condition; the maximum score is 15 and the minimum score 3. Adults scoring less than 9 have a poor prognosis. The three main areas assessed by the Glasgow coma scale are eye opening, verbal response, and motor response; 6 is the maximum score in the motor response category.

144. B: The false vocal cords or vestibular folds consist of elastic connective tissue covered by folds of mucous membranes; the false vocal cords prevent air from leaving the lungs as well as foreign materials such as liquids or food from entering the airway. The true vocal cords lie below the false vocal cords and consist of cordlike structures that vibrate to produce sound. The glottis is the slit-like opening between the vocal cords. The thyroid cartilage that comprises the main laryngeal cartilage is known as the Adam's apple.

145. C: Carbon dioxide is carried to the lungs in three ways: dissolved in plasma, combined with hemoglobin, or combined with water as carbonic acid.

146. A: A decline in oxygen saturation results in a reduction in oxygen content; thus, with 90% saturation, the partial pressure of oxygen (PO_2) falls to 60 mmHg, with 75%, to 40 mmHg, and with 50%, to 27 mmHg.

147. B: Upper airway obstruction may be caused by the tongue or teeth, vomiting, swelling due to allergic reaction or smoke inhalation, and epiglottitis. Cricoid pressure is a means of preventing gastric distention or regurgitation.

148. D: The whistle-top suctioning catheter is a small, flexible tube capable of extending into the lower respiratory tract to remove fluid, blood, vomitus, and other secretions. The tonsil tip suctioning catheter is effective in removing larger particles and larger volumes of secretions and may be useful during laryngoscopy.

149. B: Procedures and devices useful in providing assisted breathing include the demand-valve resuscitator and automatic ventilator as well as mouth-to-mouth and mouth-to-mask breathing; the whistle-top suctioning catheter is used to remove fluid, blood, vomitus, or secretions from the airway.

150. C: The esophageal-tracheal Combitube should only be used in unconscious patients; it is not indicated in responsive or semi-responsive patients with a gag reflex or in those with esophageal disease.

How to Overcome Test Anxiety

Just the thought of taking a test is enough to make most people a little nervous. A test is an important event that can have a long-term impact on your future, so it's important to take it seriously and it's natural to feel anxious about performing well. But just because anxiety is normal, that doesn't mean that it's helpful in test taking, or that you should simply accept it as part of your life. Anxiety can have a variety of effects. These effects can be mild, like making you feel slightly nervous, or severe, like blocking your ability to focus or remember even a simple detail.

If you experience test anxiety—whether severe or mild—it's important to know how to beat it. To discover this, first you need to understand what causes test anxiety.

Causes of Test Anxiety

While we often think of anxiety as an uncontrollable emotional state, it can actually be caused by simple, practical things. One of the most common causes of test anxiety is that a person does not feel adequately prepared for their test. This feeling can be the result of many different issues such as poor study habits or lack of organization, but the most common culprit is time management. Starting to study too late, failing to organize your study time to cover all of the material, or being distracted while you study will mean that you're not well prepared for the test. This may lead to cramming the night before, which will cause you to be physically and mentally exhausted for the test. Poor time management also contributes to feelings of stress, fear, and hopelessness as you realize you are not well prepared but don't know what to do about it.

Other times, test anxiety is not related to your preparation for the test but comes from unresolved fear. This may be a past failure on a test, or poor performance on tests in general. It may come from comparing yourself to others who seem to be performing better or from the stress of living up to expectations. Anxiety may be driven by fears of the future—how failure on this test would affect your educational and career goals. These fears are often completely irrational, but they can still negatively impact your test performance.

Elements of Test Anxiety

As mentioned earlier, test anxiety is considered to be an emotional state, but it has physical and mental components as well. Sometimes you may not even realize that you are suffering from test anxiety until you notice the physical symptoms. These can include trembling hands, rapid heartbeat, sweating, nausea, and tense muscles. Extreme anxiety may lead to fainting or vomiting. Obviously, any of these symptoms can have a negative impact on testing. It is important to recognize them as soon as they begin to occur so that you can address the problem before it damages your performance.

The mental components of test anxiety include trouble focusing and inability to remember learned information. During a test, your mind is on high alert, which can help you recall information and stay focused for an extended period of time. However, anxiety interferes with your mind's natural processes, causing you to blank out, even on the questions you know well. The strain of testing during anxiety makes it difficult to stay focused, especially on a test that may take several hours. Extreme anxiety can take a huge mental toll, making it difficult not only to recall test information but even to understand the test questions or pull your thoughts together.

Effects of Test Anxiety

Test anxiety is like a disease—if left untreated, it will get progressively worse. Anxiety leads to poor performance, and this reinforces the feelings of fear and failure, which in turn lead to poor performances on subsequent tests. It can grow from a mild nervousness to a crippling condition. If allowed to progress, test anxiety can have a big impact on your schooling, and consequently on your future.

Test anxiety can spread to other parts of your life. Anxiety on tests can become anxiety in any stressful situation, and blanking on a test can turn into panicking in a job situation. But fortunately, you don't have to let anxiety rule your testing and determine your grades. There are a number of relatively simple steps you can take to move past anxiety and function normally on a test and in the rest of life.

Physical Steps for Beating Test Anxiety

While test anxiety is a serious problem, the good news is that it can be overcome. It doesn't have to control your ability to think and remember information. While it may take time, you can begin taking steps today to beat anxiety.

Just as your first hint that you may be struggling with anxiety comes from the physical symptoms, the first step to treating it is also physical. Rest is crucial for having a clear, strong mind. If you are tired, it is much easier to give in to anxiety. But if you establish good sleep habits, your body and mind will be ready to perform optimally, without the strain of exhaustion. Additionally, sleeping well helps you to retain information better, so you're more likely to recall the answers when you see the test questions.

Getting good sleep means more than going to bed on time. It's important to allow your brain time to relax. Take study breaks from time to time so it doesn't get overworked, and don't study right before bed. Take time to rest your mind before trying to rest your body, or you may find it difficult to fall asleep.

Along with sleep, other aspects of physical health are important in preparing for a test. Good nutrition is vital for good brain function. Sugary foods and drinks may give a burst of energy but this burst is followed by a crash, both physically and emotionally. Instead, fuel your body with protein and vitamin-rich foods.

Also, drink plenty of water. Dehydration can lead to headaches and exhaustion, especially if your brain is already under stress from the rigors of the test. Particularly if your test is a long one, drink water during the breaks. And if possible, take an energy-boosting snack to eat between sections.

Along with sleep and diet, a third important part of physical health is exercise. Maintaining a steady workout schedule is helpful, but even taking 5-minute study breaks to walk can help get your blood pumping faster and clear your head. Exercise also releases endorphins, which contribute to a positive feeling and can help combat test anxiety.

When you nurture your physical health, you are also contributing to your mental health. If your body is healthy, your mind is much more likely to be healthy as well. So take time to rest, nourish your body with healthy food and water, and get moving as much as possible. Taking these physical steps will make you stronger and more able to take the mental steps necessary to overcome test anxiety.

Mental Steps for Beating Test Anxiety

Working on the mental side of test anxiety can be more challenging, but as with the physical side, there are clear steps you can take to overcome it. As mentioned earlier, test anxiety often stems from lack of preparation, so the obvious solution is to prepare for the test. Effective studying may be the most important weapon you have for beating test anxiety, but you can and should employ several other mental tools to combat fear.

First, boost your confidence by reminding yourself of past success—tests or projects that you aced. If you're putting as much effort into preparing for this test as you did for those, there's no reason you should expect to fail here. Work hard to prepare; then trust your preparation.

Second, surround yourself with encouraging people. It can be helpful to find a study group, but be sure that the people you're around will encourage a positive attitude. If you spend time with others who are anxious or cynical, this will only contribute to your own anxiety. Look for others who are motivated to study hard from a desire to succeed, not from a fear of failure.

Third, reward yourself. A test is physically and mentally tiring, even without anxiety, and it can be helpful to have something to look forward to. Plan an activity following the test, regardless of the outcome, such as going to a movie or getting ice cream.

When you are taking the test, if you find yourself beginning to feel anxious, remind yourself that you know the material. Visualize successfully completing the test. Then take a few deep, relaxing breaths and return to it. Work through the questions carefully but with confidence, knowing that you are capable of succeeding.

Developing a healthy mental approach to test taking will also aid in other areas of life. Test anxiety affects more than just the actual test—it can be damaging to your mental health and even contribute to depression. It's important to beat test anxiety before it becomes a problem for more than testing.

Study Strategy

Being prepared for the test is necessary to combat anxiety, but what does being prepared look like? You may study for hours on end and still not feel prepared. What you need is a strategy for test prep. The next few pages outline our recommended steps to help you plan out and conquer the challenge of preparation.

STEP 1: SCOPE OUT THE TEST

Learn everything you can about the format (multiple choice, essay, etc.) and what will be on the test. Gather any study materials, course outlines, or sample exams that may be available. Not only will this help you to prepare, but knowing what to expect can help to alleviate test anxiety.

STEP 2: MAP OUT THE MATERIAL

Look through the textbook or study guide and make note of how many chapters or sections it has. Then divide these over the time you have. For example, if a book has 15 chapters and you have five days to study, you need to cover three chapters each day. Even better, if you have the time, leave an extra day at the end for overall review after you have gone through the material in depth.

If time is limited, you may need to prioritize the material. Look through it and make note of which sections you think you already have a good grasp on, and which need review. While you are studying, skim quickly through the familiar sections and take more time on the challenging parts.

Write out your plan so you don't get lost as you go. Having a written plan also helps you feel more in control of the study, so anxiety is less likely to arise from feeling overwhelmed at the amount to cover.

STEP 3: GATHER YOUR TOOLS

Decide what study method works best for you. Do you prefer to highlight in the book as you study and then go back over the highlighted portions? Or do you type out notes of the important information? Or is it helpful to make flashcards that you can carry with you? Assemble the pens, index cards, highlighters, post-it notes, and any other materials you may need so you won't be distracted by getting up to find things while you study.

If you're having a hard time retaining the information or organizing your notes, experiment with different methods. For example, try color-coding by subject with colored pens, highlighters, or post-it notes. If you learn better by hearing, try recording yourself reading your notes so you can listen while in the car, working out, or simply sitting at your desk. Ask a friend to quiz you from your flashcards, or try teaching someone the material to solidify it in your mind.

STEP 4: CREATE YOUR ENVIRONMENT

It's important to avoid distractions while you study. This includes both the obvious distractions like visitors and the subtle distractions like an uncomfortable chair (or a too-comfortable couch that makes you want to fall asleep). Set up the best study environment possible: good lighting and a comfortable work area. If background music helps you focus, you may want to turn it on, but otherwise keep the room quiet. If you are using a computer to take notes, be sure you don't have any other windows open, especially applications like social media, games, or anything else that could distract you. Silence your phone and turn off notifications. Be sure to keep water close by so you stay hydrated while you study (but avoid unhealthy drinks and snacks).

Also, take into account the best time of day to study. Are you freshest first thing in the morning? Try to set aside some time then to work through the material. Is your mind clearer in the afternoon or evening? Schedule your study session then. Another method is to study at the same time of day that you will take the test, so that your brain gets used to working on the material at that time and will be ready to focus at test time.

STEP 5: STUDY!

Once you have done all the study preparation, it's time to settle into the actual studying. Sit down, take a few moments to settle your mind so you can focus, and begin to follow your study plan. Don't give in to distractions or let yourself procrastinate. This is your time to prepare so you'll be ready to fearlessly approach the test. Make the most of the time and stay focused.

Of course, you don't want to burn out. If you study too long you may find that you're not retaining the information very well. Take regular study breaks. For example, taking five minutes out of every hour to walk briskly, breathing deeply and swinging your arms, can help your mind stay fresh.

As you get to the end of each chapter or section, it's a good idea to do a quick review. Remind yourself of what you learned and work on any difficult parts. When you feel that you've mastered the material, move on to the next part. At the end of your study session, briefly skim through your notes again.

But while review is helpful, cramming last minute is NOT. If at all possible, work ahead so that you won't need to fit all your study into the last day. Cramming overloads your brain with more information than it can process and retain, and your tired mind may struggle to recall even previously learned information when it is overwhelmed with last-minute study. Also, the urgent nature of cramming and the stress placed on your brain contribute to anxiety. You'll be more likely to go to the test feeling unprepared and having trouble thinking clearly.

So don't cram, and don't stay up late before the test, even just to review your notes at a leisurely pace. Your brain needs rest more than it needs to go over the information again. In fact, plan to finish your studies by noon or early afternoon the day before the test. Give your brain the rest of the day to relax or focus on other things, and get a good night's sleep. Then you will be fresh for the test and better able to recall what you've studied.

STEP 6: TAKE A PRACTICE TEST

Many courses offer sample tests, either online or in the study materials. This is an excellent resource to check whether you have mastered the material, as well as to prepare for the test format and environment.

Check the test format ahead of time: the number of questions, the type (multiple choice, free response, etc.), and the time limit. Then create a plan for working through them. For example, if you have 30 minutes to take a 60-question test, your limit is 30 seconds per question. Spend less time on the questions you know well so that you can take more time on the difficult ones.

If you have time to take several practice tests, take the first one open book, with no time limit. Work through the questions at your own pace and make sure you fully understand them. Gradually work up to taking a test under test conditions: sit at a desk with all study materials put away and set a timer. Pace yourself to make sure you finish the test with time to spare and go back to check your answers if you have time.

After each test, check your answers. On the questions you missed, be sure you understand why you missed them. Did you misread the question (tests can use tricky wording)? Did you forget the information? Or was it something you hadn't learned? Go back and study any shaky areas that the practice tests reveal.

Taking these tests not only helps with your grade, but also aids in combating test anxiety. If you're already used to the test conditions, you're less likely to worry about it, and working through tests until you're scoring well gives you a confidence boost. Go through the practice tests until you feel comfortable, and then you can go into the test knowing that you're ready for it.

Test Tips

On test day, you should be confident, knowing that you've prepared well and are ready to answer the questions. But aside from preparation, there are several test day strategies you can employ to maximize your performance.

First, as stated before, get a good night's sleep the night before the test (and for several nights before that, if possible). Go into the test with a fresh, alert mind rather than staying up late to study.

Try not to change too much about your normal routine on the day of the test. It's important to eat a nutritious breakfast, but if you normally don't eat breakfast at all, consider eating just a protein bar. If you're a coffee drinker, go ahead and have your normal coffee. Just make sure you time it so that the caffeine doesn't wear off right in the middle of your test. Avoid sugary beverages, and drink enough water to stay hydrated but not so much that you need a restroom break 10 minutes into the test. If your test isn't first thing in the morning, consider going for a walk or doing a light workout before the test to get your blood flowing.

Allow yourself enough time to get ready, and leave for the test with plenty of time to spare so you won't have the anxiety of scrambling to arrive in time. Another reason to be early is to select a good seat. It's helpful to sit away from doors and windows, which can be distracting. Find a good seat, get out your supplies, and settle your mind before the test begins.

When the test begins, start by going over the instructions carefully, even if you already know what to expect. Make sure you avoid any careless mistakes by following the directions.

Then begin working through the questions, pacing yourself as you've practiced. If you're not sure on an answer, don't spend too much time on it, and don't let it shake your confidence. Either skip it and come back later, or eliminate as many wrong answers as possible and guess among the remaining ones. Don't dwell on these questions as you continue—put them out of your mind and focus on what lies ahead.

Be sure to read all of the answer choices, even if you're sure the first one is the right answer. Sometimes you'll find a better one if you keep reading. But don't second-guess yourself if you do immediately know the answer. Your gut instinct is usually right. Don't let test anxiety rob you of the information you know.

If you have time at the end of the test (and if the test format allows), go back and review your answers. Be cautious about changing any, since your first instinct tends to be correct, but make sure you didn't misread any of the questions or accidentally mark the wrong answer choice. Look over any you skipped and make an educated guess.

At the end, leave the test feeling confident. You've done your best, so don't waste time worrying about your performance or wishing you could change anything. Instead, celebrate the successful completion of this test. And finally, use this test to learn how to deal with anxiety even better next time.

> **Review Video: Test Anxiety**
> Visit mometrix.com/academy and enter code: 100340

Important Qualification

Not all anxiety is created equal. If your test anxiety is causing major issues in your life beyond the classroom or testing center, or if you are experiencing troubling physical symptoms related to your anxiety, it may be a sign of a serious physiological or psychological condition. If this sounds like your situation, we strongly encourage you to seek professional help.

Additional Bonus Material

Due to our efforts to try to keep this book to a manageable length, we've created a link that will give you access to all of your additional bonus material:

mometrix.com/bonus948/advancedemt

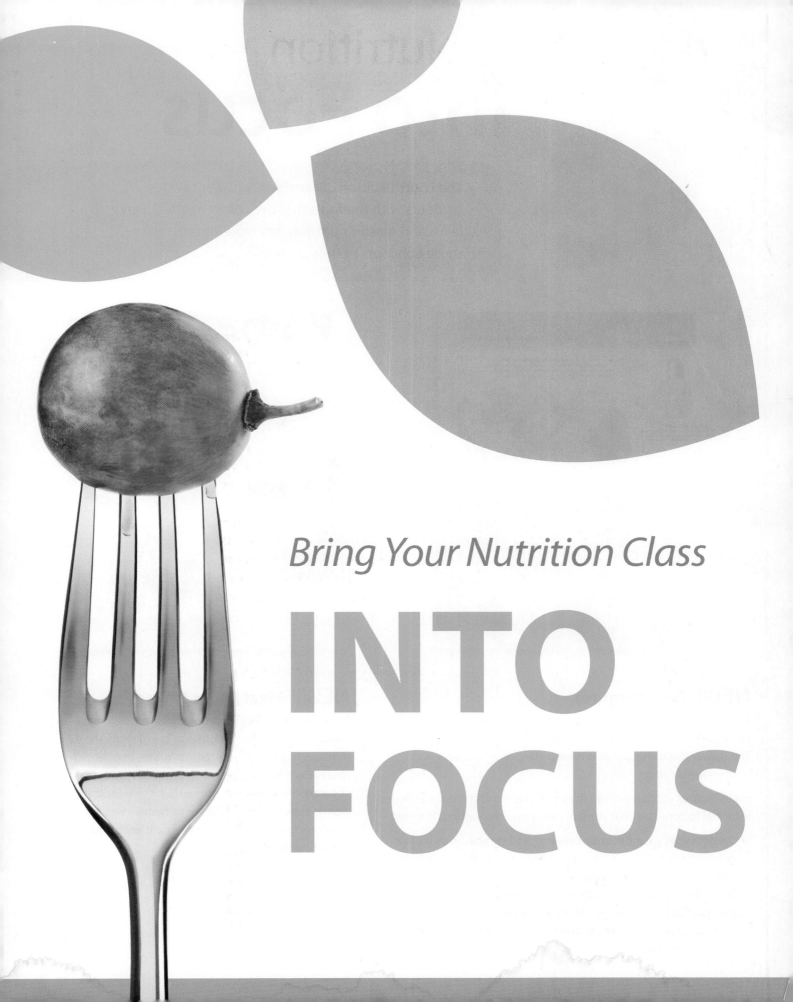

Bring Your Nutrition Class

INTO FOCUS

Bring Nutrition Into Focus

The Fourth Edition of *Nutrition for Life* provides students with the tools that they need to effectively learn and master nutrition concepts and to apply those concepts to their daily lives.

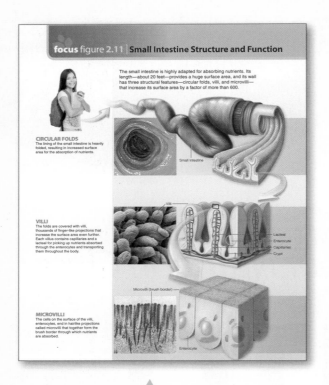

NEW! Focus Figures

These colorful, full-page figures teach students key concepts in nutrition through bold, clear, and detailed visual presentations. The dynamic new figures also have corresponding tutorials in MasteringNutrition.

Focus Figures include introductory text that explains how the figure is central to concepts that students will cover throughout the text.

* Students get clear directions via text and stepped-out art that guide the eye through complex processes, breaking them down into manageable pieces that are easy to teach and understand.
* Focus Figures provide dynamic illustrations—often paired with photographs—that make topics come alive.
* Full-page format enables micro-to-macro levels of explanation for complex topics.

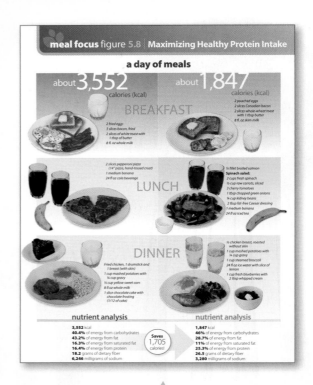

NEW! Meal Focus Figures

Students get a visual comparison of possible meal choices, ranging from high- and low-density meals to meals high in refined carbohydrates vs fiber-rich meals. Each figure offers easy-to-understand comparisons of the key nutrients for that topic as well as clear images of the foods being assessed. New coaching activities complement each figure in MasteringNutrition.

Fats
Essential Energy-Supplying Nutrients

4

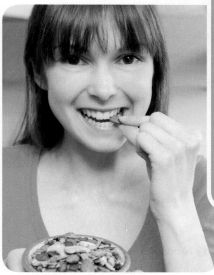

learning outcomes

After studying this chapter, you should be able to:

1. Compare and contrast the three types of lipids found in foods, pp. 101–106.

2. Discuss how the level of saturation of a fatty acid affects its shape and the form it takes, pp. 101–106.

3. Explain the health benefits and dietary sources of the essential fatty acids, pp. 101–106.

4. List five functions of fat, pp. 107–108.

5. Describe the steps involved in fat digestion, absorption, and transport, pp. 109–111.

6. Identify the dietary recommendations for intakes of total fat, saturated fat, *trans* fats, and the essential fatty acids, pp. 112–117.

7. Identify common food sources of less healthful versus more healthful fats, pp. 112–117.

8. Summarize our current understanding of the relationship between intake of dietary fats and the development of cardiovascular disease and cancer, pp. 118–124.

test yourself

Are these statements true or false? Circle your guess.

1. **T F** Dietary cholesterol is not required because our body makes all the cholesterol it needs.

2. **T F** Fat is an important fuel source during rest and exercise.

3. **T F** Certain fats protect against heart disease.

Test Yourself answers can be found at the end of the chapter.

MasteringNutrition™
Go online for chapter quizzes, pre-tests, Interactive Activities, and more!

◀ NEW! Learning Outcomes and Study Plan

Learning Outcomes now introduce every chapter, giving students a roadmap for their reading. Each chapter concludes with a Study Plan, which summarizes key points of the chapter and provides review questions to check understanding, both tied to the chapter's learning outcomes.

---

chapter summary

Scan to hear an MP3 Chapter Review in MasteringNutrition.

LO 1 Summarize the two main reasons that foodborne illness is a critical concern in the United States

- According to the CDC, about 48 million Americans report experiencing foodborne illness each year. Moreover, food production is increasingly complex, with more foods mass-produced than ever before, using a combination of ingredients from a much greater number of sources, including fields, feedlots, and a variety of processing facilities all over the world. Contamination can occur at any point from farm to table, and when it does, it can be difficult to trace.

LO 2 Identify the types of microorganisms most commonly involved in foodborne illness

- Food infections result from the consumption of food containing pathogenic microorganisms, such as bacteria, whereas food intoxications result from consuming food in which microorganisms have secreted toxins. Chemical residues in food can also cause illness.

- Food infections are most commonly caused by viruses, especially the norovirus; bacteria such as *Salmonella*; and parasites, such as helminths.

LO 3 Describe strategies for preventing foodborne illness at home, while eating out, and when traveling to other countries

- To reproduce in foods, microorganisms require a precise range of temperature, humidity, acidity, and oxygen content. You can prevent foodborne illness at home by washing your hands and kitchen surfaces often, separating foods to prevent cross-contamination, storing foods in the refrigerator or freezer, and cooking foods to their proper temperatures.

- When traveling, avoid raw foods and choose beverages that are boiled, bottled, or canned, without ice.

LO 4 Compare and contrast the different methods manufacturers use to preserve foods

- Some of the oldest techniques for food preservation include salting, sugaring, drying, smoking, and cooling.

STUDY PLAN | MasteringNutrition™

Customize your study plan—and master your nutrition!— in the Study Area of **MasteringNutrition**.

what can I do **today?**

Now that you've read this chapter, try making these three changes.

1. Before every meal, whether you're preparing it yourself or eating out, wash your hands!

2. Buy a thermometer for your refrigerator and freezer. If you eat meat, buy a meat thermometer. Then start to use them!

3. If you purchase an apple today, pay the extra cash for organic. Apples top the list of high-pesticide foods.

test yourself | *answers*

1. **False.** A majority of cases of foodborne illness are caused by just one species of virus, called norovirus. Bacteria also commonly cause foodborne illness. Mold is not usually a culprit.

2. **False.** Freezing destroys some microorganisms but only inhibits the ability of other microorganisms to reproduce. When the food is thawed, these cold-tolerant microorganisms resume reproduction.

3. **True.** In 2008 through 2012, the last five years for which data are available, more than 14% of American households have experienced food insecurity.

---

review questions

LO 1 Compare and contrast the three types of lipids found in foods

1. Cholesterol is
   a. a triglyceride.
   b. a form of saturated fatty acid.
   c. a sterol.
   d. a phospholipid.

LO 2 Discuss how the level of saturation of a fatty acid affects its shape and the form it takes

2. Triglycerides with a double carbon bond at one part of the molecule are referred to as
   a. monounsaturated fats.
   b. hydrogenated fats.
   c. saturated fats.
   d. sterols.

LO 3 Explain the health benefits and dietary sources of the essential fatty acids

3. EPA and DHA
   a. are omega-3 fatty acids.
   b. are found in fatty fish.
   c. reduce the risk of cardiovascular disease.
   d. all of the above.

LO 4 List five functions of fat

4. Fats
   a. provide energy, but less per gram than carbohydrates.
   b. provide energy for resting functions, but not for physical activity.
   c. enable the transport of proteins.
   d. enable the transport of fat-soluble vitamins.

Continuous Learning
Before, During & After Class with
MasteringNutrition™ with MyDietAnalysis

MasteringNutrition with MyDietAnalysis is the most effective and widely used online homework, tutorial, and assessment system for the sciences. It delivers self-paced tutorials that focus on your course objectives, provides individualized coaching, and responds to each student's progress.

BEFORE CLASS

Dynamic Study Modules and Pre-Class Assignments provide students with a preview of what's to come.

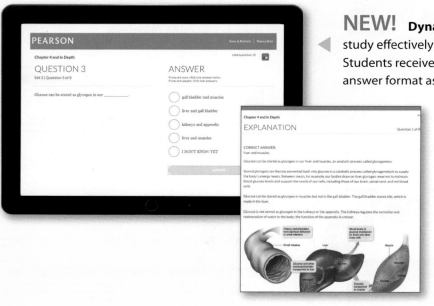

NEW! **Dynamic Study Modules** enable students to study effectively on their own in an adaptive format. Students receive an initial set of questions with a unique answer format asking them to indicate their confidence level.

Once completed, Dynamic Study Modules include explanations using materials taken directly from the text. These modules can be accessed on smartphones, tablets and computers. You can also assign an individual Dynamic Study Module for completion as a graded assignment prior to class.

Mastering offers Pre-Lecture Quiz Questions that are easy to customize and assign.

NEW! **Reading Questions** ensure that students complete the assigned reading before class and stay on track with reading assignments. Reading Questions are 100% mobile ready and can be completed by students on mobile devices.

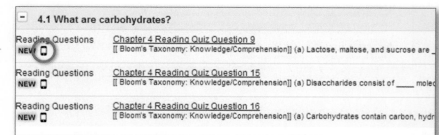

DURING CLASS

Learning Catalytics™ and Engaging Media

What has professors and students so excited? Learning Catalytics, a "bring your own device" student engagement, assessment, and classroom intelligence system, allows students to use their smartphone, tablet, or laptop to respond to questions in class. With Learning Catalytics, you can:

* Assess students in real-time using open ended question formats to uncover student misconceptions and adjust lectures accordingly.
* Automatically create groups for peer instruction based on student response patterns, to optimize discussion productivity.

> My students are so busy and engaged answering Learning Catalytics questions during lecture that they don't have time for Facebook.

Declan De Paor
Old Dominion University

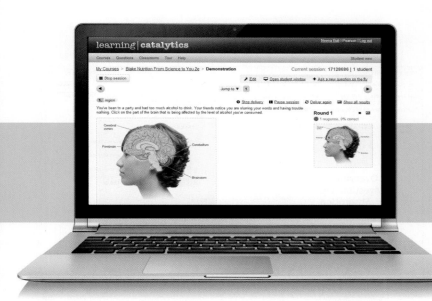

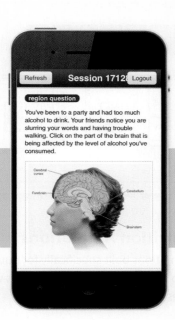

Engaging In-class Media

Instructors can also incorporate dynamic media from the **Teaching Toolkit DVD** into lecture and build class discussions and activities around Nutrition Animations, *ABC News* Lecture Launchers, NutriTools, and more. For more information, please see the last page of this walkthrough.

MasteringNutrition™

AFTER CLASS

Easy-to-Assign, Customizable, and Automatically Graded Assignments

The breadth and depth of content available to you to assign in Mastering is unparalleled, allowing you to quickly and easily assign homework to reinforce key concepts.

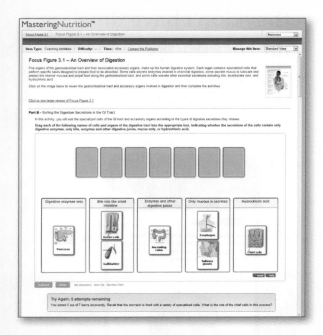

◀ Focus Figure Coaching Activities

Coaching activities guide students through key nutrition concepts with interactive mini-lessons that provide hints and feedback.

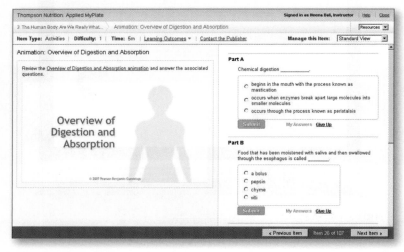

Nutrition Animations

Animations built specifically for nutrition help students master tough topics with assessment and feedback. ▶

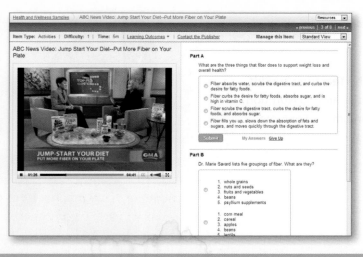

◀ *ABC News* Videos

27 *ABC News* videos with assessment and feedback help nutrition come to life and show how it's related to the real world.

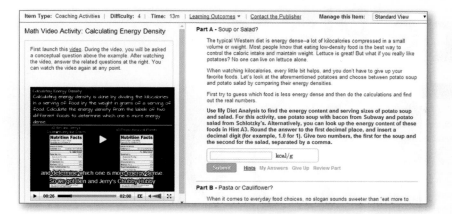

Math Video Activities

These interactive activities walk students through important calculations and provide hands-on practice with wrong-answer feedback to help students understand and apply the material.

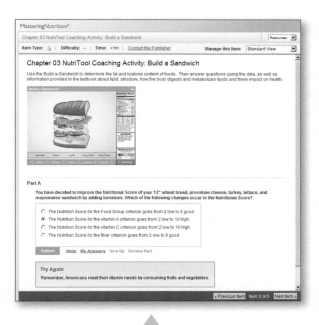

NutriTool Build-A-Meal Activities

These unique activities allow students to combine and experiment with different food options and learn first-hand how to build healthier meals.

MasteringNutrition also Includes Access to MyDietAnalysis

MyDietAnalysis is now available as a single sign on to MasteringNutrition. For smartphone users, a new mobile website version of MyDietAnalysis is available. Students can track their diet and activity intake accurately, anytime and anywhere, from their mobile device.

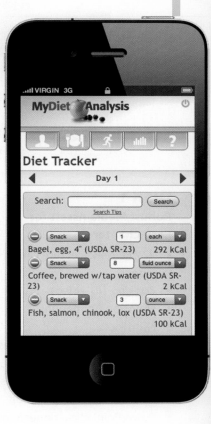

Learning Outcomes

All of the MasteringNutrition assignable content is tagged to book content and to Bloom's Taxonomy. You also have the ability to add your own outcomes, helping you track student performance against your learning outcomes. You can view class performance against the specified learning outcomes and share those results quickly and easily by exporting to a spreadsheet.

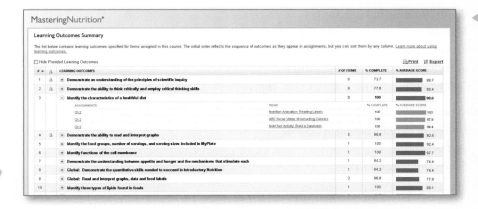

Everything You Need to Teach
In One Place

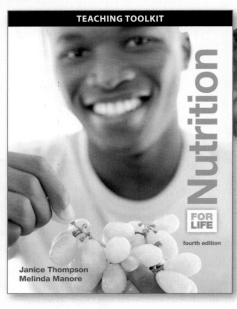

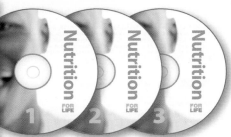

Teaching Toolkit DVD for
Nutrition for Life

The Teaching Toolkit DVD provides everything that you need to prep for your course and deliver a dynamic lecture in one convenient place. Included on 3 disks are these valuable resources:

DISK 1
Robust Media Assets for Each Chapter

- 27 *ABC News* Lecture Launcher videos
- *Cooking 101* videos
- Nutrition Animations
- NutriTools
- PowerPoint Lecture Outlines
- Media Link PowerPoint slides for easy importing of videos, animations, and NutriTools
- PowerPoint clicker questions and Jeopardy-style quiz show questions
- Files for all illustrations and tables and selected photos from the text

DISK 2
Comprehensive Test Bank

- Test Bank in Word and RTF formats
- Computerized Test Bank, which includes all of the questions from the test bank in a format that allows you to easily and intuitively build exams and quizzes

DISK 3
Additional Innovative Supplements for Instructors and Students

For Instructors
- Instructor's Resource Support Manual
- Introduction to Mastering Nutrition
- Introductory video for Learning Catalytics

For Students
- *Eat Right! Healthy Eating in College and Beyond*
- *Food Composition Table*

User's Quick Guide for *Nutrition for Life*

This easy-to-use printed supplement accompanies the Teaching Toolkit and offers easy instructions for both experienced and new faculty members to get started with rich Toolkit content, how to access assignments within MasteringNutrition, and how to "flip" the classroom with Learning Catalytics.

Nutrition 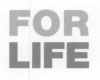 FOR LIFE

Nutrition FOR LIFE

fourth edition

Janice Thompson, PhD, FACSM

University of Birmingham, UK

Melinda Manore, PhD, RD, FACSM

Oregon State University

PEARSON

Acquisitions Editor: Sandra Lindelof/Michelle Cadden
Project Manager: Tu-Anh Dang-Tran
Program Manager: Susan Malloy
Development Editor: Laura Bonazzoli
Art Development Editor: Marie Beaugureau
Editorial Assistant: Leah Sherwood
Text Permissions Project Manager: Timothy Nicholls
Development Manager: Barbara Yien
Program Management Team Lead: Mike Early
Project Management Team Lead: Nancy Tabor
Copyeditor: Mike Rossa

Project Management and Composition: S4Carlisle Publishing Services, Lynn Steines
Design Manager: Marilyn Perry
Cover and Interior Design: Elise Lansdon
Illustrators: Precision Graphics
Photographer: Kristin Piljay
Photo Permissions Management: Eric Schrader
Photo Researcher: Jen Simmons, Steve Merland
Manufacturing Buyer: Stacey Weinberger
Executive Marketing Manager: Neena Bali

Cover Photo Credit: Ian Hooton/Science Photo Library/Corbis

Library of Congress Cataloging-in-Publication Data
Thompson, Janice, 1962- , author.
   Nutrition for life / Janice Thompson, Melinda Manore. — Fourth edition.
      p. ; cm.
   Includes bibliographical references.
   ISBN 978-0-13-385336-0 — ISBN 0-13-385336-5
   I. Manore, Melinda, 1951- , author. II. Title.
   [DNLM: 1. Nutritional Physiological Phenomena. 2. Food. QU 145]
   TX354
   613.2—dc23
                                                      2014037618

1 2 3 4 5 6 7 8 9 10—**V011**—17 16 15 14

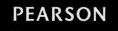

ISBN 10: 0-13-385336-5 (Student edition)
ISBN 13: 978-0-13-385336-0 (Student edition)

ISBN 10: 0-13-390245-5 (Instructor's Review copy)
ISBN 13: 978-0-13-390245-7 (Instructor's Review copy)
www.pearsonhighered.com

"To our Moms—your consistent love and support are the keys to our happiness and success. You have been incredible role models."

"To our Dads—you raised us to be independent, intelligent, and resourceful. We miss you and wish you were here to be proud of, and to brag about, our accomplishments."

about the authors

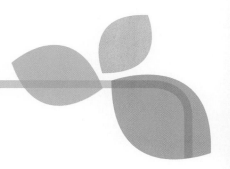

Janice Thompson, PhD, FACSM

University of Birmingham, UK

Janice Thompson earned a PhD from Arizona State University in exercise science with an emphasis in exercise physiology and nutrition. She is currently a professor of Public Health Nutrition in the School of Sport, Exercise and Rehabilitation Sciences at The University of Birmingham, UK. Her research focuses on developing nutrition and physical activity interventions to reduce the risks for obesity and type 2 diabetes in high-risk populations. Janice retains her U.S. affiliation by regularly collaborating with colleagues across the United States and maintaining strong professional links with the American College of Sport Medicine (ACSM).

Janice is a Fellow of the ACSM and recently served as Vice President of ACSM. She is also a member of the American Society for Nutrition (ASN), the British Association of Sport and Exercise Science (BASES), The Nutrition Society in the United Kingdom, and the European College of Sports Science (ECSS), where she serves as a member of the Scientific Committee. Janice won an undergraduate teaching award while at the University of North Carolina, Charlotte. In addition to *Nutrition for Life*, Janice coauthored the Pearson textbooks *Nutrition: An Applied Approach*, with Melinda Manore, and *The Science of Nutrition*, with Melinda Manore and Linda Vaughan. Janice loves traveling, yoga, hiking, and cooking and eating delicious food. She likes almost every vegetable except canned peas and believes chocolate should be listed as a food group.

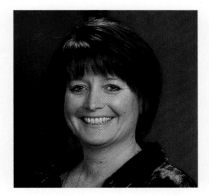

Melinda Manore, PhD, RD, FACSM

Oregon State University

Melinda Manore earned a PhD in human nutrition with a minor in exercise physiology at Oregon State University (OSU). She is the past chair of the Department of Nutrition and Food Management at OSU and is currently a professor of nutrition in the School of Population and Biological Sciences. Prior to her tenure at OSU, she was a professor at Arizona State University. Melinda's area of expertise is nutrition and exercise, especially the role of diet and exercise in health, energy balance, and weight management; chronic disease prevention; and the energy and nutrient needs of active people, especially active girls and women. She is currently engaged in two large community-based, obesity prevention projects in families with children and in high school soccer players.

Melinda is an active member of the Academy of Nutrition and Dietetics (AND). She is a current Fellow of the American College of Sports Medicine (ACSM) and a past vice president. She is the past chair of the AND Research Committee and the Research Dietetic Practice Group, and she served on the AND Obesity Steering Committee. She is an active member of SCAN, a nutrition and exercise practice group of AND. Melinda is also a member of the American Society of Nutrition (ASN) and the Obesity Society. She is also the past chair of USDA's Nutrition and Health Planning and Guidance Committee and the USDA, ACSM, and AND Energy Balance Working Group. Melinda is the past nutrition column author and associate editor for ACSM's *Health and Fitness Journal* and *Medicine and Science in Sports and Exercise*, and she serves on the editorial boards of numerous research journals. She has won awards for excellence in research and teaching. She also coauthored the Pearson textbooks *Nutrition: An Applied Approach*, with Janice Thompson, and *The Science of Nutrition*, with Janice Thompson and Linda Vaughan. Melinda is an avid walker, hiker, and former runner who loves to cook and eat great food. She is now trying her hand at cycling, gardening, and birding.

Welcome to *Nutrition for Life,* Fourth Edition!

Why We Wrote the Book

You stop at the convenience store for a snack. Blaring across the front of a bag of chips is the banner *No Trans Fats!* while a bag of pretzels claims *Now with Whole Grains!* What do these claims really mean, you wonder, and why should you care? You buy the chips and take them to a party, where a football game is on TV. It's half-time and an athlete is pushing some new protein supplement. A friend comes up and offers you a can of something called *Action!* "It's this new high-energy drink," he explains. But then your roommate snickers, "Yeah, and the caffeine in it can give you a heart attack! You know, they've banned that stuff in France!"

No doubt about it, nutrition is a hot topic, but do you ever wind up with information overload? Everybody claims to be an expert, but what's their advice based on? Is it reliable? How do you navigate through the endless recommendations and arrive at a way of eating that's right for *you*—one that energizes you, allows you to maintain a healthful weight, and helps you avoid disease and promote good health?

We Wrote This Book to Help You Answer These Questions

Nutrition for Life began with the conviction that students would benefit from an engaging, accurate, and clear textbook that links essential nutrition content to their own health and encourages them to make nutrition part of their everyday life. As authors and educators, we know that students have a natural interest in their body, their health, their weight, and their success in sports and a range of life activities. By demonstrating how nutrition relates to these interests, *Nutrition for Life*, Fourth Edition, empowers students to reach their personal health and nutritional goals. We use multiple strategies to capture students' interest, from highlighting how nutrients are critical to health, to discussing the vitamins and minerals based on their clear functions within the body, to a variety of special features and activities that bring nutrition to life. Throughout the text, material is presented in a lively narrative style that consistently links the essential facts to students' lifestyles and goals. Information on current topics and research keeps the inquisitive spark alive, illustrating that nutrition is very much a "living" science, and the source of ongoing debate, research, and interest. We present nutritional basics in an easy-to-read, friendly narrative with engaging features that reduce students' apprehensions and encourage them to apply the information directly to their lives. We've also ensured that the organization and flow of the content and the art work together to provide a learning resource that is enjoyable to engage for both instructors and students.

As educators, we're familiar with the myriad challenges of presenting nutrition information in the classroom, and we have included tools in the book and ancillary materials that will assist instructors in successfully meeting these challenges. Through broad instructor and student support with print and media supplements, we hope to contribute to the excitement of teaching and learning about nutrition: a subject that affects all of us, one so important and relevant that correct and timely information can make the difference between health and disease.

Features of *Nutrition for Life*

The following features are integrated throughout *Nutrition for Life,* Fourth Edition, to help you learn, study, and apply all the fascinating concepts of nutrition to your own life. As you read through each chapter, be sure to look at the feature boxes and test your knowledge with the Review Questions. You can also find more information, resources, and self-quizzing activities in the Study Area of MasteringNutrition.

- **Test Yourself** questions are located at the beginning of each chapter. These targeted prompts will help you dispel common myths about nutrition. The answers can be found at the end of each chapter.
- **Learning Outcomes** are a new feature to this edition and highlight key lessons students should take away from each section. The Learning Outcomes have been repeated throughout the chapter so students can regularly stop and evaluate their understanding of the main concept.
- **What About You?** feature boxes help you figure out where you stand with regard to important nutrition issues. This feature, appearing in most chapters, provides self-assessment prompts and exercises that enable you to determine whether your diet and lifestyle are as healthful as they could be, and whether you should be concerned about any particular nutrition-related issues.
- **Game Plan** feature boxes offer detailed strategies for adopting healthful eating and lifestyle changes. They have been updated and reconfigured in this edition into a consistent checklist format, making it even easier to follow the recommended tips and guidelines.
- **Nutrition Label Activities** will show you how to evaluate the labels from actual food products so that you can make educated decisions about the foods you consume. Updated for this edition, these activities have been made even more interactive, providing hands-on practice that you can apply when you do your own food shopping. Answers to Nutrition Label Activities, when applicable, can be found in MasteringNutrition.
- **Nutrition Myth or Fact?** feature boxes provide the facts behind the hype surrounding many current nutrition and dietary issues. They dispel common misconceptions and show you how to critically evaluate information you encounter every day from the Internet, media sources, and your peers.
- **Highlight** feature boxes provide deeper background into topics you'll recognize from the Internet, mass media, and popular culture, including issues such as sports beverages, alternative sweeteners, and fad diets. Highlight boxes review the facts and theories surrounding widely discussed subjects and help you sort out the core issues they relate to.
- **Foods You Don't Know You Love Yet** feature boxes describe "emerging foods" you might not be familiar with (and which pack a surprising nutritional punch) or more common foods you might have overlooked.
- **What Can I Do *Today?*** appears at the end of each chapter and prompts you to think in active, concrete ways about three key things you can do right now to incorporate your new nutritional knowledge into your life.
- **Nutrition Online** icons appear throughout each chapter, directing you to web links, videos, podcasts, and other useful online and new media resources.
- **Healthwatch** sections found throughout the text are special subject areas designed to highlight the health effects of various key nutrients and foods, illuminating the consequences of diet on your health.
- **Recaps** are placed strategically throughout each chapter to clearly review and highlight the key points, helping you to grasp the full concepts in easily understood terms.
- **Organization of vitamins and minerals** is unique in this book. Traditionally, students are taught vitamin and mineral content by memorizing each nutrient, along with its deficiency and toxicity symptoms. We've found that, with that approach, students quickly forget the information and don't truly understand why these nutrients are important and how they affect the body. In *Nutrition for Life,* Fourth Edition, we organize the vitamins and minerals based on their *functions* inside your body, giving you a framework for understanding why they're

important, what they do, and what happens when you don't get enough—or get too much!—of each one. This breakthrough approach has enjoyed enormous success and popularity with students and instructors alike.

■ **Art, photos, and tables** in this edition have been updated and designed to take you clearly through your body's processing of nutrients. Figures are constructed to show step-by-step what happens to the food you eat, as well as which foods are good sources of key nutrients. Photos illustrate various conditions created by deficiency and toxicity and identify foods that you may not immediately think of as good sources for specific nutrients.

■ **Chapter Summaries** have been added and have been correlated to Learning Outcomes so students can see what the standout lessons are for each section.

■ **Review Questions** at the end of each chapter help you assess your retention and understanding of the material covered in each chapter. Answers to Review Questions appear at the end of the book.

■ **Web Links** at the end of each chapter identify additional web-based resources for further information and study.

■ **References,** located in this edition at the end of the book, provide students with references to all the research used within the chapters.

New to the Fourth Edition

For this edition, our goal was to make the book even more practical and relevant to students in applying the information to their own lives. We also wanted to include more material on how to evaluate nutrition information and to provide the most up-to-date and accurate nutrition information currently available.

New to this edition, we have added **Learning Outcomes** to each chapter, allowing students to track their own understanding and knowledge of the key concepts of each chapter. Each Learning Outcome has been correlated to the individual sections so students know what to focus on. The **Review Questions** and **Chapter Summary** bullet points have also been correlated to Learning Outcomes in an integrated Study Plan so the message and key points are repeated throughout the chapter.

Also new to this edition are dynamic and eye-catching full-page **Focus Figures** that depict some of the most important and complex processes or concepts discussed in the chapter. These figures provide a visual, step-by-step walkthrough that will help students understand and master these topics.

Another new feature is the **Meal Focus Figures**. These figures depict one day's poor meal choices versus healthy meal choices and provide a nutrient analysis of each day's meals so that students can compare the nutritional differences. Each Meal Focus Figure shows students two different options for breakfast, lunch, and dinner.

In addition to these exciting new features in this edition, we have modified or expanded many of the existing features to be even more practical, often appearing as worksheets or checklists that students can work through. The design and art programs have been updated with dynamic colors to add to visual clarity and interest. To provide a focused and streamlined text, we've moved the **Nutri-Case** features and **Cooking 101** videos online where they will be available through **MasteringNutrition**. The visual summary of features in the front of the book provides an overview of these and other important features in the fourth edition. For specific changes to each chapter, please see below.

Chapter 1

■ Added Learning Outcomes and revised and updated Test Yourself questions
■ Updated Figure 1.4 with new statistics on obesity
■ Replaced DRI figures with a new Focus Figure
■ Replaced former Figure 1.7 comparing high- versus low-density meals with new Meal Focus Figure
■ Replaced Mediterranean diet pyramid and Latin diet pyramid with "plate" versions to correspond to MyPlate. Deleted Asian diet pyramid.

Chapter 2

- Added Learning Outcomes and revised and updated Test Yourself questions
- Deleted former Figure 2.3 on the organization of the human body
- Replaced figure of gastrointestinal tract anatomy with new Focus Figure
- Replaced figure of absorptive features of the small intestine with new Focus Figure
- Fully updated the information about nutrigenomics in the Nutrition Myth or Fact? box
- Fully updated the information about probiotics—and added prebiotics—to the Highlight box
- Expanded content discussing the importance of fiber to GI health
- Moved figure of enzyme function from the protein chapter to this chapter, where enzymes are first discussed
- Updated content on ulcers
- Updated content and figure on GERD
- Added information on non-celiac gluten sensitivity
- Updated the Review Questions

Chapter 3

- Added Learning Outcomes and revised and updated Test Yourself questions
- Moved table of terms related to grains into the Highlight on what constitutes a whole grain
- Replaced figure of carbohydrate digestion with new Focus Figure
- Updated information on glycemic index and load
- Revised information on high fructose corn syrup
- Converted the Highlight on artificial sweeteners into a narrative section and entirely updated it
- Replaced former Figure 3.14 comparing high- versus low-fiber meals with new Meal Focus Figure
- Slightly expanded the information on the consequences of uncontrolled diabetes
- Deleted former Figure 3.15 (race/ethnicity graph of type 2 diabetes)

Chapter 4

- Added Learning Outcomes and revised and updated Test Yourself questions
- Updated information on *trans* fats to reflect FDA preliminary finding on partially hydrogenated oils (PHOs) no longer being recognized as safe
- Moved information on Urquhart's research with the Inuits from the Nutrition Milestone into the narrative
- In the Nutrition Myth or Fact? box on butter versus margarine, added a table providing nutritional information
- Added information on the role of steroids in steroid hormones
- Replaced former Figure 4.7 of lipid digestion with new Focus Figure
- Added a new Meal Focus Figure comparing meals high and low in saturated fat
- Moved the information and table comparing reduced-fat, low-fat, and nonfat foods from a separate Highlight box into the Nutrition Label Activity on fat on food labels
- Deleted the discussion of fat replacers
- Added chia seeds and pumpkin seeds to the Foods You Don't Know You Love Yet on flaxseeds
- Replaced former Figure 4.12 of photos of atherosclerotic blood vessels with full-page atherosclerosis Focus Figure

Chapter 5

- Added Learning Outcomes and revised and updated Test Yourself questions
- Moved former Figure 5.5 on enzymes to Chapter 2 where enzymes are introduced
- Replaced former Figure 5.7 on protein digestion with new Focus Figure
- Slightly expanded information on the waste products of protein digestion
- Reorganized the discussion of protein deficiency and protein excess to improve flow

- Fully updated the Nutrition Myth or Fact? box on high-protein diets
- Added a new Meal Focus Figure comparing meals with poor versus healthful protein sources
- Fully updated the Highlight on soy and moved tips on increasing soy into the Game Plan on adding legumes to your diet
- Fully updated the information on protein and amino acid supplements
- Fully updated the information on vegetarian diets and replaced the vegetarian food pyramid with a link to the Vegetarian Resource Group's vegan MyPlate

Chapter 6
- Added Learning Outcomes and revised and updated Test Yourself questions
- Updated the information on vitamin DRIs
- Added a new narrative section called Vitamins Are Vulnerable on preventing excessive losses during storage and cooking
- Converted the information on dietary supplements—which had been in a Highlight box—into a narrative section and updated to include new research questioning the benefits of MVM supplements for most consumers, and removed information on functional foods (which is now mentioned in Chapter 2)
- Added a new Meal Focus Figure comparing meals poor versus rich in a variety of vitamins

Chapter 7
- Added Learning Outcomes and revised and updated Test Yourself questions
- Revised chapter-opening story to introduce both osteopenia and osteoporosis
- Expanded modestly the content on sodium in foods, specifically on sodium in fast foods
- Added a new figure identifying key components of the DASH diet
- Simplified the figure showing the structure of hemoglobin
- Added a bulleted list of tips for boosting iron intake
- Expanded the discussion on osteoporosis prevention

Chapter 8
- Added Learning Outcomes and revised and updated Test Yourself questions
- Revised the chapter opener to introduce the FDA's concerns related to energy drinks
- Fully revised and updated the discussion of sources of drinking water
- Shortened the discussion of tea
- Added a new discussion of alkaline water and black water as examples of many types of bottled water marketed with ungrounded health claims
- Fully revised, updated, and expanded the discussion of energy drinks
- Added a discussion of coconut water
- Added a discussion of the Calorie costs of alcoholic beverages

Chapter 9
- Added Learning Outcomes and revised and updated Test Yourself questions
- Updated the chapter opener
- Added information on new research into the protective effects of being modestly overweight
- Replaced the former figure on the energy balance equation with a new Focus Figure and added a brief discussion of the limitations of the energy balance equation
- Added photos for visual interest to the table on the energy costs of physical activities
- Fully updated the information on the genetic, metabolic, and social factors influencing body weight
- Added a new Meal Focus Figure comparing meals high in empty Calories versus lower Calorie meals high in nutrient density

- Deleted Figure 9.12, the graph that showed rising rates of childhood obesity
- Fully updated the information on pharmacologic and surgical treatments for obesity
- Fully revised the material on eating disorders to reflect DSM-5 classifications

Chapter 10

- Added Learning Outcomes and revised and updated Test Yourself questions
- Updated the chapter opener
- Comprehensively revised and updated the information on designing a quality fitness program
- Replaced former Figure 10.6 with a new Focus Figure on energy use during physical activity
- Condensed the narrative on dehydration, heatstroke, and other heat-related problems, because these are discussed fully in Chapter 8
- Modestly expanded the information on ergogenic aids

Chapter 11

- Added Learning Outcomes and revised and updated Test Yourself questions
- Modestly condensed the discussions of a pregnant woman's specific nutrient needs and of smoking and substance abuse during pregnancy
- Modestly condensed the section on breastfeeding
- Deleted the former Nutrition Myth or Fact? box on feeding a vegan diet to toddlers
- Replaced the MyPyramid for Kids poster with the new MyPlate food plan for preschoolers
- Revised and expanded the material on school lunches
- Revised and expanded the material on food insecurity among children
- Fully updated the discussion of obesity in children
- Replaced the old Tufts food pyramid for older adults with the new Tufts MyPlate for Older Adults
- Expanded the discussion of polypharmacy among older adults
- Fully revised the discussion of calorie restriction to boost life span

Chapter 12

- Added Learning Outcomes and revised and updated Test Yourself questions
- Replaced the chapter introduction to highlight the problem of norovirus
- Fully updated all foodborne illness statistics and governmental regulations related to food safety
- Updated and expanded discussion of the viral sources of foodborne illness
- Entirely updated Table 12.2 on the six most common bacterial causes of foodborne illness
- Updated the data in the Nutrition Myth or Fact? feature box on mad cow disease
- Revised and expanded the discussion of toxins in foods, for example, toxic algae
- Replaced FightBac figure with similar figure from foodsafety.gov
- Included link to FSIS information on thawing foods safely
- Deleted Thermy figure
- Updated information on the GRAS list, including FDA proposal to remove PHOs
- Fully updated all information on GMOs, including in the Highlight feature box
- Discussed effects of endocrine disruptors—BPA, phthalates, and dioxins—as residues in foods
- Updated research into the increased nutrients and reduced pesticide levels of organic foods
- Added EWG's "Dirty Dozen" and "Clean Fifteen" lists of pesticide levels in foods
- Comprehensively revised the chapter-closing section on the food movement, including the discussions of sustainability issues, food diversity, slow food, local food, food equity, food insecurity, and fair trade
- Moved the discussion of global food insecurity to the website

Appendices and Back Matter

- Appendix A is The USDA Food Guide Evolution, which provides an overview of the development of the USDA nutritional recommendations and MyPlate
- Appendix D is the most up to date Choose Your Food List for Diabetes from 2014 which provides a variety of meal planning choices for carbohydrates, proteins, beverages, and many more
- Available on MasteringNutrition are the Cooking 101 Videos and Glossary, with adaptations from the *Eat Right! Healthy Eating and Beyond* print ancillary, including recipes, shopping lists, tips for eating on a budget, and essential cooking terms and concepts
- The 2010 Dietary Guidelines are posted on the inside front cover of the text. Located on the inside back cover, and in adjoining back pages of this text, are the current Tolerable Upper Intake Levels (ULs) for Vitamins and Elements (minerals), and the Dietary Reference Intakes (DRIs) for Macronutrients, Vitamins, and Elements (minerals)

So Many Options for Your Students

Students today want options when it comes to their learning and especially their textbooks. **Nutrition for Life** gives students the flexibility they desire, offering a wide range of formats for the book and a large array of online learning resources. Let your students find a version that works best for them!

Whether it's on a laptop, tablet, or cell phone, *Nutrition for Life* lets students access media and other tools about nutrition.

Nutrition for Life
MasteringNutrition with eText

0-133-98327-7 / 978-0-133-98327-2

Available at no charge within MasteringHealth, the Pearson eText 2.0 version of Access to Health gives students access to the text whenever and wherever they have access to the Internet. Features of the eText now include:

- Now available on smartphones and tablets.
- Seamlessly integrated videos and other rich media.
- Accessible (screen-reader ready).
- Configurable reading settings, including resizable type and night reading mode.
- Instructor and student note-taking, highlighting, bookmarking, and search.

Nutrition for Life
CourseSmart eTextbook

0-133-90244-7 / 978-0-133-90244-0

CourseSmart eTextbooks are an exciting new choice for students looking to save money. As an alternative to purchasing the print textbook, students can subscribe to the same content online and save up to 40% off the suggested list price of the print text. Go to **www.coursesmart.com**.

Nutrition for Life Books a La Carte

0-133-99319-1 / 978-0-133-99319-6

Books a la Carte features the same exact content as *Nutrition for Life* in a convenient, three-hole-punched, loose-leaf version. Books a la Carte offers a great value for your students–this format costs 35% less than a new textbook package.

Pearson Custom Library: You Create
Your Perfect Text

www.pearsonlearningsolutions.com/custom-library

Nutrition for Life is available on the Pearson Custom Library, allowing instructors to create the perfect text for their course. Select the chapters you need, in the sequence you want. Delete chapters you don't use: Your students pay only for the materials you choose.

> No matter the format, with each new copy of the text students will receive full access to the **Study Area of MasteringNutrition**, providing a wealth of videos, MP3 study podcasts, animations, and more. Give your students all the learning options with *Nutrition for Life*.

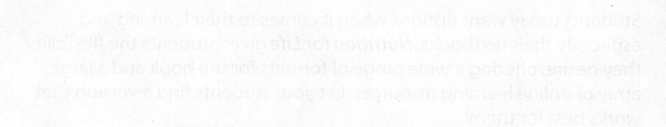

acknowledgments

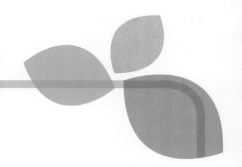

It is always eye opening to write a textbook and realize how many people actually contribute to the final, completed product!

We would like to thank the fabulous staff at Pearson Higher Education for their incredible support and dedication to this book. Frank Ruggirello, Publisher, committed extensive resources to ensuring the quality of this text, and his support and enthusiasm helped us maintain the momentum we needed to continue to enhance this project. Our Acquisitions Editor, Sandy Lindelof, encouraged us to be authors and provided unwavering support and guidance throughout the entire process of writing and publishing this book. We could never have written this text without the exceptional writing and organizational skills of Laura Bonazzoli, our Developmental Editor. Laura's energy, enthusiasm, and creativity significantly enhanced the quality of this text. Tu-Anh Dang-Tran, our dedicated Project Manager, kept us sane and focused with her excellent editorial skills. And Leah Sherwood, Editorial Assistant, managed endless critical details and tasks with grace and aplomb.

We also extend our deep gratitude to our wonderful contributor, Linda Vaughan, who expertly developed and enhanced the fluids and life cycle chapters in this and the previous editions. We would also like to gratefully acknowledge Carole Conn of the University of New Mexico for her contributions to the first edition and her efforts and research on global nutrition issues.

Multiple talented players helped build this book in the production and design process as well. Lynn Steines and the skilled team at S4Carlisle Publishing Services kept manuscripts moving through the production process and expertly tracked every minute detail. Eric Schrader supervised the art and photo programs, and Steve Merland and Jen Simmons researched photos. Elise Lansdon, with the excellent guidance of Marilyn Perry, created a beautiful interior text and cover design.

We can't go without thanking the marketing and sales teams, especially Neena Bali, Executive Marketing Manager, who has worked so hard to get this book out to those who will benefit most from it.

Our goal of meeting instructor and student needs could not have been realized without the strong team of educators and editorial staff who worked on the substantial supplements for *Nutrition for Life*. Pat Longoria adroitly updated and revised the comprehensive Test Bank, and Southern Editorial authored the wonderful Instructor Manual. Anna Page did a fabulous job updating the Lecture Outline and Quiz Show PowerPoint. Special thanks to Chelsea Logan who masterfully guided the development of the Teaching Toolkit DVD package and its assets. Additionally, thanks to Liz Winer for heading up the coordination and development of the MasteringNutrition website.

Finally, we would also like to acknowledge the many colleagues, friends, and family members who helped us along the way. Janice would especially like to thank her family and friends, who have been so wonderful throughout her career. She also thanks her colleagues and students, who continue to challenge her and contribute significantly to her deep enjoyment of teaching and nutrition-related research. Melinda would specifically like to thank her husband, Steve Carroll, for the patience and understanding he has shown through this process—once again. He has learned that there is always another chapter due! Melinda also thanks her family, friends, and professional colleagues for their support and attentive listening through this whole process. They have all helped make life a little easier during this incredibly busy time.

Reviewers

First Edition

Cassandra August, *Baldwin-Wallace College*
Gale Cohen, *Mercer County Community College*
K. Shane Croughton, *University of Wyoming*
Johanna Donnenfield, *Scottsdale Community College*
Sally Ebmeier, *Wayne State College*
Renee Finnecy, *Mercyhurst College*
Anne Holmes, *Luzerne County Community College*
Caryl Johnson, *Eastern New Mexico University*
U. Beate Krinke, *University of Minnesota*
Barbara K. McCahan, *Plymouth State University*
Anna M. Page, *Johnson County Community College*
Susan Rippy, *Eastern Illinois University*
Janet Schwartz, *Framingham State College*
Jane Burrell Uzcategui, *California State University, Los Angeles*
Andrea Villarreal, *Phoenix College*
Green T. Waggener, *Valdosta State University*
Diane Wagoner, *Indiana University of Pennsylvania*
Melissa Wdowik, *University of North Carolina, Charlotte*
Louise Whitney, *Lansing Community College*
Cynthia A. Wilson, *Seattle Central Community College*

Second Edition

Cassandra August, *Baldwin-Wallace College*
Valerie J. Benedix, *Clovis Community College*
Anne K. Black, *Austin Peay State University*
K. Shane Broughton, *University of Wyoming*
Fay C. Carpenter, *Housatonic Community College*
Gale Cohen, *Mercer County Community College*
Paula Cochrane, *New Mexico Community College*
Johanna Donnenfield, *Scottsdale Community College*
Sally Ebmeier, *Wayne State College*
Renee Finnecy, *Mercyhurst College*
Gary Fosmire, *Pennsylvania State University*
Anne Holmes, *Luzerne County Community College*
Caryl Johnson, *Eastern New Mexico University*
Jayanthi Kandiah, *Ball State University*
U. Beate Krinke, *University of Minnesota*
Barbara J. McCahan, *Plymouth State University*
Karen E. McConnell, *Pacific Lutheran University*
Karen Meyers, *University of Central Oklahoma*
Anna M. Page, *Johnson County Community College*
Roseann L. Poole, *Tallahassee Community College*
Susan Rippy, *Eastern Illinois University*
Janet Schwartz, *Framingham State College*
Jane Burrell Uzcategui, *California State University, Los Angeles*
Andrea Villarreal, *Phoenix College*
Green T. Waggener, *Valdosta State University*
Diane Wagoner, *Indiana University of Pennsylvania*
Melissa Wdowik, *University of North Carolina, Charlotte*
Louise Whitney, *Lansing Community College*
Cynthia A. Wilson, *Seattle Central Community College*
Maureen Zimmerman, *Mesa Community College*

Third Edition

Susan Asanovic, *Norwalk Community College*
Tom Brennan, *Macomb Community College*
Nancy Graves, *University of Houston*
Peg Johnston, *University of Nebraska – Kearney*
Shawnee Kelly, *Penn State University*
Michelle Pecchino, *Merced College*
Jennifer Ravia, *University of Arizona*
Beverly Roe, *Eric Community College – South Campus*
Andrea Villarreal, *Phoenix College*

MasteringNutrition™ **Faculty Advisory Board**

Brian Barthel, *Utah Valley College*
Melissa Chabot, *University at Buffalo – The State University of New York*
Julia Erbacher, *Salt Lake Community College*
Carol Friesen, *Ball State University*
Urbi Ghosh, *Oakton Community College*
Judy Kaufman, *Monroe Community College*
Michelle Konstantarakis, *University of Nevada, Las Vegas*
Milli Owens, *College of the Sequoias*
Janet Sass, *Northern Virginia Community College*
Dana Sherman, *Ozarks Technical Community College*
Priya Venkatesan, *Pasadena City College*

brief contents

Contents

contents

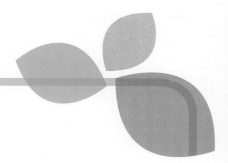

1

Nutrition: Making It Work for You 1

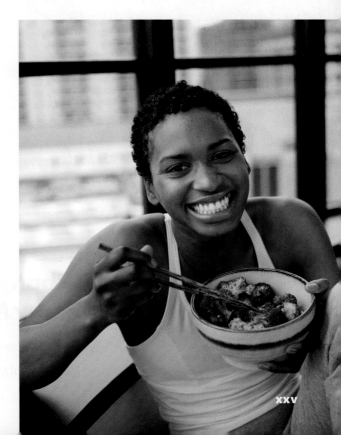

2

The Human Body: Are We Really What We Eat? 38

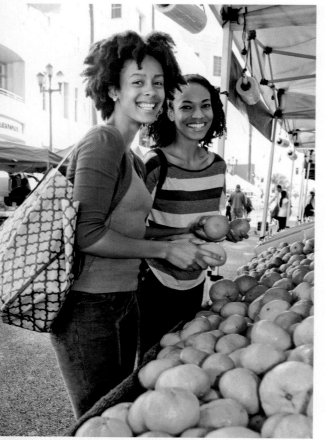

3

Carbohydrates: Plant-Derived Energy Nutrients 69

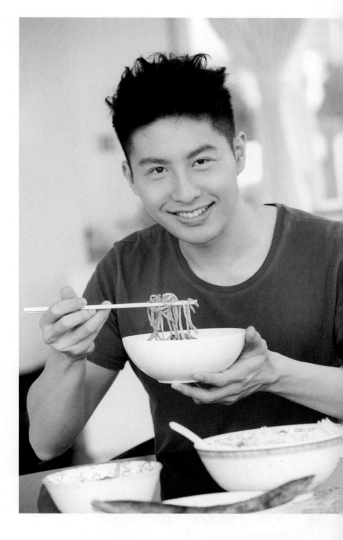

4

Fats: Essential Energy-Supplying Nutrients 100

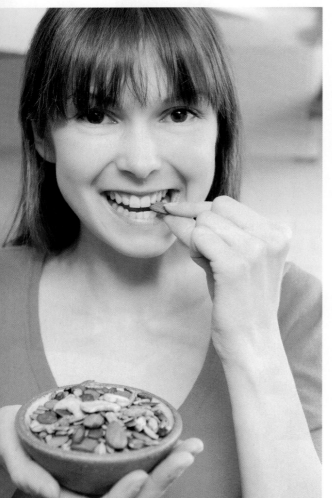

5

Proteins: Crucial Components of All Body Tissues 129

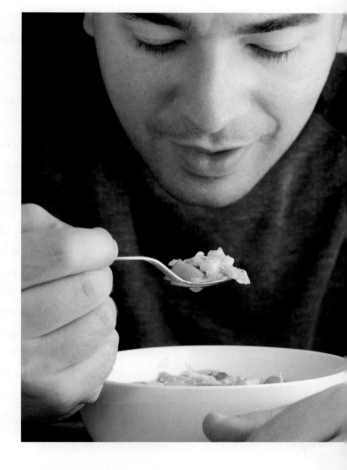

6

Vitamins: Micronutrients with Macro Powers 155

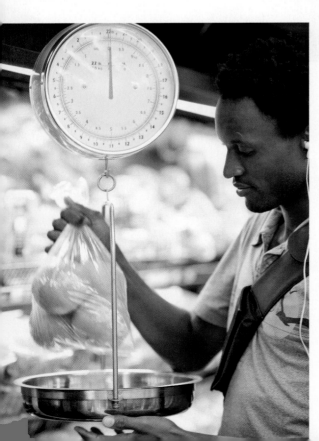

7

Minerals: Building and Moving Our Body 192

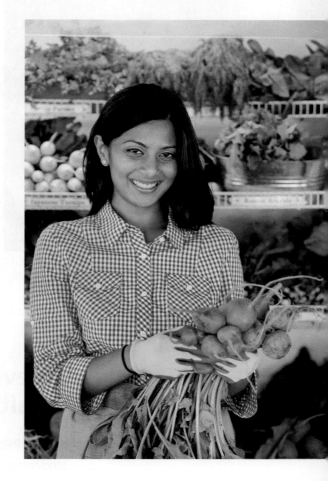

8

Fluid Balance, Water, and Alcohol 225

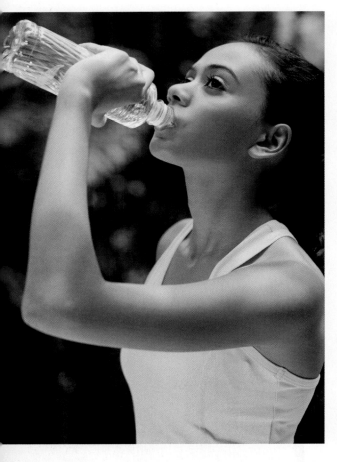

9

Achieving and Maintaining a Healthful Body Weight 250

10

Nutrition and Physical Activity: Keys to Good Health 293

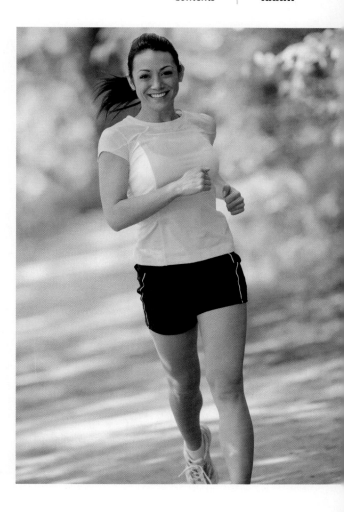

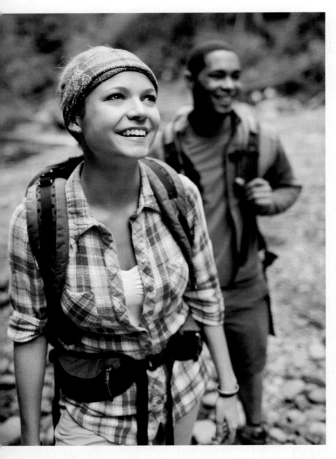

11
Nutrition Throughout the Life Cycle 326

had more than a thousand chances to influence your body's functioning! Let's take a closer look at how nutrition supports health and wellness.

Nutrition Is One of Several Factors Supporting Wellness

Wellness can be defined in many ways. Traditionally considered simply the absence of disease, wellness is now described as a multidimensional state of being that includes physical, emotional, and spiritual health (**FIGURE 1.1**). Wellness is not an end point in our lives but is an active process we work on every day.

In this book, we focus on a critical aspect of wellness: physical health, which is influenced by both our nutrition and our level of physical activity. The two are so closely related that you can think of them as two sides of the same coin: our overall state of nutrition is influenced by how much energy we expend doing daily activities, and our level of physical activity has a major impact on how we use the nutrients in our food. Several studies have even suggested that healthful nutrition and regular physical activity can increase feelings of well-being and reduce feelings of anxiety and depression. In other words, wholesome food and physical activity just plain feel good!

A Healthful Diet Can Prevent Some Diseases and Reduce Your Risk for Others

Nutrition appears to play a role—from a direct cause to a mild influence—in the development of many diseases (**FIGURE 1.2**). Poor nutrition is a direct cause of deficiency diseases such as scurvy and pellagra. Scurvy is caused by a deficiency of vitamin C, whereas pellagra is a result of a deficiency of niacin, one of the B-vitamins. Early nutrition research focused on identifying the missing nutrient

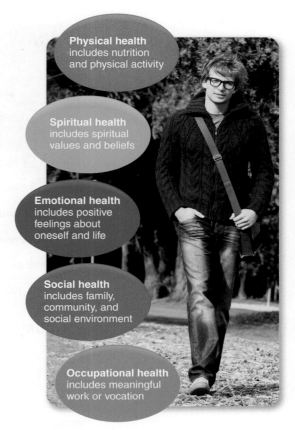

FIGURE 1.1 Many factors contribute to our wellness. Primary among these are a nutritious diet and regular physical activity.

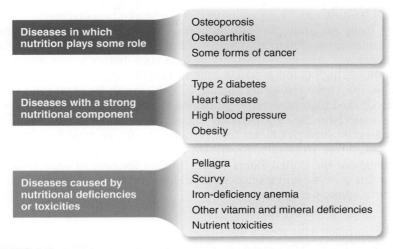

FIGURE 1.2 The relationship between nutrition and human disease. Notice that, whereas nutritional factors are only marginally implicated in the diseases of the top row, they are strongly linked to the development of the diseases in the middle row, and truly causative of those in the bottom row.

wellness A multidimensional, lifelong process that includes physical, emotional, and spiritual health.

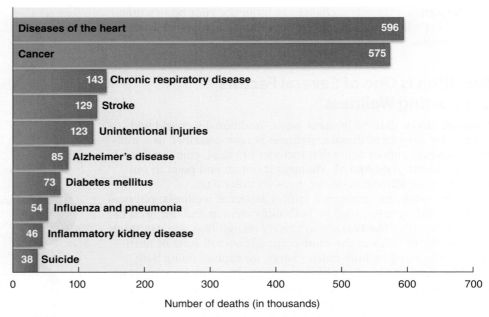

	Number of deaths (in thousands)
Diseases of the heart	596
Cancer	575
Chronic respiratory disease	143
Stroke	129
Unintentional injuries	123
Alzheimer's disease	85
Diabetes mellitus	73
Influenza and pneumonia	54
Inflammatory kidney disease	46
Suicide	38

⬆ **FIGURE 1.3** Of the ten leading causes of death in the United States in 2011, three—heart disease, stroke, and diabetes—are strongly associated with poor nutrition. In addition, nutrition plays a more limited role in the development of some forms of cancer.

Data from: "Deaths: Preliminary Data for 2011" (U.S. Department of Health and Human Services). Data from Centers for Disease Control and Prevention, NCHS. FastStats. Death and Morality. **www.cdc.gov/nchs/fastats/deaths.htm**

behind such diseases and on developing guidelines for nutrient intakes that are high enough to prevent them. Over the years, nutrition scientists successfully lobbied for fortification of foods with the nutrients of greatest concern. These measures, along with a more abundant and reliable food supply, have almost completely wiped out the majority of nutrient-deficiency diseases in developed countries. However, they are still major problems in many developing nations.

In addition to directly causing disease, poor nutrition can have a more subtle influence on our health. For instance, it can contribute to the development of brittle bones (a disease called *osteoporosis*), as well as to the progression of some forms of cancer. These associations are considered mild; however, poor nutrition is also strongly associated with three chronic diseases that are among the top ten causes of death in the United States (**FIGURE 1.3**). These are heart disease, stroke, and diabetes.

A recent study examining the burden of diseases, injuries, and risk factors in the United States from 1990 to 2010 found that the leading risk factors contributing to disability and premature mortality include poor dietary habits, physical inactivity, smoking, high blood pressure, high fasting blood glucose levels, alcohol use, and obesity.[1] These researchers identified diets low in fruits, vegetables, and nuts and seeds, and high in sodium, processed meats, and *trans* fats as the most important dietary risks facing Americans today. As you are probably aware, obesity is a well-established risk factor for heart disease, stroke, type 2 diabetes, and some forms of cancer. Unfortunately, the prevalence of obesity has dramatically increased throughout the United States during roughly the past 30 years (**FIGURE 1.4**). Throughout this text, we will discuss in detail how nutrition and physical activity affect the development of obesity.

Want to see how the prevalence of obesity has changed in the United States year-by-year for the past 25 years? Go to **www.cdc.gov** and enter "obesity data trend maps" into the search bar.

recap Nutrition is the science that studies food and how food affects our body and our health. Nutrition is an important component of wellness and is strongly associated with physical activity. One goal of a healthful diet is to prevent nutrient-deficiency diseases, such as scurvy and pellagra; a second goal is to lower the risk for chronic diseases, such as type 2 diabetes and heart disease.

1994

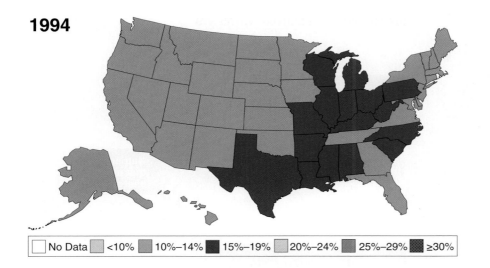

No Data | <10% | 10%–14% | 15%–19% | 20%–24% | 25%–29% | ≥30%

2012

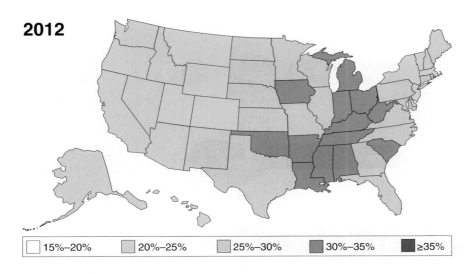

15%–20% | 20%–25% | 25%–30% | 30%–35% | ≥35%

◀ **FIGURE 1.4** These diagrams illustrate the increase in obesity rates across the United States from 1994 to 2012 as documented in the Behavioral Risk Factor Surveillance System. Obesity is defined as a body mass index greater than or equal to 30, or approximately 30 lb overweight for a 5'4" woman.

Graphics and data from: "Prevalence of Self-Reported Obesity Among U.S. Adults" and "Percent of Obese (BMI ≥ 30) in U.S. Adults: 1994" (Centers for Disease Control and Prevention).

What are nutrients?

 Identify the six classes of nutrients essential for health.

A spoonful of peanut butter may seem as if it is all one substance, but in reality most foods are made up of many different chemicals. Some of these chemicals are not useful to the body, whereas others are critical to human growth and function. These latter chemicals are referred to as **nutrients**. The following are the six groups of nutrients found in the foods we eat (**FIGURE 1.5**):

- carbohydrates
- fats (solid fats and liquid oils)
- proteins
- vitamins
- minerals
- water

Carbohydrates, Fats, and Proteins Are Macronutrients That Provide Energy

Carbohydrates, fats, and proteins are the only nutrients in foods that provide energy. By this we mean that these nutrients break down and reassemble into fuel that our body uses to support physical activity and basic functioning. Although taking

nutrients Chemicals found in foods that are critical to human growth and function.

▶ **FIGURE 1.5** The six groups of essential nutrients found in the foods we consume.

SIX GROUPS OF ESSENTIAL NUTRIENTS

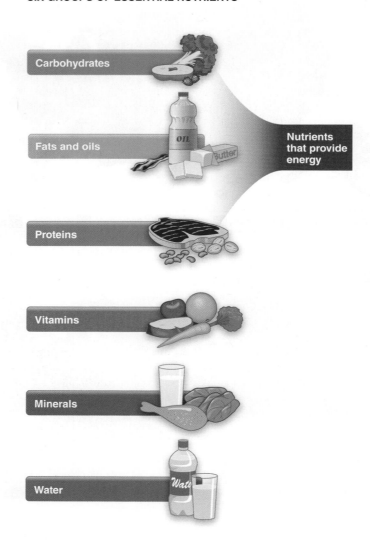

a multivitamin and a glass of water might be beneficial in other ways, it will not provide you with the energy you need to do your 20 minutes on the stair-climber! The energy nutrients are also referred to as **macronutrients**. *Macro* means "large," and our body needs relatively large amounts of these nutrients to support normal functioning. Macronutrient needs are measured in grams, metric units of weight. Grams are small: ¼ teaspoon of sugar weighs about 1 gram.

Alcohol is a chemical found in food, and it provides energy. Nevertheless, it is not technically considered a nutrient because it does not support body functions or the building or repair of tissues. In fact, the alcohol in beverages is technically classified as a narcotic drug.

Nutrition scientists describe the amount of energy in food as units of *kilocalories* (*kcal*). A kilocalorie is the amount of heat required to raise the temperature of 1 kilogram of water (the weight of about 1 quart of water) by 1 degree Celsius. *Kilo-* is a prefix used in the metric system to indicate 1,000; so a kilocalorie is technically 1,000 Calories. However, for the sake of simplicity, food labels use the term *Calories* to indicate kilocalories. Thus, if the wrapping on an ice cream bar states that it contains 150 Calories, it actually contains 150 *kilo*calories. In this textbook, we use the term *kilocalories* as a unit of energy; we use the term *Calories* when discussing food labels or for everyday usage.

macronutrients Nutrients that our body needs in relatively large amounts to support normal function and health. Carbohydrates, fats, and proteins are macronutrients.

Carbohydrates Are a Primary Fuel Source

Carbohydrates are the primary source of fuel for our active body, particularly for the brain. They provide 4 kcal per gram. Many carbohydrates are *fiber rich*; that is, they contain nondigestible parts of plants that offer a variety of health benefits. Many are also rich in *phytochemicals*, plant chemicals that are thought to reduce our risk for cancer and heart disease.

Carbohydrates encompass a wide variety of foods. Grains, fruits, and vegetables contain carbohydrates, as do legumes (a class of vegetable including lentils, dry beans, and peas), seeds and nuts, and milk and other dairy products.

Fats Provide More Energy Than Carbohydrates

Fats are also an important source of energy for our body, especially during rest and low-intensity activity. Because they pack together tightly, fats yield more energy per gram than carbohydrates, 9 kcal versus 4 kcal. Dietary fats come in a variety of forms. Solid fats include such foods as butter, lard, and margarine. Liquid fats are referred to as *oils* and include vegetable oils, such as corn, canola, and olive oils. You've probably heard about a fatty substance called *cholesterol*, which is present in animal foods such as meats and egg yolks. Cholesterol is synthesized in our body, so we don't need to consume it; thus, it's not an essential nutrient.

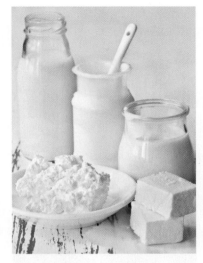

▲ Fat-soluble vitamins are found in a variety of fat-containing foods, including dairy products.

Proteins Support Tissue Growth, Repair, and Maintenance

Although **proteins** can provide energy (4 kcal per gram), they are not a primary source of energy for our body. Proteins play a major role in building new cells and tissues, maintaining the structure and strength of bone, repairing damaged structures, and assisting in many body functions. Meats and dairy products are primary sources of proteins for many Americans, but we can also obtain adequate amounts from nuts and seeds, legumes and other vegetables, and whole grains.

Vitamins and Minerals Are Micronutrients

Vitamins and minerals are referred to as **micronutrients** because we need relatively small amounts of them (*micro* means "small") to support normal health and body functions.

Vitamins Assist in Regulating Body Functions

Vitamins are compounds that contain the substance carbon and assist us in regulating the processes of our body. For example, vitamins play a critical role in building and maintaining healthy bone, blood, and muscle tissue; supporting the immune system so we can fight illness and disease; and maintaining healthy vision. Contrary to popular belief, vitamins do not provide energy (kilocalories); however, vitamins do play an important role in assisting our body with releasing and using the energy found in carbohydrates, fats, and proteins.

A vitamin's ability to dissolve in water versus fat affects how it is absorbed, transported, stored, and excreted from our body. Thus, nutrition experts classify vitamins into two groups (TABLE 1.1):

- water soluble
- fat soluble

Because our body cannot synthesize most vitamins, we must consume them in our diet. Both water-soluble and fat-soluble vitamins are essential for our health and are found in a variety of foods, from animal products, nuts, and seeds to fruits and vegetables. Many vitamins break down upon prolonged exposure to heat and/or light, which explains why vitamin supplements are not sold in clear bottles.

carbohydrates The primary fuel source for our body, particularly for the brain and for physical exercise.

fats An important energy source for our body at rest and during low-intensity exercise.

proteins Macronutrients that the body uses to build tissue and regulate body functions. Proteins can provide energy but are not a primary source.

micronutrients Nutrients needed in relatively small amounts to support normal health and body functions. Vitamins and minerals are micronutrients.

vitamins Micronutrients that contain carbon and assist us in regulating the processes of our body. They are classified as water soluble or fat soluble.

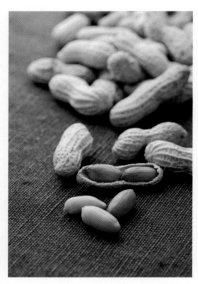

↑ Peanuts are a good source of the major minerals magnesium and phosphorus, which play important roles in the formation and maintenance of our skeleton.

TABLE 1.1 **Overview of Vitamins**

Type	Names	Characteristics
Fat soluble	A, D, E, and K	Soluble in fat
		Stored in the human body
		Toxicity can occur from consuming excess amounts, which accumulate in the body
Water soluble	C, B vitamins (thiamin, riboflavin, niacin, vitamin B_6, vitamin B_{12}, pantothenic acid, biotin, and folate)	Soluble in water
		Not stored significantly in the human body
		Excess is excreted in urine
		Toxicity generally only occurs as a result of vitamin supplementation

Minerals Are Not Broken Down During Digestion

The sodium in table salt, the calcium in milk, and the iron in red meat are all examples of minerals essential to human health and functioning. **Minerals** are substances that

- are single elements of matter, not compounds,
- are not broken down during digestion, and
- are not destroyed by heat or light.

Thus, all minerals maintain their structure no matter what environment they are in. This means that the calcium in our bones is the same as the calcium in the milk we drink, and the sodium in our cells is the same as the sodium in table salt. Among their many important functions, minerals assist in fluid regulation and energy production, are essential to the health of our bones and blood, and help rid our body of harmful chemicals. They are classified into two groups, according to the amounts we need in our diet and how much of the mineral is found in our body (**TABLE 1.2**):

- major minerals
- trace minerals

Major minerals earned their name from the fact that we need to consume at least 100 milligrams (mg) per day in our diet and because the total amount found in our body is at least 5 grams (5,000 mg). **Trace minerals** are those we need to consume in amounts less than 100 mg per day, and the total amount in our body is less than 5 grams (5,000 mg). Food sources of major and trace minerals are varied and include meats, dairy products, fruits and vegetables, and nuts and seeds.

Water Supports All Body Functions

Water is a nutrient vital for our survival. We consume water in its pure form; in juices, soups, and other liquids; and in solid foods, such as fruits and vegetables. Adequate water intake ensures the proper balance of fluid both inside and outside our cells and assists in the regulation of nerve impulses, muscle contractions, nutrient transport, and excretion of waste products.

minerals Micronutrients that are single elements of matter, not compounds, are not broken down during digestion, and are not destroyed by heat or light. Minerals assist in the regulation of many body processes and are classified as major minerals or trace minerals.

major minerals Minerals we need to consume in amounts of at least 100 mg per day and of which the total amount in our body is at least 5 grams.

trace minerals Minerals we need to consume in amounts less than 100 mg per day and of which the total amount in our body is less than 5 grams.

TABLE 1.2 **Overview of Minerals**

Type	Names	Characteristics
Major minerals	Calcium, phosphorus, sodium, potassium, chloride, magnesium, sulfur	Needed in amounts greater than 100 mg/day in our diet
		Amount present in the human body is greater than 5 grams (5,000 mg)
Trace minerals	Iron, zinc, copper, manganese, fluoride, chromium, molybdenum, selenium, iodine	Needed in amounts less than 100 mg/day in our diet
		Amount present in the human body is less than 5 grams (5,000 mg)

The six essential nutrient groups found in foods are carbohydrates, fats, proteins, vitamins, minerals, and water. Carbohydrates, fats, and proteins are macronutrients, and they provide our body with the energy necessary to thrive. Vitamins and minerals are micronutrients that do not provide energy but are essential to human functioning. Adequate water intake ensures the proper balance of fluid both inside and outside our cells.

What is a healthful diet?

> **LO3** Identify the characteristics of a healthful diet.

A **healthful diet** provides the proper combination of energy and nutrients. It has four characteristics: it is adequate, moderate, balanced, and varied. Whether you are young or old, overweight or underweight, healthy or coping with illness, if you keep in mind these characteristics of a healthful diet, you will be able to select foods that provide you with the optimal combination of nutrients and energy each day.

A Healthful Diet Is Adequate

An **adequate diet** provides enough energy, nutrients, and fiber to maintain a person's health. A diet may be inadequate in many areas or only one. For example, many people in the United States do not eat enough vegetables and therefore are not consuming enough of many of the important nutrients found in vegetables, such as fiber-rich carbohydrate, vitamin C, beta-carotene, and potassium. Other people may eat only plant-based foods. Unless they supplement or use fortified foods, their diet will be inadequate in a single nutrient, vitamin B_{12}.

A Healthful Diet Is Moderate

Moderation refers to eating the right amounts of foods to maintain a healthy weight and to optimize the functioning of our body. People who eat too much or too little of certain foods may not be able to reach their health goals. For example, let's say a person drinks 60 fluid ounces (three 20 oz bottles) of soft drinks each day. These drinks contribute an extra 765 kcal of energy to the person's diet. To avoid weight gain from these kilocalories, most people would need to reduce their food intake, probably by cutting out healthful food choices. Consuming soft drinks in moderation keeps more energy available for nourishing foods.

A Healthful Diet Is Balanced

A **balanced diet** is one that contains the combinations of foods that provide the proper balance of nutrients. As you will learn in this course, our body needs many types of foods in varying amounts to maintain health. For example, fruits and vegetables are excellent sources of fiber, vitamin C, beta-carotene, potassium, and magnesium. Meats are not good sources of these nutrients, but they are excellent sources of protein, iron, zinc, and copper. By eating a proper balance of healthful foods, we can be confident that we are consuming enough of the nutrients we need.

A Healthful Diet Is Varied

Variety refers to eating different foods each day. In many communities in the United States, there are thousands of healthful foods to choose from. By trying new foods on a regular basis, we optimize our chances of consuming the multitude of nutrients our body needs. In addition, eating a varied diet prevents boredom and avoids getting into a "food rut."

healthful diet A diet that provides the proper combination of energy and nutrients and is adequate, moderate, balanced, and varied.

adequate diet A diet that provides enough energy, nutrients, and fiber to maintain a person's health.

moderation Eating the right amounts of foods to maintain a healthy weight and to optimize our body's functioning.

balanced diet A diet that contains the combinations of foods that provide the proper proportion of nutrients.

variety Eating different foods each day.

 A healthful diet provides adequate nutrients and energy in moderate amounts. A healthful diet also includes an appropriate balance and a wide variety of foods.

▶ A diet that is adequate for one person may not be adequate for another. A woman who is lightly active may require fewer kilocalories of energy per day than a highly active male, for example.

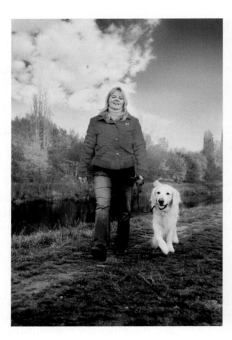
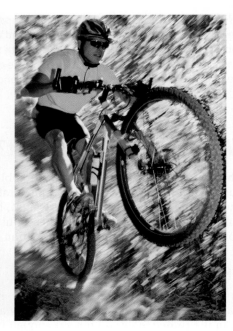

LO4 Compare and contrast the six types of Dietary Reference Intakes for nutrients.

LO5 Describe the *Dietary Guidelines for Americans* and discuss how these Guidelines can be used to design a healthful diet.

LO6 Identify the food groups in the USDA food patterns and the amounts adults should eat each day.

LO7 Explain how to read and use the Nutrition Facts panel found on food labels.

Dietary Reference Intakes (DRIs)
A set of nutritional reference values for the United States and Canada that apply to healthy people.

Estimated Average Requirement (EAR) The average daily nutrient intake level estimated to meet the requirement of half of the healthy individuals in a particular life stage and gender group.

Recommended Dietary Allowance (RDA) The average daily nutrient intake level that meets the nutrient requirements of 97% to 98% of healthy individuals in a particular life stage and gender group.

Adequate Intake (AI)
A recommended average daily nutrient intake level based on observed or experimentally determined estimates of nutrient intake by a group of healthy people.

How can you design a diet that works for you?

Now that you know what the six classes of nutrients are, you are probably wondering how much of each you need each day. To answer this question for yourself, you need to know the current recommended nutrient intakes.

Use the Dietary Reference Intakes to Figure Out Your Nutrient Needs

The lists of dietary standards in both the United States and Canada are called the **Dietary Reference Intakes (DRIs)**. These standards identify the amount of a nutrient you need to prevent deficiency disease, but they also consider how much of this nutrient may reduce your risk for chronic disease. The DRIs also establish an upper level of safety for some nutrients.

The DRIs consist of six values (**FIGURE 1.6**):

- The **Estimated Average Requirement (EAR)** represents the average daily nutrient intake level estimated to meet the requirement of half of the healthy individuals in a particular life stage or gender group.[1] Notice that it's not a recommended intake. Instead, scientists use it to determine the Recommended Dietary Allowance.
- The **Recommended Dietary Allowance (RDA)** represents the average daily nutrient intake level that meets the nutrient requirements of 97% to 98% of healthy individuals in a particular life stage and gender group.[2] For example, the RDA for iron is 18 mg per day for women between the ages of 19 and 30 years. This amount of iron will meet the nutrient requirements of almost all women in this age category. Again, scientists use the EAR to establish the RDA. In fact, if an EAR cannot be determined for a nutrient, then this nutrient cannot have an RDA. When this occurs, an Adequate Intake value is determined.
- The **Adequate Intake (AI)** value is a recommended average daily nutrient intake level based on estimates of nutrient intake by a group of healthy people.[2] These estimates are assumed to be adequate and are used when the evidence necessary to determine an RDA is not available. Several nutrients have an AI value, including vitamin K, potassium, and chloride.
- The **Tolerable Upper Intake Level (UL)** is the highest average daily intake likely to pose no risk of adverse health effects. As intake of a nutrient increases in amounts

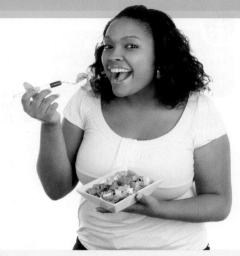

Dietary Reference Intakes (DRIs) are specific reference values for each nutrient issued by the United States National Academy of Sciences, Institute of Medicine. They identify the amounts of each nutrient that one needs to consume to maintain good health.

DRIs FOR MOST NUTRIENTS

EAR The Estimated Average Requirement (EAR) is the average daily intake level estimated to meet the needs of half the people in a certain group. Scientists use it to calculate the RDA.

RDA The Recommended Dietary Allowance (RDA) is the average daily intake level estimated to meet the needs of nearly all people in a certain group. Aim for this amount!

AI The Adequate Intake (AI) is the average daily intake level assumed to be adequate. It is used when an EAR cannot be determined. Aim for this amount if there is no RDA!

UL The Tolerable Upper Intake Level (UL) is the highest average daily intake level likely to pose no health risks. Do not exceed this amount on a daily basis!

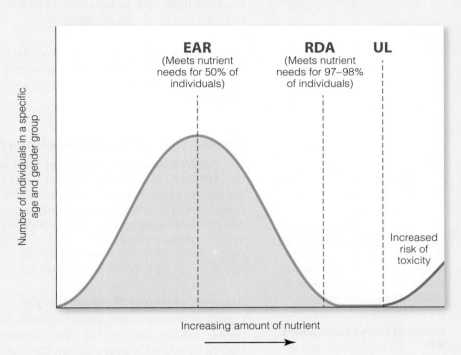

DRIs RELATED TO ENERGY

AMDR The Acceptable Macronutrient Distribution Range (AMDR) is the recommended range of carbohydrate, fat, and protein intake expressed as a percentage of total energy.

EER The Estimated Energy Requirement (EER) is the average daily energy intake predicted to meet the needs of healthy adults.

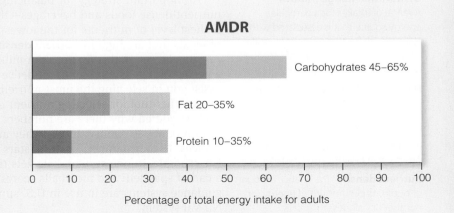

above the UL, the potential for toxic effects and health risks increases. Note that there is not enough research to define the UL for all nutrients.

■ The **Estimated Energy Requirement (EER)** is the average energy (kcal) intake that is predicted to maintain energy balance in a healthy adult. This recommendation considers a person's level of physical activity: the EER for an active person is higher than the EER for an inactive person, even if all other factors (for example, age, gender) are the same.

■ The **Acceptable Macronutrient Distribution Range (AMDR)** is a range of intakes for carbohydrate, fat, and protein that is associated with reduced risk for chronic disease and provides adequate levels of essential nutrients. The AMDR is expressed as a percentage of total energy or as a percentage of total Calories.

(*Note:* Many of the DRI values are listed in tables on the inside back covers of this book and in adjoining back pages; they are also reviewed with each nutrient as it is introduced throughout this text. To determine your nutrient needs using those tables, find your life stage group and gender in the left-hand column; then look across to see each nutrient's value that applies.) Using the DRI values in conjunction with diet-planning tools such as the *Dietary Guidelines for Americans*, discussed next, will help ensure a healthful and adequate diet.

recap The Dietary Reference Intakes (DRIs) are specific reference values for each nutrient. You can use them to find out how much of each nutrient you need to consume to avoid nutrient deficiencies and toxicities and to reduce your risk for certain chronic diseases.

Follow the Dietary Guidelines for Americans

The ***Dietary Guidelines for Americans*** are a set of principles developed by the U.S. Department of Agriculture and the U.S. Department of Health and Human Services to promote health, reduce the risk for chronic diseases, and reduce the prevalence of overweight and obesity among Americans through improved nutrition and physical activity.[3] They are updated approximately every 5 years, and are currently being revised for publication in 2015. The 2010 *Dietary Guidelines for Americans* include twenty-three recommendations for the general population, but you don't have to remember all twenty-three! Instead, focus on the following four main ideas.

Balance Calories to Maintain Weight

Consume adequate nutrients to promote your health while staying within your energy needs. This will help you maintain a healthful weight. You can achieve this by controlling your Calorie intake; if you are overweight or obese, you will need to consume fewer Calories from foods and beverages. At the same time, increase your level of physical activity and reduce the time that you spend in sedentary behaviors, such as watching television and sitting at the computer.

An important strategy for balancing your Calories is to consistently choose nutrient-dense foods and beverages—that is, foods and beverages that supply the highest level of nutrients for the lowest level of Calories. **FIGURE 1.7** compares 1 day of meals that are high in **nutrient density** to meals that are low in nutrient density. As you can see in this figure, skim milk is more nutrient dense than whole milk, and a peeled orange is more nutrient dense than an orange soft drink. This example can assist you in selecting the most nutrient-dense foods when planning your meals.

Another tool for selecting nutrient-dense foods is in your supermarket! Have you ever wondered why there are numbers or stars on the shelf labels under everything from produce to canned goods? They are there to help shoppers make more healthful choices. Higher numbers or more stars indicate foods with a higher nutrient density. For example, in one system, kale gets the highest possible numerical score, whereas a can of spaghetti and meatballs scores near the bottom. Although a few nutritional guidance systems are in use in U.S. supermarkets, by far the most common is the Nu-Val system.

Tolerable Upper Intake Level (UL) The highest average daily nutrient intake level likely to pose no risk of adverse health effects to almost all individuals in a particular life stage and gender group.

Estimated Energy Requirement (EER) The average dietary energy intake that is predicted to maintain energy balance in a healthy adult.

Acceptable Macronutrient Distribution Range (AMDR) A range of intakes for a particular energy source that is associated with reduced risk for chronic disease while providing adequate intake of essential nutrients.

Dietary Guidelines for Americans A set of principles developed by the U.S. Department of Agriculture and the U.S. Department of Health and Human Services to assist Americans in designing a healthful diet and lifestyle.

nutrient density The relative amount of nutrients per amount of energy (or number of Calories).

a day of meals

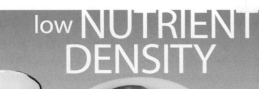

low NUTRIENT DENSITY

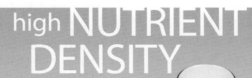

high NUTRIENT DENSITY

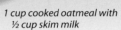

BREAKFAST

1 cup puffed rice cereal with
½ cup whole milk
1 slide white toast with
1 tsp. butter
6 fl. oz grape drink

1 cup cooked oatmeal with
½ cup skim milk
1 slice whole-wheat toast with
1 tsp. butter
6 fl. oz grapefruit juice

LUNCH

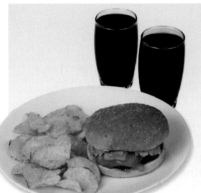

Cheeseburger
3 oz regular ground beef
1.5 oz cheddar cheese
1 white hamburger bun
2 tsp. Dijon mustard
2 leaves iceberg lettuce
1 snack-sized bag potato chips
32 fl. oz cola soft drink

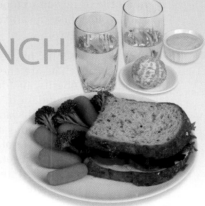

Turkey Sandwich
3 oz turkey breast
2 slices whole-grain bread
2 tsp. Dijon mustard
3 slices fresh tomato
2 leaves red leaf lettuce
1 cup baby carrots with
broccoli crowns
20 fl. oz (2.5 cups) water
1 peeled orange
1 cup nonfat yogurt

DINNER

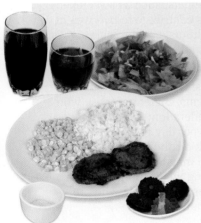

Green salad
1 cup iceberg lettuce
¼ cup diced tomatoes
1 tsp. green onions
¼ cup bacon bits
1 tbsp. regular Ranch salad dressing
3 oz beef round steak, breaded and fried
½ cup cooked white rice
½ cup sweet corn
8 fl. oz (1 cup) iced tea
3 chocolate sandwich cookies
1 12-oz can diet soft drink
10 Gummi Bears candy

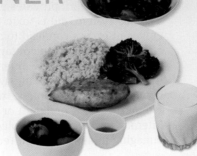

Spinach salad
1 cup fresh spinach leaves
¼ cup sliced tomatoes
¼ cup diced green pepper
½ cup kidney beans
1 tbsp. fat-free Italian salad
dressing
3 oz broiled chicken breast
½ cup cooked brown rice
½ cup steamed broccoli
8 fl. oz (1 cup) skim milk
1-1/2 cup mixed berries

nutrient analysis

3,319 kcal
11.4% of energy from saturated fat
11.6 grams of dietary fiber
3,031 milligrams of sodium
83 milligrams of vitamin C
18.2 milligrams of iron
825 milligrams of calcium

Provides
more
nutrients
and fewer
calories!

nutrient analysis

1,753 kcal
3% of energy from saturated fat
53.1 grams of dietary fiber
2,231 milligrams of sodium
372 milligrams of vitamin C
15.2 milligrams of iron
1,469 milligrams of calcium

Limit Sodium, Fat, Sugars, and Alcohol

The Dietary Guidelines suggest that we reduce our consumption of the following foods and food components. Doing so will help us maintain a healthy weight and lower our risks for chronic diseases.

Sodium Excessive consumption of sodium, a major mineral found in salt, is linked to high blood pressure in some people. Eating a lot of sodium also can cause some people to lose calcium from their bones, which can increase their risk for bone loss and bone fractures. Although table salt contains sodium and the major mineral chloride, much of the sodium we consume in our diet comes from processed and prepared foods. Key recommendations include keeping your daily sodium intake below 2,300 milligrams (mg) per day. This is the amount in just 1 teaspoon of table salt! If you are African American; have high blood pressure, diabetes, or chronic kidney disease; or are over age 50, you should aim for a daily sodium intake below 1,500 mg. Some ways to decrease your sodium intake include the following:

- Eat fresh, plain frozen, or canned vegetables without added salt.
- Limit your intake of processed meats, such as cured ham, sausage, bacon, and most canned meats.
- When shopping for canned or packaged foods, look for those with labels that say "low sodium."
- Add little or no salt to foods at home.
- Limit your intake of salty condiments, such as ketchup, mustard, pickles, soy sauce, and olives.

Fat Fat is an essential nutrient and therefore an important part of a healthful diet; however, because fats are energy dense, eating a diet high in total fat can lead to overweight and obesity. In addition, eating a diet high in cholesterol and saturated fat (a type of fat abundant in meats and other animal-based foods) is linked to an increased risk for heart disease. For these reasons, less than 10% of your total daily Calories should come from saturated fat, and you should try to consume less than 300 mg per day of cholesterol. You can achieve this goal by replacing solid fats, such as butter and lard, with vegetable oils, as well as by eating meat less often and fish or vegetarian meals more often. Finally, replace full-fat milk, yogurt, and cheeses with low-fat or nonfat versions.

Sugars Limit foods and beverages that are high in added sugars, such as sweetened soft drinks and fruit drinks, cookies, and cakes. These foods contribute to overweight and obesity, and they promote tooth decay. Moreover, doughnuts, cookies, cakes, pies, and other pastries are typically made with unhealthful fats and are high in sodium.

Alcohol Alcohol provides energy, but not nutrients. In the body, it depresses the nervous system and is toxic to the liver and other body cells. Drinking alcoholic beverages in excess can lead to serious health and social problems; therefore, those who choose to drink are encouraged to do so sensibly and in moderation: no more than one drink per day for women and no more than two drinks per day for men, and only by adults of legal drinking age. Adults who should not drink alcohol are those who cannot restrict their intake, women of childbearing age who may become pregnant, women who are pregnant or breastfeeding, individuals taking medications that can interact with alcohol, people with certain medical conditions, and people who are engaging in activities that require attention, skill, or coordination.

Consume More Healthful Foods and Nutrients

Another goal of the Dietary Guidelines is to encourage people to increase their consumption of healthful foods rich in nutrients, while keeping their Calorie intake within their daily energy needs. Key recommendations for achieving this goal include the following:

- Increase your intake of fruits and vegetables. Each day, try to eat a variety of dark-green, red, and orange vegetables, along with legumes.
- Make sure that at least half of all grain foods—for example, breads, cereals, and pasta—that you eat each day are made from whole grains.

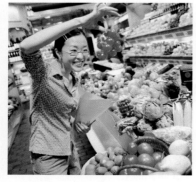

When grocery shopping, try to select a variety of fruits and vegetables.

- Choose fat-free or low-fat milk and milk products, which include milk, yogurt, cheese, and fortified soy beverages.
- When making protein choices, choose protein foods that are lower in solid fat and Calories, such as lean cuts of beef or skinless poultry. Try to eat more fish and shellfish in place of traditional meat and poultry choices. Also choose eggs, legumes, soy products, and unsalted nuts and seeds.
- Choose foods that provide an adequate level of dietary fiber and nutrients of concern in the American diet, including potassium, calcium, and vitamin D. An adequate intake of these nutrients helps reduce our risks for certain diseases. Healthful foods that are good sources of these nutrients include fruits, legumes and other vegetables, whole grains, and low-fat milk and milk products.

Follow Healthy Eating Patterns

There is no one healthy eating pattern that everyone should follow. Instead, the recommendations made in the Dietary Guidelines are designed to accommodate diverse cultural, ethnic, traditional, and personal preferences and to fit within different individuals' food budgets. Still, the Guidelines offer several flexible templates you can follow to build your healthy eating pattern, including the USDA Food Patterns and the Mediterranean diet (both discussed shortly).

Building a healthy eating pattern also involves following food safety recommendations to reduce your risk for foodborne illnesses, such as those caused by microorganisms and their toxins. The four food safety principles emphasized in the Dietary Guidelines are

- *Clean* your hands, food contact surfaces, and vegetables and fruits;
- *Separate* raw, cooked, and ready-to-eat foods while shopping, storing, and preparing foods;
- *Cook* foods to a safe temperature; and
- *Chill* (refrigerate) perishable foods promptly.

Another important tip is to avoid unpasteurized juices and milk products and raw or undercooked meats, seafood, poultry, eggs, and raw sprouts.

The **Game Plan** feature box provides examples of how you can change your current diet and physical activity habits to meet some of the recommendations in the Dietary Guidelines.

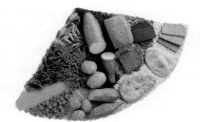

Eating a diet rich in whole-grain foods, such as whole-wheat bread and brown rice, can enhance your overall health.

recap The goals of the *Dietary Guidelines for Americans* are to promote health, reduce the risk for chronic diseases, and reduce the prevalence of overweight and obesity among Americans through improved nutrition and physical activity. This can be achieved by eating whole-grain foods, fruits, and vegetables daily; reducing intake of foods with unhealthful fats and cholesterol, salt, and added sugar; eating more foods rich in potassium, dietary fiber, calcium, and vitamin D; keeping foods safe to eat; and drinking alcohol in moderation, if at all.

The USDA Food Patterns

As just mentioned, you can use the U.S. Department of Agriculture (USDA) Food Patterns to design healthy eating patterns. The visual representation of the USDA Food Patterns is called **MyPlate** (FIGURE 1.8). MyPlate is an interactive, personalized guide that you can access on the Internet to assess your current diet and physical activity level and to plan appropriate changes. MyPlate replaces the previous MyPyramid graphic (see Appendix A). It illustrates how to

- eat in moderation to balance calories,
- eat a variety of foods,
- consume the right proportion of each recommended food group,
- personalize your eating plan,
- increase your physical activity, and
- set goals for gradually improving your food choices and lifestyle.

MyPlate The visual representation of the USDA Food Patterns.

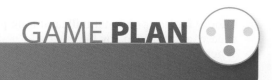

GAME **PLAN**

Ways to Incorporate the Dietary Guidelines into Your Daily Life

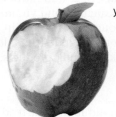

People experience a wide range of reactions when reading the *Dietary Guidelines for Americans*. Some feel satisfied that they are already following them, but many people see one or more areas where their behaviors could improve. If that sounds like you, and you'd like to make some changes, we recommend you start small. Substitute just one of these actions for your regular behavior each week, and by the time you finish this course, you'll have made the *Dietary Guidelines for Americans* part of your healthy life!

If You Normally Do This . . .	**Try Doing This Instead . . .**
Watch television when you get home at night	Do 30 minutes of stretching or lifting of hand weights in front of the television
Drive to the store down the block	Walk to and from the store
Go out to lunch with friends	Take a 15- to 30-minute walk with your friends at lunchtime 3 days each week
Eat white bread with your sandwich	Eat whole-wheat bread or some other bread made from whole grains
Eat white rice or fried rice with your meal	Eat brown rice or try wild rice
Choose cookies or a candy bar for a snack	Choose a fresh peach, apple, pear, orange, or banana for a snack
Order french fries with your hamburger	Order a green salad with low-fat salad dressing on the side
Spread butter or margarine on your white toast	Spread fresh fruit compote or peanut butter on whole-grain toast
Order a bacon double cheeseburger at your favorite restaurant	Order a turkey burger or grilled chicken sandwich without the cheese and bacon, and add lettuce and tomato
Drink non-diet soft drinks to quench your thirst	Drink iced tea, ice water with a slice of lemon, seltzer water, or diet soft drinks
Eat potato chips and pickles with your favorite sandwich	Eat carrot slices and crowns of fresh broccoli and try cauliflower dipped in low-fat or nonfat ranch dressing

MyPlate Incorporates Many of the Features of the Mediterranean Diet

MyPlate incorporates many of the features of the so-called "Mediterranean diet." This diet has received significant attention for many years, largely because the rates of cardiovascular disease in many Mediterranean countries are substantially lower than rates in the United States. There is actually not a single Mediterranean diet, because this region of the world includes Portugal, Spain, Italy, France, Greece, Turkey, and Israel. Each of these countries has different dietary patterns; however, there are many similarities. Aspects of the diet seen as more healthful than the typical U.S. diet include the following:

- Red meat is eaten only monthly, and eggs, poultry, fish, and sweets are eaten weekly, making the diet low in saturated fats and refined sugars.
- The predominant fat used for cooking and flavor is olive oil, making the diet high in monounsaturated fats.
- Foods eaten daily include grains, such as bread, pasta, couscous, and bulgur; fruits; beans and other legumes; other vegetables; nuts; and cheese and yogurt. These choices make this diet high in vitamins and minerals, fiber, phytochemicals, and probiotics (living, beneficial bacteria).
- Wine is included, in moderation.

As you'll discover shortly, MyPlate does not make specific recommendations for protein food choices. In contrast, the Mediterranean diet recommends beans, other legumes, and nuts as daily sources of protein; fish, poultry, and eggs weekly; and red meat only about once each month. Also, for dairy choices, the Mediterranean diet recommends cheese and yogurt in moderation and suggests drinking water or wine (in moderation) rather than milk. As illustrated in **FIGURE 1.9**, it's easy to create a healthy Mediterranean-style eating plan using the principles of MyPlate.

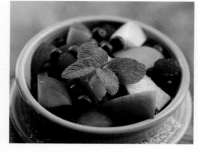

⬆ MyPlate encourages people to eat a variety of fruits.

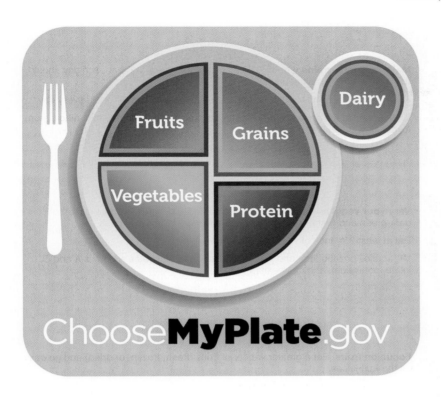

◀ **FIGURE 1.8** The USDA MyPlate graphic. MyPlate is an interactive food guidance system based on the 2010 *Dietary Guidelines for Americans* and the Dietary Reference Intakes from the National Academy of Sciences. Eating more fruits, vegetables, and whole grains and choosing foods low in fat, sugar, and sodium from the five food groups in MyPlate will help you balance your Calories and consume a healthier overall food pattern.
ChooseMyPlate.gov

Food Groups in the USDA Food Patterns

The food groups emphasized in the USDA Food Patterns are grains, vegetables, fruits, dairy, and protein foods. The food groups are represented in the plate graphic with segments of five different colors. **FIGURE 1.10** illustrates each of these food groups and provides more detailed information on the nutrients they provide and the amounts adults should eat each day.

The Concept of Empty Calories

One concept emphasized in the USDA Food Patterns is that of **empty Calories**. These are Calories from solid fats and/or added sugars that provide few or no nutrients.

empty Calories Calories from solid fats and/or added sugars that provide few or no nutrients.

◀ **FIGURE 1.9** MyPlate can be easily used to design a Mediterranean-style eating plan.

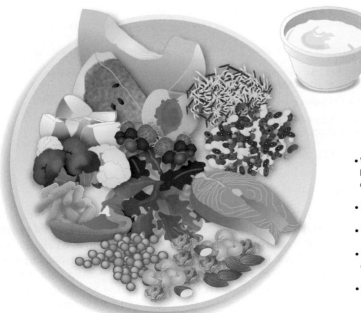

- Vegetables, fruits, nuts, beans and other legumes, whole grains, cheese and yogurt consumed daily.

- Eggs, poultry, and fish consumed weekly.

- Red meat consumed once per month.

- Olive oil is the predominant fat used for cooking and flavor.

- Wine is consumed in moderation.

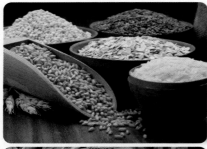

<table>
<tr><td>Grains</td><td>Make half your grains whole. At least half of the grains you eat each day should come from whole-grain sources.

Eat at least 3 oz of whole-grain bread, cereal, crackers, rice, or pasta every day.

Whole-grain foods provide fiber-rich carbohydrates, riboflavin, thiamin, niacin, iron, folate, zinc, protein, and magnesium.</td></tr>
</table>

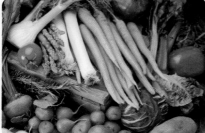

Vary your veggies. Eat a variety of vegetables and increase consumption of dark-green and orange vegetables, as well as dry beans and peas.

Eat at least 2½ cups of vegetables each day.

Vegetables provide fiber and phytochemicals, carbohydrates, vitamins A and C, folate, potassium, and magnesium.

Vegetables

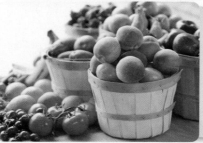

Focus on fruits. Eat a greater variety of fruits (fresh, frozen, or dried) and go easy on the fruit juices.

Eat at least 1½ cups of fruit every day.

Fruits provide fiber, phytochemicals, vitamins A and C, folate, potassium, and magnesium.

Fruits

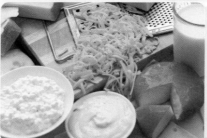

Get your calcium-rich foods. Choose low-fat or fat-free dairy products, such as milk, yogurt, and cheese. People who can't consume dairy foods can choose lactose-free dairy products or other sources, such as calcium-fortified juices and soy and rice beverages.

Get 3 cups of low-fat dairy foods, or the equivalent, every day.

Dairy foods provide calcium, phosphorus, riboflavin, protein, and vitamin B_{12} and are often fortified with vitamins D and A.

Dairy Foods

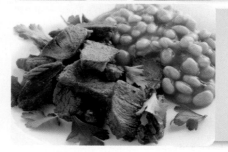

Go lean with protein. Choose low-fat or lean meats and poultry. Switch to baking, broiling, or grilling more often, and vary your choices to include more fish, processed soy products, beans, nuts, and seeds. Legumes, including beans, peas, and lentils, are included in both the protein and the vegetable groups.

Eat about 5½ oz of lean protein foods each day.

These foods provide protein, phosphorus, vitamin B_6, vitamin B_{12}, magnesium, iron, zinc, niacin, riboflavin, and thiamin.

Protein Foods

FIGURE 1.10   Food groups of the USDA Food Patterns.

The USDA recommends that you limit the empty Calories you eat to a small number that fits your Calorie and nutrient needs depending on your age, gender, and level of physical activity. Foods that contain the most empty Calories for Americans include cakes, cookies, pastries, doughnuts, soft drinks, fruit drinks, cheese, pizza, ice cream, sausages, hot dogs, bacon, and ribs. High-sugar foods, such as candies, desserts, gelatin, soft drinks, and alcoholic beverages, are called *empty Calorie foods*. However, a few foods that contain empty Calories from solid fats and added sugars also provide important nutrients. Examples are sweetened applesauce, sweetened breakfast cereals, regular ground beef, and whole milk. To reduce your intake of empty Calories but ensure you get adequate nutrients, choose the unsweetened, lean, or non-fat versions of these foods.

Number and Size of Servings in the USDA Food Patterns

The USDA Food Patterns also helps you decide *how much* of each food you should eat. The number of servings is based on your age, gender, and activity level. A term used when defining serving sizes that may be new to you is **ounce-equivalent (oz-equivalent)**. It is defined as a serving size that is 1 ounce, or is equivalent to an ounce, for the grains and meats and beans sections. For instance, both a slice of bread and ½ cup of cooked brown rice qualify as ounce-equivalents.

What is considered a serving size for the foods recommended in the USDA Food Patterns? **FIGURE 1.11** identifies the number of cups or oz-equivalent servings

ounce-equivalent (oz-equivalent) A term used to define a serving size that is 1 ounce, or equivalent to an ounce, for the grains section and the protein foods section of MyPlate.

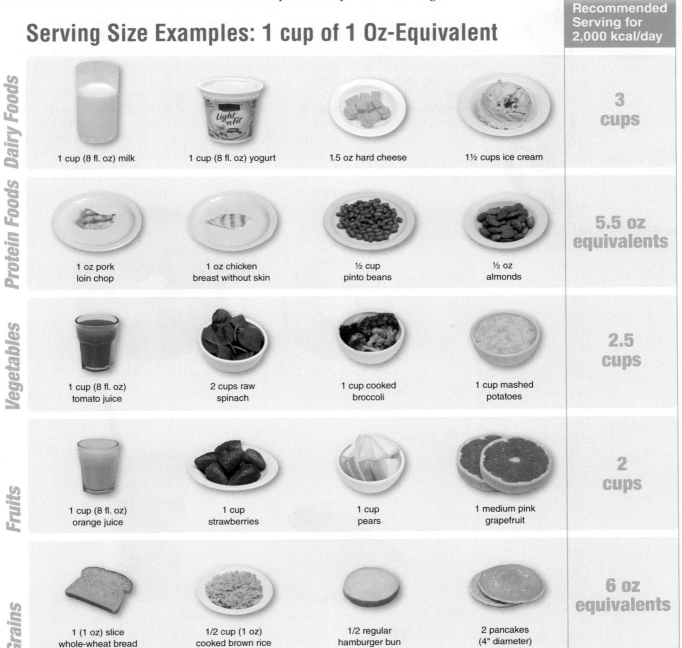

Serving Size Examples: 1 cup of 1 Oz-Equivalent

				Recommended Serving for 2,000 kcal/day
Dairy Foods	1 cup (8 fl. oz) milk	1 cup (8 fl. oz) yogurt	1.5 oz hard cheese	1½ cups ice cream → **3 cups**
Protein Foods	1 oz pork loin chop	1 oz chicken breast without skin	½ cup pinto beans	½ oz almonds → **5.5 oz equivalents**
Vegetables	1 cup (8 fl. oz) tomato juice	2 cups raw spinach	1 cup cooked broccoli	1 cup mashed potatoes → **2.5 cups**
Fruits	1 cup (8 fl. oz) orange juice	1 cup strawberries	1 cup pears	1 medium pink grapefruit → **2 cups**
Grains	1 (1 oz) slice whole-wheat bread	1/2 cup (1 oz) cooked brown rice	1/2 regular hamburger bun	2 pancakes (4" diameter) → **6 oz equivalents**

FIGURE 1.11 Examples of equivalent amounts for foods in each food group of MyPlate for a 2,000-Calorie food intake pattern. Here are some examples of household items that can help you estimate serving sizes: 1.5 oz of hard cheese is equal to four stacked dice, 3 oz of meat is equal in size to a deck of cards, and half of a regular hamburger bun is the size of a yo-yo.

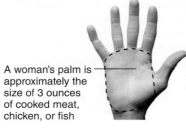

A woman's palm is approximately the size of 3 ounces of cooked meat, chicken, or fish

(a)

A woman's fist is about the size of 1 cup of pasta or vegetables (a man's fist is the size of about 2 cups)

(b)

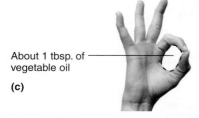

About 1 tbsp. of vegetable oil

(c)

🔺 **FIGURE 1.12** Use your hands to help estimate serving sizes of common foods.

recommended for a 2,000-Calorie diet and gives examples of amounts equal to 1 cup or 1 oz-equivalent for foods in each group. As you study this figure, notice the variety of examples for each group. For instance, an oz-equivalent serving from the grains group can mean ½ cup of cooked brown rice or two small pancakes. Because of their low density, 2 cups of raw, leafy vegetables, such as spinach, actually constitute a 1-cup serving from the vegetables group. Although an oz-equivalent serving of meat is actually 1 oz, ½ oz of nuts also qualifies. One egg, 1 tablespoon of peanut butter, and ¼ cup cooked legumes are also considered 1 oz-equivalents from the protein group. Although it may seem inconvenient to measure food servings, understanding the size of a serving is crucial to planning a nutritious diet. **FIGURE 1.12** shows you a practical way to estimate serving sizes using just your own hand.

No nationally standardized definition for a serving size exists for any food. Thus, a serving size as defined in the USDA Food Patterns may not be equal to a serving size identified on a food label. For instance, the serving size for crackers suggested in the USDA Food Patterns is three to four small crackers, whereas a serving size for crackers on a food label can range from five to eighteen crackers, depending on the size and weight of the cracker.

For food items consumed individually, such as muffins, frozen burgers, and bottled juices, the serving sizes in the USDA Food Patterns are typically much smaller than the items we actually buy and eat. In addition, serving sizes in restaurants, cafés, and movie theaters have grown substantially over the past 20 years (**FIGURE 1.13**). This "super-sizing" phenomenon, now seen even at home, indicates a major shift in

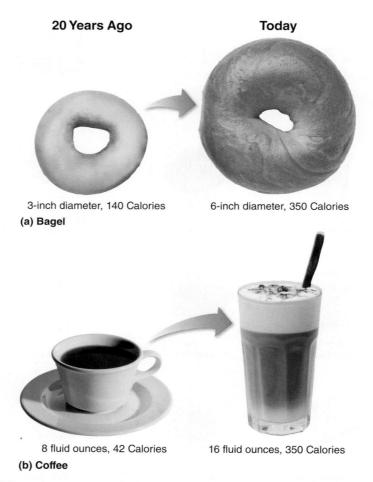

20 Years Ago   **Today**

3-inch diameter, 140 Calories   6-inch diameter, 350 Calories

(a) Bagel

8 fluid ounces, 42 Calories   16 fluid ounces, 350 Calories

(b) Coffee

🔺 **FIGURE 1.13** Examples of increases in food portion sizes over the past 20 years. **(a)** A bagel has increased in diameter from 3 inches to 6 inches; **(b)** a cup of coffee has increased from 8 fl. oz to 16 fl. oz and now commonly contains Calorie-dense flavored syrup as well as steamed whole milk.

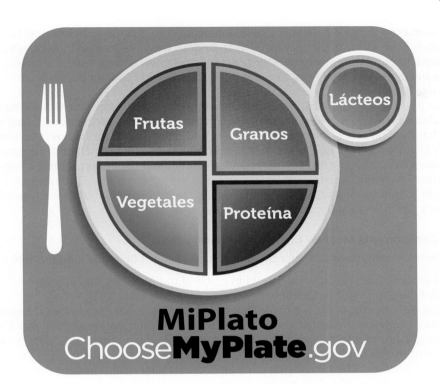

FIGURE 1.14 MiPlato is the Spanish language version of MyPlate.
ChooseMyPlate.gov

accepted eating behaviors. It is also an important contributor to the rise in obesity rates around the world. A study[4] reported that the discrepancy between USDA serving sizes and the portion size of many common foods sold outside the home is staggering—chocolate chip cookies are seven times larger than USDA standards, a serving of cooked pasta in a restaurant is almost five times larger, and steaks are more than twice as large.[5] Thus, when using diet-planning tools, such as the USDA Food Patterns, learn the definition of a serving size for the tool you're using and *then* measure your food intake to find out whether you're meeting the guidelines. If you don't want to gain weight, it's important to become informed about portion size.

> Think you understand the relationship between portion sizes and the physical activity necessary to avoid weight gain? Find out by taking the National Heart, Lung, and Blood Institute's *Portion Distortion Quiz* at www.nhlbi.nih.gov; enter "portion distortion" into the search box to get under way.

Ethnic and Other Variations of MyPlate

As you know, the population of the United States is culturally and ethnically diverse, and this diversity influences our food choices. **FIGURE 1.14** is a Spanish-language version of MyPlate. Like the English-language version, it recommends food groups, not specific food choices. As we illustrated with the Mediterranean diet, MyPlate easily accommodates foods that we may consider part of an ethnic diet. You can also incorporate into MyPlate foods that match a vegetarian diet or other lifestyle preferences.

recap The USDA Food Patterns can be used to plan a healthful, balanced diet that includes foods from the grains group, vegetables group, fruits group, dairy group, and protein foods group. As defined in the USDA Food Patterns, serving sizes typically are smaller than the amounts we normally eat or are served, so it is important to learn the definitions of serving sizes when using the USDA Food Patterns to design a healthful diet. There are many ethnic and cultural variations of the USDA Food Patterns. This flexibility enables anyone to design a diet that meets the goals of adequacy, moderation, balance, variety, and nutrient density.

Read Food Labels

If you want to take control of your food choices, then it's essential to read food labels. That's because food labels give you the facts behind the hype. The U.S. Food and Drug

Administration (FDA) requires all food manufacturers to include complete nutrition information on labels of all packaged foods. Besides fresh produce and meats, which are unpackaged or minimally packaged, the only products exempt from the labeling requirement are foods, such as coffee and most spices, that contain insignificant amounts of all nutrients.

Keep in mind that the current nutrition labeling system used in the United States is evolving. The FDA is planning to revise current regulations, so that food labels provide information that is clearer to consumers and more consistent with recent updates in the Dietary Guidelines. Proposed changes under consultation include (1) a greater emphasis on Calories, with this information in larger and bold type; (2) including information on added sugars; and (3) amount per serving listed more prominently and with the actual serving size listed (for instance, "amount per cup").[6] The following sections describe what is currently required on food labels.

Five Components Must Be Included on Food Labels

Five primary components of information must be included on food labels (**FIGURE 1.15**):

1. *A statement of identity:* The common name of the product or an appropriate identification must be prominently displayed on the label.
2. *The net contents of the package:* This information accurately describes the quantity of the food product in the entire package. This information may be listed as weight (for example, grams), volume (for example, fluid ounces), or numerical count (for example, four bars).
3. *Ingredient list:* The ingredients must be listed by their common name, in descending order by weight. This means that the first product listed in the ingredient list is the predominant ingredient in that food.

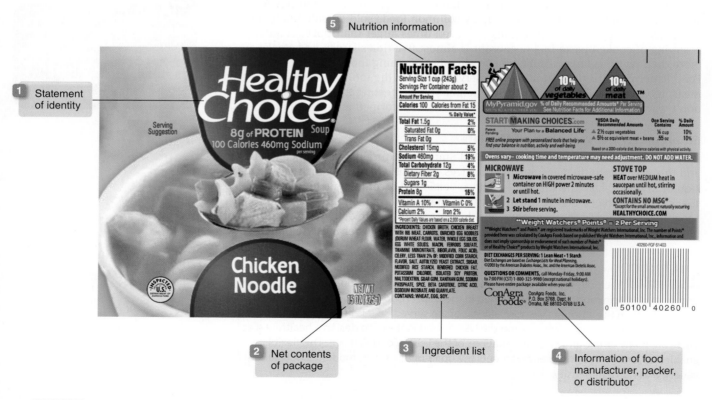

⬟ FIGURE 1.15 The five primary components that are required for food labels.
Data from Food Label © Con Agra Foods.

4. *The name and address of the food manufacturer, packer, or distributor:* This information can be used to contact the company.

5. *Nutrition Facts panel:* This panel is the primary tool to assist you in choosing more healthful foods. Let's take a closer look at the components of the Nutrition Facts panel.

How to Read and Use the Nutrition Facts Panel

FIGURE 1.16 shows an example of a **Nutrition Facts panel** and the proposed changes. This part of the label includes a variety of information that is useful when designing a healthful diet. Let's start at the top of the panel and work our way down.

1. *Serving size and servings per container:* The FDA has defined serving sizes based on the amounts people typically eat for each food. However, keep in mind that the serving size listed on the package may not be the same as the amount you eat. You must factor in how much of the food you eat when determining the amount of nutrients that this food contributes to your actual diet.

2. *Total Calories and Calories from fat per serving:* By looking at this section of the label, you can determine if this food is relatively high in fat. For example, one serving of the food on this label contains 320 total Calories, of which 90 are from fat. This means that this food contains approximately 28% of its total Calories as fat, making it relatively low in fat.

3. *List of nutrients:* Those nutrients listed toward the top, including total fat, saturated fat, cholesterol, and sodium, are generally nutrients that we strive to limit in a healthful diet. Some of the nutrients listed toward the bottom are those we try to consume more of, including fiber, vitamins A and C, calcium, and iron.

4. *The **percent daily values (%DV)**:* This information tells you how much a serving of food contributes to your overall intake of nutrients listed on the label. Because we are all individuals with unique nutritional needs, it is impossible to include nutrition information that applies to each person consuming this food. Thus, the FDA used standards based on a 2,000-Calorie diet when defining the %DV. You can use these percentages to determine whether a food is high or low in a given nutrient, even if you do not consume a 2,000-Calorie diet each day. For example, if you are trying to consume more calcium, you might compare the labels of two different brands of fortified orange juice: you read that one contains 10% DV for calcium in an 8 oz serving, whereas the other contains 25% DV for calcium in an 8 oz serving. Thus, you can make your choice between these products without having to know anything about how many Calories you need.

5. *Footnote:* The footnote includes an explanatory note and a table with Daily Values for a 2,000- and 2,500-Calorie diet. This table, which may not be present on the package if the size of the food label is too small, is always the same because the information refers to nutrients, not to a specific food. For instance, it states that someone eating 2,000 Calories should strive to eat less than 65 g of fat per day, whereas a person eating 2,500 Calories should eat less than 80 g of fat per day.

Food Labels Can Contain a Variety of Claims

Have you ever noticed a food label displaying a claim such as "This food is low in sodium" or "This food is part of a heart-healthy diet"? The claim may have influenced you to buy the food, even if you weren't sure what it meant. Let's take a look.

The FDA regulates two types of claims that food companies put on food labels: nutrient claims and health claims. Food companies are prohibited from using a nutrient or health claim that is not approved by the FDA.

The Daily Values on the food labels serve as a basis for nutrient claims. For instance, if the label states that a food is "low in sodium," the food cannot contain

Learn more about using the Nutrition Facts panel to guide your food choices. Go to www.fda.gov and type "Labeling and Nutrition" in the search box. Then click on "Nutrition Facts Label Programs and Materials."

Nutrition Facts panel The label on a food package that contains the nutrition information required by the FDA.

percent daily values (%DV) Information on a Nutrition Facts Panel that tells you how much a serving of food contributes to your overall intake of nutrients listed on the label. The information is based on an energy intake of 2,000 Calories per day.

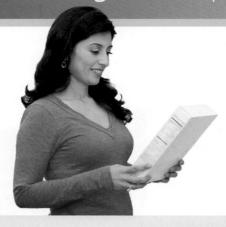

The U.S. Food and Drug Administration (FDA) is proposing new changes to the 20-year-old nutrition labels on packaged foods. The changes to the nutrition label provide information to help compare products and make healthy food choices.

Current Label

GRANOLA

Nutrition Facts

Serving Size 2/3 cup (55g)
Servings Per Container About 8

Amount Per Serving

Calories 230   Calories from Fat 72

	% Daily Value*
Total Fat 8g	**12%**
Saturated Fat 1g	**5%**
Trans Fat 0g	
Cholesterol 0mg	**0%**
Sodium 160mg	**7%**
Total Carbohydrates 37g	**12%**
Dietary Fiber 4g	**16%**
Sugars 1g	
Protein 3g	
Vitamin A	10%
Vitamin C	8%
Calcium	20%
Iron	45%

* Percent Daily Values are based on a 2,000 calorie diet. Your daily value may be higher or lower depending on your calorie needs.

	Calories:	2,000	2,500
Total Fat	Less than	65g	80g
Sat Fat	Less than	20g	25g
Cholesterol	Less than	300mg	300mg
Sodium	Less than	2,400mg	2,400mg
Total Carbohydrate		300g	375g
Dietary Fiber		25g	30g

SERVINGS

- Serving sizes are standardized, making comparison shopping easier.

NEW

- Servings and serving sizes are larger and bolder.
- "Amount per serving" will be changed to "Amount per (serving size)" such as "Amount per cup."

CALORIES

- Calories per serving and the number of servings in the package are listed.

NEW

- Calories are larger to stand out more.
- "Calories from fat" is removed.

DAILY VALUES

- Daily Values are general reference values based on a 2,000 calorie diet.
- The %DV can tell you if a food is high or low in a nutrient or dietary substance.

NEW

- Daily Values are listed first.
- The meaning of the Daily Values will be explained in a new detailed footnote.

ADDED SUGARS

NEW

- Added sugars are listed.

VITAMINS & MINERALS

- Vitamin A, vitamin C, calcium, and iron are required.
- Other vitamins and minerals are voluntary.

NEW

- Vitamin D and potassium are required, in addition to calcium and iron.
- Vitamins A and C are voluntary.
- Actual amounts of each nutrient are listed as well as the %DV.

Proposed New Label

GRANOLA

Nutrition Facts

8 servings per container

Serving size   2/3 cup (55g)

Amount per 2/3 cup

Calories   **230**

% DV*	
12%	**Total Fat** 8g
5%	**Saturated Fat** 1g
	Trans **Fat** 0g
0%	**Cholesterol** 0mg
7%	**Sodium** 160mg
12%	**Total Carbs** 37g
14%	Dietary Fiber 4g
	Sugars 1g
	Added Sugars 0g
	Protein 3g
10%	**Vitamin D** 2mcg
20%	**Calcium** 260mg
45%	**Iron** 8mg
5%	**Potassium** 235mg

* Footnote on Daily Values (DV) and calories reference to be inserted here.

TABLE 1.3 **U.S. Food and Drug Administration (FDA)–Approved Nutrient-Related Terms and Definitions**

Nutrient	Claim	Meaning
Energy	Calorie free	Less than 5 kcal per serving
	Low Calorie	40 kcal or less per serving
	Reduced Calorie	At least 25% fewer kcal than reference (or regular) food
Fat and Cholesterol	Fat free	Less than 0.5 g of fat per serving
	Low fat	3 g or less fat per serving
	Reduced fat	At least 25% less fat per serving than reference food
	Saturated fat free	Less than 0.5 g of saturated fat **AND** less than 0.5 g of *trans* fat per serving
	Low saturated fat	1 g or less saturated fat and less than 0.5 g *trans* fat per serving **AND** 15% or less of total kcal from saturated fat
	Reduced saturated fat	At least 25% less saturated fat **AND** reduced by more than 1 g saturated fat per serving as compared to reference food
	Cholesterol free	Less than 2 mg of cholesterol per serving **AND** 2 g or less saturated fat and *trans* fat combined per serving
	Low cholesterol	20 mg or less cholesterol **AND** 2 g or less saturated fat per serving
	Reduced cholesterol	At least 25% less cholesterol than reference food **AND** 2 g or less saturated fat per serving
Fiber and Sugar	High fiber	5 g or more fiber per serving*
	Good source of fiber	2.5 g to 4.9 g fiber per serving
	More or added fiber	At least 2.5 g more fiber per serving than reference food
	Sugar free	Less than 0.5 g sugars per serving
	Low sugar	Not defined; no basis for recommended intake
	Reduced/less sugar	At least 25% less sugars per serving than reference food
	No added sugars or without added sugars	No sugar or sugar-containing ingredient added during processing
Sodium	Sodium free	Less than 5 mg sodium per serving
	Very low sodium	35 mg or less sodium per serving
	Low sodium	140 mg or less sodium per serving
	Reduced sodium	At least 25% less sodium per serving than reference food
Relative Claims	Free, without, no, zero	No or a trivial amount of given nutrient
	Light (or lite)	This term can have three different meanings: (1) a serving provides ⅓ fewer kcal than or half the fat of the reference food; (2) a serving of a low-fat, low-Calorie food provides half the sodium normally present; or (3) lighter in color and texture, with the label making this clear (for example, light molasses)
	Reduced, less, fewer	Contains at least 25% less of a nutrient or kcal than reference food
	More, added, extra, or plus	At least 10% of the Daily Value of nutrient as compared to reference food (may occur naturally or be added). May only be used for vitamins, minerals, protein, dietary fiber, and potassium.
	Good source of, contains, or provides	10% to 19% of Daily Value per serving (may not be used for carbohydrate)
	High in, rich in, or excellent source of	20% or more of Daily Value per serving for protein, vitamins, minerals, dietary fiber, or potassium (may not be used for carbohydrate)

*High-fiber claims must also meet the definition of low fat; if not, then the level of total fat must appear next to the high-fiber claim.

Data adapted from "Food Labeling Guide" (U.S. Food and Drug Administration).

more than 140 mg of sodium per serving. **TABLE 1.3** defines the terms approved for use in nutrient claims.

The FDA also allows food labels to display certain claims related to health and disease **(TABLE 1.4)**. The claims listed are backed up with significant scientific agreement as to their validity.

In addition to nutrient and health claims, labels may also contain structure–function claims. These claims can be made without approval from the FDA. Although these claims can be generic statements about a food's impact on the body's structure and function, they cannot refer to a specific disease or symptom. Examples of structure–function claims include "Builds stronger bones," "Improves memory," "Slows signs of aging," and "Boosts your immune system." It is important

TABLE 1.4 U.S. Food and Drug Administration–Approved Health Claims on Labels

Disease/Health Concerns	Nutrient	Example of Approved Claim Statement
Osteoporosis	Calcium	Regular exercise and a healthy diet with enough calcium help teens and young adult white and Asian women maintain good bone health and may reduce their high risk for osteoporosis later in life.
Coronary heart disease	Saturated fat and cholesterol Fruits, vegetables, and grain products that contain fiber, particularly soluble fiber Soluble fiber from whole oats, psyllium seed husk, and beta glucan soluble fiber from oat bran, rolled oats (or oatmeal), and whole oat flour Soy protein Plant sterol/stanol esters Whole-grain foods	Diets low in saturated fat and cholesterol and rich in fruits, vegetables, and grain products that contain some types of dietary fiber, particularly soluble fiber, may reduce the risk for heart disease, a disease associated with many factors.
Cancer	Dietary fat Fiber-containing grain products, fruits, and vegetables Fruits and vegetables Whole-grain foods	Low-fat diets rich in fiber-containing grain products, fruits, and vegetables may reduce the risk for some types of cancer, a disease associated with many factors.
Hypertension and stroke	Sodium Potassium	Diets containing foods that are a good source of potassium and that are low in sodium may reduce the risk for high blood pressure and stroke.*
Neural tube defects	Folate	Healthful diets with adequate folate may reduce a woman's risk of having a child with a brain or spinal cord defect.
Dental caries	Sugar alcohols	Frequent between-meal consumption of foods high in sugars and starches promotes tooth decay. The sugar alcohols in [name of food] do not promote tooth decay.

*Required wording for this claim. Wordings for other claims are recommended model statements but not required verbatim.

Data adapted from "Food Labeling Guide" (U.S. Food and Drug Administration).

to remember that these claims can be made with no proof, and thus there are no guarantees that any benefits identified in structure–function claims are true about that food. Thus, just because something is stated on the label doesn't guarantee it is always true!

 recap The ability to read and interpret food labels is important for planning and maintaining a healthful diet. Food labels must list the identity of the food, the net contents of the package, the contact information for the food manufacturer or distributor, the ingredients in the food, and a Nutrition Facts panel. The Nutrition Facts panel provides specific information about Calories, macronutrients, and selected vitamins and minerals. Food labels may also display FDA-approved claims related to nutrients and health, but body structure and function claims can be made without approval from the FDA.

LO8 List at least four sources of reliable and accurate nutrition information.

Where can you turn for nutrition advice?

Over the past few decades, the public has become more and more interested in understanding how nutrition affects health. One result of this booming interest has been the publication of an almost overwhelming quantity of nutrition claims on television; on websites; in newspapers, magazines, and journals; and on product packages. Most consumers lack the training to evaluate the reliability of these claims and thus are vulnerable to misinformation.

Throughout this text we provide facts and activities to help you become a savvy food consumer. As you may know, **quackery** is the misrepresentation of a product, program, or service for financial gain. For example, a high-priced supplement may be marketed as uniquely therapeutic when, in fact, it is only as effective as much less expensive alternatives that are commonly available. Many manufacturers of such products describe them as "patented," but this means only that the product has been registered with the U.S. Patent Office, for a fee. It provides no guarantee of the product's effectiveness or its safety. So the question for a savvy consumer would be, Is this a legitimate product or service, or is it quackery? Armed with the information in this book, plus plenty of opportunities to test your knowledge, you'll become more confident when evaluating nutrition claims. Let's start by identifying *trustworthy* sources of nutrition information.

To learn more about how to spot quackery, go to www.quackwatch.com, enter "spot quack" in the search box, and then click on "Critiquing Quack Ads."

Trustworthy Experts Are Educated and Credentialed

Many types of healthcare professionals provide reliable and accurate nutrition information. The following are the most common:

- *Registered Dietitian (RD):* To become a registered dietitian (RD) requires, minimally, a bachelor's degree, completion of a supervised clinical experience, a passing grade on a national examination, and maintenance of registration with the Academy of Nutrition and Dietetics. There is now an optional change to the RD designation— RD/Nutritionist. This designation indicates that anyone who has earned an RD is also a qualified nutritionist; however, not all nutritionists are RDs (see below). RDs are qualified to provide nutrition counseling in a variety of settings.
- *Licensed dietitian:* A licensed dietitian is a dietitian meeting the credentialing requirement of a given state in the United States to engage in the practice of dietetics.[7] Each state has its own laws regulating dietitians. These laws specify which types of licensure or registration a nutrition professional must obtain in order to provide nutrition services or advice. Individuals who practice nutrition and dietetics without the required license or registration can be prosecuted for breaking the law.
- *Nutritionist:* This term generally has no definition or laws regulating it. In some cases, it refers to a professional with academic credentials in nutrition who may also be an RD.[7] In other cases, the term may refer to anyone who thinks he or she is knowledgeable about nutrition. Thus, there is no guarantee that a nutritionist is educated, trained, and experienced in the field of nutrition. So before taking advice from a nutritionist, ask about his or her credentials. In the chapter-opening scenario, how might Miguel have determined whether or not the "nutritionist" was qualified to give him advice?
- *Professional with a master's degree (MA or MS) or doctoral degree (PhD) in nutrition:* Many individuals hold an advanced degree in nutrition and have years of experience in a nutrition-related career. For instance, they may teach at colleges or universities or work in fitness or healthcare settings. Unless these individuals are licensed or registered dietitians, they are not certified to provide clinical dietary counseling or treatment for individuals with disease. However, they are reliable sources of information about nutrition and health.
- *Physician:* The term *physician* encompasses a variety of healthcare professionals. A medical doctor (MD) is educated, trained, and licensed to practice medicine in the United States. However, medical students in the United States are not required to take any nutrition courses throughout their academic training; thus, MDs typically have very limited knowledge of nutrition. On the other hand, a number of MDs take nutrition courses out of personal interest and thus have a solid background in nutrition. Nevertheless, if you require a dietary plan to treat an illness or a disease, most MDs will refer you to an RD. In contrast, an osteopathic physician, referred to as a doctor of osteopathy (DO), may have studied nutrition extensively, as may a naturopathic physician, a homeopathic physician, or a chiropractor. Thus, it is prudent to determine a physician's level of expertise rather than assuming that he or she has extensive knowledge of nutrition.

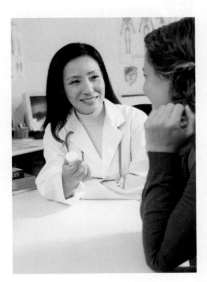

Medical doctors may have limited experience and training in the area of nutrition, but they can refer you to a registered dietitian (RD) or a licensed dietitian to help you meet your dietary needs.

quackery The promotion of an unproven remedy, such as a supplement or other product or service, usually by someone unlicensed and untrained.

Government Agencies Are Usually Trustworthy

Many government health agencies address the problem of nutrition-related disease in the United States. These organizations are publicly funded, and many provide financial support for research in the areas of nutrition and health. Two of the most recognized and respected of these government agencies are:

- *Centers for Disease Control and Prevention (CDC):* The CDC is considered the leading federal agency that protects the health and safety of people in the United States. The CDC is located in Atlanta, Georgia, and works in the areas of health promotion, disease prevention and control, and environmental health.
- *National Institutes of Health (NIH):* The NIH is the world's leading medical research center and the focal point for medical research in the United States. The NIH is one of the agencies of the Public Health Service, which is part of the U.S. Department of Health and Human Services. The NIH has many institutes, such as the National Cancer Institute and the National Center for Complementary and Alternative Medicine, that focus on a broad array of health issues. NIH headquarters are located in Bethesda, Maryland.

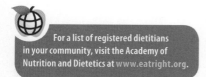

For a list of registered dietitians in your community, visit the Academy of Nutrition and Dietetics at www.eatright.org.

Professional Organizations Provide Reliable Nutrition Information

A number of professional organizations represent nutrition professionals, scientists, and educators. These organizations publish cutting-edge nutrition research studies and educational information in journals that are accessible in most university and medical libraries. Some of these organizations are:

- *The Academy of Nutrition and Dietetics:* This is the largest organization of food and nutrition professionals in the world. The mission of this organization is to promote nutrition, health, and well-being. The Canadian equivalent is Dietitians of Canada. The Academy publishes a professional journal called the *Journal of the Academy of Nutrition and Dietetics.*
- *The American Society for Nutrition (ASN):* The ASN is the premier research society dedicated to improving quality of life through the science of nutrition. The ASN fulfills its mission by fostering, enhancing, and disseminating nutrition-related research and professional education activities. The ASN publishes a professional journal called the *American Journal of Clinical Nutrition.*
- *The American College of Sports Medicine (ACSM):* The ACSM is the leading sports medicine and exercise science organization in the world. The mission of the ACSM is to advance and integrate scientific research to provide educational and practical applications of exercise science and sports medicine. Many members are nutrition professionals who combine their nutrition and exercise expertise to promote health and athletic performance. *Medicine and Science in Sports and Exercise* is the professional journal of the ACSM.
- *The North American Association for the Study of Obesity (NAASO):* NAASO is the leading scientific society dedicated to the study of obesity. It is committed to encouraging research on the causes and treatments of obesity and to keeping the medical community and public informed of new advances. The official NAASO journal is *Obesity Research,* which is intended to increase knowledge, stimulate research, and promote better treatment of people with obesity.

For more information on any of these organizations, see the **Web Links** at the end of this chapter.

If you aren't sure whether the source of your information is reliable or can't tell whether the results of a particular study apply to you, how do you find out? What if two studies seem sound but their findings contradict each other? The next section explains how to interpret nutrition-related research.

recap   Health professionals who provide reliable and accurate nutrition information include registered dietitians, licensed dietitians, professionals with an advanced degree in nutrition, and some physicians. The term *nutritionist* is not a guarantee that the individual has any training in nutrition. The Centers for Disease Control and Prevention is the leading U.S. federal agency that protects citizen's health and safety. The National Institutes of Health is the leading medical research agency in the world. The Academy of Nutrition and Dietetics is one of several professional organizations providing reliable nutrition information.

How can you interpret the results of research studies?

LO**9** Describe the steps of the scientific method used in research studies.

"Reduce your fat intake! Make sure at least 60% of your diet comes from carbohydrates!"

"Eat more protein and fat! Carbohydrates cause obesity!"

Do you ever feel overwhelmed by the abundant and often conflicting advice in media reports related to nutrition? If so, you're not alone. In addition to the "high-carb, low-carb" controversy, we've had mixed messages about the effectiveness of calcium supplements in preventing bone loss, high fluid intake in preventing constipation, and high fiber intake in preventing colon cancer. And after decades of warnings that coffee and tea could be bad for our health, it now appears that both contain chemicals that can be beneficial! When even nutrition researchers don't seem to agree, whom can we believe?

Nutrition is a relatively young science: the U.S. Congress first funded research into human nutrition in 1894. At that time, vitamins were unknown, and the role of minerals in the body was unclear.[8] Moreover, discoveries in nutrition rely in part on the discoveries of other relatively young sciences, such as biochemistry and genetics. New experiments are being designed every day to determine how nutrition affects our health, and new discoveries are being made. Viewing conflicting evidence as essential to the advancement of our understanding may help you feel more comfortable with the contradictions. In fact, controversy is what stimulates researchers to explore unknown areas and attempt to solve the mysteries of nutrition and health.

In addition, it's important to recognize that media reports rarely include a thorough review of the research findings on a given topic. Typically, they focus only on the most recent study. Thus, one report on the nightly news should never be taken as absolute fact on any topic. To become a more educated consumer and informed critic of nutrition reports in the media, you need to understand the research process and how to interpret the results of different types of studies. So let's take a closer look.

Research Involves Applying the Scientific Method

When confronted with a claim about any aspect of our world, from "The Earth is flat" to "Carbohydrates cause obesity," scientists must first consider whether the claim can be tested. In other words, can evidence be presented to substantiate the claim and, if so, what data would qualify as evidence? Scientists worldwide use a standardized method of looking at evidence called the *scientific method*. This method is a multistep process that involves observation, experimentation, and development of a theory **(FIGURE 1.17)**. Its standardized procedures minimize the influence of personal prejudices on our understanding of natural phenomena. Thus, this method is used to perform quality research studies in any discipline, including nutrition.

Observation of a Phenomenon Starts the Research Process

The first step in the scientific method is observing and describing a phenomenon. As an example, let's say you are working in a healthcare office that caters to mostly elderly clients. You have observed that many of the elderly have high blood pressure, but there are some who have normal blood pressure. After talking with a large

▶ **FIGURE 1.17** The scientific method, which forms the framework for scientific research. A researcher begins by making an observation about a phenomenon. This leads the researcher to ask a question. A hypothesis is generated to explain the observation. The researcher then conducts an experiment to test the hypothesis. Observations are made during the experiment, and data are generated and documented. The data may either support or refute the hypothesis. If the data support the hypothesis, more experiments are conducted to test and confirm support for the hypothesis. A hypothesis that is supported after repeated testing may be called a theory. If the data do not support the hypothesis, the hypothesis is either rejected or modified and then retested.

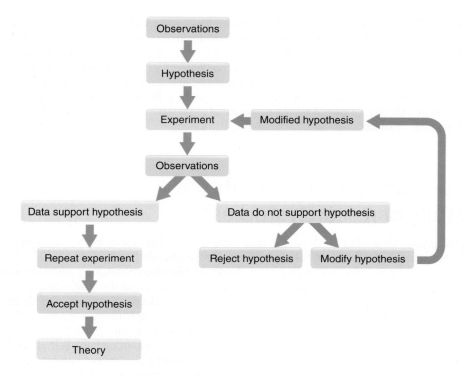

number of elderly clients, you notice a pattern developing in that the clients who report being more physically active are also those having lower blood pressure readings. This observation leads you to question the relationship that might exist between physical activity and blood pressure. Your next step is to develop a **hypothesis**, or possible explanation for your observation.

A Hypothesis Is a Possible Explanation for an Observation

A hypothesis states an assumption you want to test. It is also sometimes referred to as a research question. In this example, your hypothesis would be something like "Regular physical activity lowers blood pressure in elderly people." You must generate a hypothesis before you can conduct experiments to determine what factors may explain your observation.

An Experiment Is Designed to Test the Hypothesis

An *experiment* is a scientific process that tests a hypothesis. A well-designed experiment attempts to control for factors that may coincidentally influence the results. In the case of your research study, it is well known that weight loss can reduce blood pressure in people with high blood pressure. Thus, in designing an experiment on the effects of exercise on blood pressure, you would want to control for weight loss. You could do this by making sure people eat enough food, so that they do not lose weight during your study, and by weighing them regularly to verify weight maintenance.

It is important to emphasize that one research study does not prove or disprove a hypothesis. Ideally, multiple experiments are conducted over many years to thoroughly examine a hypothesis. Science exists to allow us to continue to challenge existing hypotheses and expand what we currently know.

A Theory May Be Developed After Extensive Research

If multiple experiments do not support a hypothesis, then the hypothesis is rejected or modified. On the other hand, if the results of multiple experiments consistently support a hypothesis, then it is possible to develop a theory. A **theory** represents a hypothesis or group of related hypotheses that have been confirmed through repeated scientific experiments. Theories are strongly accepted principles, but they can be challenged and changed as a result of applying the scientific method. Remember that, centuries ago, it was theorized that the Earth was flat. People were so convinced of

hypothesis An educated guess as to why a phenomenon occurs.

theory A conclusion, or scientific consensus, drawn from repeated experiments.

this that they refused to sail beyond known boundaries because they believed they would fall off the edge of the Earth. Only after multiple explorers challenged this theory was it discovered that the Earth is round. We continue to apply the scientific method today to test hypotheses and challenge theories.

Various Types of Research Studies Tell Different Stories

Different types of research studies yield different types of information. Let's explore the options.

Animal Versus Human Studies

In many cases, studies involving animals provide preliminary information that assists scientists in designing human studies. Animal studies also are used to conduct research that cannot be done with humans. For instance, researchers can cause a nutrient deficiency in an animal and study its adverse health effects over the animal's life span, but this type of experiment with humans is not acceptable. Drawbacks of animal studies include ethical concerns and the fact that the results may not apply directly to humans.

Over the past century, animal studies have advanced our understanding of many aspects of nutrition, from micronutrients to obesity. Still, some hypotheses can only be investigated using human subjects. The three primary types of studies conducted with humans include observational studies, case-control studies, and clinical trials.

Observational Studies

Observational studies are used in assessing nutritional habits, disease trends, or other health phenomena of large populations and determining the factors that may influence these phenomena. However, these studies can only indicate *relationships* between factors; they do not suggest that the data are linked by cause and effect. For instance, smoking and low vegetable intake appear to be related in some studies, but this does not mean that smoking cigarettes causes people to eat fewer vegetables, or that eating fewer vegetables causes people to smoke.

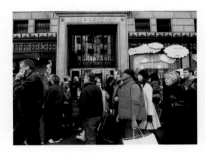

▲ Observational studies are used in assessing habits, trends, and other phenomena in large populations of people.

Case-Control Studies

Case-control studies are more complex observational studies with additional design features that allow scientists to gain a better understanding of things that may influence disease. They involve comparing a group of individuals with a particular condition (for instance, 100 elderly people with high blood pressure) to a similar group without this condition (for instance, 100 elderly people with normal blood pressure). This comparison allows the researcher to identify factors other than the defined condition that differ between the two groups. For example, researchers may find that 75% of the people in their normal blood pressure group are physically active but that only 20% of the people in their high blood pressure group are physically active. Again, this would not prove that physical activity prevents high blood pressure. It would merely suggest a significant relationship between these two factors.

Clinical Trials

Clinical trials are tightly controlled experiments in which an intervention is given to determine its effect on a particular disease or health condition. Interventions may include medications, nutritional supplements, controlled diets, or exercise programs. In clinical trials, people in an experimental group are given the intervention, and people in a control group are not. The responses of the two groups are compared. In the case of the blood pressure experiment, researchers could assign one group of elderly people with high blood pressure to an exercise program and assign a second group of elderly people with high blood pressure to a program where no exercise is done. Over the next few weeks, months, or even years, researchers could measure the blood pressure of the people in each group. If the blood pressure of those who exercised decreased and the blood pressure of those who did not exercise rose or remained the same, the influence of exercise on lowering blood pressure would be supported.

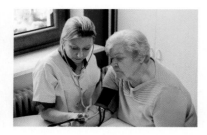

⬆ In a clinical trial, an intervention is given to determine its effect on a health condition or disease.

Two questions important to consider when evaluating the quality of a clinical trial are whether the subjects were randomly chosen and whether the researchers and subjects were *blinded*:

- *Randomized trials.* Ideally, researchers should *randomly* assign research participants to intervention groups (who get the treatment) and control groups (who do not get the treatment). Randomizing participants is like flipping a coin or drawing names from a hat; it reduces the possibility of showing favoritism toward any participants and ensures that the groups are similar on the factors you are measuring in the study. These types of studies are called *randomized clinical (controlled) trials.*
- *Single- and double-blind experiments.* If possible, it is also important to *blind* both researchers and participants to the treatment being given. A *single-blind experiment* is one in which the participants are unaware of or *blinded* to the treatment they're receiving, but the researchers know which group is getting the treatment and which group is not. A *double-blind experiment* is one in which neither researchers nor participants know which group is really getting the treatment. Double blinding helps prevent the researcher from seeing only the results he or she wants to see, even if these results do not actually occur. In the case of testing medications or nutrition supplements, the blinding process can be assisted by giving the control group a placebo. A *placebo* is an imitation treatment that has no effect on participants; for instance, a sugar pill may be given in place of a vitamin supplement. Studies like this are referred to as *double-blind randomized clinical trials.*

Use Your Knowledge of Research to Help You Evaluate Nutrition Claims

You probably wouldn't think it strange to read an ad from your favorite brand of ice cream encouraging you to "Go ahead. Indulge." It's just an ad, right? But what if you were to read about a research study in which people who ate your favorite brand of ice cream improved the density of their bones? Could you trust the study results more than you would the ad?

To answer that question, you'd have to investigate several more:

- Who conducted the research, and who paid for it?
- Was the study funded by a company that stands to profit from certain results?
- Are the researchers receiving goods, personal travel funds, or other perks from the research sponsor, or do they have investments in companies or products related to their study?

If the answer to any of these questions was yes, a *conflict of interest* would exist between the researchers and the funding agency. Whenever a conflict of interest exists, it can seriously compromise the researchers' ability to conduct impartial research and report the results in an accurate and responsible manner. That's why, when researchers submit their results for publication in scientific journals, they are required to reveal any conflicts of interest they may have that could be seen as affecting the integrity of their research. In this way, people who review the study are better able to consider whether researcher *bias* influenced the results. A bias is an inclination in advance to favor certain results.

Now that you've increased your understanding of scientific research, you're better equipped to discern the truth or fallacy of nutrition-related claims. Keep the nearby **Highlight** feature box in mind when evaluating the findings of research studies and the claims made on commercial websites.

Recent media investigations have reported widespread bias in studies funded by pharmaceutical companies testing the effectiveness of their drugs. In addition, journals in both the United States and Europe have been found less likely to publish negative results (that is, study results suggesting that a therapy is not effective). We also know that clinical trials funded by pharmaceutical companies are more likely to report positive results than are trials that were independently financed.[9,10] This has serious implications: if ineffectiveness and side effects are not fully reported,

highlight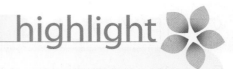

Detecting Media Hype

If you have an e-mail account, you're probably familiar with spam fads that promise weight-loss miracles for "only $19.99!" Do you delete them unread? A study from Brooklyn College of the City University of New York found that, in the course of 1 year, 42% of students with weight problems had opened spam e-mails touting weight-loss products, and almost 19% had placed an order! Lead researchers were shocked by the findings and advised physicians to discuss with patients the potential risks of using weight-loss products marketed via spam e-mails.[1]

How can you avoid being fooled by the media hype that bombards you daily? Here are some tips to help you sort nutrition fact from fallacy:

- *Consider the author of the information.* If the report is about a product on the market and is written or reported by a person or group who may financially benefit from your buying the product, you should be skeptical. Also, whatever the subject of the report, bear in mind that many people who write for popular magazines and newspapers are not trained in science and are capable of misinterpreting research results.

- *Find out who conducted the research and who paid for it.* Was the study funded by a company that stands to profit from certain results? Do the researchers have investments in such a company, or are they receiving money or other perks from the research sponsor? If the answer to these questions is yes, a conflict of interest exists between the researchers and the funding agency.

- *Evaluate the content.* Is the report based on reputable research studies? Did the research follow the scientific method, and were the results reported in a reputable scientific journal? Ideally, the journal is peer-reviewed; that is, the articles are critiqued by other specialists working in the same scientific field. A reputable report should cite the source of the information, and should identify researchers by name.

- *Watch for red flags.* Is the report based on testimonials about personal experiences? Testimonials are fraught with bias. Are sweeping conclusions made from only one study? Remember that one study cannot prove any hypothesis. Are the claims made in the report too good to be true? If something sounds too good to be true, it probably is.

---

healthcare providers may be prescribing medications that are ineffective or even harmful.

The seriousness of this issue has inspired researchers around the world to demand a global system whereby all clinical trials are registered and all research results are made accessible to the public. The development of such a system would allow for independent review of research data and work toward ensuring that healthcare decisions were fully informed. As a first step, the U.S. Food and Drug Administration in 2009 launched a Transparency Initiative with the goal of making useful and understandable information about FDA activities and decision making available to the public.

To learn more about the FDA Transparency Initiative, enter "Transparency Initiative" into the search box at www.fda.gov.

recap The steps in the scientific method are (1) observing a phenomenon, (2) creating a hypothesis, (3) designing and conducting an experiment, and (4) collecting and analyzing data that support or refute the hypothesis. Studies involving animals provide preliminary information that assists scientists in designing human studies. Human studies include observational studies, case-control studies, and clinical trials. When evaluating research studies, consider whether a conflict of interest exists.

STUDY **PLAN** | MasteringNutrition™

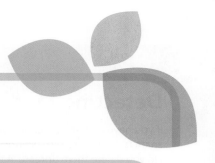

Customize your study plan—and master your nutrition!—
in the Study Area of **MasteringNutrition**.

what can I do today?

Now that you've read this chapter, try making these three changes.

1 Read the Nutrition Facts panel of your favorite snacks and change your usual selections to ones that are lower in sodium, total fat, or saturated fat.

2 Log on to the MyPlate website (www.choosemyplate.gov) and design a healthy food plan that will help you maintain your present weight or lose weight.

3 Follow the Mediterranean diet for one full day and see how you like it!

test yourself | *answers*

1. **True.** Although nutrition guidelines recommend that we consume these types of foods only occasionally, they can be included in moderation as part of a healthful diet.

2. **False.** A Calorie is a measure of energy in a food. More precisely, a kilocalorie is the amount of heat required to raise the temperature of 1 kilogram of water by 1 degree Celsius.

3. **False.** There is no minimum level of education or national certification process required for people who identify themselves as a "nutritionist."

summary

Scan to hear an MP3 Chapter Review in **MasteringNutrition**.

LO **1** **Define the term *nutrition* and explain why nutrition is important to health**

- Nutrition is the science that studies food and how food affects our bodies and our health.

- Nutrition is an important component of wellness. A healthful diet prevents nutrient-deficiency diseases, and reduces the risk for diseases like type 2 diabetes in which nutrition plays some role.

- Nutrients are chemicals found in food that are critical to human growth and function.

LO **2** **Identify the six classes of nutrients essential for health**

- The six essential nutrient groups found in foods are carbohydrates, fats, proteins, vitamins, minerals, and water.

- Carbohydrates, fats, and proteins provide our bodies with the energy we need to survive. Carbohydrates are the primary energy source for the activities of the body, whereas fats provide energy for the body at rest and during light activity. Protein contributes to tissue growth and repair and is only secondarily an energy source.

- Vitamins and minerals are micronutrients essential to human functioning. Some vitamins are water soluble, and others are fat soluble. Two groups of minerals are trace minerals and major minerals.

- Water is critical for our survival and is important for regulating nervous impulses, muscle contractions, nutrient transport, and excretion of waste products.

LO **3** **Identify the characteristics of a healthful diet**

- A healthful diet provides adequate nutrients and energy and includes only moderate amounts of sweets, fats, and salt. A healthful diet also includes an appropriate balance and variety of foods.

LO **4** **Compare and contrast the six types of Dietary Reference Intakes for nutrients**

- The Dietary Reference Intakes (DRIs) are dietary standards for nutrients established for healthy people in a particular life stage or gender group.

LO **5** **Describe the *Dietary Guidelines for Americans* and discuss how these Guidelines can be used to design a healthful diet**

- The *Dietary Guidelines for Americans* emphasize healthful food choices and physical activity behaviors. The guidelines include balancing food intake and physical activity to achieve and maintain a healthy weight; limiting sodium, fat, sugars, and alcohol; consuming nutrient-dense foods; and following healthy eating patterns, including keeping foods safe to eat.

LO **6** **Identify the food groups in the USDA food patterns and the amounts adults should eat each day**

- MyPlate is an interactive, web-based tool developed as part of the USDA food patterns to help Americans make better food choices. It can be used to assess one's current diet and physical activity levels. The food groups in the plate include grains, vegetables, fruits, dairy foods, and protein foods.

- Empty Calories from solid fats and/or added sugars provide few or no nutrients. The USDA recommends that empty Calories should be limited in a daily diet.

- Specific serving sizes are defined for foods in each group of MyPlate. There is no standard definition for a serving size, and the serving sizes defined in the plate are generally smaller than those listed on food labels and the servings generally sold to consumers.

LO **7** **Explain how to read and use the Nutrition Facts panel found on food labels**

- Food labels must list the identity of the food, the net contents of the package, the contact information for the food manufacturer or distributor, the ingredients in the food, and a Nutrition Facts panel.

- The Nutrition Facts Panel provides specific information about Calories, macronutrients, percent daily values (%DV), and select vitamins and minerals.

LO **8** **List at least four sources of reliable and accurate nutrition information**

- Quackery is the misrepresentation of a product, program, or service for financial gain.

- Health professionals who provide reliable and accurate nutrition information include registered dietitians (RDs), licensed dietitians, professionals with an advanced degree in nutrition, and some physicians. The term *nutritionist* is not a guarantee that the individual has any training in nutrition.

- Reliable nutrition information is also provided by the Centers for Disease Control and Prevention, the Academy of Nutrition and Dietetics, and many other governmental agencies and professional organizations.

LO **9** **Describe the steps of the scientific method used in research studies**

- The steps in the scientific method are (1) observing a phenomenon, (2) creating a hypothesis, (3) designing and conducting an experiment, and (4) collecting and analyzing data that support or refute the hypothesis. If the data are rejected, then an alternative hypothesis is proposed and tested. If the data support the original hypothesis, then a conclusion is drawn.

- A scientific theory represents a conclusion drawn from repeated experimentation.

review questions

LO **1** **Define the term *nutrition* and explain why nutrition is important to health**

1. Nutrition scientists might study
   a. how the human body digests and stores fats.
   b. how to increase children's consumption of fruits and vegetables.
   c. how much carbohydrate athletes should eat before competitions.
   d. any of the above.

2. Poor nutrition
   a. is a direct cause of nutrient deficiency diseases.
   b. is strongly associated with the development of most types of cancer.
   c. is a direct cause of type 2 diabetes.
   d. plays a minor role in the development of nutrient toxicity diseases.

LO **2** **Identify the six classes of nutrients essential for health**

3. Which of the following foods contains all six groups of essential nutrients?
   a. a low-fat yogurt parfait with fresh strawberries and walnuts
   b. an egg-salad sandwich with mayonnaise, lettuce, and whole-grain bread
   c. creamy tomato soup made with whole milk
   d. all of the above

LO **3** **Identify the characteristics of a healthful diet**

4. An adequate diet
   a. provides enough energy to meet minimum daily requirements.
   b. provides enough of the energy, nutrients, and fiber necessary to maintain a person's health.
   c. provides a sufficient variety of nutrients to maintain a healthy weight and to optimize the body's functioning.
   d. contains combinations of foods that provide healthful proportions of nutrients.

LO **4** **Compare and contrast the six types of Dietary Reference Intakes for nutrients**

5. The amount of a nutrient that meets the needs of 97–98% of people in a particular group is the
   a. Estimated Average Requirement.
   b. Estimated Energy Requirement.
   c. Recommended Dietary Allowance.
   d. Adequate Intake.

LO **5** **Describe the *Dietary Guidelines for Americans* and discuss how these Guidelines can be used to design a healthful diet**

6. The *Dietary Guidelines for Americans* recommend which of the following?
   a. choosing and preparing all foods without salt
   b. consuming alcohol in moderation each day
   c. being physically active each day
   d. consuming a fat-free diet

LO **6** **Identify the food groups in the USDA food patterns and the amounts adults should eat each day**

7. The USDA Food Patterns recommend
   a. eating at least 6 oz of grain foods each day.
   b. eating more dark-green and orange vegetables, beans, and peas.
   c. consuming at least one glass of fruit juice and one fresh fruit each day.
   d. eating no more than 3 oz of protein foods each day.

LO **7** **Explain how to read and use the Nutrition Facts panel found on food labels**

8. The Nutrition Facts panel on packaged foods provides information about the micronutrients
   a. vitamin D, calcium, sodium, and potassium.
   b. vitamin A, vitamin C, sodium, iron, and calcium.
   c. sodium and calcium.
   d. No micronutrient information is included on the Nutrition Facts Panel.

LO **8** **List at least four sources of reliable and accurate nutrition information**

9. Which of the following is the most reliable source of information about the health benefits of eating chocolate?
   a. a study funded by the National Institutes of Health
   b. a study funded by a company that produces chocolate
   c. a study reported on a natural-foods website
   d. a study reported in a cooking magazine

LO **9** **Describe the steps of the scientific method used in research studies**

10. After an initial experiment yields evidence that supports a hypothesis, scientists
    a. reject the hypothesis.
    b. challenge the hypothesis with further experiments.
    c. advance a theory.
    d. accept the hypothesis as fact.

Answers to Review Questions are located at the back of this text.

web links

The following websites and apps explore further topics and issues related to personal health.
Visit MasteringNutrition for links to the websites and RSS feeds.

www.acsm.org
American College of Sports Medicine (ACSM)
Obtain information about the leading sports medicine and exercise science organization in the world.

www.cdc.gov
Centers for Disease Control and Prevention (CDC)
Visit this site for additional information about the leading federal agency in the United States that protects the health and safety of people.

www.chooseMyPlate.gov
USDA's MyPlate Homepage

Use the SuperTracker on this website to assess the overall quality of your diet and level of physical activity based on the USDA MyPlate.

www.cnpp.usda.gov
2010 *Dietary Guidelines for Americans*

Use these guidelines to make changes in your food choices and physical activity habits to help reduce your risk for chronic disease. Scroll down to "dietaryguidelines" for details.

www.eatright.org
Academy of Nutrition and Dietetics

Obtain a list of registered dietitians in your community from the largest organization of food and nutrition professionals in the United States. You can also visit the Public Information Center section of this website for additional resources to help you achieve a healthful lifestyle.

www.fda.gov
U.S. Food and Drug Administration

Learn more about the government agency that regulates our food and first established regulations for nutrition information on food labels.

www.hsph.harvard.edu
Harvard School of Public Health

Visit this site for reliable nutrition information on a variety of topics. For instance, type in "nutrition source" in the A to Z index to learn more about the Healthy Eating Plate, an alternative to the USDA MyPlate.

www.iom.edu
Institute of Medicine of the National Academies

Learn about the Institute of Medicine's history of examining the nation's nutritional well-being and providing sound information about food and nutrition.

www.nih.gov
National Institutes of Health (NIH)

Find out more about the National Institutes of Health, an agency under the U.S. Department of Health and Human Services.

www.nutrition.org
American Society for Nutrition (ASN)

Learn more about the American Society for Nutrition and its goal to improve quality of life through the science of nutrition.

www.obesity.org
The Obesity Society

Learn about this interdisciplinary society and its work to develop, extend, and disseminate knowledge in the field of obesity.

www.pcrm.org
Physicians Committee for Responsible Medicine

Click on Health and Nutrition to access a variety of nutrition-related resources. For instance, to view the Power Plate, a vegetarian alternative to the USDA MyPlate, go to Vegetarian and Vegan Diets, then choose "The Power Plate" icon.

2

The Human Body
Are We Really What We Eat?

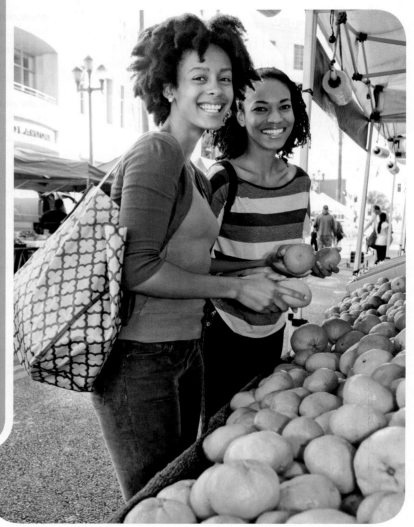

test yourself

Are these statements true or false? Circle your guess.

1. T F Your stomach is the primary organ responsible for telling you when you are hungry.

2. T F The entire process of digestion and absorption of one meal takes about 24 hours.

3. T F Some types of bacteria actually help keep us healthy.

Test Yourself answers can be found at the end of the chapter.

Two months ago, Andrea's lifelong dream of becoming a lawyer came one step closer to reality: she moved out of her parents' home in the Midwest to attend law school in Boston. Unfortunately, the adjustment to a new city, new friends, and her intensive coursework has been more stressful than she'd imagined, and Andrea has been experiencing insomnia and exhaustion. What's more, her always "sensitive stomach" has been getting worse: after almost every meal, she gets cramps so bad she can't stand up, and twice she has missed classes because of sudden attacks of pain and diarrhea. She suspects that the problem is related to stress, and wonders if she is going to experience it throughout her life. She is even thinking of dropping out of school if that would make her feel well again.

Almost everyone experiences brief periods of abdominal pain, diarrhea, or other symptoms of gastrointestinal distress from time to time. Such episodes are usually caused by food poisoning. But do you know anyone who experiences these symptoms periodically for days, weeks, or even years? If so, has it made you wonder why? What are the steps in normal digestion and absorption of food, and at what points can the process break down?

We begin this chapter with a look at some of the factors that make us feel as if we want to eat. We'll then take a tour of the organs of the body that help us digest food, absorb nutrients, and eliminate wastes. Finally, we'll discuss some common disorders that affect these functions.

Why do we want to eat what we want to eat?

 Compare and contrast the feelings of hunger and appetite, and the factors contributing to each.

You've just finished eating at your favorite Thai restaurant. As you walk back to the block where you parked your car, you pass a bakery window displaying several cakes and pies, each of which looks more enticing than the last; through the door wafts a complex aroma of coffee, cinnamon, and chocolate. You stop. You know you're not hungry, but you go inside and buy a slice of chocolate torte and an espresso, anyway. Later that night, when the caffeine from the chocolate and espresso keeps you awake, you wonder why you succumbed.

Two mechanisms prompt us to seek food: hunger and appetite. **Hunger** is a physical drive for food that occurs when our bodies sense that we need to eat. The drive is *nonspecific;* when you're hungry, a variety of foods could satisfy you. If you've recently finished a nourishing meal, then hunger probably won't compel you toward a slice of chocolate torte. Instead, the culprit is likely to be **appetite**, a psychological desire for *specific* foods. It is aroused when environmental cues—such as the sight of chocolate cake or the smell of coffee—stimulate your senses, triggering pleasant emotions and memories.

People commonly experience appetite in the absence of hunger. That's why you can crave cake and coffee even after eating a full meal. On the other hand, it is possible to have a physical need for food yet have no appetite. This state, called *anorexia,* can accompany a variety of illnesses. It can also occur as a side effect of certain medications, such as the chemotherapy used in treating cancer patients. Although the following sections describe hunger and appetite as separate entities, ideally the two states coexist: we seek specific, appealing foods to satisfy a physical need for nutrients.

The Hypothalamus Prompts Hunger in Response to Various Signals

Because hunger occurs when we physically need to eat, we often feel it as a negative or unpleasant sensation. The primary organ producing that sensation is the brain.

hunger A physical sensation that prompts us to eat.

appetite A psychological desire to consume specific foods.

▶ FIGURE 2.1

The hypothalamus triggers hunger by integrating signals from nerve cells throughout the body, as well as from messages carried by hormones.

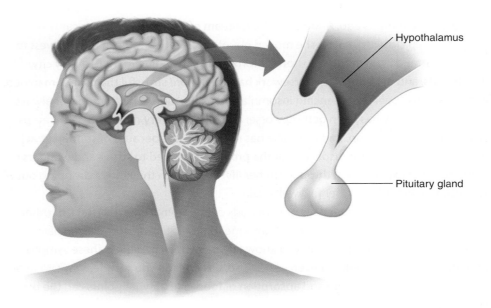

Hypothalamus

Pituitary gland

That's right—it's not our stomach but our brain that tell us when we're hungry. The region of brain tissue responsible for prompting us to seek food is called the **hypothalamus** **(FIGURE 2.1)**. It's located above the pituitary gland in a part of the brain that regulates many types of involuntary activity. The hypothalamus triggers feelings of either hunger or satiation (fullness) by integrating signals from three sources: nerve cells, chemicals called *hormones,* and the amount and type of food we eat. Let's review these three types of signals.

The Role of Nerve Cells

One important signal comes from nerve cells lining the stomach and small intestine that detect changes in pressure according to whether the organ is empty or filled with food. The cells relay these data to the hypothalamus. For instance, if you have not eaten for many hours, nerve cells in your stomach and small intestine send a signal to your hypothalamus, which in turn prompts you to feel the sensation of hunger.

The Role of Hormones

Our body has several *glands* that release chemicals called **hormones** into the bloodstream. From there, hormones travel to distant parts of the body and influence its functions. Insulin and glucagon are two hormones that can trigger the sensation of hunger. Here's how. Glucose is our body's most readily available fuel. When we have not eaten for a while, our blood glucose levels fall. This decrease in turn triggers a change in the blood's level of insulin and glucagon. This chemical message reaches the hypothalamus, which then prompts us to feel hungry so that we eat and supply our bodies with more glucose.

After we eat, the hypothalamus picks up signals from nerve cells sensing our full stomach, other signals from the gut, and a rise in blood glucose levels. When it integrates these signals, you have the experience of feeling full, or *satiated*. However, as we have noted, even though our brain sends us clear signals about hunger, most of us become adept at ignoring them and eat when we are not truly hungry.

In addition to insulin and glucagon, a variety of other hormones and hormone-like substances signal the hypothalamus to cause us to feel hungry or satiated. So it's not surprising that many nutrition researchers are exploring the role of hormones in weight management.

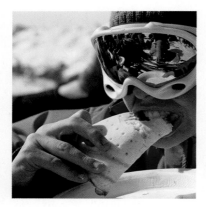

◀ Our body feels hunger when we haven't eaten for many hours or our blood glucose is low.

hypothalamus A brain region where sensations such as hunger and thirst are regulated.

hormones Chemical messengers secreted into the bloodstream by one of the many glands of the body.

The Role of the Amount and Type of Food

Although the reason behind this observation is not fully understood, researchers have long recognized that foods containing protein have the highest satiety value.[1] This means that a ham and egg breakfast will cause us to feel satiated for a longer period of time than will pancakes with maple syrup, even if both meals have exactly the same number of Calories.

Another factor affecting hunger is how bulky the meal is—that is, how much fiber and water is within the food. Bulky meals tend to stretch the stomach and small intestine, which sends signals back to the hypothalamus telling us that we are full, so we stop eating. This is one reason that people who want to lose weight are encouraged to increase the amount of fiber in their diet. In addition, beverages tend to be less satisfying than solid foods. For example, if you were to eat a bunch of grapes, you would feel a greater sense of fullness than if you drank a glass of grape juice.

recap In contrast to appetite, hunger is a physical sensation triggered by the hypothalamus in response to cues from nerve cells about stomach and intestinal fullness and the levels of certain hormones and hormone-like substances. High-protein foods make us feel satiated for longer periods of time, and bulky meals fill us up quickly, causing us to stop eating sooner.

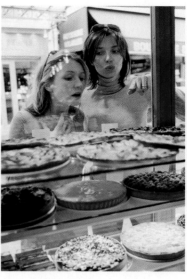

Food stimulates our senses.

Environmental Cues Trigger Appetite

Whereas hunger is prompted by internal signals, appetite is triggered by aspects of our environment. The most significant factors influencing our appetite are sensory data, social and cultural cues, and learning (**FIGURE 2.2**).

The Role of Sensory Data

Foods stimulate our five senses. Foods that are artfully prepared, arranged, or ornamented, with several different shapes and colors, appeal to our sense of sight. The aromas of foods such as freshly brewed coffee and baked goods can also be powerful stimulants. Much of our ability to taste foods actually comes from our sense of smell. This is why foods are not as appealing when we have a stuffy nose due to

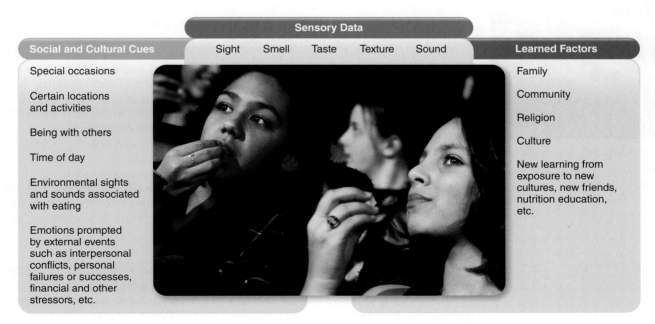

Social and Cultural Cues	Sensory Data					Learned Factors
	Sight	Smell	Taste	Texture	Sound	

Social and Cultural Cues:
- Special occasions
- Certain locations and activities
- Being with others
- Time of day
- Environmental sights and sounds associated with eating
- Emotions prompted by external events such as interpersonal conflicts, personal failures or successes, financial and other stressors, etc.

Learned Factors:
- Family
- Community
- Religion
- Culture
- New learning from exposure to new cultures, new friends, nutrition education, etc.

FIGURE 2.2 Appetite is a drive to consume specific foods, such as popcorn at the movies. It is aroused by social and cultural cues and sensory data and is influenced by learning.

a cold. Certain tastes, such as sweetness, are almost universally appealing, whereas others, such as the astringent taste of spinach and kale, are quite individual. Texture, or "mouth feel," is also important in food choices, as it stimulates nerve endings sensitive to touch in our mouth and on our tongue. Even our sense of hearing can be stimulated by foods, from the fizz of cola to the crunch of pretzels.

The Role of Social and Cultural Cues

In addition to sensory cues, our brain's association with certain social events, such as birthday parties and holiday gatherings, can stimulate our appetite. At these times, our culture gives us permission to eat more than usual or to eat "forbidden" foods. Even when we feel full, these cues can motivate us to accept a second helping.

For some people, being in a certain location, such as at a baseball game or a movie theater, can trigger appetite. Others may be triggered to eat when they engage in certain activities, such as watching television or studying. Many people feel an increase or a decrease in appetite according to whom they are with; for example, they may eat more when at home with family members and less when out on a date.

In some people, appetite masks an emotional response to an external event. For example, a person might experience a desire for food rather than a desire for emotional comfort after receiving a failing grade or arguing with a close friend. Many people crave food when they're frustrated, worried, or bored or when they're at a gathering where they feel anxious or awkward. Others subconsciously seek food as a "reward." For example, have you ever found yourself heading out for a burger and fries after handing in a term paper?

The Role of Learning

Pigs' feet, anyone? What about blood sausage, stewed octopus, or snakes? These are delicacies in various cultures. Would you eat grasshoppers? If you'd grown up in certain parts of Africa or Central America, you might. That's because your preference for particular foods is largely a learned response. The culture in which you are raised teaches you what plant and animal products are appropriate to eat. If your parents fed you cubes of plain tofu throughout your toddlerhood, then you are probably still eating tofu.

That said, early introduction to foods is not essential: we can learn to enjoy new foods at any point in our life. For instance, many immigrants adopt a diet typical of their new home, especially when their traditional foods are not readily available. This happens temporarily when we travel: the last time you were away from home, you probably sampled a variety of dishes that are not normally part of your diet.

Food preferences also change when people learn what foods are most healthful. Since the first day of your nutrition class, has your diet changed at all? Chances are, as you learn more about the health benefits of specific types of carbohydrates, fats, and proteins, you'll start incorporating more of these foods in your diet.

We can also "learn" to dislike foods we once enjoyed. For example, if we experience an episode of food poisoning after eating undercooked scrambled eggs, we might develop a strong distaste for all types of eggs. Many adults who become vegetarians do so after learning about the treatment of animals in slaughterhouses: they might have eaten meat daily when young but no longer have any appetite for it.

Now that you understand the differences between appetite and hunger, and the influence of learning on food choices, you might be curious to investigate your own reasons for eating what and when you do. If so, check out the self-assessment box *What About You?*

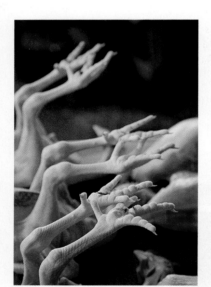

⬆ Our preference, or distaste, for certain foods is something we learn from our culture.

recap In contrast to hunger, appetite is a psychological desire to consume specific foods. It is triggered when external stimuli arouse our senses, and it often occurs in combination with social and cultural cues. Our preference for certain foods is largely learned from the culture in which we were raised, but our food choices can change with exposure to new foods or through new learning experiences.

WHAT ABOUT **YOU?**

Do You Eat in Response to External or Internal Cues?

Whether you're trying to lose or gain weight, or simply to eat more healthfully, you might find it intriguing to keep a log of the reasons behind your decisions about what, when, where, and why you eat. Are you eating in response to internal sensations telling you that your body needs food, or in response to your emotions, your situation, or a prescribed diet? Keeping a "cues" log for 1 full week would give you the most accurate picture of your eating habits, but even logging 2 days of meals and snacks should increase your cue awareness.

Each day, every time you eat a meal, snack, or beverage other than water, make a quick note of the following:

- *When you eat:* Many people eat at certain times (for example, 6 PM) whether they are hungry or not.
- *What you eat, and how much:* Do you choose a cup of yogurt and a 6 oz glass of orange juice or a candy bar and a 20 oz cola?
- *Where you eat:* home, watching television; on the subway; and so on.
- *With whom you eat:* Are you alone or with others? If with others, are they eating as well? Have they offered you food?
- *Your sensations—what you see, hear, or smell:* Are you eating because you just saw a TV commercial for pizza, smelled homemade cookies, or the like?
- *Your emotions:* Some people indulge in a "treat" when they feel happy. Others binge on carbs when they're anxious, depressed, bored, or frustrated. Still others refuse to eat as a way of denying feelings they don't want to identify and deal with.

- *Any dietary restrictions:* Are you choosing a particular food because it is allowed on your current diet plan? Or are you hungry for a meal but drinking a diet soda to stay within a certain allowance of Calories? Are you restricting yourself because you feel guilty about having eaten too much at another time?
- *Your physiologic hunger:* Finally, rate your hunger on a scale from 1 to 5 as follows:
  - 1 = you feel uncomfortably full or even stuffed
  - 2 = you feel satisfied but not uncomfortably full
  - 3 = neutral; you feel no discernible satiation or hunger
  - 4 = you feel hungry and want to eat
  - 5 = you feel strong physiologic sensations of hunger and need to eat.

After keeping a log for 2 or more days, you might become aware of patterns you'd like to change. For example, maybe you notice that you often eat when you are not actually hungry but are worried about homework or personal relationships. Or maybe you notice that you can't walk past the snack bar without going in. This self-awareness may prompt you to change those patterns. For instance, instead of stifling your worries with food, you could write down exactly what you are worried about, including steps you can take to address your concerns. And the next time you approach the snack bar, you could check with your gut: are you truly hungry? If so, then purchase a healthful snack, maybe a piece of fruit or a bag of peanuts. If you're not really hungry, then take a moment to acknowledge the strength of this visual cue—and then walk on by.

Are we really what we eat?

LO2 Identify the relationship between the foods we eat and the structures and functions of our cells.

You've no doubt heard the saying that "you are what you eat." But is this scientifically true? To answer that question, and to better understand how we digest and process foods, we'll need to look at how our body is organized.

Like all substances on Earth, our body is made up of *atoms*. Atoms are the smallest units of matter, and almost constantly bind to each other in nature to form groups called *molecules*. For example, a molecule of water is composed of two atoms of hydrogen and an atom of oxygen, which is abbreviated H_2O. Every bite of food we eat is composed of molecules. When we digest food, we break it down into molecules small enough for our body to easily use. The chemical reactions that join atoms and molecules into larger compounds, and break compounds apart into smaller molecules and atoms, are collectively called **metabolism**. Energy metabolism is the set of chemical reactions that break down and convert food into energy.

Cells are the smallest units of life. That is, cells can grow, reproduce themselves, take in nutrients, and excrete wastes. The human body is composed of more than 37 trillion cells that are continually being replaced.[2] To support the construction of new cells, we need a steady supply of nutrient molecules to serve as building blocks.

metabolism The chemical reactions occurring in the body in order to maintain life.

cells The smallest units of matter that exhibit the properties of living things, such as growth, reproduction, and the taking in of nutrients.

▶ FIGURE 2.3 Representative cell of the small intestine, showing the cell membrane, the cytoplasm, the nucleus, and several mitochondria.

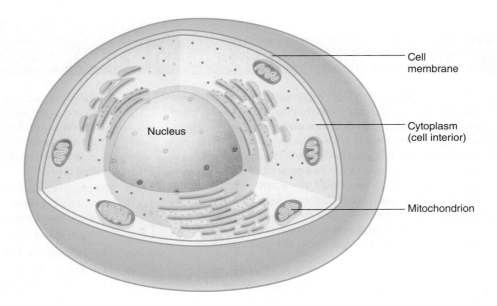

Cell membrane

Nucleus

Cytoplasm (cell interior)

Mitochondrion

Again, we get these from metabolizing the foods we eat. Nutrient molecules also provide the fuel and other chemicals that cells need to perform their functions.

Cells of a single type, such as muscle cells, join together to form tissues, which in turn make up organs. Organs are structures that perform a unique body function. The stomach, for example, is an organ that holds and partially digests a meal. Organs work together in systems that perform integrated functions. The gastrointestinal system is responsible for digesting food, absorbing nutrients, and excreting wastes. The stomach and several other organs work together to perform these functions, as we'll see shortly.

The contents of a cell are enclosed by a **cell membrane** (FIGURE 2.3). This thin, outer coat defines the cell's boundaries. Cell membranes are *semipermeable:* some molecules can easily flow through them, whereas others cannot. This quality enables the cell membrane to act as a gatekeeper, controlling what goes into and out of the cell.

Inside the cell is a fluid called **cytoplasm**. Floating in the cytoplasm are many tiny structures that accomplish some surprisingly sophisticated functions. These include:

- *Mitochondria:* Cells that have high energy needs, such as muscle cells, contain lots of mitochondria. You can think of mitochondria as a cell's "powerhouse," because they convert food molecules into energy.
- *A nucleus:* Nearly all body cells have a nucleus, where genetic information, in the form of DNA (deoxyribonucleic acid), is located. Segments of DNA, called genes, contain the instructions the cell uses to assemble structural proteins—components of the body's tissues—and functional proteins involved in everything from immunity to digestion.

Reflecting our growing understanding of the importance of genetics in human health, a new field of research called *nutrigenomics* is seeking to uncover links between our genes, our environment, and our diet. Some even claim that our diet should be personalized to our unique DNA! But is the idea of personalized nutrition just wishful thinking? Find out in the ***Nutrition Myth or Fact?*** feature box.

cell membrane The boundary of an animal cell that separates its internal cytoplasm, nucleus, and other structures from the external environment.

cytoplasm The fluid within an animal cell, enclosed by the cell membrane.

recap Atoms, the smallest units of matter, group together to form molecules. Digestion breaks down food into molecules small enough to be easily used by cells. The smallest units of life, cells are encased in a cell membrane, which acts as a gatekeeper. Cells of the same type join together to make tissues. Different tissues combine to form different kinds of organs. Body systems, such as the gastrointestinal system, depend on many different organs to carry out their functions.

nutrition myth or fact?

Nutrigenomics: Personalized Nutrition or Pie in the Sky?

Imagine a patient with high blood pressure visiting his physician. The physician consults the genetic information in the patient's electronic medical record, then hands the patient a prescription: *2 servings of citrus fruits and 2 servings of onions, garlic, leeks, or shallots daily*. The patient accepts the prescription gratefully, assuring his physician as he says goodbye, "I'll stop at the market on my way home!"

This scenario might sound unreal, but as researchers explore the link between genes and diet, could such prescriptions become routine? Let's examine the evidence.

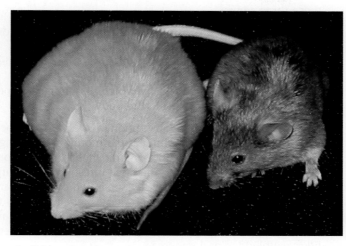

⬥ With only a change in diet, inbred agouti mice (left) gave birth to young mice (right) that differed not only in their appearance but also in their susceptibility to disease.

Look at the photo on this page of the obese mother mouse, on the left, and her offspring, on the right. The offspring is obviously brown and of normal weight, but what you can't see is that it did not inherit its mother's susceptibility to chronic disease. What caused these dramatic differences? The answer is diet! Before allowing the mother mouse to breed, researchers fed her a diet that was high in a compound they suspected would affect the gene responsible for her fur color and poor health. Sure enough, this dietary compound attached to the gene and, in essence, turned it off. When the mother conceived, her offspring still carried the gene on their DNA, but their cells no longer used the gene to make proteins. So the traits that were linked to the gene did not appear. The mice were born brown and healthy. This study was one of the first in the emerging science of *nutrigenomics*, which studies the interactions between genes, the environment, and nutrition.

Scientists have long recognized that diet can contribute to disease, but what has not been understood before is *how*. A key theory behind nutrigenomics is that foods can act like a "switch" in body cells, turning genes on or off. When a gene is activated, it instructs the cell to assemble a protein that will show up as a physical characteristic or function, such as the ability to store fat. When a gene is switched off, the cell will not create that protein, and the organism's form or function will differ. In addition, as we saw in the study of mice, switching a gene on or off can cause changes in the individual's offspring. Not only foods, but alcohol, tobacco, exercise, and other factors are thought to affect gene activation.

Nutrigenomics is an intriguing theory—and many studies suggest that the theory has merit. For example, it has long been noted that people following the same diet and exercise program will lose very different amounts of weight. The varying results may reflect how the foods in the diet affect the study participants' genes. Scientists also point to evidence from population studies of cardiovascular disease risk. Moderate alcohol intake reduces the risk in people with a particular set of genes, but it doesn't benefit people who don't have these genes.[1] Similarly, when different ethnic groups are exposed to a high-fat Western diet, the percentage of cardiovascular disease increases in some populations significantly more than in others.[1] Still other population studies suggest that when pregnant women experience either a famine or a food surplus during critical periods of fetal development, their offspring are more likely to develop obesity-related diseases.[2]

One promise of nutrigenomics is that a change in diet can help people reduce their risk of developing certain diseases and possibly even treat existing diseases. For example, researchers are now studying how chemical components of certain vegetables may regulate genes that inhibit the spread of cancer.[3] In the future, genetic analysis might guide your healthcare provider in creating a diet tailored to your specific genetic makeup. By identifying both foods to eat and foods to avoid, this personalized diet would help you to turn on genes that could be beneficial to you and turn off genes that could be harmful.

If the promises of nutrigenomics strike you as pie in the sky, you're not alone. Many researchers caution that dietary "prescriptions" to prevent or treat chronic diseases are unrealistic for several reasons. First, our DNA contains about 25,000 genes, and we don't yet know the function of many thousands of them. Second, our thousands of genes affect our metabolism in ways that are almost unimaginably complex. Third, other factors such as age, gender, and lifestyle also affect how foods interact with genetic pathways. In short, the number of variables that have to be considered is staggering.[4] This means that nutrigenomics is—for now—more dream than reality.

digestion The process by which foods are broken down into their component molecules, both mechanically and chemically.

absorption The physiologic process by which molecules of food are taken from the GI tract into the body.

elimination The process by which the undigested portions of food and waste products are removed from the body.

gastrointestinal (GI) tract A long, muscular tube consisting of several organs: the mouth, esophagus, stomach, small intestine, and large intestine.

sphincters Tight rings of muscle separating organs of the GI tract; they open in response to nerve signals, indicating that food is ready to pass into the next section.

accessory organs Organs that assist in digestion but are not anatomically part of the GI tract; they include the salivary glands, liver, gallbladder, and pancreas.

saliva A mixture of water, mucus, enzymes, and other chemicals that moistens the mouth and food, binds food particles together, and begins the digestion of carbohydrates.

salivary glands A group of glands that together act as an accessory organ of digestion, releasing saliva continually as well as in response to the thought, sight, smell, or presence of food.

enzymes Chemicals, usually proteins, that act on other chemicals to speed up body processes.

What happens to the food we eat?

When we eat, the food is digested, then the useful nutrients are absorbed, and finally the waste products are eliminated. Here are some useful definitions for these three steps:

- **Digestion** is the process by which foods are broken down into their component molecules, either mechanically or chemically.
- **Absorption** is the process of taking the products of digestion through the wall of the intestine.
- **Elimination** is the process by which the undigested portions of food and waste products are removed from the body.

The processes of digestion, absorption, and elimination occur within the **gastrointestinal (GI) tract**, a long tube beginning at the mouth and ending at the anus (**FIGURE 2.4**). It is composed of several distinct organs, including the mouth, the esophagus, the stomach, the small intestine, and the large intestine. These organs work together to process foods but are kept somewhat separated by muscular **sphincters**, which are tight rings of muscle that open when a nerve signal indicates that food is ready to pass into the next section. Four other organs assist digestion but are not part of the gastrointestinal tract. These are called the **accessory organs**. They include the salivary glands, liver, gallbladder, and pancreas.

The nerves serving the GI tract are known as *enteric nerves* (*entero-* is a prefix referring to the intestine). Enteric nerves can often work independently; in other words, they don't need to relay signals produced within the GI tract to the brain for interpretation or assistance. One of their most important functions is to regulate the secretion of digestive juices, mucus, and water by glands located all along the GI tract. These substances promote gastrointestinal functioning, as described next.

Imagine that you eat a turkey sandwich for lunch today. It contains two slices of bread spread with mayonnaise, some turkey, two lettuce leaves, and a slice of tomato. Let's travel along with the sandwich and see what changes it undergoes within your GI tract.

Digestion Begins in the Mouth

Believe it or not, your body starts preparing to digest food even before you take your first bite. In response to the sight, smell, or thought of food, the nervous system stimulates the release of digestive juices that help prepare the GI tract for the breakdown of food. Sometimes we even experience some involuntary movement of the GI tract, commonly called "hunger pangs."

Now it's time to take that first bite and chew. Chewing is very important because it moistens the food and mechanically breaks it down into pieces small enough to swallow (**FIGURE 2.5**). The tough lettuce fibers and tomato seeds are also broken open. Thus, chewing initiates the mechanical digestion of food.

As our teeth cut and grind the different foods in the sandwich, more surface area is exposed to the digestive juices in our mouth. The most important of these is **saliva**, a fluid we secrete from **salivary glands** found under and behind the tongue and beneath the jaw. Saliva moistens food with mucus and water and contains antibiotics that protect the body from germs entering the mouth and help keep the oral cavity free from infection. Another component of saliva is *salivary amylase*, a chemical that begins to break apart the carbohydrate molecules in food.

Salivary amylase is the first of many *enzymes* that assist the body in digesting and absorbing food. Because we will encounter many enzymes on our journey through the GI tract, let's discuss them briefly here. **Enzymes** are chemicals, usually proteins, that induce chemical changes in other substances to speed up body

The digestive system consists of the organs of the gastrointestinal (GI) tract and associated accessory organs. The processing of food in the GI tract involves ingestion, mechanical digestion, chemical digestion, propulsion, absorption, and elimination.

ORGANS OF THE GI TRACT

MOUTH

Ingestion Food enters the GI tract via the mouth.

Mechanical digestion Mastication tears, shreds, and mixes food with saliva.

Chemical digestion Salivary amylase begins carbohydrate breakdown.

PHARYNX AND ESOPHAGUS

Propulsion Swallowing and peristalsis move food from mouth to stomach.

STOMACH

Mechanical digestion Mixes and churns food with gastric juice into a liquid called chyme.

Chemical digestion Pepsin begins digestion of proteins, and gastric lipase begins to break lipids apart.

Absorption A few fat-soluble substances are absorbed through the stomach wall.

SMALL INTESTINE

Mechanical Digestion and **Propulsion** Segmentation mixes chyme with digestive juices; peristaltic waves move it along tract.

Chemical digestion Digestive enzymes from pancreas and brush border digest most classes of nutrients.

Absorption Nutrients are absorbed into blood and lymph through enterocytes.

LARGE INTESTINE

Chemical digestion Some remaining food residues are digested by bacteria.

Absorption Reabsorbs salts, water, and vitamins.

Propulsion Compacts waste into feces and propels it toward the rectum.

RECTUM

Elimination Temporarily stores feces before voluntary release through the anus.

ACCESSORY ORGANS

SALIVARY GLANDS

Produce saliva, a mixture of water, mucus, enzymes, and other chemicals.

LIVER

Produces bile to emulsify fats.

GALLBLADDER

Stores bile before release into the small intestine through the bile duct.

PANCREAS

Produces digestive enzymes and bicarbonate, which are released into the small intestine via the pancreatic duct.

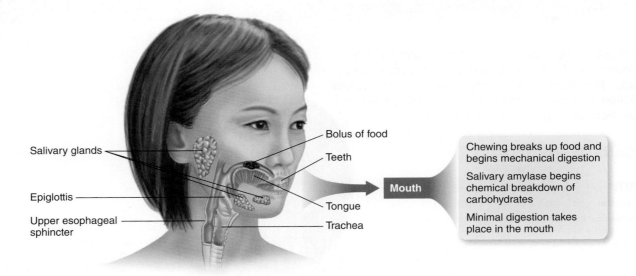

Salivary glands

Bolus of food

Teeth

Epiglottis

Tongue

Upper esophageal
sphincter

Trachea

Mouth

Chewing breaks up food and
begins mechanical digestion

Salivary amylase begins
chemical breakdown of
carbohydrates

Minimal digestion takes
place in the mouth

◆ **FIGURE 2.5** Where your food is now: the mouth. Chewing moistens food and mechanically breaks it down into pieces small enough to swallow, while salivary amylase and lingual lipase begin chemical digestion.

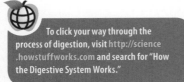

To click your way through the process of digestion, visit http://science .howstuffworks.com and search for "How the Digestive System Works."

processes (**FIGURE 2.6**). Imagine them as facilitators: a chemical reaction that might take hours to occur independently can happen in seconds with the help of one or more enzymes. Also, because enzymes are not changed by the processes they assist, they can be used over and over again. Digestion—and other metabolic functions— couldn't happen without enzymes. By the way, enzyme names typically end in *ase* (as in amylase), so they'll be easy for you to recognize as we discuss the digestive process. A few of the many digestive enzymes active in the GI tract are identified in **TABLE 2.1**.

In reality, very little chemical digestion occurs in the mouth. We don't hold food in our mouth for long, and few of the enzymes needed to break down food are present. Lingual lipase secreted by tongue cells (*lingua-* means tongue) mixes with saliva and begins to digest fats. Also, as noted earlier, salivary amylase begins the digestion of carbohydrates; however, this ends when food reaches the stomach, because the acidic environment of the stomach destroys this enzyme.

▶ **FIGURE 2.6** Enzymes speed up the body's chemical reactions, including many reactions essential to the digestion and absorption of food. Here, an enzyme joins two small compounds to create a larger compound. Notice that the enzyme itself is not changed in the process.

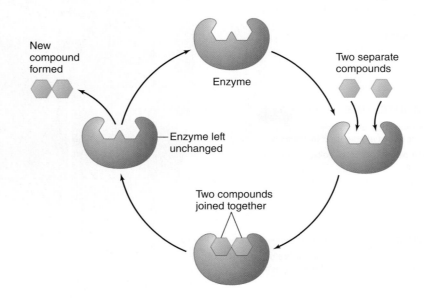

New
compound
formed

Enzyme

Two separate
compounds

Enzyme left
unchanged

Two compounds
joined together

TABLE 2.1 **Some Digestive Enzymes and Their Actions**

Site of Production	Enzyme	Site of Action	Primary Action
Mouth	Salivary amylase	Mouth	Digests carbohydrates
	Lingual lipase		Digests lipids
Stomach	Pepsin	Stomach	Digests proteins
	Gastric lipase		Digests lipids
Pancreas	Various proteases	Small intestine	Digest proteins
	Pancreatic lipase		Digests lipids
	Pancreatic amylase		Digests carbohydrates
Small intestine	Variety of peptidases	Small intestine	Digest proteins
	Lipase		Digests lipids
	Sucrase		Digests sucrose
	Maltase		Digests maltose
	Lactase		Digests lactose

The Esophagus Transports Food into the Stomach

Now that our sandwich is soft and moist, it's time to swallow (**FIGURE 2.7**). Most of us take swallowing for granted, but it's a very complex process. As the bite of sandwich moves to the *pharynx*, the space at the very back of the mouth, nerve cells signal the brain to raise the soft palate. This temporarily closes the openings to the nasal passages, preventing aspiration of food or liquid into the sinuses. The brain also receives a signal to close off the *epiglottis*, a tiny flap of tissue that is like a trapdoor covering the entrance to the trachea ("windpipe"). The epiglottis is normally open, allowing us to breathe freely. When it closes during swallowing, food and liquid cannot enter the trachea. Sometimes this protective mechanism goes awry—for instance, when we try to eat and talk at the same time and food or liquid "goes down the wrong way." When this happens, we experience the sensation of choking, and we cough until the offending food or liquid is expelled.

As the trachea closes, the *upper esophageal sphincter* opens. This allows food to pass from the pharynx into the **esophagus**, the muscular tube that propels food toward

esophagus Muscular tube of the GI tract connecting the back of the mouth to the stomach.

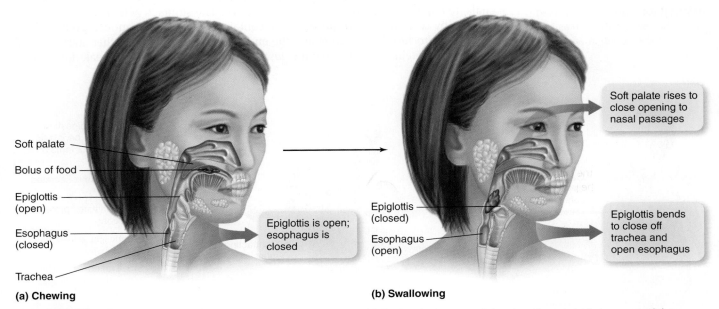

Soft palate
Bolus of food
Epiglottis (open)
Esophagus (closed)
Trachea

Epiglottis is open; esophagus is closed

(a) Chewing

Soft palate rises to close opening to nasal passages

Epiglottis (closed)
Esophagus (open)

Epiglottis bends to close off trachea and open esophagus

(b) Swallowing

⬆ **FIGURE 2.7** Chewing and swallowing are complex processes. **(a)** During the process of chewing, the epiglottis is open and the esophagus is closed so that we can continue to breathe as we chew. **(b)** During swallowing, the epiglottis closes so that food does not enter the trachea and obstruct our breathing. Also, the soft palate rises to seal off our nasal passages to prevent aspiration of food or liquid into the sinuses.

▶ **FIGURE 2.8**
Where your food is now: the esophagus. Peristalsis, the rhythmic contraction and relaxation of muscles in the esophagus, propels food toward the stomach. Peristalsis occurs throughout the GI tract.

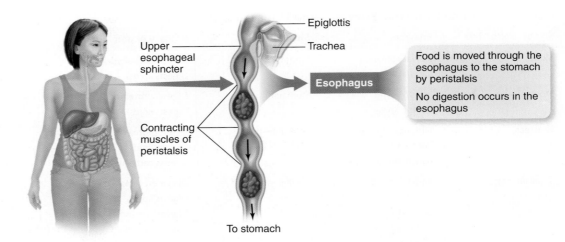

the stomach (**FIGURE 2.8**). It does this by contracting two sets of muscles: inner sheets of circular muscle squeeze the food, while outer sheets of longitudinal muscle push food along. Together, these rhythmic waves of squeezing and pushing are called **peristalsis**. We will see shortly that peristalsis occurs throughout the GI tract.

Gravity also helps food move down the esophagus. Together, peristalsis and gravity can transport a bite of food from the mouth to the opening of the stomach in 5 to 8 seconds. At the end of the esophagus is another sphincter muscle, the *gastroesophageal sphincter* (*gastro-* indicates the stomach; also called the *lower esophageal sphincter*), that is normally tightly closed. When food reaches the end of the esophagus, this sphincter relaxes to allow it to pass into the stomach. In some people, this sphincter is continually somewhat relaxed. Later in the chapter, we'll discuss this disorder and why it causes the sensation of heartburn.

The Stomach Mixes, Digests, and Stores Food

The J-shaped **stomach** is a saclike organ that can expand in some people to hold several cups of food (**FIGURE 2.9**). Before any food reaches the stomach, the brain sends signals, telling it to be ready for the food to arrive. The stomach gets ready for your sandwich by secreting **gastric juice**, which contains several important compounds, including *hydrochloric acid (HCl)* and the enzyme *pepsin*, which together start to break down proteins, and the enzyme *gastric lipase*, which begins to break down fats.

peristalsis Waves of squeezing and pushing contractions that move food in one direction through the length of the GI tract.

stomach A J-shaped organ in which food is partially digested, churned, and stored until released into the small intestine.

gastric juice Acidic liquid secreted within the stomach that contains hydrochloric acid, pepsin, and other chemicals.

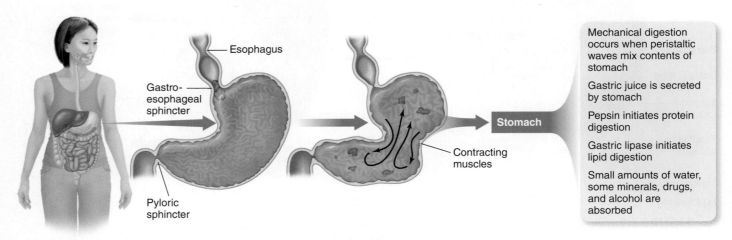

▲ **FIGURE 2.9** Where your food is now: the stomach. In the stomach, the protein and fat in your sandwich begin to be digested. Your meal is churned into chyme and stored until released into the small intestine.

The stomach also secretes mucus, which protects its lining from being digested by the hydrochloric acid and pepsin.

In addition to chemical digestion, the stomach performs mechanical digestion, mixing and churning the food until it becomes a liquid called **chyme**. Enzymes can access this liquid chyme more easily than solid food.

Although most absorption occurs in the small intestine, the stomach lining does begin absorbing a few substances. These include water, some minerals and some fats, and certain drugs, including aspirin and alcohol.

Another of your stomach's jobs is to store your sandwich until the next part of the digestive tract, the small intestine, is ready for it. Remember that the stomach can hold several cups of food. This amount would overwhelm the small intestine if it were released all at once. Instead, food stays in your stomach about 2 hours before it is released a little at a time, as chyme, into the small intestine. The *pyloric sphincter* regulates this release.

recap Chewing initiates mechanical and chemical digestion. During swallowing, our nasal passages close and the epiglottis covers the trachea. The esophagus is a muscular tube that transports food from the mouth to the stomach via rhythmic waves called peristalsis. The stomach secretes gastric juice, which begins the breakdown of proteins and fats, as well as mucus to protect its lining. It mixes food into chyme, which is released into the small intestine through the pyloric sphincter.

Most Digestion and Absorption Occurs in the Small Intestine

The **small intestine** is the longest portion of the GI tract, accounting for about two-thirds of its length. However, at only an inch in diameter, it is comparatively narrow.

The small intestine is composed of three sections **(FIGURE 2.10)**:

- The first section is the *duodenum*. It is connected via the pyloric sphincter to the stomach.
- The *jejunum* is the middle portion of the small intestine.
- The *ileum* is the last portion. It is connected to the large intestine at another sphincter, called the *ileocecal valve*.

chyme Semifluid mass consisting of partially digested food, water, and gastric juice.

small intestine The largest portion of the GI tract, in which most digestion and absorption take place.

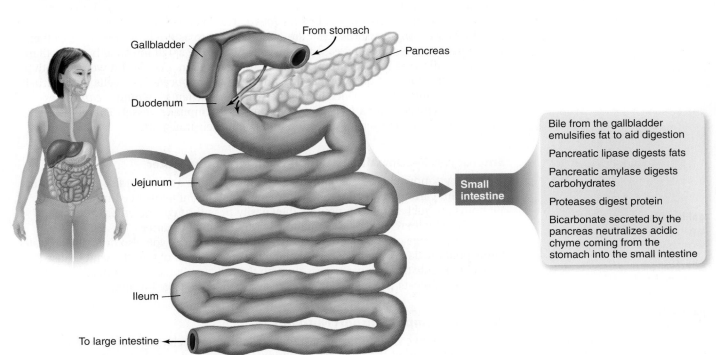

▲ **FIGURE 2.10**   Where your food is now: the small intestine. Here, most of the digestion and absorption of the nutrients in your sandwich take place.

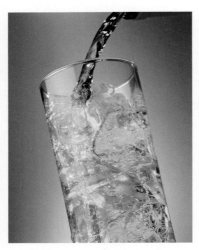

← Water is readily absorbed along the entire length of the GI tract, especially in the large intestine.

Most digestion and absorption takes place in the small intestine. Here, food is broken down into its smallest components, molecules that the body can then absorb into its internal environment. As we explore these processes of digestion and absorption, notice the roles played by three accessory organs—the gallbladder, pancreas, and liver—and the variety of enzymes involved.

The Gallbladder and Pancreas Aid in Digestion

As the fat from the turkey and mayonnaise enters the small intestine, the **gallbladder** contracts. An accessory organ, the gallbladder is located beneath the liver (see Figures 2.4 and 2.10) and stores a greenish fluid produced by the liver called **bile**. Contraction of the gallbladder sends bile into the duodenum via the bile duct. Bile then *emulsifies* the fat—that is, it breaks it up into smaller particles that are more accessible to digestive enzymes. If you've ever noticed how a drop of liquid dish soap breaks up a film of fat floating at the top of a basin of greasy dishes, you understand the function of bile.

The **pancreas**, an accessory organ located behind the stomach, manufactures, holds, and releases digestive enzymes into the duodenum via the pancreatic duct. These enzymes include pancreatic amylase, which breaks down carbohydrates; pancreatic lipase, which breaks down fats; and a variety of proteases, which break down proteins (see Table 2.1). The pancreas is also responsible for manufacturing hormones that are important in the conversion of food into energy. Finally, the pancreas secretes bicarbonate—a base—into the duodenum, where it neutralizes the acidity of the chyme entering from the stomach.

Now the macronutrients in your sandwich have been processed into a liquid that contains molecules small enough for absorption. This molecular "soup" continues to move along the small intestine via peristalsis, encountering the absorptive cells of the intestinal lining all along the way.

A Specialized Lining Enables the Small Intestine to Absorb Food

The lining of the small intestine is especially well suited for absorption. If you looked at it under a microscope, you would notice that it is heavily folded **(FIGURE 2.11)**. Within these circular folds are small, finger like projections called *villi*, whose constant movement helps them encounter and trap nutrient molecules. Covering the villi are even tinier, hairlike structures called *microvilli*. The microvilli form a surface somewhat like the bristles on a hairbrush and are often referred to as the *brush border*. Together, these absorptive features increase the surface area of the small intestine by more than 600 times, allowing it to absorb many more nutrients than it could if it were smooth.

Nutrients enter the body by passing through the *enterocytes*, the cells of the brush border (*-cyte* means cell). Once inside the villi, the nutrients encounter *capillaries* (tiny blood vessels) and a *lacteal*, which is a small lymphatic vessel. These vessels soak up the final products of digestion and begin their transport.

Enterocytes Readily Absorb Vitamins, Minerals, and Water

The turkey sandwich you ate contained several vitamins and minerals in addition to the protein, carbohydrate, and fat. These vitamins and minerals need no digestion. Vitamins are such small compounds they easily pass through the enterocytes, as do minerals, which are already the smallest possible units of matter.

Finally, a large component of food is water, and, of course, you also drink lots of water throughout the day. Water is absorbed along the entire length of the GI tract, because it is a small molecule that can easily pass through the cell membrane. However, as we will see shortly, a significant percentage of water is absorbed in the large intestine.

Blood and Lymph Transport Nutrients

Our body has two main fluids that transport nutrients (including water) and waste products throughout the body. These fluids are blood and lymph. Blood travels through the cardiovascular system, and lymph travels through the lymphatic system **(FIGURE 2.12)**.

gallbladder A sac like accessory organ of digestion that stores bile and secretes it into the small intestine.

bile Fluid produced by the liver and stored in the gallbladder that emulsifies fats in the small intestine.

pancreas Accessory organ of digestion that secretes digestive enzymes into the small intestine via the pancreatic duct; certain pancreatic cells secrete the hormones insulin and glucagon into the bloodstream.

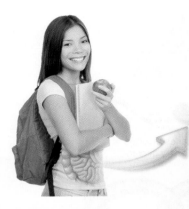

The small intestine is highly adapted for absorbing nutrients. Its length—about 20 feet—provides a huge surface area, and its wall has three structural features—circular folds, villi, and microvilli—that increase its surface area by a factor of more than 600.

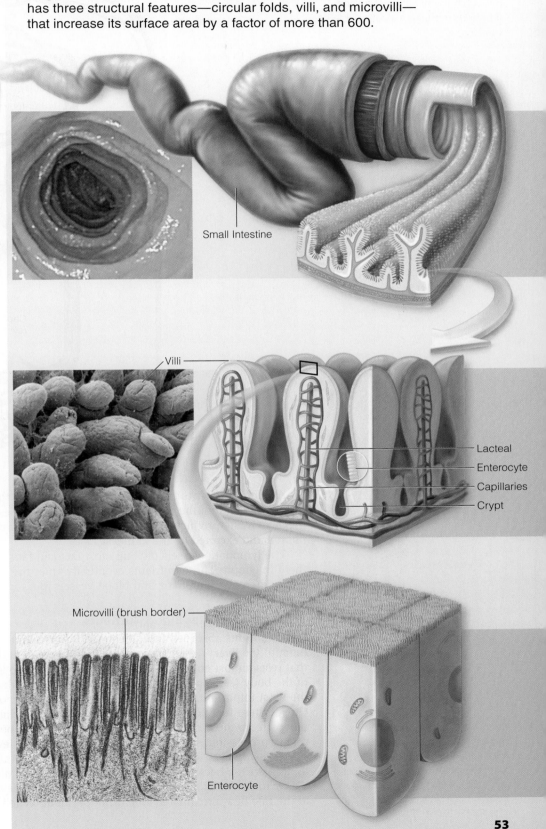

CIRCULAR FOLDS
The lining of the small intestine is heavily folded, resulting in increased surface area for the absorption of nutrients.

Small Intestine

VILLI
The folds are covered with villi, thousands of finger like projections that increase the surface area even further. Each villus contains capillaries and a lacteal for picking up nutrients absorbed through the enterocytes and transporting them throughout the body.

Villi

Lacteal

Enterocyte

Capillaries

Crypt

Microvilli (brush border)

MICROVILLI
The cells on the surface of the villi, enterocytes, end in hairlike projections called microvilli that together form the brush border through which nutrients are absorbed.

Enterocyte

▶ **FIGURE 2.12** Blood travels through the cardiovascular system to transport nutrients and fluids and pick up waste products. Lymph travels through the lymphatic system and transports most fats and fat-soluble vitamins.

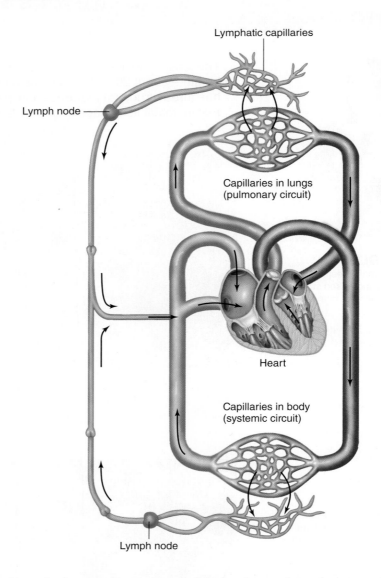

Lymphatic capillaries

Lymph node

Capillaries in lungs (pulmonary circuit)

Heart

Capillaries in body (systemic circuit)

Lymph node

As blood travels through the GI tract, it picks up the nutrients that were absorbed through the villi of the small intestine and then carries them to the liver for processing. The waste products picked up by the blood as it circulates around the body are filtered and excreted by the kidneys.

The lymphatic vessels pick up most fats and fat-soluble vitamins and transport them in lymph. These nutrients eventually enter the bloodstream at an area near the heart where the lymphatic and blood vessels join together.

The Liver Regulates Blood Nutrients

Most nutrients absorbed from the small intestine enter the *portal vein,* which carries them to the **liver**. Another accessory digestive organ, the liver is a triangular wedge that rests almost entirely within the protection of the lower rib cage, on the right side of the body (see Figure 2.4). The liver is the largest digestive organ; it is also one of the most important organs in the body, performing more than 500 discrete functions. One of these functions is to receive the products of digestion and then release into the bloodstream those nutrients needed throughout the body. The liver also plays a major role in processing, storing, and regulating the blood levels of the energy nutrients.

Have you ever wondered why people who abuse alcohol are at risk for damaging their liver? It's because another of its functions is to filter the blood, removing potential toxins, such as alcohol and other drugs. The liver can filter alcohol from the blood at the rate of approximately one drink per hour. When someone exceeds this rate, the

liver The largest accessory organ of digestion and one of the most important organs of the body. Its functions include production of bile and processing of nutrient-rich blood from the small intestine.

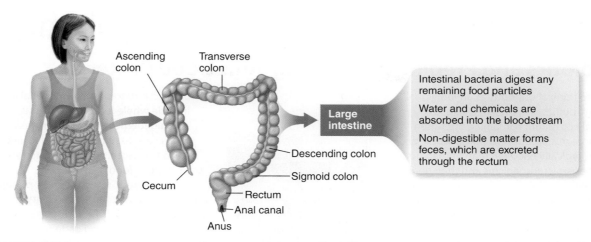

Intestinal bacteria digest any remaining food particles

Water and chemicals are absorbed into the bloodstream

Non-digestible matter forms feces, which are excreted through the rectum

◆ **FIGURE 2.13** Where your food is now: the large intestine. Most water absorption occurs here, as does the formation of food wastes into feces. Peristalsis propels the feces to the body exterior.

liver becomes overwhelmed by the excessive alcohol, which damages its cells. With chronic alcohol abuse, scar tissue forms. The scar tissue blocks the free flow of blood through the liver, so that any further toxins accumulate in the blood. This can lead to confusion, coma, and even death.

Another important job of the liver is to synthesize many of the chemicals the body uses in carrying out digestion. For example, the liver synthesizes bile, which, as we just discussed, is then stored in the gallbladder until needed to emulsify fats.

The Large Intestine Stores Food Waste Until It Is Excreted

The **large intestine** is a thick, tubelike structure that frames the small intestine on three and a half sides (**FIGURE 2.13**). It begins with a sack of tissue called the *cecum*. From the cecum, it continues up the right side of the abdomen as the *ascending colon*. The *transverse colon* runs across the top of the small intestine, and then the *descending colon* comes down on the left side of the abdomen. The *sigmoid colon* is the last segment of the colon. It extends from the bottom left corner to the *rectum*. The rectum ends in the *anal canal*, which is just over an inch long.

What has happened to your turkey sandwich? When any undigested and unabsorbed food components and water in the chyme finally reach the large intestine, they mix with intestinal bacteria. These "probiotic" (life-promoting) bacteria are normal and helpful residents, digesting any remaining particles left from your sandwich, manufacturing certain vitamins, and performing other beneficial functions. In fact, the probiotic bacteria living in the large intestine are so helpful that, as discussed in the *Highlight* feature box, many people consume them deliberately!

No other digestion occurs in the large intestine. Its main functions are to store the chyme for 12 to 24 hours and during that time to absorb chemicals and water from it, leaving a semisolid mass called *feces*. Weak waves of peristalsis move the feces through the colon, except for one or more stronger waves each day that force the feces more powerfully toward the rectum for elimination.

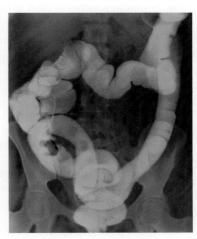

◆ The large intestine is a thick, tubelike structure that stores the undigested mass leaving the small intestine and absorbs much of the remaining water, as well as other nutrients.

recap Most digestion and absorption occurs in the small intestine with the help of bile, which emulsifies fats, and pancreatic enzymes that break down carbohydrates, fats, and proteins. The lining of the small intestine contains villi and microvilli that trap and absorb nutrients. The liver processes nutrients absorbed from the small intestine. Bacteria in the large intestine assist with digestion of any remaining digestible food products. The large intestine stores chyme, from which it absorbs water and any other remaining nutrients, leaving a semisolid mass, called feces, which is then eliminated from the body.

large intestine Final organ of the GI tract consisting of the cecum, colon, rectum, and anal canal and in which most water is absorbed and feces are formed.

highlight

Probiotics and Prebiotics: Boosting Your Good Bacteria

We like to think of our body as an individual organism, but it's not. Each of us is a lush microbial ecosystem containing about ten times more *microorganisms* (microscopic organisms, typically bacteria) than human body cells.[5] These microorganisms and their genes interact with our human cells and genes in a dizzying number of ways that affect our health. Although microorganisms live on our skin, in our urinary tract, and elsewhere in our body, here we'll focus on the probiotic bacteria in our GI tract.

Researchers have identified many ways in which probiotic bacteria benefit human health. For example, genes carried by these bacteria enable humans to digest foods and absorb nutrients that otherwise would be unavailable to us.[5] It seems likely that these bacterial genes complement the functions of human genes required for healthy digestion.[6] Moreover, probiotic bacteria directly:[7,8]

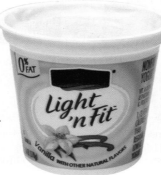

⬆ Probiotics can be found in yogurt and other fermented milk products.

- Manufacture chemicals (called enzymes) that help us digest our food and absorb nutrients from food
- Supply key nutrients used to replace worn-out components of the GI tract
- Produce certain essential vitamins
- Degrade potential carcinogens (cancer-causing agents) in foods
- Oppose excessive inflammation and thereby protect against infectious diarrhea, inflammatory bowel disorders, asthma, and allergies

Furthermore, some studies suggest a link between depletion of our probiotic bacteria and the development of obesity as well as type 2 diabetes.[8,9] And recent research suggests that a healthy level of probiotic bacteria, by regulating the inflammatory response, can even reduce stress and improve mood.[10]

Given this research, you're probably wondering how to maintain a large and healthy population of probiotic bacteria in your GI tract. The answer is—eat them! Probiotic foods like yogurt contain billions per serving. These foods are one type of *functional foods*, defined as components of the usual diet that may have biologically active ingredients with the potential to provide health benefits beyond basic nutrition.[11]

Also called *nutraceuticals*, functional foods include whole foods such as nuts, oats, and blueberries, as well as processed foods such as juices with added calcium, breads and cereals enriched with folate, and probiotic foods.

In the United States, the most popular probiotic foods are fermented dairy products such as regular and "Greek" yogurts, a creamy beverage called *kefir*, and certain fermented, soft cheeses such as Gouda. Nondairy probiotic foods include miso soup, sourdough bread, some types of sauerkraut, and fermented soybean cakes called *tempeh*. Probiotics are also sold in supplement form.

When a person consumes probiotics, the bacteria adhere to the intestinal wall, but survive for only a few days. This means that probiotic foods and supplements should be consumed daily to be most effective. They must also be properly stored and consumed within a relatively brief period of time to confer maximal benefit. In general, refrigerated foods containing probiotics have a shelf life of 3 to 6 weeks, whereas refrigerated supplements keep about 12 months. However, because the probiotic content of foods is much more stable than that of supplements, yogurt and other probiotic foods may be a better health bet.

One way to keep your body's population of probiotic microorganisms thriving is to feed them! That's where *prebiotics* come in. These are nondigestible substances, typically carbohydrates, that stimulate the growth and/or activity of probiotic bacteria.[11] An example is inulin, a carbohydrate found in a few fruits, garlic, onions, certain green vegetables, some tubers, and some grains. Like other prebiotics, inulin travels through the GI tract without being digested or absorbed until it reaches the colon, where it nourishes the bacteria living there.

In addition to whole prebiotic foods, many processed foods claim to be prebiotics. For example, inulin is added to certain brands of yogurt, milk, and cottage cheese, some fruit juices, cookies, and fiber bars and supplements. Watch out, though, that your desire to feed your microbes doesn't cause you to overindulge. Products touted as prebiotics may have just as many Calories as regular versions of the same foods.

What disorders are related to digestion, absorption, and elimination?

LO7 Discuss the causes, symptoms, and treatment of gastroesophageal reflux disease and peptic ulcers.

LO8 Distinguish between food intolerance and food allergy, and between celiac disease and non-celiac gluten sensitivity.

LO9 Compare and contrast diarrhea, constipation, and irritable bowel syndrome.

Considering the complexity of digestion, absorption, and elimination, it's no wonder that sometimes things go wrong. Let's look at some GI tract disorders and what you can do if any of these problems affect you.

Belching and Flatulence Are Common

Many people complain of problems with belching and/or flatulence (passage of intestinal gas). The primary cause of belching is swallowed air. Eating too fast, wearing improperly fitting dentures, chewing gum, sucking on hard candies or a drinking straw, and gulping food or fluid can increase the risk for swallowing air. To prevent or reduce belching, avoid these behaviors.

Although many people find *flatus* (intestinal gas) uncomfortable and embarrassing, its presence in the GI tract is completely normal, as is its expulsion. Flatus is a mixture of many gases, including nitrogen, hydrogen, oxygen, methane, and carbon dioxide. Interestingly, all of these are odorless. It is only when flatus contains sulfur that it causes the embarrassing odor associated with flatulence.

Foods most commonly reported to cause flatus include those rich in fibers, starches, and sugars, such as dairy products, and beans and some other vegetables. The partially digested carbohydrates from these foods pass into the large intestine, where they are acted on by bacteria, producing gas. Other food products that may cause flatus, intestinal cramps, and diarrhea include products made with the fat substitute olestra, sugar alcohols, and quorn (a meat substitute made from fungus).

Since many of the foods that can cause flatus are healthful, it is important not to avoid them. Eating smaller portions can help reduce the amount of flatus produced and passed. In addition, some preventive products, such as Beano, can offer some relief. These over-the-counter supplements contain alpha-galactosidase, an enzyme that digests the complex sugars in gas-producing foods. Although flatus is generally normal, some people have malabsorption diseases that cause painful bloating and require medical treatment. Some of these disorders are described later in this section.

Gastroesophageal Reflux Is Backflow of Gastric Juice

We noted earlier that, even as you're chewing your first bite of food, your stomach is beginning to secrete gastric juice to prepare for digestion. As the gastroesophageal sphincter relaxes to permit food to enter the stomach, it's normal for a small amount of this gastric juice to flow "backward" into the lower esophagus for a moment. This phenomenon is technically known as gastroesophageal reflux, or GER.

However, in some people, peristalsis in the esophagus is weak, so food enters the stomach too slowly, or the gastroesophageal sphincter is overly relaxed and stays partially open. In either case, the result is that gastric juice isn't cleared from the lower esophagus quickly and completely (**FIGURE 2.14**).

Although the stomach is protected from the highly acidic gastric juice by a thick coat of mucus, the esophagus does not have this coating. Thus, the gastric juice burns it. When this happens, the person experiences a painful sensation in the region of the chest behind the sternum (breastbone). This symptom is commonly called *heartburn*. Many people take over-the-counter antacids to raise the pH of the gastric juice, thereby relieving the heartburn. A non-drug approach is to repeatedly swallow: this action causes any acid pooled in the esophagus to be swept down into the stomach, eventually relieving the symptoms.

▶ **FIGURE 2.14** The mechanism of heartburn and gastroesophageal reflux disease is the same: acidic gastric juice seeps backward through the gastroesophageal sphincter into the lower portion of the esophagus and pools there, burning its lining. The pain is felt behind the sternum (breastbone), over the heart.

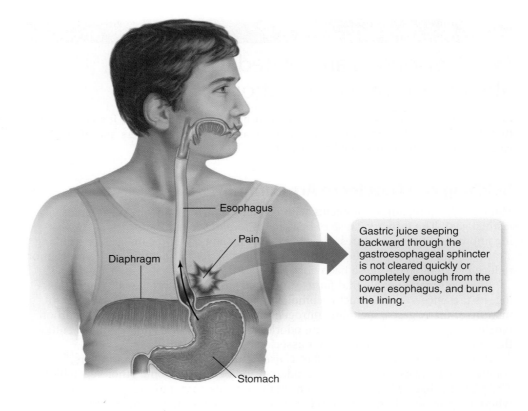

Esophagus

Pain

Diaphragm

Gastric juice seeping backward through the gastroesophageal sphincter is not cleared quickly or completely enough from the lower esophagus, and burns the lining.

Stomach

Search for "GERD and hernia" to access a video explaining the relationship between GERD and a hiatal hernia at www.mayoclinic.com.

Occasional heartburn is common and not a cause for concern; however, heartburn is also the most common symptom of **gastroesophageal reflux disease (GERD)**, a chronic disease in which episodes of reflux cause heartburn or other symptoms more than twice per week. These other symptoms include chest pain, trouble swallowing, burning in the mouth, the feeling that food is stuck in the throat, and hoarseness in the morning.[3]

The exact causes of GERD are unknown. However, a number of factors may contribute, including the following:[3]

- A hiatal hernia, which occurs when the upper part of the stomach lies above the diaphragm muscle. Normally, the horizontal diaphragm muscle separates the stomach from the chest cavity and helps keep gastric juice from seeping into the esophagus. Gastric juice can more easily enter the esophagus in people with a hiatal hernia.
- Overweight, obesity, or pregnancy.
- Cigarette smoking.
- Alcohol use.
- Certain foods such as citrus fruits, garlic, onions, spicy foods, and tomato-based foods.
- Large, high-fat meals.
- Lying down soon after a meal. This positions the body so it is easier for the gastric juice to back up into the esophagus.

One way to reduce the symptoms of GERD is to identify the types of foods or situations that trigger episodes, and then avoid them. Eat smaller meals and wait at least 3 hours before lying down. Sleep with the head of the bed raised 4 to 6 inches—for instance, by placing a wedge between the mattress and the box spring. People with GERD who smoke should stop, and, if they are overweight, they should lose weight. Taking an antacid before a meal can help prevent symptoms, and many other medications are now available.

gastroesophageal reflux disease (GERD) A chronic disease in which painful episodes of gastroesophageal reflux cause heartburn or other symptoms more than twice per week.

It is important to treat GERD because it can lead to bleeding, ulcers, and the development of scar tissue in the esophagus. Some people can develop a condition called Barrett's esophagus, which can lead to cancer. Asthma can also be aggravated or even caused by GERD.

An Ulcer Is an Area of Erosion in the GI Tract

A **peptic ulcer** is an area of the GI tract that has been eroded away by a combination of hydrochloric acid and the enzyme pepsin **(FIGURE 2.15)**. In almost all cases, it is located in the stomach area (*gastric ulcer*) or the part of the duodenum closest to the stomach (*duodenal ulcer*). It causes a burning pain in the abdominal area, typically 1 to 3 hours after eating a meal. In serious cases, eroded blood vessels bleed into the GI tract, causing vomiting of blood and/or blood in the stools, as well as anemia. If the ulcer entirely perforates the tract wall, stomach contents can leak into the abdominal cavity, causing a life-threatening infection called *peritonitis*.

For decades, physicians believed that experiencing high levels of stress, drinking alcohol, and eating spicy foods were the primary factors responsible for ulcers. But in 1982, Australian gastroenterologists Robin Warren and Barry Marshall detected the same species of bacterium, *Helicobacter pylori* (*H. pylori*), in the majority of their ulcer patients' stomachs. Treatment with an antibiotic effective against the bacterium cured the ulcers. It is now known that *H. pylori* plays a key role in the development of most peptic ulcers. The hydrochloric acid in gastric juice kills most bacteria, but *H. pylori* is unusual in that it thrives in acidic environments. Intriguingly, many people who have this bacterium in their stomach do not develop ulcers. The reason for this is not known.[4]

Prevention of infection with *H. pylori,* as with any infectious microorganism, includes regular hand washing and safe food-handling practices. Because of the role of *H. pylori* in ulcer development, treatment usually involves antibiotics and acid-suppressing medications. Special diets and stress-reduction techniques are no longer typically recommended, because they do not reduce acid secretion. However, people with ulcers should avoid specific foods they identify as causing them discomfort.

Although most peptic ulcers are caused by *H. pylori* infection, some are caused by prolonged use of nonsteroidal anti-inflammatory drugs (NSAIDs); these drugs include

Watch a video on peptic ulcers by entering "ulcers video" in the search box at www.medlineplus.gov.

peptic ulcer An area of the GI tract that has been eroded away by the acidic gastric juice of the stomach.

◀ **FIGURE 2.15** Ulcer formation. **(a)** The *Helicobacter pylori* bacterium plays a key role in the development of most peptic ulcers. **(b)** A peptic ulcer.

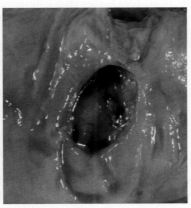

(a) The *Helicobacter pylori* (*H. pylori*) bacterium plays a key role in the development of most peptic ulcers.

(b) A peptic ulcer.

pain relievers such as aspirin, ibuprofen, and naproxen sodium. They appear to cause ulcers by suppressing the secretion of a substance that normally protects the stomach from its acidic gastric juice and helps control bleeding.[5] Ulcers caused by NSAID use generally heal once a person stops taking the medication.[5]

recap Gastroesophageal reflux (GER) is seepage of gastric juice into the esophagus. Gastroesophageal reflux disease (GERD) is a chronic disease in which gastric juice pools in the esophagus, causing symptoms such as heartburn more than twice per week. A peptic ulcer is an area of the stomach lining that has been eroded by gastric juice.

Some People Experience Disorders Related to Specific Foods

You check out the ingredients list on your energy bar, and you notice that it says "Produced in a facility that processes peanuts." The package on your microwave dinner cautions "Contains wheat, milk, and soy." Why all the warnings about these foods? The reason is that, to some people, consuming these foods can be dangerous, even life threatening. To learn more about product labeling for potential food offenders, see the *Nutrition Label Activity*.

Disorders related to specific foods can be clustered into three main groupings: food intolerances, food allergies, and a genetic disorder called celiac disease. We discuss these separately.

Food Intolerance

A **food intolerance** is a cluster of GI symptoms (often gas, pain, and diarrhea) that occurs following consumption of a particular food. The immune system plays no role in intolerance, and although episodes are unpleasant, they are usually transient, resolving after the offending food has been eliminated from the body. An example is lactose intolerance. It occurs in people whose bodies do not produce sufficient quantities of the enzyme lactase, which is needed for the breakdown of the milk sugar lactose. People can also have an intolerance to wheat, soy, and other foods, but as with lactose intolerance, the symptoms pass once the offending food is out of the person's system.

Food Allergy

A **food allergy** is a hypersensitivity reaction of the immune system to a particular component (usually a protein) in a food. This reaction causes the immune cells to release chemicals that cause either limited or body-wide inflammation. Although they are much less common than food intolerances, food allergies can be far more serious. Approximately 30,000 consumers require emergency room treatment and 150 Americans die each year because of allergic reactions to such common foods as peanuts, shellfish, eggs, or milk.[6]

In food allergies, the immune response begins when even a trace amount of the offending food enters the body and stimulates immune cells to release their inflammatory chemicals. In some people, the inflammation is localized. For instance, oral allergy syndrome (OAS) is an allergic reaction to certain raw fruits and vegetables, including apples, celery, and green peppers. It occurs most commonly in people who also experience hay fever and typically causes itching and swelling of the lips, mouth, and throat.[7] In other people, the inflammation can be widespread, producing, for example, a rash on the chest and arms. In a minority of people, the immune response is life-threatening, rapidly affecting the whole body and producing a state called *anaphylaxis* in which breathing is constricted, blood pressure plummets, and the person's heart may stop beating. Left untreated, anaphylaxis is nearly always fatal, so many people with known food allergies carry with them an "EpiPen" containing an injection of a powerful stimulant called epinephrine. This drug can reduce symptoms long enough to buy the victim time to get emergency medical care.

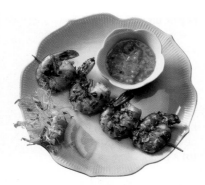

For some people, eating a meal of grilled shrimp with peanut sauce would cause a severe allergic reaction.

food intolerance A cluster of GI symptoms that occurs following consumption of a particular food but is not caused by an immune system response.

food allergy An inflammatory reaction caused by an immune system hypersensitivity to a protein component of a food.

nutrition label activity

Recognizing Common Allergens in Foods

The U.S. Food and Drug Administration (FDA) requires food labels to clearly identify any ingredients containing protein derived from the eight major allergenic foods.[12] Manufacturers must identify "in plain English" the presence of ingredients that contain protein derived from

- milk,
- eggs,
- fish,
- crustacean shellfish (crab, lobster, shrimp, and so on),
- tree nuts (almonds, pecans, walnuts, and so on),
- peanuts,
- wheat, and
- soybeans.

Although more than 160 foods have been identified as causing food allergies in sensitive individuals, the FDA requires labeling for only these eight foods because together they account for over 90% of all documented food allergies in the United States and represent the foods most likely to result in severe or life-threatening reactions.[12]

These eight allergenic foods must be indicated in the list of ingredients; alternatively, adjacent to the ingredients list, the label must say "Contains" followed by the name of the food. For example, the label of a product containing the milk-derived protein casein would have to use the term *milk* in addition to the term *casein*, so that those with milk allergies would clearly understand the presence of an allergen they need to avoid.[12] Any food product found to contain an undeclared allergen is subject to recall by the FDA.

Look at the ingredients list from an energy bar, shown below, and try the following questions:

- Which of the FDA's eight allergenic foods does this bar definitely contain? _____

- If you were allergic to peanuts, would eating this bar pose any risk to you?
    YES or NO

- If you were allergic to almonds, would eating this bar pose any risk to you?
    YES or NO

(See MasteringNutrition for answers.)

Ingredients: Soy protein isolate, rice flour, oats, milled flaxseed, brown rice syrup, evaporated cane juice, sunflower oil, soy lecithin, cocoa, nonfat milk solids, salt.

Contains soy and dairy. May contain traces of peanuts and other nuts.

Physicians use a variety of tests to diagnose food allergies. Usually, the physician orders a skin test, commonly known as a "skin prick test," in which a clinician injects a small amount of fluid containing the suspected allergen just below the surface of the patient's skin. After a few minutes, the clinician checks the area: redness and/or swelling indicates that the patient is allergic to the substance. However, people can have a positive skin response yet not have any problems when the substance is consumed.[7] Thus, both a positive skin test and a history of allergic reactions to the food are needed for diagnosis. Some physicians perform a blood test, in which a sample of the patient's blood is tested for the presence of proteins called *antibodies* that the immune system produces in a person with an allergy. But once again, the presence of antibodies does not necessarily mean the person will react to consumption of the food. The only test that can definitively establish the presence of a food allergy is an *oral challenge*, in which the patient consumes the suspected food and the healthcare provider monitors the reaction.

Beware of e-mail spam, Internet websites, and ads in popular magazines attempting to link a vast assortment of health problems to food allergies. Typically, these ads offer allergy-testing services for exorbitant fees, then make even more money by selling "nutritional counseling" and sometimes supplements and other products they say will help you cope with your allergies. If you experience symptoms that cause you to suspect you might have a food allergy, consult an MD.

> Watch a video providing an overview of food allergies by searching for "Food Allergies: What You Need to Know" at www.fda.gov.

Celiac Disease and Other Gluten-Related Disorders

Celiac disease is an immune disease that severely damages the lining of the small intestine and interferes with absorption of nutrients. Because there is a strong genetic

celiac disease An immune disease in which consumption of gluten triggers damage to the lining of the small intestine that interferes with the absorption of nutrients.

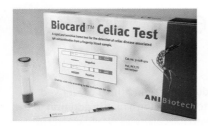

⬆ A simple blood test can identify celiac disease.

predisposition to celiac disease, with the risk now linked to specific gene markers, it is also classified as a genetic disorder.[8,9] Once thought to be rare, celiac disease is now known to occur in about 1 of 141 Americans.[10]

In celiac disease, the offending food component is *gluten*, a protein found in wheat, rye, and barley. When people with celiac disease eat gluten, their immune system triggers an inflammatory response that erodes the villi of the small intestine. If the person is unaware of the disorder and continues to eat gluten, repeated immune reactions cause the villi to become greatly decreased. As a result, the person becomes unable to absorb certain nutrients properly—a condition known as *malabsorption*. Over time, malabsorption can lead to malnutrition (poor nutrient status).

Symptoms of celiac disease can mimic those of other intestinal disturbances, so the condition is often misdiagnosed. Some of the characteristic symptoms include fatty stools (due to poor fat absorption); diarrhea; and weight loss. Other symptoms that do not involve the GI tract may also occur. These include an intensely itchy rash called *dermatitis herpetiformis*, osteoporosis (poor bone density), anemia, infertility, seizures, anxiety, depression, and fatigue, among others.[9]

Diagnostic tests for celiac disease include a variety of blood tests that screen for the presence of certain antibodies to gluten or for the genetic markers of the disease. However, the "gold standard" for diagnosis is a biopsy of the small intestine showing atrophy of the intestinal villi. Because long-term complications of undiagnosed celiac disease include an increased risk for liver disease and for cancer of the small intestine, early diagnosis can be life-saving. Unfortunately, celiac disease is thought to be widely underdiagnosed and misdiagnosed in the United States.[8]

Currently, there is no cure for celiac disease. Treatment is with a special gluten-free diet that excludes all forms of wheat, rye, and barley. The diet is challenging, but many gluten-free foods are now available, including breads, pasta, and other products made from corn, rice, soy, and even garbanzo bean flours. The FDA allows food manufacturers to identify their products as gluten-free if they contain less than 20 parts per million of gluten, which is the lowest amount detectable by scientific analysis. This labeling is important because many processed foods not obviously made from

foods you don't know you love YET

Job's Tears

One grain on the "no" list for people with celiac disease is barley, a popular ingredient in soups and stews. Fortunately, a pleasing, gluten-free barley substitute called Job's tears is available in many Asian markets and natural food stores, where you might find it labeled as Asian barley. Job's tears, the seeds of an Asian grass, are the color of pearl barley but much larger, with a brown groove splitting the seed on one side. Cooked Job's tears have a sweet taste somewhat like corn. They can be used in any recipe calling for barley, including soups and stews, or served on their own as a side dish instead of rice. They can even be cooked as a gluten-free breakfast porridge.

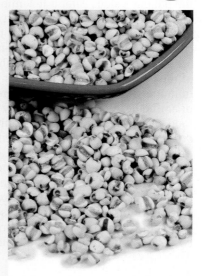

grains—such as packaged meals, soups, and some beverages—may contain sweeteners or other ingredients derived from gluten.

Notice that celiac disease is not the same as a gluten allergy. Many people believe they are allergic to gluten because they experience symptoms (a runny nose, a skin rash, and so on) when they eat foods containing gluten. Diagnostic testing can help these people find out whether or not they have a gluten allergy. In some cases, the healthcare provider might also recommend testing for celiac disease.

What about "gluten sensitivity," which has been blamed for everything from abdominal bloating to depression? Currently, researchers recognize that some people experience a variety of symptoms that do appear to be related to gluten consumption even though they have been tested for celiac disease and don't have the intestinal damage, characteristic antibodies, or genetic markers. They classify these cases under the umbrella term *non-celiac gluten sensitivity (NCGS)*.[9] However, the condition is thought to be rare, and the mechanisms are unknown. Researchers speculate that patients' symptoms might arise from reactions to different components of the gluten protein, or even to other proteins in grain products besides gluten. The bottom line? If you're experiencing symptoms you suspect may be due to the gluten in your diet, see your doctor.

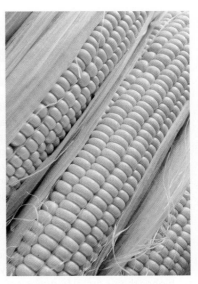

▲ For people with celiac disease, corn is a gluten-free source of carbohydrates.

recap Food intolerance is a condition in which a person experiences gastrointestinal discomfort following consumption of certain foods, but the symptoms are not prompted by the immune system. In contrast, both food allergies and celiac disease are caused by an immune response. Food allergies can cause a range of problems from minor discomfort to a life-threatening anaphylactic reaction. Celiac disease is an immune disorder that causes damage to the intestinal villi following consumption of gluten, a protein found in wheat, rye, and barley. It is associated with antibodies to gluten and specific genetic markers. Non-celiac gluten sensitivity is a recognized gluten-related disorder characterized by a variety of symptoms following consumption of gluten; however, the precise mechanisms are unknown.

Diarrhea Results When Stools Are Expelled Too Quickly

Diarrhea is the passage of loose, watery stools, often three or more times a day. Other symptoms may include cramping, abdominal pain, bloating, nausea, fever, and bloody stools. Diarrhea occurs when increased peristalsis moves chyme too quickly through the intestines, and as a result, too little water is absorbed.

Acute diarrhea lasts less than 3 weeks and is usually caused by an infection from bacteria, a virus, or a parasite. Chronic diarrhea is usually caused by undiagnosed food intolerances or allergies, celiac disease, irritable bowel syndrome (discussed shortly), or some other disorder.[11] It may also be due to certain medications and supplements. Whatever the cause, diarrhea can be harmful because the person can lose large quantities of water and minerals, such as sodium, and become severely dehydrated. Diarrhea is particularly dangerous in infants and young children. In fact, each year millions of children worldwide die from dehydration caused by diarrhea. Oral rehydration with specially formulated fluids can reverse dehydration and allow for the introduction of yogurt, rice, banana, and other mild foods.

A condition referred to as *traveler's diarrhea* has become a common health concern because of the expansion in global travel. The accompanying *Game Plan* provides tips for avoiding traveler's diarrhea.

Constipation Results When Stools Are Expelled Too Slowly

Constipation is typically defined as a condition in which no stools are passed for 2 or more days; however, it is important to recognize that many people normally experience bowel movements only every second or third day. Thus, the definition of constipation varies from one person to another. In addition to being infrequent, the

diarrhea A condition characterized by the frequent passage of loose, watery stools.

constipation A condition characterized by the absence of bowel movements for a period of time that is significantly longer than normal for the individual. When a bowel movement does occur, stools are usually small, hard, and difficult to pass.

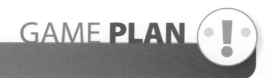

Tips for Avoiding Traveler's Diarrhea

Diarrhea is the rapid movement of fecal matter through the large intestine, often accompanied by large volumes of water. *Traveler's diarrhea* (also called *dysentery*), which is experienced by people traveling to regions where clean drinking water is not readily available, is usually caused by viral or bacterial infections. Diarrhea represents the body's way of ridding itself of the invasive agent. The large intestine and even some of the small intestine become irritated by the microbes and the body's defense against them. This irritation leads to increased secretion of fluid and increased peristalsis of the large intestine, causing watery stools and a higher-than-normal frequency of bowel movements.

People generally get traveler's diarrhea from consuming water or food that is contaminated with fecal matter. Travelers to developing countries are at increased risk; however, hikers and others traveling in remote regions anywhere are at risk if they drink untreated water from lakes, rivers, and streams.

Traveler's diarrhea usually starts within the first week of travel, but it can be delayed, sometimes even until you've returned home. Symptoms include fatigue, lack of appetite, abdominal cramps, and watery diarrhea. In some cases, you may also experience nausea, vomiting, and low-grade fever. Usually, the diarrhea passes within 2 days, and people recover completely. What can you do to prevent traveler's diarrhea? The following tips should help.[13]

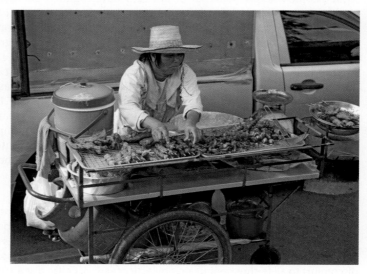

When traveling in developing countries, it is wise to avoid food from street vendors.

☐ Drink only hot beverages such as coffee and tea made with water that has been boiled, and brand-name bottled or canned beverages, including bottled water, soft drinks, beer, and wine. Use bottled water even for brushing your teeth. In general, it is smart to assume that all local water is unsafe.

☐ Wipe the bottle or can clean before drinking the beverage.

☐ Do not drink beverages over ice. Freezing does not kill all bacteria.

☐ Avoid foods and beverages exposed to or cleaned with local water.

☐ Avoid drinking unpasteurized milk and eating raw or rare meat, poultry, fish, or shellfish. Avoid raw vegetables, including salad greens. Do not eat raw fruits unless they've been washed in boiled or bottled water, then peeled. Do not eat fruits without peels, such as berries.

☐ Avoid eating food purchased from street vendors and any cooked food that is no longer hot in temperature.

☐ Prior to traveling to a high-risk country, discuss your trip with your physician for current recommendations for prevention and treatment.

If you do suffer from traveler's diarrhea, drink a specially formulated oral rehydration solution to help replenish vital nutrients; these solutions are available in most countries at local pharmacies and stores. Researchers are currently investigating the effectiveness of probiotic foods such as yogurt in speeding recovery.[13] If the diarrhea persists for more than 10 days after the initiation of treatment, or if there is blood in your stools, you should see a physician immediately to determine the cause and avoid serious medical consequences. Antibiotics or other prescription medications may be needed.

stools are difficult to pass and usually hard and small, because their slower transit has allowed the colon more time to absorb water from them.

Many people experience temporary constipation at various times in their life in response to a variety of factors. Often, people have trouble with it when they travel, when their schedule is disrupted, if they change their diet, or if they are on certain medications or supplements. Neural factors are thought to be responsible in some people, as explained in the following discussion of irritable bowel syndrome. Treatment with a short course of laxatives or bowel stimulants is often effective. Many healthcare professionals recommend increasing the consumption of fiber-rich foods such as fruits, vegetables, nuts and seeds, and whole-grain breads and cereals (such as oatmeal). Fiber not only increases the bulk of the stools, making them easier to move, but also holds water in the stools. Along with fiber, an adequate fluid intake is essential, and physical activity may also be helpful.

Irritable Bowel Syndrome Can Cause Either Diarrhea or Constipation

Irritable bowel syndrome (IBS) is a bowel disorder that interferes with normal functions of the colon. Symptoms include painful abdominal cramps, bloating, and either diarrhea or constipation. Approximately 10–15% of Americans have symptoms of IBS, and it is more commonly diagnosed in women than men.[12] IBS typically first appears before the age of 45.[12]

Although no definitive cause of IBS is known, recent studies indicate that the syndrome may arise from an abnormality in the way the brain interprets information from the colon or from abnormal functioning of chemicals called neurotransmitters that transmit messages within the nervous system—including the enteric nervous system.[13] Researchers also theorize that IBS may be triggered by a GI infection (gastroenteritis) or by bacterial overgrowth in the small intestine. In some cases, undiagnosed celiac disease is determined to be the cause.

Emotional and physiologic stress are currently thought to contribute to symptoms of IBS. Foods linked to physiologic stress include caffeinated beverages, alcohol, dairy products, wheat, large meals, and certain medications.

Whatever the cause, normal peristalsis appears to be disrupted. In some people with IBS, food moves too quickly through the colon and fluid cannot be absorbed fast enough, which causes diarrhea. In others, the movement of the colon is too slow and too much fluid is absorbed, leading to constipation. Therefore, treatment options include medications that treat diarrhea or constipation, as well as antispasmodics and antidepressants. Psychological counseling, hypnotherapy, and mindfulness training have also been shown to help. Recommended lifestyle changes include regular physical activity and dietary strategies such as eating smaller meals with increased fiber and fluids, especially plain water. Finally, probiotic foods and supplements have been found to improve symptoms of IBS.[13]

For a video providing ten tips for preventing episodes of irritable bowel syndrome (IBS), visit www.youtube.com and type "IBS Health Recommendations" in the search box. Click the video by WGOFoundations to get started.

recap Diarrhea is the frequent passage of loose or watery stools, whereas constipation is the failure to have a bowel movement for 2 or more days or within a time period that is normal for the individual. Irritable bowel syndrome (IBS) causes abdominal cramps, bloating, and diarrhea or constipation. The causes of IBS are unknown; however, both physiologic and emotional factors are thought to play a role.

irritable bowel syndrome (IBS)
A bowel disorder that interferes with normal functions of the colon. IBS causes abdominal cramps, bloating, and diarrhea or constipation.

STUDY **PLAN** | MasteringNutrition™

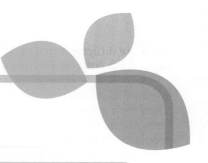

Customize your study plan—and master your nutrition!—
in the Study Area of **MasteringNutrition.**

what can I do **today?**

Now that you've read this chapter, try making these three changes:

1 At mealtimes today, select nourishing foods that provide dietary fiber. Take smaller portions. Eat slowly. Savor each bite.

2 Take better care of your GI tract! If you smoke, stop. If you drink alcohol, do so in moderation. Drink water and other healthful fluids throughout the day and stay active.

3 If you're experiencing GI pain, unexplained weight loss, or problems with bowel function, make an appointment with your healthcare provider or student health services center. Do it today!

test yourself | *answers*

1. **False.** Your brain, not your stomach, is the primary organ responsible for telling you when you are hungry.

2. **True.** Although there are individual variations in how we respond to food, the entire process of digestion and absorption of one meal usually takes about 24 hours.

3. **True.** Certain bacteria are normal and helpful residents of the large intestine, where they assist in digestion. They also appear to protect the tissue lining the intestinal walls and may improve health in other ways as well. Foods and supplements containing these bacteria are called *probiotics.*

summary

Scan to hear an MP3 Chapter Review in **MasteringNutrition.**

LO **1** **Compare and contrast the feelings of hunger and appetite, and the factors contributing to each**

- Hunger is a physical sensation triggered by the hypothalamus in response to cues from nerve cells about stomach and intestinal fullness; the levels of certain hormones, chemical messengers secreted by glands in response to changes in internal conditions; and the amount and type of food we eat. High-protein foods make us feel satiated for longer periods of time, and bulky meals fill us up quickly, causing us to stop eating sooner.

- Appetite is a psychological desire to consume specific foods. The most significant factors influencing our appetite are sensory data, social and cultural cues, and learning.

LO **2** **Identify the relationship between the foods we eat and the structures and functions of our cells**

- Atoms are the smallest units of matter. They bond together to form molecules.

- The food we eat is composed of molecules. The chemical reactions that join atoms and molecules into larger compounds, and break compounds apart into smaller molecules and atoms, are collectively called metabolism.

- Cells are the smallest units of life. We build cells from the nutrients we absorb as a result of digesting food. The primary goal of digestion is to break food into molecules small enough to be absorbed and transported throughout the body.

- Cells are encased in a cell membrane, which acts as a gatekeeper to determine which substances go into and out of the cell. Cells of a single type join together to form tissues. Several types of tissues join together to form organs, such as the liver. Organs group together to form systems that perform integrated functions. The gastrointestinal system is an example.

LO **3** **Name and state the function of each of the major organs of the gastrointestinal tract and the four accessory organs**

- Digestion is the process of breaking down foods into molecules; absorption is the process of taking molecules of food into the body; and elimination is the process of removing undigested food and waste products from the body.

- The gastrointestinal tract begins at the mouth, where chewing starts mechanical digestion of food. Food moves from the mouth through the esophagus via a process called peristalsis. It enters the stomach, which mixes it with gastric juices. Hydrochloric acid and the enzyme pepsin initiate protein digestion, and a minimal amount of fat digestion begins through the action of gastric lipase. The stomach releases the partially digested food, referred to as chyme, periodically into the small intestine, where most digestion and absorption of nutrients occurs. The remaining semisolid waste moves into the large intestine, which digests any remaining food particles, absorbs water and chemicals, and moves feces to the rectum for elimination.

- The salivary glands, gallbladder, pancreas, and liver are accessory digestive organs. The salivary glands secrete saliva, which contains salivary amylase, which begins the breakdown of carbohydrate. The gallbladder stores bile and secretes it into the small intestine, where it emulsifies fats. The pancreas manufactures and secretes digestive enzymes into the small intestine. The liver processes and stores all absorbed nutrients and synthesizes bile.

LO **4** **Explain how the food you eat is broken down mechanically and chemically**

- Mechanical digestion occurs in the mouth, via chewing; in the stomach, which mixes and churns food; and all along the GI tract via peristalsis, which helps break food apart as it moves it along. Chemical digestion also occurs in several organs of the GI tract. It is accomplished largely through the action of several digestive enzymes, hydrochloric acid secreted from the stomach, and bile synthesized by the liver.

LO **5** **Identify the unique features of the small intestine that contribute to its ability to absorb nutrients**

- The lining of the small intestine has thousands of folds, finger like projections called villi, and hairlike lining cells called microvilli, all of which increase its surface area more than 500 times. This in turn significantly increases the absorptive capacity of the small intestine.

LO **6** **Describe how the body eliminates food wastes**

- Bacteria in the large intestine assist with digestion of any remaining digestible food products.

The large intestine stores chyme, from which it absorbs water and any other remaining nutrients, leaving a semisolid mass, called feces, which is then eliminated from the body.

LO **7** **Discuss the causes, symptoms, and treatment of gastroesophageal reflux disease and peptic ulcers**

- Heartburn—or gastroesophageal reflux—occurs when hydrochloric acid seeps into the esophagus and is not quickly cleared, thus burning its lining. Gastroesophageal reflux disease (GERD) is a more painful type of heartburn that occurs more than twice per week.

- A peptic ulcer is an area in the stomach or duodenum that has been eroded away by hydrochloric acid and pepsin. The primary cause of peptic ulcers is a bacterium called *Helicobacter pylori*.

LO **8** **Distinguish between food intolerance and food allergy, and between celiac disease and non-celiac gluten sensitivity**

- A food intolerance is gastrointestinal discomfort caused by foods. It does not result from an immune system reaction. In contrast, symptoms of food allergies occur when the immune system releases inflammatory chemicals in response to the presence of an offending food substance, usually a protein.

- Celiac disease is a genetic disorder caused by an immune response to a wheat protein called gluten that damages the lining of the small intestine. The person experiences malabsorption of nutrients. Undiagnosed celiac disease increases the risk for liver disease and cancer of the small intestine. Non-celiac gluten sensitivity is a disorder in which people who do not have celiac disease nevertheless experience a variety of symptoms that appear to be related to gluten consumption.

LO **9** **Compare and contrast diarrhea, constipation, and irritable bowel syndrome**

- Diarrhea is the frequent passage of loose, watery stools. Constipation is a condition in which no stools are passed for a length of time considered abnormally long for the individual. Irritable bowel syndrome is a disorder that interferes with normal functions of the colon, causing abdominal pain and either diarrhea or constipation.

review questions

LO **1** **Compare and contrast the feelings of hunger and appetite, and the factors contributing to each**

1. Which of the following statements about hunger is true?
   a. The most significant triggers of hunger are social and cultural cues.
   b. Hunger is a psychological drive to consume specific foods.
   c. A region of the brain called the hypothalamus triggers hunger.
   d. Beverages are likely to satisfy hunger more effectively than solid foods.

LO **2** **Identify the relationship between the foods we eat and the structures and functions of our cells**

2. Cells are
   a. the smallest units of life.
   b. enclosed by a semipermeable membrane.
   c. the building blocks of tissues and organs.
   d. All of the above are true.

LO **3** **Name and state the function of each of the major organs of the gastrointestinal tract and the four accessory organs**

3. The liver
   a. is an accessory organ of digestion.
   b. stores bile.
   c. synthesizes hydrochloric acid (HCl).
   d. All of the above are true.

LO **4** **Explain how the food you eat is broken down mechanically and chemically**

4. Most digestion of carbohydrates, fats, and proteins takes place in the
   a. mouth.
   b. stomach.
   c. small intestine.
   d. large intestine.

5. The pancreas
   a. releases digestive enzymes into the small intestine.
   b. releases bile into the small intestine.
   c. releases bicarbonate into the large intestine.
   d. releases chyme into the large intestine.

LO **5** **Identify the unique features of the small intestine that contribute to its ability to absorb nutrients**

6. The circular folds, villi, and microvilli of the small intestine
   a. increase peristalsis.
   b. increase nutrient absorption.
   c. protect against bacterial infection.
   d. None of the above is true.

LO **6** **Describe how the body eliminates food wastes**

7. Food wastes
   a. are eliminated from the body through the ileocecal valve.
   b. are acted on by trillions of resident bacteria that finish digestion.
   c. are propelled through the colon by almost continuous, strong waves of peristalsis.
   d. absorb additional water secreted by the large intestine as they move toward the rectum.

LO **7** **Discuss the causes, symptoms, and treatment of gastroesophageal reflux disease and peptic ulcers**

8. Gastroesophageal reflux disease is caused by
   a. regurgitation of undigested food into the pharynx.
   b. pooling of gastric juice in the esophagus.
   c. backflow of bicarbonate into the esophagus.
   d. seepage of gastric juice into the chest cavity.

LO **8** **Distinguish between food intolerance and food allergy, and between celiac disease and non-celiac gluten sensitivity**

9. Celiac disease
   a. occurs when the body cannot manufacture an enzyme that digests gluten.
   b. is characterized by an allergic response to gluten ranging from mild itchiness to anaphylaxis.
   c. is an immune response to gluten that erodes the lining of the small intestine.
   d. is a sensitivity to gluten in the absence of gluten-specific antibodies and certain genetic markers.

LO **9** **Compare and contrast diarrhea, constipation, and irritable bowel syndrome**

10. Normal peristalsis is disrupted in
    a. diarrhea.
    b. constipation.
    c. irritable bowel syndrome.
    d. all of the above.

Answers to Review Questions are located at the back of this text.

web links

The following websites and apps explore further topics and issues related to personal health.
Visit **MasteringNutrition** for links to the websites and RSS feeds.

http://americanceliac.org
American Celiac Disease Alliance

www.csaceliacs.org
Celiac Support Association

www.digestive.niddk.nih.gov
National Digestive Diseases Information Clearinghouse (NDDIC)

www.foodallergy.org
Food Allergy Research & Education

www.ibsassociation.org
Irritable Bowel Syndrome Association

www.isapp.net
International Scientific Association for Probiotics and Prebiotics

Carbohydrates
Plant-Derived Energy Nutrients

3

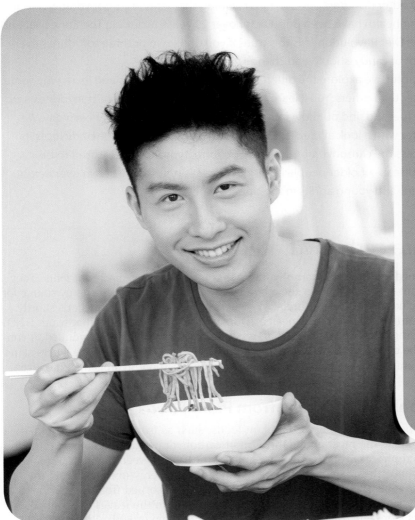

test yourself

Are these statements true or false? Circle your guess.

1. **T F** The terms *carbohydrate* and *sugar* mean the same thing.

2. **T F** Diets high in sugar cause hyperactivity in children.

3. **T F** Carbohydrates are fattening.

Test Yourself answers can be found at the end of the chapter.

MasteringNutrition™

Go online for chapter quizzes, pre-tests, Interactive Activities, and more!

Jasmine skipped school again today. When her Mom asked her why, she said she had a headache. That is only partly true: her real "headache" is the thought of explaining to her friends why, all of a sudden, she can't have the sodas and snacks they've always consumed at school. She and her friends admit they're overweight, but they've always had fun together, so their weight hasn't bothered them. Jasmine doesn't want her friends to find out that things are different now—that she has to change her diet, exercise regularly, and lose weight. She doesn't want to admit that she's just been diagnosed with the same disease her grandmother has: type 2 diabetes.

Does consuming sugary foods and drinks lead to diabetes, or, for that matter, to obesity or any other disorder? Several diets claiming that refined carbohydrates can be harmful to your health have been popular for over 20 years, including The Zone Diet and Dr. Atkins' New Diet Revolution.[1,2] Is this true? If you drink two or three soft drinks every day, or eat a lot of candy, should you change your ways?

In this chapter, we explore the different types of carbohydrates and learn why some really are better than others. You'll learn how the body breaks down carbohydrates and uses them for fuel and find out how much carbohydrate you should eat each day. We end the chapter with a look at diabetes, a disease that occurs when the body loses its ability to process the carbohydrates we eat. One form, type 2 diabetes, used to be considered a disease of older people but is now increasingly diagnosed in overweight and obese teens and young adults in the United States.

LO1 Distinguish between simple and complex carbohydrates

What are carbohydrates?

As we mentioned in Chapter 1, **carbohydrates** are one of the three macronutrients. They are an important energy source for the entire body and are the preferred energy source for nerve cells, including those of the brain. We will say more about their functions shortly.

The term *carbohydrate* literally means "hydrated carbon." You know that water (H_2O) is made of hydrogen and oxygen and that, when something is said to be hydrated, it contains water. The chemical abbreviation for carbohydrate is CHO. These three letters stand for the three components of a molecule of carbohydrate: carbon, hydrogen, and oxygen.

Most Carbohydrates Come from Plant Foods

We obtain carbohydrates mainly from plant foods, such as fruits, vegetables, and grains. Plants make the most abundant form of carbohydrate, called glucose, through a process called **photosynthesis**. During photosynthesis, the green pigment of plants, called chlorophyll, absorbs sunlight, which provides the energy needed to fuel the manufacture of glucose. As shown in **FIGURE 3.1**, water absorbed from the Earth by the roots of plants combines with carbon dioxide present in the leaves to produce glucose. Plants store glucose and use it to support their own growth. When we eat plant foods, that stored glucose is available to us.

The only non-plant sources of carbohydrates are foods derived from milk. For instance, breast milk, cow's milk, and ice cream all contain a carbohydrate called lactose.

Simple Carbohydrates Are Sugars

Carbohydrates can be classified as *simple* or *complex*. These terms describe carbohydrates based on the number of molecules of sugar present. Simple carbohydrates contain either one or two molecules, whereas complex carbohydrates contain hundreds to thousands of molecules.

Simple carbohydrates are commonly called *sugars*. Six sugars are common in our diet. Three of these are called **monosaccharides** because they consist of only a single sugar

carbohydrate One of the three macronutrients, a compound made up of carbon, hydrogen, and oxygen. It is derived from plants and provides energy.

photosynthesis The process by which plants use sunlight to fuel a chemical reaction that combines carbon and water into glucose, which is then stored in their cells.

simple carbohydrate A monosaccharide or disaccharide, such as glucose; commonly called *sugar*.

monosaccharide The simplest of carbohydrates; consists of one sugar molecule, the most common form of which is glucose.

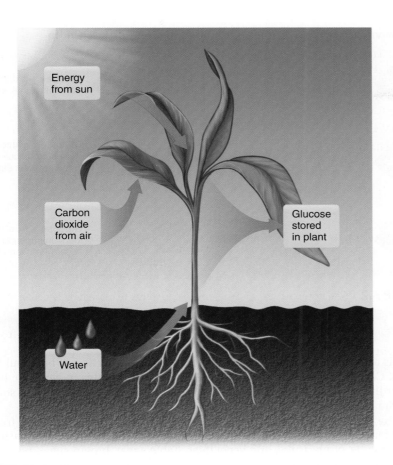

⬆ **FIGURE 3.1** Plants make carbohydrates through the process of photosynthesis. Water, carbon dioxide, and energy from the sun are combined to produce glucose.

molecule (*mono* means "one," and *saccharide* means "sugar"). The other three sugars are **disaccharides** and consist of two molecules of sugar joined together (*di* means "two").

The Three Monosaccharides Are Glucose, Fructose, and Galactose

Glucose, *fructose*, and *galactose* are the three monosaccharides in our diet **(FIGURE 3.2)**. Because plants manufacture **glucose**, it probably won't surprise you to discover that glucose is the most abundant sugar in our diet and in our body. Glucose does not generally occur by itself in foods; instead, it is usually attached to other sugars in larger molecules. In our body, glucose is the preferred source of energy for the brain, and it is a very important source of energy for all cells.

Fructose, the sweetest natural sugar, is found in fruits and vegetables. Fructose is also called *fruit sugar*. In many processed foods, it comes in the form of *high-fructose corn syrup*. This syrup is made from corn and is used to sweeten many common foods including soft drinks, desserts, candies, and jellies.

Galactose does not occur alone in foods. It joins with glucose to create lactose, one of the three most common disaccharides.

The Three Disaccharides Are Lactose, Maltose, and Sucrose

The three most common disaccharides found in foods are *lactose*, *maltose*, and *sucrose* (Figure 3.2). **Lactose** (also called *milk sugar*) is made up of glucose and galactose. Interestingly, human breast milk has a higher amount of lactose than cow's milk and therefore tastes sweeter.

Maltose (also called *malt sugar*) consists of two molecules of glucose. It does not generally occur by itself in foods but, rather, is bound together with other molecules. As our body breaks these larger molecules down, maltose results as a by-product.

disaccharide A carbohydrate compound consisting of two sugar molecules joined together.

glucose The most abundant sugar molecule; a monosaccharide generally found in combination with other sugars. The preferred source of energy for the brain and an important source of energy for all cells.

fructose The sweetest natural sugar; a monosaccharide that occurs in fruits and vegetables. Also called *fruit sugar*.

galactose A monosaccharide that joins with glucose to create lactose, one of the three most common disaccharides.

lactose A disaccharide consisting of one glucose molecule and one galactose molecule; also called *milk sugar*. Found in milk, including human breast milk.

maltose A disaccharide consisting of two molecules of glucose. Does not generally occur independently in foods but results as a by-product of digestion. Also called *malt sugar*.

Monosaccharides　　　　　　　　　**Disaccharides**

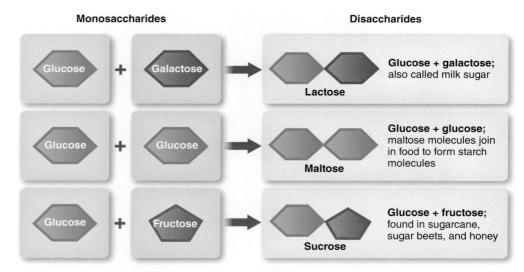

FIGURE 3.2 Galactose, glucose, and fructose join together to make the disaccharides lactose, maltose, and sucrose.

Maltose is also the sugar that is fermented during the production of beer and liquor products. Contrary to popular belief, very little maltose remains in alcoholic beverages after the fermentation process; thus, alcoholic beverages are not good sources of carbohydrate.

Sucrose is composed of glucose and fructose. Because sucrose contains fructose, it is sweeter than lactose or maltose. Sucrose provides much of the sweet taste found in honey, maple syrup, fruits, and vegetables. Table sugar, brown sugar, powdered sugar, and many other products are made by refining the sucrose found in sugarcane and sugar beets. Are naturally occurring forms of sucrose more healthful than manufactured forms? The ***Nutrition Myth or Fact?*** box investigates the common belief that honey is more nutritious than table sugar.

Complex Carbohydrates Are Polysaccharides

Complex carbohydrates, the second major type of carbohydrate, generally consist of long chains of glucose molecules. The technical name for complex carbohydrates is **polysaccharides** (*poly* means "many"). Complex carbohydrates exist in foods as either starches or fiber. A third complex carbohydrate, glycogen, is not obtained from our diet (**FIGURE 3.3**). Let's look at each of these three types.

sucrose A disaccharide composed of one glucose molecule and one fructose molecule. It is sweeter than lactose or maltose.

complex carbohydrate A nutrient compound consisting of long chains of glucose molecules, such as starch, glycogen, and fiber.

polysaccharide A complex carbohydrate consisting of long chains of glucose.

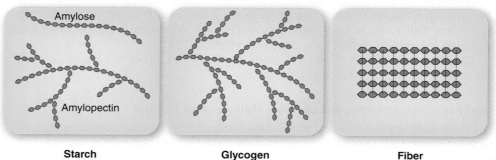

Starch	**Glycogen**	**Fiber**
Storage form of glucose in plants; found in grains, legumes, and tubers	Storage form of glucose in animals; stored in liver and muscles	Forms the support structures of leaves, stems, and plants

FIGURE 3.3 Polysaccharides include starch, glycogen, and fiber.

nutrition myth or fact?

Is Honey More Nutritious than Table Sugar?

Liz's friend Tiffany is dedicated to eating healthful foods. She advises Liz to avoid white sugar and to eat foods that contain honey, molasses, or raw sugar. Like many people, Tiffany believes these sweeteners are more natural and nutritious than refined table sugar. How can Liz sort sugar fact from fiction?

Remember that sucrose consists of one glucose molecule and one fructose molecule joined together. From a chemical perspective, honey is almost identical to sucrose, because honey also contains glucose and fructose molecules in almost equal amounts. However, enzymes in the "honey stomachs" of bees separate some of the glucose and fructose molecules. Also, bees use their wings to fan the honey stored in combs, reducing its moisture content. These factors alter the taste, appearance, and texture of honey.

Honey does not contain any more nutrients than sucrose, so it is not a more healthful choice than sucrose. In fact, per tablespoon, honey has more Calories (energy) than table sugar. This is because the crystals in table sugar take up more space on a spoon than the liquid form of honey, so a tablespoon contains less sugar. However, some people argue that honey is sweeter, so you use less.

It's important to note that honey commonly contains bacteria that can cause fatal food poisoning in infants. The more mature digestive system of older children and adults is immune to the effects of these bacteria, but babies younger than 12 months should *never* be given honey.

Are raw sugar and molasses more healthful than table sugar? Actually, the "raw sugar" available in the United States is not really raw. Truly raw sugar is made up of the first crystals obtained when sugar is processed. Sugar in this form contains dirt, parts of insects, and other by-products that make it illegal to sell in the United States. The raw sugar products in American stores have actually gone through more than half of the same steps in the refining process used to make table sugar.

Molasses is the syrup that remains when sucrose is made from sugarcane. Molasses is darker and less sweet than table sugar. It does contain some iron, but this iron does not occur naturally; it is a contaminant from the machines that process the sugarcane!

The truth is, no added sugars contain many nutrients that are important for health. This is why highly sweetened products are referred to as "empty Calories."

Starch Is a Polysaccharide Stored in Plants

Plants store glucose not as single molecules but as polysaccharides in the form of **starch**. Excellent food sources include grains (wheat, rice, corn, oats, and barley), legumes (peas, beans, and lentils), and tubers (potatoes and yams). Our cells cannot use starch molecules exactly as they occur in plants. Instead, our body must break them down into the monosaccharide glucose, from which we can then fuel our energy needs.

Fiber Is a Polysaccharide That Gives Plants Their Structure

Fiber is the nondigestible part of plants that forms leaves, stems, and seeds. Like starches, fiber consists of long polysaccharide chains. The body easily breaks apart the chains in starches; however, the bonds that connect fiber molecules are not easily broken. This means that most forms of fiber pass through the digestive system without being broken down and absorbed, so fiber contributes little or no energy to our diet. However, fiber offers many health benefits, which we will discuss shortly.

Nutrition experts and food producers use several terms to distinguish among different types of fiber. We discuss these terms here, because they're important for understanding the contribution of fiber to our health.

Dietary vs. Functional Fiber Fiber that occurs naturally in foods is called **dietary fiber**. In a sense, you can think of dietary fiber as the plant's "skeleton." Good food

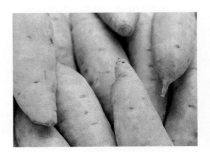

⬆ Tubers, such as these sweet potatoes, are excellent food sources of starch.

starch A polysaccharide stored in plants; the storage form of glucose in plants.

fiber The nondigestible carbohydrate parts of plants that form the support structures of leaves, stems, and seeds.

dietary fiber The type of fiber that occurs naturally in foods.

sources of dietary fiber include fruits, vegetables, seeds, legumes, and whole grains. We often hear the recommendation to eat *whole* grains, but is grain ground into flour and baked into bread still whole? Maybe, maybe not! So what does the term *whole grain* really mean? Find out in the **Highlight** feature box.

Another type of fiber, called **functional fiber**, is manufactured and added to foods and fiber supplements. Examples of functional fiber sources you might see on nutrition labels are cellulose, guar gum, pectin, and psyllium.

Total fiber is the sum of dietary fiber and functional fiber in a particular food. On the Nutrition Facts Panel, the term *Dietary Fiber* actually represents the total amount of fiber in that food. It includes the dietary fiber that occurs naturally in addition to any functional fiber that may have been added.

Soluble vs. Insoluble Fiber   Fiber can also be classified, according to its chemical and physical properties, as soluble or insoluble. **Soluble fibers** dissolve in water. They are also *viscous*, which means they form a gel when wet. Although the digestive tract cannot independently digest soluble fibers, they are easily digested by bacteria present in the colon. Soluble fibers are typically found in citrus fruits, berries, oat products, and beans. Research suggests that consuming soluble fibers regularly reduces the risks for cardiovascular disease and type 2 diabetes by lowering blood cholesterol and blood glucose levels.

Insoluble fibers are those that don't typically dissolve in water and can't easily be digested by bacteria in the colon. Insoluble fibers are generally found in whole grains, such as wheat, rye, and brown rice, as well as in many vegetables. These fibers are not associated with reducing cholesterol levels but are known for promoting regular bowel movements, alleviating constipation, and reducing the risk for a disorder called diverticulosis (discussed later in this chapter).

Fiber-Rich Carbohydrates   Materials written for the general public usually don't refer to the carbohydrates found in foods as complex or simple; instead, resources such as the *Dietary Guidelines for Americans* 2010 emphasize eating **fiber-rich carbohydrates**, such as fruits, vegetables, and whole grains.[3] This term is important because fiber-rich carbohydrates are known to contribute to good health, but not all complex carbohydrate foods are fiber-rich. For example, potatoes that have been processed into frozen hash browns retain very little of their original fiber. On the other hand, some foods rich in simple carbohydrates (such as fruits) are also fiber-rich. So when you're reading labels, it pays to check the grams of dietary fiber per serving. And if the food you're considering is fresh produce, that almost guarantees it's fiber-rich.

Check the **Nutrition Label Activity** to learn how to recognize various carbohydrates on food labels.

Glycogen Is a Polysaccharide Stored by Animals

Glycogen is the storage form of glucose for animals (including humans). We store glycogen in our muscles and liver, and we can break it down very quickly into glucose when we need it for energy. Very little glycogen exists in food; thus, glycogen is not a dietary source of carbohydrate.

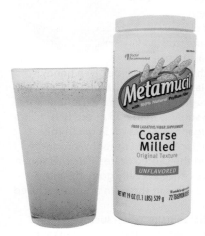

▲ Dissolvable laxatives are examples of soluble fibers.

functional fiber The nondigestible forms of carbohydrate that are extracted from plants or manufactured in the laboratory and have known health benefits.

total fiber The sum of dietary fiber and functional fiber.

soluble fibers Fibers that dissolve in water.

insoluble fibers Fibers that do not dissolve in water.

fiber-rich carbohydrates A group of foods containing either simple or complex carbohydrates that are rich in dietary fiber. These foods, which include most fruits, vegetables, and whole grains, are typically fresh or only moderately processed.

glycogen A polysaccharide stored in animals; the storage form of glucose in animals.

recap   Carbohydrates are energy-providing macronutrients that contain carbon, hydrogen, and oxygen. Plants make one type of carbohydrate, glucose, through the process of photosynthesis. Simple carbohydrates include the monosaccharides glucose, fructose, and galactose and the disaccharides lactose, maltose, and sucrose. All complex carbohydrates are polysaccharides. They include starch, glycogen, and fiber. Starch is the storage form of glucose in plants, whereas glycogen is the storage form of glucose in animals. Fiber forms the support structures of plants; fiber-rich carbohydrates are known to contribute to good health.

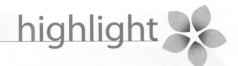

What Makes a Whole Grain Whole?

Grains are grasses that produce edible kernels. A kernel of grain is the seed of the grass: if you were to plant a kernel of barley, a blade of grass would soon shoot up. Kernels of different grains all share a similar design. As shown in **FIGURE 3.4**, they consist of three parts:

- The outermost covering, called the *bran,* is very high in fiber and contains most of the grain's vitamins and minerals.
- The *endosperm* is the grain's midsection and contains most of the grain's carbohydrates and protein.
- The *germ* sits deep in the base of the kernel, surrounded by the endosperm, and is rich in healthful fats and some vitamins.

Whole grains are kernels that retain all three of these parts.

The kernels of some grains also have a *husk* (hull): a thin, dry coat that is inedible. Removing the husk is always the

first step in milling (grinding) these grains for human consumption. People worldwide have milled grain for centuries, usually using heavy stones. A little milling removes only a small amount of the bran, leaving a crunchy grain suitable for cooked cereals. For example, cracked wheat and hulled barley retain much of the kernel's bran.

Whole-grain flours are produced when whole grains are ground and then recombined. Because these hearty flours retain a portion of the bran, endosperm, and germ, foods such as breads made with them are rich in fiber and a wide array of vitamins and minerals.

With the advent of modern technology, processes for milling grains became more sophisticated, with seeds being repeatedly ground and sifted into increasingly finer flours, retaining little or no bran and therefore little fiber and few vitamins and minerals. For instance, white wheat flour, which consists almost entirely of endosperm, is high in carbohydrate but retains only about 25% of the wheat's fiber, vitamins, and minerals. In the United States, manufacturers of breads and other baked goods made with white flour are required by law to enrich their products with vitamins and minerals to replace some of those lost in processing. However, enrichment replaces only a handful of nutrients and leaves the bread low in fiber.

When shopping for whole-grain breads, crackers, and other baked goods, don't be fooled. A loaf of "wheat bread" may contain no whole grains at all. Although many labels for breads and cereals list wheat flour as the first ingredient, this term actually refers to enriched white flour, which is made when wheat flour is processed. Look for the word "whole" on the ingredient list: whole wheat, whole oats, or similar whole grains. This ensures that the product contains the fiber and micronutrients that nature packed into the plant's seed. Refer to **TABLE 3.1** below for terms used to describe grains and cereals on nutrition labels.

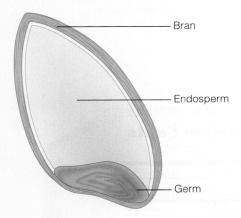

FIGURE 3.4 A whole grain includes the bran, endosperm, and germ.

TABLE 3.1 Terms Used to Describe Grains and Cereals on Nutrition Labels

Term	Definition
Brown bread	Bread that may or may not be made using whole-grain flour. Many brown breads are made with white flour with brown (caramel) coloring added.
Enriched (or fortified) flour or grain	Enriching or fortifying grains involves adding nutrients back to refined foods. In order to use this term in the United States, a minimum amount of iron, folate, niacin, thiamin, and riboflavin must be added. Other nutrients can also be added.
Refined flour or grain	Refining involves removing the coarse parts of food products; refined wheat flour is flour in which all but the internal part of the kernel has been removed. Refined sugar is made by removing the outer portions of sugar beets or sugarcane.
Stone ground	Refers to a milling process in which limestone is used to grind any grain. Stone ground does not mean that bread is made with whole grain, because refined flour can be stone ground.
Unbleached flour	Flour that has been refined but not bleached; it is very similar to refined white flour in texture and nutritional value.
Wheat flour	Any flour made from wheat; includes white flour, unbleached flour, and whole-wheat flour.
White flour	Flour that has been bleached and refined. All-purpose flour, cake flour, and enriched baking flour are all types of white flour.
Whole-grain flour	A grain that is not refined; whole grains are milled in their complete form, with only the husk removed.
Whole-wheat flour	An unrefined whole-grain flour made from whole-wheat kernels.

nutrition label activity

Recognizing Carbohydrates on the Label

FIGURE 3.5 shows labels for two breakfast cereals. The cereal on the left **(a)** is processed and sweetened, whereas the one on the right **(b)** is a whole-grain product with no added sugar. Which is the better breakfast choice? Fill in the label data below to find out!

■ **Check the center of each label to locate the amount of total carbohydrate.**

1. For the sweetened cereal, the total carbohydrate is _____ *gram(s)*.
2. For the whole-grain cereal, the total carbohydrate is _____ *gram(s)* for a smaller serving size.

■ **Look at the information listed as subgroups under Total Carbohydrate. The label for the sweetened cereal lists all types of carbohydrates in the cereal: dietary fiber, sugars, and other carbohydrate (which refers to starches). Notice that this cereal contains 13 grams of sugar—half of its total carbohydrates.**

3. How many grams of dietary fiber does the sweetened cereal contain? _____

■ **The label for the whole-grain cereal lists only 1 gram of sugar, which is less than 4% of its total carbohydrates.**

4. How many grams of dietary fiber does the whole-grain cereal contain? _____

(Answers can be found on the Study Area of MasteringNutrition.)

Which cereal should you choose to increase your fiber intake? Check the ingredients list for the sweetened cereal. Remember that they're listed in order from highest to lowest amount. The second and third ingredients listed are sugar and brown sugar, and the corn and oat flours are not whole-grain flours. Now look at the ingredients for the other cereal—it contains whole-grain oats. Although the sweetened product is enriched with B-vitamins, iron, and zinc, the whole-grain cereal packs 4 grams of fiber per serving and contains no added sugars. Overall, it is a more healthful choice.

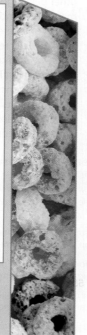

Nutrition Facts

Serving Size: 3/4 cup (30g)
Servings Per Package: About 14

Amount Per Serving	Cereal	Cereal With 1/2 Cup Skim Milk
Calories	120	160
Calories from Fat	15	15
	% Daily Value**	
Total Fat 1.5g*	2%	2%
Saturated Fat 0g	0%	0%
Trans Fat 0g		
Polyunsaturated Fat 0g		
Monounsaturated Fat 0.5g		
Cholesterol 0mg	0%	1%
Sodium 220mg	9%	12%
Potassium 40mg	1%	7%
Total Carbohydrate 26g	9%	11%
Dietary Fiber 1g	3%	3%
Sugars 13g		
Other Carbohydrate 12g		
Protein 1g		

INGREDIENTS: Corn Flour, Sugar, Brown Sugar, Partially Hydrogenated Vegetable Oil (Soybean and Cottonseed), Oat Flour, Salt, Sodium Citrate (a flavoring agent), Flavor added [Natural & Artificial Flavor, Strawberry Juice Concentrate, Malic Acid (a flavoring agent)], Niacinamide (Niacin), Zinc Oxide, Reduced Iron, Red 40, Yellow 5, Red 3, Yellow 6, Pyridoxine Hydrochloride (Vitamin B6), Riboflavin (Vitamin B2), Thiamin Mononitrate (Vitamin B1), Folic Acid (Folate) and Blue 1.

(a)

Nutrition Facts

Serving Size: 1/2 cup dry (40g)
Servings Per Container: 13

Amount Per Serving	
Calories	150
Calories from Fat	25
	% Daily Value*
Total Fat 3g	5%
Saturated Fat 0.5g	2%
Trans Fat 0g	
Polyunsaturated Fat 1g	
Monounsaturated Fat 1g	
Cholesterol 0mg	0%
Sodium 0mg	0%
Total Carbohydrate 27g	9%
Dietary Fiber 4g	15%
Soluble Fiber 2g	
Insoluble Fiber 2g	
Sugars 1g	
Protein 5g	

INGREDIENTS: 100% Natural Whole Grain Rolled Oats.

(b)

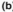

▲ **FIGURE 3.5** Labels for two breakfast cereals: **(a)** processed and sweetened cereal and **(b)** whole-grain cereal with no added sugar.

Why do we need to eat carbohydrates?

LO2   List four functions of carbohydrates in our body

We have seen that carbohydrates are an important energy source for our body. Let's learn more about this and some other functions of carbohydrates.

Carbohydrates Provide Energy

Carbohydrates, an excellent source of energy for all our cells, provide 4 kilocalories (kcal) of energy per gram. Some of our cells can also use fat and even protein for energy if necessary. However, our red blood cells, as well as our brain and our nerve cells, rely on glucose. This is why you get tired, irritable, and shaky when you have not eaten carbohydrates for a prolonged period of time.

As shown in **FIGURE 3.6**, our body always uses some combination of carbohydrates and fat to fuel daily activities. Fat is the primary energy source used by most of our cells at rest and during low-intensity activities, such as sitting, standing, and walking. Even during rest, however, our brain cells and red blood cells still rely on glucose.

When we exercise briskly or perform any activity that causes us to breathe harder and sweat, we begin to use more glucose than fat. When you are exercising at maximal effort, carbohydrates are providing almost 100% of the energy your body requires.

If the diet does not provide enough carbohydrate, the body will make glucose from protein. This involves breaking down the proteins in blood and tissues, then converting the components to glucose. This process is called **gluconeogenesis** ("generating new glucose").

Using proteins for energy reduces the level of proteins available to make new cells, repair tissues, or perform any of their other functions. Also, over a prolonged period of time, deriving proteins from the breakdown of tissues such as the muscles, heart, liver, and kidneys can seriously damage these organs. So, carbohydrates are also important in the diet to "spare," or preserve, body protein.

gluconeogenesis The generation of glucose from the breakdown of proteins.

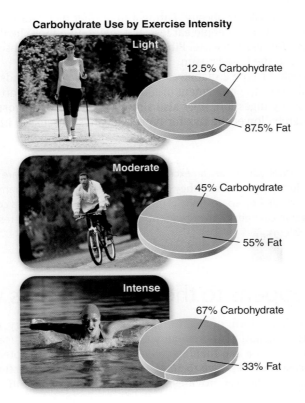

Carbohydrate Use by Exercise Intensity

Light
- 12.5% Carbohydrate
- 87.5% Fat

Moderate
- 45% Carbohydrate
- 55% Fat

Intense
- 67% Carbohydrate
- 33% Fat

◀ **FIGURE 3.6** Amounts of carbohydrate and fat used during light, moderate, and intense exercise.

Romijn, J. A., E. F. Coyle, L. S. Sidossis, A. Gastaldelli, J. F. Horowitz, E. Endert, and R. R. Wolfe. 1993. Regulation of endogenous fat and carbohydrate metabolism in relation to exercise intensity and duration, from the *American Journal of Physiological Endocrinology and Metabolism*, vol. 265, no. 3, Sept. 1993. Copyright © 1993 the American Physiological Society. Reprinted by permission.

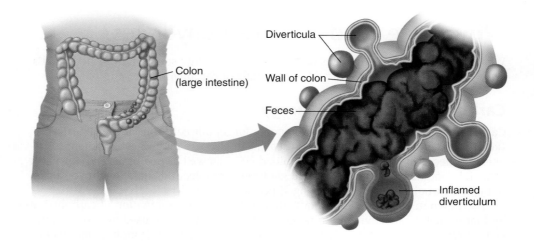

▶ **FIGURE 3.7** Diverticulosis occurs when bulging pockets form in the wall of the large intestine (colon). These pockets become infected and inflamed, demanding proper treatment.

Fiber-Rich Carbohydrates Have Health Benefits

A diet rich in fiber may reduce the risk for gastrointestinal diseases, such as colon cancer, and help prevent hemorrhoids, constipation, and similar problems by keeping stools moist and soft. Fiber gives gut muscles "something to push on" and makes it easier to eliminate stools. For the same reason, fiber reduces the risk for *diverticulosis*, a condition that is caused in part by trying to eliminate small, hard stools. A great deal of pressure must be generated in the large intestine (colon) to pass hard stools. This increased pressure weakens intestinal walls, causing them to bulge outward and form pockets **(FIGURE 3.7)**. Feces and fibrous materials can get trapped in these pockets, which become infected and inflamed. Diverticulitis is a painful condition that must be treated with antibiotics or surgery.

Other health benefits of eating fiber-rich carbohydrates include:

- Reduced overall risk for obesity. Eating a high-fiber diet causes a person to feel fuller, which may help people eat less and maintain a more healthful weight.
- Reduced risk for heart disease. Fiber can delay or block the absorption of dietary cholesterol into the bloodstream.
- Decreased risk for type 2 diabetes. Fiber absorbs water, expands in the large intestine, and slows the movement of food through the upper part of the digestive tract. In slowing digestion, fiber also slows the release of glucose into the blood and may thereby lower the risk for type 2 diabetes (discussed in detail later in this chapter).

recap Carbohydrates are an excellent energy source while we are at rest and during exercise, and they provide 4 kcal of energy per gram. Carbohydrates are necessary in the diet to "spare" body protein. Complex carbohydrates contain fiber and phytochemicals that can reduce the risk for obesity, heart disease, diabetes, colon cancer, and other health problems.

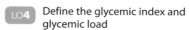 Explain how carbohydrates are digested and absorbed by our body

LO4 Define the glycemic index and glycemic load

What happens to the carbohydrates we eat?

Because glucose is the form of sugar that our body uses for energy, the primary goal of carbohydrate digestion is to break down polysaccharides and disaccharides into monosaccharides, which can then be converted to glucose. (Chapter 2 provided an overview of digestion.) Here, we focus in more detail on the digestion and absorption of carbohydrates. **FIGURE 3.8** provides a visual tour of carbohydrate digestion.

The primary goal of carbohydrate digestion is to break down polysaccharides and disaccharides into monosaccharides that can then be converted to glucose.

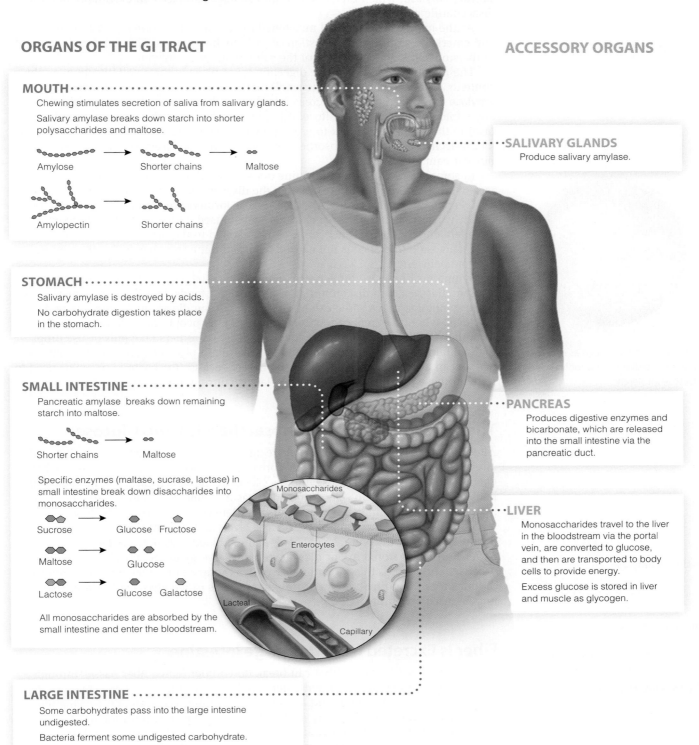

ORGANS OF THE GI TRACT

MOUTH

Chewing stimulates secretion of saliva from salivary glands.

Salivary amylase breaks down starch into shorter polysaccharides and maltose.

Amylose → Shorter chains → Maltose

Amylopectin → Shorter chains

STOMACH

Salivary amylase is destroyed by acids.

No carbohydrate digestion takes place in the stomach.

SMALL INTESTINE

Pancreatic amylase breaks down remaining starch into maltose.

Shorter chains → Maltose

Specific enzymes (maltase, sucrase, lactase) in small intestine break down disaccharides into monosaccharides.

Sucrose → Glucose Fructose

Maltose → Glucose

Lactose → Glucose Galactose

All monosaccharides are absorbed by the small intestine and enter the bloodstream.

LARGE INTESTINE

Some carbohydrates pass into the large intestine undigested.

Bacteria ferment some undigested carbohydrate.

Remaining fiber is excreted in feces.

ACCESSORY ORGANS

SALIVARY GLANDS

Produce salivary amylase.

PANCREAS

Produces digestive enzymes and bicarbonate, which are released into the small intestine via the pancreatic duct.

LIVER

Monosaccharides travel to the liver in the bloodstream via the portal vein, are converted to glucose, and then are transported to body cells to provide energy.

Excess glucose is stored in liver and muscle as glycogen.

Monosaccharides

Enterocytes

Lacteal

Capillary

Digestion Breaks Down Most Carbohydrates into Monosaccharides

Carbohydrate digestion begins in the mouth (see Figure 3.8). The starch in the foods you eat mixes with your saliva during chewing. Saliva contains an enzyme called **salivary amylase**, which breaks starch into smaller particles and eventually into the disaccharide maltose.

As the mass of chewed and moistened food (called the *bolus*) leaves the mouth and enters the stomach, all digestion of carbohydrates stops. This is because the acid in the stomach inactivates most of the salivary amylase enzyme.

The majority of carbohydrate digestion takes place in the small intestine. As the contents of the stomach enter the small intestine, an enzyme called **pancreatic amylase** is released by the pancreas into the small intestine. This enzyme digests any remaining starch into maltose. Additional enzymes (maltase, sucrase, and lactase) in the enterocytes work to break down disaccharides into monosaccharides. All monosaccharides are then absorbed into the enterocytes, from which they enter the bloodstream.

In some people, the small intestine does not produce enough of the enzyme lactase, which is necessary to break down the disaccharide lactose, found in milk products. People with this condition, called **lactose intolerance**, cannot digest dairy foods properly. Lactose intolerance should not be confused with a milk allergy: people who are allergic to milk experience an immune reaction to the proteins found in cow's milk. Lactose intolerance is not caused by an immune response but, rather, by an enzyme deficiency.

Symptoms of lactose intolerance include intestinal gas, bloating, cramping, nausea, diarrhea, and discomfort after eating dairy foods. Not everyone experiences these symptoms to the same extent. Some people can digest small amounts of dairy products, whereas others cannot tolerate any. Many people can tolerate specially formulated milk products that are low in lactose, but others take pills or use drops that contain the lactase enzyme when they eat dairy products. Some lactose-intolerant people can also digest yogurt and aged cheese, because the bacteria or molds used to ferment these products break down the lactose during processing.

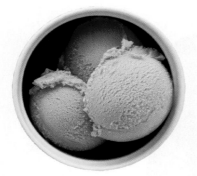

▲ Milk products, such as ice cream, are hard to digest for people who are lactose intolerant.

The Liver Converts All Monosaccharides into Glucose

After they are absorbed into the bloodstream, monosaccharides travel to the liver, where any non-glucose monosaccharides are converted to glucose. If needed immediately for energy, the liver releases glucose into the bloodstream, which carries it throughout the body to provide energy to cells. If the body has no immediate demand for glucose, it is stored as glycogen in the liver and muscles. Between meals, the body draws on liver glycogen reserves to maintain blood glucose levels and support the needs of cells, including those of the brain, spinal cord, and red blood cells (**FIGURE 3.9**).

The glycogen stored in our muscles provides energy to the muscles during intense exercise. Endurance athletes can increase their storage of muscle glycogen from two to four times the normal amount through a process called *glycogen loading*, also known as *carbohydrate loading* (see Chapter 10).

Fiber Is Excreted from the Large Intestine

We do not possess enzymes that can break down fiber. Thus, fiber passes through the small intestine undigested and enters the large intestine, or colon. There, bacteria break down the soluble fiber and any previously undigested starches, causing the production of gas and a few fatty acids. The cells of the large intestine use these fatty acids for energy. The fiber remaining in the colon adds bulk to stools and is excreted in feces. In this way, fiber helps to maintain bowel regularity.

salivary amylase An enzyme in saliva that breaks starch into smaller particles and eventually into the disaccharide maltose.

pancreatic amylase An enzyme secreted by the pancreas into the small intestine that digests any remaining starch into maltose.

lactose intolerance A disorder in which the body does not produce sufficient lactase enzyme and therefore cannot digest foods that contain lactose, such as cow's milk.

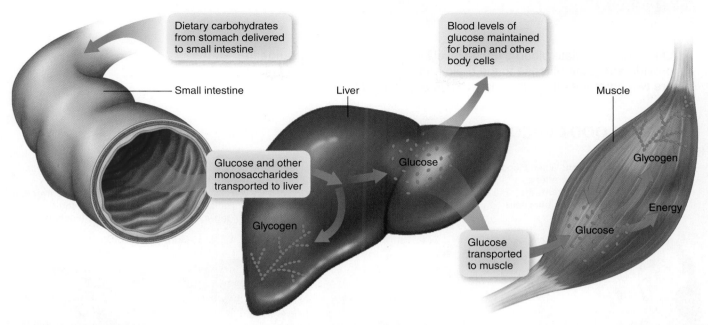

Dietary carbohydrates from stomach delivered to small intestine

Small intestine

Glucose and other monosaccharides transported to liver

Glycogen

Liver

Glucose

Glycogen

Blood levels of glucose maintained for brain and other body cells

Glucose transported to muscle

Muscle

Glycogen

Energy

Glucose

▲ **FIGURE 3.9**   Glucose is stored as glycogen in both the liver and in muscle. The glycogen stored in the liver maintains blood glucose between meals; muscle glycogen provides immediate energy to the muscle during exercise.

recap   Carbohydrate digestion starts in the mouth and continues in the small intestine. Glucose and other monosaccharides are absorbed into the bloodstream and travel to the liver, where non-glucose sugars are converted to glucose. Glucose is either used by the cells for energy or is converted to glycogen and stored in the liver and muscle for later use. Lactose intolerance results from the inability to digest lactose due to insufficient amounts of lactase. Insoluble fiber adds bulk to stools.

Insulin and Glucagon Regulate the Level of Glucose in Blood

Our body continually regulates the level of glucose in the blood within a fairly narrow range that meets the body's needs. Two hormones, insulin and glucagon, assist the body in maintaining blood glucose. Special cells in the pancreas synthesize, store, and secrete both hormones.

When we eat a meal, our blood glucose level rises. However, glucose in the blood cannot help nerve, muscle, and other cells function unless it can cross into them. Glucose molecules are too large to cross cell membranes independently. To get in, glucose needs assistance from the hormone **insulin**, which is secreted by the beta cells of the pancreas (**FIGURE 3.10a**). Insulin increases the movement of proteins, called *glucose transporters*, from the inside of the cell to the cell membrane; these transporters allow glucose to enter the cell. Insulin also stimulates the liver and muscles to take up glucose and store it as glycogen.

When you have not eaten for some time, your blood glucose levels decline. This decrease in blood glucose stimulates the alpha cells of the pancreas to secrete another hormone, **glucagon** (**FIGURE 3.10b**). Glucagon acts in an opposite way to insulin: it causes the liver to convert its stored glycogen into glucose, which is then secreted into the bloodstream and transported to the cells for energy. Glucagon also assists in the breakdown of body proteins, so that the liver can stimulate *gluconeogenesis*, discussed earlier.

insulin A hormone secreted by the beta cells of the pancreas in response to increased blood levels of glucose; facilitates uptake of glucose by body cells.

glucagon A hormone secreted by the alpha cells of the pancreas in response to decreased blood levels of glucose; causes breakdown of liver stores of glycogen into glucose.

Our bodies regulate blood glucose levels within a fairly narrow range to provide adequate glucose to the brain and other cells. Insulin and glucagon are two hormones that play a key role in regulating blood glucose.

HIGH BLOOD GLUCOSE

(a)

1 **Insulin secretion:** When blood glucose levels increase after a meal, the pancreas secretes the hormone insulin from the beta cells into the bloodstream.

2 **Cellular uptake:** Insulin travels to the tissues. There, it stimulates glucose transporters within cells to travel to the cell membrane, where they facilitate glucose transport into the cell to be used for energy.

3 **Glucose storage:** Insulin also stimulates the storage of glucose in body tissues. Glucose is stored as glycogen in the liver and muscles (glycogenesis), and is stored as triglycerides in adipose tissue (lipogenesis).

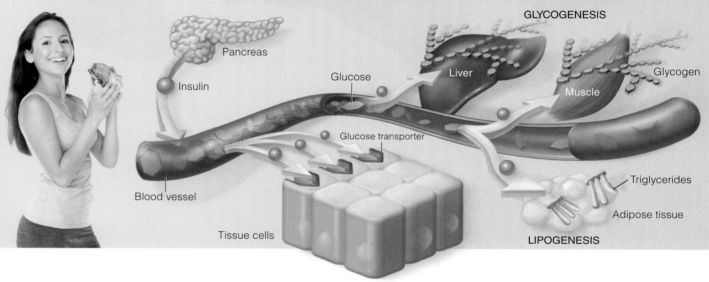

GLYCOGENESIS
Pancreas
Insulin
Glucose
Liver
Muscle
Glycogen
Glucose transporter
Blood vessel
Triglycerides
Adipose tissue
Tissue cells
LIPOGENESIS

LOW BLOOD GLUCOSE

(b)

1 **Glucagon secretion:** When blood glucose levels are low, the pancreas secretes the hormone glucagon from the alpha cells into the bloodstream.

2 **Glycogenolysis:** Glucagon stimulates the liver to convert stored glycogen into glucose, which is released into the blood and transported to the cells for energy.

3 **Gluconeogenesis:** Glucagon also assists in the breakdown of proteins and the uptake of amino acids by the liver, which creates glucose from amino acids.

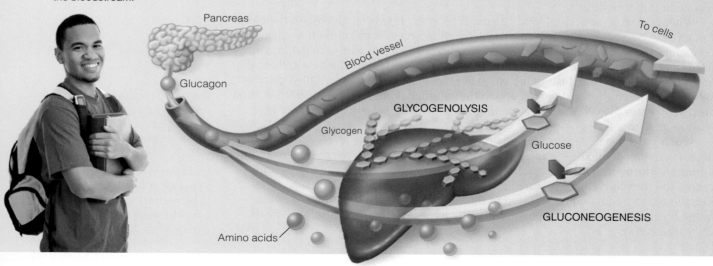

Pancreas
To cells
Glucagon
Blood vessel
GLYCOGENOLYSIS
Glycogen
Glucose
GLUCONEOGENESIS
Amino acids

Typically, the effects of insulin and glucagon balance each other to maintain blood glucose within a healthy range. If this balance is altered, it can lead to negative health conditions such as diabetes or hypoglycemia. In **hypoglycemia**, blood glucose falls to lower-than-normal levels. One cause of hypoglycemia is excessive production of insulin, which lowers blood glucose too far. The symptoms usually appear about 1 to 3 hours after a meal and include nervousness, shakiness, anxiety, sweating, irritability, headache, weakness, and rapid or irregular heartbeat. Although many people believe they experience these symptoms, true hypoglycemia is rare. People with diabetes can develop hypoglycemia if they inject too much insulin or when they exercise and fail to eat enough carbohydrates. It can also be caused by a pancreatic tumor, liver infection, or other underlying disorder.

recap Two hormones, insulin and glucagon, are involved in regulating blood glucose. Insulin lowers blood glucose levels by facilitating the entry of glucose into cells. Glucagon raises blood glucose levels by stimulating gluconeogenesis and the breakdown of glycogen stored in the liver. Hypoglycemia is a condition characterized by lower-than-normal blood glucose level.

The Glycemic Index Shows How Foods Affect Our Blood Glucose Levels

The **glycemic index** is a measurement of the potential of foods to raise blood glucose levels. Foods with a high glycemic index cause a sudden spike in blood glucose. This in turn triggers a surge in insulin, which may be followed by a dramatic drop in blood glucose. Foods with a low glycemic index cause low to moderate fluctuations in blood glucose. When foods are assigned a glycemic index value, they are often compared with the glycemic effect of pure glucose.

The glycemic index of a food is not always easy to predict. **FIGURE 3.11** ranks certain foods according to their glycemic index. Do any of these rankings surprise you?

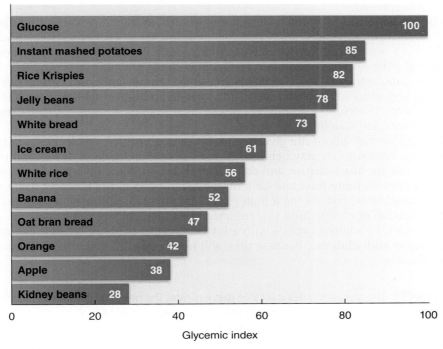

Food	Glycemic index
Glucose	100
Instant mashed potatoes	85
Rice Krispies	82
Jelly beans	78
White bread	73
Ice cream	61
White rice	56
Banana	52
Oat bran bread	47
Orange	42
Apple	38
Kidney beans	28

◆ FIGURE 3.11 Glycemic index values for various foods as compared with pure glucose.

Data from Foster-Powell, K., S. H. A. Holt, and J. C. Brand-Miller. 2002. International table of glycemic index and glycemic load values. *Am. J. Clin. Nutr.* 76: 5–56.

hypoglycemia A condition marked by blood glucose levels that are below normal fasting levels.

glycemic index A value that rates the potential of a given food to raise blood glucose and insulin levels.

foods you don't know you love YET

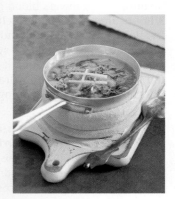

Dhal

Have you heard of dhal? If you enjoy foods from India, Pakistan, Nepal, Sri Lanka, or Bangladesh, you've probably tried it. If not, it's time to find out about this healthy dish! Dhal (also spelled *dal*, *dahl*, or *daal*) is a spicy dish traditionally made with lentils, dried peas, or beans that have been stripped of their outer hull. The processed legumes themselves are also referred to as dhal. They've been used in foods since prehistoric times and are high in protein and fiber, with a low glycemic index.

Like dry beans, most varieties of dhal are cooked slowly in water for 30–60 minutes. A variety of spices, as well as tomatoes, onions, and other vegetables, can be added, and the resulting fragrant dish—the consistency of a thick soup—is typically served with rice or breads, such as chapatti or naan.

Most people assume that foods containing simple sugars have a higher glycemic index than starches, but this is not the only factor involved. The presence of other components in the food, including dietary fiber, and the food form and particle size, also play a role. For instance, compare the glycemic index for apples and instant mashed potatoes. Although instant potatoes are a starchy food, they have a glycemic index value of 85, whereas the value for an apple is only 38! Nutritious, low-glycemic-index foods include beans and lentils, fresh vegetables and fruits, and whole-wheat bread.

The **glycemic load** of a food is the amount of carbohydrate it contains multiplied by its glycemic index value (number). Some nutrition experts believe that the glycemic load is a better indicator than the glycemic index value of the effect of food on a person's glucose response, because it factors in both the glycemic index and the total grams of carbohydrate in the food that is consumed. For instance, raw carrots have a relatively high glycemic index but very little total carbohydrate and thus have a low glycemic load. Therefore, a serving of raw carrots is unlikely to cause a significant rise in glucose and insulin.

Why do we care about the glycemic load? Among healthy people, consuming a low-glycemic-load diet may help maintain healthy blood glucose levels and reduce the risk for heart disease and colon cancer, because low-glycemic-load foods generally contain more fiber and help decrease fat levels in the blood.[4,5] Among endurance athletes, consuming a high-glycemic-load meal following a vigorous training session or competition can enhance the replenishment of glycogen in their muscles. In addition, meals with a lower glycemic load are a better choice for someone with diabetes, because they will not trigger dramatic fluctuations in blood glucose.

To find out the glycemic index and glycemic load of over 100 foods, visit www.health.harvard.edu and type in "glycemic index" into the search box.

glycemic load The amount of carbohydrate contained in a given food, multiplied by its glycemic index value.

recap The glycemic index is a value that indicates the potential of foods to raise blood glucose and insulin levels. The glycemic load of a food is the amount of carbohydrate it contains multiplied by its glycemic index value (number).

How much carbohydrate should we eat?

Carbohydrates are an important part of a balanced, healthy diet. The Recommended Dietary Allowance (RDA) for carbohydrate is based on the amount of glucose the brain uses.[6] The current RDA for carbohydrate for adults age 19 and older is 130 grams per day. It is important to emphasize that this RDA does not cover the amount of carbohydrate needed to support daily activities; it covers only the amount of carbohydrate needed to supply adequate glucose to the brain.

As we mentioned earlier (in Chapter 1), carbohydrates and the other macronutrients are also assigned an Acceptable Macronutrient Distribution Range (AMDR). This is the intake range associated with a decreased risk for chronic diseases. The AMDR for carbohydrates is 45% to 65% of total energy intake. **TABLE 3.2** compares the carbohydrate recommendations from the Institute of Medicine with the *Dietary Guidelines for Americans* related to carbohydrate-containing foods.[3,6] As you can see, the Institute of Medicine provides specific numeric recommendations, whereas the *Dietary Guidelines for Americans* are general suggestions for foods high in whole grains and fiber and low in refined grains and added sugars. Most health agencies agree that most of the carbohydrates you eat each day should be fiber rich and unprocessed. Eating the recommended amount of whole grains and fruits and vegetables every day will ensure that you get enough fiber and other complex carbohydrates that your body needs.

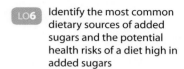
LO5 Identify the RDA and the AMDR for carbohydrates, and the AI for fiber

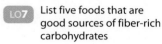
LO6 Identify the most common dietary sources of added sugars and the potential health risks of a diet high in added sugars

LO7 List five foods that are good sources of fiber-rich carbohydrates

> **recap** The RDA for carbohydrate is 130 grams per day; this amount is only sufficient to supply adequate glucose to the brain. The AMDR for carbohydrate is 45% to 65% of total energy intake.

Most Americans Eat Too Much Refined Carbohydrate

On average, half of the Calories that Americans consume daily come from carbohydrates. And for some people, most of these carbohydrates consist of simple sugars. Some of this sugar comes from healthful food sources, such as fruits and milk. Some comes from foods made with refined grains, such as soft white breads and saltine crackers. Much of the rest comes from **added sugars**—that is, sugars and syrups that are added to foods during processing or preparation.[6] For example, many processed foods include high-fructose corn syrup (HFCS), an added sugar.

The most common source of added sugars in the U.S. diet is sodas and soft drinks; we drink an average of 40 gallons per person each year. If you drink this average amount, you consume more than 16,420 grams of sugar (about 267 cups) every year.

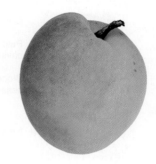
◄ Eating the recommended amount of whole grains, vegetables, and fruit each day ensures that you'll get enough fiber and other complex carbohydrates in your diet.

added sugars Sugars and syrups that are added to food during processing or preparation.

TABLE 3.2 Dietary Recommendations for Carbohydrates

Institute of Medicine Recommendations*	Dietary Guidelines for Americans†
Recommended Dietary Allowance (RDA) for adults 19 years of age and older is 130 grams of carbohydrate per day.	Increase vegetable and fruit intake.
	Eat a variety of vegetables, especially dark-green and red and orange vegetables and beans and peas.
The Acceptable Macronutrient Distribution Range (AMDR) for carbohydrate is 45% to 65% of total daily energy intake.	Consume at least half of all grains as whole grains. Increase whole-grain intake by replacing refined grains with whole grains.
Added sugar intake should be 25% or less of total energy intake each day.	Limit the consumption of foods that contain refined grains, especially refined-grain foods that contain solid fats, added sugars, and sodium.
	Reduce intake of sugar-sweetened beverages.
	Monitor intake of 100% fruit juice for children and adolescents, especially those who are overweight or obese.

*Data from Dietary Reference Intakes for Energy, Carbohydrates, Fiber, Fat, Fatty Acids, Cholesterol, Protein, and Amino Acids (Macronutrients). © 2005, National Academy of Sciences, courtesy of the National Academies Press, Washington, DC.
†U.S. Department of Agriculture and U.S. Department of Health and Human Services. 2010. *Dietary Guidelines for Americans, 2010*. 7th ed. Washington, DC: U.S. Government Printing Office.

That's a lot of sugar! Other common sources of added sugars include cookies, cakes, pies, fruit drinks, fruit punches, and candy. Even many non-dessert items, such as peanut butter, yogurt, and even salad dressing, contain added sugars.

If you want a quick way to figure out the amount of sugar in a processed food, check the Nutrition Facts panel on the box for the line that identifies "Sugars." You'll notice that the amount of sugar in a serving is identified in grams. Divide the total grams by 4 to get teaspoons. For instance, one national brand of yogurt contains 21 grams of sugar in a half-cup serving. That's more than 5 teaspoons of sugar! Doing this simple math before you buy may help you choose between different, more healthful versions of the same food.

Added sugars are not chemically different from naturally occurring sugars. However, foods and beverages with added sugars do have lower levels of vitamins, minerals, and fiber than fruits and other foods that naturally contain sugars. That's why most health-care organizations recommend that we limit our consumption of added sugars.

The Atkins Diet and many other diet plans blame sugar for a variety of health problems, from tooth decay to hyperactivity to obesity. Does sugar deserve its bad reputation? Let's examine the facts behind the accusations.

Sugar Causes Tooth Decay

Simple carbohydrates, both naturally occurring and in processed foods, play a clear role in dental problems, because the bacteria that cause tooth decay thrive on them. These bacteria produce acids that eat away at tooth enamel and can eventually cause cavities and gum disease (**FIGURE 3.12**).

Eating sticky foods that cling to teeth, such as caramels, crackers, pretzels, breads, sugary cereals, marshmallows, and licorice, and sipping sweetened beverages over a given time period, increase the risk for tooth decay. Babies should not be put to sleep with a bottle in their mouth unless it contains water. As we have seen, even breast milk contains sugar, which can slowly drip onto the baby's gums. As a result, infants should not be routinely allowed to fall asleep at their mother's breast.

To reduce your risk for tooth decay, brush your teeth after every meal and especially after drinking sugary drinks or after eating candy and other sticky foods. Drinking fluoridated water and using a fluoride toothpaste will also help protect your teeth.

There Is No Proven Link Between Sugar and Hyperactivity in Children

Although many people believe that eating sugar causes hyperactivity and other behavioral problems in children, there is little scientific evidence to support this claim. Some children actually become *less* active shortly after a high-sugar meal! However, it is important to emphasize that most studies of sugar and children's behavior have only looked at the effects of sugar a few hours after ingestion. We know very little about the long-term effects of sugar intake on the behavior of children. Behavioral and learning problems are complex issues, most likely caused by a multitude of factors. Because of this complexity, the Institute of Medicine has stated that, overall, there currently does not appear to be enough evidence to suggest that eating too much sugar causes hyperactivity or other behavioral problems in children.[6] Thus, a Tolerable Upper Intake Level for sugar has not been set.

High Sugar Intake Can Lead to Unhealthful Levels of Blood Lipids

Many low-carbohydrate diet plans claim that North Americans' overconsumption of simple sugars is partly responsible for our high rates of heart disease. Is this claim valid? Research evidence does suggest that consuming a diet high in added sugars is associated with unhealthful changes in blood lipids.[7] (You will learn more about blood lipids, including cholesterol and lipoproteins, in Chapter 4.) For example, higher intakes of added sugars are associated with higher levels of blood lipids that contribute to heart disease and associated with lower levels of blood lipids that are considered protective against heart disease. Two recent studies have shown that people who consume sugar-sweetened beverages have an increased risk of heart disease.[8,9] Although these recent findings don't provide enough evidence to prove that eating a diet high in sugar directly causes higher levels of heart disease, they do suggest that it is prudent to eat a diet low in added sugars. Because added sugars are a component of many processed foods and beverages, careful label reading is advised.

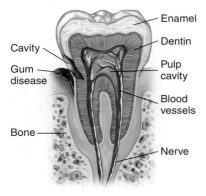

FIGURE 3.12 Eating simple carbohydrates can cause an increase in cavities and gum disease. This is because bacteria in the mouth consume simple carbohydrates present on the teeth and gums and produce acids, which eat away at these tissues.

High Sugar Intake Is Associated with Diabetes and Obesity

Recent studies suggest that eating a diet high in added sugars is associated with a higher risk for diabetes; this relationship is particularly strong between higher intakes of sugar-sweetened beverages and diabetes.[10-12] A recent study examined the relationship between diabetes and sugar intake across 175 countries and found that for every 150 kcal per person per day increase in availability of sugar (equivalent to about one can of soft drink per day), the prevalence of diabetes increased by 1.1%.[13] Although the exact mechanisms explaining this relationship are not clear, experts have speculated that the dramatic increase in glucose and insulin levels that occur when we consume high amounts of rapidly absorbable carbohydrates (which includes any forms of sugar or high-fructose corn syrup) may stimulate appetite, increase food intake, and promote weight gain, which increases our risk for diabetes. High-fructose corn syrup in particular has negative effects on how we metabolize and store body fat; this can lead to us being more resistant to the normal actions of insulin and increase our risk for diabetes.[14]

There is also evidence linking sugar intake with obesity. For example, a recent systematic review of various studies found that reducing intake of sugars in adults results in weight loss, and increasing intake of sugars results in weight gain.[15] This increase in weight is due to the excess Calorie intake and not due to the sugars per se. This same review found that children who consume one or more servings of sugar-sweetened beverages per day had a 1.55 times higher risk of being overweight than those children consuming none or very little.

We know that if you consume more energy than you expend, you will gain weight. It makes intuitive sense that people who consume extra energy from high-sugar foods are at risk for obesity, just like people who consume extra energy from fat or protein. In addition to the increased potential for obesity, another major concern about high-sugar diets is that they tend to be low in nutrient density because the intake of high-sugar foods tends to replace that of more nutritious foods. The relationship between added sugars and obesity is highly controversial and will likely be the focus of research for years to come.

> To watch a CBS News video on the HFCS controversy, visit www.cbsnews.com. Search for the video, "High Fructose Corn Syrup," in the search box and click on the video.

recap Added sugars include sucrose, high-fructose corn syrup, and other sugars and syrups added to foods during processing or preparation. Sugar causes tooth decay but does not appear to cause hyperactivity in children. Higher intakes of simple sugars are associated with increases in unhealthful blood lipids and increased risks for heart disease, diabetes, and obesity.

Most Americans Eat Too Little Fiber-Rich Carbohydrate

If you're like most people in the United States, you eat only about 2 servings of fruits or vegetables daily, which is far below the amount recommended in the USDA Food Plans. Do you eat whole grains every day? Many people eat lots of breads, pastas, and cereals, but most don't consistently choose whole-grain products. As we explained earlier, whole-grain foods have a lower glycemic index and provide more fiber than foods made with enriched flour.

We Need at Least 25 Grams of Fiber Daily

How much fiber do we need? The Adequate Intake for fiber is 25 grams per day for women and 38 grams per day for men, or 14 grams of fiber for every 1,000 kcal per day that a person eats.[6] Most people in the United States eat only 12 to 18 grams of fiber each day, getting only half of the fiber they need. Although fiber supplements are available, it is *best to get fiber from food* because foods contain additional nutrients, such as vitamins and minerals.

Eating the amounts of whole grains, legumes and other vegetables, fruits, and nuts recommended in the USDA Food Patterns will ensure that you eat adequate fiber. **FIGURE 3.13** lists some common foods and their fiber content. Think about how you can design your own diet to include high-fiber foods.

It is also important to drink more water as you increase your fiber intake, because fiber binds with water to soften stools. Inadequate water intake with a high-fiber diet can result in hard, dry stools that are difficult to pass through the colon. Thus, eating a high-fiber diet without consuming adequate water can result in constipation.

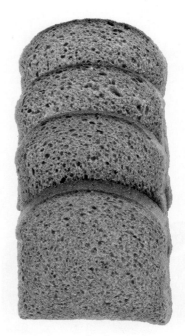

Whole-grain foods provide more nutrients and fiber than foods made with enriched flour.

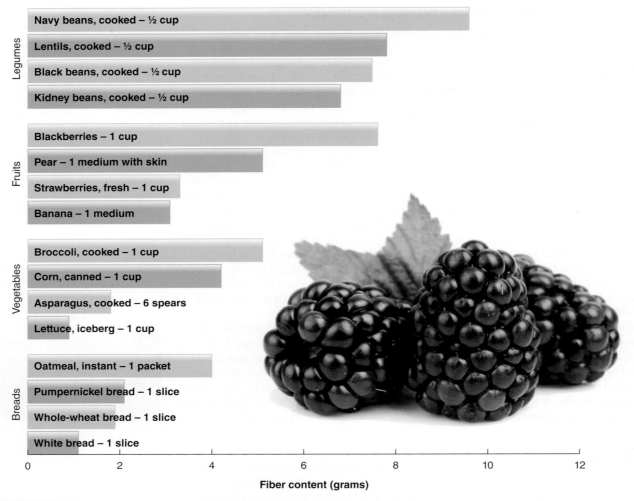

FIGURE 3.13 Fiber content of common foods. *Note:* The Adequate Intake for fiber is 25 grams per day for women and 38 grams per day for men.

Data from U.S. Department of Agriculture, Agricultural Research Service. 2013. USDA National Nutrient Database for Standard Reference, Release 26. Nutrient Data Laboratory Home Page, www.ars.usda.gov/ba/bhnrc/ndl.

Excessive Fiber Intake

Can you eat too much fiber? Excessive fiber consumption can lead to problems such as the following:

- Intestinal gas and bloating.
- Dehydration: because fiber binds with water, it causes the body to eliminate more water, so a very-high-fiber diet can result in dehydration.
- Reduced absorption of certain nutrients: because fiber binds many vitamins and minerals, a high-fiber diet can reduce the absorption of important nutrients, such as iron, zinc, and calcium.
- Malnutrition in groups such as children, some elderly, the chronically ill, and other at-risk populations: in these groups, excess fiber intake can lead to malnutrition, because they feel full before they have eaten enough to provide adequate energy and nutrients.

If you want to increase the amount of fiber you consume each day, go slowly, giving your system time to adjust. Otherwise, you might experience some of the symptoms of excessive fiber consumption. To avoid stressing your body, check out the ***Game Plan*** for tips on increasing your fiber intake one step at a time.

To see a vast menu of high-fiber choices for each meal of the day, and find out how much fiber the foods you eat provide, visit www.webmd.com. Type in "fiber meter" in the search box, then select the Health Tool Fiber-O-Meter link to begin.

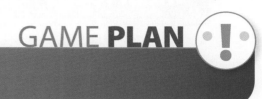

GAME **PLAN**

Tips for Increasing Your Fiber Intake One Step at a Time

Gradually increasing your fiber intake gives your gastrointestinal organs time to adjust to the increased bulk in your diet. This is especially important if you've been eating a very-low-fiber diet (fewer than 10 grams of fiber per day) for many years. Here's how to increase your fiber intake one step at a time:

Step 1 Incorporate just one of the strategies listed below each day for 1 week.

Step 2 Make sure you drink plenty of fluids. The best way to make sure you're well hydrated is to track your output: if your urine is clear to pale yellow, you're getting enough fluid.

Step 3 Keep a record of your total daily fiber intake and of how you're feeling.

Step 4 If you adjust well to the increased fiber, then go ahead and incorporate two strategies a day the following week.

Step 5 Continue until you reach your optimal daily fiber intake.

Here are some strategies to choose from:

☐ Switch from a low-fiber breakfast cereal to one that has at least 4 grams of fiber per serving.

☐ Switch to whole-grain bread for morning toast or lunchtime sandwiches. Two slices of whole-grain bread provide 4–6 grams of fiber. (Check the Nutrition Facts Panel of the whole-grain bread you're using.)

☐ For a midmorning snack, mix 1–2 tablespoons of bran or whole ground flaxseed meal (4 grams of fiber) into a cup of low-fat yogurt. These products are available at most health-food stores and many large supermarkets.

☐ Instead of chips with your sandwich, have a side of carrot sticks or celery sticks (approximately 2 grams of fiber per serving).

☐ For an afternoon snack, choose an apple or a pear, with the skin on (approximately 5 grams of fiber). Or munch ¼ cup of almonds (4 grams of fiber).

☐ Eat 1 serving of beans or other legumes at dinner (approximately 6 grams of fiber).

☐ Don't forget the vegetables! A cup of boiled chopped okra or beet greens provides about 4 grams of fiber, and acorn squash a whopping 9 grams! Raw veggies are fiber-rich, too, so a large salad is a good source of fiber.

☐ For dessert, switch from cookies, cake, or ice cream to a serving of fresh, frozen, or dried fruit. A half cup of fresh or frozen blackberries or raspberries provides 4–5 grams of fiber, and a single ounce of dried mixed fruit (for example, prunes, apricots) provides 2 grams.

☐ For an evening snack, try a mixture of plain, air-popped popcorn, peanuts, and raisins: 1 cup of popcorn (1 gram of fiber) with ¼ cup of peanuts (3 grams) and ¼ cup of raisins (2 grams) provides a total of 6 grams of fiber.

If you incorporate these strategies and experience diarrhea, constipation, or excess intestinal gas, then your body may not be adjusting well to the increased fiber. Try cutting the serving size or incorporating a strategy only every other day. And make sure to drink plenty of fluids! Try this for 2 weeks; then increase gradually again.

Shopper's Guide: Hunting for Fiber

FIGURE 3.14 compares the food and fiber content of two diets: one high in fiber-rich carbohydrates and one high in refined carbohydrates. Here are some hints for selecting healthful carbohydrate sources:

- Select breads and cereals made with whole grains, such as wheat, oats, barley, and rye (make sure the label says *whole* before the word *grain*). Choose foods that have at least 2 to 3 grams of fiber per serving.
- Buy fresh fruits and vegetables whenever possible. When appropriate, eat foods such as potatoes, apples, and pears with the skin left on.
- Frozen vegetables and fruits can be a healthful alternative when fresh produce is not available. Check frozen selections to make sure there is no extra sugar or salt added.

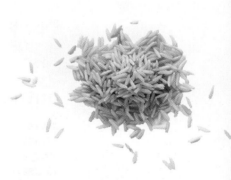

◀ Brown rice is a good food source of dietary fiber.

a day of meals

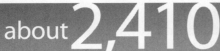

about **2,410** calories (kcal)

about **2,182** calories (kcal)

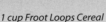

BREAKFAST

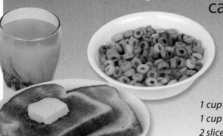

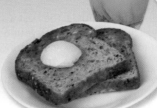
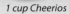

1 cup Froot Loops Cereal
1 cup skim milk
2 slices of white bread with
1 tbsp of butter
8 fl. oz orange juice

1 cup Cheerios
1 cup skim milk
1 medium banana
2 slices whole-wheat toast with
1 tbsp light margarine
8 fl. oz orange juice

LUNCH

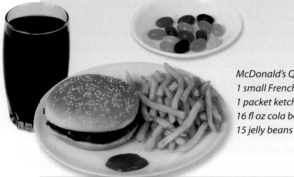

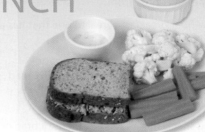

McDonald's Quarter Pounder
1 small French Fries
1 packet ketchup
16 fl oz cola beverage
15 jelly beans

Tuna Sandwich with:
2 slices of whole wheat bread
3 oz tuna packed in water,
drained
1 tsp Dijon mustard
1 tbsp reduced-calorie
mayonnaise
1 large carrot, sliced
1 cup raw cauliflower
2 tbsp fat-free ranch dressing
8 fl oz non-fat fruit yogurt

DINNER

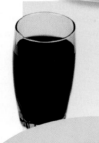
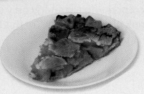
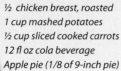
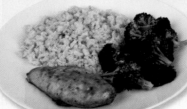

½ chicken breast, roasted
1 cup mashed potatoes
½ cup sliced cooked carrots
12 fl oz cola beverage
Apple pie (1/8 of 9-inch pie)

1/2 chicken breast, roasted
1 cup brown rice
1 cup steamed broccoli
Spinach salad:
1 cup chopped spinach
1 boiled egg
2 slices turkey bacon
3 cherry tomatoes
2 tbsp cream poppyseed
dressing
1 cup fresh blueberries with
½ cup whipped cream
8 fl oz cranberry juice

nutrient analysis

nutrient analysis

2,410 kcal
58.3% of energy from carbohydrates
29.2% of energy from fat
12.5% of energy from protein
15.6 grams of dietary fiber

Double the fiber intake!

2,181 kcal
58.5% of energy from carbohydrates
22.3% of energy from fat
19.2% of energy from protein
32 grams of dietary fiber

- Be careful when buying canned fruits and vegetables, because many are high in sodium and added sugar. Foods that are packed in their own juice are more healthful than those packed in syrup.
- Eat legumes frequently—every day if possible. Canned or fresh beans, peas, and lentils are excellent sources of complex carbohydrates, fiber, vitamins, and minerals. Add them to soups, casseroles, and other recipes—it's an easy way to eat more of them. If you're trying to consume less sodium, rinse canned beans to remove extra salt or choose low-sodium alternatives.

recap The Adequate Intake for fiber is 25 grams per day for women and 38 grams per day for men. Most Americans eat only half of the fiber they need each day. Foods high in fiber include whole grains and cereals, fruits, some nuts, and legumes and other vegetables. The more processed the food, the less fiber it is likely to contain.

What's the story on alternative sweeteners?

 Compare and contrast a variety of alternative sweeteners

Most of us love sweets but want to avoid the extra Calories and tooth decay that go along with them. Remember that all carbohydrates, whether simple or complex, contain 4 kcal of energy per gram. Because sweeteners such as sucrose, fructose, honey, and brown sugar contribute energy, they are called **nutritive sweeteners**.

Other nutritive sweeteners include the *sugar alcohols* such as mannitol, sorbitol, isomalt, and xylitol. Popular in sugar-free gums, mints, and diabetic candies, sugar alcohols are less sweet than sucrose. Foods with sugar alcohols have health benefits that foods made with sugars do not have, such as a reduced glycemic response and decreased risk of dental caries. Also, because sugar alcohols are absorbed slowly and incompletely from the intestine, they provide less energy than sugar, usually 2 to 3 kcal of energy per gram. However, because they are not completely absorbed from the intestine, they can attract water into the large intestine and cause diarrhea.

A number of other products have been developed to sweeten foods without promoting tooth decay and weight gain. Because these products provide little or no energy, they are called **non-nutritive,** or *alternative*, **sweeteners**.

Limited Use of Alternative Sweeteners Is Not Harmful

Research has shown alternative sweeteners to be safe for adults, children, and individuals with diabetes. Women who are pregnant should discuss the use of alternative sweeteners with their healthcare provider. In general, it appears safe for pregnant women to consume alternative sweeteners in amounts within the Food and Drug Administration (FDA) guidelines.[16] These amounts, known as the **Acceptable Daily Intake (ADI)**, are estimates of the amount of a sweetener that someone can consume each day over a lifetime without adverse effects. The estimates are based on studies conducted on laboratory animals, and they include a 100-fold safety factor. It is important to emphasize that actual intake by humans is typically well below the ADI.

Saccharin

Discovered in the late 1800s, *saccharin* is about 300 times sweeter than sucrose. Concerns arose in the 1970s that saccharin could cause cancer; however, more than 20 years of subsequent research failed to link saccharin to cancer in humans. Based on this evidence, in May 2000 the National Toxicology Program of the U.S. government removed saccharin from its list of products that may cause cancer. No ADI has been set for saccharin, and it is used in foods and beverages and as a tabletop sweetener. It is sold as Sweet n' Low (also known as "the pink packet") in the United States.

Acesulfame-K

Acesulfame-K (acesulfame potassium) is marketed under the names Sunette and Sweet One. It is a Calorie-free sweetener that is 200 times sweeter than sugar. It is

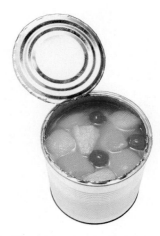

◆ Check to make sure that canned fruits are packed in their own juices, not syrup.

nutritive sweeteners Sweeteners, such as sucrose, fructose, honey, and brown sugar, that contribute calories (energy).

non-nutritive sweeteners Manufactured sweeteners that provide little or no energy; also called *alternative sweeteners*.

Acceptable Daily Intake (ADI) An estimate made by the Food and Drug Administration of the amount of a non-nutritive sweetener that someone can consume each day over a lifetime without adverse effects.

used to sweeten gums, candies, beverages, instant tea, coffee, gelatins, and puddings. The taste of acesulfame-K does not change when it is heated, so it can be used in cooking. The body does not metabolize acesulfame-K, so it is excreted unchanged by the kidneys. The ADI for acesulfame-K is 15 mg per kg body weight per day. For example, the ADI in an adult weighing 150 pounds (or 68 kg) would be 1,020 mg.

Aspartame

Aspartame, also called Equal ("the blue packet") and NutraSweet, is one of the most popular alternative sweeteners currently in use. Aspartame is composed of two amino acids: phenylalanine and aspartic acid. When these amino acids are separate, one is bitter and the other has no flavor—but joined together, they make a substance that is 180 times sweeter than sucrose. Although aspartame contains 4 kcal of energy per gram, it is so sweet that only small amounts are used; thus, it ends up contributing little or no energy. Heat destroys the bonds that bind the two amino acids in aspartame. Thus, it cannot be used in cooking because it loses its sweetness.

Although there are numerous claims that aspartame causes headaches and dizziness, and can increase a person's risk for cancer and nerve disorders, studies do not support these claims.[17] A significant amount of research has been done to test the safety of aspartame.

The ADI for aspartame is 50 mg per kg body weight per day. For an adult weighing 150 pounds (or 68 kg), the ADI would be 3,400 mg. TABLE 3.3 shows how many servings of aspartame-sweetened foods would have to be consumed to exceed the ADI. Because the ADI is a very conservative estimate, it would be difficult for adults or children to exceed this amount of aspartame intake. However, drinks sweetened with aspartame, which are extremely popular among children and teenagers, are very low in nutritional value. They should not replace more healthful beverages such as milk and water.

There are some people who should not consume aspartame at all: those with the disease *phenylketonuria (PKU).* This is a genetic disorder that prevents the breakdown of the amino acid phenylalanine. Because the person with PKU cannot metabolize phenylalanine, it builds up to toxic levels in the tissues of the body and causes irreversible brain damage. In the United States, all newborn babies are tested for PKU; those who have it are placed on a phenylalanine-limited diet. Some foods that are common sources of protein and other nutrients for many growing children, such as meats and milk, contain phenylalanine. Thus, it is critical that children with PKU not waste what little phenylalanine they can consume on nutrient-poor products sweetened with aspartame.

TABLE 3.3 **The Amount of Food That a 50-lb Child and a 150-lb Adult Would Have to Consume Each Day to Exceed the ADI for Aspartame**

Food	50 lb Child	150 lb Adult
12 fl. oz carbonated soft drink	7	20
8 fl. oz powdered soft drink	11	34
4 fl. oz gelatin dessert	14	42
Packets of tabletop sweetener	32	97

Data from International Food Information Council. 2003. Food safety and nutrition information. Sweeteners. Everything you need to know about aspartame. www.foodinsight.org/Resources/Detail.aspx?topic=Everything_You_Need_to_Know_About_Aspartame.

Sucralose

Sucralose is marketed under the brand name Splenda and is known as "the yellow packet." It is made from sucrose, but chlorine atoms are substituted for the hydrogen and oxygen normally found in sucrose, and it passes through the digestive tract unchanged, without contributing any energy. It is 600 times sweeter than sucrose and is stable when heated, so it can be used in cooking. It has been approved for use in many foods, including chewing gum, salad dressings, beverages, gelatin and pudding products, canned fruits, frozen dairy desserts, and baked goods. Studies have shown sucralose to be safe. The ADI for sucralose is 5 mg per kg body weight per day. For example, the ADI of sucralose in an adult weighing 150 pounds (or 68 kg) would be 340 mg.

Neotame and Stevia

Neotame is an alternative sweetener that is 7,000 times sweeter than sugar. Manufacturers use it to sweeten a variety of products, such as beverages, dairy products, frozen desserts, and chewing gums.

Stevia was approved as an alternative sweetener by the FDA in 2008. It is produced from a purified extract of the stevia plant, native to South America. Stevia is 200 times sweeter than sugar. It is currently used commercially to sweeten beverages and is available in powder and liquid for tabletop use. Stevia is also called Rebiana, Reb-A, Truvia, and Purevia.

Using Artificial Sweeteners Does Not Necessarily Prevent Weight Gain

A recent scientific statement from the American Heart Association and the American Diabetes Association concludes that existing evidence is insufficient to support the claims that consuming artificial sweeteners reduces appetite, energy intake, body weight, or risks for heart disease and diabetes.[18] Remember that to prevent weight gain, you need to balance the total number of Calories you consume against the number you expend. If you're expending an average of 2,000 kcal a day and you consume about 2,000 kcal per day, then you'll neither gain nor lose weight. But if, in addition to your normal diet, you regularly indulge in "treats," you're bound to gain weight, whether they are sugar free or not. Consider the Calorie count of these artificially sweetened foods:

- One cup of nonfat chocolate frozen yogurt with artificial sweetener = 199 Calories
- One sugar-free chocolate cookie = 100 Calories
- One serving of no-sugar-added hot cocoa = 55 Calories

Does the number of Calories in these foods surprise you? *Remember, sugar free doesn't mean Calorie free.* Make it a habit to check the Nutrition Facts panel to find out how much energy is really in your food!

recap Alternative sweeteners can be used in place of sugar to sweeten foods. Most of these products do not promote tooth decay and contribute little or no energy. The alternative sweeteners approved for use in the United States are considered safe when consumed in amounts less than the acceptable daily intake.

HEALTHWATCH

What is diabetes, and why has it become a public health concern?

Diabetes is a serious chronic disease in which the body can no longer regulate glucose within normal limits and blood glucose levels become dangerously high or fall dangerously low. Diabetes causes disease when chronic exposure to elevated blood glucose levels damages the body's blood vessels, and this in turn damages other body tissues. As the concentration of glucose in the blood increases, a shift in the body's chemical balance allows glucose to attach to certain body proteins, including ones that make up blood vessels. Glucose coats these proteins like a sticky glaze,

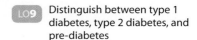
LO9 Distinguish between type 1 diabetes, type 2 diabetes, and pre-diabetes

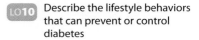
LO10 Describe the lifestyle behaviors that can prevent or control diabetes

diabetes A serious, chronic disease in which the body can no longer regulate glucose.

causing damage and dysfunction. If not controlled, diabetes can lead to blindness, seizures, kidney failure, nerve disease, amputations, stroke, and heart disease. In severe cases, it can be fatal.

Approximately 25.8 million people in the United States—8.3% of the total population, including adults and children—live with diabetes. Of these, 18.8 million have been diagnosed, and it is speculated that another 7 million people have the disease but don't know it. There are two main forms of diabetes: type 1 and type 2. Some women develop a third form, *gestational diabetes,* during pregnancy; we discuss this in more detail later in this text (Chapter 11). Type 2 diabetes is more common in ethnic minority groups. Although approximately 7% of Caucasians live with type 2 diabetes, it is estimated that 12.6% of African Americans, 11.8% of Hispanic/Latino individuals, and 16.1% of American Indians/Alaska Natives have type 2 diabetes.[19] It is also more common in older adults than in younger adults and children.

In Type 1 Diabetes, the Body Does Not Produce Enough Insulin

Approximately 10% of people with diabetes have **type 1 diabetes**, in which the pancreas produces little to no insulin. When people with type 1 diabetes eat a meal and their blood glucose rises, the pancreas is unable to secrete insulin in response. Glucose levels soar, and the body tries to expel the excess glucose by excreting it in the urine. In fact, the medical term for the disease is *diabetes mellitus* (from the Greek *diabainein,* "to pass through," and the Latin *mellitus,* "sweetened with honey"), and frequent urination is one of its warning signs (see **TABLE 3.4** for other symptoms). If blood glucose levels are not controlled, a person with type 1 diabetes will become confused and lethargic and have trouble breathing. This is because the person's brain is not getting enough glucose to function properly.

Uncontrolled diabetes can lead to *ketoacidosis*, a condition that occurs when inadequate glucose levels prompt the body to break down stored fat for energy. The fuels produced from fat breakdown, called ketones, are acidic. Their production therefore raises the level of acidity of the blood (a condition called *acidosis*). Any form of acidosis—including ketoacidosis—interferes with basic body functions and damages many body tissues; left untreated, the ultimate results are coma and death.

The cause of type 1 diabetes is unknown, but it may be an *autoimmune disease.* This means that the body's immune system attacks and destroys its own tissues—in this case, the beta cells of the pancreas.

Most cases of type 1 diabetes are diagnosed in adolescents around 10 to 14 years of age, although the disease can appear in younger children and adults. It occurs more often in families, so siblings and children of people with type 1 diabetes are at greater risk.

The only treatment for type 1 diabetes is daily insulin injections. Insulin is a hormone composed of protein, so it would be digested in the small intestine if taken as a pill. People with type 1 diabetes must monitor their blood glucose levels closely, using a

TABLE 3.4 Symptoms of Type 1 and Type 2 Diabetes

Type 1 Diabetes	Type 2 Diabetes*
Increased or frequent urination	Any of the type 1 signs and symptoms
Excessive thirst	Greater frequency of infections
Constant hunger	Sudden vision changes
Unexplained weight loss	Slow healing of wounds or sores
Extreme fatigue	Tingling or numbness in the hands or feet
Blurred vision	Very dry skin

*Some people with type 2 diabetes experience no symptoms.
Data adapted from: U.S. Dept. of Health and Human Services, National Diabetes Information Clearinghouse (NDIC). Available online at Your Guide to Diabetes: Type 1 and Type 2: Learn about Diabetes—National Diabetes Information Clearinghouse.

type 1 diabetes The form of diabetes in which the pancreas produces little or no insulin.

device called a *glucometer*, and must give themselves injections of insulin several times a day to maintain their blood glucose levels within a healthful range (**FIGURE 3.15**).

In Type 2 Diabetes, Cells Become Less Responsive to Insulin

In **type 2 diabetes**, body cells become *resistant,* or less responsive, to insulin. This type of diabetes develops progressively, meaning that the biological changes resulting in the disease occur over a long period of time.

In most cases, obesity is the trigger for a cascade of changes that eventually result in the disorder. Specifically, the cells of many obese people exhibit a condition called *insulin insensitivity* (or *insulin resistance*). The pancreas attempts to compensate for this by secreting more insulin. Over time, a person who is insulin insensitive will have to circulate very high levels of insulin to use glucose for energy. Eventually, this excessive production of insulin becomes insufficient for preventing a rise in fasting blood glucose. The resulting condition is referred to as **impaired fasting glucose**, meaning glucose levels are higher than normal but not high enough to indicate a diagnosis of type 2 diabetes. Some health professionals refer to this as *pre-diabetes*, because people with impaired fasting glucose are more likely to develop type 2 diabetes. Ultimately, the pancreas becomes incapable of secreting such excessive amounts of insulin, and the beta cells stop producing the hormone altogether.

As noted, obesity is the most common trigger for type 2 diabetes. However, many other factors also play a role. For instance, relatives of people with type 2 diabetes are at increased risk, as are people with a sedentary lifestyle.

A cluster of risk factors referred to as the *metabolic syndrome* is also known to increase the risk for type 2 diabetes. The criteria for metabolic syndrome are

- a waist circumference of or greater than 35 inches (88 cm) for women, and 40 inches (102 cm) for men,
- elevated blood pressure,
- unhealthful levels of certain blood lipids, and
- abnormally high blood glucose levels.

Increased age is another risk factor for type 2 diabetes: most cases develop after age 45, and 23% of Americans 60 years and older have diabetes. Once commonly known as *adult-onset diabetes,* type 2 diabetes in children was virtually unheard of until recently. Unfortunately, the disease is increasing dramatically among children and adolescents, posing serious health consequences for them and their future children. In a 2012 study, more than 7% of college students were found to have pre-diabetes.[20] In addition, each year about 3,600 people under age 20 are newly diagnosed with full-blown type 2 diabetes.[19]

Lifestyle Choices Can Help Control or Prevent Type 2 Diabetes

Type 2 diabetes can be treated in a variety of ways. Losing weight, establishing healthful eating patterns, and exercising regularly can control the symptoms in many people. More severe cases may require oral medications, such as pills. These drugs work in one of two ways: they improve the sensitivity of body cells to insulin or reduce the amount of glucose the liver produces. However, if a person with type 2 diabetes can no longer secrete enough insulin, the patient must have daily injections of insulin just like a person with type 1 diabetes.

People with diabetes should follow most of the same dietary guidelines recommended for those without diabetes. One difference is that people with diabetes may need to eat less carbohydrate, and slightly more fat or protein, to help regulate their blood glucose levels. Like people without diabetes, those with diabetes should choose high-fiber carbohydrate food sources when they do consume carbohydrates. Typically, a registered dietitian develops an individualized diet plan based on each patient's responses to foods.

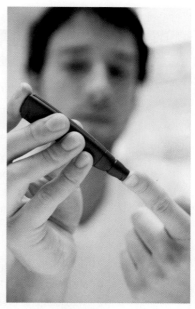

FIGURE 3.15 Monitoring blood glucose typically requires pricking a finger each day and measuring the blood using a device called a glucometer.

To find out your risk for type 2 diabetes, go to www.diabetes.org. Type "risk test" in the search bar, then click on the test.

type 2 diabetes The form of diabetes in which body cells progressively become less responsive to insulin, or the pancreas does not produce enough insulin.

impaired fasting glucose Fasting blood glucose levels that are higher than normal but not high enough to lead to a diagnosis of type 2 diabetes; also called *pre-diabetes*.

WHAT ABOUT **YOU?** ⸮

Calculate Your Risk for Type 2 Diabetes

To calculate your risk for developing type 2 diabetes, circle your answers to the following questions:

I am overweight.	YES or NO
I am sedentary (I exercise fewer than three times a week).	YES or NO
I have a close family member with type 2 diabetes.	YES or NO
I am a member of one of the following groups:	YES or NO
• African American	
• Hispanic American (Latino)	
• Native American	
• Pacific Islander	
I have had gestational diabetes, or I gave birth to at least one baby weighing more than 9 lb.	YES or NO
My blood pressure is 140/90 or higher, or I have been told that I have high blood pressure.	YES or NO
My cholesterol levels are not normal. (See a fuller discussion of cholesterol in Chapter 4.)	YES or NO

The more "yes" responses you give, the higher your risk of developing type 2 diabetes. You cannot change your ethnicity or your family members' health, but you can take steps to maintain a healthful weight and increase your physical activity. For tips, see Chapters 9 and 10.

Data from The National Diabetes Information Clearinghouse (NDIC). http://diabetes.niddk.nih.gov.

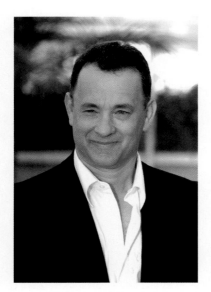

⬆ Actor Tom Hanks has type 2 diabetes.

In addition, people with diabetes should avoid alcoholic beverages, which can cause hypoglycemia. The symptoms of alcohol intoxication and hypoglycemia are very similar. The person with diabetes, his or her companions, and healthcare professionals may confuse these conditions; this can result in a potentially life-threatening situation.

Although there is no cure for type 2 diabetes, many cases could be prevented or their onset delayed. We cannot control our family history, but we can use the following strategies to decrease our risk:

- Eat a balanced diet with plenty of whole grains, fruits, and legumes and other vegetables.
- Exercise regularly: moderate daily exercise may prevent the onset of type 2 diabetes more effectively than dietary changes alone.
- Maintain an appropriate body weight: studies show that losing only 10 to 30 lb can reduce or eliminate the symptoms of type 2 diabetes.

What's your risk of developing diabetes? Check out the *What About You?* feature box to find out.

recap Diabetes is a serious disease that results in dangerously high levels of blood glucose. In type 1 diabetes, the pancreas secretes little or no insulin, so insulin injections are required to manage the disease. Type 2 diabetes develops over time and may be triggered by obesity: body cells are no longer sensitive to the effects of insulin, or the pancreas no longer secretes sufficient insulin for the body's needs. Supplemental insulin, usually in the form of injections, may or may not be needed. Diabetes causes tissue damage and increases the risk for heart disease, blindness, kidney disease, and amputations. Many cases of type 2 diabetes could be prevented or delayed by eating a balanced diet, getting regular exercise, and maintaining a healthful body weight.

STUDY **PLAN** | MasteringNutrition™

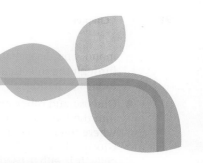

Customize your study plan—and master your nutrition!—
in the Study Area of **MasteringNutrition.**

what can I do **today?**
Now that you've read this chapter, try making these three changes.

1 Eat more high-fiber foods with each meal—including fruits, vegetables, legumes, and whole-grain cereals and breads.

2 Drink fewer sweetened beverages and more water with every meal to reduce your energy intake and help with digesting the higher amount of fiber you are eating.

3 Brush your teeth more often throughout the day, particularly after eating sweet foods or sticky, starchy foods. This will reduce your risk for dental caries.

test yourself | *answers*

1. **False.** The term *carbohydrate* refers to both simple and complex carbohydrates. The term *sugar* refers to the simple carbohydrates: monosaccharides and disaccharides.

2. **False.** There is no evidence that diets high in sugar cause hyperactivity in children.

3. **False.** At 4 kcal per gram, carbohydrates have less than half the energy of a gram of fat. Eating a high-carbohydrate diet will not cause people to gain body fat unless their total diet contains more energy (Calories) than they expend. In fact, eating a diet high in fiber-rich carbohydrates is associated with a lower risk for obesity.

summary

Scan to hear an MP3 Chapter Review in **MasteringNutrition.**

LO 1 Distinguish between simple and complex carbohydrates

- Carbohydrates contain carbon, hydrogen, and oxygen. Plants make the carbohydrate glucose during photosynthesis.

- Simple carbohydrates include mono- and disaccharides. The three primary monosaccharides are glucose, fructose, and galactose. Two monosaccharides joined together are called disaccharides. Glucose and fructose join to make sucrose; glucose and glucose join to make maltose; and glucose and galactose join to make lactose.

- Complex carbohydrates include starches, which are polysaccharides. They are the storage form of glucose in plants. Other complex carbohydrates are dietary fiber, the nondigestible parts of plants present in foods, and glycogen, the storage form of glucose in humans. Glycogen is stored in the liver and in muscles.

LO 2 List four functions of carbohydrates in our body

- Glucose provides 4 kcal/gram to fuel the functions of our body cells. Our red blood cells, brain, and central nervous system prefer to use glucose exclusively for energy. Moreover, using glucose for energy helps spare body proteins. Glucose is an especially important fuel for the body during exercise. Exercising regularly trains our muscles to become more efficient at using both glucose and fat for energy.

- Fiber-rich carbohydrates help us maintain the healthy elimination of waste products. Eating adequate fiber may possibly reduce the risk of colon cancer, type 2 diabetes, obesity, heart disease, hemorrhoids, and diverticulosis.

LO 3 Explain how carbohydrates are digested and absorbed by our body

- Carbohydrate digestion starts in the mouth, where chewing and the secretion of salivary amylase start breaking down the carbohydrates in food. It continues in the small intestine, where enzymes break starches into smaller mono- and disaccharides. As disaccharides pass through the intestinal cells, they are digested into monosaccharides.

- Glucose and other monosaccharides are absorbed into the bloodstream and travel to the liver, where the molecules are converted to glucose. Glucose is transported in the bloodstream to the cells. It is either used for energy or stored in the liver or muscles as glycogen.

- Insulin and glucagon are hormones secreted by the pancreas in response to changes in blood glucose. Insulin is secreted when blood glucose levels are high, and it assists with the transport of glucose into cells. Glucagon is secreted when blood glucose levels are low, and it assists with the conversion of glycogen to glucose and with gluconeogenesis.

LO 4 Define the glycemic index and glycemic load

- The glycemic index is a value that indicates how much a food increases glucose levels. The glycemic load of a food is the amount of carbohydrate it contains multiplied by its glycemic index.

LO 5 Identify the RDA and the AMDR for carbohydrates, and the AI for fiber

- The RDA for carbohydrate for adults age 19 and older is 130 grams per day. The AMDR is 45% to 65% of total energy intake. The AI for fiber is 25 grams per day for women and 38 grams per day for men, or 14 grams of fiber for every 1,000 kcal per day that a person eats.

LO 6 Identify the most common dietary sources of added sugars and the potential health risks of a diet high in added sugars

- Common sources of added sugars in the U.S. diet are sweetened soft drinks, other sugary drinks, and candy, pastries, cookies, and other sweets. High added-sugar intake can cause tooth decay, can contribute to elevated levels of blood lipids thought to promote heart disease, and is associated with obesity and type 2 diabetes. It does not appear to cause hyperactivity in children.

LO 7 List five foods that are good sources of fiber-rich carbohydrates

- Fiber-rich foods include whole-grain breads and cereals, fruits, legumes and other vegetables, nuts, and seeds. Eating the recommended amount of these foods helps ensure that you meet your goals for fiber intake.

LO 8 Compare and contrast a variety of alternative sweeteners

- Acesulfame-K and stevia are about 200 times sweeter than sucrose, a level slightly higher than that of aspartame, which is one of the most popular alternative sweeteners currently in use. Saccharin is the oldest non-nutritive sweetener, and is about 300 times sweeter than sucrose. Sucralose is 600 times sweeter than sucrose and is stable when heated, so it can be used in cooking. Neotame is 7,000 times sweeter than sucrose and is used in a variety of processed foods.

LO 9 Distinguish between type 1 diabetes, type 2 diabetes, and pre-diabetes

- Diabetes is a disease that results in dangerously high levels of blood glucose. In type 1 diabetes, the pancreas cannot secrete sufficient insulin. In type 2 diabetes, body cells are no longer sensitive to the effects of insulin, or the pancreas no longer secretes sufficient insulin for bodily needs. Pre-diabetes is a condition characterized by impaired fasting glucose and increases the risk for type 2 diabetes.

LO 10 Describe the lifestyle behaviors that can prevent or control diabetes

- Diabetes causes tissue damage and increases the risk of heart disease, blindness, kidney disease, and amputations. Many cases of type 2 diabetes could be prevented or delayed with a balanced diet, regular exercise, and achieving and maintaining a healthful body weight.

review questions

LO 1 Distinguish between simple and complex carbohydrates

1. Glucose, fructose, and galactose are
   a. monosaccharides.
   b. disaccharides.
   c. polysaccharides.
   d. complex carbohydrates.

LO 2 List four functions of carbohydrates in our body

2. Carbohydrates
   a. are the body's sole source of energy.
   b. provide 4 kilocalories of energy per gram.
   c. can be converted to protein when protein stores are low.
   d. All of the above are true.

LO **3** **Explain how carbohydrates are digested and absorbed by our body**

3. Maltase, sucrase, and lactase
   a. are salivary enzymes destroyed in the stomach.
   b. are gastric enzymes that break down soluble fiber.
   c. are intestinal enzymes that break down disaccharides.
   d. are pancreatic enzymes that break down polysaccharides.

LO **4** **Define the glycemic index and glycemic load**

4. The glycemic index rates
   a. the acceptable amount of alternative sweeteners to consume in 1 day.
   b. the potential of foods to raise blood glucose and insulin levels.
   c. the risk of a given food for causing diabetes.
   d. the ratio of soluble to insoluble fiber in a complex carbohydrate.

LO **5** **Identify the RDA and the AMDR for carbohydrates, and the AI for fiber**

5. Which of the following DRIs for carbohydrates for adults is correct?
   a. The AMDR for carbohydrate intake is 35–45%.
   b. The RDA for carbohydrates is 60 grams per day.
   c. The RDA for fiber is 12 grams for every 1,000 kilocalories a person eats.
   d. The AI for fiber is 25 grams per day for women and 38 grams per day for men.

LO **6** **Identify the most common dietary sources of added sugars and the potential health risks of a diet high in added sugars**

6. The most common source of added sugar in the American diet is
   a. table sugar.
   b. white flour.
   c. alcohol.
   d. sweetened soft drinks.

LO **7** **List five foods that are good sources of fiber-rich carbohydrates**

7. Which of the following meals provides the most fiber-rich carbohydrates?
   a. stir-fry with brown rice, black beans, and broccoli
   b. cobb salad with iceberg lettuce, ham, cheddar cheese, and ranch dressing
   c. scrambled eggs, salsa, and wheat-bread toast
   d. sesame-seed bagel, cream cheese, and a glass of orange juice

LO **8** **Compare and contrast a variety of alternative sweeteners**

8. Stevia is
   a. a sugar alcohol.
   b. marketed as NutraSweet.
   c. derived from a South American plant.
   d. 7,000–13,000 times sweeter than sugar.

LO **9** **Distinguish between type 1 diabetes, type 2 diabetes, and pre-diabetes**

9. Type 1 diabetes
   a. is characterized by insulin resistance.
   b. is typically diagnosed in adolescents.
   c. progresses to type 2 diabetes if left untreated.
   d. is most commonly triggered by obesity.

LO **10** **Describe the lifestyle behaviors that can prevent or control diabetes**

10. Abnormally high blood glucose levels can sometimes be reduced with
    a. regular exercise and modest weight loss.
    b. a diet rich in high-glycemic-index foods.
    c. moderate alcohol intake.
    d. oral insulin intake.

Answers to Review Questions are located at the back of this text.

web links

The following websites and apps explore further topics and issues related to personal health.
Visit **MasteringNutrition** for links to the websites and RSS feeds.

www.ada.org
American Dental Association

www.diabetes.org
American Diabetes Association

www.eatright.org
Academy of Nutrition and Dietetics

www2.niddk.nih.gov
National Institute of Diabetes and Digestive and Kidney Diseases (NIDDK)

4 Fats
Essential Energy-Supplying Nutrients

learning outcomes

After studying this chapter, you should be able to:

1 Compare and contrast the three types of lipids found in foods, pp. 101–107.

2 Discuss how the level of saturation of a fatty acid affects its shape and the form it takes, pp. 101–107.

3 Explain the health benefits and dietary sources of the essential fatty acids, pp. 101–107.

4 List five functions of fat, pp. 107–109.

5 Describe the steps involved in fat digestion, absorption, and transport, pp. 109–112.

6 Identify the dietary recommendations for intakes of total fat, saturated fat, *trans* fats, and the essential fatty acids, pp. 112–118.

7 Identify common food sources of less healthful versus more healthful fats, pp. 112–118.

8 Summarize our current understanding of the relationship between intake of dietary fats and the development of cardiovascular disease and cancer, pp. 118–125.

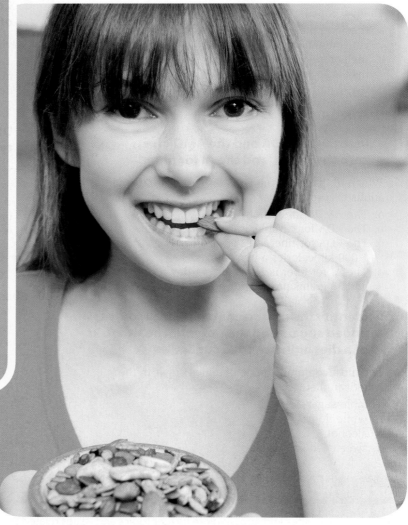

test yourself

Are these statements true or false? Circle your guess.

1. **T** **F** Dietary cholesterol is not required because our body makes all the cholesterol it needs.

2. **T** **F** Fat is an important fuel source during rest and exercise.

3. **T** **F** Certain fats protect against heart disease.

Test Yourself answers can be found at the end of the chapter.

MasteringNutrition™

Go online for chapter quizzes, pre-tests, Interactive Activities, and more!

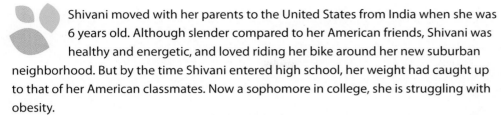

Shivani moved with her parents to the United States from India when she was 6 years old. Although slender compared to her American friends, Shivani was healthy and energetic, and loved riding her bike around her new suburban neighborhood. But by the time Shivani entered high school, her weight had caught up to that of her American classmates. Now a sophomore in college, she is struggling with obesity.

Shivani explains, "In India, the diet is mostly rice, *dhal*, and vegetables. Many people are vegetarians, or they eat only fish and poultry. Breakfast might be fruit and yogurt, not eggs and sausage. And for most families, desserts are only for special occasions. When we moved to America, I wanted to eat like all the other kids: hamburgers, french fries, ice cream, cookies . . . I gained a lot of weight, and now my doctor says I weigh too much, my blood pressure is high, and I need to have a cholesterol test to see if I'm at risk for heart disease. It freaks me out thinking that some day I might have a heart attack! I wish I could start eating like my relatives back in India again, but they don't serve rice and *dhal* in the cafeteria."

Is a high-fat diet always to blame for heart disease? Can a low-fat diet prevent it? When was the last time you heard anything good about dietary fat?

Although some people think they should avoid eating any fatty foods, a certain amount of fat is absolutely essential for good health. In this chapter, we'll discuss the function of fat in the human body and help you distinguish between beneficial and harmful types of dietary fat. You'll also learn how much fat you need in your diet, and find out how dietary fat influences your risk for cardiovascular disease and cancer.

What are fats?

Fats are just one form of a much larger and more diverse group of substances called **lipids** that are distinguished by the fact that they are *insoluble* (do not dissolve) in water. Think of a salad dressing made with vinegar and olive oil—a lipid. Shaking the bottle *disperses* the oil but doesn't *dissolve* it: that's why it separates back out again so quickly. Lipids are found in all sorts of living things, including plants, animals, and you. In fact, their presence on your skin explains why you can't clean your face with water alone: you need some type of soap to break down the insoluble lipids before you can wash them away.

We consume lipids in either of two forms: fats, such as butter, which are solid at room temperature, and oils, such as olive oil, which are liquid at room temperature. In this chapter, we focus on three types of lipids found in foods:

- triglycerides
- phospholipids
- sterols

Most of the fat we eat (95%) is in the form of triglycerides, which is the same way most of the fat in our body is stored. So although this chapter discusses phospholipids and sterols briefly, our main focus is on triglycerides. Also, because most people are familiar with the term *fats*, we'll use that term throughout this book whenever we're discussing triglycerides, whether we're referring to solid fats or liquid oils.

Triglycerides Can Contain Saturated or Unsaturated Fatty Acid Chains

As reflected in the prefix *tri*, a **triglyceride** is a molecule consisting of *three* fatty acids attached to a *three*-carbon glycerol backbone (**FIGURE 4.1**). **Fatty acids** are long chains

LO1 Compare and contrast the three types of lipids found in foods.

LO2 Discuss how the level of saturation of a fatty acid affects its shape and the form it takes.

LO3 Explain the health benefits and dietary sources of the essential fatty acids.

lipids A diverse group of organic substances that are insoluble in water; lipids include triglycerides, phospholipids, and sterols.

triglyceride A molecule consisting of three fatty acids attached to a three-carbon glycerol backbone.

fatty acids Long chains of carbon atoms bound to each other as well as to hydrogen atoms.

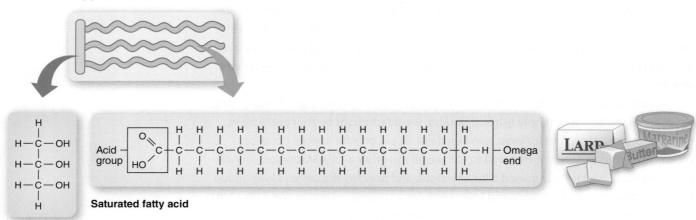

Triglyceride

Glycerol

Saturated fatty acid

FIGURE 4.1 A triglyceride consists of three fatty acid chains attached to a three-carbon glycerol backbone. The fatty acid chain shown here is a saturated fatty acid. Saturated fatty acid chains stack well together to make solids, like butter and lard.

of carbon atoms bound to each other as well as to hydrogen. They are classified as acids because they contain an acid group at one end of their chain. As we'll see momentarily, fatty acid chains can vary in their structure. In contrast, **glycerol**, the backbone of a triglyceride molecule, never varies in structure.

Saturated and Unsaturated Fats Differ in Hydrogen Content

An atom of carbon has four "attachment sites." For each carbon in a **saturated fatty acid (SFA)**, two of these four sites are bound to adjacent carbon atoms and the two remaining sites are bound to hydrogen atoms. You can see this in Figure 4.1. Because the carbons in this chain have the maximum amount of hydrogen bound to them—two hydrogen atoms—the fatty acid is said to be *saturated* with hydrogen.

In contrast, look at the fatty acid chains shown in **FIGURE 4.2**. Notice that, at one or more points, these chains have a *double bond* between adjacent carbon atoms. (Chemists indicate double bonds between atoms with two parallel lines, like an equal sign [$C=C$].) This double bond fills two attachment sites, one of which would otherwise be filled by hydrogen. As a result, each of the carbons participating in a double bond has just one hydrogen attached, not two. Thus, the total amount of hydrogen is lower in these fatty acid chains. In other words, they are unsaturated. *Mono-* means "one," and a **monounsaturated fatty acid (MUFA)** has one double carbon bond in which hydrogen is excluded (see Figure 4.2a). *Poly-* means "many," and a **polyunsaturated fatty acid (PUFA)** has two or more double carbon bonds (see Figure 4.2b and c).

Saturated and Unsaturated Fats Differ in Form

Notice in Figure 4.2 that the double carbon bonds give fatty acids chains a "kink" wherever they occur. SFAs have no such bonds, so they always form straight, rigid chains. This quality allows them to pack together densely in solids like butter, lard, cheese, and beef fat, as well as coconut and palm oil, which are semisolid at room temperature. To understand why, it might help to imagine SFAs as toothpicks, hundreds of which can pack together into a small box.

Now imagine breaking a bunch of toothpicks into V shapes. They're like MUFAs and PUFAs—kinked—and unable to pack together. Because they take up a lot of space, MUFAs and PUFAs are usually liquid at room temperature. Olive and canola oils are high in MUFAs, as is the fat in cashew nuts and nut butters. Good sources of PUFAs include peanut, corn, and safflower oils.

glycerol An alcohol composed of three carbon atoms; it is the backbone of a triglyceride molecule.

saturated fatty acid (SFA) A fatty acid that has no carbons joined together with a double bond; these types of fatty acids are generally solid at room temperature.

monounsaturated fatty acid (MUFA) A fatty acid that has two carbons in the chain bound to each other with one double bond; these types of fatty acids are generally liquid at room temperature.

polyunsaturated fatty acids (PUFAs) Fatty acids that have more than one double bond in the chain; these types of fatty acids are generally liquid at room temperature.

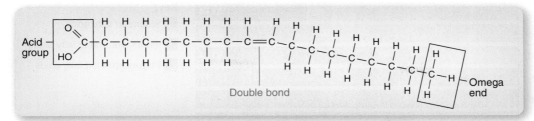
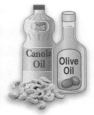

(a) Monounsaturated fatty acid

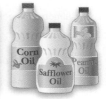

(b) Polyunsaturated omega-6 fatty acid (linoleic acid)

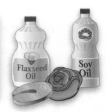

(c) Polyunsaturated omega-3 fatty acid (alpha-linolenic acid)

⬥ **FIGURE 4.2** Unsaturated fatty acids have one or more double carbon bonds that kink the chain. **(a)** Monounsaturated fatty acid chains have one double carbon bond. Olive oil, canola oil, and certain nuts, like cashews, are rich in monounsaturated fatty acids. **(b)** Polyunsaturated fatty acid chains have two or more double carbon bonds. The polyunsaturated fatty acid shown here is an omega-6 fatty acid called linoleic acid. Notice that the second of the two double carbon bonds is located between the sixth and seventh carbon counting from the omega end of the chain. Many plant oils are good sources of omega-6 fatty acids. **(c)** The polyunsaturated fatty acid shown here is an omega-3 fatty acid called alpha-linolenic acid. The third of the three double carbon bonds is located between the third and fourth carbon from the omega end. Fatty fish, dark green, leafy vegetables, and certain plant oils are good sources of omega-3 fatty acids.

As shown in **FIGURE 4.3**, foods typically contain a variety of fatty acids. For example, animal fats provide approximately 40% to 60% of their energy from saturated fats but also provide some unsaturated fats. Most plant fats provide 80% to 90% of their energy from monounsaturated and polyunsaturated fats. For this reason, diets higher in plant foods (fruits, vegetables, grains, nuts, and seeds) will usually be lower in saturated fats than diets high in animal products.

Do the rigid versus kinked forms of the fatty acid chains make any difference to our health? Although the answer to this question is currently the subject of controversy, decades of research suggest that a diet high in SFAs increases our risk for cardiovascular disease, whereas a diet in which the majority of fat is consumed as MUFAs and PUFAs decreases the risk. We'll discuss these relationships in more detail later in this chapter.

recap Three lipids are found in foods: triglycerides, phospholipids, and sterols. Triglycerides, or fats, are the most common. They are made up of a glycerol backbone attached to three fatty acid chains. Saturated fatty acids are solid at room temperature and are plentiful in butter, lard, cheese, and coconut and palm oils. Monounsaturated and polyunsaturated fatty acids are liquid at room temperature and are plentiful in vegetable oils, nuts, and many fish.

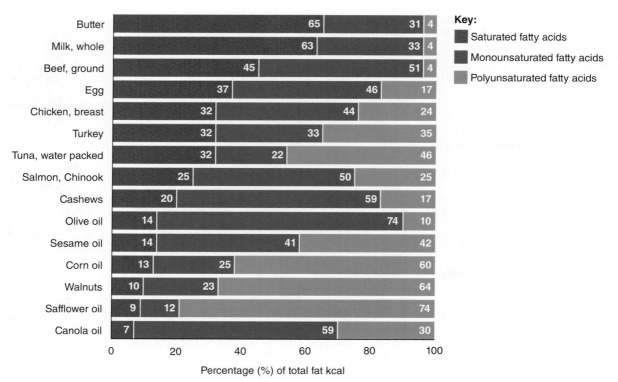

FIGURE 4.3 Major sources of dietary fat.

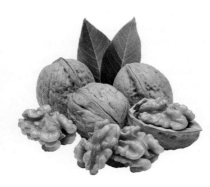

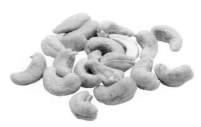

Walnuts and cashews are high in monounsaturated fatty acids.

hydrogenation The process of adding hydrogen to unsaturated fatty acids, making them more saturated and therefore more solid at room temperature.

Trans Fats Are Harmful to Health

In November, 2013, the U.S. Food and Drug Administration announced that it had made a preliminary determination that partially hydrogenated oils (PHOs), the main source of *trans* fatty acids in the U.S. food supply, were no longer recognized as safe to consume. If the FDA makes a final determination to this effect, then food manufacturers will no longer be allowed to use PHOs in their foods. What's behind this announcement? What are *trans* fats and PHOs, and why are they harmful?[1]

Trans fats are rigid, just like saturated fats. They occur rarely in nature; extremely small amounts are found only in dairy foods, beef, and lamb. In contrast, they are abundant in many margarines, commercial frying fats, shortenings, and any processed foods or fast foods made with these products. Health concerns about *trans* fats began to arise with research that linked high-*trans*-fat diets with heart disease and early death.

The trouble began in the late 1800s, when food manufacturers identified the need for a fat that could be produced cheaply and abundantly from vegetable oils, that could be sold in a solid form, and that had a long shelf life. (As you may know, most fats and oils cannot be stored for long without going rancid.) They developed a process called **hydrogenation**, in which pressurized hydrogen is inserted into the double carbon bonds in the unsaturated fatty acid chains of vegetable oils. The result is a partially hydrogenated oil—a PHO. Hydrogenation straightens out the chains, making the liquid fat more solid at room temperature—as well as more saturated. In addition, the extra hydrogen helps the fat resist rancidity.

Research has shown that *trans* fats are harmful to our health because they change the way our cell membranes function and reduce the removal of cholesterol from the blood. For these reasons, the 2010 *Dietary Guidelines for Americans* and the Institute of Medicine recommend keeping consumption of *trans* fats to an absolute minimum.[2,3] In addition, the FDA requires food manufacturers to list the amount of *trans* fatty acids per serving on the Nutrition Facts panel. However, some products labeled as having "zero" *trans* fats still contain them! That's because—as of this writing—the FDA allows products that have less than 1 gram of *trans* fat per serving to claim that they are *trans* fat free. If you're determined to keep *trans* fats out of your diet, check the ingredients list: if it states that the product contains PHOs (partially hydrogenated corn oil, for example), that means it contains *trans* fats.

Essential Fatty Acids Protect Our Health

Two groups of PUFAs are called "essential" because they must be consumed in the diet; our body cannot make them. These **essential fatty acids (EFAs)** are incorporated into the many phospholipids in our body (described shortly) and are needed to make a number of important biological compounds called *eicosanoids*. In the body, eicosanoids help regulate some key functions, including gastrointestinal tract motility, blood clotting, blood pressure, and inflammation—just to name a few. The two EFAs are linoleic acid and alpha-linolenic acid (see Figure 4.2b and c).

Linoleic Acid

Linoleic acid is found in vegetable and nut oils, such as sunflower, safflower, corn, soy, flax, and peanut oils. If you eat lots of vegetables or use vegetable oil–based margarines or vegetable oils, you're probably getting adequate amounts of this essential fatty acid in your diet. In the body, linoleic acid is transformed into arachidonic acid, which is in turn used to make compounds that regulate body functions such as blood clotting and blood pressure.

Linoleic acid is a type of *omega-6 fatty acid*. To understand the reason for this name, you need to know that chemists call the final carbon in a fatty acid chain the *omega carbon*. (Omega [Ω] is the last letter in the Greek alphabet.) *Omega-6* refers to the sixth carbon in a fatty acid chain when counting back from the omega carbon. In omega-6 fatty acids, the endmost double carbon bond occurs at this carbon. You can see this in Figure 4.2b. The body cannot make fatty acids with double carbon bonds this close to the omega end of the chain, and so linoleic acid is an essential fatty acid.

Alpha-Linolenic Acid

The second essential fatty acid is **alpha-linolenic acid**, an *omega-3 fatty acid*. Its outermost double carbon bond is even further along the chain, at the omega-3 carbon. In addition, its many double carbon bonds make this fatty acid highly kinked and therefore highly fluid. Alpha-linolenic acid is found mainly in leafy green vegetables, flaxseeds and flaxseed oil, soy oil and foods, canola oil, and fatty fish and fish oils.

As early as 1935, population studies began to show a link between high fish consumption and a significantly reduced risk for cardiovascular disease. That year, J. A. Urquhart, a physician working among the Inuit people of the Arctic Circle in Canada, reported that in 7 years of working with the Inuit—whose diets were made up of as much as 75% fat—he had encountered no cases of cardiovascular disease. The key, researchers soon discovered, was in the *type* of fat the Inuit consume. The cold-water fish and sea mammals that are staples of their diet are low in saturated fats and high in unsaturated fats, especially two types of omega-3 fatty acids, **eicosapentaenoic acid (EPA)** and **docosahexaenoic acid (DHA)**. The high degree of unsaturation of EPA and DHA helps keep the cell membranes of these animals flexible even in extremely cold temperatures. Research indicates that EPA and DHA protect against cardiovascular disease by improving the function of blood vessels and reducing inflammation, blood-clotting, blood pressure, irregularities in the heartbeat, and the level of triglycerides circulating in the bloodstream.[4,5]

Getting enough of these essential fatty acids is important for health. Dietary recommendations for the EFAs are discussed later in this chapter.

> **re**cap *Trans* fatty acids are associated with an increased risk for cardiovascular disease. In contrast, essential fatty acids are critical to our health. The body cannot synthesize essential fatty acids, so we must consume them. Research suggests that two omega-3 essential fatty acids—EPA and DHA—protect against cardiovascular disease.

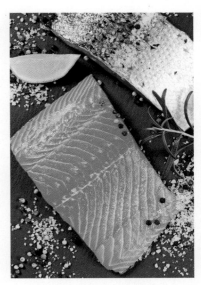

Salmon is high in omega-3 fatty acid content.

essential fatty acids (EFAs) Fatty acids that must be consumed in the diet because they cannot be made by our body. The two essential fatty acids are linoleic acid and alpha-linolenic acid.

linoleic acid An essential fatty acid found in vegetable and nut oils; also known as omega-6 fatty acid.

alpha-linolenic acid An essential fatty acid found in leafy green vegetables, flaxseed oil, soy oil, fish oil, and fish products; an omega-3 fatty acid.

eicosapentaenoic acid (EPA) A type of omega-3 fatty acid that can be made in the body from alpha-linolenic acid and found in our diet primarily in marine plants and animals.

docosahexaenoic acid (DHA) A type of omega-3 fatty acid that can be made in the body from alpha-linolenic acid and found in our diet primarily in marine plants and animals; together with EPA, it appears to reduce our risk for a heart attack.

▶ **FIGURE 4.4** Structure of a phospholipid. Phospholipids consist of a glycerol backbone attached to two fatty acids and a compound that contains phosphate. They are an important component of our cell membranes and are found in certain foods, such as peanuts, egg yolks, and some processed foods that contain dispersed fats.

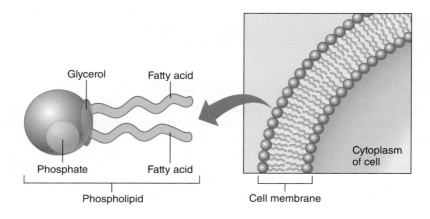

Phospholipids Combine Lipids with Phosphate

Along with the triglycerides just discussed, two other types of fats—phospholipids and sterols—are present in the foods we eat. **Phospholipids** consist of a glycerol backbone bound to two fatty acids. In place of the third fatty acid found in triglycerides, phospholipids have a compound that contains *phosphate*, a chemical that is soluble (dissolves) in water **(FIGURE 4.4)**. This substitution of a phosphate compound makes phospholipids soluble in water, a property that enables them to assist in transporting fats in our bloodstream (blood is about 50% water). Also, as shown in Figure 4.4, phospholipids are an important component of the outer membrane of every cell in the body and thus help regulate the transport of substances into and out of our cells.

Phospholipids are present in peanuts, egg yolk, and some processed foods with dispersed fats, such as salad dressings. However, because our body manufactures them, they are not essential for us to include in our diet.

Sterols Have a Ring Structure

phospholipid A type of lipid in which a fatty acid is combined with another compound that contains phosphate; unlike other lipids, phospholipids are soluble in water.

sterol A type of lipid found in foods and the body that has a ring structure; cholesterol is the most common sterol that occurs in our diet.

Sterols are also a type of lipid found both in foods and in the body, but their multiple ring structure is different from that of triglycerides or phospholipids **(FIGURE 4.5a)**. Sterols are found in both plant and animal foods and are also produced in the body.

Cholesterol is the most commonly occurring sterol in our diet **(FIGURE 4.5b)**. Cholesterol is found only in the fatty part of animal products, such as butter, egg yolks, whole milk, meats, and poultry. Egg whites, skim milk, and lean meats have little or no cholesterol. Dietary cholesterol (cholesterol that comes from foods) has a bad reputation: As you will read later in this chapter, elevated blood cholesterol levels suggest an increased risk for cardiovascular disease.

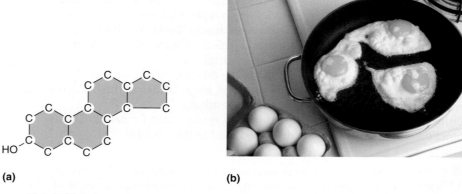

(a)   (b)

◀ **FIGURE 4.5** Sterol structure. **(a)** Cholesterol and other sterols are lipids that contain multiple ring structures. **(b)** Cholesterol is the most commonly occurring sterol in the diet. It is found in meats, fish, egg yolks, butter, and dairy products.

nutrition myth or fact?

Is Margarine More Healthful Than Butter?

Your toast just popped up! Which topping will you use: butter or margarine? Butter is 65% saturated fat: 1 tablespoon provides 30 grams of cholesterol! In contrast, corn oil margarine is just 2% saturated fat, with no cholesterol. But how much *trans* fat does that margarine contain? And which is better—the more natural and more saturated butter or the more processed and less saturated margarine?

You're not the only one asking this question. Until recently, vegetable-based oils were hydrogenated to make margarines. These products were filled with *trans* fats that could increase the risk for heart disease, as well as harm cell membranes, weaken immune function, and inhibit the body's natural anti-inflammatory hormones. Some margarines also contained harmful amounts of toxic metals, such as nickel and aluminum, as by-products of the hydrogenation process. These are among some of the reasons researchers began warning consumers against using margarines years ago.

So does that mean that the saturated-fat, cholesterol-rich butter is the better choice? A decade ago, that may have been true, but, over the last 10 years, food manufacturers have introduced "*trans* fat-free margarines and spreads" that contain no cholesterol or *trans* fats and low amounts of saturated fats. The American Heart Association advises consumers to reduce saturated fats,[1] so choose *trans* fat–free margarines and spreads over butter. Other groups point out that such manufactured products are still "non-foods" and recommend choosing unprocessed nut butters (peanut, walnut, cashew, and almond butters) instead. Although they are still about as high in Calories as butter, these alternatives are rich in essential fatty acids and other heart-healthy unsaturated fats.

Remember, a label claiming that a margarine has zero *trans* fat or *trans* fatty acids doesn't guarantee that the product is actually free of them. You'll need to look for margarines with no partially hydrogenated oils: that's the only way to know that your spread is entirely free of *trans* fatty acids.

We don't need to consume cholesterol in our diet because our body continually produces it, mostly in the liver and intestines. This continuous production (or *synthesis*) is vital because cholesterol is part of every cell membrane, where it works with fatty acids to help maintain cell membrane integrity. Cholesterol is particularly plentiful in the neural cells that make up the brain, spinal cord, and nerves. Thus, despite cholesterol's bad reputation, it is absolutely essential to our health.

We said earlier that many margarines contain *trans* fats, but butter contains cholesterol! So which is a better spread for your bread? See the **Nutrition Myth or Fact?** box to find out.

recap Phospholipids combine two fatty acids and a glycerol backbone with a phosphate-containing compound that makes them soluble in water. They help transport fats in our bloodstream and are found in the cell membrane. Sterols have a multiple-ring structure; cholesterol is the most commonly occurring sterol in our diet.

Why do we need to eat fats?

LO4   List five functions of fat.

Dietary fat provides energy and helps our body perform some essential internal functions.

Fats Provide Energy

Dietary fat is a primary source of energy. Fat provides 9 kcal per gram, while carbohydrate and protein provide only 4 kcal per gram. This means that fat is much more energy-dense. For example, just 1 tablespoon of butter or oil contains about 100 kcal, whereas it takes 2.5 cups of steamed broccoli or 1 slice of whole-wheat bread to provide 100 kcal.

When we are at rest, approximately 30% to 70% of the energy used by our muscles and organs comes from fat.[6] The exact amount of fat you burn when you are at rest depends on how much fat you eat in your diet, how physically active you are, and whether you are gaining or losing weight.

Fat is also a major energy source during physical activity. In fact, one of the best ways of losing body fat is through regular aerobic exercise. During exercise, the body begins to break down fat stores to fuel the working muscles. The amount and source of the fat used depend on your level of fitness; the type, intensity, and duration of the exercise; and what and how much you've eaten before you exercise. Because the body has only a limited supply of stored carbohydrate (as glycogen) in muscle tissue, the longer you exercise, the more fat you use for energy.

Fats Store Energy for Later Use

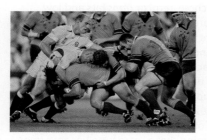

▲ Adipose tissue pads our body and protects our organs when we fall or are bruised.

Our bodies store extra energy as fat in our *adipose tissue,* which then can be used for energy at rest, during exercise, or during periods of low energy intake. Adipose tissue provides the body with an energy source even when we choose not to eat (or are unable to eat), when we are exercising, and while we are sleeping. Our body has relatively little stored carbohydrate—only enough to last about 1 to 2 days—and there is no place that our body can store extra protein. We cannot consider our muscles and organs as a place where "extra" protein is stored! For these reasons, although we don't want too much stored adipose tissue, some is essential to keep the body going.

Fats Enable the Transport of Fat-Soluble Vitamins

Dietary fat enables the transport of the fat-soluble vitamins. These are vitamins A, D, E, and K. Vitamin A is important for vision, vitamin D helps maintain bone health, vitamin E prevents and repairs damage to cells, and vitamin K is important for blood clotting and bone health. Without an appropriate intake of dietary fat, our body can become deficient in these important vitamins.

Fats Support Body Functions and Structures

Fats are a critical part of every cell membrane. There, they help determine what substances are transported into and out of the cell and regulate what substances can bind to the cell; thus, fats strongly influence the function of the cell. In addition, fats help maintain cell fluidity and other physical properties of the cell membrane. Fats enable our red blood cells, for example, to be flexible enough to bend and move through the smallest capillaries in our body, delivering oxygen to all our cells.

Fats also provide the materials needed to make cholesterol, which is then used to synthesize steroid reproductive hormones such as testosterone, estrogens, and progesterone. The adrenal glands also make over twenty different hormones called corticosteroids, which are involved in the stress response, metabolism, fluid balance, and many other functions.

Finally, stored body fat pads the body and protects our organs, such as the kidneys and liver, when we fall or are bruised. The fat under our skin acts as insulation to help us retain body heat. Although we often think of all body fat as "bad," it does play an important role in keeping our body healthy and functioning properly.

Fats Contribute to the Flavor, Texture, and Satiety of Foods

Dietary fat adds texture and flavor to foods. Fat makes salad dressings smooth and ice cream "creamy," and it gives cakes and cookies their moist, tender texture. Frying foods in fat, as with doughnuts or french fries, gives them a crisp, flavorful coating. On the other hand, foods containing fats, such as cookies, crackers, chips, and breads, become rancid quickly if they are not stored properly. Manufacturers add preservatives to increase the shelf life of foods with fats.

Fats in foods help us feel *satiated*—satisfied—more quickly during a meal, so we end up consuming less food. They also help us avoid hunger for a longer period of time afterward. Two factors probably contribute to this effect: first, as noted earlier, fat has a much higher energy density than carbohydrate or protein. An amount of butter weighing the same number of grams as a medium apple would contain 840 kcal! Second, fat takes longer to digest than protein or carbohydrate because more steps are involved in the digestion process. You may feel satisfied longer because energy is being released into your body more slowly.

recap Dietary fats provide twice the energy of protein and carbohydrate, at 9 kcal per gram, and the majority of energy required while we are at rest. Fats are also a major fuel source during exercise. Dietary fats help transport the fat-soluble vitamins into the body and help regulate cell function and maintain membrane integrity. Stored body fat in the adipose tissue helps protect vital organs and pad the body. Fats contribute to the flavor and texture of foods and the satiety we feel after a meal.

What happens to the fats we eat?

 LO5 Describe the steps involved in fat digestion, absorption, and transport.

Because fats are not soluble in water, they cannot enter the bloodstream easily from the digestive tract. Thus, fats must be digested, absorbed, and transported within the body differently than are carbohydrates and proteins, which are water soluble. Let's review the process here (**FIGURE 4.6**).

The Mouth and Stomach Have Limited Roles in Fat Digestion

Dietary fats usually come mixed with other foods in our diet, which we chew and then swallow. Water, mucus, and a salivary enzyme called lingual lipase mix with the fats in the mouth, but this enzyme has a limited role in the breakdown of fats until they reach the stomach (Figure 4.6, mouth).

Once in the stomach, lingual lipase and gastric lipase, which is secreted by the stomach, can digest about 10% of fats present. But the primary role of the stomach in fat digestion is to mix and break up the fat into droplets (Figure 4.6, stomach). Because they are not soluble in water, these fat droplets typically float on top of the watery digestive juices in the stomach until they are passed into the small intestine.

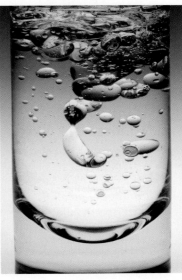

◄ Fats and oils do not dissolve readily in water.

The Gallbladder, Liver, and Pancreas Assist in Fat Breakdown

Because fat is not soluble in water, its digestion requires the help of mixing compounds from the gallbladder and digestive enzymes from the pancreas. Recall that the gallbladder is a sac attached to the underside of the liver, and the pancreas is an oblong-shaped organ sitting below the stomach. Both have a duct connecting them to the small intestine.

As fat enters the small intestine from the stomach, the gallbladder contracts and releases a substance called *bile* (Figure 4.6, liver and gallbladder). Bile is produced in the liver from cholesterol and is stored in the gallbladder until needed. Bile contains salts that are detergents and, much like soap, break up the fat into smaller and smaller droplets. At the same time, lipid-digesting enzymes produced in the pancreas travel through the pancreatic duct into the small intestine. Once bile has broken the fat into small droplets, these pancreatic enzymes take over, breaking up the triglycerides by removing some of the fatty acids from the glycerol backbone. Each triglyceride molecule is eventually broken down into two free fatty acids and one *monoglyceride,* which is the glycerol backbone with one fatty acid still attached.

Most Fat Is Absorbed in the Small Intestine

The free fatty acids and monoglycerides next need to be transported to the entero-cytes that line the small intestine (Figure 4.6, small intestine), so that they can be absorbed into the body. This trip requires the help of *micelles,* globules of bile

focus figure 4.6 | Lipid Digestion Overview

The majority of lipid digestion takes place in the small intestine, with the help of bile from the liver and digestive enzymes from the pancreas. Micelles transport the end products of lipid digestion to the enterocytes for absorption and eventual transport via the blood or lymph.

ORGANS OF THE GI TRACT

MOUTH
Lingual lipase secreted by tongue cells and mixed with saliva digests some triglycerides.

Little lipid digestion occurs here.

STOMACH
Most fat arrives intact at the stomach, where it is mixed and broken into droplets.

Gastric lipase digests some triglycerides.

SMALL INTESTINE
Bile from the gallbladder breaks fat into smaller droplets.

Lipid-digesting enzymes from the pancreas break triglycerides into monoacylglycerides and fatty acids.

Lipid-digesting enzymes from the pancreas break dietary cholesterol and phospholipids into their components.

Products of fat digestion combine with bile salts to form micelles.

Micelles transport lipid digestion products to the enterocytes.

Within enterocytes, components from micelles reform triglycerides and are repackaged as chylomicrons for transport into the lymphatic system.

Shorter fatty acids can be absorbed directly into the bloodstream.

ACCESSORY ORGANS

SALIVARY GLANDS
Produce saliva.

LIVER
Produces bile, which is stored in the gallbladder.

GALLBLADDER
Contracts and releases bile into the small intestine.

PANCREAS
Produces lipid-digesting enzymes, which are released into the small intestine.

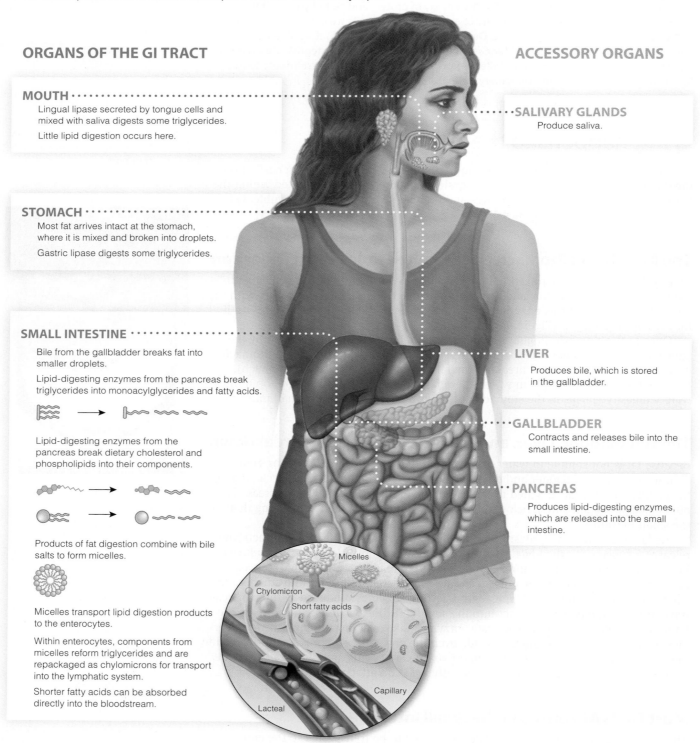

Micelles

Chylomicron

Short fatty acids

Capillary

Lacteal

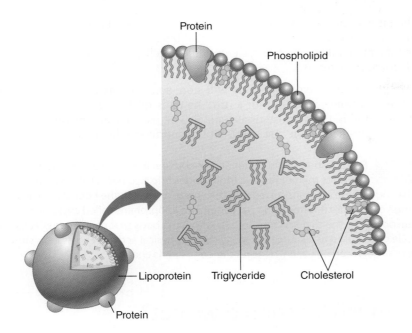

FIGURE 4.7 Structure of a lipoprotein. Notice that the fat clusters in the center of the molecule and the phospholipids and proteins, which are water soluble, form the outside of the sphere. This enables lipoproteins to transport fats in the bloodstream.

and phospholipids that trap the free fatty acids and monoglycerides and transport them to the intestinal cells. Once there, shorter fatty acids can pass directly across the intestinal cell membrane. Longer fatty acids first bind to a special carrier protein and then are absorbed into the cells.

After absorption into the enterocytes, the shortest fatty acids cross unassisted into the bloodstream and are then transported to the liver. In contrast, the longer fatty acids and monoglycerides are reformulated back into triglycerides. As you know, triglyceride molecules don't mix with water, so they can't cross independently into the bloodstream. Once again, their movement requires special packaging, this time in the form of lipoproteins. A **lipoprotein** is a spherical (round-shaped) compound in which triglycerides cluster deep in the center and phospholipids and proteins, which are water soluble, form the surface of the sphere (**FIGURE 4.7**). The specific lipoprotein that transports fat from a meal is called a **chylomicron**. Once chylomicrons are formed, they are transported from the enterocytes into the lymphatic system, and from there, released into the bloodstream.

Now that you know how fats are absorbed into the body, you may be wondering if there's any way to block the process so you could enjoy french fries and ice cream without getting the Calories. Manufacturers of weight-loss supplements called "fat-blockers" claim their products do precisely this, and current research provides some evidence to back up their claim. The main ingredient in one group of fat-blockers is *chitosan*, a nondigestible substance from marine crustaceans that is said to bind fat.[7] Research has shown that consumption of chitosan can produce modest weight loss: an average of 1.7–3.7 pounds over 8–9 weeks.[8–11]

Another fat-blocker, an over-the-counter medication called Alli®, doesn't bind fat but blocks the enzymes that break it down. Research shows that, like chitosan, Alli® can produce modest weight loss, although only when combined with a low-fat diet.[12] A common side effect of fat-blockers is gastrointestinal distress. If you're trying to lose weight, consult your healthcare provider to learn about the options that make the most sense for you.

Fat Is Stored for Later Use

There are three primary fates of the dietary fat in the chylomicrons:

- If your body needs the fat for energy, it can be quickly transported to your body cells and used as fuel.

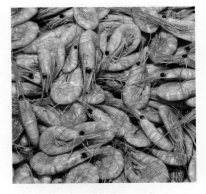

Chitosan, which comes from marine crustaceans, such as these shrimp, is the main ingredient in one group of fat-blockers.

lipoprotein A spherical (round-shaped) compound in which fat clusters in the center and phospholipids and proteins form the outside of the sphere.

chylomicron A lipoprotein produced in the enterocyte; transports dietary fat out of the intestinal tract.

- If the fat isn't needed for energy, the liver can use it to make lipid-containing compounds, such as certain hormones and bile.
- The fat can be taken up by muscle or adipose cells, repackaged as triglyceride, and stored for later use.

If you are physically active, your body will store some of this fat in your muscle cells, so that the next time you go out for a run, the fat is readily available for energy. Of course, fat stored in the adipose tissue can also be used for energy during exercise, but it must be broken down first and then transported to the muscle cells.

recap Fat digestion begins when fats are broken into droplets by bile. Pancreatic enzymes then digest the triglycerides into two free fatty acids and one monoglyceride. These are transported into the enterocytes with the help of micelles. Once inside, triglycerides are reformed and packaged into lipoproteins called chylomicrons. Dietary fat is transported by the chylomicrons to cells within the body that need energy. Fat stored in the muscle cells is used as a source of energy during physical activity. Excess fat is stored in the adipose tissue and can be used whenever the body needs energy.

LO6 Identify the dietary recommendations for intakes of total fat, saturated fat, *trans* fats, and the essential fatty acids.

LO7 Identify common food sources of less healthful versus more healthful fats.

How much fat should we eat?

Without a doubt, Americans agree that dietary fat is bad! Yet, because fat plays such an important role in keeping our body healthy, our diet should include a moderate amount of energy from fat. But what, exactly, is a moderate amount? And what foods contain healthful fats? We'll explore these questions here.

Dietary Reference Intake for Total Fat

The Acceptable Macronutrient Distribution Range (AMDR) for fat is 20% to 35% of total energy intake.[3] For a diet of 2,000 kcal per day, this amounts to 400 to 700 kcal, or approximately 45 to 77 grams of fat. For reference, a tablespoon of butter is 11 grams of fat and about 100 kcal.

Athletes and other physically active people typically eat a lower percentage of fat than sedentary people, because their carbohydrate and protein needs are often higher. However, it's still recommended that athletes consume 20% to 35% of their total energy from fat. Consuming less than 20% of energy from fat does not benefit performance.[13] This level of fat intake represents about 45 to 78 grams per day of fat for an athlete consuming 2,000 kcal per day, and 78 to 136 grams per day of fat for an athlete consuming 3,500 kcal per day.

Although many people trying to lose weight greatly restrict their consumption of fat, this practice may do more harm than good, especially if they are also eating fewer than 1,500 kcal per day. Research suggests that very-low-fat diets (those with less than 15% of energy from fat) do not provide additional health or performance benefits over moderate-fat diets, and are often very difficult to follow.[14] In fact, most people find that they feel better, are more successful in maintaining weight, and are less preoccupied with food if they keep their fat intakes at 20% to 25% of their total energy intake.

Additionally, people trying to reduce their dietary fat often eliminate entire food groups such as meat, dairy, eggs, and nuts. In doing so, they also eliminate important potential sources of protein and many essential vitamins and minerals needed for maintaining good health and an active lifestyle. Diets very low in fat may also be deficient in essential fatty acids.

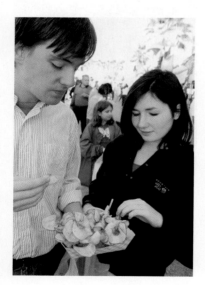

◆ In the United States, we eat too many saturated and *trans* fats.

Dietary Reference Intakes for Specific Fatty Acids

Dietary Reference Intakes (DRIs) for the two essential fatty acids were set in 2005.[3] The adequate intakes are as follows:

- Linoleic acid: 14 to 17 grams per day for adult men and 11 to 12 grams per day for women 19 years and older. Using the typical energy intakes for adult men and women, this translates into an AMDR of 5% to 10% of total energy.

- Alpha-linolenic acid: 1.6 grams per day for adult men and 1.1 grams per day for adult women. This translates into an AMDR of 0.6% to 1.2% of total energy.

For example, a person consuming 2,000 kcal per day should consume about 11 to 22 grams per day of linoleic acid and about 1.3 to 2.6 grams per day of alpha-linolenic acid.

Although the body converts some alpha-linolenic acid to DHA and EPA, the extent of this conversion is limited. Thus, some public health authorities, such as the World Health Organization, are now making formal recommendations for DHA and EPA specifically. These recommendations typically range from 0.25 to 0.5 grams per day of EPA/DHA, and 0.8 to 1.1 grams per day of alpha-linolenic acid.[5,15,16]

We said earlier that, of the dietary fat we eat, MUFAs and PUFAs, including EFAs, are associated with a reduced risk for cardiovascular disease, whereas SFAs and *trans* fats are associated with an increased risk. Thus, the majority of our fat intake should be from unsaturated fats. The American Heart Association recommends intake of saturated fat between 5% and 6% of total energy.[17] Additionally, the 2010 *Dietary Guidelines for Americans* and the Institute of Medicine recommend that we keep our intake of *trans* fatty acids to an absolute minimum.[2]

recap The Acceptable Macronutrient Distribution Range (AMDR) for total fat is 20% to 35% of total energy. The adequate intake (AI) for linoleic acid is 14 to 17 grams per day for adult men and 11 to 12 grams per day for adult women. The AI for alpha-linolenic acid is 1.6 grams per day for adult men and 1.1 grams per day for adult women. Because saturated and *trans* fatty acids are associated with an increased risk for heart disease, health professionals recommend that we reduce our intake of saturated fat to 5–6% of our total energy intake and reduce our intake of *trans* fatty acids to the absolute minimum.

Shopper's Guide: Choosing Foods with Healthful Fats

FIGURE 4.8 compares a day's meals on two diets: one high in healthful unsaturated fats and one high in saturated fats and cholesterol. Ahead are helpful strategies for choosing foods with healthful fats.

Visible Versus Invisible Fats

At breakfast this morning, did you add cream to your coffee? Spread butter on your toast? These added fats, such as oils, butter, margarine, cream, shortening, mayonnaise, or salad dressings, are called **visible fats** because we can easily see that we are adding them to our food.

When we add fat to foods ourselves, we know how much we are adding and what kind. When fat is added in the preparation of a frozen dinner or a fast-food burger and fries, we are less aware or unaware of how much or what type of fat is actually there. In fact, unless we read food labels carefully, we might not know that a food contains any fat at all. We call fats in prepared and processed foods **invisible fats** because they are effectively hidden within the food. In fact, their invisibility often tricks us into choosing them over more healthful foods. For example, a slice of yellow cake is much higher in fat (40% of total energy) than a slice of angel food cake (1% of total energy). Yet many people would assume the fat content of these foods is the same, because both are cake. For most of us, the majority of the fat in our diet comes from invisible fat. Foods that can be high in invisible fats are baked goods, regular-fat dairy products, processed meats or meats that are not trimmed, and most convenience and fast foods, such as hamburgers, hot dogs, chips, ice cream, french fries, and other fried foods.

Food Sources of Beneficial Fats

In addition to limiting your total fat consumption to no more than 35% of your diet, it's essential to choose healthful forms of fat. Substituting unsaturated fats for saturated

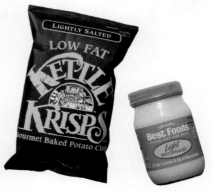

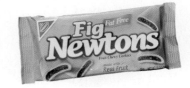

visible fats Fats that we can see in our foods or see added to foods, such as butter, margarine, cream, shortening, salad dressings, chicken skin, and untrimmed fat on meat.

invisible fats Fats that are hidden in foods, such as those found in baked goods, regular-fat dairy products, marbling in meat, and fried foods.

a day of meals

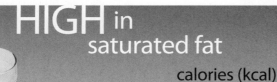

HIGH in
saturated fat
calories (kcal)

LOW in
saturated fat
calories (kcal)

BREAKFAST

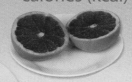

1 egg, fried
2 slices bacon
2 slices white toast with
   2 tsp. butter
8 fl. oz whole milk

2 egg whites, scrambled
2 slices whole-wheat toast
   with 2 tsp. olive oil spread
1 grapefruit
8 fl. oz skim milk

McDonald's Quarter Pounder
   with cheese
McDonald's French fries, small
12 fl. oz cola beverage

Tuna Sandwich
3 oz tuna (packed in water)
2 tsp. reduced fat mayonnaise
2 leaves red leaf lettuce
2 slices rye bread
1 large carrot, sliced with
   1 cup raw cauliflower with
   2 tbsp. low-fat Italian salad
   dressing
1 1-oz bag of salted potato chips
24 fl. oz water

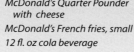

LUNCH

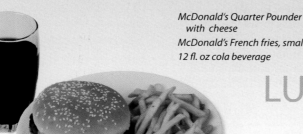

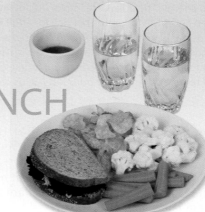

DINNER

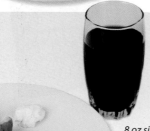

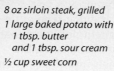

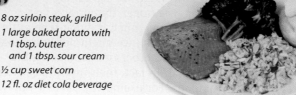

1 cup minestrone soup
4 oz grilled salmon
1 cup brown rice with 2 tsp.
   slivered almonds
1 cup steamed broccoli
1 dinner roll with 1 tsp. butter
12 fl. oz iced tea

8 oz sirloin steak, grilled
1 large baked potato with
   1 tbsp. butter
   and 1 tbsp. sour cream
½ cup sweet corn
12 fl. oz diet cola beverage

nutrient analysis

nutrient analysis

2,316 kcal
36.6% of energy from carbohydrates
39.1% of energy from fat
16% of energy from saturated fat
15.3% of energy from unsaturated fat
23% of energy from protein
15.3 grams of dietary fiber
2,713 milligrams of sodium

11%
LESS
saturated
fat

2,392 kcal
46.6% of energy from carbohydrates
28.1% of energy from fat
5% of energy from saturated fat
18.8% of energy from unsaturated fat
17.5% of energy from protein
28 grams of dietary fiber
2,713 milligrams of sodium

TABLE 4.1   Omega-3 Fatty Acid Content of Selected Foods

Food Item	Total Omega-3	DHA* g/Serving	EPA†
Flaxseed oil, 1 tbsp.	7.25	0.00	0.00
Salmon oil (fish oil), 1 tbsp.	4.39	2.48	1.77
Sardine oil, 1 tbsp.	3.01	1.45	1.38
Flaxseed, whole, 1 tbsp.	2.50	0.00	0.00
Chia seeds, whole, 1 tbsp.	1.87	0.00	0.00
Herring, Atlantic, broiled, 3 oz	1.83	0.94	0.77
Salmon, Coho, steamed, 3 oz	1.34	0.71	0.46
Canola oil, 1 tbsp.	1.28	0.00	0.00
Sardines, Atlantic, w/bones & oil, 3 oz	1.26	0.43	0.40
Trout, rainbow fillet, baked, 3 oz	1.05	0.70	0.28
Walnuts, English, 1 tbsp.	0.66	0.00	0.00
Halibut, fillet, baked, 3 oz	0.53	0.31	0.21
Shrimp, canned, 3 oz	0.47	0.21	0.25
Tuna, white, in oil, 3 oz	0.38	0.19	0.04
Crab, Alaska King, steamed, 3 oz	0.36	0.10	0.25
Scallops, broiled, 3 oz	0.31	0.14	0.17
Smart Balance Omega-3 Buttery Spread (1 tbsp.)	0.32	0.01	0.01
Tuna, light, in water, 3 oz	0.23	0.19	0.04
Avocado, Calif., fresh, whole	0.22	0.00	0.00
Spinach, cooked, 1 cup	0.17	0.00	0.00
Egglands Best, 1 large egg, with omega-3	0.12	0.06	0.03

*DHA = docosahexaenoic acid.
†EPA = eicosapentaenoic acid.
Data from Food Processor SQL, Version 10.3, ESHA Research, Salem, OR and manufacturer labels.

or *trans* fats isn't difficult. **TABLE 4.1** identifies the omega-3 fatty acid content of various foods. In addition, the following are some general guidelines for finding healthful fats.

Eat More Fish   Americans appear to get adequate amounts of omega-6 fatty acids, probably because of the high amount of salad dressings, vegetable and nut oils, margarine, and mayonnaise we eat. In contrast, our consumption of omega-3 fatty acids—and especially EPA/DHA—varies and can be low in the diets of people who don't eat fish, one of the most reliable dietary sources of these fatty acids (Table 4.1). So, to increase your consumption of EPA/DHA, choose fish or shellfish at least twice a week. At the deli, grab a tuna sandwich instead of roast beef. Out for Mexican food? Order fish tacos. Asian food? Try a stir-fry with prawns. Burgers? A haddock or salmon burger makes a nice change from beef.

You may be aware of warnings associated with eating large amounts of certain types of fish on a regular basis. These include sport-caught fish and predator fish such as shark, swordfish, and king mackerel, which can contain high levels of environmental contaminants, such as mercury and polychlorinated biphenyls (PCBs). Women who are pregnant or breastfeeding, women who may become pregnant, and small children are at particularly high risk for toxicity from these contaminants. Fortunately, many types of fish that provide EPA/DHA are considered safe to consume. These include salmon (except from the Great Lakes region), farmed trout, flounder, sole, mahi mahi, and cooked shellfish.

Choose Plants   Of course, healthful fats include not only the essential fatty acids but also polyunsaturated and monounsaturated fats in general. An easy way to shift

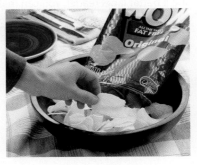

Baked goods are often high in invisible fats.

Low-Fat, Reduced-Fat, Nonfat . . . What's the Difference?

Although most of us enjoy high-fat foods, we also know that eating a lot of fat isn't good for our health or our waistline. Because of this concern, food manufacturers have produced thousands of modified fat foods—so you can have your cake and eat it, too!

The Food and Drug Administration and the U.S. Department of Agriculture have set specific regulations on allowable product descriptions for reduced-fat products. The following claims are defined for 1 serving:

Fat-free: less than 0.5 grams of fat

Low-fat: 3 grams or less of fat

Reduced or less fat: at least 25% less fat as compared to a standard serving

Light: one-third fewer Calories or 50% less fat as compared with a standard serving size.

TABLE 4.2 lists a number of full-fat foods with their lower-fat alternatives. If you incorporate these products into your diet on a regular basis, you can significantly reduce the amount of fat you consume, but watch out! You might not be reducing the number of Calories you consume.

Check it out for yourself. As shown in the first row of the table, drinking nonfat milk (86 Calories and 0.5 grams of fat per serving) instead of whole milk (150 Calories and 8.2 grams of fat per serving) will significantly reduce both fat and Calorie intake. Now look at the last row. If you eat 3 fat-free Fig Newton cookies, you won't consume any fat, but how many Calories will you take in? And how does this compare to the Calorie count for 3 regular Fig Newton cookies?

How do you know if a food you're buying is high in fat or Calories? Read the Nutrition Facts panel on the label! By becoming a better label reader, you can make more healthful food selections. For some practice, look at the "reduced fat" cracker label shown in **FIGURE 4.9**. Notice the total fat per serving. Does this product qualify as a low-fat food? Now look at the number of Calories and the grams of dietary fiber. Would you consider this a healthful choice for snacking? Why or why not?

TABLE 4.2 **Comparison of Full-Fat, Reduced-Fat, and Low-Fat Foods**

Product and Serving Size	Version	Energy (kcal)	Fat (g)
Milk, 8 oz	Whole, 3.3% fat	150	8.2
	2% fat	121	4.7
	Skim (nonfat)	86	0.5
Mayonnaise, 1 tbsp.	Regular	100	11.0
	Light	50	5.0
Margarine, corn oil, 1 tbsp.	Regular	100	11.0
	Reduced-fat	60	7.0
Peanut butter, 1 tbsp.	Regular	95	8.2
	Reduced-fat	81	5.4
Wheat Thins, 18 crackers	Regular	158	6.8
	Reduced-fat	120	4.0
Cookies, Oreo, 3 cookies	Regular	160	7.0
	Reduced-fat	130	3.5
Cookies, Fig Newton, 3 cookies	Regular	210	4.5
	Fat-free	204	0.0

Data from Food Processor-SQL, Version 9.9, ESHA Research, Salem, OR.

your diet toward these healthful fats—without increasing your total fat intake—is to replace animal-based foods with versions derived from plants. For example, drink soy milk or almond milk instead of cow's milk. Order your Chinese takeout with tofu instead of beef. Plant oils are excellent sources of unsaturated fats, so cook with olive, canola, soybean, or walnut oil instead of butter. Use thin slices of avocado in a sandwich in place of cheese, or serve tortilla chips with just guacamole instead of nacho-cheese.

Nuts and seeds provide another way to increase the healthful fats in your diet. They are rich in unsaturated fats and provide protein, minerals, vitamins, and fiber. Yet they are also high in energy: a 1 oz serving of nuts (about 4 tablespoons) contains 160–180 kcal. So eat them in moderation—for instance, by sprinkling a few on your salad, yogurt, or breakfast cereal. Spread a nut butter on your morning toast (try something new, like almond butter), or pack a peanut butter sandwich for lunch. Or add some pumpkin or sunflower seeds to raisins and pretzel sticks for a quick trail mix.

nutrition label activity

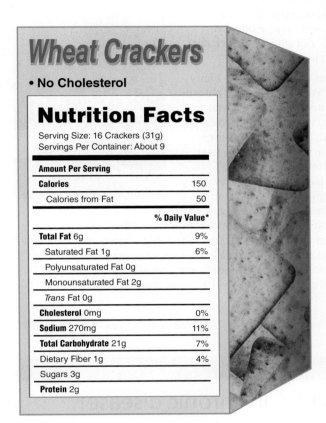

(a)

Wheat Crackers

- No Cholesterol

Nutrition Facts

Serving Size: 16 Crackers (31g)
Servings Per Container: About 9

Amount Per Serving

Calories	150
Calories from Fat	50

	% Daily Value*
Total Fat 6g	9%
Saturated Fat 1g	6%
Polyunsaturated Fat 0g	
Monounsaturated Fat 2g	
Trans Fat 0g	
Cholesterol 0mg	0%
Sodium 270mg	11%
Total Carbohydrate 21g	7%
Dietary Fiber 1g	4%
Sugars 3g	
Protein 2g	

(b)

Reduced-Fat Wheat Crackers

- **No Cholesterol**
- **Low Saturated Fat**
  Contains 4g Fat Per Serving

Nutrition Facts

Serving Size: 16 Crackers (29g)
Servings Per Container: About 9

Amount Per Serving

Calories	130
Calories from Fat	35

	% Daily Value*
Total Fat 4g	6%
Saturated Fat 1g	4%
Polyunsaturated Fat 0g	
Monounsaturated Fat 1.5g	
Trans Fat 0g	
Cholesterol 0mg	0%
Sodium 260 mg	11%
Total Carbohydrate 21g	7%
Dietary Fiber 1g	4%
Sugars 3g	
Protein 2g	

FIGURE 4.9 Nutrition Facts panel of reduced-fat wheat crackers.

Opt for Low-Fat When you are consuming animal-based foods, choose those lower in fat. Select lean meats, poultry, and fish. When preparing these foods at home or ordering them at a restaurant, make sure they're broiled or grilled rather than fried. Select low-fat or nonfat milk and yogurt, and reduce your intake of full-fat cheeses and cheese spreads. When shopping, look for lower-fat versions of all processed foods you buy. However, bear in mind that these lower-fat foods may not necessarily have fewer Calories. Read the ***Nutrition Label Activity*** to learn how to compare the fat and Calorie content of packaged foods.

Concerned about the saturated fat and cholesterol in the meat you eat? Use this guide to choosing the leanest cuts of beef at www.mayoclinic.com. Go to the search box and type in "cuts of beef" to get in-depth information.

recap Visible fats can be easily recognized, such as fat on meats. Invisible fats are those fats added to food during the manufacturing or cooking process. Common food sources of omega-6 fatty acids include vegetables and vegetable oils, nuts and nut oils, salad dressings, margarine, and mayonnaise. Food sources of omega-3 fatty acids include fish, walnuts, soy milk, and soybean, canola, or flaxseed oil. However, certain fish and shellfish are the best sources of EPA/DHA specifically.

foods you don't know you love YET

Seeds

Seeds are generally high in plant protein and heart-healthy unsaturated fatty acids. They also tend to be a good source of fiber and certain minerals. You're probably already accustomed to eating sesame seeds on your bagel, or sunflower seeds in your trail mix, but why not branch out? Here are a few more healthful choices:

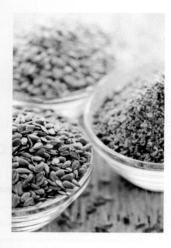

- Pumpkin seeds are a delicious source of omega-3 fatty acids and plant sterols, which reduce the body's absorption of cholesterol. They're also very high in several minerals, including magnesium and zinc. But avoid the packaged brands loaded with salt. Instead, buy them raw, in bulk, and roast them in your oven on low heat (200° F or lower) for 15 to 20 minutes.
- Chia seeds are from a desert plant grown in Mexico. They have a nutty taste and are high in omega-3 fatty acids, protein, and fiber. Sprinkle some on cereal, in yogurt, or on stir-fried vegetables, or toss some into the batter of muffins or other baked goods.
- Flaxseeds are largely undigestible, but when ground they provide omega-6 and omega-3 fatty acids as well as fiber and phytochemicals called *lignans* associated with a reduced risk for cardiovascular disease.[2] Mix ground flaxseeds into yogurt and other creamy foods. You can also sprinkle them on breakfast cereal or mix them into the batter of baked goods for an added nutritional boost.

 HEALTHWATCH

LO8 Summarize our current understanding of the relationship between intake of dietary fats and the development of cardiovascular disease and cancer.

What role do fats play in chronic disease?

We know that a diet high in saturated and *trans* fatty acids can contribute to chronic diseases, including cardiovascular disease and cancer. But just how significant a factor is diet, and what other factors also play a role?

What Is Cardiovascular Disease?

Cardiovascular disease is a general term used to describe any abnormal condition involving dysfunction of the heart (*cardio* means "heart") and blood vessels. There are many forms of the disease, but the three most common forms are listed here:

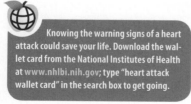
Knowing the warning signs of a heart attack could save your life. Download the wallet card from the National Institutes of Health at www.nhlbi.nih.gov; type "heart attack wallet card" in the search box to get going.

cardiovascular disease A general term referring to abnormal conditions (dysfunction) of the heart and blood vessels; cardiovascular disease can result in heart attack or stroke.

- *Coronary heart disease* occurs when blood vessels supplying the heart (the *coronary arteries*) become blocked or constricted; such blockage reduces the flow of blood—and the oxygen and nutrients it carries—to the heart. This can result in chest pain and lead to a heart attack.
- *Stroke* is caused by blockage or rupture of one of the blood vessels supplying the brain (the *cerebral arteries*). When this occurs, the region of the brain depending on that artery for oxygen and nutrients cannot function. As a result, the movement, speech, or other body functions controlled by that part of the brain suddenly stop.
- *Hypertension*, also called *high blood pressure*, is a condition that may not cause any immediate symptoms but increases your risk for a heart attack or stroke. If your blood pressure is high, it means the force of the blood flowing through your arteries is above normal.

According to the Centers for Disease Control and Prevention, cardiovascular disease (in its various forms) is the leading cause of death in the United States across racial and ethnic groups and is a major cause of permanent disability (see Figure 1.3).

Dietary Fats Play an Important Role in Cardiovascular Disease

Recall that lipids are transported in the blood by lipoproteins made up of a lipid center and a protein outer coat. Because lipoproteins are soluble in blood, they are commonly called *blood lipids*. In addition to the chylomicrons discussed earlier in this chapter, three lipoproteins are important to consider in any discussion of cardiovascular health and disease:

- very-low-density lipoproteins (VLDLs)
- low-density lipoproteins (LDLs)
- high-density lipoproteins (HDLs)

The density of a lipoprotein refers to its *ratio* of lipid (less dense) to protein (very dense). Thus, a VLDL contains mostly lipid and little protein. The chemical composition of various lipoproteins is compared in **FIGURE 4.10**. Our blood contains a mixture of these blood lipids according to our diet, our fitness level, and whether we have been eating or fasting. Let's look at each of these blood lipids in more detail to determine how they are linked to heart disease risk.

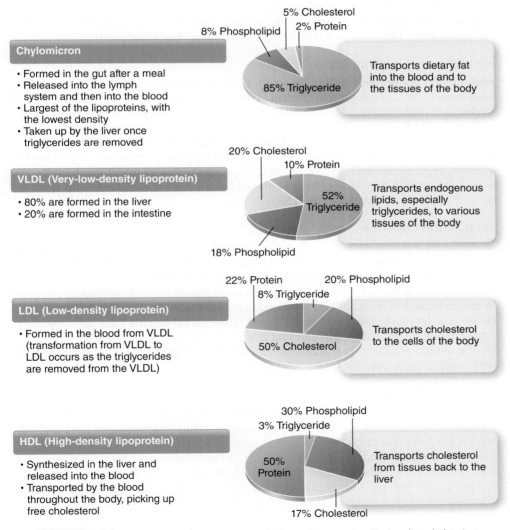

Chylomicron
- Formed in the gut after a meal
- Released into the lymph system and then into the blood
- Largest of the lipoproteins, with the lowest density
- Taken up by the liver once triglycerides are removed

5% Cholesterol
2% Protein
8% Phospholipid
85% Triglyceride

Transports dietary fat into the blood and to the tissues of the body

VLDL (Very-low-density lipoprotein)
- 80% are formed in the liver
- 20% are formed in the intestine

20% Cholesterol
10% Protein
52% Triglyceride
18% Phospholipid

Transports endogenous lipids, especially triglycerides, to various tissues of the body

LDL (Low-density lipoprotein)
- Formed in the blood from VLDL (transformation from VLDL to LDL occurs as the triglycerides are removed from the VLDL)

22% Protein
8% Triglyceride
20% Phospholipid
50% Cholesterol

Transports cholesterol to the cells of the body

HDL (High-density lipoprotein)
- Synthesized in the liver and released into the blood
- Transported by the blood throughout the body, picking up free cholesterol

30% Phospholipid
3% Triglyceride
50% Protein
17% Cholesterol

Transports cholesterol from tissues back to the liver

FIGURE 4.10 The chemical components of various lipoproteins. Notice that chylomicrons contain the highest proportion of triglycerides, making them the least dense, while HDLs have the highest proportion of protein, making them the most dense.

Very-Low-Density Lipoproteins

Very-low-density lipoproteins (VLDLs) are made up mostly of triglyceride. The liver is the primary source of VLDLs, but they are also produced in the intestines. VLDLs are mainly transport vehicles that carry triglycerides, which are produced in the liver or intestine, to other cells of the body. If their triglyceride load is not needed for fuel, the fatty acids can be released and taken up by the adipose cells for storage.

Diets high in saturated fat, simple sugars, and extra energy tend to increase blood levels of VLDLs, because they increase the production of triglycerides in the liver. Conversely, diets high in omega-3 fatty acids can help reduce VLDL levels, because they inhibit the production of triglycerides, which are the primary component of VLDLs.[5] In addition, exercise can reduce VLDLs because the triglycerides transported in the VLDLs can be used for energy instead of remaining to circulate in the blood.

Low-Density Lipoproteins

The lipoproteins that result when VLDLs release their triglyceride load are much higher in cholesterol, phospholipids, and protein and therefore somewhat more dense. These **low-density lipoproteins (LDLs)** circulate in the blood until they are absorbed by the body's cells, thereby delivering their cholesterol to the cells. Diets high in saturated and *trans* fats decrease the removal of LDLs by body cells and therefore increase LDL levels in the blood. The more LDLs circulating in the blood, the greater the risk that some of their cholesterol will be taken up into the walls of the blood vessels. This is one step in a complex process known as atherosclerosis, which greatly increases the risk for a heart attack or stroke (**FIGURE 4.11**). For this reason, LDL-cholesterol is often referred to as "bad cholesterol."

High-Density Lipoproteins

High-density lipoproteins (HDLs) are small, dense lipoproteins with a very low cholesterol content and a high protein content. They are produced in the liver, then released to circulate in the blood, picking up cholesterol from dying cells and arterial plaques or transferring it to other lipoproteins. When HDLs deliver their newly acquired cholesterol to the liver, they remove it from the cardiovascular system. That's why high blood levels of HDLs are associated with a lower risk for coronary artery disease and why HDL-cholesterol is often referred to as "good cholesterol."[16] Incidentally, one of the ways in which diets high in omega-3 fatty acids may decrease our risk for heart disease is by increasing HDL-cholesterol.[15,18]

Total Serum Cholesterol

Normally, as the level of dietary cholesterol increases, the body decreases the amount of cholesterol it makes, which keeps the body's level of cholesterol fairly constant. Unfortunately, this feedback mechanism does not work well in everyone. For some people, eating dietary cholesterol doesn't decrease the amount of cholesterol produced in the body, and as a result their total body cholesterol levels rise. This in turn increases the levels of cholesterol in the blood. They would benefit from reducing their intake of dietary cholesterol, by limiting their intake of animal products or selecting low-fat animal products. Research also shows that high intakes of saturated and *trans* fatty acids can increase the total serum cholesterol.

The Role of *Trans* Fatty Acids

Research indicates that *trans* fatty acids can raise blood LDL-cholesterol levels.[17,19] Thus, to reduce the risk for heart disease, we must reduce our intake of both high-fat animal products and foods that contain vegetable shortening or partially hydrogenated oils (PHOs). Foods fried in PHOs, such as French fries and doughnuts, are also high in *trans* fatty acids, so these types of foods should be avoided as well. Finally, if you use margarine and shortening, look for products that contain no *trans* fatty acids. Choose olive oil, nut butters, and other healthful fats instead.

Calculate Your Risk for Cardiovascular Disease

A simple laboratory analysis of your blood can reveal your blood lipid levels, specifically your LDL-cholesterol, HDL-cholesterol, and total serum cholesterol. If you

⬆ Foods fried in hydrogenated vegetable oils, such as French fries, are high in *trans* fatty acids and should be avoided.

very-low-density lipoprotein (VLDL) A large lipoprotein made up mostly of triglyceride. Functions primarily to transport triglycerides from their source to the body's cells, including to adipose tissues for storage.

low-density lipoprotein (LDL) A molecule resulting when a VLDL releases its triglyceride load. Higher cholesterol and protein content makes LDLs somewhat more dense than VLDLs.

high-density lipoprotein (HDL) A small, dense lipoprotein with a very low cholesterol content and a high protein content.

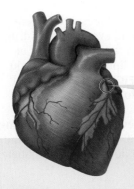

Plaque accumulation within coronary arteries narrows their interior and impedes the flow of oxygen-rich blood to the heart.

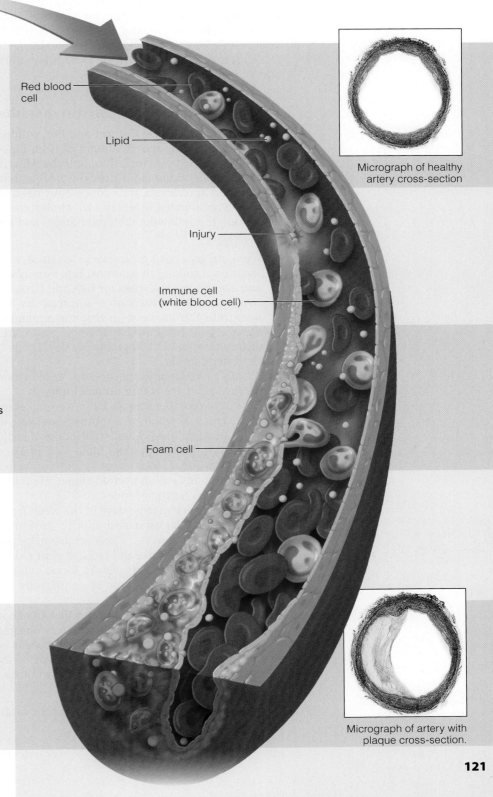

HEALTHY ARTERY

Blood flows unobstructed through normal, healthy artery.

ARTERIAL INJURY

The artery's lining is injured, attracting immune cells, and prompting inflammation.

LIPIDS ACCUMULATE IN WALL

Lipids, particulary cholesterol-containing LDLs, seep beneath the wall lining. The LDLs become oxidized. Immune cells, attracted to the site, engulf the oxidized LDLs and are transformed into foam cells.

FATTY STREAK

The foam cells accumulate to a form a fatty streak, which releases more toxic and inflammatory chemicals.

PLAQUE FORMATION

The foam cells, along with platelets, calcium, protein fibers, and other substances, form thick deposits of plaque, stiffening and narrowing the artery. Blood flow through the artery is reduced or obstructed.

Red blood cell

Lipid

Injury

Immune cell (white blood cell)

Foam cell

Micrograph of healthy artery cross-section

Micrograph of artery with plaque cross-section.

do not know this information about yourself, there are easy ways to find out. Many college health centers offer blood lipid screenings at low cost or for free to students. Or the next time you visit your physician, ask to have your blood lipids measured. You should also get your blood pressure checked regularly. Blood pressure screening is often offered at student health centers, at health fairs, and even in many drug stores. It is especially important to take these steps if you have a family history of heart disease. Once you know your blood pressure and blood lipid levels, then you can estimate your risk of developing cardiovascular disease (**FIGURE 4.12**). You can also do this quick assessment on family members or friends to help them become more aware of their risk factors for cardiovascular disease.

Your healthcare provider also considers your blood lipid levels when determining your risk for *metabolic syndrome*. As you learned in Chapter 3, metabolic syndrome is a cluster of factors more likely to be present in people who develop type 2 diabetes and/or cardiovascular disease.

Reduce Your Risk for Cardiovascular Disease

The Centers for Disease Control and Prevention (CDC), the Expert Panel on Detection, Evaluation, and Treatment of High Blood Cholesterol in Adults (ATP III), the American Heart Association, and the American College of Cardiology have all made recommendations for diet, physical activity, and lifestyle factors that can improve blood lipid levels and reduce your risk for cardiovascular disease.[17,20,21] Aim for the recommended levels of LDL-cholesterol, HDL-cholesterol, and triglycerides by making the following dietary changes and incorporating physical activity into your lifestyle:

- *Maintain your total fat intake* to within 20% to 35% of energy.[3]
- *Focus on including unsaturated fats* from plant oils, nuts, and seeds in your diet, and eat fish twice a week for EPA and DHA.
- *Decrease your consumption of saturated fat* to 5–6% of total energy intake and keep *trans* fats intake at an absolute minimum.[17]
- *Increase your consumption of whole grains, fruits, and vegetables*, so that total dietary fiber is 20 to 30 grams per day. Foods high in fiber decrease blood LDL-cholesterol levels.
- *Schedule regular physical checkups* to help monitor your lipid levels and determine if your values are within normal limits.
- *Eat a healthful diet overall.* Eat fewer processed foods and more foods that are *whole* (such as whole-wheat breads and cereals, fruits and vegetables, and beans and legumes). Limit your intake of sodium, which is often present in high amounts in processed food. Limit your intake of high-sugar foods (for example, sweetened sodas, cookies, and candy) to help maintain blood glucose and insulin concentrations within normal ranges. High blood glucose levels are associated with high blood triglycerides.
- *Be active.* Exercise most days of the week for 30 to 60 minutes whenever possible, and make regular exercise a priority. Research shows that aerobic exercise lowers LDL-cholesterol levels.[17] Exercise also helps you maintain a healthy body weight, lowers blood pressure, and reduces your risk for diabetes.
- *Maintain a healthy body weight.* Blood lipids and glucose levels typically improve when people who are obese or significantly overweight lose weight and engage in regular physical activity.
- *Avoid tobacco.* Research indicates that smokers have a 70% greater chance of developing cardiovascular disease than nonsmokers. Without question, stopping smoking or never starting in the first place is one of the best ways to reduce your risk for cardiovascular disease. A 15-year period of nonsmoking will reduce your risk factors for cardiovascular disease to those of a nonsmoker. You should also avoid secondhand smoke.

For more strategies for reducing your risk for cardiovascular disease, check out the **Game Plan** feature box.

WHAT IS YOUR AGE?

Female:

Age	Points
20–34	–7
35–39	–3
40–44	0
45–49	3
50–54	6
55–59	8
60–64	10
65–69	12
70–74	14
75–79	16

Male:

Age	Points
20–34	–9
35–39	–4
40–44	0
45–49	3
50–54	6
55–59	8
60–64	10
65–69	11
70–74	12
75–79	13

Enter your points ☐

WHAT IS YOUR TOTAL CHOLESTEROL NUMBER?

Female:

Age	Total Cholesterol					
	<160	160–199	200–239	240–279	≥280	
20–39	0	4	8	11	13	Points
40–49	0	3	6	8	10	
50–59	0	2	4	5	7	
60–69	0	1	2	3	4	
70–79	0	1	1	2	2	

Male:

Age	Total Cholesterol					
	<160	160–199	200–239	240–279	≥280	
20–39	0	4	7	9	11	Points
40–49	0	3	5	6	8	
50–59	0	2	3	4	5	
60–69	0	1	1	2	3	
70–79	0	0	0	1	1	

Enter your points ☐

DO YOU SMOKE?

Nonsmoker, Female:

Age	Points
20–39	0
40–49	0
50–59	0
60–69	0
70–79	0

Nonsmoker, Male:

Age	Points
20–39	0
40–49	0
50–59	0
60–69	0
70–79	0

Smoker, Female:

Age	Points
20–39	9
40–49	7
50–59	4
60–69	2
70–79	1

Smoker, Male:

Age	Points
20–39	8
40–49	5
50–59	3
60–69	1
70–79	1

Enter your points ☐

WHAT IS YOUR HIGH-DENSITY LIPOPROTEIN NUMBER (HDL)?

Female:

HDL (mg/dL)	Points
≥60	–1
50–59	0
40–49	1
<40	2

Male:

HDL (mg/dL)	Points
≥60	–1
50–59	0
40–49	1
<40	2

Enter your points ☐

WHAT IS YOUR TOTAL NUMBER OF POINTS (what is your 10-year risk)?

Female:

Point total	10-Year risk %
<9	<1
9	1
10	1
11	1
12	1
13	2
14	2
15	3
16	4
17	5
18	6
19	8
20	11
21	14
22	17
23	22
24	27
≥25	≥30

Male:

Point total	10-Year risk %
<0	<1
0	1
1	1
2	1
3	1
4	1
5	2
6	2
7	3
8	4
9	5
10	6
11	8
12	10
13	12
14	16
15	20
16	25
≥17	≥30

Enter your 10-year risk percentage ☐

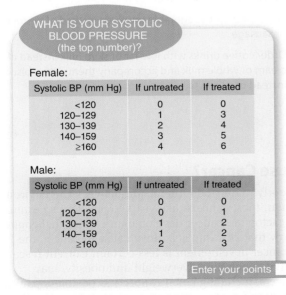

WHAT IS YOUR SYSTOLIC BLOOD PRESSURE (the top number)?

Female:

Systolic BP (mm Hg)	If untreated	If treated
<120	0	0
120–129	1	3
130–139	2	4
140–159	3	5
≥160	4	6

Male:

Systolic BP (mm Hg)	If untreated	If treated
<120	0	0
120–129	0	1
130–139	1	2
140–159	1	2
≥160	2	3

Enter your points ☐

FIGURE 4.12 Calculation matrix to estimate the 10-year risk for cardiovascular disease for men and women.

Data from National Institutes of Health. 2001. *Third Report of the National Cholesterol Education Program: Detection, Evaluation and Treatment of High Blood Cholesterol in Adults (ATP: III).* Bethesda, MD: National Cholesterol Education Program, National Heart, Lung, and Blood Institute. https://www.nhlbi.nih.gov/guidelines/cholesterol/risk_tbl.htm

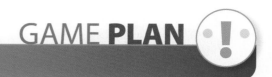

GAME **PLAN**

Tips for Heart-Healthy Eating

When shopping for and preparing meals at home, as well as when eating out, try these simple strategies to tip the balance of your diet toward heart-healthy fats.

At Home

☐ Boost the nutrients in your breakfast cereal by adding 1 tablespoon of ground flaxseed meal.

☐ Select whole-grain breads, and try peanut, almond, cashew, or walnut butter as a spread for your toast.

☐ If you normally eat two eggs for breakfast, remove the yolk from one egg for half the cholesterol. Do the same in recipes calling for two eggs.

☐ Select low-fat or nonfat milk, coffee creamers, yogurt, cream cheese, cottage cheese, sour cream, mayonnaise, and salad dressings.

☐ Substitute lower-fat cheeses, such as parmesan, for higher-fat cheeses, such as cheddar.

☐ If you use margarine, choose one made from a high-omega-3 oil, such as canola oil, and free of PHOs.

☐ Start meals with a salad dressed with olive oil and vinegar, or a fat-free soup.

☐ Select lean cuts of meat. Load your plate with vegetables, and make meat a "condiment."

☐ Instead of frying meats, fish, and vegetables, bake or broil them.

☐ Trim visible fat from meats and poultry before cooking. Eat poultry without the skin.

☐ Instead of buttering your bread, dip it in a mixture of olive oil with a dribble of balsamic vinegar.

☐ If you buy crackers, make sure they're low in saturated fats, high in fiber, and free of PHOs.

☐ Choose ice milk, sorbet, or low-fat or nonfat yogurt and fruit for dessert instead of high-fat ice cream.

☐ For snacks, munch on air-popped popcorn, raw vegetables, or a mixture of whole and dried fruits, nuts, seeds, and pretzels.

☐ Choose water, skim milk, soy milk, almond milk, or unsweetened beverages over sugar-sweetened beverages.

☐ Read the labels of packaged foods and select only versions made without PHOs.

☐ Control your portion size, especially when eating high-fat foods.

Eating Out

☐ When eating out, select a high-omega-3 fatty acid fish, such as salmon, or try a vegetarian entrée made with tofu or tempeh. If you do choose meat, ask for it to be trimmed of fat and broiled rather than fried.

☐ Consider splitting an entrée with a friend and complement it with a side salad.

☐ On your salad, choose olive oil and vinegar instead of a cream-based dressing. Also use olive oil and vinegar instead of butter for your bread.

☐ Order a baked potato or rice instead of french fries or potatoes with cheese toppings.

☐ Consider splitting a dessert or selecting fruit for dessert.

☐ The next time you order a fast-food meal, skip the french fries or order the kid's meal to help your portion control.

☐ Order pizza with vegetable toppings instead of pepperoni or sausage.

☐ Order coffee drinks with low-fat or skim milk instead of cream or whole milk and accompany them with a biscotti instead of a brownie.

Does a High-Fat Diet Cause Cancer?

Cancer develops as a result of a poorly understood interaction between the environment and genetic factors. In addition, most cancers take years to develop, so examining the impact of specific lifestyle factors on cancer development can be challenging. For example, whereas we now know that smoking is a direct cause of cancer, the contribution of dietary factors to cancer development is less certain. Current research shows that diet and physical inactivity, including overweight and obesity, may account for 25% to 30% of all cancers, including colon cancer and postmenopausal breast cancer.[22] Of course, a diet high in fat can contribute to obesity.

Three types of cancer have been studied extensively for their possible relationship to dietary fat intake: breast cancer, colon cancer, and prostate cancer.

- Breast cancer. Currently, research does not support a link between the amount or type of fat consumed and increased risk for breast cancer.[23] There is some evidence to suggest that a higher saturated fat intake may be associated with increased risk of breast cancer.[24]
- Colon cancer. Research shows that the typical American diet characterized by high red and processed meat consumption increases the risk of colon cancer, while diets higher in fruits and vegetables decrease risk.[25]
- Prostate cancer. As with other cancers, dietary animal fat intake has been associated with prostate cancer,[26] but there is no strong evidence or exact mechanism to support this link.[26,27] Currently there is no conclusive evidence showing that a single dietary factor reduces the risk of prostate cancer.[26]

Until we know more about the link between diet (especially fat) and cancer, the American Cancer Society recommends the following diet and lifestyle changes to reduce your risks.[22]

- Achieve and maintain a healthy body weight throughout life.
- Adopt a physically active lifestyle.
- Consume a healthy diet, with an emphasis on plant sources (fruits, vegetables, and whole grains) and limited consumption of processed meat and red meats.
- If you drink alcohol, limit consumption. Drink no more than 1 drink per day for women and 2 per day for men.

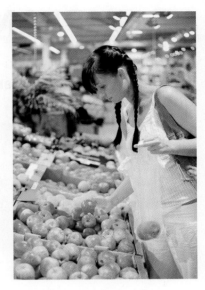

Eating whole fruits and vegetables can reduce your risk for colon cancer.

recap The types of fats we eat can significantly affect our risk for disease. Saturated and *trans* fatty acids increase our risk for heart disease, whereas the omega-3 fatty acids EPA and DHA can reduce our risk. High levels of LDL-cholesterol and low levels of HDL-cholesterol increase your risk for heart disease. Other risk factors for heart disease include being overweight, being physically inactive, smoking, having high blood pressure, and having diabetes. Consuming a healthful diet and making recommended lifestyle choices may also reduce your risk for some cancers.

STUDY **PLAN** | MasteringNutrition™

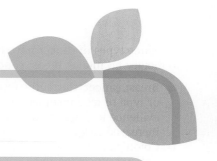

Customize your study plan—and master your nutrition!—
in the Study Area of **MasteringNutrition**.

what can I do **today?**

Now that you've read this chapter, try making these four changes.

1 Instead of having meat at both lunch and dinner today, choose fish or shellfish. Or, have a vegetarian meal that might include beans, whole grains, or a low-fat cheese.

2 Select low-fat dairy products.

3 Check the ingredients list on food labels to make sure there are no PHOs in the food.

4 Get at least 30 minutes of physical activity today, and see how it makes you feel.

test yourself | *answers*

1. **True.** The body can manufacture all the cholesterol it needs from nutrients, so we don't need to consume it in our diet. Eating a diet low in saturated fat will also keep intake of dietary cholesterol within recommended levels.

2. **True.** Fat is our primary source of energy, both at rest and during low-intensity exercise. Fat is also an important fuel source during prolonged exercise.

3. **True.** Certain essential fatty acids reduce inflammation, blood clotting, and other risk factors associated with heart disease.

summary

Scan to hear an MP3 Chapter Review in **MasteringNutrition**.

LO **1** **Compare and contrast the three types of lipids found in foods**

- Fats and oils are forms of a larger and more diverse group of substances called lipids. Most lipids are insoluble in water. The three types of lipids commonly found in foods are triglycerides, phospholipids, and sterols.

- Triglycerides have a glycerol backbone attached to three fatty-acid chains. They are the most abundant lipid in our diet and our body. Phospholipids have a glycerol backbone with two fatty acids and a phosphate group. Phospholipids are soluble in water and assist with transporting fats in our bloodstream. Sterols have a ring structure. Cholesterol is the most common sterol in our diet, and is found only in animal foods.

LO **2** **Discuss how the level of saturation of a fatty acid affects its shape and the form it takes**

- Saturated fatty acids have no carbons attached together with a double bond, which means that every carbon atom in the fatty acid chain is saturated with hydrogen. Saturated fats are straight in shape, allowing the fatty acid chains to pack tightly together and making them solid at room temperature.

- Monounsaturated fatty acids contain one double bond between two carbon atoms; polyunsaturated fatty acids contain more than one double bond between carbon atoms. Their double bonds give unsaturated fats a kink along their length, which prevents them from packing tightly together, making them liquid at room temperature.

- A *trans* fatty acid has hydrogen atoms located on opposite sides of the double carbon bond. This positioning causes *trans* fatty acids to be straighter and more rigid like saturated fats. The *trans* positioning results when oils are hydrogenated during food processing. A high intake of *trans* fats is associated with increased LDL-cholesterol and total serum cholesterol and decreased HDL-cholesterol concentrations in the blood.

LO **3** **Explain the health benefits and dietary sources of the essential fatty acids**

- The essential fatty acids are linoleic acid, a type of omega-6 fatty acid, and alpha-linolenic acid, a type of omega-3 fatty acid. They cannot be synthesized by the body and must be consumed in our diet. Linoleic acid is found in vegetable and nut oils, such as sunflower, safflower, corn, soy, flax, and peanut oils. Alpha-linolenic acid is found mainly in leafy green vegetables, flaxseed and flaxseed oil, soy oil and foods, canola oil, and fatty fish and fish oils. Two omega-3 fatty acids found in oily fish, EPA and DHA, are thought to protect against cardiovascular disease.

LO 4 List five functions of fat

- Fats are a primary energy source during rest and exercise, are our major source of stored energy, enable the transport of fat-soluble vitamins, help maintain cell function and structures, and contribute to the flavor, texture, and satiety of foods.

LO 5 Describe the steps involved in fat digestion, absorption, and transport

- The majority of fat digestion and absorption occurs in the small intestine. Fat is broken into droplets by bile, which is produced by the liver and stored in the gallbladder. Monoglycerides and free fatty acids are transported across the enterocytes of the small intestine in micelles.

- These are reformed into triglycerides, which are packaged into lipoproteins called chylomicrons before being released into the lymphatic system then bloodstream for transport to cells.

LO 6 Identify the dietary recommendations for intakes of total fat, saturated fat, *trans* fats, and the essential fatty acids

- The AMDR for fat is 20% to 35% of total energy. Our intake of saturated fats and *trans* fatty acids should be kept to a minimum. Individuals who limit fat intake to less than 15% of energy intake need to make sure that essential fatty acid needs are met, as well as protein and energy needs.

- For the essential fatty acids, the adequate intake (AI) for linoleic acid is 14 to 17 grams per day for adult men and 11 to 12 grams per day for adult women. The AI for alpha-linolenic acid is 1.6 grams per day for adult men and 1.1 grams per day for adult women.

- The recommended intake of saturated fat is 5% to 6% of total energy, and *trans* fat intake should be kept to an absolute minimum.

LO 7 Identify common food sources of less healthful versus more healthful fats

- Saturated fats are found in butter, cream, cheese, poultry skin, and meats, as well as cakes, cookies, and other desserts, and fried foods. More healthful unsaturated fats are found in fish and plant foods such as nuts and seeds, soy milk and tofu, salad dressings, and plant oils.

LO 8 Summarize our current understanding of the relationship between intake of dietary fats and the development of cardiovascular disease and cancer

- Diets high in saturated fat and *trans* fatty acids can increase our risk for cardiovascular disease. Other risk factors for cardiovascular disease are excess weight or obesity, physical inactivity, smoking, high blood pressure, and diabetes mellitus.

- High levels of circulating low-density lipoproteins, or LDLs, which are rich in cholesterol, increase the formation of plaque on arterial walls, leading to an increased risk for cardiovascular disease. This is why LDL-cholesterol is sometimes called "bad cholesterol."

- High levels of circulating high-density lipoproteins, or HDLs, reduce our risk for cardiovascular disease. This is why HDL-cholesterol is sometimes called "good cholesterol."

- Some studies suggest that diets high in fat may increase our risk for cancer of the breast, colon, or prostate; however, the role of dietary fat in cancer is still controversial.

review questions

LO 1 Compare and contrast the three types of lipids found in foods

1. Cholesterol is
   a. a triglyceride.
   b. a form of saturated fatty acid.
   c. a sterol.
   d. a phospholipid.

LO 2 Discuss how the level of saturation of a fatty acid affects its shape and the form it takes

2. Triglycerides with a double carbon bond at one part of the molecule are referred to as
   a. monounsaturated fats.
   b. hydrogenated fats.
   c. saturated fats.
   d. sterols.

LO **3** **Explain the health benefits and dietary sources of the essential fatty acids**

3. EPA and DHA
   a. are omega-3 fatty acids.
   b. are found in fatty fish.
   c. reduce the risk of cardiovascular disease.
   d. all of the above.

LO **4** **List five functions of fat**

4. Fats
   a. provide energy, but less per gram than carbohydrates.
   b. provide energy for resting functions, but not for physical activity.
   c. enable the transport of proteins.
   d. enable the transport of fat-soluble vitamins.

LO **5** **Describe the steps involved in fat digestion, absorption, and transport**

5. Micelles assist in the
   a. transport of dietary fat to the enterocytes of the small intestine.
   b. emulsification of dietary fat in the small intestine.
   c. production of cholesterol in the liver.
   d. storage of excess fat in adipose tissue.

6. Dietary fat not immediately used by the body is repackaged
   a. as glycogen and stored in the liver.
   b. as triglyceride and stored in the adipose tissue.
   c. as cholesterol and stored in the blood vessels.
   d. as bile and excreted from the body in stools.

LO **6** **Identify the dietary recommendations for intakes of total fat, saturated fat, *trans* fats, and the essential fatty acids**

7. The Acceptable Macronutrient Distribution Range (AMDR) for fat is
   a. less than 15% of total energy.
   b. 15–25% of total energy.
   c. 20–35% of total energy.
   d. 25–40% of total energy.

LO **7** **Identify common food sources of less healthful versus more healthful fats**

8. Which of the following lunch choices is rich in both unsaturated fats and fiber?
   a. A serving of macaroni and cheese
   b. A peanut butter and jelly sandwich on whole-wheat bread
   c. A garlic bagel with low-fat cream cheese
   d. A hamburger on a sesame-seed bun

LO **8** **Summarize our current understanding of the relationship between intake of dietary fats and the development of cardiovascular disease and cancer**

9. The risk for cardiovascular disease is lower in people who have high blood levels of
   a. triglycerides.
   b. very-low-density lipoprotein (VLDL)-cholesterol.
   c. low-density lipoprotein (LDL)-cholesterol.
   d. high-density lipoprotein (HDL)-cholesterol.

10. Which of the following statements is true?
    a. A diet high in saturated fats, *trans* fats, and cholesterol is thought to increase the risk of cancer by 25–30%.
    b. A low-fat diet is thought to increase the risk of cancer by 25–30%.
    c. A poor diet and physical inactivity together may account for 25–30% of all cancers.
    d. A poor diet, physical inactivity, and smoking together may account for 25–30% of all cancers.

Answers to Review Questions are located at the back of this text.

web links

The following websites and apps explore further topics and issues related to personal health.
Visit MasteringNutrition for links to the websites and RSS feeds.

www.heart.org
American Heart Association

www.hsph.harvard.edu
Harvard University's Nutrition Source: Knowledge for Healthy Eating

www.nih.gov
National Institutes of Health (NIH)

www.nlm.nih.gov
MEDLINE Plus Health Information

5

Proteins
Crucial Components of All Body Tissues

learning outcomes

After studying this chapter, you should be able to:

1 Describe how proteins differ from carbohydrates and fats, pp. 130–132.

2 Describe the processes by which DNA directs protein synthesis and proteins organize into levels of structure, pp. 132–134.

3 Explain the significance of mutual supplementation and identify non-meat food combinations that are complete protein sources, pp. 132–134.

4 Identify at least four functions of proteins in our body, pp. 134–136.

5 Explain how our body digests and absorbs protein, pp. 136–138.

6 Calculate your recommended dietary allowance for protein, pp. 138–148.

7 Describe two disorders related to inadequate protein intake, pp. 138–148.

8 Identify several healthful food sources of animal and plant protein, pp. 138–148.

9 List the types, benefits, and potential challenges of vegetarian diets, pp. 148–151.

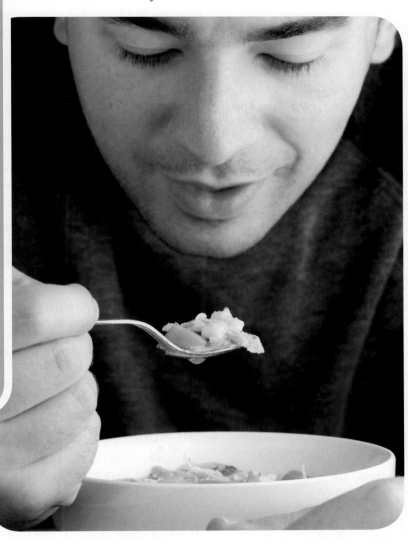

MasteringNutrition™

Go online for chapter quizzes, pre-tests, Interactive Activities, and more!

test yourself

Are these statements true or false? Circle your guess.

1. **T F** Protein is a primary source of energy for our body.

2. **T F** Any protein eaten in excess is excreted in your urine.

3. **T F** Most people in the United States consume more protein than they need.

Test Yourself answers can be found at the end of the chapter.

What do tennis star Venus Williams, Olympic gold medalist skier Bode Miller, Olympic silver medalist cyclist Lizzie Armitstead, and dozens of other athletes have in common? They're all vegetarians! Although precise statistics on the number of vegetarian athletes aren't available, a total of 3.4% of the U.S. population—approximately 6–8 million Americans—are estimated to be vegetarians.[1]

What exactly is a vegetarian? Do you qualify? If so, how do you plan your diet to include sufficient protein, especially if you play competitive sports? Are there real advantages to eating meat, or is plant protein just as good?

It seems as if everybody has an opinion about protein, both how much you should consume and from what sources. In this chapter, we address these and other questions to clarify the importance of protein in the diet and dispel common myths about this crucial nutrient.

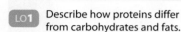 Describe how proteins differ from carbohydrates and fats.

What are proteins?

Proteins are large, complex molecules found in the cells of all living things. Although best known as part of our muscle mass, proteins are critical components of all body tissues. In certain circumstances, they can also provide energy. These and many more functions of proteins will be discussed later in this chapter.

How Do Proteins Differ from Carbohydrates and Lipids?

Proteins are one of the three macronutrients and are found in a wide variety of foods. Our body is able to manufacture (*synthesize*) all the macronutrients. But **DNA**, the genetic material in our cells, dictates the structure only of protein molecules, not of carbohydrates or lipids. We'll explore how our body synthesizes proteins and the role that DNA plays in this process shortly.

Another key difference between proteins and the other macronutrients lies in their chemical makeup. In addition to the carbon, hydrogen, and oxygen also found in carbohydrates and lipids, proteins contain a special form of nitrogen that our body can readily use. When we digest protein-containing plant and animal foods, nitrogen is released for use in many important body processes. Carbohydrates and lipids do not provide this critical form of nitrogen.

The Building Blocks of Proteins Are Amino Acids

Proteins are long, chainlike compounds made up of unique molecules called **amino acids**. If you were to imagine proteins as beaded necklaces, each bead would be an amino acid (**FIGURE 5.1**). The links that bind the amino acid "beads" to each other are unique chemical bonds called **peptide bonds**.

Most of the proteins in our body are made from varying combinations of just 20 amino acids, identified in **TABLE 5.1**. By "stringing together" dozens to hundreds of copies of these 20 amino acids in different sequences, our cells manufacture an estimated 10,000 to 50,000 unique proteins.

Now let's look at the structure of these amino acid "beads." At the core of every amino acid molecule is a central carbon atom. As you learned in the previous chapter, carbon atoms have four attachment sites. In amino acids, the central carbon's four attachment sites are filled by the following (**FIGURE 5.2A**):

1. a *hydrogen atom*.
2. an *acid group:* all acid groups in amino acids are identical.
3. an *amine group:* the word *amine* means "nitrogen-containing," and nitrogen is indeed the essential component of the amine portion of the molecule; like acid groups, all amine groups in amino acids are identical.

proteins Large, complex molecules made up of amino acids and found as essential components of all living cells.

DNA A molecule present in the nucleus of all body cells that directs the assembly of amino acids into body proteins.

amino acids Nitrogen-containing molecules that combine to form proteins.

peptide bonds Unique types of chemical bonds in which the amine group of one amino acid binds to the acid group of another to manufacture dipeptides and all larger peptide molecules.

TABLE 5.1 Amino Acids of the Human Body

Essential Amino Acids	Nonessential Amino Acids
These amino acids must be obtained from food.	*These amino acids can be manufactured by the body.*
Histidine	Alanine
Isoleucine	Arginine
Leucine	Asparagine
Lysine	Aspartic acid
Methionine	Cysteine
Phenylalanine	Glutamic acid
Threonine	Glutamine
Tryptophan	Glycine
Valine	Proline
	Serine
	Tyrosine

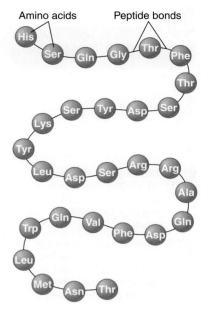

Glucagon

◂ **FIGURE 5.1** Structure of proteins. Proteins are chains of amino acids linked together by special chemical bonds called peptide bonds. This illustration shows a molecule of glucagon, a protein important in regulating blood glucose level. Notice that glucagon contains sixteen different amino acids. Some of these occur more than once, for a total of twenty-nine amino acids in this protein.

4. a *side chain:* this is the portion of the amino acid that makes each unique; as shown in Figure 5.2b, variations in the structure of the side chain give each amino acid its distinct properties.

Of the 20 amino acids in our body, 9 are classified as essential. This does not mean that they are more important than the 11 nonessential amino acids. Instead, **essential amino acids** are those that our body cannot produce at all or cannot produce in sufficient quantities to meet our physiologic needs. Thus, we must obtain essential amino acids from food. If we do not consume enough of the essential amino acids, we lose our ability to make the proteins and other nitrogen-containing compounds our body needs.

Nonessential amino acids are just as important to our body as essential amino acids, but it can make them in sufficient quantities, so we do not need to consume them in our diet. We make nonessential amino acids by combining parts of different amino acids and the breakdown products of carbohydrates and fats.

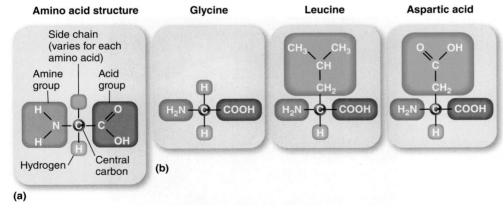

(a)

(b)

◂ **FIGURE 5.2** Structure of an amino acid. **(a)** All amino acids contain five parts: a central carbon atom, an amine group around the atom that contains nitrogen, an acid group, a hydrogen atom, and a side chain. **(b)** Only the side chain differs for each of the twenty amino acids, giving each its unique properties.

essential amino acids Amino acids not produced by the body that must be obtained from food.

nonessential amino acids Amino acids that can be manufactured by the body in sufficient quantities and therefore do not need to be consumed regularly in our diet.

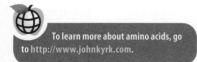

To learn more about amino acids, go to http://www.johnkyrk.com.

recap Proteins are critical components of all tissues of the human body. Like carbohydrates and lipids, they contain carbon, hydrogen, and oxygen. Unlike the other macronutrients, they also contain nitrogen, and their structure is dictated by DNA. The building blocks of proteins are amino acids. The amine group of the amino acid contains nitrogen. The portion of the amino acid that changes, giving each amino acid its distinct identity, is the side chain. The body cannot make essential amino acids, so we must obtain them from our diet. Our body can make nonessential amino acids from parts of other amino acids, carbohydrates, and fats.

LO2 Describe the processes by which DNA directs protein synthesis and proteins organize into levels of structure.

LO3 Explain the significance of mutual supplementation and identify non-meat food combinations that are complete protein sources.

How are proteins made?

You are unique because you inherited a unique set of genes from your parents. **Genes** are segments of DNA that carry the instructions for assembling available amino acids into your body's unique proteins. Slight differences in amino acid sequencing lead to slight differences in proteins. These differences in proteins result in the unique physical and physiologic characteristics you possess.

Protein Shape Determines Function

Two amino acids joined together form a *dipeptide,* and three amino acids joined together are called a *tripeptide.* The term *oligopeptide* is used to identify a string of four to nine amino acids. Proteins are made up of *polypeptides,* which are chains of ten or more amino acids linked together by peptide bonds. As a polypeptide chain grows longer, it begins to fold into any of a variety of complex shapes that give proteins their sophisticated structure.

The three-dimensional shape of a protein is critically important, because it determines that protein's function in the body. For example, the proteins that form tendons are much longer than they are wide. Tendons are connective tissues that attach bone to muscle, and their long, rodlike structure provides strong, fibrous connections. In contrast, the proteins that form red blood cells are globular in shape, and they result in the red blood cells being shaped like flattened disks with depressed centers, similar to a microscopic doughnut (**FIGURE 5.3**). This structure and the flexibility of the proteins in the red blood cells permit them to change shape and flow freely through even the tiniest blood vessels to deliver oxygen and still return to their original shape.

Proteins can uncoil and lose their shape when they are exposed to heat, acids, bases, heavy metals, alcohol, and other damaging substances. The term used to describe this change in the shape of proteins is *denaturation.* When a protein is

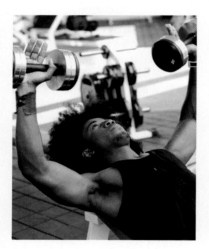

Proteins are an integral part of body tissues, including muscle tissue.

gene A segment of DNA that carries the instructions for assembling available amino acids into a unique protein.

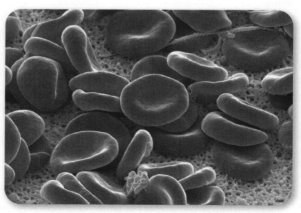

FIGURE 5.3 Protein shape determines function. The globular shape of the protein in red blood cells contributes to the flexible-disk shape of the cells. This in turn enables their passage through the tiniest blood vessels of the body.

denatured, its function is lost. Familiar examples of protein denaturation are the stiffening of egg whites when they are whipped, the curdling of milk when lemon juice or another acid is added, and the solidifying of eggs as they cook. Denaturation also occurs during protein digestion as a response to body heat and stomach acids.

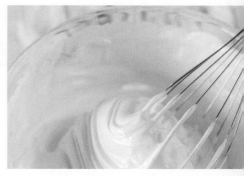

⬥ Stiffening egg whites denatures some of the proteins within them.

Protein Synthesis Can Be Limited by Missing Amino Acids

Our body synthesizes proteins by selecting the needed amino acids from the pool of all amino acids available at any given time. For protein synthesis to occur, all essential amino acids must be available to the cell. If this is not the case, the amino acid that is missing or in the smallest supply is called the **limiting amino acid**. Without the proper combination and quantity of essential amino acids, protein synthesis slows to the point at which proteins cannot be generated. For instance, the protein hemoglobin contains the essential amino acid histidine. If we do not consume enough histidine, our body will be unable to make hemoglobin, and we will lose the ability to transport oxygen to our cells. Without oxygen, our cells cannot function and will eventually die.

Proteins can be described as incomplete or complete:

- **Incomplete proteins** do not contain all the essential amino acids in sufficient quantities to support growth and health. They are also called *low-quality proteins*. Lentils, for example, are an incomplete protein.
- **Complete proteins** have all nine of the essential amino acids. They are also called *high-quality proteins*. These include proteins derived from animal products, such as egg whites, beef, poultry, fish, and dairy products such as milk and cheese. Soybeans also contain all nine essential amino acids and are the only complete vegetable protein.

Protein Synthesis Can Be Enhanced by Mutual Supplementation

Many people believe that we must consume meat or dairy products to obtain complete proteins. Not true! Consider a meal of black beans and rice. Black beans are low in the amino acids methionine and cysteine but have adequate amounts of isoleucine and lysine. Rice is low in isoleucine and lysine but contains sufficient methionine and cysteine. By combining black beans and rice, we create a complete protein source.

Mutual supplementation is the process of combining two or more incomplete protein sources to make a complete protein. The foods involved provide **complementary proteins** that, when combined, provide all nine essential amino acids (**FIGURE 5.4**). Thus, mutual supplementation is important for people who consume no animal products.

Complementary proteins do not need to be eaten at the same meal. We maintain a free "pool" of amino acids in the blood; these amino acids come from food and sloughed-off cells. When we eat an incomplete protein, its amino acids join those in the free amino acid pool. These free amino acids can then combine to synthesize complete proteins. However, to maximize protein synthesis, it is wise to eat complementary-protein foods during the same day.

recap Amino acids bind together to form proteins. Genes regulate the amino acid sequence, and thus the structure, of all proteins. The shape of a protein determines its function. When a protein is denatured by damaging substances, such as heat and acids, it loses its shape and its function. For protein synthesis to occur, all nine essential amino acids must be available to the cell. A complete protein provides all nine essential amino acids. Mutual supplementation combines two complementary-protein sources to make a complete protein.

limiting amino acid The essential amino acid that is missing or in the smallest supply in the amino acid pool and is thus responsible for slowing or halting protein synthesis.

incomplete proteins Foods that do not contain all the essential amino acids in sufficient amounts to support growth and health.

complete proteins Foods that contain all nine essential amino acids.

mutual supplementation The process of combining two or more incomplete protein sources to make a complete protein.

complementary proteins Two or more foods that together contain all nine essential amino acids necessary for a complete protein. It is not necessary to eat complementary proteins at the same meal.

Combining Complementary Foods

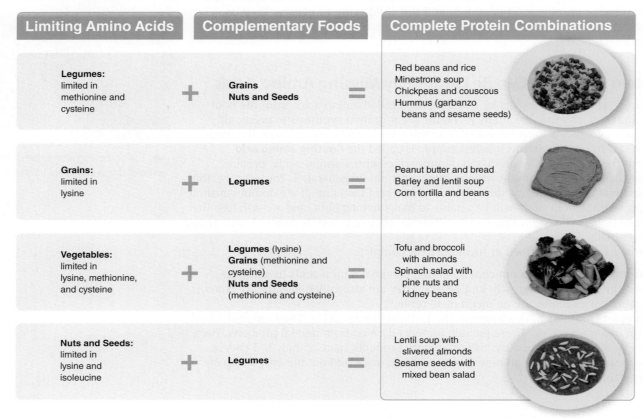

Limiting Amino Acids		Complementary Foods		Complete Protein Combinations
Legumes: limited in methionine and cysteine	+	**Grains** **Nuts and Seeds**	=	Red beans and rice Minestrone soup Chickpeas and couscous Hummus (garbanzo beans and sesame seeds)
Grains: limited in lysine	+	**Legumes**	=	Peanut butter and bread Barley and lentil soup Corn tortilla and beans
Vegetables: limited in lysine, methionine, and cysteine	+	**Legumes** (lysine) **Grains** (methionine and cysteine) **Nuts and Seeds** (methionine and cysteine)	=	Tofu and broccoli with almonds Spinach salad with pine nuts and kidney beans
Nuts and Seeds: limited in lysine and isoleucine	+	**Legumes**	=	Lentil soup with slivered almonds Sesame seeds with mixed bean salad

FIGURE 5.4 Complementary food combinations.

LO4 Identify at least four functions of proteins in our body.

Why do we need to eat proteins?

The functions of proteins in the body are so numerous that only a few can be described in detail here. Note that proteins function most effectively when we also consume adequate amounts of energy as carbohydrates and fat. When there is not enough energy available, the body uses proteins as an energy source, limiting their availability for other functions.

Proteins Contribute to Cell Growth, Repair, and Maintenance

The proteins in our body are dynamic, meaning that they are constantly being broken down, repaired, and replaced. When proteins are broken down, many amino acids are recycled into new proteins. Think about all the new proteins that are needed to allow an embryo to develop and grow into a 9-month-old fetus. In this case, an entire human body is being made! In fact, a newborn baby has more than 10 trillion body cells.

Even in the mature adult, our cells are constantly turning over, meaning old cells are broken down and parts are used to create new cells. Our red blood cells live for only 3 to 4 months, and the cells lining our intestinal tract are replaced every 3 to 6 days. In addition, cellular damage that occurs must be repaired in order to maintain our health. The constant turnover of proteins from our diet is essential for such cell growth, repair, and maintenance.

Proteins Act as Enzymes and Hormones

You may remember that *enzymes* are small chemicals, usually proteins, that act on other chemicals to speed up body processes but are not apparently changed during those processes. Enzymes can bind substances together or break them apart, and they can transform one substance into another. Each cell contains thousands of enzymes that facilitate specific cellular reactions. For example, the enzyme phosphofructokinase (PFK) speeds up the conversion of carbohydrates to energy during physical exercise. Without PFK, we would be unable to generate energy at a fast enough rate to allow us to be physically active.

You may also recall that *hormones* are substances that act as chemical messengers in the body. They are stored in various glands, which release them in response to changes in the body's environment. They then signal the body's organs and tissues to restore the body to normal conditions. Whereas many hormones are made from lipids, some are made from amino acids. These include insulin and glucagon, which play a role in regulating blood glucose levels, and thyroid hormone, which helps control the rate at which glucose is used for fuel.

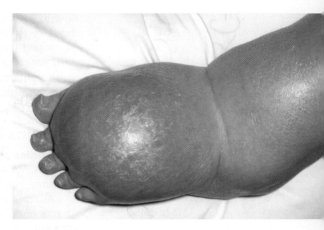

FIGURE 5.5 Edema can result from deficient protein intake. This foot with edema is swollen because of fluid imbalance.

Proteins Help Maintain Fluid and Electrolyte Balance

For our body to function properly, fluids and *electrolytes* (minerals, such as sodium and potassium, that are able to carry an electrical charge) must be maintained at healthy levels inside and outside cells and within blood vessels. Proteins help maintain fluid and electrolyte balance in two ways:

- They attract fluids. Proteins in the bloodstream, the cells, and the spaces surrounding the cells work together to keep both fluids and electrolytes moving across these spaces.
- They move and retain fluids in the proper quantities to help us maintain both fluid balance and blood pressure.

When protein intake is deficient, the concentration of proteins in the bloodstream is insufficient to draw fluid from the tissues and across the blood vessel walls; fluid then collects in the tissues, causing **edema** (**FIGURE 5.5**). In addition to being uncomfortable, edema can lead to serious medical problems.

The conduction of nerve signals and contraction of muscles also depend on a proper balance of electrolytes. If protein intake is deficient, we lose our ability to maintain these functions, resulting in potentially fatal changes in the rhythm of the heart. Other consequences of chronically low protein intakes include muscle weakness and spasms, kidney failure, and, if conditions are severe enough, death.

Proteins Transport Nutrients and Other Substances

Proteins play a key role in transporting nutrients and other important substances throughout the body. Some examples of these **transport proteins** include the following:

- Transport proteins within the cell membrane help maintain fluid and electrolyte balance. These proteins act as pumps to assist in the movement of the electrolytes sodium and potassium into and out of the cell.
- Transport proteins also carry vitamins and minerals through the bloodstream to the organs and cells that need them. For example, retinol-binding protein transports fat-soluble vitamin A (also called retinol) in the blood.
- Transport proteins also move glucose from the bloodstream into the cells, where it can be used for energy.

Proteins Help Maintain Acid–Base Balance

The body's cellular processes result in the constant production of acids and bases. *Acids* are substances that contain significant amounts of hydrogen, whereas *bases* are

edema A disorder in which fluids build up in the tissue spaces of the body, causing fluid imbalances and a swollen appearance.

transport proteins Protein molecules that help transport substances throughout the body and across cell membranes.

low in hydrogen. Some hydrogen is essential to life, but too much can be harmful to body cells. Thus, the body maintains very tight control over the **pH**, or the level of hydrogen (H), in the blood. Proteins are excellent **buffers**, meaning they help maintain proper acid–base balance. They do this by attracting hydrogen and neutralizing it. Proteins can also release hydrogen when the blood becomes too basic. By buffering acids and bases, proteins help maintain acid–base balance.

Proteins Help Maintain a Strong Immune System

Antibodies are special proteins that help our body defend itself against foreign substances. When bacteria, viruses, toxins, and other harmful agents enter our body, our immune system produces antibodies that attach to and neutralize the invaders.

Adequate protein is necessary to support the increased production of antibodies that occurs in response to a cold, the flu, or any other infectious illness. If we do not consume enough protein, our resistance is weakened. On the other hand, eating more protein than we need does not improve immune function.

Proteins Serve as an Energy Source

The body's primary energy sources are carbohydrate and fat. So it's not surprising that both these macronutrients have specialized storage forms that can be used for energy—carbohydrate as glycogen and fat as triglycerides. Proteins do not have a specialized storage form for energy. This means that, when proteins need to be used for energy, they are taken from the blood and body tissues, such as the liver and skeletal muscle.

Adequate intake of carbohydrate and fat spares protein. During times of low carbohydrate and fat intake, the body breaks down proteins into individual amino acids, which are degraded further to provide the building blocks for the production of glucose, which provides needed energy to the brain. This process is called *gluconeogenesis*. In well-nourished people, proteins contribute very little to energy needs. Because we are efficient at recycling amino acids, our protein needs are relatively low compared to our needs for carbohydrate and fat.

 Proteins serve many important functions, including (1) enabling growth, repair, and maintenance of body tissues; (2) acting as enzymes and hormones; (3) maintaining fluid and electrolyte balance; (4) transporting nutrients and other substances; (5) maintaining acid–base balance; (6) making antibodies, a component of our immune system; and (7) providing energy when carbohydrate and fat intakes are inadequate. Proteins function best when we also consume adequate amounts of carbohydrate and fat.

LO5 Explain how our body digests and absorbs protein.

pH Stands for "percentage of hydrogen." It is a measure of the acidity—or level of hydrogen—of any solution, including human blood.

buffers Proteins that help maintain proper acid–base balance by attaching to, or releasing, hydrogen ions as conditions change in the body.

antibodies Defensive proteins of the immune system. Their production is prompted by the presence of bacteria, viruses, toxins, or allergens.

What happens to the proteins we eat?

Our body does not directly use proteins from the foods we eat to make the proteins we need. Dietary proteins are first digested and broken into smaller particles, such as amino acids, dipeptides, and tripeptides, so that they can pass through the cells of the intestinal lining. In this section, we will review how proteins are digested and absorbed. As you read about each step in this process, refer to **FIGURE 5.6**.

- The mechanical digestion of proteins in food occurs through chewing, crushing, and moistening the food with saliva. These actions ease swallowing and increase the surface area for more efficient digestion farther down the digestive tract. There is no chemical digestive action on proteins in the mouth.
- When proteins reach the stomach, they are broken apart by *hydrochloric acid*, which denatures the strands of protein. Hydrochloric acid also converts the

focus figure 5.6 | Protein Digestion Overview

Digestion of dietary proteins into single amino acids occurs primarily in the stomach and small intestine. The single amino acids are then transported to the liver, where they may be converted to glucose or fat, used for energy or to build new proteins, or transported to cells as needed.

ORGANS OF THE GI TRACT

MOUTH

Proteins in foods are crushed by chewing and moistened by saliva.

STOMACH

Proteins are denatured by hydrochloric acid.

Pepsin is activated to break proteins into single amino acids and smaller polypeptides.

SMALL INTESTINE

Proteases are secreted to digest polypeptides into smaller units.

Cells in the wall of the small intestine complete the breakdown of dipeptides and tripeptides into single amino acids, which are absorbed into the bloodstream.

ACCESSORY ORGANS

PANCREAS

Produces proteases, which are released into the small intestine.

LIVER

Amino acids are transported to the liver, where they are converted to glucose or fat, used for energy or to build new proteins, or sent to the cells as needed.

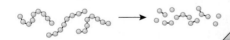

Amino acids

Enterocytes

Lacteal

Capillary

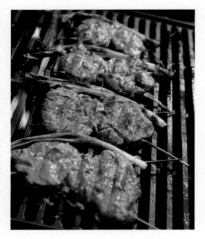

 Meats are highly digestible sources of dietary protein.

inactive enzyme *pepsinogen* into its active form, **pepsin**. Although pepsin is a protein, it is not denatured by stomach acid because it has evolved to work optimally in an acidic environment. Pepsin begins breaking proteins into single amino acids and smaller polypeptides, which then travel to the small intestine for further digestion.

■ In the small intestine, the polypeptides encounter enzymes called **proteases**, which digest them into single amino acids, dipeptides, and tripeptides. The cells in the wall of the small intestine then absorb these molecules. Enzymes in the intestinal cells complete digestion by breaking the dipeptides and tripeptides into single amino acids.

■ The amino acids are transported into the bloodstream to the liver and on to cells throughout our body as needed. The main waste product resulting from the breakdown of amino acids is *urea*, which contains nitrogen and is generated from the amine group. Urea is transported to the kidneys via the bloodstream, where it is then excreted in our urine.

As discussed earlier, the number of essential amino acids in a protein affects its quality: higher-quality-protein foods contain more of the essential amino acids needed to build proteins. Another factor to consider when determining protein quality is *digestibility,* or how efficiently our body can digest and absorb a protein. Animal foods and legumes, including soy products, have high digestibility, and we absorb almost all of their proteins. Grains and many vegetable proteins are less digestible.

recap   In the stomach, hydrochloric acid denatures proteins and pepsin breaks proteins into single amino acids and smaller polypeptides. In the small intestine, proteases break down polypeptides. Enzymes in the cells in the wall of the small intestine break the remaining peptide fragments into single amino acids, which are then transported to the liver for distribution to the body.

LO6 Calculate your recommended dietary allowance for protein.

LO7 Describe two disorders related to inadequate protein intake.

LO8 Identify several healthful food sources of animal and plant protein.

How much protein should we eat?

Consuming adequate protein is a major concern for many people. In fact, one of the most common concerns among athletes is that their diet is deficient in protein (see the *Nutrition Myth or Fact?* box for a discussion of this topic). In developed nations, concerns about people getting sufficient dietary protein are generally unnecessary, because we can easily consume the protein our body needs by eating an adequate amount and variety of foods. However, many people in developing nations are at risk for protein deficiency. The diseases resulting from protein deficiency are discussed in detail shortly.

Recommended Dietary Allowance (RDA) for Protein

How much protein should we eat? **TABLE 5.2** lists the daily recommendations for protein intake for sedentary adults and for athletes. It also provides a calculation for converting the recommendation, which is stated in grams per kilogram of body weight, into total grams of protein per day. If you are sedentary and weigh 140 pounds, you need about 50 grams of protein a day. If you're an athlete who weighs 140 pounds, you need about 75 to 108 grams. Protein needs are higher for children, adolescents, and pregnant/lactating women, because more protein is needed during times of growth and development.

When you consider that a small serving (3 oz) of canned tuna or ground beef provides about 16 to 22 grams of protein and a glass of low-fat milk another 8 grams, you can see how easy it is to meet this recommendation. In fact, it shouldn't surprise you to learn that most Americans eat 1.5 to 2 times their RDA for protein without any effort!

The recommended percentage of energy that should come from protein is 12% to 20% of your total daily energy intake. Many high-protein, low-carbohydrate diets recommend that a much greater percentage of your diet be derived from protein, but as we discuss next, excessive protein intake has some health costs.

pepsin An enzyme in the stomach that begins the breakdown of proteins into shorter polypeptide chains and single amino acids.

proteases Enzymes that continue the breakdown of polypeptides in the small intestine.

nutrition myth or fact?

Do Athletes Need More Protein than Inactive People?

At one time, it was believed that the Recommended Dietary Allowance (RDA) for protein, which is 0.8 gram per kilogram of body weight, was sufficient for both inactive people and athletes. Recent studies, however, show that the protein needs of athletes are higher.

Athletes need more protein for several reasons:

- Regular exercise increases the transport of oxygen to body tissues, requiring changes in the oxygen-carrying capacity of the blood. To carry more oxygen, we need to produce more of the protein that carries oxygen in the blood (that is, hemoglobin, which is a protein).
- During intense exercise, we use a small amount of protein directly for energy.
- We also use protein to make glucose to prevent hypoglycemia (low blood sugar) during exercise.
- Regular exercise stimulates tissue growth and causes tissue damage, which must be repaired by additional proteins.

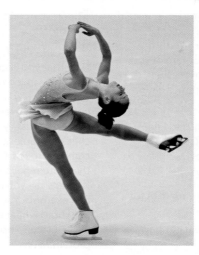

⬆ Some athletes who persistently diet are at risk for low protein intake.

As a result of these increased demands for protein, strength athletes (such as weightlifters) need 1.8 to 2 times more protein than the current RDA, and endurance athletes (such as distance runners) need 1.5 to 1.75 times more protein.[1] More recent research suggests that optimal protein needs for both these types of athletes could be as high as 1.6 to 2.25 times the current RDA.[2]

Does this mean that, if you are an athlete, you should add more protein to your diet? Not necessarily. Contrary to popular belief, most Americans, including athletes, already consume more than twice the RDA for protein. Thus, they are already more than fulfilling their protein needs. In fact, eating more protein or taking amino acid supplements does not cause muscles to become bigger or stronger. Only regular strength training, combined with an adequate protein intake, can achieve these goals. By eating a balanced diet and consuming a variety of foods, athletes can easily meet their protein requirements.

TABLE 5.2 **Recommended Protein Intakes**

Group	Recommended Protein Intake (g/kg body weight/day)*
Most adults[†]	0.8
Nonvegetarian endurance athletes[‡]	1.2 to 1.4
Nonvegetarian strength athletes[‡]	1.2 to 1.7
Vegetarian endurance athletes[‡]	1.3 to 1.5
Vegetarian strength athletes[‡]	1.3 to 1.8

*To convert body weight to kilograms, divide weight in pounds by 2.2.
Weight (lb) ÷ 2.2 = Weight (kg). For example, 150 lb ÷ 2.2 = 68 kg.
Weight (kg) × recommended protein intake = protein intake (grams per day). For example, for a non-athlete, 68 kg × 0.8 = 54.4 grams per day.

[†]Data from Food and Nutrition Board, Institute of Medicine. 2005. *Dietary Reference Intakes for Energy, Carbohydrate, Fiber, Fat, Fatty Acids, Cholesterol, Protein, and Amino Acids (Macronutrients)*. Washington, DC: National Academies Press.

[‡]Data from: American College of Sports Medicine, American Dietetic Association, and Dietitians of Canada. 2009. Joint Position Statement. Nutrition and athletic performance. *Med. Sci. Sports Exerc. 41*(3):709–731.

To find out whether you're meeting—or exceeding—your protein needs, complete the calculation in the feature box *What About You?*.

recap The RDA for protein for most nonactive, nonpregnant, nonlactating, nonvegetarian adults is 0.8 gram per kilogram of body weight. Children, pregnant women, nursing mothers, vegetarians, and athletes need more. Most people who eat enough energy and carbohydrates have no problem meeting their RDA for protein.

Are You Meeting Your Protein Needs?

Before you can figure out whether you're meeting your protein needs, you have to know what those needs are. Look at Table 5.2. Unless you qualify as an endurance or strength athlete, your protein needs are 0.8 gram per kilogram of your body weight. If you're not familiar with the metric system, the following steps will help you translate this recommendation into the number of grams right for you:

1. Start by converting your weight from pounds to kilograms. For example, let's say you weigh 150 pounds. To convert this value to kilograms, divide by 2.2:

    150 pounds ÷ 2.2 pounds/kg = 68 kg.

2. Next, multiply your weight in kilograms by your RDA for protein:

    68 kg × 0.8 g/kg = 54 grams of protein per day.

    If you work out vigorously for an hour or more 5 or 6 days a week, you might want to use a protein intake level of 1 gram per kilogram of body weight. This calculation is easier!

1. Start by converting your weight from pounds to kilograms. For example, let's say you weigh 200 pounds. To convert this value to kilograms, divide by 2.2:

    200 pounds ÷ 2.2 pounds/kg = 91 kg.

2. Next, multiply your weight in kilograms by your RDA for protein:

    91 kg × 1 g/kg = 91 grams of protein per day.

Now that you know how many grams of protein you need each day, you can log on to www.choosemyplate.gov/supertracker-tools/supertracker.html to see how much protein you're getting in an average day and whether that amount meets—or even exceeds—your needs. Or you can get a rough estimate by checking Table 5.3, which identifies grams of protein for many common foods. Circle the foods you eat most days and add up the protein per serving.

Let's say you need 68 grams of protein per day, as in our first example. You typically eat either a ham or tuna sandwich on whole-wheat bread with a glass of skim milk for lunch. Either of these options would meet more than half of your daily protein needs—in one meal! As you can see, it's easy for most Americans to get enough protein every day.

Protein–Energy Malnutrition Can Lead to Debility and Death

When a person consumes too little protein and energy, the result is **protein–energy malnutrition** (also called *protein–Calorie malnutrition*). Two diseases that can follow are marasmus and kwashiorkor **(FIGURE 5.7)**.

Marasmus Results from Grossly Inadequate Energy Intake

Marasmus is a disease that results from a grossly inadequate intake of total energy, especially protein. Essentially, marasmus is starvation. It is most common in young children (6 to 18 months of age) living in impoverished conditions who are severely undernourished. For example, the children may be fed diluted cereal drinks that are inadequate in energy, protein, and most nutrients.

People suffering from marasmus have the look of "skin and bones" because their body fat and tissues are wasting. The consequences of marasmus include the following:

- Wasting and weakening of muscles, including the heart muscle
- Stunted physical and mental growth and development
- *Anemia* (abnormally low levels of hemoglobin in the blood)
- Severely weakened immune system
- Fluid and electrolyte imbalances

If marasmus is left untreated, death from dehydration, heart failure, or infection will result. Treatment begins with careful correction of fluid and electrolyte imbalances. Protein and carbohydrates are provided once the body's condition has stabilized. Fat is introduced much later, because the protein levels in the blood must improve to the point at which the body can use them to carry fat, so that it can be safely metabolized by the body.

protein–energy malnutrition
A disorder caused by inadequate consumption of protein. It is characterized by severe wasting.

marasmus A form of protein–energy malnutrition that results from grossly inadequate intake of energy and protein and other nutrients and is characterized by extreme tissue wasting and stunted growth and development.

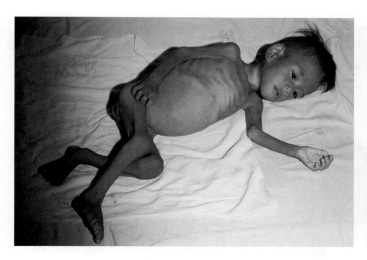
(a)

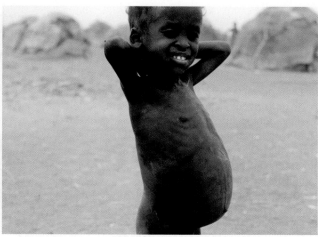
(b)

⬥ **FIGURE 5.7** Two forms of protein–energy malnutrition: **(a)** marasmus and **(b)** kwashiorkor.

Kwashiorkor Results from a Low-Protein Diet

Kwashiorkor often occurs in developing countries where infants are weaned early due to the arrival of a subsequent baby. This deficiency disease is typically seen in young children (1 to 3 years of age) who no longer drink breast milk. Instead, they often are fed a low-protein, starchy cereal. Recent research suggests that dysfunctional GI bacteria combined with a low-protein diet interact to contribute to the development of kwashiorkor.[2] Unlike marasmus, kwashiorkor often develops quickly and causes the person to look swollen, particularly in the belly. This edema occurs because the low protein content of the blood is inadequate to keep fluids from seeping into the tissue spaces. These are some other symptoms of kwashiorkor:

- Some weight loss and muscle wasting, with some retention of body fat
- Retarded growth and development but less severe than that seen with marasmus
- Loss of appetite, sadness, irritability, apathy
- Development of sores, hair loss, and other skin and hair problems

Kwashiorkor can be reversed if adequate protein and energy are given in time. Because of their severely weakened immune systems, many individuals with kwashiorkor die from infectious diseases. Of those who are treated, many return home to the same impoverished conditions, only to develop this deficiency once again.

Although children in developing countries are at highest risk for these diseases, protein–energy malnutrition occurs in all countries and affects both children and adults. In the United States, poor people living in inner cities and isolated rural areas are especially affected. Others at risk include the elderly, the homeless, people with eating disorders, those addicted to alcohol and other drugs, and individuals with wasting diseases, such as AIDS or cancer.

Can Too Much Dietary Protein Be Harmful?

Over the last few decades, many people seeking to lose weight have turned to high-protein diets. Are such diets the key to weight loss? The ***Nutrition Myth or Fact?*** feature box explores this question. One concern associated with such diets is that they may increase the risk for health problems. Three health conditions that have received particular attention are heart disease, bone loss, and kidney disease. Here is the state of current research into these three claims:

- *Heart disease:* High-protein diets composed of predominantly animal sources are associated with higher blood cholesterol levels. Until recently, this was assumed to be due to the saturated fat in animal products, which has been shown to increase

To find out what you can do to take action against hunger, go to http://www.actionagainsthunger.org.

kwashiorkor A form of protein–energy malnutrition that is typically seen in malnourished infants and toddlers and is characterized by wasting, edema, and other signs of protein deficiency.

nutrition myth or fact?

Are High-Protein Diets the Key to Weight Loss?

The promotional photo shows a juicy steak on the grill. If you're a meat eater and want to lose weight, chances are you've at least flirted with the idea of following a high-protein diet. Do these diets work, and are they safe?

Supporters of high-protein diets propose that our high-simple-carbohydrate diet (including refined grains and sugars) has caused the alarming rise in obesity in the United States in the past few decades. They claim that high-protein diets, such as the Atkin's Diet, result in substantial weight loss. They also say that, despite the high saturated-fat content of animal sources of protein, meat-based high-protein diets do not cause unhealthful changes in blood cholesterol.

Are there any research studies to support these claims? A review published in 2008 of the studies on high-protein, low-carbohydrate diets concluded that the increase in energy expenditure and satiety that occurs with eating a higher protein diet does contribute to weight loss and improvements in cardiovascular disease risk factors at least comparable to, if not better than, that seen with lower protein diets up to 12 months.[3] The authors of this review emphasized that these benefits are observed with diets that are moderately higher in protein and moderately restricted in carbohydrate and saturated fat. A more recent study in obese adults found that a moderately high protein diet was more acceptable than a diet with a lower protein content, and those eating the higher protein diet were less likely to drop out of the study and regain the weight.[4]

Detractors of high-protein weight-loss diets contend that the U.S. population is substantially overweight because we eat too many Calories, not because we eat too much carbohydrate or fat, specifically. Nutrition experts have long agreed that the key to weight loss is eating less energy than you expend. Thus, any type of diet that contains fewer Calories than the person expends will result in weight loss. Additionally, concerns about potential health risks have prevented many nutrition experts from endorsing high-protein diets for weight loss. These include the following:

- Low blood glucose levels leading to low energy levels, diminished cognitive functioning, and elevated ketones. Despite this concern, recent evidence shows that these problems do not occur in people eating a high-protein diet that is modestly restricted in carbohydrate and fat.

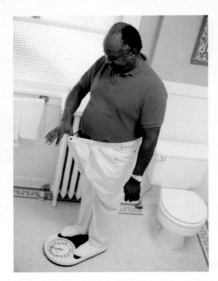

▲ Many people will try any diet to lose weight, but is it worth it in the long run?

- Increased risk for heart disease because high-protein diets that rely on animal sources of protein are typically high in saturated fat. As just discussed, until recently the established opinion of most nutrition experts was that eating a diet high in saturated fat increases a person's LDL-cholesterol, which in turn increases the risk for heart disease, but this view has recently been challenged.[5] Nevertheless, as just discussed, research shows that high-protein diets that are lower in saturated fat and contain lean meat choices and low-fat dairy products do not cause unhealthful changes in blood lipids. In fact, these types of diets can improve blood lipids.[6]

- Increased risk for some forms of cancer due to eating a diet that is high in fat and low in fiber. Some high-protein diet plans recommend few foods that contain fiber and antioxidants, yet some research suggests that eating this type of a diet over many years will increase a person's risk for some forms of cancer, particularly colon cancer. In a recent study, for example, seventeen obese men ate weight-loss diets high in protein and low in carbohydrate and fiber for 4 weeks.[7] At the end of this study, the men were found to have a decrease in cancer-protective substances and an increase in cancer-promoting substances in their feces. However, revised versions of some high-protein diets promote the consumption of many foods that are high in fiber and antioxidants and lower in saturated fat. The effects of these revised diets on cancer risk have yet to be explored.

Should you adopt a high-protein diet? This is not an easy question to answer. Each of us must decide on the type of diet to consume based on our own needs, preferences, health risks, and lifestyle. At the present time, there is not enough evidence to state with any certainty that high-protein diets are always better than higher-carbohydrate plans, and we still need to learn much more about the safety of eating a high-protein diet over many years. Based on what we currently know, the most sound weight-loss plans are those that are moderately reduced in energy intake and contain ample fruits, vegetables, and whole grains; adequate lean protein; moderate amounts of total fat; and relatively low amounts of saturated fat. It is also important to choose a food plan that you can follow throughout your lifetime.

blood cholesterol levels and the risk for heart disease. Interestingly, a recent review draws into question these widely-held assumptions, because it found that eating more saturated fat was *not* associated with an increased risk for heart disease.[3] The authors of this study suggest that this may be due to two reasons: (1) the LDL cholesterol linked with saturated fat intake is of a subtype that is not associated with increasing a person's risk for heart disease; and (2) saturated fat also increases a person's HDL cholesterol, which is protective against heart disease. This topic is still highly contentious, and nutrition experts stress that eating less saturated fat, and replacing it with more healthful foods higher in polyunsaturated fats, such as nuts, avocados, fish, whole grains, and olive oil, is the best approach to reducing one's risk for heart disease. Also, vegetarians have been shown to have a greatly reduced risk for heart disease.[4]

- *Bone loss:* Proteins from animal products contain more of the sulfur amino acids (methionine and cysteine). Metabolizing these amino acids makes the blood more acidic, and calcium is pulled from the bone to buffer these acids. Nevertheless, we do not know whether a diet high in animal proteins actually causes bone loss. In contrast, we do know that eating too little protein causes bone loss, which increases the risk for fractures and osteoporosis. Higher intakes of animal and soy protein have been shown to protect bone in middle-aged and older women. A recent systematic review of the literature has concluded that there is no evidence to support the contention that high-protein diets lead to bone loss, except in people consuming inadequate calcium.[5]

- *Kidney disease:* The more protein we eat, the more protein the body has to break down. Recall that a waste product of protein digestion is the chemical *urea:* the kidneys form urea when the nitrogen-containing amine group is removed during amino acid breakdown. A high protein intake can therefore be stressful to kidneys that aren't functioning properly, so people with kidney disease are advised to eat a low-protein diet. On the other hand, experts agree that eating up to 2 grams of protein per kilogram of body weight each day is safe for healthy people.[6] Still, people who consume a lot of protein should also consume more fluid to flush the excess urea from their kidneys.

recap Protein–energy malnutrition can lead to marasmus and kwashiorkor. These diseases primarily affect impoverished children in developing nations. However, residents of developed countries are also at risk, especially the elderly, the homeless, people struggling with substance abuse, and people with AIDS, cancer, and other wasting diseases. Although eating too much protein, particularly protein sources high in saturated fat, has previously been shown to increase your risk for heart disease, recent evidence suggests this may not be the case. More research is needed in this area.

Shopper's Guide: Good Food Sources of Protein

TABLE 5.3 compares the protein content of a variety of foods. In general, good sources of protein include meats (lean cuts of beef, pork, poultry, and seafood), low-fat dairy products, egg whites, soy products, legumes, nuts, and certain whole grains. Refer to **FIGURE 5.8** to see a comparison of meals that are either poor or healthful sources of protein.

Although most people are aware that meats are an excellent source of protein, many are surprised to learn that the quality of the protein in some legumes rivals that of meat. As noted earlier, soy is a complete protein, providing all essential amino acids. For more information about the nutrients and health benefits of soy, check out the ***Highlight*** box.

Other legumes include kidney beans, pinto beans, black beans, garbanzo beans (chickpeas), lentils, green peas, black-eyed peas, and lima beans. In addition to being excellent sources of protein, legumes are high in fiber, iron, calcium, and many of the B-vitamins (although they do not contain vitamin B_{12}). They are also low in saturated fat and have no cholesterol. Because legumes other than soy are deficient in methionine, an essential amino acid, they are often served with grains, which supply it.

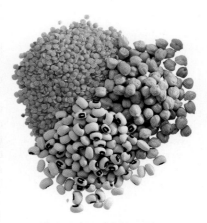

The quality of the protein in some legumes is almost equal to that of meat.

TABLE 5.3 Protein Content of Commonly Consumed Foods

Food	Serving Size	Protein (g)	Food	Serving Size	Protein (g)
Beef			**Beans**		
Ground, lean, baked (15% fat)	3 oz	22	Refried	½ cup	6
Beef tenderloin steak, broiled (1/8 in. fat)	3 oz	22.5	Kidney, red	½ cup	8
Top sirloin, broiled (1/8 in. fat)	3 oz	23	Black	½ cup	7.6
Poultry			**Nuts**		
Chicken breast, broiled, no skin (bone removed)	½ breast	27	Peanuts, dry roasted	1 oz	6.7
Chicken thigh, bone and skin removed	1 thigh	28	Peanut butter, creamy	2 tbsp.	8
Turkey breast, roasted, Louis Rich	3 oz	13	Almonds, blanched	1 oz	6
Seafood			**Cereals, Grains, and Breads**		
Cod, cooked	3 oz	19	Oatmeal, quick instant	1 cup	6
Salmon, Chinook, baked	3 oz	22	Cheerios	1 cup	3.4
Shrimp, steamed	3 oz	19	Grape Nuts	½ cup	7.2
Tuna, in water, drained	3 oz	16.5	Raisin Bran	1 cup	4.7
Pork			Brown rice, cooked	1 cup	5
Pork loin chop, broiled	3 oz	22	Whole-wheat bread	1 slice	3.6
Ham, roasted, extra lean (5% fat)	3 oz	18	Bagel, 3½ in. diameter	1 each	10.5
Dairy			**Vegetables**		
Whole milk (3.25% fat)	8 fl. oz	7.7	Carrots, raw (7.25 to 8.5 in. long)	1 each	0.7
1% milk	8 fl. oz	8.2	Broccoli, raw, chopped	1 cup	2.6
Skim milk	8 fl. oz	8.3	Collards, cooked from frozen	1 cup	5
Low-fat, plain yogurt	8 fl. oz	13	Spinach, raw	1 cup	0.9
American cheese, processed	1 oz	5			
Cottage cheese, low-fat (2%)	1 cup	27			
Soy Products					
Tofu, firm	½ cup	10			
Tempeh, cooked	3 oz	5.5			
Soy milk beverage	1 cup	8			

Data from U.S. Department of Agriculture (USDA). 2013. National Nutrient Database for Standard Reference, Release 26. www.ars.usda.gov/ba/bhnrc/ndl

Eating legumes regularly, including foods made from soybeans, may help reduce your risk for heart disease by lowering blood cholesterol levels. A recent review found that eating approximately ¾ cup of legumes each day resulted in a 5% reduction in LDL cholesterol, and this degree of change could reduce the risk of a heart attack by 5% to 6%.[7] Diets high in legumes and soy products are also associated with lower rates of some cancers. If you're not used to eating beans and lentils, the *Game Plan* box provides tips for incorporating these nourishing foods into your daily diet.

Nuts are another healthful high-protein food. In fact, the USDA Food Patterns counts ⅓ cup of nuts or 2 tablespoons of peanut butter as equivalent to 1 ounce—about one-third of a serving—of meat! Moreover, as you learned previously (see Chapter 4), studies show that consuming about 2 to 5 oz of nuts per week significantly reduces people's risk for cardiovascular disease.[8,9] Additional evidence suggests that eating nuts, and in particular walnuts, is associated with a lower risk of type 2 diabetes.[10] Although the exact mechanism behind this is not known, nuts contain many nutrients and other substances that are associated with health benefits, including fiber, unsaturated fats, potassium, folate, plant sterols, and antioxidants.

A popular source of non-meat protein that is available in most supermarkets is *quorn*, a protein product derived from fermented fungus. It is mixed with a variety of other foods to produce various types of meat substitutes. Some "new" foods high in protein include some very ancient grains! For instance, you may have heard of pastas and other products made with *quinoa*, a plant so essential to the diet of the ancient Incas that they considered it sacred. No wonder: quinoa, cooked much like rice,

a day of meals

about **3,552**
calories (kcal)

BREAKFAST

2 fried eggs
3 slices bacon, fried
2 slices of white toast with
  1 tbsp. of butter
8 fl. oz whole milk

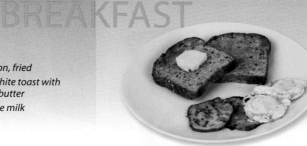

about **1,847**
calories (kcal)

2 poached eggs
2 slices Canadian bacon
2 slices whole-wheat toast
  with 1 tbsp. butter
8 fl. oz skim milk

LUNCH

2 slices pepperoni pizza
  (14" pizza, hand-tossed crust)
1 medium banana
24 fl. oz cola beverage

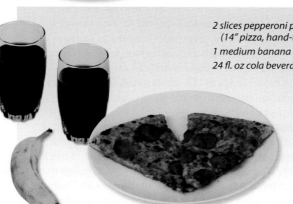
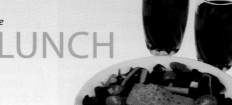

½ fillet broiled salmon
Spinach salad:
2 cups fresh spinach
½ cup raw carrots, sliced
3 cherry tomatoes
1 tbsp. chopped green onions
¼ cup kidney beans
2 tbsp. fat-free Caesar dressing
1 medium banana
24 fl. oz iced tea

DINNER

Fried chicken, 1 drumstick and
  1 breast (with skin)
1 cup mashed potatoes with
  ¼ cup gravy
½ cup yellow sweet corn
8 fl. oz whole milk
1 slice chocolate cake with
  chocolate frosting
  (1/12 of cake)

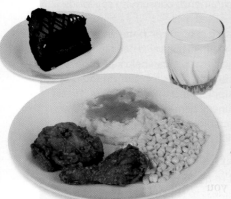
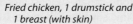
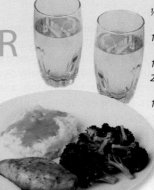

½ chicken breast, roasted
  without skin
1 cup mashed potatoes with
  ¼ cup gravy
1 cup steamed broccoli
24 fl. oz ice water with slice of
  lemon
1 cup fresh blueberries with
  2 tbsp. whipped cream

nutrient analysis

3,552 kcal
40.4% of energy from carbohydrates
43.2% of energy from fat
16.3% of energy from saturated fat
16.4% of energy from protein
18.2 grams of dietary fiber
6,246 milligrams of sodium

**Saves
1,705
calories!**

nutrient analysis

1,847 kcal
46% of energy from carbohydrates
28.7% of energy from fat
11% of energy from saturated fat
25.3% of energy from protein
26.5 grams of dietary fiber
3,280 milligrams of sodium

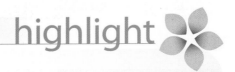

What's So Great About Soy?

Twenty years ago, if you were able to find a soy-based food in a traditional grocery store in the United States or Canada, it was probably soy milk. Now, it seems there are soy products in almost every aisle, from marinated tofu and tempeh to miso soup to soy-based cheeses, cereals, hot dogs, burgers, frozen dinners, and even tofu ice cream. Why the explosion? What's so great about soy, and should you give it a try?

What Is Soy?

Before we explore the many health claims tied to soy-based foods, let's define some terms. First, all soy-based foods start with soybeans, a staple in many Asian countries. Soybeans provide all essential amino acids and have almost twice as much protein as any other legume (7–10 grams of protein in 1 cup of soy milk). Although they also pack three to ten times as much fat as other beans, almost all of it is unsaturated, and soy has no cholesterol. Soy is also rich in several types of phytochemicals. Here are some common varieties of soy-based foods you might find in your local supermarket:

- *Soy milk* is a beverage produced when soybeans are ground with water. Flavorings are added to make the drink palatable, and many brands of soy milk are fortified with calcium and vitamin D.
- *Tofu* is made from soy milk coagulated to form curds. If the coagulant used is calcium sulfate, the resulting product is high in calcium. Tofu is usually sold in blocks, like cheese, and is used as a meat substitute. Although many people object to its bland taste and mushy texture, tofu adapts well to many seasonings, and when drained and frozen before cooking it develops a chewy texture similar to meat.
- *Tempeh* is a more flavorful and firmer-textured meat substitute made from soybeans fermented with grains. It is often used in stir-fried dishes.
- *Miso* is a paste made from fermented soybeans and grains. It is used sparingly as a base for soups and sauces, because it is very high in sodium.
- *Edamame* are precooked, frozen soybeans eaten as a snack or in salads and other dishes.

Soy May Reduce Your Risk for Chronic Disease

Proponents say that a diet high in soy protein can reduce your risk for heart disease, certain types of cancer, and osteoporosis (loss of bone density). Let's review the research behind each of these claims.

The U.S. Food and Drug Administration (FDA) allows food manufacturers to put labels on products high in soy protein stating that a daily diet containing 25 grams of soy protein and low in saturated fat and cholesterol may reduce the risk for heart disease.[8] The FDA reviewed twenty-seven relevant clinical studies before concluding that diets providing four servings a day of soy-based foods (not supplements) can provoke a modest reduction in blood levels of LDL-cholesterol. The American Heart Association therefore recommends consuming soy milk and tofu as part of a heart-healthy diet.[9]

Many studies suggest that soy protects against prostate cancer, which is the most common cancer in men.[10] It is unclear, however, whether or not soy reduces a woman's risk for breast cancer. The American Cancer Society (ACS) states that "a number of laboratory and animal experiments and human observational studies suggest that soy may reduce the risk for several types of cancer, including breast, prostate, ovarian, and uterine cancer," and recommends consuming soy foods as part of a balanced, plant-based diet.[11]

Published studies of the effect of soy on bone density, a particular concern for older women, have also been inconclusive. Whereas some suggest that soy can help keep bones strong, others suggest little benefit. A recent study found that taking soy phytochemical supplements over a period of 3 years modestly improved bone mineral density in certain groups of post-menopausal women, but did not significantly increase bone mineral density overall.[12] More research is needed.

Adding Soy to Your Diet

If you decide that you want to try soy, how do you go about it? A first step for many people is to substitute soy milk for cow's milk on its own, on cereal, in smoothies, or in recipes for baked goods. Different brands of soy milk can have very different flavors, so try a few before you decide you don't like the taste. Refer to the ***Game Plan*** feature box for more tips on adding soy—and other legumes—to your diet.

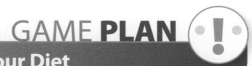

GAME **PLAN**

Tips for Adding Soy and Other Legumes to Your Diet

They're high in protein and fiber and low in fat, and they fill you up with fewer calories than meat sources of protein. What's more, they taste good! Maybe that's why nutrition experts consider soy and other legumes almost perfect foods. From main dishes to snacks, here are some simple ways to add them to your daily diet. By the way, some people experience uncomfortable intestinal gas after eating legumes. This is produced when bacteria in the colon break down the starches. If you're one of those people, make sure you soak legumes thoroughly, changing the water once or twice, before cooking. You can also try using enzyme supplements available in most grocery stores, such as Beano. Taken before meals, they reduce the occurrence of intestinal gas.

Breakfast

- Instead of cereal, eggs, or a muffin, microwave a frozen bean burrito for a quick, portable breakfast.
- Make your pancakes with soy milk or pour soy milk on your cereal.
- If you normally have a side of bacon, ham, or sausage with your eggs, have a side of black beans.

Lunch and Dinner

- Try a sandwich made with hummus (a garbanzo bean spread), cucumbers, tomato, avocado, and/or lettuce on whole-wheat bread or in a whole-wheat pocket.
- Add garbanzo beans, kidney beans, edamame, or fresh peas to tossed salads, or make a three-bean salad with kidney beans, green beans, and garbanzo beans.
- Make a side dish using legumes, such as peas, with pearl onions or succotash (lima beans, corn, and tomatoes).
- Make black-bean soup, lentil soup, pea soup, minestrone soup, or a batch of dhal (a type of yellow lentil used in Indian cuisine) and serve over brown rice. Top with plain yogurt, a traditional accompaniment in many Asian cuisines.
- Make tacos or burritos with black or pinto beans instead of shredded meat.

- Make a "meatloaf" using cooked, mashed lentils instead of ground beef.
- For fast food at home, keep canned beans on hand. Serve over rice with a salad for a complete and hearty meal.
- Use soy nut butter (similar to peanut butter), soy deli meats, or soy cheese in sandwiches.
- Try soy sausages, bacon, hot dogs, burgers, ground "beef," and "chicken" patties.
- Toss cubes of prepackaged flavored, baked tofu or tempeh or a handful of edamame into stir-fried vegetables and serve over Chinese noodles or rice.
- Order soy-based dishes, such as spicy bean curd and miso soup, at Asian restaurants.

Snacks

- Instead of potato chips or pretzels, try one of the new bean chips.
- Dip fresh vegetables in bean dip.
- Have hummus on wedges of pita bread.
- Add roasted soy "nuts" to your trail mix.
- Keep frozen tofu desserts, such as tofu ice cream, in your freezer.

provides 8 grams of protein in a 1-cup serving. It's highly digestible, and unlike many more familiar grains, provides all nine essential amino acids. See the feature **Foods You Don't Know You Love Yet** for more on quinoa. A similar grain called amaranth also provides complete protein. Teff, millet, and sorghum are grains long cultivated in Africa as rich sources of protein. They are now widely available in the United States. Although these three grains are low in the essential amino acid lysine, combining them with legumes produces a complete-protein meal.

Most other types of grains, as well as fruits and vegetables, are not particularly high in protein; however, these foods provide fiber and many vitamins and minerals and are excellent sources of carbohydrates. Thus, eating fruits, vegetables, and grains can help spare protein for use in building and maintaining our body rather than using it for energy.

Protein and Amino Acid Supplements: Any Truth to the Hype?

"Amino acid supplements—you can't gain without them!" This is just one of the countless headlines found in bodybuilding magazines and on Internet sites touting amino acid supplements as the key to achieving power, strength, and performance

foods you don't know you love YET

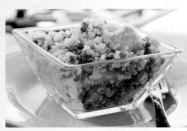

Quinoa

Quinoa (pronounced KEEN-wa) is a South American plant related to spinach and chard. Like these greens, its leaves are edible. However, quinoa is grown for its delicious, high-protein seeds, which are used in dishes the same way we use rice and other grains. Botanically, quinoa is considered a *pseudocereal*, which means it is not a member of the grass family and therefore not a grain at all.

Quinoa is an excellent plant source of complete protein and a good source of fiber and minerals, including phosphorus, magnesium, and iron. It is also gluten free, so it's a safe grain choice for people who are allergic to gluten or have celiac disease.

Because quinoa has a bitter coating in its natural state, it needs to be soaked and rinsed prior to cooking. However, many stores sell quinoa that has been pre-rinsed; check the package instructions. Once cooked, quinoa is light and fluffy, with a nutty taste. You can use quinoa as a substitute for rice or couscous in dishes such as stuffing, pilaf, salads, and soups. Quinoa pasta is also available in various shapes. Quinoa can be found in most major supermarkets and health food stores, and it can be bought online through websites such as Amazon.com.

"perfection." Many athletes who read these claims believe that taking amino acid supplements will boost their energy during performance, replace proteins metabolized for energy during exercise, enhance muscle growth and strength, and hasten recovery from intense training or injury. Should you believe the hype?

Until recently, it was stated by most nutrition experts that taking amino acids supplements and consuming excess protein in the diet do not result in enhancing muscle mass or strength gains. This is due to the fact that we use very little protein for energy during exercise. In addition, as already discussed earlier in this chapter, most Americans already consume more than two times the RDA for protein. Thus, scientific consensus was that most of us already get more than enough protein to support either strength or endurance exercise training and performance. Although many amino acid supplements do not enhance muscle building and strength, recent evidence suggests that dietary protein, and particularly the amino acid leucine, are important triggers to enhance the synthesis of protein in the muscle.[11] However, there is no need to put a dent in your wallet by taking expensive protein powders and amino acid supplements, because these benefits can be derived by consuming a glass of milk after exercise![11]

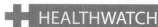 Good sources of protein include meats, eggs, dairy products, soy products, legumes, nuts, quorn, and certain grains. Consuming the amino acid leucine has been shown to enhance muscle building and strength; this amino acid can be easily and inexpensively consumed in adequate quantities by drinking milk.

HEALTHWATCH

 LO9 List the types, benefits, and potential challenges of vegetarian diets.

Can a vegetarian diet provide adequate protein?

vegetarianism The practice of restricting the diet to food substances of plant origin, including vegetables, fruits, grains, and nuts.

Vegetarianism is the practice of restricting the diet to food substances of vegetable origin, including fruits, grains, and nuts. To address the question of whether a vegetarian diet can provide adequate protein, let's begin with a look at the different types of vegetarian diets.

TABLE 5.4   Terms and Definitions of a Vegetarian Diet

Type of Diet	Foods Consumed	Comments
Semivegetarian (also called a flexitarian or plant-based diet)	Vegetables, grains, nuts, fruits, legumes, eggs, dairy products, and occasionally seafood and/or poultry	Typically excludes or limits red meat; may also avoid other meats.
Pescovegetarian	Similar to a semivegetarian but excludes poultry	*Pesco* means "fish," the only nonplant source of protein in this diet
Lacto-ovo-vegetarian	Vegetables, grains, nuts, fruits, legumes, dairy products (*lacto*), and eggs (*ovo*)	Excludes animal flesh and seafood
Lacto-vegetarian	Similar to a lacto-ovo-vegetarian but excludes eggs	Relies on milk and cheese for animal sources of protein
Ovovegetarian	Vegetables, grains, nuts, fruits, legumes, and eggs	Excludes dairy, flesh, and seafood products
Vegan (also called strict vegetarian)	Only plant-based foods (vegetables, grains, nuts, seeds, fruits, and legumes)	May not provide adequate vitamin B_{12}, zinc, iron, or calcium
Macrobiotic diet	Vegan-type of diet; becomes progressively more strict until almost all foods are eliminated; at the extreme, only brown rice and small amounts of water or herbal tea are consumed	When taken to extremes, can cause malnutrition and death
Fruitarian	Only raw or dried fruit, seeds, nuts, honey, and vegetable oil	Extremely restrictive; deficient in protein, calcium, zinc, iron, vitamin B_{12}, riboflavin, and other nutrients

There Are Many Types of Vegetarian Diets

There are almost as many types of vegetarian diets as there are vegetarians. Some people who consider themselves vegetarians regularly eat fish. Others avoid the flesh of animals but consume eggs, milk, and cheese liberally. Still others strictly avoid all products of animal origin, including milk and eggs, and even by-products, such as candies and puddings made with gelatin. A type of "vegetarian" diet receiving significant media attention recently has been the *flexitarian* diet. Flexitarians are considered semivegetarians who eat mostly plant foods, eggs, and dairy but occasionally eat red meat, poultry, and/or fish; hence, they are flexible about occasionally adding some meat-based protein to their diet. Vegetarian diets are also referred to as *plant-based* diets and are recognized for having many health benefits compared to diets that contain more meat and fewer plant-based foods.

TABLE 5.4 identifies the various types of vegetarian diets, ranging from the broadest to the most restrictive. Notice that the more restrictive the diet, the more challenging it becomes to get adequate dietary protein.

Why Do People Become Vegetarians?

When discussing vegetarianism, one of the most often-asked questions is why people make this food choice. The most common responses are included here.

Religious, Ethical, and Food-Safety Reasons

Some make the choice for religious reasons. Several religions prohibit or restrict the consumption of animal flesh; however, generalizations can be misleading. For example, although certain sects within Hinduism observe nonviolence, including toward animals, scanning the menu at an Indian restaurant will reveal that many Hindus regularly consume small quantities of meat, poultry, and fish. Many Buddhists are vegetarians, as are some Christians, including most Seventh-Day Adventists.

Many vegetarians are guided by their personal philosophy to choose vegetarianism. These people feel that it is wrong to consume animals and any products from animals (such as dairy or egg products), because they view the practices in the modern animal industries as inhumane. They may consume milk and eggs but choose to purchase them only from family farms where they believe animals are treated humanely.

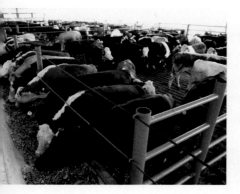

(a)

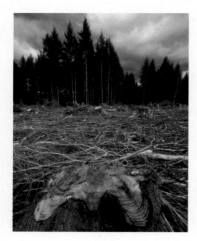

(b)

⬆ **FIGURE 5.9** Both **(a)** livestock production and **(b)** aggressive deforestation contribute to greenhouse gases.

Interested in trying a vegetarian diet but don't know where to begin? Check out the Vegetarian Starter Kit from the Physicians Committee for Responsible Medicine, at http://pcrm.org.

carcinogens Cancer-causing agents, such as certain pesticides, industrial chemicals, and pollutants.

There is also a great deal of concern about meat-handling practices, because outbreaks of foodborne illness occur frequently and can have serious consequences. For example, in recent years, outbreaks of severe bloody diarrhea have been traced to a bacterium called *E. coli* in hamburgers and steaks prepared at home or served in restaurants. Many people have had to be hospitalized, some with kidney failure, which in a few victims proved fatal. Contaminated poultry products—from ground turkey to frozen chicken pies and dinners—have also caused disease outbreaks, typically because of a bacterium called *Salmonella*.

Ecological Reasons

Many people choose vegetarianism because of their concerns about the effect of the meat industries on the global environment. They argue that cattle consume large quantities of grain and water, require grazing areas that could be used for plant food production, destroy vulnerable ecosystems (including rain forests), produce wastes that run off into surrounding bodies of water, and belch methane, a greenhouse gas associated with global warming **(FIGURE 5.9)**. Meat industry organizations argue that such effects are minor and greatly exaggerated. One area of agreement that has recently emerged focuses the argument not on *whether* we eat meat but on *how much* meat we consume. The environmental damage caused by the raising of livestock is due in part to the large number of animals produced. When a population reduces its consumption of meat, reduced production follows. The United Nations Intergovernmental Panel on Climate Change (IPCC) therefore recommends that we increasingly replace meat-based meals with vegetarian meals.

Health Benefits

Still others practice vegetarianism because of its health benefits. Research over several years has consistently shown that a varied and balanced vegetarian diet can reduce the risk for many chronic diseases. Its health benefits include the following:[12]

- reduced risk for obesity, type 2 diabetes, high blood pressure, and heart disease, most likely due to the lower saturated-fat content of vegetarian diets
- fewer intestinal problems, most likely due to the higher fiber content of vegetarian diets
- reduced risk for some cancers, particularly colon cancer; many components of a vegetarian diet can contribute to reducing cancer risks, including higher fiber, lower dietary fat, lower consumption of **carcinogens** (cancer-causing agents) that are formed when cooking meat, and higher consumption of soy protein, which may have anticancer properties
- reduced risk for kidney disease, kidney stones, and gallstones; the lower protein content of vegetarian diets, plus the higher intake of legumes and vegetables, may be protective against these conditions.

What Are the Challenges of a Vegetarian Diet?

Although a vegetarian diet can be healthful, it also presents some challenges. With reduced consumption of flesh and dairy products, there is a potential for inadequate intakes of certain nutrients. **TABLE 5.5** lists the nutrients that can be deficient in a vegan type of diet plan and describes good non-animal sources of these nutrients. Supplementation may be necessary for certain individuals if they cannot include adequate amounts in their diet.

Can a vegetarian diet provide enough protein? Because high-quality protein sources are quite easy to obtain in developed countries, a well-balanced vegetarian diet can provide adequate protein. In fact, the American Dietetic Association endorses

TABLE 5.5   Nutrients of Concern in a Vegan Diet

Nutrient	Functions	Non-Meat/Non-Dairy Food Sources
Vitamin B_{12}	Assists with DNA synthesis; protection and growth of nerve fibers	Vitamin B_{12}–fortified cereals, yeast, soy products, and other meat analogs; vitamin B_{12} supplements
Vitamin D	Promotes bone growth	Vitamin D–fortified cereals, margarines, and soy products; adequate exposure to sunlight; supplementation may be necessary for those who do not get adequate exposure to sunlight
Riboflavin (vitamin B_2)	Promotes release of energy; supports normal vision and skin health	Whole and enriched grains, green leafy vegetables, mushrooms, beans, nuts, and seeds
Iron	Assists with oxygen transport; involved in making amino acids and hormones	Whole-grain products, prune juice, dried fruits, beans, nuts, seeds, and leafy vegetables (such as spinach)
Calcium	Maintains bone health; assists with muscle contraction, blood pressure, and nerve transmission	Fortified soy milk and tofu, almonds, dry beans, leafy vegetables, calcium-fortified juices, and fortified breakfast cereals
Zinc	Assists with DNA and RNA synthesis, immune function, and growth	Whole-grain products, wheat germ, beans, nuts, and seeds

an appropriately planned vegetarian diet as healthful, nutritionally adequate, and beneficial in reducing and preventing various diseases.[12]

As you can see, the emphasis is on a *balanced* and *adequate* vegetarian diet; thus, it is important for vegetarians to consume soy products, eat complementary proteins, and obtain enough energy from other macronutrients to spare protein from being used as an energy source. Although the digestibility of a vegetarian diet is potentially lower than that of an animal-based diet, there is no separate protein recommendation for vegetarians who consume complementary plant proteins.[13]

Using MyPlate on a Vegetarian Diet

Although the USDA has not designed a version of MyPlate specifically for people following a vegetarian diet, healthy eating tips for vegetarians are available at MyPlate online (see the Web resources at the end of this chapter). For example, to meet their needs for protein and calcium, lacto-vegetarians can consume low-fat or nonfat dairy products. Vegans and ovovegetarians can consume calcium-fortified soy milk or one of the many protein bars fortified with calcium.

Vegans need to consume vitamin B_{12} either from fortified foods or supplements, because this vitamin is found naturally only in animal foods. They should also pay special attention to consuming food high in vitamin D, riboflavin (B_2), and the minerals zinc and iron. Supplementation of these micronutrients may be necessary for certain individuals if they cannot consume adequate amounts in their diet.

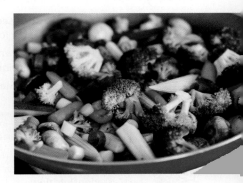

◆ A well-balanced vegetarian diet can provide adequate protein and other nutrients.

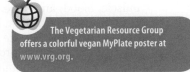

The Vegetarian Resource Group offers a colorful vegan MyPlate poster at www.vrg.org.

recap   A balanced vegetarian diet may reduce the risk for obesity, type 2 diabetes, heart disease, digestive problems, some cancers, kidney disease, kidney stones, and gallstones. Although varied vegetarian diets can provide enough protein, vegetarians who consume no animal products need to supplement their diet with good sources of vitamin B_{12}, vitamin D, riboflavin, iron, calcium, and zinc.

STUDY **PLAN** | MasteringNutrition™

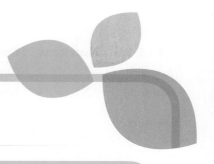

Customize your study plan—and master your nutrition!—
in the Study Area of **MasteringNutrition**.

what can I do **today?**

Now that you've read this chapter, try making these three changes.

1 Try adding soy milk to your breakfast cereal.

2 Make it a goal today to consume meals that provide adequate protein from sources low in saturated fats and cholesterol, such as fish, poultry without the skin, lean beef, egg whites, legumes, nuts and nut butters, and tofu.

3 If you regularly eat meat at both lunch and dinner, try replacing one of these meat-based meals for the next 7 days with a plant-based meal including legumes, nuts, quorn, veggie burgers/sausages, or tofu or tempeh.

test yourself | *answers*

1. **False.** Although protein can be used for energy in certain circumstances, fats and carbohydrates are the primary sources of energy for our body.

2. **False.** Excess protein is broken down and its component parts are either stored as fat or used for energy or tissue building and repair. Only the nitrogen component of protein is excreted in the urine.

3. **True.** Most people in the United States consume 1.5 to 2 times more protein than they need.

summary

Scan to hear an MP3 Chapter Review in **MasteringNutrition**.

LO **1** **Describe how proteins differ from carbohydrates and fats**

- Proteins are large, complex molecules that are critical components of all tissues, including muscle, blood, and bone. Like carbohydrates and fat, they contain carbon, hydrogen, and oxygen. In contrast, however, the structure of proteins is dictated by DNA, and proteins contain nitrogen.

- Amino acids are the building blocks of proteins; they are made up of a hydrogen atom, an acid group, an amine group containing nitrogen, and a unique side chain.

- There are 20 amino acids in our bodies: 9 are essential amino acids, meaning that our bodies cannot produce them, and we must obtain them from food; and 11 are nonessential, meaning our bodies can make them, so they do not need to be consumed in the diet.

LO **2** **Describe the processes by which DNA directs protein synthesis and proteins organize into levels of structure**

- Our genetic makeup determines the sequence of amino acids in our proteins. Genes carry the instructions that cells use to make proteins.

- The three-dimensional shape of proteins determines their function in the body. When proteins are exposed to damaging substances such as heat, acids, bases, and alcohol, they are denatured, meaning they lose their shape and function.

- A limiting amino acid is one that is missing or in limited supply, preventing the synthesis of adequate proteins.

- Incomplete proteins, also known as low-quality proteins, do not contain all the essential amino acids in sufficient quantities to support growth and health. Complete proteins, also known as high-quality proteins, have all nine of the essential amino acids and can therefore support growth and health.

LO **3** **Explain the significance of mutual supplementation and identify non-meat food combinations that are complete protein sources**

- Mutual supplementation is the process of combining two incomplete protein sources to make a complete protein. The two foods in this process are called complementary proteins. Non-meat food combinations that provide complete proteins include legumes when served with either grains or nuts and seeds.

LO 4 **Identify at least four functions of proteins in our body**

- Proteins are needed to promote cell growth, repair, and maintenance. They act as enzymes and hormones; help maintain the balance of fluids, electrolytes, acids, and bases; transport nutrients and other substances; and support healthy immune function. They can be used for energy if intake of carbohydrate and fat is inadequate to support energy needs.

LO 5 **Explain how our body digests and absorbs protein**

- In the stomach, proteins are denatured by hydrochloric acid, and pepsin begins breaking the proteins into smaller polypeptides and single amino acids. Most digestion of proteins occurs in the small intestine with the help of proteases. These break the polypeptides into tripeptides, dipeptides, and single amino acids, which are absorbed into the enterocytes. These break the remaining peptides into amino acids.
- The amino acids are transported into the bloodstream to the liver and on to cells throughout our body as needed.
- Protein digestibility affects its quality, with those proteins that are more digestible being of a higher quality. Animal sources, soy protein, and legumes are highly digestible forms of protein.

LO 6 **Calculate your recommended dietary allowance for protein**

- The RDA for protein for sedentary people is 0.8 grams of protein per kilogram body weight per day. To calculate your protein needs, start by converting your weight from pounds to kilograms by dividing your weight in pounds by 2.2. Next, multiply by 0.8. The AMDR for protein is 10% to 35% of total energy.
- Most people in the United States routinely eat 1.5 to 2 times the RDA for protein.

LO 7 **Describe two disorders related to inadequate protein intake**

- Protein-energy malnutrition can lead to marasmus and kwashiorkor. These diseases primarily affect impoverished children in developing nations. However, residents of developed countries are also at risk, especially the elderly, the homeless, people struggling with substance abuse, and people with AIDS, cancer, and other wasting diseases.

LO 8 **Identify several healthful food sources of animal and plant protein**

- Healthful sources of protein include lean meats, poultry, fish, low-fat dairy products, eggs, soy and other legumes, quinoa, and nuts, as well as plant-based meals combining complementary proteins.

LO 9 **List the types, benefits, and potential challenges of vegetarian diets**

- There are many forms of vegetarianism, from flexitarians (semivegetarians) who may occasionally eat meat, to vegans, who eat no form of animal product. Consuming a well-planned vegetarian diet may reduce the risk of obesity, high blood pressure, heart disease, type 2 diabetes, certain intestinal problems, kidney disorders, and gallstones. Some research suggests that it may also reduce the risk for some forms of cancer.
- Vegans may need to supplement their diet with vitamins B_{12} and D, riboflavin, iron, calcium, and zinc.

review questions

LO 1 **Describe how proteins differ from carbohydrates and fats**

1. One way that proteins differ from carbohydrates and fats is that only proteins
   a. can be synthesized by our body.
   b. contain nitrogen.
   c. can be used for energy.
   d. contain carbon, oxygen, and hydrogen.

LO 2 **Describe the processes by which DNA directs protein synthesis and proteins organize into levels of structure**

2. Proteins are synthesized following instructions dictated by
   a. enzymes.
   b. DNA.
   c. amino acids.
   d. ketones.

LO 3 **Explain the significance of mutual supplementation and identify non-meat food combinations that are complete protein sources**

3. The process of combining peanut butter and whole-wheat bread to make a complete protein is called
   a. deamination.
   b. vegetarianism.
   c. transamination.
   d. mutual supplementation.

LO 4 **Identify at least four functions of proteins in our body**

4. Proteins
   a. do not have a specialized storage form for energy.
   b. repel fluids, thereby reducing our risk for edema.
   c. help destroy antibodies, toxic by-products of our immune response to infection.
   d. None of the above is true.

LO **5** **Explain how our body digests and absorbs protein**

5. In the small intestine,
   a. pepsinogen begins the breakdown of proteins into polypeptides.
   b. polypeptides are absorbed into the bloodstream, where they travel to the liver for breakdown into single amino acids.
   c. enzymes break polypeptides into single amino acids.
   d. amino acids are broken down and urea, a by-product of amine digestion, moves to the large intestine for excretion in feces.

LO **6** **Calculate your recommended dietary allowance for protein**

6. If you are moderately active, but not an athlete, and you weigh 165 pounds, how many grams of protein do you need to eat each day?
   a. 60 grams
   b. 70 grams
   c. 80 grams
   d. 90 grams

LO **7** **Describe two disorders related to inadequate protein intake**

7. Marasmus is
   a. a form of protein–energy malnutrition.
   b. sometimes seen in people who consume diets with sufficient Calories but insufficient protein.
   c. initially treated with balanced fluid and electrolytes and a high-fat diet.
   d. all of the above.

LO **8** **Identify several healthful food sources of animal and plant protein**

8. Which of the following foods provides the most protein?
   a. 1 cup of raw broccoli
   b. 2 slices of whole-wheat bread
   c. 1 cup of soy milk
   d. 1 cup of low-fat, plain yogurt

LO **9** **List the types, benefits, and potential challenges of vegetarian diets**

9. Which of the following meals is typical of a vegan diet?
   a. Rice, pinto beans, acorn squash, soy butter, and almond milk
   b. Veggie dog, bun, and a banana blended with yogurt
   c. Raw lean beef and green tea
   d. Egg salad on whole-wheat toast, broccoli, carrot sticks, and soy milk

10. Vegetarian meals
    a. are typically low in vitamin C, niacin, iron, zinc, omega-6 fatty acids, and protein.
    b. are recommended by many climate change experts because they reduce production of greenhouse gases as compared with meat-based meals.
    c. must be carefully planned to include complementary proteins.
    d. all of the above.

Answers to Review Questions are located at the back of this text.

web links

The following websites and apps explore further topics and issues related to personal health.
Visit **MasteringNutrition** for links to the websites and RSS feeds.

www.choosemyplate.gov
The USDA's MyPlate Website

This section of the MyPlate website contains useful, healthy eating tips for vegetarians.

www.eatright.org
Academy of Nutrition and Dietetics

Search for "vegetarian diets" to learn how to plan healthful meat-free meals.

http://fnic.nal.usda.gov
USDA Food and Nutrition Information Center

Click on "food consumption" in the left navigation bar to find a searchable database of the nutrient values of foods.

www.meatlessmonday.com
Meatless Monday Campaign

Find out how to start going meatless one day a week with this innovative campaign's website.

www.vrg.org
The Vegetarian Resource Group

Visit this site for additional information on how to build a balanced vegetarian diet.

www.who.int
World Health Organization Nutrition

Visit this site to find out more about the worldwide scope of protein-deficiency diseases and related topics.

Vitamins
Micronutrients
with Macro Powers

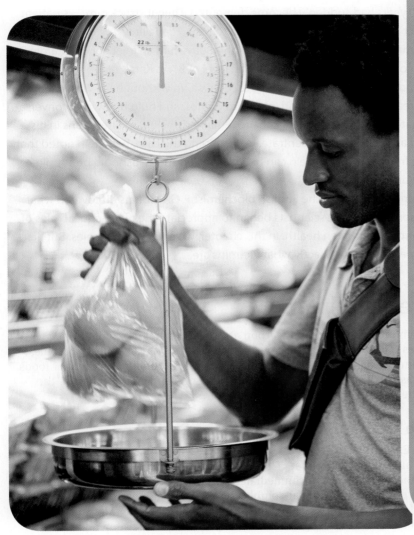

test yourself

Are these statements true or false? Circle your guess.

1. **T F** Vitamin D is called the "sunshine vitamin" because our body can make it by using energy obtained from sunlight.

2. **T F** Taking vitamin C supplements helps prevent colds.

3. **T F** The B-vitamins are an important source of energy for our body.

Test Yourself answers can be found at the end of the chapter.

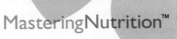

MasteringNutrition™

Go online for chapter quizzes, pre-tests, Interactive Activities, and more!

Dr. Leslie Bernstein looked in astonishment at the 80-year-old man in his office. A leading gastroenterologist and professor of medicine at Albert Einstein College of Medicine in New York City, he had admired Pop Katz for years as one of his most healthy patients, a strict vegetarian and athlete who just weeks before had been going on 3-mile runs. Now he could barely stand. He was confused, cried easily, was wandering away from his home, and had lost control of his bladder. Tests showed that he had not had a stroke; did not have a tumor, an infection, or Alzheimer's disease; and had no evidence of exposure to pesticides or other toxins. A neurologist diagnosed dementia, but Bernstein was skeptical that a man who hadn't been sick for 80 years had suddenly become demented. Then it struck him. His patient had been a strict vegetarian for 38 years. He had to be B_{12} deficient.[1]

Bernstein immediately tested Katz's blood, then gave him an injection of vitamin B_{12}. The blood test confirmed Bernstein's hunch: the level of B_{12} in Katz's blood was too low to detect. The morning after his injection, Katz could sit up without help. Within a week of continuing treatment, he could read, play card games, and hold his own in conversations. Unfortunately, some neurologic damage remained, including alterations in his personality and an inability to concentrate. In describing the case, Bernstein noted that, although a diet free of animal protein can be healthful and safe, it should be supplemented with vitamin B_{12}.[1]

It was not until 1906, when the English biochemist F. G. Hopkins discovered what he called *accessory factors* that scientists began to appreciate the many critical roles of vitamins in maintaining human health. In this chapter, we explore these roles. But first, let's take a moment to define exactly what vitamins are.

LO1 Compare and contrast fat-soluble and water-soluble vitamins.

What are vitamins?

Vitamins are compounds that contain carbon and are essential in regulating our body's processes **(FIGURE 6.1)**. Because our body cannot synthesize most vitamins, we must consume them in our diet. Fortunately, most are found in a variety of foods. Vitamins are classified as either fat soluble or water soluble. Here, we discuss the general properties of these two groups.

Fat-Soluble Vitamins Are Stored in the Body

Vitamins A, D, E, and K are **fat-soluble vitamins**. These vitamins are absorbed in our small intestine along with dietary fat. They are then transported to the liver or other organs, where they are either used immediately or stored in fatty tissues for later use. Because we are capable of storing fat-soluble vitamins, we do not have to consume the recommended intakes every single day. As long as our diet provides the average amounts recommended over any given time period, we won't develop deficiencies.

Our ability to store fat-soluble vitamins has a distinct disadvantage. If we consume more of these vitamins than our body can use, they can build up to toxic levels in our fatty tissues. Symptoms of toxicity include damage to our hair, skin, bones, eyes, and nervous system. **Megadosing**—that is, taking ten or more times the recommended amount of a nutrient—can even lead to death when it involves the fat-soluble vitamins A and D.

Even though we can store fat-soluble vitamins, deficiencies sometimes occur, especially in people with diseases that prevent the normal absorption of fat and in people who consume very little fat. Using mineral oil as a laxative can result in a significant loss of fat-soluble vitamins in our feces. Deficiencies of fat-soluble vitamins can lead to serious health problems, such as night blindness, fragile bones, and even death in the most severe cases.

vitamins Micronutrients that contain carbon and assist us in regulating our body's processes. They are classified as water soluble or fat soluble.

fat-soluble vitamins Vitamins that are not soluble in water but soluble in fat. These include vitamins A, D, E, and K.

megadosing Taking a dose of a nutrient that is ten or more times greater than the recommended amount.

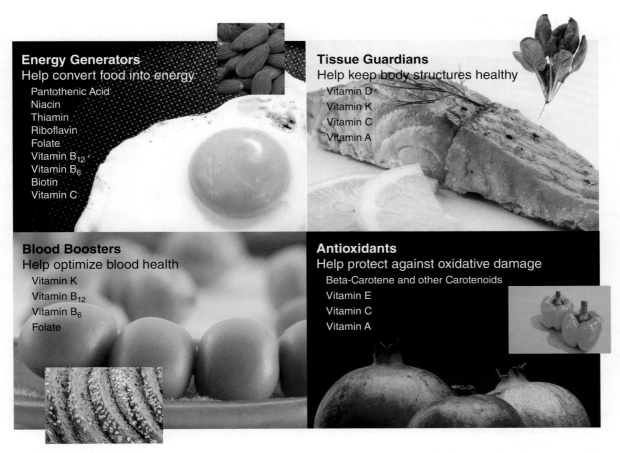

Energy Generators
Help convert food into energy
Pantothenic Acid
Niacin
Thiamin
Riboflavin
Folate
Vitamin B$_{12}$
Vitamin B$_6$
Biotin
Vitamin C

Tissue Guardians
Help keep body structures healthy
Vitamin D
Vitamin K
Vitamin C
Vitamin A

Blood Boosters
Help optimize blood health
Vitamin K
Vitamin B$_{12}$
Vitamin B$_6$
Folate

Antioxidants
Help protect against oxidative damage
Beta-Carotene and other Carotenoids
Vitamin E
Vitamin C
Vitamin A

◆ **FIGURE 6.1** The functions of fat-soluble and water-soluble vitamins and related compounds, such as beta-carotene and biotin. Good food sources are also shown for each functional group.

The potential for toxicity from supplements is one reason it's wise to get your vitamins from foods whenever possible. Fat-soluble vitamins are found in a variety of fat-containing foods. Meats, dairy products, vegetable oils, avocados, nuts, and seeds are all potentially good sources. **TABLE 6.1** identifies major functions and recommended intakes.

Water-Soluble Vitamins Should Be Consumed Daily or Weekly

Vitamin C and the B-vitamins (thiamin, riboflavin, niacin, vitamin B$_6$, vitamin B$_{12}$, pantothenic acid, biotin, and folate) are the **water-soluble vitamins**. Because they dissolve in water, these vitamins are readily absorbed through the enterocytes directly into the bloodstream. They then travel to cells, where they are needed.

We cannot store large amounts of water-soluble vitamins, because our kidneys filter out from our bloodstream any that are unneeded. We then excrete them in our urine. Because we don't store them efficiently, we rarely experience toxicity when we consume excess amounts of these vitamins from foods. We *can* develop toxic levels through supplementation, however, if we consume more than our body can eliminate.

A disadvantage of our inability to store large amounts of water-soluble vitamins is that, if we don't consume adequate amounts regularly, we can develop deficiency symptoms and even disease fairly quickly. Still, most people don't need to use supplements: the water-soluble vitamins are abundant in many foods, including whole grains, fruits, vegetables, meats, and dairy products. **TABLE 6.2** identifies major functions and recommended intakes.

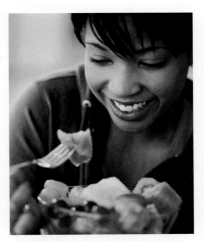

◆ Because we cannot store large amounts of water-soluble vitamins, we need to consume foods that contain them, such as fruits and vegetables, daily.

water-soluble vitamins Vitamins that are soluble in water. These include vitamin C and the B-vitamins.

TABLE 6.1 Fat-Soluble Vitamins

Vitamin Name	Primary Functions	Recommended Intake*	Reliable Food Sources	Toxicity/Deficiency Symptoms
A (retinol, retinal, retinoic acid)	Required for ability of eyes to adjust to changes in light Protects color vision Assists cell differentiation Required for sperm production in men and fertilization in women Contributes to healthy bone Contributes to healthy immune system	RDA: Men = 900 µg Women = 700 µg UL = 3,000 µg/day	Preformed retinol: beef and chicken liver, egg yolks, milk Carotenoid precursors: spinach, carrots, mango, apricots, cantaloupe, pumpkin, yams	*Toxicity:* fatigue; bone and joint pain; spontaneous abortion and birth defects of fetuses in pregnant women; nausea and diarrhea; liver damage; nervous system damage; blurred vision; hair loss; skin disorders *Deficiency:* night blindness, xerophthalmia; impaired growth, immunity, and reproductive function
D (cholecalciferol)	Regulates blood calcium levels Maintains bone health Assists cell differentiation	RDA (assumes that person does not get adequate sun exposure): Adult aged 19 to 50 = 600 IU/day Adult aged 51 to 70 = 600 IU/day Adult aged >70 = 800 U/day UL = 4,000 IU/day	Canned salmon and mackerel, milk, fortified cereals	*Toxicity:* hypercalcemia *Deficiency:* rickets in children; osteomalacia and/or osteoporosis in adults
E (tocopherol)	As a powerful antioxidant, protects cell membranes, polyunsaturated fatty acids, and vitamin A from oxidation Protects white blood cells Enhances immune function Improves absorption of vitamin A	RDA: Men = 15 mg/day Women = 15 mg/day UL = 1,000 mg/day	Sunflower seeds, almonds, vegetable oils, fortified cereals	*Toxicity:* rare *Deficiency:* hemolytic anemia; impairment of nerve, muscle, and immune function
K (phylloquinone, menaquinone, menadione)	Serves as a coenzyme during production of specific proteins that assist in blood coagulation and bone metabolism	AI: Men = 120 µg/day Women = 90 µg/day	Kale, spinach, turnip greens, Brussels sprouts	*Toxicity:* none known *Deficiency:* impaired blood clotting; possible effect on bone health

*Abbreviations: RDA, Recommended Dietary Allowance; UL, upper limit; AI, Adequate Intake.

For a helpful overview of vitamins, check out the FDA video *Fortify Your Knowledge About Vitamins*. Go to www.fda.gov and click the expandable menu on the far left and choose "Consumer Updates" to search for the video.

Vitamins Are Vulnerable!

Because all vitamins are organic compounds, they are all more or less vulnerable to decay from exposure to heat, oxygen, or other factors. Follow these tips for preserving the vitamins in the foods you eat:

- Watch the water. Soak and cook foods in as little water as possible to minimize the loss of water-soluble vitamins. For the best possible outcome, steam vegetables in a steamer basket over half an inch of water.
- Lower the heat. Avoid high temperatures for long periods of time. Heat causes some loss of nutrients, especially vitamin C, thiamin, and riboflavin. Cook vegetables only until tender.
- Limit the light. Riboflavin is destroyed by light. Because milk is an excellent source of riboflavin, it is typically packaged in light-obstructing containers, such as coated cardboard or opaque bottles.
- Avoid air. Vitamins A, C, E, K, and B are destroyed by exposure to air. Ways to minimize losses are to cut fruits and vegetables in large pieces and store them in airtight containers or covered in plastic wrap. Peel and cut produce immediately

TABLE 6.2   Water-Soluble Vitamins

Vitamin Name	Primary Functions	Recommended Intake*	Reliable Food Sources	Toxicity/Deficiency Symptoms
Thiamin (vitamin B$_1$)	Required as enzyme cofactor for carbohydrate and amino acid metabolism	RDA: Men = 1.2 mg/day Women = 1.1 mg/day	Pork, fortified cereals, enriched rice and pasta, peas, tuna, legumes	*Toxicity:* none known *Deficiency:* beriberi; fatigue, apathy, decreased memory, confusion, irritability, muscle weakness
Riboflavin (vitamin B$_2$)	Required as enzyme cofactor for carbohydrate and fat metabolism	RDA: Men = 1.3 mg/day Women = 1.1 mg/day	Beef liver, shrimp, milk and other dairy foods, fortified cereals, enriched breads and grains	*Toxicity:* none known *Deficiency:* ariboflavinosis; swollen mouth and throat; seborrheic dermatitis; anemia
Niacin, nicotinamide, nicotinic acid	Required for carbohydrate and fat metabolism Plays role in DNA replication and repair and cell differentiation	RDA: Men = 16 mg/day Women = 14 mg/day UL = 35 mg/day	Beef liver, most cuts of meat/fish/poultry, fortified cereals, enriched breads and grains, canned tomato products	*Toxicity:* flushing, liver damage, glucose intolerance, blurred vision differentiation *Deficiency:* pellagra; vomiting, constipation, or diarrhea; apathy
Pyridoxine, pyridoxal, pyridoxamine (vitamin B$_6$)	Required as enzyme cofactor for carbohydrate and amino acid metabolism Assists synthesis of blood cells	RDA: Men and women aged 19 to 50 = 1.3 mg/day Men aged >50 = 1.7 mg/day Women aged >50 = 1.5 mg/day UL = 100 mg/day	Chickpeas (garbanzo beans), most cuts of meat/fish/poultry, fortified cereals, white potatoes	*Toxicity:* nerve damage, skin lesions *Deficiency:* anemia; seborrheic dermatitis; depression, confusion, convulsions; elevated homocysteine levels
Folate (folic acid)	Required as enzyme cofactor for amino acid metabolism Required for DNA synthesis Involved in metabolism of homocysteine	RDA: Men = 400 µg/day Women = 400 µg/day UL = 1,000 µg/day	Fortified cereals, enriched breads and grains, spinach, legumes (lentils, chickpeas, pinto beans), greens (spinach, romaine lettuce), liver	*Toxicity:* masks symptoms of vitamin B$_{12}$ deficiency, specifically signs of nerve damage *Deficiency:* macrocytic anemia; neural tube defects in a developing fetus; elevated homocysteine levels
Cobalamin (vitamin B$_{12}$)	Assists with formation of blood Required for healthy nervous system function Involved as enzyme cofactor in metabolism of homocysteine	RDA: Men = 2.4 µg/day Women = 2.4 µg/day	Shellfish, all cuts of meat/fish/poultry, milk and other dairy foods, fortified cereals	*Toxicity:* none known *Deficiency:* macrocytic anemia; tingling and numbness of extremities; nerve damage; memory loss, disorientation, dementia; elevated homocysteine levels
Pantothenic acid	Assists with fat metabolism	AI: Men = 5 mg/day Women = 5 mg/day	Meat/fish/poultry, shiitake mushrooms, fortified cereals, egg yolk	*Toxicity:* none known *Deficiency:* rare
Biotin	Involved as enzyme cofactor in carbohydrate, fat, and protein metabolism	AI: Men = 30 µg/day Women = 30 µg/day	Nuts, egg yolk	*Toxicity:* none known *Deficiency:* rare
Ascorbic acid (vitamin C)	Antioxidant in extracellular fluid and lungs Regenerates oxidized vitamin E Assists with collagen synthesis Enhances immune function Assists in synthesis of hormones, neurotransmitters, and DNA Enhances iron absorption	RDA: Men = 90 mg/day Women = 75 mg/day Smokers = 35 mg more per day than RDA UL = 2,000 mg	Sweet peppers, citrus fruits and juices, broccoli, strawberries, kiwi	*Toxicity:* nausea and diarrhea, nosebleeds, increased oxidative damage, increased formation of kidney stones in people with kidney disease *Deficiency:* scurvy; bone pain and fractures, depression, anemia

*Abbreviations: RDA, Recommended Dietary Allowance; UL, upper limit; AI, Adequate Intake.

before cooking and eat them as soon after cooking as possible. Finally, eat vegetables and fruits whole, unpeeled, and raw whenever possible.

■ Don't disturb the pH. Adding baking soda to vegetables to help them retain their color is not smart. Baking soda makes cooking water alkaline, and thiamin, riboflavin, vitamin K, and vitamin C are destroyed.

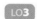 Vitamins are carbon-containing compounds that are essential in regulating a multitude of body processes. Vitamins A, D, E, and K are fat soluble and are present in certain fat-containing foods. We store fat-soluble vitamins in the fatty tissues of our body. Water-soluble vitamins include vitamin C and the B-vitamins (thiamin, riboflavin, niacin, vitamin B_6, vitamin B_{12}, pantothenic acid, biotin, and folate). Because these vitamins are soluble in water, the body cannot store large amounts, so it excretes excesses in the urine. The vitamin content of foods can be preserved by reducing the amount of water used in cooking, lowering cooking heat, limiting exposure of foods to light, avoiding exposure of foods to air, and not adding baking soda to vegetables in an effort to maintain their color.

LO2 Explain the role of vitamin A in vision and cell differentiation, and its relationship to beta-carotene.

LO3 Identify the primary functions and food sources of vitamins D and K.

Tissue guardians: Vitamins A, D, and K

The fat-soluble vitamins A, D, and K are important for the health of certain body tissues. Vitamin A protects the retina of the eyes, vitamin D is required for healthy bone, and vitamin K guards against blood loss. Let's take a closer look at these three fat-soluble vitamins.

Vitamin A Protects Our Sight

Vitamin A is multitalented: its known functions are numerous, and researchers speculate that many are still to be discovered. Most would agree, though, that vitamin A's starring role is in the maintenance of healthy vision. Vitamin A enables us to see images and to distinguish different colors. Let's take a closer look at this process.

Light enters our eyes through the cornea, travels through the lens, and then hits the **retina**, a delicate membrane lining the back of the inner eyeball (**FIGURE 6.2**). Indeed, the primary form that vitamin A takes in our body is *retinal*, which got its name because it is found in—and is integral to—the retina. When light hits the retina, it reacts with the retinal within it. This reaction sparks the transmission of a signal along the optic nerve to the brain that is interpreted as a black-and-white image. If the light hitting the retina is bright enough, retinal can also enable the retina to distinguish the different wavelengths of light as different colors. These processes go on continually, allowing us to perceive moment-by-moment changes in our visual field, such as green and yellow leaves fluttering in the wind.

Our abilities to adjust to dim light and recover from a bright flash of light are also critically dependent on adequate levels of retinal in our eyes. That's why deficiency of vitamin A causes vision disorders, including night blindness, discussed shortly.

retina The delicate, light-sensitive membrane lining the inner eyeball and connected to the optic nerve. It contains retinal.

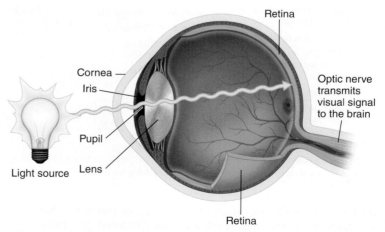

FIGURE 6.2 Vitamin A is necessary to maintain healthy vision. Light enters the eye through the cornea, travels through the lens, and hits the retina, located in the back of the eye. The light reacts with the retinal stored in the retina, which allows us to see images.

How Else Do We Use Vitamin A?

Vitamin A also contributes to **cell differentiation**, the process by which immature cells develop into highly specialized cells that perform unique functions. This process is critical to the development of healthy *epithelial tissues* (the skin and the tissues that line the respiratory and gastrointestinal tracts) and specialized immune cells called *T lymphocytes,* which help us fight infections.

Vitamin A also

- helps break down old bone tissue, so that new bone can develop,
- is involved in sperm production in men and in fertilization in women, and
- is associated with lower risks of some forms of cancer and heart disease when blood levels of this vitamin are adequate.

Two popular treatments for acne contain derivatives of vitamin A. Retin-A, or tretinoin, is a treatment applied to the skin. Accutane, or isotretinoin, is taken orally. These medications should be used carefully and only under the supervision of a physician. Both medications increase a person's sensitivity to the sun, and it is recommended that exposure to the sun be limited while using them. They also can cause birth defects in infants whose mothers used them while pregnant. It is recommended that a woman discontinue use at least 2 years prior to conceiving. Women of childbearing age who are using one of these medications must use reliable contraceptives to avoid becoming pregnant. Both medications have also been associated with other toxicity problems in some patients. Interestingly, vitamin A itself has no effect on acne; thus, vitamin A supplements are not recommended in its treatment.

What Is the Role of Beta-Carotene?

Beta-carotene is a water-soluble *provitamin* found in many fruits and vegetables. **Provitamins** are inactive forms of vitamins that the body cannot use until they are converted to their active form. Our body converts beta-carotene to an active form of vitamin A called *retinol.* For this reason, beta-carotene is also referred to as a *precursor* of retinol.

Beta-carotene is also classified as a **carotenoid**, one of a group of more than 600 plant pigments that are the basis for the red, orange (think *carrots*), and deep-yellow colors of many fruits and vegetables. (Even dark-green leafy vegetables contain plenty of carotenoids, but the green pigment, chlorophyll, masks their color.) We are just beginning to learn about the many functions of carotenoids in the body and how they influence our health. We do know that carotenoids

- defend against damage to our cell membranes,
- enhance our immune system,
- protect our skin from the damage caused by the sun's ultraviolet rays, and
- prevent or delay age-related vision impairment.

Interestingly, taking beta-carotene supplements has been shown to *increase* the risk for lung and stomach cancers.[2] In contrast, consuming carotenoids in foods is associated with a *decreased* risk for certain types of cancer, as well as cardiovascular disease. Still, it's possible to overdo it! Although harmless and reversible, eating large amounts of foods high in beta-carotene can turn your skin yellow or orange. Carotenoids and other beneficial plant chemicals (called *phytochemicals*) are discussed in detail shortly.

How Much Vitamin A Should We Consume?

Table 6.1 identifies the RDA for vitamin A. Nutrition scientists do not classify beta-carotene and other carotenoids as micronutrients, because they play no known essential roles in our body and are not associated with any deficiency symptoms. Thus, no formal dietary reference intake (DRI) for beta-carotene has been determined.

Because the body converts vitamin A and beta-carotene into retinol, you may also see the expression *retinol activity equivalents (RAE)* or *retinol equivalents (RE)* for

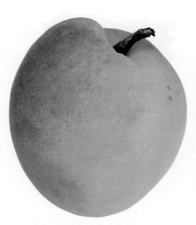

Apricots are high in carotenoids.

cell differentiation The process by which immature, undifferentiated cells develop into highly specialized functional cells of discrete organs and tissues.

provitamin An inactive form of a vitamin that the body can convert to an active form. An example is beta-carotene.

carotenoid Fat-soluble plant pigment that the body stores in the liver and adipose tissues. The body is able to convert certain carotenoids to vitamin A.

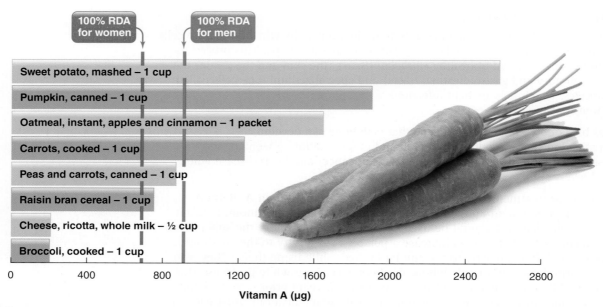

100% RDA for women

100% RDA for men

Sweet potato, mashed – 1 cup

Pumpkin, canned – 1 cup

Oatmeal, instant, apples and cinnamon – 1 packet

Carrots, cooked – 1 cup

Peas and carrots, canned – 1 cup

Raisin bran cereal – 1 cup

Cheese, ricotta, whole milk – ½ cup

Broccoli, cooked – 1 cup

0   400   800   1200   1600   2000   2400   2800

Vitamin A (μg)

🔺 **FIGURE 6.3** Common food sources of vitamin A or beta-carotene. The RDA for vitamin A is 900 μg per day for men and 700 μg per day for women.

Data from U.S. Department of Agriculture, Agricultural Research Service. 2013. USDA Nutrient Database for Standard Reference, Release 26. Nutrient Data Laboratory Home Page. **www.ars.usda.gov/ba/bhnrc/ndl**

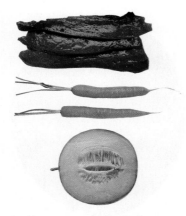

🔺 Liver, carrots, and cantaloupe are all good sources of vitamin A.

night blindness A vitamin A–deficiency disorder that results in the loss of the ability to see in dim light.

vitamin A on food labels and dietary supplements. Sometimes, the vitamin A content of foods and supplements is expressed in International Units (IU).

We consume vitamin A from animal foods, such as beef liver, chicken liver, eggs, and dairy products. Vitamin A is also available from foods high in beta-carotene and other carotenoids, which the body can convert to vitamin A. These include dark-green, orange, and deep-yellow fruits and vegetables, such as spinach, carrots, mango, and cantaloupe. Common food sources of vitamin A and beta-carotene are also identified in **FIGURE 6.3**.

Vitamin A is highly toxic, and toxicity symptoms develop after consuming only three to four times the RDA. Toxicity rarely results from food sources, but vitamin A supplements are known to have caused severe illness and even death. That's why single-nutrient vitamin A supplements should never be taken unless prescribed by your healthcare provider. Consuming excess vitamin A while pregnant can cause serious birth defects and spontaneous abortion. Other toxicity symptoms include fatigue, loss of appetite, blurred vision, hair loss, skin disorders, bone and joint pain, abdominal pain, nausea, diarrhea, and damage to the liver and nervous system. If caught in time, many of these symptoms are reversible once vitamin A supplementation is stopped. However, permanent damage can occur to the liver, eyes, and other organs. Because liver contains such a high amount of vitamin A, children and pregnant women should not consume liver on a daily or weekly basis.

What happens if we don't consume enough vitamin A? **Night blindness**, the inability to see in dim light, is a major vitamin A–deficiency concern in developing nations. Color blindness and other vision impairments can also occur. If night blindness progresses, it can result in irreversible total blindness due to hardening of the cornea (the transparent membrane covering the front of the eye). This is why it is critical to catch night blindness in its early stages and treat it either with the regular consumption of fruits and vegetables that contain beta-carotene or with vitamin A supplementation.

Other deficiency symptoms include impaired immunity, increased risk for illness and infections, reproductive system disorders, and stunted bone growth. According to the World Health Organization, as many as 250,000 to 500,000 vitamin A–deficient children become permanently blind each year, with half of them dying within 1 year of losing their sight.[3]

Vitamin D Guards Our Bones

Vitamin D is different from other nutrients in that it does not always need to come from the diet. This is because our body can synthesize vitamin D using energy from sunlight: when the ultraviolet rays of the sun hit our skin, they react with a cholesterol compound in skin cells. This reaction converts the compound into a precursor of vitamin D, which travels to the liver and then to the kidneys for further conversion into the form of vitamin D our body can use.

Functions of Vitamin D

Vitamin D can be considered not only a nutrient but also a *hormone* because it is made in one part of the body, yet it regulates various activities in other parts of the body. One of its most important functions is to work with other hormones to regulate blood calcium levels. You probably know that calcium is the primary mineral in our bones. According to our body's changing needs for calcium, vitamin D causes more or less calcium to be absorbed from the small intestine and signals the kidneys to excrete more or less in our urine. Vitamin D also assists the process by which calcium is crystallized into bone tissue and assists in cell differentiation.

How Much Vitamin D Should We Consume?

Table 6.1 identifies the RDA for vitamin D, which is based on the assumption that an individual does not get adequate sun exposure. If your exposure to the sun is adequate, then you do not need to consume any vitamin D in your diet. But how do you know whether or not you are getting enough sunshine?

Of the many factors that affect our ability to synthesize vitamin D from sunlight, latitude and time of year are most significant. Individuals living in very sunny climates close to the equator, such as the southern United States and Mexico, may synthesize enough vitamin D from the sun to meet their needs throughout the year—as long as they spend a few minutes out of doors each day with at least their arms and face exposed. However, vitamin D synthesis from the sun is not possible in the winter months in Canada and the northern United States, from northern Virginia in the East to northern California in the West. This is because, at northern latitudes during the winter, the sun never rises high enough in the sky to provide the direct sunlight needed. Thus, people living in northern states and Canada need to consume vitamin D in the winter.

In addition, vitamin D synthesis is decreased in older adults and in people with darkly pigmented skin, which puts them at increased risk for vitamin D deficiency. Other individuals at increased risk include people 65 years of age or older, because their capacity to synthesize vitamin D from the sun is reduced, and they are more likely to spend more time indoors and have inadequate dietary intakes.[4] Vitamin D deficiency has been shown to be on the rise, and since the Institute of Medicine set its vitamin D recommendations in 1997, new information has been published about vitamin D metabolism and its potential role in reducing the risks for diseases such as type 1 diabetes, some cancers, multiple sclerosis, and metabolic syndrome.[5,6] These discussions have resulted in a full review of the current research on vitamin D.[7]

Most foods naturally contain very little vitamin D. Thus, our primary source of vitamin D in the diet is fortified foods, such as milk. As identified in **FIGURE 6.4**, other common food sources of vitamin D include fatty fish—such as salmon, mackerel, and sardines—and certain fortified cereals. Because plants contain very little vitamin D, vegetarians who consume no dairy products need to obtain their vitamin D from sun exposure, from fortified soy or cereal products, or from supplements.

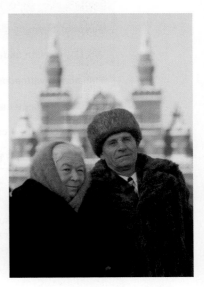

Vitamin D synthesis from the sun is not possible during most of the winter months for people living in high latitudes. Therefore, many people need to consume vitamin D in their diet, particularly during the winter.

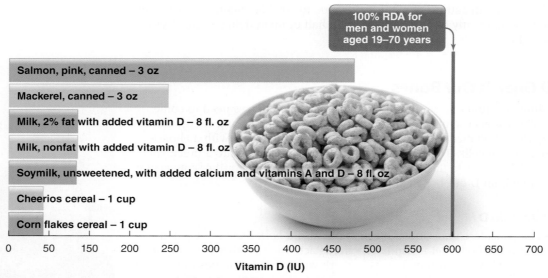

🔺 **FIGURE 6.4** Common food sources of vitamin D. For men and women aged 19 to 70 years, the RDA for vitamin D is 600 IU per day. The RDA increases to 800 IU per day for adults over the age of 70 years.

Data from U.S. Department of Agriculture, Agricultural Research Service. 2013. USDA Nutrient Database for Standard Reference, Release 26. Nutrient Data Laboratory Home Page. www.ars.usda.gov/ba/bhnrc/ndl

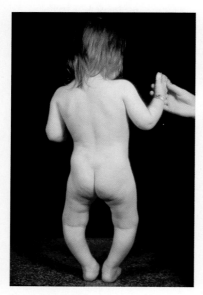

🔺 **FIGURE 6.5** A vitamin D deficiency causes a bone-deforming disease in children called rickets.

rickets A vitamin D–deficiency disease in children. Symptoms include deformities of the skeleton, such as bowed legs and knocked knees.

osteomalacia Vitamin D–deficiency disease in adults, in which bones become weak and prone to fractures.

We cannot get too much vitamin D from sun exposure, because our skin has the ability to limit its production. The only way we can consume too much vitamin D is through supplementation. Toxicity of vitamin D causes the bones to leach calcium into the bloodstream. High blood calcium concentrations cause weakness, loss of appetite, diarrhea, mental confusion, vomiting, and the formation of calcium deposits in soft tissues, such as the kidneys, liver, and heart.

What Happens If We Don't Get Enough Vitamin D?

The primary deficiency associated with inadequate vitamin D is loss of bone mass. Calcium is a key component of bones, but when vitamin D levels are inadequate, our intestines can absorb only 10% to 15% of the calcium we consume. Vitamin D–deficiency disease in children, called **rickets**, causes deformities of the skeleton, such as bowed legs and knocked knees **(FIGURE 6.5)**. However, severe cases can be fatal. Rickets is not common in the United States because of the fortification of milk products with vitamin D. The risk is increased in children with darker skin (their need for adequate sun exposure is higher than that of light-skinned children), in breastfed children who do not receive adequate vitamin D supplementation, in children with illnesses that cause fat malabsorption, and in children who drink no milk and get limited sun exposure.[8,9]

Vitamin D–deficiency disease in adults is called **osteomalacia**, a term meaning "soft bones." With osteomalacia, bones become weak and prone to fractures, and the person typically experiences diffuse bone pain. Today, osteomalacia occurs most often in individuals who have diseases that cause intestinal malabsorption of fat, and thus of the fat-soluble vitamins.

Vitamin D deficiency can also contribute to *osteoporosis*, a condition in which the bones are overly porous and prone to fractures. Although the symptoms of osteomalacia and osteoporosis are similar, the symptoms of osteomalacia are reversed after treatment with vitamin D, whereas many factors are typically involved in the development and treatment of osteoporosis. Vitamin D deficiencies have recently been found to be more common among American adults than previously thought. This may be partly due to jobs and lifestyle choices that keep people indoors for most of the day.

WHAT ABOUT **YOU?** ❓

Do You Get Enough Vitamin D?

After reading this chapter, you may wonder whether you're getting enough vitamin D to keep your tissues healthy and strong. Take the following simple quiz to find out. For each question, circle YES or NO.

- I live south of 37° latitude (see **FIGURE 6.6**) and expose my bare arms and face to sunlight (without sunscreen) for at least a few minutes 2 or 3 times per week all year.

     YES or NO

- I consume a multivitamin supplement or vitamin D supplement that provides at least 5 µg or 200 IU per day.

     YES or NO

- I consume a diet high in fatty fish, fortified milk or milk alternatives, and/or fortified cereals that provides at least 5 µg or 200 IU per day.

     YES or NO

If you answered *No* to all three of these statements, you are at high risk for vitamin D deficiency. You are probably getting enough vitamin D if you answered *Yes* to at least one. Notice, though, that if you rely on sun exposure for your vitamin D, you must make sure that you expose your bare skin to sunlight for an adequate length of time. What's adequate varies for each person: the darker your skin tone, the more time you need in the sun. A general guideline is to expose your skin for one-third to one-half the amount of time in which you would get sunburned. This means that, if you normally sunburn in 1 hour, you should get 30 minutes of sun two or three times a week. Expose your skin when the sun is high in the sky (generally between the hours of 10 AM and 3 PM). Put on sunscreen only *after* your skin has had its daily dose of sunlight.[1]

     Remember: if you live in the northern United States or Canada, you cannot get adequate sun exposure to synthesize

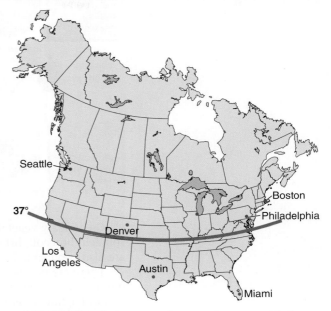

🔺 **FIGURE 6.6**   This map illustrates the geographical location of 37° latitude in the United States. In southern cities below 37° latitude, such as Los Angeles, Austin, and Miami, the sunlight is strong enough to allow for vitamin D synthesis throughout the year. In northern cities above 37° latitude, such as Seattle, Chicago, and Boston, the sunlight is too weak from about mid-October through mid-March to allow for adequate vitamin D synthesis.

vitamin D from approximately mid-October through mid-March, no matter how long you expose your bare skin to the sun. If you are not regularly consuming fortified foods, fatty fish, or cod liver oil, you need to supplement vitamin D during those months.

Now that you've read about the "sunshine vitamin," you might be wondering whether or not you should supplement this nutrient, especially if you live in a northern climate. If so, check out the accompanying *What About You?* feature box.

Vitamin K Protects Against Blood Loss

Vitamin K is a fat-soluble vitamin required for blood clotting. It acts as a **coenzyme**—that is, a compound that combines with an inactive enzyme to form an active enzyme. **FIGURE 6.7** illustrates how coenzymes work. As a coenzyme, vitamin K assists in the synthesis of a number of proteins involved in the coagulation of blood. Without adequate vitamin K, blood cannot clot quickly and adequately. This can lead to increased bleeding from even minor wounds, as well as internal hemorrhaging. Vitamin K also acts as a coenzyme to facilitate the production of osteocalcin, a protein associated with bone turnover.

Our needs for vitamin K are relatively small, as shown in Table 6.1, but vitamin K is found in few foods. Probiotic bacteria produce vitamin K in the large intestine, providing us with an important nondietary source.

coenzyme A compound that combines with an inactive enzyme to form an active enzyme.

▶ **FIGURE 6.7** Coenzymes combine with enzymes to activate them, ensuring that the chemical reactions that depend on these enzymes can occur.

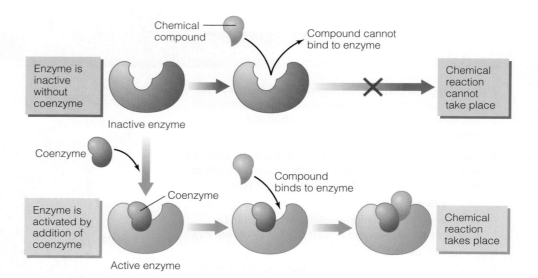

Green leafy vegetables are good sources of vitamin K, including collard greens, spinach, broccoli, brussels sprouts, and cabbage (**FIGURE 6.8**). Soybean and canola oils are also good sources.

There are no known side effects associated with consuming large amounts of vitamin K from supplements or from food.[10] People with diseases that cause malabsorption of fat can suffer secondarily from a deficiency of vitamin K. In the United States, physicians typically give newborns an injection of vitamin K at birth, because they lack the intestinal bacteria necessary to produce this nutrient.

recap   Vitamin A and its precursor, beta-carotene, are essential for healthy vision, cell differentiation, bone growth, and immune and reproductive functions. Single-nutrient supplementation with vitamin A can lead to life-threatening toxicity. Vitamin D regulates blood calcium levels and maintains bone health. Unless we have adequate sun exposure, we need to consume vitamin D in foods or supplements. Vitamin K is essential for blood clotting.

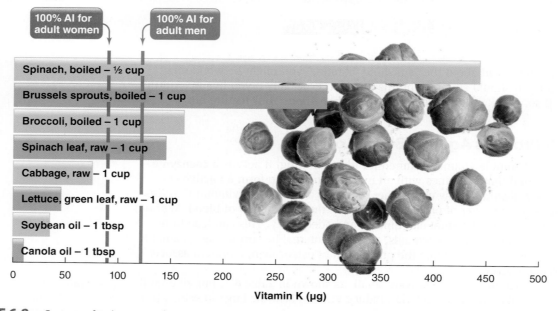

▲ **FIGURE 6.8** Common food sources of vitamin K. The AIs for adult men and women are 120 μg/day and 90 μg/day, respectively.

Data from U.S. Department of Agriculture, Agricultural Research Service. 2013. USDA Nutrient Database for Standard Reference, Release 26. Nutrient Data Laboratory Home Page. **www.ars.usda.gov/ba/bhnrc/ndl**

The antioxidants: Vitamins E and C

Fitness and health magazines, supplement companies, and even food manufacturers tout the benefits of antioxidants. But what exactly does this term mean, and why are antioxidant micronutrients important to our health?

What Are Antioxidants, and How Does Our Body Use Them?

As we discussed earlier in the text (Chapter 2), chemical reactions occur continuously in our body to break down the food we eat and reassemble its smaller molecules into the substances we need to live. Many of these chemical reactions involve the exchange of oxygen. Such reactions are collectively referred to as *oxidation*. *Anti* means "against"; thus, **antioxidants** are vitamins and minerals that protect our cells against oxidation.

Our cells need the protection of antioxidants because, although necessary to our functioning, oxidation results in the production of **free radicals**, unstable atoms with an unpaired electron. Free radicals are harmful because, like chemical thieves, they attempt to "steal" electrons from stable molecules. When they do, they transform those molecules into new free radicals. This prompts a dangerous chain reaction as the generated free radicals, in turn, damage more and more cells.

One of the most significant sites of free-radical damage is within the lipid portion of the cell membrane. When lipid molecules are damaged by free radicals, they no longer repel water, and the cell membrane loses its integrity. It can no longer regulate the movement of fluids and nutrients into and out of the cell. Free radicals also damage our low-density lipoproteins (LDLs), cell proteins, and DNA. Not surprisingly, oxidation is one of the factors thought to cause our body to age. In addition, many diseases are linked to free-radical production, including cancer, heart disease, stroke, and diabetes.

Antioxidant vitamins, especially vitamins E and C, work by stabilizing free radicals, thereby halting the chain reaction of cell membrane injury **(FIGURE 6.9)**. When our intake of these vitamins is not sufficient, free-radical damage can be significant. Note that the carotenoids discussed earlier, and the mineral selenium, also play roles in antioxidant functioning.

Vitamin E Maintains Healthy Cells

About 90% of the vitamin E in our body is stored in our adipose (fat) tissues; the rest is found in our cell membranes, protecting them from oxidation. Vitamin E also

 LO4 Discuss the process of oxidation and explain how it can damage cells.

 LO5 Discuss the interrelated roles of vitamins E and C in protecting cells from oxidation.

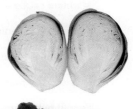
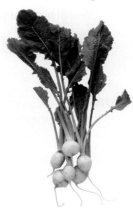

Green leafy vegetables, including brussels sprouts and turnip greens, are good sources of vitamin K.

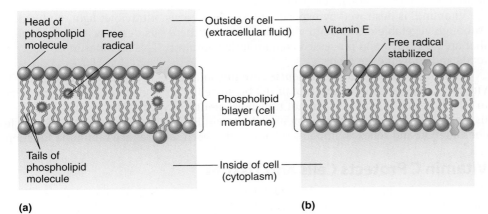

(a)

(b)

FIGURE 6.9 **(a)** The formation of free radicals in the lipid portion of our cell membranes can cause a dangerous chain reaction that damages the integrity of the membrane and can cause cell death. **(b)** Vitamin E is stored in the lipid portion of our cell membranes. By donating an electron to free radicals, it protects the lipid molecules in our cell membranes from being oxidized and stops the chain reaction of oxidative damage.

antioxidant A compound that has the ability to prevent or repair the damage caused by oxidation.

free radical A highly unstable atom with an unpaired electron.

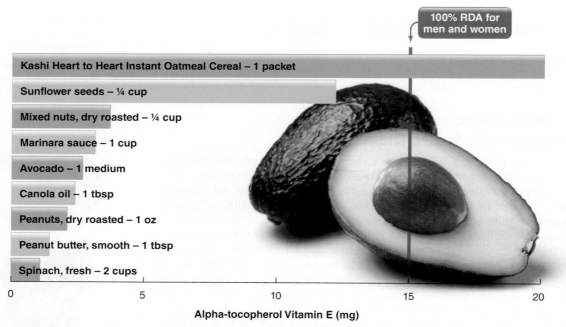

100% RDA for men and women

Kashi Heart to Heart Instant Oatmeal Cereal – 1 packet

Sunflower seeds – ¼ cup

Mixed nuts, dry roasted – ¼ cup

Marinara sauce – 1 cup

Avocado – 1 medium

Canola oil – 1 tbsp

Peanuts, dry roasted – 1 oz

Peanut butter, smooth – 1 tbsp

Spinach, fresh – 2 cups

0   5   10   15   20

Alpha-tocopherol Vitamin E (mg)

FIGURE 6.10 Common food sources of vitamin E. The RDA for vitamin E is 15 mg alpha-tocopherol per day for men and women.

Data from U.S. Department of Agriculture, Agricultural Research Service. 2013. USDA Nutrient Database for Standard Reference, Release 26. Nutrient Data Laboratory Home Page. **www.ars.usda.gov/ba/bhnrc/ndl**

protects LDLs, red blood cells, and the cells of our lungs, which are continuously exposed to oxygen from the air we breathe.

In addition to its role as an antioxidant, vitamin E is critical for normal fetal and early-childhood development of nerves and muscles and for neuromuscular function throughout life. It protects white blood cells and other components of the immune system, thereby helping defend our body against infection and disease. Vitamin E also improves the absorption of vitamin A if dietary intake of vitamin A is low.

Considering the importance of vitamin E to our health, you might think that you need to consume a huge amount daily. In fact, as you can see in Table 6.1, the RDA for vitamin E for men and women is modest.

Vitamin E is widespread in foods **(FIGURE 6.10)**. Much of the vitamin E we consume comes from vegetable oils and the products made from them. Safflower oil, sunflower oil, canola oil, and soybean oil are good sources. Nuts, seeds, some vegetables, wheat germ, and soybeans also contribute vitamin E to our diet. Cereals are often fortified with vitamin E, and other grain products contribute modest amounts. Animal and dairy products are poor sources of vitamin E.

Vitamin E is destroyed by exposure to oxygen, metals, ultraviolet light, and heat. Although vegetable oils contain vitamin E, heating these oils destroys it. Thus, foods that are deep-fried and processed contain little vitamin E. This includes most fast foods and convenience foods.

Vitamin E toxicities and deficiencies are uncommon. One result of significant vitamin E deficiency is a rupturing of red blood cells that leads to *anemia,* a condition in which our red blood cells cannot transport enough oxygen to our tissues, leaving us weak and fatigued. Other symptoms of vitamin E deficiency include loss of muscle coordination and reflexes, impaired vision and speech, and reduced immune function.

Vitamin C Protects Cells and Tissues

Vitamin C is also known as *ascorbic acid.* Like vitamin E, it's a potent antioxidant, but because it's water soluble, it primarily acts within the fluid outside of cells. There, it binds with free radicals, keeping them from destroying cell membranes. It plays a key role in defending our lung tissues from the damage caused by ozone, cigarette smoke, and other airborne pollutants. Indeed, smoking increases a person's need for vitamin C to combat oxidative damage to the lungs. In the stomach, vitamin C reduces the formation of *nitrosamines,* cancer-causing agents found in foods such as cured and processed meats. Vitamin C also regenerates vitamin E after it has been oxidized, enabling vitamin E to "get back to work."

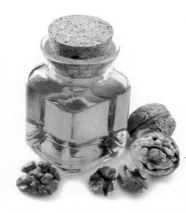

Vegetable oils, nuts, and seeds are good sources of vitamin E.

nutrition myth or fact?

Can Vitamin C Prevent the Common Cold?

What do you do when it seems as if everyone around you is suffering from a cold? If you are like many people, you drink a lot of orange juice or take vitamin C supplements to ward it off. But do these approaches really help prevent a cold?

It is well known that vitamin C is important for a healthy immune system. Deficiency of vitamin C can seriously weaken the ability of immune cells to detect and destroy invading microbes, increasing our susceptibility to many diseases and illnesses, including the common cold. It's not surprising, then, that many people turn to vitamin C supplements to prevent colds. When they do, they find their local drug store stocking at least a dozen forms of vitamin C, from lozenges to tablets and even packets of powder to mix with water into a cold-fighting cocktail. But do these products work?

Unfortunately, it appears they do not. A recent review of many of the studies of vitamin C and the common cold reported that people who took vitamin C experienced as many colds as people who took a placebo. However, the *duration* of their colds may be somewhat reduced.[2] Interestingly, taking vitamin C supplements regularly did seem to provide some benefit in reducing the number of colds experienced by marathon runners, skiers, and soldiers participating in exercises done under extreme environmental conditions.

The amount of vitamin C taken in these studies was at least 200 mg per day, with many using doses as high as 4,000 mg per day (more than forty times the RDA), with no harmful effects noted in those studies that reported adverse events.

In summary, it appears that, for most people, taking vitamin C supplements regularly will not prevent colds but may reduce their duration. Consuming a healthful diet that includes excellent sources of vitamin C will also help you maintain a strong immune system. Taking vitamin C after the onset of cold symptoms does not appear to help.

So what *can* you do to prevent a cold? The National Institute of Allergy and Infectious Diseases suggests the following:[3]

- Because most cold germs enter the body via the eyes or the nose, try to keep from touching or rubbing your eyes and nose.
- If possible, avoid being close to people who have colds.
- Wash your hands frequently with soap and warm (not hot) water throughout cold season and whenever you have had contact with many people (throughout the workday or school day, when returning home from shopping, and so on). Hand-washing is one of the most effective ways to keep from getting colds or giving them to others. When water isn't available, use an alcohol-based waterless hand sanitizer.
- Cold viruses can live for up to 3 hours on your skin or on objects, such as telephones and desks. Clean environmental surfaces with a virus-killing disinfectant when feasible.

One word of caution: if you're thinking of taking vitamin C supplements, bear in mind that vitamin C enhances the absorption of iron. It is recommended that people with low iron stores consume vitamin C–rich foods along with iron sources to improve absorption of the iron. For people with high iron stores, however, this practice can be dangerous and lead to iron toxicity. Before you begin supplementing, check with your healthcare provider.

How Else Do We Use Vitamin C?

Another important role of vitamin C is to synthesize **collagen**, a structural protein in bone, teeth, skin, tendons, and blood vessels. Without adequate vitamin C, the body cannot form collagen; thus, bones become brittle, blood vessels leak, wounds fail to heal, and teeth fall out. These symptoms characterize the disease called *scurvy*, which centuries ago was responsible for more than half the deaths that occurred at sea **(FIGURE 6.11)**. During long sea voyages, the crew ate all the fruits and vegetables early in the trip. These foods are high in vitamin C. Later in the voyage, only grain and animal products were available. These foods do not provide vitamin C. In 1740 in England, Dr. James Lind discovered that the consumption of citrus fruits can prevent scurvy. Thus, British sailors were given rations of lime juice, earning them the nickname "limeys."

Vitamin C assists in the synthesis of other important compounds as well, including DNA, neurotransmitters (chemicals that transmit messages via the nervous system), and various hormones. Vitamin C also enhances our immune response and thus protects us from illness and infection. Indeed, you might have heard that vitamin C supplements can prevent the common cold. See the **Nutrition Myth or Fact?** box to find out if this claim is true.

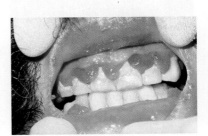

▲ **FIGURE 6.11** Bleeding gums are one symptom of scurvy, the most common vitamin C–deficiency disease.

collagen A protein found in all connective tissues in our body.

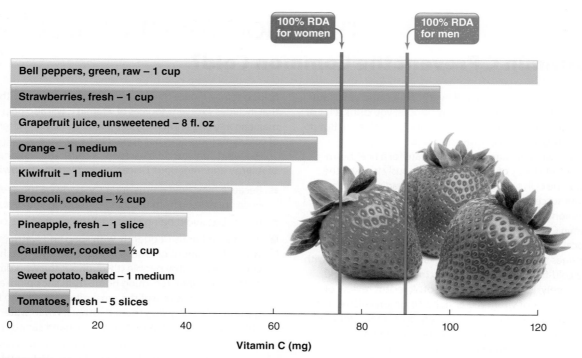

FIGURE 6.12 Common food sources of vitamin C. The RDA for vitamin C is 90 mg per day for men and 75 mg per day for women.

Data from U.S. Department of Agriculture, Agricultural Research Service. 2013. USDA Nutrient Database for Standard Reference, Release 26. Nutrient Data Laboratory Home Page. www.ars.usda.gov/ba/bhnrc/ndl

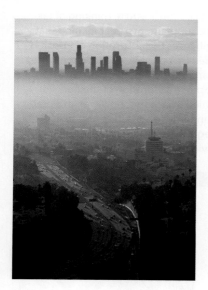

Vitamin C helps protect our lung tissue from airborne pollutants.

Finally, vitamin C enhances the absorption of iron. It is recommended that people with low iron stores consume vitamin C–rich foods along with iron sources to improve absorption. For people with high iron stores, this practice can lead to iron toxicity.

How Much Vitamin C Should We Consume?

The RDA for vitamin C is listed in Table 6.2. Many fruits and vegetables are excellent sources (**FIGURE 6.12**). Because heat and oxygen destroy vitamin C, fresh, raw foods have the highest content. Cooking foods, especially boiling, leaches them of their vitamin C, which is then lost when we strain them. Forms of cooking that are least likely to compromise the vitamin C content of foods include steaming, microwaving, and stir-frying.

Because vitamin C is water soluble, excess amounts are easily excreted and do not lead to toxicity. Even taking megadoses of vitamin C is not fatally harmful. However, side effects of doses exceeding 2,000 mg per day include nausea, diarrhea, abdominal cramps, and nosebleeds and may increase the risk for kidney stones in some people.

recap Vitamin E protects the fatty portion of our cell membranes from oxidation, enhances immune function, and improves our absorption of vitamin A if dietary intake is low. Vitamin C scavenges free radicals and regenerates vitamin E after it has been oxidized. It is required for the synthesis of collagen and assists in the synthesis of certain hormones, neurotransmitters, and DNA. Vitamin C boosts the absorption of iron.

 LO6 Explain how our body uses the B vitamins to generate energy.

 LO7 Discuss the importance of adequate folate intake for women of childbearing age.

The energy generators: B-vitamins

Contrary to popular belief, vitamins and minerals do not contain energy (Calories). Only the macronutrients (carbohydrates, fats, and proteins) contain energy. However, vitamins and minerals do assist the body in *generating* energy. **Metabolism** is the sum of all the chemical and physical processes by which the body breaks down and builds up molecules. The B-vitamins play a critical role in energy metabolism, because they assist the chemical reactions that release energy from carbohydrates, fats, and proteins. This group of water-soluble vitamins includes thiamin, riboflavin, vitamin B₆, niacin, folate, vitamin B₁₂, pantothenic acid, and biotin.

LO8 Describe the interrelationship of vitamin B_6, folate, and vitamin B_{12} in homocysteine metabolism and cardiovascular disease.

How Does Our Body Use B-Vitamins to Produce Energy?

B-vitamins help us access the energy in the food we eat by acting as coenzymes. Recall that a coenzyme is a molecule that combines with an enzyme to activate it and help it do its job (see Figure 6.7). Without the B-vitamins working as coenzymes, we would be unable to produce the energy necessary to stay alive.

For instance, thiamin combines with another enzyme to assist in the breakdown of glucose. Riboflavin is a part of two coenzymes that help break down glucose and fatty acids. The specific functions of each B-vitamin are described in detail next. Their DRIs are identified in Table 6.2.

In addition to the B-vitamins and a vitamin-like substance called choline, the minerals iodine, chromium, manganese, copper, and sulfur are also involved in energy metabolism. (Minerals are discussed in Chapter 7.)

Thiamin (Vitamin B₁) Helps Metabolize Glucose

Thiamin was the first B-vitamin discovered, hence its designation as vitamin B_1. Thiamin is part of a coenzyme that plays a critical role in the breakdown of glucose for energy. It also acts as a coenzyme in the metabolism of a few amino acids. Thiamin is also used in producing DNA and plays a role in the synthesis of neurotransmitters.

Good food sources of thiamin include enriched cereals and grains, whole-grain products, ready-to-eat cereals, and ham and other pork products (**FIGURE 6.13**). There are no known adverse effects from consuming excess amounts of thiamin.

Thiamin-deficiency disease is called **beriberi**. In this disease, the body's inability to metabolize energy leads to muscle wasting and nerve damage; in later stages,

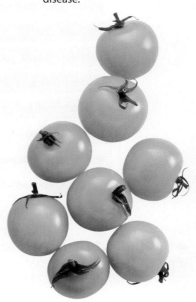

Many fruits, such as these yellow tomatoes, are high in vitamin C.

metabolism The sum of all the chemical and physical processes by which the body breaks down and builds up molecules.

beriberi A disease caused by thiamin deficiency.

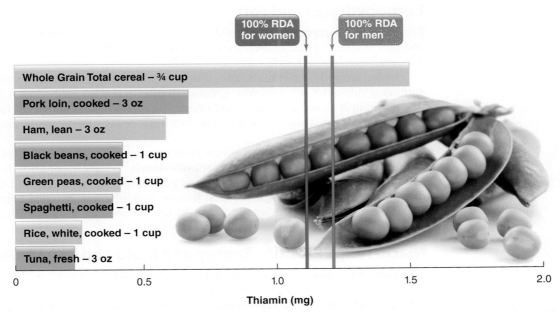

FIGURE 6.13 Common food sources of thiamin. The RDA for thiamin is 1.2 mg/day for men and 1.1 mg/day for women 19 years and older.

Data from U.S. Department of Agriculture, Agricultural Research Service. 2013. USDA Nutrient Database for Standard Reference, Release 26. Nutrient Data Laboratory Home Page. **www.ars.usda.gov/ba/bhnrc/ndl**

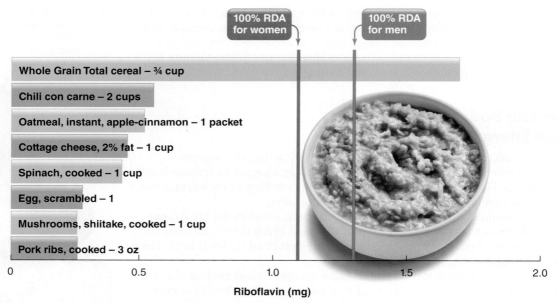

FIGURE 6.14 Common food sources of riboflavin. The RDA for riboflavin is 1.3 mg/day for men and 1.1 mg/day for women 19 years and older.

Data from U.S. Department of Agriculture, Agricultural Research Service. 2013. USDA Nutrient Database for Standard Reference, Release 26. Nutrient Data Laboratory Home Page. **www.ars.usda.gov/ba/bhnrc/ndl**

patients may be unable to move at all. The heart muscle may also be affected, and the patient may die of heart failure. Beriberi occurs when unenriched, processed grains are a primary food source; for instance, it was widespread throughout Asia a century ago when rice was first processed and refined. Rice and many other staples are now enriched with thiamin, and beriberi is rarely seen except among people displaced by wars and natural disasters receiving inadequate food aid. In these populations, symptoms can begin to develop within 2 to 3 months. Beriberi is also seen in people with heavy alcohol consumption and limited food intake.

Riboflavin (Vitamin B₂) Helps Break Down Carbohydrates and Fats

Riboflavin is an important component of coenzymes that break down carbohydrates and fats. It is also a part of an antioxidant enzyme that helps cells defend against oxidative damage.

Flavins are yellow pigments, and, indeed, riboflavin is found in egg yolks. Milk is another good source of riboflavin. Because riboflavin is destroyed when it is exposed to light, milk is stored in opaque containers. Other good food sources of riboflavin include yogurt, enriched bread and grain products, ready-to-eat cereals, and organ meats **(FIGURE 6.14)**.

There are no known adverse effects from consuming excess amounts of riboflavin. Riboflavin deficiency is referred to as **ariboflavinosis**. Symptoms of ariboflavinosis include sore throat, swelling of the mucous membranes in the mouth and throat, lips that are dry and scaly, a purple-colored tongue, and inflamed, irritated patches on the skin. Severe riboflavin deficiency can impair the metabolism of vitamin B₆.

Niacin Helps Produce Energy and Build and Repair DNA

As a coenzyme, niacin assists in the metabolism of carbohydrates and fatty acids and thus is essential in helping our body derive the energy from these foods. Niacin also plays an important role in DNA replication and repair and in the process of cell differentiation. Good food sources include meat, fish, poultry, enriched grain products, and tomato paste **(FIGURE 6.15)**.

ariboflavinosis A condition caused by riboflavin deficiency.

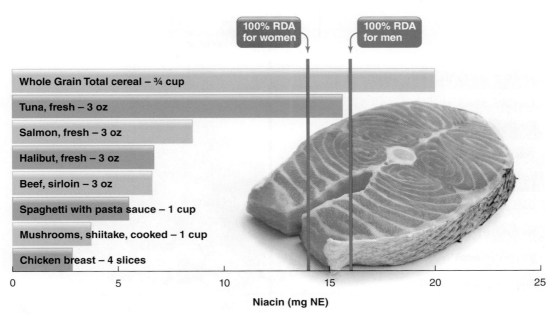

100% RDA for women

100% RDA for men

Whole Grain Total cereal – ¾ cup

Tuna, fresh – 3 oz

Salmon, fresh – 3 oz

Halibut, fresh – 3 oz

Beef, sirloin – 3 oz

Spaghetti with pasta sauce – 1 cup

Mushrooms, shiitake, cooked – 1 cup

Chicken breast – 4 slices

0   5   10   15   20   25

Niacin (mg NE)

FIGURE 6.15 Common food sources of niacin. The RDA for niacin is 16 mg niacin equivalents (NE)/day for men and 14 mg NE/day for women 19 years and older.

Data from U.S. Department of Agriculture, Agricultural Research Service. 2013. USDA Nutrient Database for Standard Reference, Release 26. Nutrient Data Laboratory Home Page. **www.ars.usda.gov/ba/bhnrc/ndl**

Megadoses of niacin have been shown to reduce LDL-cholesterol and raise HDL-cholesterol; therefore, some physicians prescribe a pharmacologic form of niacin for patients with unhealthful blood lipid levels. It is typically prescribed in a time-release preparation to prevent an uncomfortable side effect called *flushing,* which is defined as burning, tingling, and itching sensations accompanied by a reddened flush primarily on the face, arms, and chest. Unfortunately, some prescription forms of niacin can cause liver damage. Niacin toxicity can also cause glucose intolerance, blurred vision, and edema of the eyes.

Pellagra results from a severe niacin deficiency. It is characterized by a skin rash, diarrhea, mental impairment, and in severe cases death (**FIGURE 6.16**). It commonly occurred in the southern United States and parts of Europe in the early 20th century and was originally thought to be caused by infection. In 1914, a physician named Dr. Joseph Goldberger noticed that pellagra struck only impoverished people who ate a limited, corn-based diet. Goldberger began conducting experiments to test his theory that pellagra is caused by a nutrient deficiency and eventually found brewer's yeast to be a cure. After his death, researchers identified niacin and linked it to pellagra. Brewer's yeast is a rich source of niacin. Today, pellagra is rarely seen, except in cases of chronic alcoholism and in impoverished regions of the world.

FIGURE 6.16 Pellagra is often characterized by a scaly skin rash.

Vitamin B₆ (Pyridoxine) Helps Manufacture Nonessential Amino Acids

You can think of vitamin B_6 as the "protein vitamin" because it is needed for more than 100 enzymes involved in protein metabolism.[11] Without adequate vitamin B_6, all amino acids become essential and must be consumed in our diet, because our body cannot make them in sufficient quantities. Vitamin B_6 also assists in the synthesis of hemoglobin, a protein in red blood cells that transports oxygen, and it helps maintain normal blood glucose levels. In addition, vitamin B_6 is needed for the synthesis of neurotransmitters, which enable nerve cells to communicate.

Good food sources of vitamin B_6 include enriched ready-to-eat cereals, beef liver, fish, poultry, garbanzo beans, and fortified soy-based meat substitutes (**FIGURE 6.17**). White potatoes and other starchy vegetables are also good sources.

pellagra A disease that results from severe niacin deficiency.

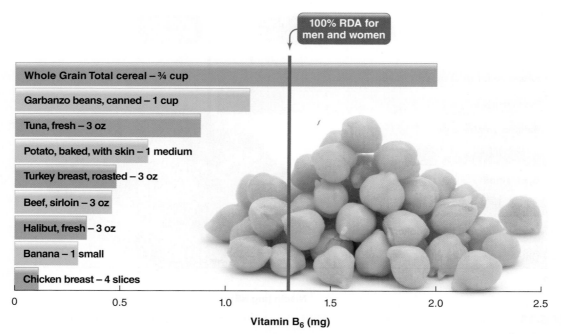

100% RDA for men and women

Whole Grain Total cereal – ¾ cup
Garbanzo beans, canned – 1 cup
Tuna, fresh – 3 oz
Potato, baked, with skin – 1 medium
Turkey breast, roasted – 3 oz
Beef, sirloin – 3 oz
Halibut, fresh – 3 oz
Banana – 1 small
Chicken breast – 4 slices

0   0.5   1.0   1.5   2.0   2.5

Vitamin B$_6$ (mg)

FIGURE 6.17 Common food sources of vitamin B$_6$. The RDA for vitamin B$_6$ is 1.3 mg/day for men and women aged 19 to 50 years.

Data from U.S. Department of Agriculture, Agricultural Research Service. 2013. USDA Nutrient Database for Standard Reference, Release 26. Nutrient Data Laboratory Home Page. www.ars.usda.gov/ba/bhnrc/ndl

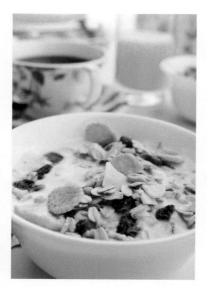

Because of its critical role in the first few weeks of pregnancy, folate is added to all ready-to-eat cereals.

homocysteine An amino acid that requires adequate levels of folate, vitamin B$_6$, and vitamin B$_{12}$ for its metabolism. High levels of homocysteine in the blood are associated with an increased risk for cardiovascular disease.

People taking vitamin B$_6$ supplements to treat conditions such as premenstrual syndrome (PMS) and carpal tunnel syndrome need to use caution. Whereas consuming excess vitamin B$_6$ from food sources does not cause toxicity, a condition called sensory neuropathy (damage to the sensory nerves) has been documented in individuals taking high-dose B$_6$ supplements. The symptoms of sensory neuropathy include numbness and tingling involving the face, neck, hands, and feet, and difficulty manipulating objects and walking.

Vitamin B$_6$ deficiency is rare in the United States except among people who chronically abuse alcohol and children taking the asthma drug theophylline, which decreases body stores of vitamin B$_6$. Deficiency symptoms include anemia, convulsions, depression, confusion, and inflamed, irritated patches on the skin. A deficiency of vitamin B$_6$ may also increase the level of the amino acid **homocysteine** in the blood. High homocysteine levels may damage coronary arteries or promote the formation of clots within arteries, increasing the risk for a heart attack or stroke. However, research to date provides little evidence that taking supplemental vitamin B$_6$ reduces the risk for a heart attack or stroke.[11]

Folate Is Critical During the Earliest Weeks of Pregnancy

All women of childbearing age need to consume adequate folate. This is because folate, which promotes DNA synthesis and cell division, is a critical nutrient during the first few weeks of pregnancy—typically before a woman even knows she is pregnant—when the combined sperm–egg cell is dividing rapidly to form the primitive tissues of the human body. When folate intake is inadequate in the first weeks of pregnancy, the fetus can develop a *neural tube defect,* a malformation affecting the spinal cord that can cause impaired movement, neurologic problems, and even death.

In everyone, folate is essential for healthy blood. Without sufficient folate, the red blood cells become unable to carry sufficient oxygen to all our body cells, and we become weak and exhausted. This condition is called *macrocytic anemia.* Folate is also important in amino acid metabolism. Like B$_6$ deficiency, folate deficiency can cause too high a level of the amino acid homocysteine in the blood, a risk factor for heart disease and stroke.

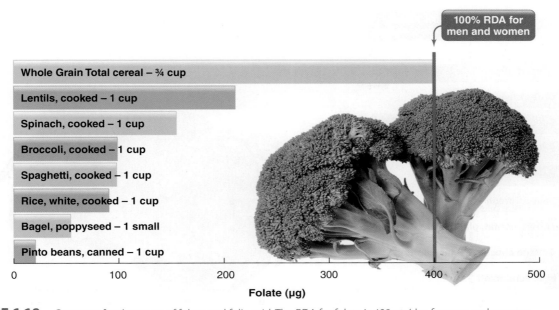

100% RDA for men and women

Whole Grain Total cereal – ¾ cup

Lentils, cooked – 1 cup

Spinach, cooked – 1 cup

Broccoli, cooked – 1 cup

Spaghetti, cooked – 1 cup

Rice, white, cooked – 1 cup

Bagel, poppyseed – 1 small

Pinto beans, canned – 1 cup

0   100   200   300   400   500

Folate (µg)

FIGURE 6.18   Common food sources of folate and folic acid. The RDA for folate is 400 µg/day for men and women.

Data from U.S. Department of Agriculture, Agricultural Research Service. 2013. USDA Nutrient Database for Standard Reference, Release 26. Nutrient Data Laboratory Home Page. **www.ars.usda.gov/ba/bhnrc/ndl**

Because of its critical role during the first few weeks of pregnancy, and the fact that many women of childbearing age do not consume adequate amounts, folate has been added to ready-to-eat cereals and bread products. Thus, these two foods are among the primary sources of folate in the United States. Other good food sources include liver, spinach, lentils, oatmeal, asparagus, and romaine lettuce (**FIGURE 6.18**).

Toxicity can occur when taking supplemental folate. One especially frustrating problem with folate toxicity is that it can mask a simultaneous vitamin B_{12} deficiency. As you saw in the chapter-opening case, a delay in the diagnosis of B_{12} deficiency can permanently damage the nervous system. There do not appear to be any clear symptoms of folate toxicity independent from its interaction with vitamin B_{12} deficiency.

Vitamin B_{12} (Cobalamin) Maintains Healthy Nerves and Blood

In the chapter-opening scenario, you saw the effects of vitamin B_{12} deficiency on Mr. Katz's nervous system. His nerve function deteriorated, because adequate levels of vitamin B_{12} are necessary to maintain the sheath that coats nerve fibers. When this sheath is damaged or absent, nerves fire inappropriately, causing numerous physical and cognitive problems. Vitamin B_{12} is also part of coenzymes that assist with the formation of blood.

In addition, as with folate and vitamin B_6, adequate levels of vitamin B_{12} are necessary to break down the amino acid homocysteine. When vitamin B_{12} consumption is inadequate, homocysteine levels—and your risk for heart disease or stroke—rise.

Vitamin B_{12} occurs naturally only in animal-based foods, so individuals consuming a vegan diet need to eat foods that are fortified with vitamin B_{12} or take vitamin B_{12} supplements or periodic injections (**FIGURE 6.19**). This is also recommended for people older than 50 years of age. That's because, as we age, we have an increased risk for a condition referred to as **atrophic gastritis**, which results in low stomach acid secretion. Stomach acid separates food-bound vitamin B_{12} from dietary proteins. Therefore, if stomach acid declines, the body cannot free up enough vitamin B_{12} from food sources alone. The prevalence of atrophic gastritis is highly variable across the world, ranging from 1% to close to 100% in some populations.[12,13]

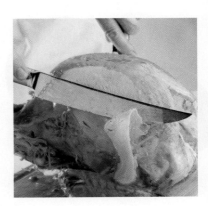

Turkey contains vitamin B_{12}.

atrophic gastritis A condition that results in low stomach acid secretion, estimated to occur in about 10% to 30% of adults older than 50 years of age.

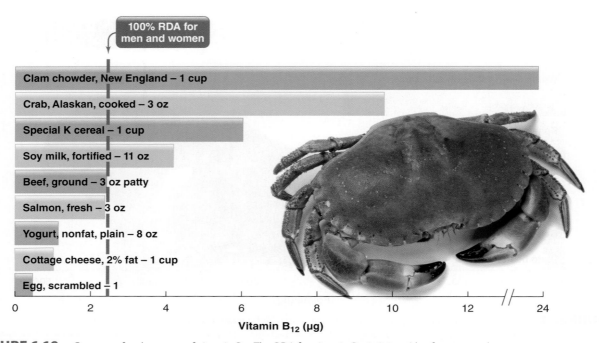

FIGURE 6.19 Common food sources of vitamin B₁₂. The RDA for vitamin B₁₂ is 2.4 μg/day for men and women.

Data from U.S. Department of Agriculture, Agricultural Research Service. 2013. USDA Nutrient Database for Standard Reference, Release 26. Nutrient Data Laboratory Home Page. **www.ars.usda.gov/ba/bhnrc/ndl**

Another important cause of vitamin B₁₂ deficiency is *pernicious anemia*, a disorder in which the body lacks adequate amounts of a protein called *intrinsic factor*. This protein, which is secreted by the stomach, helps vitamin B₁₂ be absorbed into the bloodstream.

Vitamin B₁₂ deficiency, like folate deficiency, causes macrocytic anemia, which reduces strength, energy, and exercise tolerance, and the neurologic symptoms described in the chapter-opening scenario. There are no known adverse effects from consuming excess amounts of vitamin B₁₂.

Pantothenic Acid and Biotin Help Metabolize Macronutrients

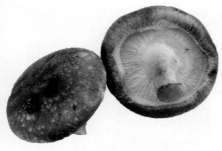

Shiitake mushrooms contain pantothenic acid.

Pantothenic acid is a component of coenzymes that assist with the metabolism of fatty acids. It is also critical for building new fatty acids. The prefix *pan* means "widespread," and indeed pantothenic acid is found in a wide variety of foods, from beef, chicken, organ meats, and egg yolk to potatoes, tomato products, and whole grains. Thus, deficiencies are very rare. There are no known adverse effects from consuming excess amounts of pantothenic acid.

Biotin is a component of coenzymes that help the body break down all the macronutrients. It also plays an important role in gluconeogenesis. The biotin content has been determined for very few foods, and these values are not reported in food composition tables or dietary analysis programs. Biotin appears to be widespread in foods. There are no known adverse effects from consuming excess amounts, and biotin deficiencies are rare.

Choline Is a Vitamin-Like Substance Found in Foods

The carbon-containing compound choline, although not classified as a vitamin, is typically grouped with the B-vitamins because of its role in assisting homocysteine metabolism. Choline also accelerates the synthesis and release of *acetylcholine,* a neurotransmitter involved in movement and other functions. It is also necessary for healthy cell membranes, and it plays an important role in the transport and metabolism of fats and cholesterol.

Choline has an AI of 550 mg per day for men ages 19 and older and an AI of 425 mg per day for women ages 19 and older. The choline content of foods is not typically reported in nutrient databases. However, we do know that choline is widespread in foods, especially milk, liver, eggs, and peanuts. Inadequate intakes of choline can eventually lead to liver damage. Excessive intake of supplemental choline results in various toxicity symptoms, including a fishy body odor, vomiting, sweating, diarrhea, and low blood pressure. In addition, a recent study suggests a potential link between the digestion of choline (derived from lecithin, which is a type of phospholipid), from foods such as meat and egg yolks, and intestinal bacteria that may increase our risk for cardiovascular disease.[14] The Upper Limit (UL) for choline for adults 19 years of age and older is 3.5 grams/day.

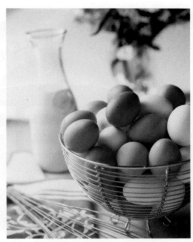

recap Water-soluble B-vitamins include thiamin, riboflavin, niacin, pyridoxine (vitamin B_6), folate, cobalamin (vitamin B_{12}), pantothenic acid, and biotin. Acting as coenzymes, the B-vitamins assist in breaking down food to produce energy. They are commonly found in enriched breads and cereals, meats, dairy products, and some fruits and vegetables. B-vitamin toxicity is rare unless a person consumes large doses in supplements. Deficiencies of most B vitamins are not common except in individuals with another health problem, such as alcohol abuse. However, folate deficiency during early pregnancy can lead to a neural tube defect in the developing fetus, and vitamin B_{12} deficiency, which leads to macrocytic anemia and nervous system damage, is sometimes seen in older adults with atrophic gastritis or pernicious anemia, and people consuming a vegan diet. Choline is a carbon-containing compound that assists in homocysteine metabolism.

 Choline is widespread in foods and can be found in eggs and milk.

What about supplements?

Dietary supplements are products taken by mouth that contain a "dietary ingredient" intended to supplement the diet. They may contain vitamins, minerals, amino acids, essential fatty acids, enzymes, herbs, or other ingredients. Multivitamin/multimineral supplements, including pills, capsules, liquids, and powders, are the most popular type of dietary supplement sold: approximately 40% of Americans report using them.[15] Do we really need all these vitamins? Let's take a look at the evidence.

LO9 Explain how dietary supplements are regulated in the United States, and the recommendations for and against their use.

Dietary Supplements Are Not Strictly Regulated

Dietary supplements are categorized by the FDA within the general group of foods, not drugs. This means that, as long as all ingredients are recognized as safe for consumption, the product is allowed on the market. Thus, the regulation of such products is much less rigorous than for drugs. As an informed consumer, you should know the following:

- Supplements do not need approval from the FDA before they are marketed.
- The manufacturer is responsible for determining that the product is safe; the FDA does not test it for safety prior to marketing.
- Companies do not have to provide the FDA with any evidence that their supplements are safe, unless the company is marketing a new dietary ingredient that was not sold in the United States prior to 1994.
- There are currently no federal guidelines on practices to ensure the purity, quality, safety, and composition of supplements.
- There are no rules to limit the serving size or amount of a nutrient in any supplement.
- Once a supplement is marketed, it is the FDA's responsibility to prove that a product is unsafe before it can be removed from the market.

Over the years, many consumer advocacy groups have petitioned the FDA to reevaluate the way it regulates dietary supplements. They contend that many companies are making unsubstantiated health claims for their products, and that the use of such products could have adverse health effects on vulnerable consumers. In response to these and other concerns, the FDA is considering a new regulatory system

How can you tell whether a dietary supplement sold online is legit? Go to www .fda.gov and click on the "Foods" tab then scroll down to select "Dietary Supplements" from the Navigate section. In the box at left, choose "Using Dietary Supplements." Then click on "Tips for Dietary Supplement Users."

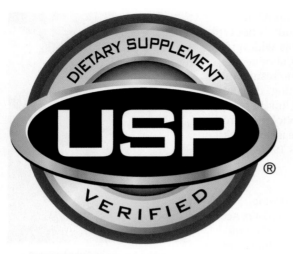

◆ **FIGURE 6.20** The USP Verified Mark indicates that the manufacturer has followed certain standards for features such as purity, strength, and quality.

by which any product bearing health claims would be subject to FDA oversight. But until such a system is in effect, you should remain skeptical about the safety and effectiveness of dietary supplements. To avoid purchasing fraudulent or dangerous supplements, keep these tips in mind:

- Look for the United States Pharmacopeia (USP) Verified Mark on the label (**FIGURE 6.20**). This mark indicates that the manufacturer followed the standards that the USP has established for features such as purity, strength, quality, packaging, labeling, and acceptable length of storage.
- Consider buying nationally recognized brands of supplements, which are more likely to have well-established manufacturing standards.
- Do not assume that the word "natural" on the label means that the product is safe. Arsenic, lead, and mercury are all natural substances that can kill you if consumed in large enough quantities.

Who Might Benefit from Taking Micronutrient Supplements?

Contrary to what some people believe, the U.S. food supply is not void of nutrients. Foods contain a diverse combination of compounds that are critical to our health and cannot be packaged in a pill. Thus, supplements are not substitutes for whole foods. To see this difference for yourself, compare the nutrient content of the two sets of meals in **FIGURE 6.21**.

That said, nutritional needs change over time, and certain groups of people do benefit from taking supplements. Some examples of widely recommended vitamin or mineral supplements include

- a single dose of vitamin K for newborns at birth,
- vitamin D supplements for breastfed infants from birth to age 6 months and iron-fortified cereal for breastfed infants 6 months of age and older,
- Fluoride supplements for children not drinking fluoridated water,
- multivitamin/multimineral supplements for people on prolonged energy-restricted diets and for people with HIV/AIDS or other wasting diseases,
- calcium and vitamin D supplements for people at risk for low bone mass, and
- vitamin B_{12} supplements for elderly people and vegans.

If you identify with one or more of these groups, you should analyze your diet to determine whether you actually need supplements. In addition, it is always a good idea to check with your healthcare provider or a registered dietitian (RD) before taking any supplements.

When Can Taking a Vitamin or Mineral Supplement Be Harmful?

Instances in which taking vitamin and mineral supplements is unnecessary or potentially harmful include the following:

- Providing fluoride supplements to children who already drink fluoridated water.
- Taking supplements in the belief that they will cure a disease such as cancer, diabetes, or heart disease.
- Taking supplements without checking with your healthcare provider to determine their reaction with medications you are taking.
- Taking beta-carotene supplements if you are a smoker. Evidence suggests that beta-carotene supplementation may increase the risk for cancer in smokers.[2]
- Taking vitamins and minerals in an attempt to improve physical appearance, athletic performance, or energy level. There is no evidence that vitamin and mineral supplements enhance appearance, athletic performance, or energy level in healthy adults who consume a varied diet with adequate energy.

a day of meals

low in MICRONUTRIENTS

high in MICRONUTRIENTS

BREAKFAST

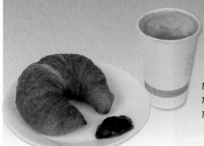

1 large butter croissant
1 tbsp. strawberry jam
1 16 fl. oz latte with whole milk

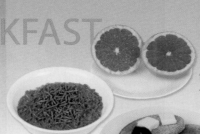

1 cup All-Bran cereal
1 cup skim milk
1 grapefruit
8 fl. oz low-fat plain yogurt
2 slices rye toast with 2 tsp. butter and 1 tbsp. blackberry preserves

LUNCH

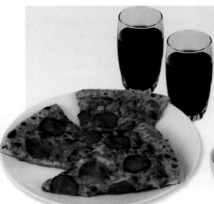

3 slices pepperoni pizza (14-inch pizza)
1.5 oz potato chips
24 fl. oz cola beverage

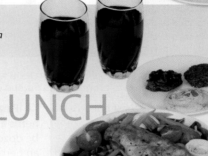

1 chicken breast, boneless, skinless, grilled
Spinach salad
2 cups spinach leaves
1 boiled egg
1 tbsp. chopped green onions
4 cherry tomatoes
½ medium carrot, chopped
1 tbsp. pine nuts
2 tbsp. Ranch dressing (reduced fat)
2 falafels (2-¼ inch diameter) with 2 tbsp. hummus

DINNER

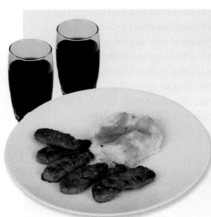
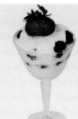

6 fried chicken tenders
1 cup mashed potatoes with ½ cup chicken gravy
24 fl. oz diet cola beverage
1 yogurt and fruit parfait

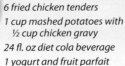

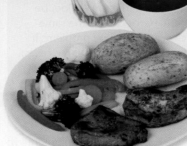
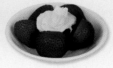

2 cups minestrone soup, reduced sodium
2 whole-grain dinner rolls with 2 tsp. margarine
2 pork loin chops, roasted
1 cup mixed vegetables, cooked
8 fl. oz skim milk
1 cup fresh strawberries (sliced) with 1 tbsp. low-fat whipped cream

nutrient analysis

nutrient analysis

2,789 kcal
46 milligrams of vitamin C
28.6 milligrams of niacin
929 milligrams of calcium
13.4 milligrams of iron
490 mcg of folate
1,300 milligrams of sodium

Provides
more
nutrients!

2,528 kcal
255 milligrams of vitamin C
42.8 milligrams of niacin
1,780 milligrams of calcium
27.5 milligrams of iron
1,335 mcg of folate
3,368 milligrams of sodium

highlight

Herbal Supplements: Use with Caution

A common saying in India cautions "A house without ginger is a sick house." Indeed, ginger, garlic, echinacea, and many other herbs have been used by cultures throughout the world for centuries to promote health and ward off disease. The National Center for Complementary and Alternative Medicine (NCCAM) defines an *herb* (also called a *botanical*) as a plant or plant part used for its scent, flavor, and/or therapeutic properties.[4] As you would suspect, with a definition this broad there are hundreds of different herbs on the market. Currently, 20% of adults in the United States use a dietary supplement with at least one botanical ingredient, either in combination with another dietary supplement, such as a vitamin/mineral supplement with echinacea, or alone.[5]

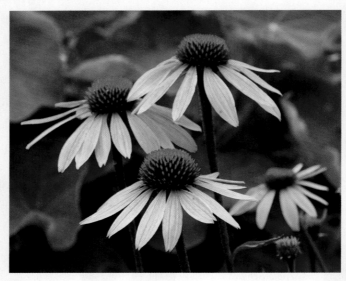

⬆ Echinacea, commonly known as purple coneflower, has been used for centuries to prevent colds, flu, and other infections.

It is clear that some herbs are effective medicines, but for what disorders, in what forms, and at what dosages? And are some herbs promoted as medicines ineffective, or even dangerous? To answer these questions about herbs you might be considering, the NCCAM evaluates dozens of the most commonly used herbs in "Herbs at a Glance" fact sheets, available at its website. See **Web Links** at the end of this chapter.

There are a number of precautions you should consider before taking herbal supplements. The most essential of these precautions is to consult your healthcare provider before using any herbal supplement. Herbs can act the same way as drugs; therefore, they can cause medical problems if not used correctly or if taken in large amounts. In some cases, people have experienced negative effects, even though they

followed the instructions on a supplement label. It's especially important to check with your healthcare provider if you are taking any prescription medications. Some herbal supplements are known to interact with medications in ways that cause health problems.

It is critical to avoid using herbs if you are pregnant or nursing, unless your physician has approved their use. Some can promote miscarriage or birth defects or can enter breast milk. This caution also applies to treating children with herbal supplements.

Finally, be aware that the active ingredients in many herbs and herbal supplements are not known. There may be dozens, even hundreds, of unknown compounds in an herbal supplement. Also, published analyses of herbal supplements have found differences between what's listed on the label and what's in the bottle. This means you may be taking less—or more—of the supplement than what the label indicates or ingesting substances not mentioned on the label. Some herbal supplements have been found to be contaminated with metals, unlabeled prescription drugs, microorganisms, and other substances. An investigation by the United States Government Accountability Office reported in 2010 that nearly all the herbal supplements it had tested contained traces of lead and other contaminants.[6] Be aware that the word *standardized*, *certified*, or *verified* on a label is no guarantee of product quality; in the United States, these terms have no legal definition for supplements.

■ Taking supplements in excess of the tolerable upper limit (UL), unless your healthcare provider prescribes them for a diagnosed medical condition. Taking amounts of the fat-soluble vitamin A above the UL can quickly lead to toxicity. In addition, excessive supplementation of some B-vitamins can lead to liver damage or nerve damage, and megadoses of vitamin C can cause severe diarrhea and other symptoms.

As advised by the American Dietetic Association, the ideal nutritional strategy is to eat a healthful diet that contains a variety of foods.[16] If you determine that you still need to supplement, make sure that together the sources don't provide more than 100% of the recommended levels of any nutrients these products contain. Avoid taking single-nutrient supplements unless advised by your healthcare provider.

In addition to micronutrient supplements, many Americans take one or more herbs, in powders, teas, tinctures, and tablets. If you're among them, check out the accompanying *Highlight: Herbal Supplements: Use with Caution*.

recap Federal regulation of dietary supplements is much less rigorous than regulation of drugs. Focus on getting your micronutrients from foods and avoid taking single-nutrient supplements unless advised by your healthcare provider.

✚ HEALTHWATCH

Do antioxidants protect against cancer?

LO10 Discuss the three stages of cancer progression and the role of dietary factors in influencing cancer risk.

Beta-carotene and the antioxidant vitamins E and C protect our cell membranes, proteins, lipoproteins, and DNA from damage by free radicals. So does that mean they protect us against cancer? Before we answer that question, let's take a closer look at precisely what cancer is and how it spreads. **Cancer** is actually a group of diseases that are all characterized by cells that grow "out of control." By this we mean that cancer cells reproduce spontaneously and independently and don't stay within the boundaries of the tissue or organ in which they grow. Instead, they aggressively invade tissues and organs, sometimes far away from those in which they originally formed.

Most forms of cancer result in one or more **tumors**, which are masses of immature cells that have no useful function. Although the word *tumor* sounds frightening, it is important to note that not every tumor is *malignant,* or cancerous. Many are *benign* (not harmful) and are made up of cells that will not spread widely.

Cancer Develops in Three Stages

FIGURE 6.22 shows how changes to normal cells prompt a series of other changes that can progress into cancer. There are three primary steps of cancer development: initiation, promotion, and progression:

1. *Initiation:* The initiation of cancer occurs when a cell's DNA is *mutated* (changed). This mutation, which can be caused by a variety of factors, including exposure to a virus, toxic chemical, or other agent, causes permanent changes in the cell that make it susceptible to promotion. Substances that prompt such mutations are called *carcinogens*.
2. *Promotion:* During this phase, the cell repeatedly divides. The mutated DNA is locked into each new cell's genetic instructions. These cells also avoid normal cell aging and death. Note that during this phase, the tumor is not yet exhibiting malignant behavior.
3. *Progression:* During this phase, the cancerous cells grow their own blood vessels, which supply them with blood and nutrients, and invade adjacent tissues. If not destroyed or removed surgically, the malignant tumor will disrupt body functions at the primary site and may shed malignant cells that invade the bloodstream and lymphatic system to *metastasize* (spread) to other sites of the body.

In the United States, cancer is the second leading cause of death across all age groups combined, accounting for nearly one in four deaths. Researchers estimate that about half of all men and one-third of all women will develop cancer during their lifetime; however, a majority of people who develop cancer survive. In 2014, the American Cancer Society reported that the 5-year survival rate for all cancers was 68%.[17]

A Diet High in Antioxidants May Help Prevent Cancer and Other Diseases

Your genes, your age, and your previous exposure to carcinogens all influence your cancer risk. You can't change these factors, of course, but a growing body of evidence suggests

cancer A group of diseases characterized by cells that reproduce spontaneously and independently and may invade other tissues and organs.

tumor Any newly formed mass of undifferentiated cells.

▶ **FIGURE 6.22** **(a)** Cancer cells develop as a result of a genetic mutation in the DNA of a normal cell. **(b)** The mutated cell replicates uncontrollably, eventually resulting in a tumor. **(c)** If not destroyed or removed, the cancerous tumor grows its own blood supply, invades nearby tissues, and metastasizes to other parts of the body.

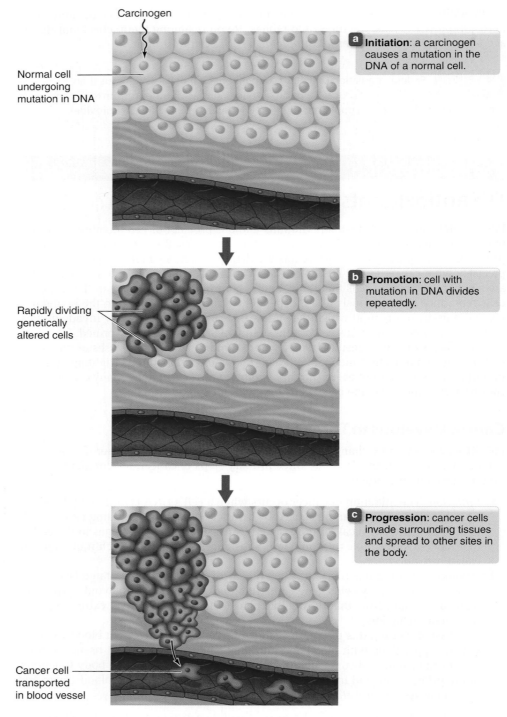

Carcinogen

Normal cell undergoing mutation in DNA

a **Initiation**: a carcinogen causes a mutation in the DNA of a normal cell.

Rapidly dividing genetically altered cells

b **Promotion**: cell with mutation in DNA divides repeatedly.

c **Progression**: cancer cells invade surrounding tissues and spread to other sites in the body.

Cancer cell transported in blood vessel

that lifestyle choices—including what you choose to eat—also play a role. Research currently suggests that a diet rich in antioxidants may reduce your risk for cancer, as well as cardiovascular disease and certain other diseases. Specifically, antioxidants are thought to:

- Enhance the immune system, which assists in the destruction and removal of precancerous cells from the body.
- Inhibit the growth of cancer cells and tumors.
- Prevent oxidative damage to the cells' DNA by seeking out and stabilizing free radicals.
- Reduce inflammation in blood vessel walls and protect against the formation and release of blood clots that can cause heart attack and stroke.

foods you don't know you love YET

Blueberries

Recently touted as a "superfood," blueberries have received a great deal of attention for their contribution to good health. Blueberries are mostly native to North America, with the state of Maine being the largest producer of wild blueberries in the world. Blueberries are actually the fruit of the flowering blueberry plant, and have a deep purple color when ripe.

Blueberries are packed with antioxidant nutrients and phytochemicals and have been shown to reduce the risk for heart disease, high blood pressure, urinary tract infections, and the cognitive decline that can occur with aging. Frozen blueberries are just as healthy as fresh, and they can be eaten in a fruit salad, with breakfast cereals, in a blended fruit smoothie, as a topping for whole-grain pancakes, or, of course, in blueberry pie. Dried blueberries can be added to trail mix and used as a substitute for raisins in recipes. Sweet with a bit of tartness, blueberries are a delicious addition to a healthy diet.

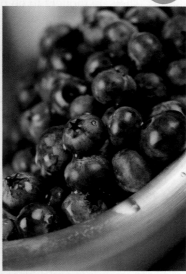

Eating whole foods high in antioxidant nutrients, such as vitamins E and C and beta-carotene—especially fruits and vegetables—is consistently shown to be associated with decreased cancer risk.[17] Additional studies show that populations eating diets low in antioxidant nutrients have a higher risk for cancer. These studies show a strong *association* between diet and disease risk, but they do not prove cause and effect. Nutrition experts agree that there are important interactions between antioxidant nutrients and other substances in foods, such as fiber and phytochemicals (discussed next), which work together to reduce the risk for many diseases.

Growing evidence over the past 20 years indicates that antioxidant supplementation does not reduce cancer risk; in fact, it may increase risks for various cancers and other chronic diseases. For example, a recent systematic review of the available published studies reports that beta-carotene supplementation has no effect on the incidence of all cancers combined, pancreatic cancer, colorectal cancer, prostate cancer, breast cancer, and skin cancer. However, the incidence of lung and stomach cancers was significantly increased in those taking higher doses (20–30 mg per day) as well as in smokers and asbestos workers.[2]

Why might foods high in antioxidants reduce cancer risk, whereas supplements do not and may even be harmful? First, it is possible that, although antioxidants appear to be beneficial at the lower doses we consume in plant foods, they may become toxic at the higher doses present in supplements. Second, other components of antioxidant-rich foods may contribute to their healthful effects. Let's learn more about these now.

Eating more fruits and vegetables high in antioxidants has been associated with reduced cancer risk.

Other Factors May Influence Cancer Risk

Many studies indicate that a diet rich in fiber can help to reduce the risk for colorectal cancer.[18] In addition, there is some evidence that a high fiber intake is associated with a reduced risk for prostate cancer and breast cancer.[19,20]

Phytochemicals have also been proposed to decrease cancer risk. These are naturally occurring chemicals in plants (*phyto* means "plant"), such as the carotenoid

phytochemicals Chemicals such as pigments that are present in plants and are believed to have health-promoting effects in humans.

pigments discussed earlier. They are found in abundance in fruits, vegetables, whole grains, legumes, seeds, soy products, garlic, onion, and green and black teas.

Phytochemicals exhibit clear cancer-prevention properties under laboratory conditions. They are thought to do this in part by moderating the damage done by free radicals. Some may enhance the body's ability to destroy cancer cells or slow or stop their growth. Although we don't yet understand precisely how phytochemicals might perform these functions, a growing body of research suggests that a diet supplying ample amounts of the following phytochemicals may play a role in reducing the risk of some forms of cancer:[21-23]

- Carotenoids, especially lycopene
- Flavonoids
- Organosulfur compounds

FIGURE 6.23 lists these and other phytochemicals linked to disease prevention and identifies their food sources.

Given the many benefits of phytochemicals, you're probably wondering how to be sure you're getting all you need each day. Check out the ***Game Plan*** box for information on the number of servings you need, preparation guidelines, and tips for phytochemically charged meals and snacks.

What else can you do to reduce your cancer risk? Here are some tips:

- Eat a variety of colorful fruits, vegetables, and whole grains daily, because these foods are rich in antioxidant nutrients and phytochemicals.
- Limit your consumption of saturated and *trans* fats. Some studies suggest that diets high in saturated fat can increase our risk for some cancers.
- Limit your consumption of red meats, processed meats, meats high in fat, and cured meats such as sausage, ham, bacon, and many lunch meats. Cured meats are high in nitrates and nitrites, which are known carcinogens.
- If you eat meat, avoid cooking methods that require high temperatures, such as broiling, frying, and barbecuing. High-temperature cooking methods prompt the development of carcinogens called *heterocyclic amines*.
- Maintain a healthful weight. Obesity appears to increase the risk for certain cancers, possibly because of hormonal changes that occur in people with excess body fat.
- If you drink alcohol, limit your consumption. Alcohol is a carcinogen, and intake is linked with an increased risk for many types of cancer.
- If you smoke cigarettes or cigars or use smokeless tobacco, stop. It is an established fact that these behaviors significantly increase the risk for many forms of cancer. More than forty compounds identified in tobacco and tobacco smoke are known carcinogens.
- Limit your sun exposure and avoid sunburn. Skin cancer is the most common form of cancer in the United States. After a few minutes of sun exposure during midday (from about 10 AM to 3 PM) to build up your vitamin D stores, apply sunscreen.
- Limit your exposure to environmental carcinogens. These include secondhand cigarette and cigar smoke and pollutants in the air, the food and water supply, and the workplace.
- Adopt a physically active lifestyle. Studies conducted over the past 10 years have shown a possible link between lower cancer risk and higher levels of physical activity. Specifically, the American Cancer Society recommends that you engage in at least moderate activity for 30 minutes or more on 5 or more days of the week.[24]
- Follow cancer screening recommendations. Screening can detect cancer at an early stage, when it is more responsive to treatment.

Are you living smart? Take this nutrition and activity quiz from the American Cancer Society to see how your choices might be affecting your cancer risk. Go to www.cancer.org and click on "Stay Healthy." Then, under "Tools and Calculators," click "Nutrition and Activity Quiz."

recap   Cancer is a group of diseases in which genetically mutated cells grow out of control. Tobacco use, sun exposure, nutritional factors, radiation and chemical exposures, and low physical activity levels are related to a higher risk for some cancers. Eating foods high in antioxidants is associated with lower rates of cancer. Phytochemicals are substances in plants that, together with the nutrients and fiber in plant-based foods, may play a role in reducing our risk for cancer.

Phytochemical	Health Claims	Food Source	
Carotenoids: alpha-carotene, beta-carotene, lutein, lycopene, zeaxanthin, etc.	Diets with foods rich in these phytochemicals may reduce the risk for cardiovascular disease, certain cancers (e.g., prostate), and age-related eye diseases (cataracts, macular degeneration).	Red, orange, and deep-green vegetables and fruits, such as carrots, cantaloupe, sweet potatoes, apricots, kale, spinach, pumpkin, and tomatoes	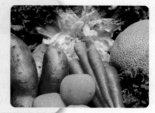
Flavonoids:[1] flavones, flavonols (e.g., quercetin), catechins (e.g., epigallocatechin gallate or EGCG), anthocyanidins, isoflavonoids, etc.	Diets with foods rich in these phytochemicals are associated with lower risk for cardiovascular disease and cancer, possibly because of reduced inflammation, blood clotting, and blood pressure and increased detoxification of carcinogens or reduction in replication of cancerous cells.	Berries, black and green tea, chocolate, purple grapes and juice, citrus fruits, olives, soybeans and soy products (soy milk, tofu, soy flour, textured vegetable protein), flaxseed, whole wheat	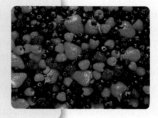
Phenolic acids:[1] ellagic acid, ferulic acid, caffeic acid, curcumin, etc.	Similar benefits as flavonoids.	Coffee beans, fruits (apples, pears, berries, grapes, oranges, prunes, strawberries), potatoes, mustard, oats, soy	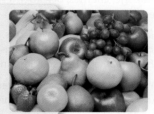
Phytoestrogens:[2] genistein, diadzein, lignans	Foods rich in these phytochemicals may provide benefits to bones and reduce the risk for cardiovascular disease and cancers of reproductive tissues (e.g., breast, prostate).	Soybeans and soy products (soy milk, tofu, soy flour, textured vegetable protein), flaxseed, whole grains	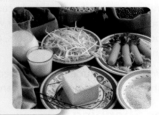
Organosulfur compounds: allylic sulfur compounds, indoles, isothiocyanates, etc.	Foods rich in these phytochemicals may protect against a wide variety of cancers.	Garlic, leeks, onions, chives, cruciferous vegetables (broccoli, cabbage, cauliflower), horseradish, mustard greens	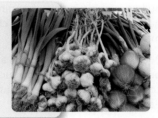

[1] Flavonoids, phenolic acids, and stilbenes are three groups of phytochemicals called phenolics. The phytochemical Resveratrol is a stilbene. Flavonoids and phenolic acids are the most abundant phenolics in our diet.
[2] Phytoestrogens include phytochemicals that have mild or anti-estrogenic action in our body. They are grouped together based on this similarity in biological function, but they also can be classified into other phytochemical groups, such as isoflavonoids.

FIGURE 6.23 Health claims and food sources of phytochemicals.

Tips for Increasing Your Phytochemical Intake

As we explained, phytochemicals (pronounced "fight-o-chemicals") may help your body fight chronic disease. So it makes sense to include an appropriate variety of them in your daily diet. But what's appropriate for you? And how can you select and prepare them in ways that work for your busy lifestyle?

Start by reviewing Figure 6.23, which identifies the largest groups of phytochemicals. Because most of these are plant pigments, and many fruits and vegetables contain several different types, you can be sure you are getting a wide variety if you eat 5 to 12 servings of brightly colored fruits and vegetables every day.

Next check out the Fruits & Veggies—More Matters health initiative, which was created by the Centers for Disease Control and Prevention and the Produce for Better Health Foundation to demonstrate that eating more fruits and vegetables can fit in with your busy schedule and help keep you healthy. The initiative offers cooking advice, nutrition information, and shopping and storage tips, and all this and more can be found at www.fruitsandveggiesmorematters.org.

The goal is to eat at least 5 servings of colorful fruits and vegetables each day to help fight cancer, heart disease, and the effects of aging. Here are only a few examples of the wide variety of foods in each group:

- ☐ Blue-purple foods include eggplant, red onions, purple cabbage, cherries, blackberries, blueberries, raspberries, red grapes, and plums.

- ☐ Green foods include avocados, broccoli, Brussels sprouts, chives, cabbage, collard greens, green peppers, kale, swiss chard, leaf lettuces, spinach, and kiwifruit.

- ☐ White foods include cauliflower, bok choy, white turnips, mushrooms, garlic, onions, leeks, scallions, and bananas.

- ☐ Yellow-orange foods include carrots, corn, yellow peppers, pumpkin, butternut and other winter squashes, sweet potatoes, cantaloupe, apricots, oranges, papaya, and mangoes.

- ☐ Red foods include tomatoes, red peppers, apples, strawberries, pink grapefruit, and watermelon.

When Shopping

- ☐ Build a rainbow in your shopping cart. That way, you'll have on hand several colorful choices to incorporate into meals and snacks each day.

- ☐ Because fruits and vegetables are perishable, purchase only an amount of fresh produce that you know you can consume within a few days. Nutrient losses increase with each day of storage.

- ☐ Purchase some less perishable forms of fruits and vegetables, such as dried fruits, 100% fruit and vegetable juices, soups, canned fruits and vegetables (check for no-sugar and no-sodium added), and frozen vegetables.

In the Kitchen

- ☐ Wash fresh fruits and vegetables thoroughly, except for berries, which should be washed immediately before eating to discourage spoilage.

- ☐ Store tomatoes, garlic, and bananas at room temperature.

- ☐ Store unripened avocados, pears, and other fruits in a lightly closed paper bag until ripe. Add a banana to the bag to speed ripening time. Once ripe, consume or refrigerate.

- ☐ Store potatoes and onions in a cool, dark location, such as a cellar or cool cupboard.

- ☐ Nutrients become depleted when exposed to air, so peel and cut fruits and vegetables only when you are ready to eat them. Many fruits and vegetables have edible peels that contain important nutrients and fiber, so wash them and eat them unpeeled when possible.

- ☐ To reduce nutrient loss in cooking water, eat vegetables raw, or zap coarsely chopped vegetables in the microwave for 2–4 minutes with approximately 1 tablespoon of water. Alternatively, stir-fry them in a small amount of oil

GAME **PLAN** !

or steam them in a basket over simmering water. Always cook vegetables for as short a time as necessary to make them palatable.

☐ Store leftovers in an airtight container in the refrigerator. If you don't plan to eat the leftovers within a few days, freeze them.

☐ Top your breakfast cereal with sliced banana, berries, or raisins or other dried fruits.

☐ Make a quick fruit salad with one can of mandarin orange slices, one can of pineapple chunks, a sliced banana, a chopped apple, and some berries, grapes, or raisins. Serve with yogurt.

☐ Add fresh vegetables to salads, soups, homemade pizza, and pasta.

☐ Add dark-green leaf lettuce, tomato, and onion to sandwiches, or make a veggie sandwich using avocado slices in place of meat.

☐ Next time you're at a barbecue, grill fruits or vegetables on skewers.

☐ For homemade salsa, combine chopped tomatoes, avocado, red onions, cilantro (coriander), and lime juice.

fruits & veggies more matters®

Data from Produce for Better Health Foundation.

☐ For shared meals, try a veggie-burrito buffet: set out a plate of warmed corn or whole-wheat tortillas with bowls of warm black or pinto beans, chopped tomatoes, chopped avocado, chopped black olives, minced onion or scallions, and plain yogurt or nonfat sour cream. Invite your friends to assemble their own!

☐ Make gazpacho! In a blender, combine 1–3 cups tomato juice, chunks of green pepper, red onion, a cucumber with seeds removed (no need to peel), the juice of one lime, a garlic clove, a splash each of red wine vinegar and olive oil, a half teaspoon each of basil and cumin, and salt and pepper to taste. Seed and dice two to three fresh tomatoes and add to blended ingredients. Chill for several hours. Serve very cold.

On the Run

☐ Buy ready-to-eat vegetables, such as baby carrots, cherry tomatoes, and celery sticks, or take a minute to wash and slice a red pepper or broccoli crowns. Toss some in a zip-lock bag to take to school or work.

☐ Throw a single-serving container of unsweetened applesauce, mandarin orange slices, pineapple chunks, or other fruit into your backpack for an afternoon snack. Don't forget the spoon!

☐ Make up small bags of fresh or dried fruits (grapes, raisins, apricots, cherries, prunes, figs, dates, banana chips, and so on) with nuts to take along.

☐ Pack a banana, an apple, a plum, an orange, or other fruit you can eat whole.

☐ Store some juice boxes in your freezer to take along. A frozen juice box will remain cold for several hours.

Data from some suggestions from Centers for Disease Control and Prevention (CDC) and Produce for Better Health Foundation at http://www.cdc.gov/nutrition/everyone/fruitsvegetables/index .html and www.fruitsandveggiesmorematters.org; and Phytochemical Information Center at www.pbhfoundation.org.

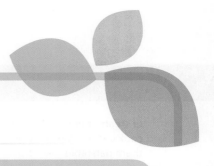

Customize your study plan—and master your nutrition!—
in the Study Area of **MasteringNutrition**

what can I do **today?**

Now that you've read this chapter, try making these three changes.

1 Try eating at least 2 servings of fruit and 3 servings of vegetables every day for 1 week—if you already eat this amount regularly, try to eat 1 more serving of each.

2 Add 1 serving of almonds or sunflower seeds to your next salad.

3 For breakfast, eat 1 serving of a high-fiber cereal that is fortified with B-vitamins, and add to that a cup of vitamin D–fortified milk or soy milk.

test yourself | *answers*

1. **True.** Our body can use energy from sunlight to convert a cholesterol compound in our skin into vitamin D.

2. **False.** Extensive research on vitamin C and colds does not support the theory that taking vitamin C supplements reduces our risk of catching a cold.

3. **False.** B-vitamins do not directly provide energy for our body. However, they enable our body to generate energy from carbohydrates, fats, and proteins.

summary

Scan to hear an MP3 Chapter Review in **MasteringNutrition**.

LO 1 Compare and contrast fat-soluble and water-soluble vitamins

- Vitamins are carbon-containing compounds that assist with regulating a multitude of body processes. Fat-soluble vitamins are soluble in fat and include vitamins A, D, E, and K. We can store fat-soluble vitamins in our liver, adipose, and other fatty tissues. Water-soluble vitamins are soluble in water and include vitamin C and the B vitamins (thiamin, riboflavin, niacin, vitamin B_6, vitamin B_{12}, pantothenic acid, biotin, and folate). Our bodies excrete excess amounts of water-soluble vitamins in our urine.

- Megadosing—taking a dose of a nutrient that is ten or more times greater than the recommended amount—can lead to serious toxicity symptoms. This is especially true for the fat-soluble vitamins A and D.

LO 2 Explain the role of vitamin A in vision and cell differentiation, and its relationship to beta-carotene

- Vitamin A is a fat-soluble vitamin that is extremely important for healthy vision. Adequate vitamin A allows us to see images and colors and to adjust to changes in the level of light.

- Other functions of vitamin A include assistance in cell differentiation, sexual reproduction, and proper bone growth. Vitamin A and its precursor, beta-carotene, also function as antioxidants. Beta-carotene is a provitamin to vitamin A. A provitamin is an inactive form of a vitamin that the body can convert to an active form. Beta-carotene is found in red, yellow, orange, and dark-green fruits and vegetables.

LO 3 Identify the primary functions and food sources of vitamins D and K

- Vitamin D is a fat-soluble vitamin that we can produce from the cholesterol in our skin using the energy from sunlight. It regulates blood calcium levels and helps maintain healthy bone. We can make vitamin D if our exposure to sunlight is adequate, and we consume it in fortified milk, soy milk, and other fortified products, as well as in fatty fish such as salmon.

- Vitamin K is a fat-soluble vitamin that serves as a coenzyme for blood clotting and bone metabolism. Probiotic bacteria in the large intestine synthesize vitamin K, and we consume it in green leafy vegetables, soybeans, and canola oil.

LO 4 Discuss the process of oxidation and explain how it can damage cells

- Oxidation refers to metabolic reactions involving the exchange of oxygen. Although these reactions are normal and necessary, they result in the production of free radicals, which are dangerous because they can damage the lipid portion of cell membranes, destroying their integrity. Free radicals also damage LDL-cholesterol, cell proteins, and DNA. The oxidative damage caused by free radicals may increase our risk for several diseases, including heart disease and some forms of cancer. Antioxidants are compounds that protect our cells from oxidative damage.

LO 5 Discuss the interrelated roles of vitamins E and C in protecting cells from oxidation

- Vitamin E is a fat-soluble vitamin that acts as an antioxidant that protects the fatty components of cell membranes, as well as LDL-cholesterol, vitamin A, and our lungs, from oxidative damage. It also assists the development of nerves and muscles, enhances immune function, and improves the absorption of vitamin A, if intake of vitamin A is low.

- Vitamin C is a water-soluble vitamin that acts as an antioxidant by scavenging free radicals and regenerating vitamin E after it has been oxidized. Other functions include the synthesis of collagen, various hormones, neurotransmitters, DNA, enhancing immune function, and increasing the absorption of iron.

LO 6 Explain how our body uses the B vitamins to generate energy

- The B vitamins include thiamin, riboflavin, vitamin B_6, niacin, folate, vitamin B_{12}, pantothenic acid, and biotin. Their primary role is to act as

coenzymes; that is, they activate enzymes. In this way, they assist in the metabolism of carbohydrates, fats, and amino acids; the repair and replication of DNA; cell differentiation; the formation and maintenance of the central nervous system; and the formation of blood.

- Deficiencies of the B vitamins can cause beriberi (thiamin), pellagra (niacin), macrocytic anemia (folate), pernicious anemia (vitamin B_{12}), and an elevated homocysteine level (folate and vitamins B_6 and B_{12}), which increases the risk for a heart attack or stroke.

LO 7 Discuss the importance of adequate folate intake for women of childbearing age

- Neural tube defects can result from inadequate folate intake during the first few weeks of pregnancy. All women of childbearing age are advised to consume an additional 400 µg/day from supplements, fortified foods, or both.

LO 8 Describe the interrelationship of vitamin B_6, folate, and vitamin B_{12} in homocysteine metabolism and cardiovascular disease

- Deficiencies of the B vitamins can cause beriberi (thiamin), pellagra (niacin), macrocytic anemia (folate), and pernicious anemia (vitamin B_{12}). Deficiency of folate, vitamin B_6, or vitamin B_{12} can disrupt the metabolism of homocysteine, an amino acid. This can promote an elevated level of homocysteine in the blood, a condition that increases the risk for a heart attack or stroke.

LO 9 Explain how dietary supplements are regulated in the United States, and the recommendations for and against their use

- Dietary supplements are products taken by mouth that contain a "dietary ingredient" intended to supplement the diet. Dietary supplements and functional foods are not strictly regulated by the Food and Drug Administration (FDA) and do not need approval prior to marketing. Although certain populations do benefit from taking certain vitamin/mineral supplements, consumers should consult their physician before using any dietary supplement. Taking megadoses of any supplement should be avoided unless they have been prescribed for a diagnosed condition.

LO 10 **Discuss the three stages of cancer progression and the role of dietary factors in influencing cancer risk**

■ Cancer is a group of diseases characterized by cells that reproduce spontaneously and independently and don't stay within the boundaries of the tissue or organ where they grow. Instead, they aggressively invade tissues and organs, sometimes far away from those in which they originally formed. Its three stages include initiation, in which a cell's DNA undergoes a mutation; promotion, in which the cell repeatedly divides; and progression, in which the mutated cells develop a blood supply and invade nearby tissues. They can then metastasize to distant sites.

■ Antioxidants are thought to play a role in cancer prevention. A diet of whole foods high in antioxidant nutrients and phytochemicals is associated with lower rates of some cancers, but supplementing with antioxidants can cause cancer in some situations. Phytochemicals are naturally occurring components in food that may reduce our risk for diseases, such as cancer and heart disease. They are found in fruits, vegetables, nuts, seeds, whole grains, soy products, garlic, onions, and tea.

review questions

LO 1 **Compare and contrast fat-soluble and water-soluble vitamins**

1. The fat-soluble vitamins
   a. are absorbed directly into the bloodstream.
   b. are only found in animal-based foods.
   c. can accumulate over time in body tissues.
   d. include the B-vitamins and vitamin C.

LO 2 **Explain the role of vitamin A in vision and cell differentiation, and its relationship to beta-carotene**

2. Vitamin A
   a. is a precursor of retinol.
   b. is essential to maintain healthy vision.
   c. is recommended in supplement form for the treatment of acne.
   d. is also classified as a carotenoid.

LO 3 **Identify the primary functions and food sources of vitamins D and K**

3. Vitamins D and K
   a. are both fat-soluble vitamins.
   b. both play a role in maintaining healthy bone.
   c. are both available from nondietary sources.
   d. all of the above.

LO 4 **Discuss the process of oxidation and explain how it can damage cells**

4. Oxidation is
   a. a chemical reaction involving the exchange of oxygen.
   b. a process in which free radicals are stabilized.
   c. an abnormal type of metabolism that occurs only in disease states such as cancer.
   d. a process in which oxygen is transported across a cell membrane.

LO 5 **Discuss the interrelated roles of vitamins E and C in protecting cells from oxidation**

5. Which of the following is a characteristic of vitamin E?
   a. It acts as an antioxidant within the fluid outside of cells.
   b. It regenerates vitamin C after it has been oxidized, enabling vitamin C to "get back to work."
   c. It is stored in adipose tissues and cell membranes.
   d. Smokers require it in increased amounts.

LO 6 **Explain how our body uses the B vitamins to generate energy**

6. The B-vitamins
   a. provide energy.
   b. regulate the body's storage of energy.
   c. are enzymes involved in energy metabolism.
   d. help activate enzymes involved in energy metabolism.

LO 7 **Discuss the importance of adequate folate intake for women of childbearing age**

7. Adequate folate intake is critical for women of childbearing age because
   a. it reduces the risk for giving birth to an infant with a neural tube defect.
   b. it reduces the risk for giving birth to an infant with pernicious anemia.
   c. it reduces the woman's risk for pernicious anemia.
   d. it helps speed up the woman's production of red blood cells following menstruation.

LO **8** **Describe the interrelationship of vitamin B$_6$, folate, and vitamin B$_{12}$ in homocysteine metabolism and cardiovascular disease**

8. Increased blood levels of the amino acid homocysteine
   a. can offer protection against deficiencies of vitamins B$_6$, folate, and B$_{12}$.
   b. can offer protection against atrophic gastritis.
   c. can increase the risk for a heart attack or stroke.
   d. can increase the risk for macrocytic anemia.

LO **9** **Explain how dietary supplements are regulated in the United States, and the recommendations for and against their use**

9. Dietary supplements
   a. are categorized by the FDA within the general group of drugs.
   b. are evaluated for safety and effectiveness by the United States Pharmacopeia before being allowed onto the market.
   c. are necessary to ensure a healthy diet.
   d. are not substitutes for a nourishing diet.

LO **10** **Discuss the three stages of cancer progression and the role of dietary factors in influencing cancer risk**

10. A carcinogen is
   a. a newly formed mass of undifferentiated cells.
   b. a factor that causes a mutation in the DNA of a normal body cell.
   c. a type of cancer cell capable of invading surrounding tissues.
   d. a cancer cell that has leaked into the bloodstream and can be carried to distant tissues.

Answers to Review Questions are located at the back of this text.

web links

The following websites and apps explore further topics and issues related to personal health. Visit **MasteringNutrition** for links to the websites and RSS feeds.

www.cancer.org
American Cancer Society (ACS)

www.cdc.gov
Centers for Disease Control and Prevention

www.fda.gov
Food and Drug Association (FDA)

lpi.oregonstate.edu
Linus Pauling Institute

www.fruitsandveggiesmorematters.org
Fruits & Veggies—More Matters

www.cancer.gov
National Cancer Institute

nccam.nih.gov
National Center for Complementary and Alternative Medicine

www.nlm.nih.gov
MEDLINE Plus Health Information

http://ods.od.nih.gov
National Institutes of Health Office of Dietary Supplements

7

Minerals
Building and Moving Our Body

learning outcomes

After studying this chapter, you should be able to:

1 Distinguish between major, trace, and ultra-trace minerals, p. 194.

2 Explain why certain minerals are referred to as electrolytes and identify their primary functions in the body, pp. 194–202.

3 Explain how the level of sodium in your blood can affect your blood pressure, pp. 194–202.

4 Identify two trace minerals important in energy metabolism, pp. 202–204.

5 Identify two trace minerals essential for the body's synthesis of thyroid hormones, pp. 202–204.

6 Explain how the body uses iron, and identify dietary sources and factors affecting its absorption, pp. 205–210.

7 Discuss the role of zinc in metabolism and immune function, and identify common food sources, pp. 205–210.

8 Identify the four mineral components of bone and explain how bone is formed and maintained, pp. 210–217.

9 State the four primary functions of calcium, pp. 210–217.

10 Discuss the risk factors and available treatments for osteoporosis, pp. 218–220.

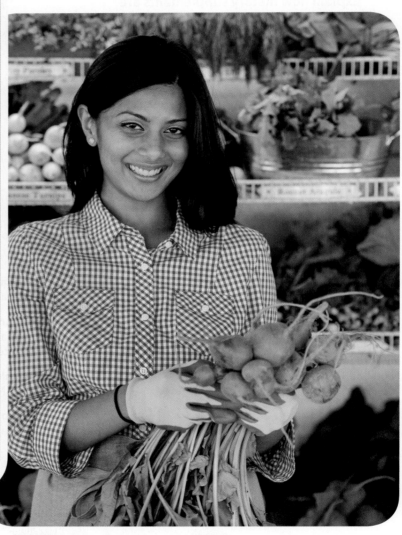

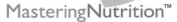

MasteringNutrition™

Go online for chapter quizzes, pre-tests, Interactive Activities, and more!

test yourself

Are these statements true or false? Circle your guess.

1. **T F** The majority of sodium in our diet comes from the table salt we sprinkle on our food.

2. **T F** Iron deficiency is the most common nutrient deficiency in the world.

3. **T F** Osteoporosis, or "porous bones," is a disease that only affects elderly women.

Test Yourself answers can be found at the end of the chapter.

Mother-daughter actresses Blythe Danner and Gwyneth Paltrow have to stay slender for the screen. But did their diet contribute to their low bone density—or was the culprit genetics, ethnicity, or level of physical activity? Whereas Paltrow has a more modest thinning of the bones not characterized as a disease, Danner has osteoporosis (meaning "porous bones"), a disease that sharply increases the risk for fractures. As you might suspect, the less dense the bone, the more likely it is to break, even during minor weight-bearing activities, such as carrying groceries. In advanced cases, bones in the hip and spine fracture spontaneously, merely from the effort of holding the body erect.

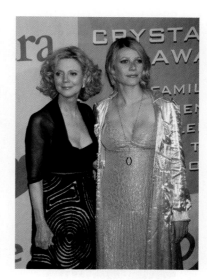

In this chapter, we discuss the minerals that form our bones and explore how mineral deficiencies lead to bone disease. We also explain how minerals called *electrolytes* provide the electrical charge that enables our body to move, think—indeed, to perform any activity at all. Still other minerals work with the B-vitamins to metabolize food into energy, and some help transport oxygen within our blood. As you can see, minerals are indispensable to our functioning (**FIGURE 7.1**). Still, you don't have to take supplements to get the minerals you need. Just make sure to eat a variety of nutrient-dense foods, especially fruits, vegetables, whole grains, legumes, and low-fat dairy products. Before we discuss individual minerals, let's pause to explore exactly what minerals are.

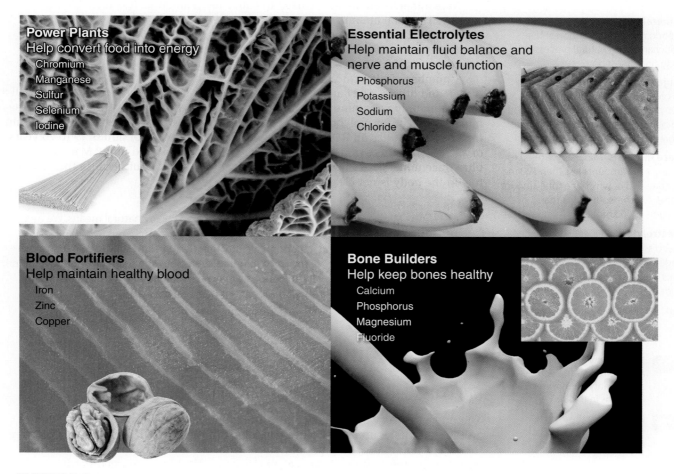

Power Plants
Help convert food into energy
Chromium
Manganese
Sulfur
Selenium
Iodine

Essential Electrolytes
Help maintain fluid balance and nerve and muscle function
Phosphorus
Potassium
Sodium
Chloride

Blood Fortifiers
Help maintain healthy blood
Iron
Zinc
Copper

Bone Builders
Help keep bones healthy
Calcium
Phosphorus
Magnesium
Fluoride

FIGURE 7.1   The functions of the major and trace minerals. Good food sources are also shown for each functional group.

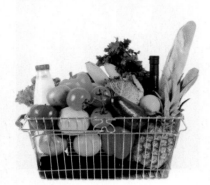

Many different foods provide minerals.

minerals Solid, crystalline substances that do not contain carbon and are not changed by natural processes, including digestion.

major minerals Minerals we need to consume in amounts of at least 100 mg per day, and of which the total amount present in the body is at least 5 grams (5,000 mg).

trace minerals Minerals we need to consume in amounts less than 100 mg per day, and of which the total amount present in the body is less than 5 grams (5,000 mg).

electrolyte A (mineral) substance that dissolves in solution into positively and negatively charged ions and is thus capable of carrying an electrical current.

ion An electrically charged particle.

What are minerals?

Whereas vitamins are compounds made up of carbon and several other types of atoms, **minerals** are elemental substances. Thus, they are not broken down during digestion or by any natural means. Minerals exist not only in foods but also in the environment: the zinc in meats is the same as the zinc in the Earth's crust.

One of the most important properties of minerals is their ability to carry an electrical charge. Like magnets, minerals with opposite electrical charges bond tightly together to form durable compounds—for instance, in our bones. The electrical charge of minerals also attracts water, so the minerals inside our cells help them retain the amount of water they need to function. And in both our cells and tissues, the electrical charges of various minerals stimulate our nerves to fire and our muscles to contract.

Minerals are classified according to the amounts we need in our diet and according to how much of the mineral is found in our body. The two categories of minerals in our diet and our body are the major minerals and the trace minerals.

Major minerals earned their name from the fact that we need to consume at least 100 mg of each per day in our diet. In addition, the total amount of each major mineral present in the body is at least 5 grams (5,000 mg). For instance, the major mineral calcium is a primary component of our bones. In addition to calcium, the major minerals include sodium, potassium, phosphorus, chloride, magnesium, and sulfur. **TABLE 7.1** identifies the primary functions, recommended intakes, and food sources of these minerals.

Trace minerals are those we need to consume in amounts less than 100 mg per day. The total amount of any trace mineral in the body is less than 5 grams (5,000 mg). The trace minerals include selenium, fluoride, iodine, chromium, manganese, iron, zinc, and copper. **TABLE 7.2** identifies major functions, recommended intakes, and food sources of these minerals.

A number of *ultra-trace minerals* are also found in our body, including boron, nickel, and others. They are classified as ultra-trace because researchers estimate that we require only very minute amounts. No DRI has been established for any of these minerals except for molybdenum.[1] This mineral is important for key enzymes within the body, and it has an RDA of 45 micrograms (µg) per day for adults 19 to 70 years of age.[2] Rich sources of molybdenum are legumes, grains, and nuts.[3] Many other ultra-trace minerals are thought to be important for health, but because their exact role in the body is not clear, they have no DRI.

recap Minerals are elements and are not changed by any natural means. We need to consume at least 100 mg per day of the major minerals, which include sodium, potassium, phosphorus, chloride, calcium, magnesium, and sulfur. We need to consume less than 100 mg per day of the trace minerals, which include selenium, fluoride, iodine, chromium, manganese, iron, zinc, and copper. Ultra-trace minerals are required in minute amounts, but no DRI for most of these minerals has been established.

Essential electrolytes: sodium, potassium, chloride, and phosphorus

The interior of all body cells contains fluid, and many cells anchored together in a fluid bath make up body tissues. Dissolved in these cellular and tissue fluids are four major minerals: sodium, potassium, chloride, and phosphorus. There, these minerals are referred to as **electrolytes**, because they form charged particles called **ions**, which carry an electrical current. This electricity is the "spark" that stimulates nerves to transmit impulses, so electrolytes are critical to nervous system functioning. Serious electrolyte disturbances can lead to seizures, loss of consciousness, and

TABLE 7.1 **Major Minerals**

Mineral	Primary Functions	Recommended Intake*	Reliable Food Sources	Toxicity/Deficiency Symptoms
Sodium	Fluid balance Acid–base balance Transmission of nerve impulses Muscle contraction	AI: adults = 1.5 g/day (1,500 mg/day)	Table salt, pickles, most canned soups, snack foods, cured lunch meats, canned tomato products	*Toxicity:* water retention, high blood pressure, loss of calcium *Deficiency:* muscle cramps, dizziness, fatigue, nausea, vomiting, mental confusion and seizures
Potassium	Fluid balance Transmission of nerve impulses Muscle contraction	AI: adults = 4.7 g/day (4,700 mg/day)	Most fresh fruits and vegetables: potatoes, bananas, tomato juice, orange juice, melons	*Toxicity:* muscle weakness, vomiting, irregular heartbeat *Deficiency:* muscle weakness, paralysis, mental confusion, irregular heartbeat
Phosphorus	Fluid balance Bone formation Component of ATP, which provides energy for our body	RDA: adults = 700 mg/day	Milk/cheese/yogurt, soy milk and tofu, legumes (lentils, black beans), nuts (almonds, peanuts, and peanut butter), poultry	*Toxicity:* muscle spasms, convulsions, low blood calcium *Deficiency:* muscle weakness, muscle damage, bone pain, dizziness
Chloride	Fluid balance Transmission of nerve impulses Component of stomach acid (HCl) Antibacterial	AI: adults = 2.3 g/day (2,300 mg/day)	Table salt	*Toxicity:* none known *Deficiency:* dangerous blood acid–base imbalances, irregular heartbeat
Calcium	Primary component of bone Acid–base balance Transmission of nerve impulses Muscle contraction	RDAs: Adults aged 19–50 = 1,000 mg/day Men aged 51–70 = 1,000 mg/day; men aged >70 = 1,200 mg/day Women aged >50 = 1,200 mg/day UL = 2,500 mg/day	Milk/yogurt/cheese (best-absorbed form of calcium), sardines, collard greens and spinach, calcium-fortified juices	*Toxicity:* mineral imbalances, shock, kidney failure, fatigue, mental confusion *Deficiency:* osteoporosis, convulsions, heart failure
Magnesium	Component of bone Muscle contraction Assists more than 300 enzyme systems	RDAs: Men aged 19–30 = 400 mg/day; men aged >30 = 420 mg/day Women aged 19–30 = 310 mg/day; women aged >30 = 320 mg/day UL = 350 mg/day	Greens (spinach, kale, collard greens), whole grains, seeds, nuts, legumes (navy and black beans)	*Toxicity:* none known *Deficiency:* low blood calcium, muscle spasms or seizures, nausea, weakness, increased risk for chronic diseases (such as heart disease, hypertension, osteoporosis, type 2 diabetes)
Sulfur	Component of certain B-vitamins and amino acids Acid–base balance Detoxification in liver	No DRI	Protein-rich foods	*Toxicity:* none known *Deficiency:* none known

*Abbreviations: RDA, Recommended Dietary Allowance; UL, upper limit; AI, Adequate Intake; DRI, Dietary Reference Intake.

cardiac arrest. The major mineral calcium is also an electrolyte. It is discussed later in this chapter.

Electrolytes are also critical to maintaining our fluid balance; that is, they keep our cells from becoming swollen with too much fluid or dehydrated from too little. Two qualities help electrolytes work together to control fluid balance: First, they all strongly attract water. Second, they are not able to move freely from one side of the cell membrane to the other. Instead, potassium and phosphate tend to remain inside our cells, and sodium and chloride tend to remain outside, in the tissue spaces. Although none of the electrolytes can move freely across the cell membrane, water can. Thus, the equal attraction for water of the electrolytes on either side of the cell membrane keeps our body in fluid balance **(FIGURE 7.2)**.

TABLE 7.2 **Trace Minerals**

Mineral	Primary Functions	Recommended Intake*	Reliable Food Sources	Toxicity/Deficiency Symptoms
Selenium	Required for carbohydrate and fat metabolism	RDA: adults = 55 μg/day UL = 400 μg/day	Nuts, shellfish, meat/fish/poultry, whole grains	*Toxicity:* brittle hair and nails, skin rashes, nausea and vomiting, weakness, liver disease *Deficiency:* specific forms of heart disease and arthritis, impaired immune function, muscle pain and wasting, depression, hostility
Fluoride	Development and maintenance of healthy teeth and bones	RDAs: Men = 4 mg/day Women = 3 mg/day UL: 2.2 mg/day for children aged 4 to 8; children aged >8 = 10 mg/day	Fish, seafood, legumes, whole grains, drinking water (variable)	*Toxicity:* fluorosis of teeth and bones *Deficiency:* dental caries, low bone density
Iodine	Synthesis of thyroid hormones Temperature regulation Reproduction and growth	RDA: Adults = 150 μg/day UL = 1,100 μg/day	Iodized salt, saltwater seafood	*Toxicity:* goiter *Deficiency:* goiter, hypothyroidism, cretinism in infant of mother who is iodine deficient
Chromium	Glucose transport Metabolism of DNA and RNA Immune function and growth	AI: men aged 19–50 = 35 μg/day; men aged >50 = 30 μg/day Women aged 19–50 = 25 μg/day; women aged >50 = 20 μg/day	Whole grains, brewer's yeast	*Toxicity:* None known *Deficiency:* Elevated blood glucose and blood lipids, damage to brain and nervous system
Manganese	Assists many enzyme systems Synthesis of protein found in bone and cartilage	AIs: Men = 2.3 mg/day Women = 1.8 mg/day UL = 11 mg/day for adults	Whole grains, nuts, leafy vegetables, tea	*Toxicity:* impairment of neuromuscular system *Deficiency:* impaired growth and reproductive function, reduced bone density, impaired glucose and lipid metabolism, skin rash
Iron	Component of hemoglobin in blood cells Component of myoglobin in muscle cells Assists many enzyme systems	RDAs: Adult men = 8 mg/day Women aged 19–50 = 18 mg/day; women aged >50 = 8 mg/day	Meat/fish/poultry (best-absorbed form of iron), fortified cereals, legumes, spinach	*Toxicity:* nausea, vomiting, and diarrhea; dizziness, confusion; rapid heartbeat, organ damage, death *Deficiency:* iron-deficiency microcytic anemia (small red blood cells), hypochromic anemia
Zinc	Assists more than 100 enzyme systems Immune system function Growth and sexual maturation Gene regulation	RDAs: Men = 11 mg/day Women = 8 mg/day UL = 40 mg/day	Meat/fish/poultry (best-absorbed form of zinc), fortified cereals, legumes	*Toxicity:* nausea, vomiting, diarrhea, headaches, depressed immune function, reduced absorption of copper *Deficiency:* growth retardation, delayed sexual maturation, eye and skin lesions, hair loss, increased incidence of illness and infection
Copper	Assists many enzyme systems Iron transport	RDA: Adults = 900 μg/day UL = 10 mg/day	Shellfish, organ meats, nuts, legumes	*Toxicity:* nausea, vomiting, diarrhea, liver damage *Deficiency:* anemia, reduced levels of white blood cells, osteoporosis in infants and growing children

*Abbreviations: RDA, Recommended Dietary Allowance; UL, upper limit; AI, Adequate Intake.

When our electrolytes go out of balance, body fluids soon go out of balance as well. For instance, imagine a shipwrecked sailor in a lifeboat. With no freshwater to drink, he drinks seawater, which is, of course, high in sodium. This heavy load of sodium remains in the tissue spaces outside his cells, where it strongly attracts water. Because the level of electrolytes inside the cells has not been increased, there is now a much greater concentration of electrolytes outside the cells. This higher concentration of electrolytes pulls water out of the cells into the tissue spaces (Figure 7.2c).

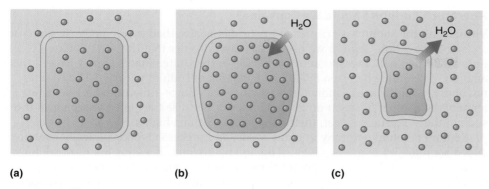

(a)   (b)   (c)

▲ **FIGURE 7.2**   The health of the body's cells depends on maintaining the proper balance of fluids and electrolytes on both sides of the cell membrane. **(a)** The concentration of electrolytes is the same on both sides of the cell membrane. **(b)** The concentration of electrolytes is much greater inside the cell, drawing water into the cell and making it swell. **(c)** The concentration of electrolytes is much greater outside the cell, drawing water out of the cell and making it shrink.

This leaves the cells dehydrated. The sailor's body then excretes the salty tissue fluid as urine, decreasing the total amount of water in his body. If the sailor continues to drink seawater, he will become so dehydrated that he will die.

Similarly, food poisoning, eating disorders, and other illnesses involving repeated vomiting and diarrhea can threaten the delicate balance of fluid inside and outside our cells. With diarrhea or vomiting, the body loses a great deal of fluid from the intestinal tract and the tissue spaces outside the cells. This heavy fluid loss causes the electrolyte concentration outside the cells to become very high. In response, a great deal of the interior fluid of the cells flows out. The resulting fluid and electrolyte imbalance alters the flow of electrical impulses through the heart, causing an irregular heart rate that can lead to death if left untreated.

The recommended intakes of the electrolytes and other major minerals are identified in Table 7.1.

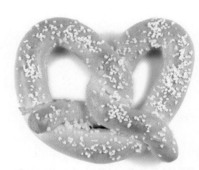

▲ Many popular snack foods are high in sodium.

recap   The major minerals sodium, potassium, chloride, and phosphorus are called electrolytes, because when they dissolve in water they form electrically charged particles called ions, which can carry an electrical current. Electrolytes assist in nerve transmission and regulation of fluid balance. Repeated diarrhea or vomiting can threaten fluid balance.

Sodium Is Part of Table Salt

Many people equate sodium with table salt, but in truth, those crystals in your salt shaker are made up of both sodium and chloride. Over the past 20 years, researchers have linked high sodium intake to an increased risk for high blood pressure. Because of this link, many people have come to believe that sodium is harmful to the body. This simply is not true: sodium is an essential nutrient that the body needs to survive. We'll explore the link between sodium and high blood pressure shortly.

Why Do We Need Sodium?

Sodium is a major mineral with many functions. As discussed, it helps cells maintain proper fluid balance. It also helps regulate blood pressure and acid–base balance, plays a leading role in the transmission of nerve signals, and is an important component of gastric secretions. Finally, sodium assists in the absorption of certain nutrients, such as glucose.

In addition to its functions in the body, sodium in table salt enhances the flavor of foods. It is also a powerful antimicrobial: for thousands of years, it has been used to preserve meats and other foods.

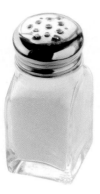

← Almost all sodium is consumed through table salt.

How Much Sodium Should We Consume?

Virtually all the sodium we consume in our diet is absorbed by the body. To give you a sense of how little sodium we need each day, consider that the AI (1,500 mg) is a little more than half a teaspoon! Most people in the United States greatly exceed this amount, consuming between 3,000 and 6,000 mg of sodium per day.[4] The AI does not apply to highly active individuals, such as endurance athletes, who lose large amounts of sodium in sweat on a regular basis.[5] Because they need to replenish the sodium they excrete in sweat, their daily intakes can be higher.

Sodium is found naturally in many foods, and processed foods typically contain added sodium. Try to guess which of the following foods contains the most sodium: 1 cup of tomato juice, 1 oz of potato chips, or four saltine crackers. Now look at **TABLE 7.3** to find the answer. Are you surprised to discover that, of these three food items, the tomato juice has the most sodium? Lots of processed foods, such as lunch meats, canned soups and beans, vegetable juices, and prepackaged rice, ramen, and pasta dishes, are very high in sodium, as are many snack foods and fast foods, not to mention many dishes served in college cafeterias!

Does Sodium Play a Role in High Blood Pressure?

Consuming excessive sodium causes water retention (bloating), because water is drawn out of the interior of cells to dilute the sodium in the tissue fluids. A high level of sodium in the fluid portion of blood (called *plasma*) similarly attracts water, and when it does, the total volume of blood circulating in the blood vessels increases. This, in turn, increases the level of pressure inside the blood vessels. This condition, commonly called high blood pressure, is clinically known as *hypertension*. Although it is one of the major chronic diseases in the United States, hypertension often causes no symptoms. Instead, it's typically diagnosed when a routine blood pressure screening reveals above-average readings. Early detection and treatment is essential, because

TABLE 7.3 High-Sodium Foods and Lower-Sodium Alternatives

High-Sodium Foods	Sodium (mg)	Lower-Sodium Food	Sodium (mg)
Dill pickle (1 large, 4 in.)	1,181	Low-sodium dill pickle (1 large, 4 in.)	12
Ham, cured, roasted (3 oz)	1,168	Pork, loin roast (3 oz)	48
Corn beef (3 oz)	1,110	Beef chuck roast, cooked (3 oz)	40
Turkey pastrami (3 oz)	915	Roasted Turkey, cooked (3 oz)	54
Tomato juice, regular (1 cup)	680	Tomato juice, lower-sodium (1 cup)	141
Tomato sauce, canned (½ cup)	642	Fresh tomato (1 medium)	6
Canned cream corn (1 cup)	730	Cooked corn, fresh (1 large ear), boiled	0
Tomato soup, canned (1 cup)	675	Low-sodium tomato soup, canned (1 cup)	60
Potato chips, salted (1 oz)	149	Baked potato, unsalted (1 medium)	17
Saltine crackers (4 each)	256	Saltine crackers, unsalted (4 each)	92
Macaroni and cheese (1 cup)	800	Spanish rice (1 cup)	5
Teriyaki chicken (1 cup)	3,210	Stir-fried pork/rice/vegetables (1 cup)	575
Ramen noodle soup (chicken flavor) (1 pkg [85 g])	1,950	Ramen noodle soup with sodium-free chicken broth (1 cup)	0
Burger King, Double Whopper, with cheese (1 item)	1,544	Fast Food Chicken Salad (1.5 c)	209
Digiorno Thin Crust Supreme Topping Pizza (1 slice)	1,616	Kashi Pizza, Basil Pesto (1/3 pizza)	593
Taco Bell, Taco Salad (1 item)	1,935	Taco Bell, Original beef taco, cheese and lettuce (1 taco)	274

*Data from U.S. Department of Agriculture, Agricultural Research Service. 2014. USDA Nutrient Database for Standard Reference, Release 26. Nutrient Data Laboratory Home Page. http://ndb.nal.usda.gov/

hypertension is a warning sign that the person is at an increased risk for a heart attack or stroke.

When we define hypertension as blood pressure above the average range, what exactly do we mean? Well, blood pressure measurements are recorded in millimeters of mercury (mm Hg) in two phases, systolic and diastolic:

- *Systolic blood pressure* represents the pressure exerted in our arteries at the moment that the heart contracts, sending blood into our blood vessels. Optimal systolic blood pressure is *less than* 120 mm Hg.
- *Diastolic blood pressure* represents the pressure in our arteries between contractions, when our heart is relaxed. Optimal diastolic blood pressure is *less than* 80 mm Hg.

For example, a healthy blood pressure reading might be 110 mm Hg systolic and 70 mm Hg diastolic—which a clinician would report to you as "110 over 70 mm Hg." *Prehypertension* is defined as a systolic blood pressure between 120 and 139 mm Hg, or a diastolic blood pressure between 80 and 89 mm Hg. So "120 over 85 mm Hg" indicates prehypertension. You would be diagnosed with true hypertension if your systolic blood pressure were greater than or equal to 140 mm Hg or your diastolic blood pressure were greater than or equal to 90 mm Hg.

Hypertension is more common in people who consume high-sodium diets, but whether high-sodium diets can actually *cause* hypertension is the subject of some controversy. In most people who consume too much sodium, the body can compensate and the kidneys will excrete the excess sodium in the urine. But in some people, the body is unable to compensate for a high sodium intake and blood pressure increases.

Research into hypertension funded by the National Institutes of Health (NIH) has led to the development of the DASH Diet, an eating plan shown to reduce hypertension. DASH stands for "Dietary Approaches to Stop Hypertension" and includes recommendations for consuming 8 to 10 servings of fruits and vegetables daily, as well as limiting dietary sodium.[6] The version of the DASH diet providing about 2,300 mg of sodium per day has been shown to significantly reduce blood pressure. Blood pressure drops even more, however, in people who follow the lowest-sodium version of the DASH diet, which provides about 1,500 mg of sodium per day.[5,6] **FIGURE 7.3** gives an overview of the DASH diet. For tips on shopping for and preparing foods with less salt, check out the *Game Plan* box.

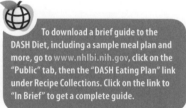

To download a brief guide to the DASH Diet, including a sample meal plan and more, go to www.nhlbi.nih.gov, click on the "Public" tab, then the "DASH Eating Plan" link under Recipe Collections. Click on the link to "In Brief" to get a complete guide.

Potassium Helps Maintain Healthful Blood Pressure

The major mineral potassium is a component of all living cells and is found in both plants and animals. About 85% of the potassium you consume is absorbed, and as with sodium, the kidneys work to regulate its level in the blood.

Potassium is a primary electrolyte within cells, where it balances the sodium outside the cell membrane to maintain proper fluid balance. It also plays a role in regulating the transmission of nerve impulses and, in contrast to sodium, eating a diet high in potassium helps maintain a lower blood pressure.

The best sources of potassium are fresh foods, particularly fresh fruits and vegetables (**FIGURE 7.4**). Processing foods generally increases their sodium and decreases their potassium. You can boost your potassium intake by eating more fresh fruits, vegetables, and whole grains. Most salt substitutes are made from potassium chloride, and these products contain relatively high amounts of potassium.

People with healthy kidneys are able to excrete excess potassium effectively, so toxicity in healthy people is rare. Because potassium is widespread in many foods, a dietary potassium deficiency is also rare. However, potassium deficiency is not uncommon among people who have serious medical disorders, including kidney disease. Extreme dehydration, vomiting, and diarrhea can also cause deficiency, as can abuse of alcohol or laxatives, and use of certain types of diuretics (medications that increase the body's excretion of fluid). Symptoms of potassium deficiency include confusion, loss of appetite, and muscle weakness. Severe deficiency results in fatal changes in heart rate; many deaths attributed to extreme dehydration or to an eating disorder are caused by abnormal heart rhythms due to potassium deficiency.

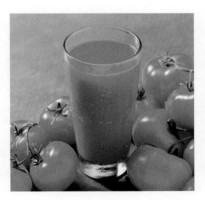

◆ Tomato juice is an excellent source of potassium. Make sure you choose the low-sodium variety!

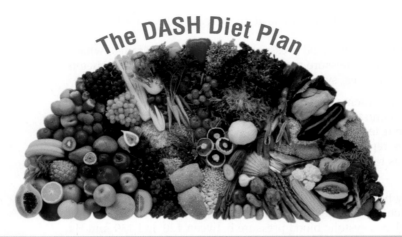

The DASH Diet Plan

Food Group	Daily Servings	Serving Size
Grains and grain products	7–8	1 slice bread 1 cup ready-to-eat cereal* ½ cup cooked rice, pasta, or cereal
Vegetables	4–5	1 cup raw leafy vegetables ½ cup cooked vegetable 6 fl. oz vegetable juice
Fruits	4–5	1 medium fruit ¼ cup dried fruit ½ cup fresh, frozen, or canned fruit 6 fl. oz fruit juice
Low-fat or fat-free dairy foods	2–3	8 fl. oz milk 1 cup yogurt 1½ oz cheese
Lean meats, poultry, and fish	2 or less	3 oz cooked lean meats, skinless poultry, or fish
Nuts, seeds, and dry beans	4–5 per week	⅓ cup or 1½ oz nuts 1 tbsp. or ½ oz seeds ½ cup cooked dry beans
Fats and oils†	2–3	1 tsp. soft margarine 1 tbsp. low-fat mayonnaise 2 tbsp. light salad dressing 1 tsp. vegetable oil
Sweets	5 per week	1 tbsp. sugar 1 tbsp. jelly or jam ½ oz jelly beans 8 fl. oz lemonade

*Serving sizes vary between ½ and 1¼ cups. Check the product's nutrition label.

†Fat content changes serving counts for fats and oils: for example, 1 tablespoon of regular salad dressing equals 1 serving; 1 tablespoon of a low-fat dressing equals ½ serving; 1 tablespoon of a fat-free dressing equals 0 servings.

FIGURE 7.3 **The DASH Eating Plan.** This plan is based on a 2,000 kcal/day diet. The number of servings in a food group may differ from the number listed here, depending on your individual energy needs.

Data adapted from Healthier Eating with DASH. The National Institutes of Health.

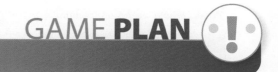

GAME **PLAN**

Tips for Sparing the Salt

If you've decided to try to reduce your intake of sodium, you're probably thinking that the first step is to hide the salt shaker. You're right—limiting the salt you add to foods *is* important! You can train your taste buds to prefer less salt by gradually reducing the amount you use over a period of several days. If you try this, you'll be surprised at how quickly chips, soups, and other foods you once enjoyed start to taste much too salty.

Still, the majority of the sodium in our diet comes from processed food—in other words, from salt that you might not even realize is there. So the next step in reducing your sodium consumption is to shop for fresh, whole foods and cook them with less salt. Here are some tips to get you started.

When Shopping

Next time you stock up on processed foods, keep the following shopping tips in mind:

☐ Look for the words "low sodium" on the label, as well as a sodium amount no higher than 200 mg per serving on the Nutrition Facts panel.

☐ When possible, choose low-sodium alternatives to the following high-sodium foods:

- canned beans, soups, gravies, pasta sauces, soy sauce, other sauces, vegetables, and vegetable juices
- packaged ramen noodle soups and pasta, rice, and potato dishes
- frozen entrées, dinners, pizza, and other frozen meals
- smoked meats and fish
- cheese
- pickles, olives, three-bean salad, salad dressing
- snack foods such as crackers, cookies, potato chips, pretzels, popcorn, and salted nuts

When Cooking

When you have time for a home-cooked meal, take these steps to limit your sodium intake:

☐ Challenge yourself to use primarily fresh ingredients. For instance, try preparing pasta with fresh tomatoes, instead of prepared pasta sauce.

☐ When using canned beans, rinse them with cold water before heating.

☐ Experiment with salt substitutes.

☐ Substitute herbs or spices for salt. The following are particularly useful in low-sodium cooking:

- *basil, oregano, or thyme:* fish, lamb, soups, and sauces
- *black pepper, cayenne pepper, or chili powder:* soups, casserole, cheese sauces, baked egg dishes, barbequed poultry, and lean meats
- *cumin or curry:* meat, chicken, fish, stews, lentils, and beans
- *garlic:* lean meats, fish, poultry, soups, salads, vegetables, and pasta dishes
- *lemon or lime juice:* fish, poultry, salads, vegetables, and sauces

☐ Add ginger or chilies to a stir-fry.

☐ Use cooking wine for meat, poultry, or fish.

☐ Avoid using the "salt" version of any spice, such as garlic salt.

At the Table

- Put the salt shaker out of reach.
- Limit your use of condiments such as catsup, mustard, or pickles.
- When eating out, ask that your food be prepared without salt.
- Don't order soup in a restaurant. Many are loaded with sodium.
- If you order a salad, skip the prepared dressing; use lemon juice and olive oil instead.

Chloride and Phosphorus Also Assist Fluid Balance

Chloride is a major mineral that we obtain almost exclusively from consuming sodium chloride, or table salt. It should not be confused with *chlorine*, which is a poisonous gas used to kill bacteria and other germs in our water supply.

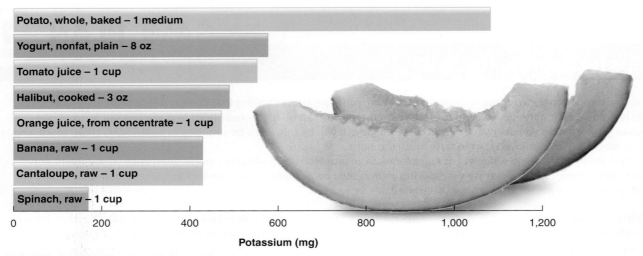

Potato, whole, baked – 1 medium

Yogurt, nonfat, plain – 8 oz

Tomato juice – 1 cup

Halibut, cooked – 3 oz

Orange juice, from concentrate – 1 cup

Banana, raw – 1 cup

Cantaloupe, raw – 1 cup

Spinach, raw – 1 cup

Potassium (mg)

FIGURE 7.4 Common food sources of potassium. The AI for potassium is 4.7 grams (or 4,700 mg) per day.

Data from U.S. Department of Agriculture, Agricultural Research Service. 2011. USDA Nutrient Database for Standard Reference, Release 24.

Coupled with sodium in the fluid outside cells, chloride assists with the maintenance of fluid balance and in the transmission of nerve impulses. Chloride is also a part of hydrochloric acid in the stomach, which aids in digesting food, and it assists white blood cells during an immune response to help kill bacteria.

Although chloride is found in some fruits and vegetables, our primary dietary sources are table salt and the salt in processed foods. There is no known toxicity symptom, and deficiency is rare except during conditions of severe dehydration and frequent vomiting.

Phosphorus is pooled with potassium in the fluid inside cells, where it helps maintain proper fluid balance. As we discuss later in this chapter, phosphorus also plays a critical role in bone formation.

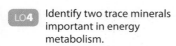 Sodium is a major mineral and is prominent in the fluid outside cells. It helps regulate fluid balance, blood pressure, and nerve function. Excessive sodium intake has been related to hypertension. Potassium is a major mineral in the fluid within cells. Like sodium, it helps regulate fluid balance, blood pressure, and nerve function. Chloride and phosphorus are major minerals that also help maintain fluid balance.

LO4 Identify two trace minerals important in energy metabolism.

LO5 Identify two trace minerals essential for the body's synthesis of thyroid hormones.

Mineral power plants: chromium, manganese, sulfur, iodine, and selenium

Many minerals help our body access the nutrients in foods by assisting their transport into cells or by helping the enzymes essential to energy metabolism. Others assist in the production of hormones that regulate metabolic processes. These minerals are discussed here, and their recommended intakes are listed in Tables 7.1 and 7.2.

Chromium and Manganese Are Important in Metabolism

Chromium is a trace mineral that plays an important role in the breakdown of carbohydrates. It does this by enhancing the ability of insulin to transport glucose from the bloodstream into cells. Chromium also assists in the metabolism of RNA and DNA, in immune function, and in growth. You may be interested to learn that the chromium in our body is the same metal used in the chrome plating for cars!

Chromium supplements have been marketed with claims that they reduce body fat and enhance muscle mass. This marketing has targeted bodybuilders and other athletes interested in improving their body composition. Refer to the ***Nutrition Myth or Fact?*** box to find out if taking supplemental chromium is effective in improving body

nutrition myth or fact?

Do Chromium Supplements Help You Gain Muscle and Lose Weight?

Chromium is one of the most popular additives to weight loss supplements, typically in the form of chromium picolinate. That's because manufacturers claim that chromium increases muscle mass and muscle strength and decreases body fat and weight. What's behind this claim?

More than 20 years ago, a study of chromium supplementation found that chromium use in both untrained men and football players decreased body fat and increased muscle mass, yet a subsequent study found no effect.[1,2]

These contradictory reports led scientists to design more sophisticated studies to assess the effect of chromium on body composition and weight. The early studies had a number of methodological flaws. One major concern was that chromium status was not assessed in the research participants prior to the study. Chromium deficiency at the onset of the study could cause a more positive reaction to chromium than would be expected in people with normal chromium status.

A second major concern was that body composition was measured using the skinfold technique, in which calipers are used to measure the thickness of the skin and fat at various sites on the body. While this method gives a good general estimate of body fat in young, lean, healthy people,

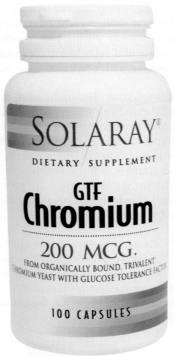

it is not sensitive to small changes in muscle mass. Thus, more sophisticated methods of measuring body composition were necessary.

The results of subsequent research studies have consistently shown that chromium supplementation has no effect on muscle mass, body fat, or muscle strength in a variety of groups, including untrained college males and females, collegiate wrestlers, and older men and women engaged in exercise programs.[3-9] Research has also carefully examined the effect of chromium supplements on weight loss in overweight or obese individuals and found little effect. Two recent reviews of randomized clinical trials (RCT) involving 622–974 participants found that those consuming chromium supplements lost only 1–2 pounds over 8–26 weeks compared to the placebo group.[10,11] Adverse responses to these chromium supplements (in doses ranging from 137–1,000 μg/day) included watery stools, dizziness, headaches, and hives.[11]

As you can see, there is little evidence behind the claims that chromium supplements enhance strength and muscle mass and reduce body fat and weight. Yet these claims result in millions of dollars of sales each year. Don't be fooled: chromium supplementation is nothing more than an expensive nutrition myth.

---

composition. There appears to be no toxicity related to consuming chromium supplements, and chromium deficiency appears to be uncommon in the United States.

A trace mineral, manganese, is involved in energy metabolism and in the formation of urea, the primary component of urine. It also assists in the synthesis of bone tissue and cartilage, a tissue supporting our joints. Manganese also helps protect the body from oxidative damage.

Sulfur Is a Component of Other Nutrients

Sulfur is a major mineral and a component of the B-vitamins thiamin and biotin. In addition, as part of the amino acids methionine and cysteine, sulfur helps the body's proteins maintain their three-dimensional shapes. The liver requires sulfur to assist in the detoxification of alcohol and various drugs, and sulfur helps maintain acid–base balance.

Our body is able to make all the sulfur we need using the amino acids in the protein-containing foods we eat; as a result, we do not need to consume sulfur in the diet, and there is no DRI for it. There are no known toxicity or deficiency symptoms associated with sulfur.

Iodine and Selenium Help Make Thyroid Hormones

Iodine and selenium are trace minerals necessary for the synthesis of thyroid hormones. The body requires thyroid hormones to grow, reproduce, regulate body temperature, and maintain resting metabolic rate.

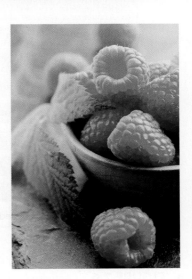

◀ Raspberries are one of the many foods that contain manganese.

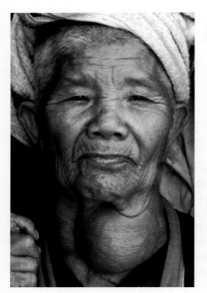

FIGURE 7.5 Goiter, or enlargement of the thyroid gland, occurs with both iodine toxicity and deficiency.

goiter A condition marked by enlargement of the thyroid gland, which can be caused by iodine toxicity or deficiency.

cretinism A form of mental retardation that occurs in people whose mothers experienced iodine deficiency during pregnancy.

Very few foods naturally contain iodine. Saltwater fish do have high amounts, because marine animals concentrate iodine from seawater. In foods, iodine is mostly found in the form of iodide. Good sources include iodized salt and breads made with iodized salt, as well as milk and other dairy products. In the United States, iodine has been added to salt since early in the 20th century to combat iodine deficiency resulting from the poor iodine content of soils in this country. Approximately ½ teaspoon of iodized salt meets the entire adult RDA for iodine.

If you consume either too much or too little iodine, your body will stop manufacturing thyroid hormones, leading to *hypothyroidism,* or low levels of thyroid hormones. This causes enlargement of the thyroid gland, called **goiter**, which occurs when the thyroid gland attempts to produce more thyroid hormones (**FIGURE 7.5**). Other symptoms of hypothyroidism are decreased body temperature, inability to tolerate cold, weight gain, fatigue, and sluggishness. If a woman experiences iodine deficiency during pregnancy, her infant has a high risk of being born with a form of mental retardation referred to as **cretinism**. In addition to mental retardation, people with cretinism may suffer from stunted growth, deafness, and muteness.

The body's selenium is contained in amino acids. In addition to its role in the production of thyroid hormones, selenium works as an antioxidant to spare vitamin E and prevent oxidative damage to cell membranes. Its role in preventing heart disease and certain types of cancer is under investigation.

Selenium is found in varying amounts in soil and thus in foods. Organ meats and nuts are good sources, but the selenium content of fruits and vegetables depends on the level in the soil in which they are grown. Selenium toxicity is rare.[7] Deficiency is associated with rare forms of heart disease and arthritis. See **FIGURE 7.6** for a list of common food sources of selenium.

recap Chromium enhances the ability of insulin to transport glucose from the bloodstream into cells. Manganese is involved in energy metabolism and in the formation of urea, the primary component of urine. Sulfur is a major mineral and a component of the B-vitamins thiamin and biotin. Iodine and selenium assist in the synthesis of thyroid hormones, and selenium has antioxidant properties.

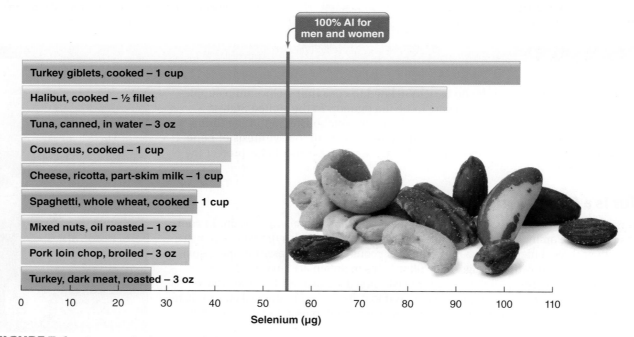

FIGURE 7.6 Common food sources of selenium. The RDA for selenium is 55 μg per day.

Data from U.S. Department of Agriculture, Agricultural Research Service. 2012. USDA Nutrient Database for Standard Reference, Release 25.

The blood fortifiers: iron, zinc, and copper

Without healthy blood to transport nutrients and oxygen to our cells and to remove cellular wastes, we could not survive. Our health and our ability to perform daily activities are compromised if the quantity and quality of our blood are diminished.

Blood is made up of four components (**FIGURE 7.7**):

- Red blood cells (*erythrocytes*) are the cells that transport oxygen.
- White blood cells (*leukocytes*) protect us from infection and illness.
- Platelets are cell fragments that assist in the formation of blood clots and help stop bleeding.
- Plasma is the fluid portion of the blood that carries the blood cells and platelets through the blood vessels.

In addition to vitamin K, the micronutrients recognized as playing a critical role in maintaining blood health include iron, zinc, and copper. Recommended intakes of these three minerals are identified in Table 7.2.

Iron Is a Key Component of Hemoglobin

Iron is a trace mineral that is needed in very small amounts in our diet; nevertheless, it is present in every one of the millions of red blood cells in a single drop of blood.

Why Do We Need Iron?

Iron is critical to healthy blood because it is a key component of **hemoglobin**, which is the oxygen-carrying protein in our red blood cells. As shown in **FIGURE 7.8a**, the hemoglobin molecule consists of four protein strands studded with four iron-containing **heme** groups. Hemoglobin depends on the iron in its heme groups to carry oxygen. In the bloodstream, iron acts as a shuttle, picking up oxygen from the air we breathe, binding it during its transport in the bloodstream, and then dropping it off again in our tissues. Figure 7.8b shows the flattened-disc shape of the red blood cells, which helps them move through the small blood vessels of the body delivering oxygen.

LO6 Explain how the body uses iron, and identify dietary sources and factors affecting its absorption.

LO7 Discuss the role of zinc in metabolism and immune function, and identify common food sources.

Watch a video of red blood cell production from the National Library of Medicine at www.medlineplus.gov. Search on "anatomy videos red blood cell production," then click on "Blood" and locate the video camera icon in the encyclopedia list on the right.

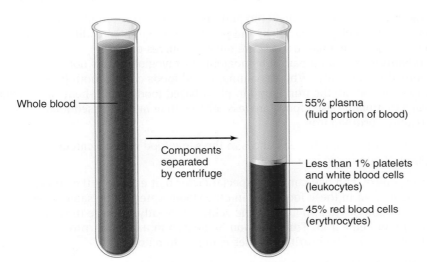

Whole blood

Components separated by centrifuge

55% plasma (fluid portion of blood)

Less than 1% platelets and white blood cells (leukocytes)

45% red blood cells (erythrocytes)

FIGURE 7.7 Blood has four components, which are visible when the blood is drawn into a test tube and spun in a centrifuge. The bottom layer is the red blood cells. The milky layer above the red blood cells contains the white blood cells and the platelets. The yellow fluid on top is the plasma.

hemoglobin The oxygen-carrying protein found in our red blood cells; almost two-thirds of all the iron in our body is found in hemoglobin.

heme The iron-containing molecule found in hemoglobin.

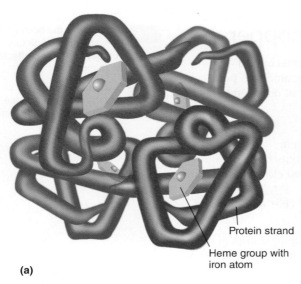

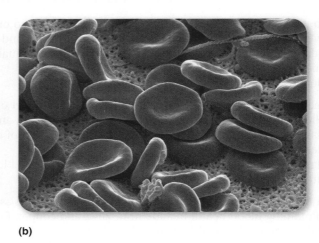

Protein strand

Heme group with
iron atom

(a)

(b)

◆ **FIGURE 7.8**   Hemoglobin. **(a)** Iron is contained in the heme portion of hemoglobin, the protein that forms red blood cells. **(b)** The flattened disc-shape of red blood cells enables them to move more easily through the body's blood vessels.

In addition to being a part of hemoglobin, iron is a component of **myoglobin**, an oxygen-binding protein that functions similarly to hemoglobin but is found in muscle cells. As a part of myoglobin, iron assists in the transport of oxygen into muscle cells, which need oxygen to function.

Finally, iron is found in the body in certain enzymes. As a component of enzymes, it assists energy production from carbohydrates, fats, and protein. Also, iron is part of an antioxidant enzyme system that fights free radicals. Interestingly, excessive iron in the body can also promote the production of free radicals.

What Factors Affect Iron Absorption?

The type of iron in the foods you eat is a major factor influencing your iron absorption—and therefore how much you need to eat. Two types of iron are found in foods:

- **Heme iron** is a part of hemoglobin and myoglobin and is found only in animal-based foods, such as meat, fish, and poultry. Heme iron is readily absorbed by the body. Thus, animal-based foods are reliable sources of iron.
- **Non-heme iron** is not a part of hemoglobin or myoglobin. It is not as easily absorbed by the body. Whereas animal-based foods contain both heme and non-heme iron, all the iron found in plant-based foods is non-heme iron. This means that plant-based foods are less reliable than animal-based foods as sources of readily absorbed iron.

Consumption of certain substances in the same food or meal can enhance the absorption of non-heme iron:

- Meat, poultry, and fish contain a special factor that enhances the absorption of the non-heme iron in these foods and in other foods eaten at the same meal.
- Consumption of vitamin C (ascorbic acid) can greatly increase the body's absorption of non-heme iron. Thus, the non-heme iron in a bean burrito will be more fully absorbed if the burrito includes chopped tomatoes.

Chemicals in certain foods impair iron absorption. These include phytates, which are binding factors found in legumes, rice, and whole grains, and polyphenols, chemicals present in black tea, coffee, and red wine. Soybean protein and calcium also inhibit iron absorption; thus, it is best to avoid drinking soy milk or cow's milk or taking calcium supplements when eating iron-rich foods.

myoglobin An iron-containing protein similar to hemoglobin, except that it is found in muscle cells.

heme iron Iron that is part of hemoglobin and myoglobin; found only in animal-based foods, such as meat, fish, and poultry.

non-heme iron The form of iron that is not a part of hemoglobin or myoglobin; found in animal- and plant-based foods.

Because of these dietary factors, it is estimated that only about 10% of the iron consumed in a vegan diet is absorbed by the body, whereas absorption averages 18% for a mixed Western diet.[2] For this reason, iron requirements are 1.8 times higher for vegetarians than for those who eat a mixed diet. This also means that people who eliminate meat, poultry, and fish from their diet are at a higher risk for anemia than those who eat animal-based foods. This risk is compounded for menstruating females; thus, supplementation or careful meal planning in consultation with a registered dietitian is advised.

What Are Iron Needs and Sources?

The iron requirement for young women is higher than for young men because of the iron in the blood women lose during menstruation each month. Those at the highest risk for iron-deficiency anemia in the United States are toddlers and menstruating girls and women, among whom the prevalence is approximately 2% to 5%.[8] Pregnancy is also a time of very high iron needs, and the RDA for pregnant women is 27 mg per day. A number of other circumstances can reduce iron status, including high levels of vigorous physical activity and any significant blood loss, such as from traumatic injury or blood donation.

Good food sources of heme iron include meats, poultry, and fish, especially clams and oysters. Enriched breakfast cereals and breads and some vegetables and legumes are good sources of non-heme iron. Your body's ability to absorb this non-heme iron can be enhanced by eating these foods with small amounts of meat, fish, or poultry or eating them with vitamin C–rich foods or beverages. **FIGURE 7.9** identifies common food sources of iron. If you need to increase your iron intake, here are some easy ways you can do it:

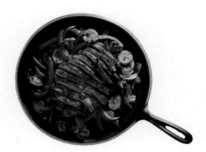

Cooking foods in cast-iron pans significantly increases their iron content.

- Shop for iron-fortified breads and cereals. Check the Nutrition Facts panel!
- Consume a food or beverage that is high in vitamin C along with plant or animal sources of iron.
- Add a small amount of meat, poultry, or fish to baked beans, vegetable soups, stir-fried vegetables or salads to enhance the absorption of the non-heme iron in the plant-based foods.

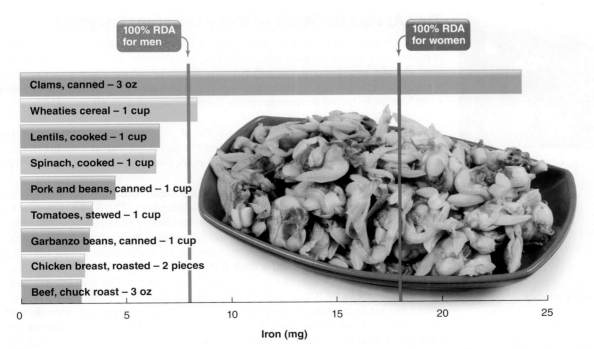

FIGURE 7.9 Common food sources of iron. The RDA for iron is 8 mg/day for men and 18 mg/day for women aged 19 to 50 years.

Data from U.S. Department of Agriculture, Agricultural Research Service. 2014. USDA Nutrient Database for Standard Reference, Release 26.

- Avoid drinking red wine, coffee, tea, cow's milk, or soy milk when eating iron-rich foods because compounds in these beverages reduce iron absorption.
- Avoid taking calcium or zinc supplements with iron-rich foods because these minerals decrease iron absorption.
- Cook foods in cast-iron pans to increase their iron content.

What Happens If We Consume Too Much or Too Little Iron?

Some iron-containing supplements resemble colorful candies, and accidental iron overdose is the most common cause of poisoning deaths in children younger than 6 years of age in the United States.[9] It is important for parents to take the same precautions with dietary supplements that they would take with other drugs, keeping them in a locked cabinet or well out of reach of children. Symptoms of iron toxicity include nausea, vomiting, diarrhea, dizziness, confusion, and rapid heartbeat. If iron toxicity is not treated quickly, significant damage to the heart, central nervous system, liver, and kidneys can result in death.

Adults who take iron supplements even at prescribed doses commonly experience constipation. Taking vitamin C with the iron supplement not only enhances absorption but also can help reduce constipation.

Iron deficiency is the most common nutrient deficiency in the world. It results in **iron-deficiency anemia**, a disorder in which the red blood cells are not able to deliver to the body's cells and tissues all the oxygen they need. Symptoms include exhaustion, increased risk for infection, and impaired thinking. Severe, chronic iron deficiency can cause premature death. People at particularly high risk include infants and young children, menstruating girls and women, and pregnant women. Sensible choices for meals and snacks can help you get all the iron you need all day—and avoid deficiency.

recap Iron is a trace mineral that, as part of the hemoglobin protein, transports oxygen in our blood. Meat, fish, and poultry are good sources of heme iron, which is more absorbable than non-heme iron. Iron deficiency is the most common nutrient deficiency in the world.

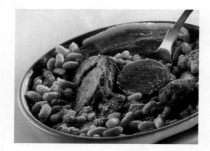

⬥ Zinc can be found in pork and beans.

iron-deficiency anemia A disorder in which the production of normal, healthy red blood cells decreases and hemoglobin levels are inadequate to fully oxygenate the body's cells and tissues.

Zinc Assists the Work of Many Different Enzymes

Zinc is a trace mineral that assists the work of approximately 100 different enzymes involved in many different tasks, including metabolism, the production of hemoglobin, and the activation of vitamin A in the retina of the eye. Zinc is also critical for normal growth. In fact, zinc deficiency was discovered in the early 1960s when researchers were trying to determine the cause of severe growth retardation in a group of Middle Eastern men.

Zinc also supports the proper development and functioning of the immune system. This role in immune functioning is behind the development of zinc lozenges, which manufacturers say help fight the common cold. See the ***Nutrition Myth or Fact?*** box to find out whether these are effective.

As with iron, our need for zinc is relatively small, but our absorption is variable. High non-heme iron intake can inhibit zinc absorption. This is a serious concern for anyone taking iron supplements (which are composed of non-heme iron), but especially for pregnant women, in whom zinc is essential for normal fetal growth. Thus, consultation with a registered dietitian may be advisable. Zinc absorption is also a concern for many vegetarians, whose diets are typically rich in non-heme iron. In addition, vegetarians tend to consume plentiful whole grains and beans: these foods contain phytates and fiber, both of which also inhibit zinc absorption. When whole grains are made into bread using yeast, the yeast produces an enzyme that breaks down the phytates. Thus, the zinc in whole-grain breads is more available for absorption than that found in breakfast cereals. In contrast, high intakes of heme iron appear to have no effect on zinc absorption, and dietary protein, especially animal-based protein, enhances zinc absorption.

nutrition myth or fact?

Do Zinc Lozenges Help Fight the Common Cold?

The common cold has plagued human beings since the beginning of time, with approximately 1 billion cases of the common cold occurring each year in the United States.[12] Children suffer from 6 to 10 colds each year, and adults average 2 to 4 per year.[13] Although colds are typically benign, they result in significant absenteeism from school and work and cause discomfort and stress. It is estimated that more than 200 different viruses can cause a cold, so developing vaccines or treatments for colds is extremely challenging.[13] Nevertheless, researchers continue to attempt to search for a cure for the common cold.

The role of zinc in the health of our immune system is well known, and zinc has been shown to inhibit the reproduction of viruses that cause the common cold. These findings led to the formulation of zinc supplements to reduce the length and severity of colds.[14,15] Consequently, zinc lozenges were formulated as a means of providing potential relief from cold symptoms. These lozenges are readily found in most drugstores.

Does taking zinc in lozenge form actually reduce the length and severity of a cold? During the past 25 years, numerous research studies have been conducted to try to answer this question. Unfortunately, the results of these studies have been mixed. Two recent reviews examined thirteen randomized controlled trials with over 966 participants.[16,17] They found a reduction of the duration of the common cold with zinc lozenges or syrups (30–160 mg/day) if administered within 24 hours of the onset of cold symptoms.[18] Overall, the duration of the cold was reduced by about 1 day. Assessment of the severity of cold symptoms is more difficult, because there is no objective measure for assessing severity. However, study participants reported significant negative effects from zinc supplementation as well, including a bad taste and nausea.

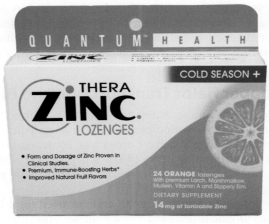

▲ Zinc lozenges come in various formulations and dosages.

Unfortunately, we will probably never know the true effect of zinc lozenges on colds for the following reasons:

- *It is difficult to truly "blind" participants to the treatment.* Because zinc lozenges have a unique taste, research participants may know whether they are getting zinc lozenges or a placebo. This could bias the study results.
- *Self-reported symptoms are subject to inaccuracy.* Many studies had the research participants self-report changes in symptoms, which may be inaccurate and influenced by mood and other emotional factors.
- *A wide variety of viruses cause the common cold.* Because more than 200 viruses can cause a cold, it is possible that people who do not respond favorably to zinc lozenges are suffering from a cold virus that does not respond to zinc.
- *Zinc formulations and dosages differ.* It is estimated that, for zinc lozenges to be effective, at least 80 mg of zinc should be consumed each day and people should begin them within 24 hours of the onset of cold symptoms, yet the studies varied in how subjects took the lozenges.[18] Also, sweeteners and flavorings found in zinc lozenge formulations may bind the zinc, limiting its absorption and effectiveness.

Have you ever tried zinc lozenges, and did you find them effective? Even if you were certain you could reduce the length of your cold by 1 day by taking zinc lozenges, next time you felt a cold coming on, would you try them?

One word of caution: if you decide to use zinc lozenges, more is not better. Excessive or prolonged zinc supplementation can depress immune function and cause other mineral imbalances. Check the label of the product you are using, and do not exceed its recommended dosage or duration of use.

Good food sources of zinc include red meats, some seafood, whole-grain breads, and enriched foods. As shown in **FIGURE 7.10**, zinc is significantly more absorbable from animal-based foods; thus, zinc deficiency is a concern for vegetarians.

Zinc toxicity is unlikely unless a person is consuming zinc in supplements and in highly fortified foods. Toxicity symptoms include intestinal pain and cramps, nausea, vomiting, loss of appetite, diarrhea, and headaches. Excessive zinc supplementation has also been shown to depress immune function. High intakes of zinc can also reduce the absorption of copper.

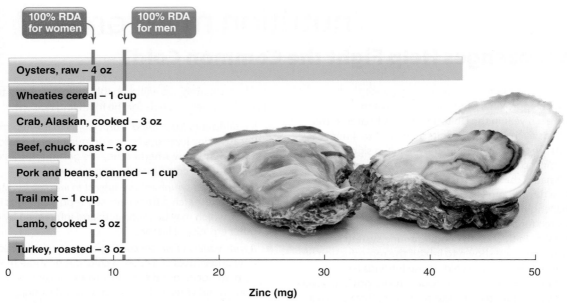

FIGURE 7.10 Common food sources of zinc. The RDA for zinc is 11 mg/day for men and 8 mg/day for women.

Data from U.S. Department of Agriculture, Agricultural Research Service. 2011. USDA Nutrient Database for Standard Reference, Release 24.

In addition to growth retardation, symptoms of zinc deficiency include diarrhea, delayed sexual maturation and impotence, eye and skin lesions, hair loss, and impaired appetite. Because zinc is critical to a healthy immune system, zinc deficiency also results in increased incidence of infections and illnesses.

Copper Helps Transport Iron and Build Tissues

Copper is a component of *ceruloplasmin*, a protein that is critical for the proper transport of iron. If ceruloplasmin levels are inadequate, iron accumulation results and can lead to iron toxicity. Copper also contributes to blood tissue, collagen, and the tissue surrounding nerve fibers. It is part of several enzyme systems and contributes to chemicals called *neurotransmitters*, which are important for transmitting nerve signals.

Copper is a trace mineral, and our need for it is very small. Nevertheless, high intakes of zinc or iron can reduce copper absorption and, subsequently, copper status. Food sources of copper include organ meats, seafood, nuts, seeds, and whole-grain products. The long-term effects of copper toxicity are not well studied in humans. Copper deficiency is rare.

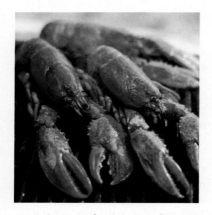

Lobster is a food source of copper.

recap Zinc is a trace mineral that is a part of almost 100 enzymes that affect virtually every body system. Zinc plays a critical role in hemoglobin synthesis, physical growth, sexual maturation, and immune function and assists in fighting the oxidative damage caused by free radicals. Copper is a trace mineral that is important in the transport of iron. It also contributes to several tissues and is part of several enzyme systems.

LO8 Identify the four mineral components of bone and explain how bone is formed and maintained.

LO9 State the four primary functions of calcium.

The bone builders: calcium, phosphorus, magnesium, and fluoride

Contrary to what most people think, our skeleton is not an inactive collection of bones that simply holds the body together. Bones are living organs with many functions. Structurally, they provide physical support, attachments for muscle movement, and protection for vulnerable organs. Think of the hard shell that our skull forms around our eyes and our brain, or the bony cage of ribs that protects the heart and lungs. Bones also act as "mineral banks," storing calcium, phosphorus, magnesium, and fluoride. When these minerals are needed for body processes, bone is broken down, so that they can be released into our bloodstream. Also, did you know that most of our blood cells are formed deep within bones?

You've learned that both vitamin D and vitamin K play roles in bone health. In addition, four minerals—calcium, phosphorus, magnesium, and fluoride—help us maintain strong bones.

Bones Are Made of Minerals and Proteins

We tend to think of bones as totally rigid, but if they were, how could we play basketball or even carry an armload of books up a flight of stairs? Bones need to be both strong and flexible, so that they can resist the crunching, stretching, and twisting that occur throughout our daily activities. Fortunately, the composition of bone is ideally suited for its complex job. About 65% of bone tissue is made up of an assortment of minerals (mostly calcium and phosphorus) that provide hardness. These minerals form tiny crystals that cluster around *collagen fibers*—protein fibers that provide strength, durability, and flexibility. Collagen fibers are phenomenally strong; they are actually stronger than steel fibers of similar size. They enable bones to bear weight while responding to demands for movement.

If you examine a bone very closely, you will notice two distinct types of tissue **(FIGURE 7.11)**: cortical bone and trabecular bone. **Cortical bone**, which is also called *compact bone*, is very dense. It composes approximately 80% of the skeleton. The outer surface of all bones is cortical; in addition, many small bones of the body, such as the bones of the wrists, hands, and feet, are made entirely of cortical bone.

In contrast, **trabecular bone** makes up only 20% of the skeleton. It is found in the ends of the long bones (such as the bones of the arms and legs) and inside the spinal vertebrae, skull, pelvis, and several other bones. Trabecular bone is sometimes referred to as *spongy bone,* because to the naked eye it looks like a sponge. The microscope reveals that trabecular bone is, in fact, aligned in a precise network of columns that protects the bone from extreme stress. You can think of trabecular bone as the bone's scaffolding.

How Do Bones Stay Healthy?

Although the shape and size of bones do not significantly change after puberty, **bone density**—the compactness and strength of bones—continues to develop into early adulthood. *Peak bone density* is the point at which bones are strongest because they are at their highest density. About 90% of a woman's bone density is built by 17 years of age. For men, peak bone density occurs during their twenties. However, male or female, before we reach the age of 30 years, our bones have reached peak density, and by age 40, our bone density has begun its irreversible decline.

Just as other body cells die off and are continually replaced, bone mass is regularly recycled. This process, called **remodeling**, involves two steps: the breakdown of existing bone and the formation of new bone **(FIGURE 7.12)**. Bone is broken down by cells called **osteoclasts**, which erode the bone surface by secreting enzymes and acids that dig grooves into the bone matrix (Figure 7.12a). New bone is formed through the action of cells called **osteoblasts**, or "bone builders" (Figure 7.12b). These cells work to synthesize new bone matrix in the eroded areas.

In young, healthy adults, bone building and bone breakdown occur at equal rates, resulting in bone mass being maintained. Around 40 years of age, bone breakdown begins to outpace bone formation, and this imbalance results in a gradual loss in bone density.

Achieving a high peak bone density requires adequate intake of the four minerals discussed in this section, and recommended intakes are identified in Tables 7.1 and 7.2. Adequate protein and vitamins D and K are also essential. In addition to nutrients, healthy bone density requires regular weight-bearing exercise, such as weight

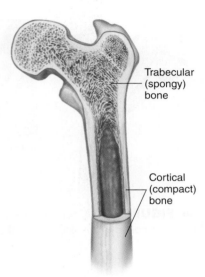

Trabecular (spongy) bone

Cortical (compact) bone

FIGURE 7.11 The structure of bone. Notice the difference in density between the trabecular (spongy) bone and the cortical (compact) bone.

cortical bone A dense bone tissue that makes up the outer surface of all bones as well as the entirety of most small bones of the body; also called compact bone.

trabecular bone A porous bone tissue found within the ends of the long bones, as well as inside the spinal vertebrae, flat bones (breastbone, ribs, and most bones of the skull), and bones of the pelvis; also called spongy bone.

bone density The degree of compactness of bone tissue, reflecting the strength of the bones. *Peak bone density* is the point at which a bone is strongest.

remodeling The two-step process by which bone tissue is recycled; includes the breakdown of existing bone and the formation of new bone.

osteoclasts Cells that break down the surface of bones by secreting enzymes and acids that dig grooves into the bone matrix.

osteoblasts Cells that prompt the formation of new bone matrix by laying down the collagen-containing component of bone, which is then mineralized.

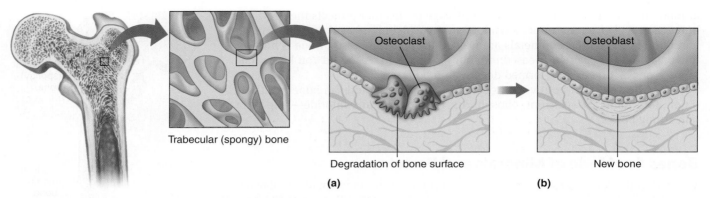

▲ FIGURE 7.12 Bone remodeling involves breakdown and formation. **(a)** Osteoclasts break down bone, releasing minerals, which are then transported to the bloodstream. **(b)** Osteoblasts work to build new bone by filling the pit formed by the erosion process with new bone.

lifting, strength training, rope jumping, tennis, jogging and walking, and even jumping jacks, all of which appropriately stress the bones and stimulate their growth.

recap Bones are composed of mineral crystals that cluster around collagen fibers. Bone tissue is recycled through a process called remodeling, in which osteoclasts break down old bone and osteoblasts lay down new bone.

Calcium Is a Key Component of Bones

Calcium is by far the most abundant major mineral in the body, composing about 2% of our entire body weight! Not surprisingly, it plays many critical roles in maintaining overall function and health.

Why Do We Need Calcium?

Calcium has four primary roles in the body. First, it provides structure to the bones and teeth. About 99% of the calcium in the body is stored in the bones, packed into crystals built up on the collagen foundation. The remaining 1% is found in the blood and soft tissues.

Calcium is alkaline, or basic, and because of this property it plays a critical role in assisting with acid–base balance. If the blood becomes acidic, osteoclasts begin to break down bone. This releases calcium into the bloodstream, making it more alkaline. It's important to consume enough dietary calcium to make sure it balances the calcium taken from the bones.

Calcium is an electrolyte critical for the normal transmission of nerve impulses. When it flows into nerve cells, it stimulates the release of neurotransmitters, chemicals that transfer nerve impulses across the gap (synapse) separating one nerve cell from the next. Without adequate calcium, the ability of nerves to transmit messages is inhibited. Not surprisingly, when blood calcium levels fall dangerously low, a person can experience seizures.

A fourth role of calcium is to assist in muscle contraction. Contraction of muscles is stimulated when calcium flows into the muscle cell. Muscles relax when calcium is pumped back outside the muscle cell.

Other roles of calcium include the maintenance of healthy blood pressure, the initiation of blood clotting, and the regulation of various hormones and enzymes. As you can see, calcium is a versatile micronutrient.

How Much Calcium Is Absorbed?

The term **bioavailability** refers to the degree to which the body can absorb and use any given nutrient. Healthy men and non-pregnant women, across a wide age range, absorb about 30% of the calcium they consume; however, absorption may decrease slightly

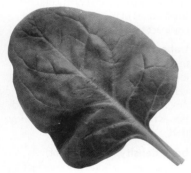

▲ Although spinach contains high levels of calcium, binding factors in the plant prevent much of its absorption.

bioavailability The degree to which our body can absorb and use any given nutrient.

with age.[10] This decrease in calcium absorption with aging and the need to maintain bone as one ages explain the higher calcium recommendations for older adults.

The body is limited in the amount of calcium it can absorb at any one time, and as the amount of calcium in a single meal or supplement goes up, the fraction that is absorbed goes down. Thus, it is important to consume calcium-rich foods throughout the day, rather than relying on a single high-dose supplement.

As with iron, dietary factors can affect the absorption of calcium. Binding factors, such as phytates and oxalates, occur naturally in some calcium-rich seeds, nuts, grains, and vegetables (such as spinach and Swiss chard). Such factors can limit calcium absorption. Additionally, consuming calcium at the same time as iron, zinc, magnesium, or phosphorus has the potential to interfere with the absorption and use of all of these minerals. Finally, because vitamin D is necessary for the absorption of calcium, lack of vitamin D severely limits the bioavailability of calcium. To learn more about how calcium absorption rates vary for select foods, see the *Nutrition Label Activity* box.

What Are Calcium Needs and Sources?

The DRIs for calcium are listed in Table 7.1. Many people in the United States do not meet the DRI, because they consume very few dairy-based foods and calcium-rich vegetables. At particular risk are menstruating women and growing girls. There are quick, simple tools available to assist you in estimating your daily calcium intake.

Dairy products are among the most common and best-absorbed sources of calcium in the U.S. diet. Skim milk, low-fat cheeses, and nonfat yogurt are excellent sources of calcium, and they are low in fat and energy. Greek yogurt provides calcium, although less than regular varieties. Cottage cheese is one dairy product that is a relatively poor source of calcium, most of which is lost in processing. Other food sources of absorbable calcium are canned fish with bones (providing that you eat the bones) and green leafy vegetables, such as kale, turnip greens, collard greens, broccoli, and Chinese cabbage (bok choy). These vegetables contain low levels of oxalates. Many beverages are fortified with calcium. For example, you can buy calcium-fortified orange juice, fruit punch, soy milk, almond milk, and rice milk. Some dairies have even boosted the amount of calcium in their brand of milk. See **FIGURE 7.13** for other common food sources of calcium.

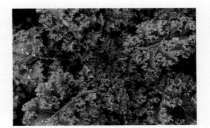

Kale is a good source of calcium.

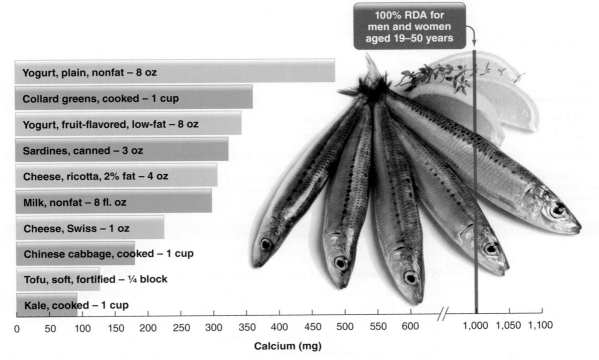

FIGURE 7.13 Common food sources of calcium. The RDA for calcium is 1,000 mg/day for men and women aged 19 to 50.

Data from U.S. Department of Agriculture, Agricultural Research Service. 2012. USDA Nutrient Database for Standard Reference, Release 25.

nutrition label activity

How Much Calcium Am I Really Getting?

As you have learned in this chapter, we do not absorb 100% of the calcium contained in foods. This is particularly true for individuals who eat lots of foods high in fiber, oxalates, and phytates, such as whole grains and certain vegetables. So if you want to design an eating plan that contains adequate calcium, it's important to understand how the rate of calcium absorption differs for the foods you include.

Although the absorption rate of calcium has not been determined for all foods, estimates have been established for common foods that are considered good sources of calcium. The accompanying table shows some of these foods, their calcium content per serving, their calcium absorption rate, and the estimated amount of calcium absorbed.

As you can see from this table, many dairy products have a similar calcium absorption rate, just over 30%. Interestingly, many green, leafy vegetables have a higher absorption rate of around 60%; however, because a typical serving of these foods contains less calcium than a serving of dairy foods, you

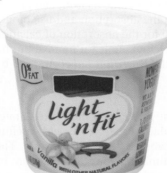

⬆ Low-fat and nonfat yogurts are excellent sources of calcium.

would have to eat more vegetables to get the same calcium as you would from a standard serving of dairy foods. Note the relatively low absorption rate for spinach, even though it contains a relatively high amount of calcium. This is due to the high levels of oxalates in spinach, which bind with calcium and reduce its bioavailability.

Remember that the DRIs for calcium take these differences in absorption rate into account. Thus, the 300 mg of calcium in a glass of milk counts as 300 mg toward your daily calcium goal. In general, you can trust that dairy products such as milk and yogurt (but not cottage cheese) are good, absorbable sources of calcium, as are most dark-green, leafy vegetables. Other dietary sources of calcium with good absorption rates include calcium-fortified orange juice, soy milk, almond milk, and rice milk; tofu processed with calcium; and fortified breakfast cereals.[19] Armed with this knowledge, you will be better able to select food sources that can optimize your calcium intake and support your bone health.

Food	Serving Size	Calcium per Serving (mg)*	Absorption Rate (%)[†]	Estimated Amount of Calcium Absorbed (mg)
Yogurt, plain skim milk	6 fl. oz	338	32	108
Yogurt, Greek skim milk	6 fl. oz	187	32	60
Milk, skim	8 fl. oz	306	32	98
Milk, 2%	8 fl. oz	285	32	91
Soymilk, calcium fortified	8 fl. oz	300	24	72
Kale, frozen, cooked	1 cup	179	59	106
Turnip greens, boiled	1 cup	197	52	103
Broccoli, frozen, chopped, cooked	1 cup	61	61	37
Cauliflower, boiled	1 cup	20	69	14
Spinach, frozen, cooked	1 cup	291	5	14

*Data from U.S. Department of Agriculture, Agricultural Research Service. 2009–2014. USDA National Nutrient Database for Standard Reference, Release 22–26. http://ndb.nal.usda.gov/

[†]Keller J. L., A. J. Lanou, and N. D. Barnard. 2002. The consumer cost of calcium from food and supplements. *JAND* 102:1669–1671; Weaver, C. M., W. R. Proulx, and R. Heaney. 1999. Choices for achieving adequate dietary calcium with a vegetarian diet. *Am. J. Clin. Nutr.* 70(suppl.):543S–548S; Weaver, C. M., and K. L. Plawecki. 1994. Dietary calcium: adequacy of a vegetarian diet. *Am. J. Clin. Nutr.* 59(suppl.):1238S–1241S.

What Happens If We Consume Too Much or Too Little Calcium?

In general, consuming extra calcium from food sources does not lead to significant toxicity symptoms in healthy people, because much of the excess calcium is excreted in urine and feces. However, excessive intake of calcium from supplements can lead to various mineral imbalances, because calcium interferes with the absorption of other minerals, including iron, zinc, and magnesium. It can also cause constipation, as the body attempts to eliminate the excess calcium via the feces. Severe hypercalcemia (excessive calcium in the blood) can lead to death.

foods you don't know you love YET

Kefir

A slightly tart, fermented beverage, kefir (commonly pronounced KEE-fer) is like a drinkable yogurt—only some claim it's better! That's because—depending on the way it's formulated—it can contain more strains of helpful bacteria in a greater quantity than is found in traditional yogurts, as well as beneficial yeasts that can compete with species that cause illness. Its curd size is smaller than that of yogurt, so people may find it even easier to digest. Moreover, some brands of kefir provide more calcium than the same-size serving of milk or yogurt and are rich in magnesium, phosphorus, and several vitamins, making kefir an excellent choice for supporting bone health. Kefir is sold in most large supermarkets in plain or fruit flavors. It's naturally thick, so you can blend it with chunks of banana, strawberries, or other sweet fruits for a delicious and easy smoothie.

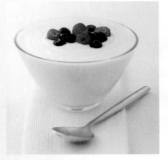

There are no short-term symptoms associated with consuming too little calcium. When dietary calcium is low, the body maintains blood calcium levels by taking calcium from the bones. The long-term consequence of inadequate calcium intake is osteoporosis. This disease is discussed in more detail shortly. To keep your bones as dense as possible, it's important to make calcium-rich menu choices, that are also low in fat and Calories, throughout the day.

recap Calcium is the most abundant mineral in the body and a significant component of bones. Bone calcium is used to maintain normal blood calcium if dietary intake is inadequate. Calcium is also necessary for acid–base balance and normal nerve and muscle function. Dairy foods, calcium-fortified juices and soy milk, and some dark-green leafy vegetables are excellent sources of calcium.

Phosphorus Is Part of the Mineral Complex of Bone

As we mentioned earlier, the major mineral phosphorus is an electrolyte that works with potassium inside cells to help regulate fluid balance and nerve and muscle function. It also plays a critical role in bone formation, because it is a part of the mineral crystals that provide the hardness of bone. About 85% of the body's phosphorus is stored in bones, with the rest stored in soft tissues, such as muscles and organs.

Additionally, phosphorus is a primary component of adenosine triphosphate (ATP), the energy molecule. It also helps activate and deactivate enzymes and is a component of the genetic material in the cells (including both DNA and RNA), cell membranes, and lipoproteins.

Phosphorus is widespread in many foods and is found in high amounts in foods that contain protein **(FIGURE 7.14)**. Milk, meats, and eggs are good sources. Phosphorus is also added to many processed foods, where it enhances smoothness, binding, and moisture retention. In the form of phosphoric acid, it is also a major component of soft drinks. Many researchers have linked the consumption of soft drinks to poor bone density. The most likely explanation for this link appears to be the *milk-displacement effect;* that is, soft drinks take the place of milk in our diet, depriving us of calcium and vitamin D.[11]

Severely high levels of phosphorus in the blood can cause muscle spasms and convulsions. Phosphorus deficiencies are rare but can occur in people who abuse alcohol, in premature infants, and in elderly people with a poor diet.

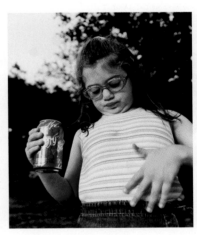

Phosphorus, in the form of phosphoric acid, is a major component of soft drinks.

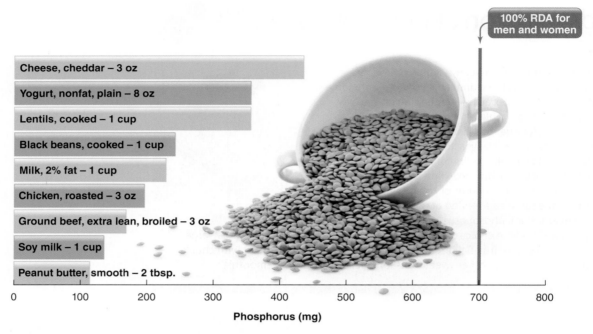

100% RDA for men and women

Cheese, cheddar – 3 oz
Yogurt, nonfat, plain – 8 oz
Lentils, cooked – 1 cup
Black beans, cooked – 1 cup
Milk, 2% fat – 1 cup
Chicken, roasted – 3 oz
Ground beef, extra lean, broiled – 3 oz
Soy milk – 1 cup
Peanut butter, smooth – 2 tbsp.

0   100   200   300   400   500   600   700   800

Phosphorus (mg)

FIGURE 7.14 Common food sources of phosphorus. The AI for phosphorus is 700 mg/day.

Data from U.S. Department of Agriculture, Agricultural Research Service. 2011. USDA Nutrient Database for Standard Reference, Release 24.

Magnesium Is Found in Bones and Soft Tissues

Magnesium is a major mineral. About 50% to 60% of the magnesium in the body is found in bones, and the rest is in soft tissues. Magnesium influences the crystallization of bone through its regulation of calcium balance and its interactions with vitamin D and parathyroid hormone.

Magnesium assists more than 300 enzyme systems with roles in the production of ATP, as well as DNA and protein synthesis and repair. It also supports muscle contraction and blood clotting.

Magnesium is found in green leafy vegetables, such as spinach, and in whole grains, seeds, and nuts. Other good sources include seafood, beans, and some dairy products (**FIGURE 7.15**). The magnesium content of drinking water varies considerably: the "harder" the water, the higher its content of magnesium.

Considering magnesium's role in bone formation, it is not surprising that long-term magnesium deficiency is associated with osteoporosis. Magnesium deficiency can also cause muscle cramps, spasms or seizures, nausea, weakness, irritability, and confusion. It may result from kidney disease, chronic diarrhea, or chronic alcohol abuse but is uncommon in healthy adults, except those who regularly consume too much fiber. As you know, dietary fiber is important to health; however, fiber binds magnesium, reducing the ability of the small intestine to absorb it. Thus, magnesium deficiency can occur in people who consume a diet with excessive fiber. To avoid magnesium deficiency, consume the recommended amount of fiber each day (19 to 38 grams per day, depending on life stage and gender).

Magnesium toxicity is rare except in people consuming high-potency supplements. Symptoms of magnesium toxicity include diarrhea, nausea, and abdominal cramps. In extreme cases, toxicity can result in acid–base imbalances, massive dehydration, cardiac arrest, and death.

Fluoride Supports Our Teeth and Bones

Fluoride is a trace mineral. About 99% of the fluoride in the body is stored in teeth and bones. During the development of both baby teeth and permanent teeth, fluoride combines with calcium and phosphorus to make teeth more

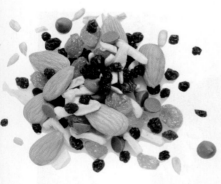

Trail mix with chocolate chips, nuts, and seeds is one common food source of magnesium.

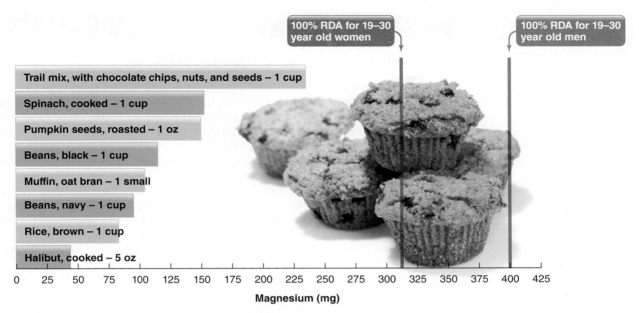

Trail mix, with chocolate chips, nuts, and seeds – 1 cup

Spinach, cooked – 1 cup

Pumpkin seeds, roasted – 1 oz

Beans, black – 1 cup

Muffin, oat bran – 1 small

Beans, navy – 1 cup

Rice, brown – 1 cup

Halibut, cooked – 5 oz

100% RDA for 19–30 year old women

100% RDA for 19–30 year old men

0 25 50 75 100 125 150 175 200 225 250 275 300 325 350 375 400 425

Magnesium (mg)

FIGURE 7.15 Common food sources of magnesium. For adult men 19 to 30 years of age, the RDA for magnesium is 400 mg/day; the RDA increases to 420 mg per day for men 31 years of age and older. For adult women 19 to 30 years of age, the RDA for magnesium is 310 mg per day; this value increases to 320 mg per day for women 31 years of age and older.

Data from U.S. Department of Agriculture, Agricultural Research Service. 2012. USDA Nutrient Database for Standard Reference, Release 25.

resistant to destruction by acids and bacteria. Thus, teeth that have been treated with fluoride are better protected against dental caries (cavities) than teeth that have not been treated. Fluoride also stimulates new bone growth, and it is currently being researched as a potential treatment for osteoporosis.

The two primary sources of fluoride for people in the United States are fluoridated water and fluoridated dental products, such as toothpastes and mouthwashes. Fluoride supplements are available only by prescription, and they are generally given only to children who do not have access to fluoridated water. Tea also contains significant amounts of fluoride independent of whether it was made with fluoridated water. There is epidemiological evidence that people who habitually consume tea (for more than 6 years) have significantly higher bone density values than people who are not habitual tea drinkers.[12,13]

Consuming too much fluoride increases the protein content of tooth enamel, resulting in a condition called **fluorosis**. Because increased protein makes the enamel more porous, the teeth become stained and pitted (**FIGURE 7.16**). Teeth seem to be at highest risk for fluorosis during the first 8 years of life. Mild fluorosis generally causes white patches on the teeth. However, neither mild nor moderate fluorosis appears to impair tooth function.[2]

The primary result of fluoride deficiency is an increased risk for dental caries.[10] Adequate fluoride intake appears necessary at an early age and throughout adult life to reduce the risk for tooth decay. Inadequate fluoride intake may also be associated with lower bone density, but there is not enough research currently available to support the widespread use of fluoride to prevent osteoporosis.

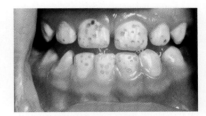

FIGURE 7.16 Consuming too much fluoride causes fluorosis, leading to staining and pitting of the teeth.

recap The major mineral phosphorus helps maintain fluid balance and bone health and is found in many high-protein foods. Magnesium is a major mineral important for bone health, energy production, and nerve and muscle function and is found in a wide variety of foods. Fluoride is a trace mineral that supports the health of teeth and bones. Primary sources of fluoride are fluoridated dental products and fluoridated water.

fluorosis A condition marked by staining and pitting of the teeth; caused by an abnormally high intake of fluoride.

LO10 Discuss the risk factors and available treatments for osteoporosis.

Are you at risk for osteoporosis?

Of the many disorders associated with poor bone health, the most prevalent one in the United States is **osteoporosis**. The bone tissue of a person with osteoporosis is more porous and thinner than that of a person with healthy bone. These structural changes weaken the bone, leading to a significantly reduced ability to bear weight and a high risk for fractures **(FIGURE 7.17)**.

Osteoporosis is the single most important cause of fractures of the hip and spine in older adults. These fractures are extremely painful and can be debilitating, with many individuals requiring nursing home care. In addition, they cause an increased risk for infection and other illnesses that can lead to premature death. Osteoporosis of the spine also causes a generalized loss of height and can be disfiguring: gradual compression fractures in the vertebrae of the upper back lead to a shortening and rounding of the spine called *kyphosis,* commonly referred to as *dowager's hump* **(FIGURE 7.18)**.

Unfortunately, osteoporosis is a common disease: worldwide, one in two women and one in four men over the age of 50 are affected, and in the United States, more than 10 million people have been diagnosed.[14]

Risk Factors for Osteoporosis

The following factors influence the risk for osteoporosis:

- *Age:* Bone density declines with age, so low bone mass and osteoporosis are significant health concerns for both older men and women. Reproductive hormones in men and women play important roles in promoting the deposition of new bone and limiting the activity of osteoclasts. With aging, the production of reproductive hormones decreases. This makes bone more sensitive to osteoclasts, and a gradual loss of bone mass occurs. Although both men and women are affected, the change is more dramatic in women, who can lose 20% of their bone mass during the first 5 to 7 years following menopause.[14,15] In addition, reduced levels of physical activity in older people and a decreased ability to metabolize vitamin D with age exacerbate hormone-related bone loss.

- *Gender:* About 80% of Americans with osteoporosis are women. This greater prevalence is due not only to women's more dramatic age-related decline in

osteoporosis A disease characterized by low bone mass and deterioration of bone tissue, leading to increased bone fragility and fracture risk.

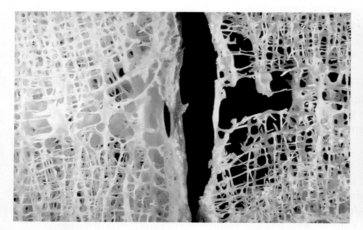

⬆ **FIGURE 7.17** The vertebra of a person with osteoporosis (right) is thinner and more collapsed than the vertebra of a healthy person (left), in which the bone is more dense and uniform.

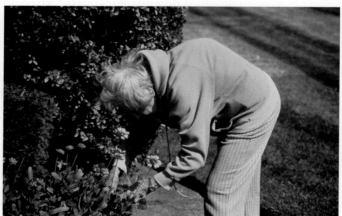

⬆ **FIGURE 7.18** Gradual compression of the vertebrae in the upper back causes a shortening and rounding of the spine called *kyphosis.*

reproductive hormones. It's also explained by the fact that women have a lower bone density than men to begin with, and they live longer than men. Secondary factors include social pressure on girls to be thin, which can lead to extreme dieting. This in turn can result in poor nutrition and amenorrhea (no menstrual period), which reduces the positive impact of reproductive hormones on bone. Extreme dieting is particularly harmful in adolescence, when bone mass is building and adequate consumption of nutrients is critical. In contrast, men experience pressure to "bulk up," typically by lifting weights. This puts healthful stress on the bones, resulting in increased density.

- *Genetics:* A family history of osteoporosis increases the risk for this disease. Particularly at risk are Caucasian women of low body weight who have a first-degree relative (mother or sister) with osteoporosis. Asian women are also at high risk.
- *Smoking:* Cigarette smoking is known to decrease bone density because of its effects on the hormones that influence bone remodeling; thus, cigarette smoking increases the risk for osteoporosis.
- *Nutrition:* Nutritional factors that appear to affect the risk for osteoporosis include total energy intake, protein, calcium, vitamin D, and fruits and vegetables.[16] Excess dieting and inadequate energy also appear to be bad for bone. There seems to be an interaction between dietary calcium and protein, in that adequate amounts of each nutrient are needed together to support bone health. Also, diets high in fruits and vegetables are associated with improved bone health.[17] This is most likely due to the fact that fruits and vegetables are good sources of the nutrients that play a role in bone and collagen health, including magnesium, vitamin C, and vitamin K. Finally, chronic alcohol abuse is detrimental to bone health and is associated with high rates of fractures.[16]
- *Physical activity:* Regular exercise is highly protective against bone loss and osteoporosis. Athletes are consistently shown to have denser bones than non-athletes, and regular participation in a variety of weight-bearing exercises, such as walking, jogging, tennis, and strength training, can help increase and maintain bone mass. Exercise causes the muscles to contract and pull on bones; this stresses bone tissue in a healthful way that stimulates increases in bone density. Intense physical activity can be harmful, however, in people who are not eating enough to maintain a healthful body weight.

Do you have a greater than average risk for osteoporosis? What about your older relatives? See the ***What About You?*** feature and find out.

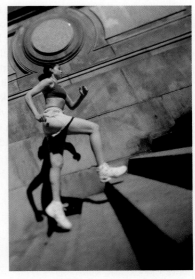

For a helpful video overview of osteoporosis, go to www.methodisthealthsystem.org. Type "osteoporosis animation" in the search bar, then click on "Osteoporosis."

⬥ Regular weight-bearing exercise, such as jogging, can help increase and maintain our bone mass.

Treatments for Osteoporosis

Although there is no cure for osteoporosis, a variety of treatments can slow and even reverse bone loss. First, individuals with osteoporosis are encouraged to consume a diet that provides adequate calcium, vitamin D, vitamin K, and other bone-building nutrients and to exercise regularly. Studies have shown that the most effective exercise programs include weight-bearing exercises such as jogging, stair climbing, and resistance training.[16]

In addition, several medications are available that slow or stop bone breakdown but do not affect bone formation. This results in an overall reduction or cessation in the rate of bone loss. *Hormone replacement therapy (HRT)* has been used for the prevention of osteoporosis in women but is controversial. HRT reduces bone loss, increases bone density, and reduces the risk for hip and spinal fractures. However, side effects include breast tenderness, changes in mood, vaginal bleeding, and an increased risk for gallbladder disease. In 2002 a federally funded study found that one type of HRT increases a woman's risk for heart disease, stroke, and breast cancer. Thus, a woman's decision regarding appropriate therapy must weigh the benefits of HRT in reducing fracture risk with the drawbacks of increased risk for other diseases.

Many people take dietary supplements—typically ones providing calcium and vitamin D—to reduce their osteoporosis risk. Now that so many foods are fortified with these nutrients, from breakfast cereals to orange juice and soy milk, it's not difficult for most people, even vegans, to get sufficient calcium and vitamin D from their

WHAT ABOUT **YOU?** ⬤❓

Are You at Risk for Osteoporosis?

One in three women and one in five men will develop osteoporosis in their lifetime. But if you know you're at risk, you can take the steps identified in this chapter, such as increasing your amount of weight bearing exercise and making sure you get enough calcium and vitamin D, to maintain the maximum amount of bone mass possible. That's why it's important to assess your risk. To the right is the International Osteoporosis Foundation's One-Minute Osteoporosis Risk Test. The more Yes answers you have, the greater likelihood that you're in a higher-risk group than the general population.

If you answered Yes to any of these questions, it does not mean you have osteoporosis. Positive answers simply mean that you have clinically proven risk factors that may lead to osteoporosis and fractures. Discuss your results with your doctor, who can advise you on whether a fracture risk assessment and/or bone density test is recommended.

1. Has either of your parents been diagnosed with osteoporosis or broken a hip after a minor fall (a fall from standing height or less)?	Yes/No
2. Have you broken a bone after a minor fall as an adult?	Yes/No
3. Have you taken corticosteroid tablets (such as cortisone or prednisone) for more than 3 consecutive months?	Yes/No
4. After the age of 40, have you lost more than 3 cm (just over 1 in.) in height?	Yes/No
5. Do you regularly drink heavily (in excess of safe drinking limits)?	Yes/No
6. Do you currently, or have you ever, smoke cigarettes?	Yes/No
7. Do you suffer frequently from diarrhea (caused by problems such as celiac disease or Crohn's disease)?	Yes/No
8. Did you undergo menopause before the age of 45?	Yes/No
For women:	
9. Have your periods stopped for 12 months or more (other than because of pregnancy)?	Yes/No
For men:	
10. Have you ever suffered from impotence, lack of libido, or other symptoms related to low testosterone levels?	Yes/No

*Data adapted from *Are You at Risk of Osteoporosis? Take the One-Minute Osteoporosis Risk Test.* International Osteoporosis Foundation. 2013.

diet. Still, you may need more of these nutrients than you're obtaining from your diet and, if that's the case, supplements may be warranted. The benefits and risks of dietary supplements for osteoporosis prevention are the subject of continuing research, and consultation with your healthcare provider is suggested.

recap Osteoporosis increases the risk for fractures and premature death from subsequent illness. Factors that increase the risk for osteoporosis include genetics, being female, being of the Caucasian or Asian race, cigarette smoking, alcohol abuse, a sedentary lifestyle, and diets low in calcium and vitamin D. Medications are available to slow bone loss.

STUDY **PLAN** | MasteringNutrition™

Customize your study plan—and master your nutrition!—
in the Study Area of **MasteringNutrition**.

what can I do **today?**

Now that you've read this chapter, try making these three changes.

1 Today, try eating 8 to 10 servings of fruits and vegetables, as recommended in the DASH diet plan.

2 Three times today, choose a beverage that provides calcium, such as calcium-fortified orange juice, milk, a yogurt smoothie, a coffee latte, or calcium-fortified soy, almond, or rice milk.

3 Exercise for at least 30 minutes today!

test yourself | *answers*

1. **False.** In the typical American diet, the majority of sodium comes from salt (sodium chloride) added to processed foods and restaurant foods.

2. **True.** Worldwide, iron deficiency is particularly common in infants, children, and women of childbearing age.

3. **False.** Osteoporosis is more common among elderly women, but elderly men are also at increased risk, and some women develop osteoporosis in their middle-adult years. Young women who suffer from an eating disorder and menstrual cycle irregularity, referred to as the *female athlete triad,* also commonly develop osteoporosis.

summary

 Scan to hear an MP3 Chapter Review in **MasteringNutrition**.

LO **1** **Distinguish between major, trace, and ultra-trace minerals**

- Minerals are essential nutrients that function in four major categories: electrolytes, power plants, blood fortifiers, and bone builders.

- Minerals are classified according to the amounts we need in our diet and according to how much of the mineral is found in our body. We need at least 100 mg of each major mineral per day in our diet. In addition, the total amount of each major mineral present in the body is at least 5 grams (5,000 mg). We need less than 100 mg per day of trace minerals, and the total amount of any trace mineral in the body is less than 5 grams. Researchers estimate that we have a dietary requirement of less than 1 mg per day of body weight for ultra-trace minerals.

LO **2** **Explain why certain minerals are referred to as electrolytes and identify their primary functions in the body**

- Electrolytes are minerals that dissolve into ions, which are capable of carrying an electrical charge. They assist in maintaining fluid balance and in the normal functioning of nerves and muscles.

- Sodium, potassium, chloride, phosphorus, and calcium are major minerals/electrolytes that help our bodies maintain fluid balance, blood pressure, transmission of nerve impulses, and muscle contraction. Phosphorus and calcium are also components of bone.

LO **3** **Explain how the level of sodium in your blood can affect your blood pressure**

- Consuming excess sodium is associated with hypertension, or high blood pressure, because sodium draws water into the fluid portion of blood, increasing its volume and pressure. Hypertension increases the risk for a heart attack or stroke.

- The DASH diet is an effective way to reduce blood pressure.

LO **4** **Identify two trace minerals important in energy metabolism**

- Chromium is a trace mineral that assists in carbohydrate metabolism by enhancing the ability of insulin to transport glucose from the bloodstream into the cell.

- Manganese, another trace mineral, assists energy metabolism and the synthesis of the protein matrix found in bone.

LO **5** **Identify two trace minerals essential for the body's synthesis of thyroid hormones**

- Iodine and selenium are trace minerals needed for the synthesis of thyroid hormones. Selenium is also an antioxidant mineral.

LO **6** **Explain how the body uses iron, and identify dietary sources and factors affecting its absorption**

- Blood is the only fluid tissue in our bodies. It has four components: erythrocytes (red blood cells); leukocytes (white blood cells); platelets, which are involved in blood clotting; and plasma, the fluid portion of our blood. Erythrocytes transport oxygen and nutrients to our cells. This function depends on adequate levels of iron.

- Iron is a trace mineral found in hemoglobin, the oxygen-carrying protein in our blood. Iron acts as a shuttle, picking up oxygen from the air we breathe, binding it during its transport in the bloodstream, and then dropping it off again in our tissues. It is also involved in the metabolism of carbohydrates, fats, and protein and is part of an antioxidant enzyme system. Meat, poultry, and fish are excellent sources of iron; however, many plant foods, including enriched breakfast cereals and breads, also provide iron.

- Consuming iron with a source of vitamin C, such as a fruit or vegetable, improves absorption. Iron absorption is inhibited by consumption of phytates, which are binding factors found in legumes, rice, and whole grains; polyphenols, which are chemicals present in black tea, coffee, and red wine; soybean protein; and calcium.

- Severe iron deficiency results in iron-deficiency anemia, in which the production of normal, healthy red blood cells decreases and hemoglobin levels are inadequate. Iron deficiency is the most common nutrient deficiency in the world.

LO **7** **Discuss the role of zinc in metabolism and immune function, and identify common food sources**

- Zinc is a trace mineral and blood fortifier that assists more than 100 enzyme systems. It is critical for hemoglobin production, cell reproduction and growth, and the proper development and functioning of the immune system. Good food sources of zinc include red meats, some seafood, whole-grain breads, and enriched foods.

LO **8** **Identify the four mineral components of bone and explain how bone is formed and maintained**

- Bones are organs that are constantly active, breaking down old bone via osteoclasts and building new bone via osteoblasts. In this process, called remodeling, bone building and bone breakdown occur at equal rates, resulting in bone mass being maintained. Around 40 years of age, bone breakdown begins to outpace bone formation, and this imbalance results in a gradual loss in bone density.

- Calcium, magnesium, phosphorus, and fluoride are the major mineral components of bone. These minerals form tiny crystals that cluster around collagen fibers—protein fibers that provide strength, durability, and flexibility.

LO **9** **State the four primary functions of calcium**

- Calcium is critical for normal nerve transmission, muscle contraction, healthy blood pressure, and blood clotting. The body maintains adequate calcium levels in the blood at all times.

LO **10** **Discuss the risk factors and available treatments for osteoporosis**

- Osteoporosis is a disease characterized by low bone density. This leads to increased risk of bone fractures and premature disability and death due to subsequent illness.

- Factors that increase the risk for osteoporosis include increased age, being female, being of the Caucasian or Asian race, cigarette smoking, alcohol abuse, vitamin D deficiency, low lifetime calcium intake, and a sedentary lifestyle. Prescription medications are available to slow bone loss but cannot cure the disease.

review questions

LO **1** **Distinguish between major, trace, and ultra-trace minerals**

1. Which of the following is true of major minerals?
   a. They are more important to our health and functioning than trace minerals.
   b. Our body can synthesize them, so they do not have to be consumed in the diet.
   c. The total amount of each major mineral in our body is 5 grams or more.
   d. We need to consume at least 5 milligrams a day of each major mineral.

LO **2** **Explain why certain minerals are referred to as electrolytes and identify their primary functions in the body**

2. Which of the following statements about electrolytes is true?
   a. They form charged particles called ions.
   b. They are critical to fluid balance and nerve impulse transmission.
   c. They include sodium and potassium.
   d. all of the above

LO **3** **Explain how the level of sodium in your blood can affect your blood pressure**

3. A diet high in sodium can increase your risk for high blood pressure because
   a. sodium can draw water into your red blood cells.
   b. sodium can draw water into your blood plasma.
   c. sodium can push potassium into your red blood cells.
   d. sodium can push chloride into your blood plasma.

LO **4** **Identify two trace minerals important in energy metabolism**

4. Two trace minerals important in energy metabolism are
   a. chromium and manganese.
   b. chromium and magnesium.
   c. chloride and manganese.
   d. chloride and magnesium.

LO **5** **Identify two trace minerals essential for the body's synthesis of thyroid hormones**

5. Hypothyroidism, goiter, and cretinism are conditions associated with a deficiency of
   a. sulfur.
   b. iron.
   c. iodine.
   d. all of the above.

LO **6** **Explain how the body uses iron, and identify dietary sources and factors affecting its absorption**

6. Which of the following statements about iron is true?
   a. Iron is stored primarily in the heart muscle and skeletal muscles.
   b. Iron is a component of hemoglobin, myoglobin, and certain enzymes.
   c. Iron is a component of red blood cells, white blood cells, platelets, and plasma.
   d. Iron needs are higher for elderly women than for young women.

LO **7** **Discuss the role of zinc in metabolism and immune function, and identify common food sources**

7. Zinc is
   a. a major mineral and a component of the amino acids methionine and cysteine.
   b. a trace mineral important to growth and immune function.
   c. more abundant in and more easily absorbed from plant-based foods.
   d. capable of increasing copper absorption and prompting copper toxicity.

LO **8** **Identify the four mineral components of bone and explain how bone is formed and maintained**

8. Which of the following statements about trabecular bone is true?
   a. It accounts for about 80% of the skeleton.
   b. It forms the outer surface of all bones.
   c. It is also called compact bone.
   d. It provides scaffolding that protects bones from extreme stress.

LO **9** **State the four primary functions of calcium**

9. Calcium is necessary for several body functions, including
   a. hemoglobin production, nerve-impulse transmission, and immune responses.
   b. the structure of cartilage, nerve-impulse transmission, and muscle contraction.
   c. the structure of bone and blood, immune responses, and muscle contraction.
   d. the structure of bone, nerve-impulse transmission, and muscle contraction.

LO **10** **Discuss the risk factors and available treatments for osteoporosis**

10. Which of the following behaviors is associated with an increased risk for osteoporosis?
    a. Smoking
    b. Overeating
    c. Consumption of alcohol
    d. All of the above

Answers to Review Questions are located at the back of this text.

web links

The following websites and apps explore further topics and issues related to personal health.
Visit MasteringNutrition for links to the websites and RSS feeds.

www.americanheart.org
American Heart Association

http://www.nhlbi.nih.gov
The National Heart, Lung, and Blood Institute's guide to lowering high blood pressure.

www.niams.nih.gov
National Institutes of Health: Osteoporosis and Related Bone Diseases—National Resource Center

www.nof.org
National Osteoporosis Foundation

Fluid Balance, Water, and Alcohol

8

learning outcomes

After studying this chapter, you should be able to:

1 Describe the location and functions of body fluid, pp. 226–229.

2 Identify two mechanisms by which our body gains fluid, pp. 229–233.

3 Identify five mechanisms by which our body loses fluid, pp. 229–233.

4 Discuss three potentially fatal consequences of fluid imbalance, pp. 229–233.

5 Compare and contrast sources of drinking water, pp. 233–237.

6 Debate the health benefits and potential concerns of at least four popular beverages, pp. 233–237.

7 Explain briefly how the body absorbs, breaks down, and excretes alcohol, pp. 237–245.

8 Discuss the health effects of moderate alcohol intake, pp. 237–245.

9 Describe how excessive alcohol use increases the risks of illness, injury, and death, pp. 237–245.

10 Explain how alcohol intake during pregnancy can affect the fetus, pp. 245–246.

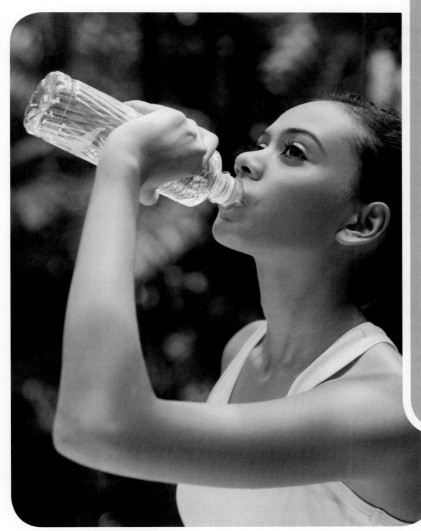

test yourself

Are these statements true or false? Circle your guess.

1. **T F** About 50% to 70% of our body weight is made up of water.

2. **T F** Although persistent vomiting is uncomfortable, it does not have any harmful health effects.

3. **T F** Carbonated alcoholic beverages are absorbed more rapidly than noncarbonated varieties.

Test Yourself answers can be found at the end of the chapter.

MasteringNutrition™

Go online for chapter quizzes, pre-tests, Interactive Activities, and more!

In December 2011, 14-year-old Anais Fournier died of cardiac arrest after consuming a 24-ounce can of a popular energy drink. An autopsy found that caffeine toxicity had caused a cardiac arrhythmia—an abnormal heart rhythm—that impaired her heart's ability to pump. Seven months later, after drinking two 16-ounce cans of the same energy drink, 19-year-old Alex Morris also suffered a cardiac arrhythmia, went into cardiac arrest, and died. In 2013, the U.S. Food and Drug Administration (FDA) released records of nearly 150 adverse events between 2004 and 2012 that were linked to three popular energy drinks. The reports included incidents of vomiting, difficulty breathing, cardiac arrests, seizures, miscarriages, and at least 18 deaths.[1]

All beverages provide water, our body's most basic nutrient. Water keeps our body hydrated, and hydration is essential to our survival. But some beverages—like energy drinks—are dangerously high in caffeine, whereas others are loaded with added sugars, and some are surprising sources of sodium or saturated fat. And then there's alcohol, which in excess, is the third leading preventable cause of death in the United States.[2] Does this mean that, when you're thirsty, the only healthful choice is plain water? Not exactly.

This chapter explains the importance of fluid balance, how our body maintains it, and the problems that can occur when our body fluids are out of balance. We then review a variety of popular beverages, from kefir to coconut water, that may or may not live up to their hype. Finally, we discuss the effects of alcohol, including the benefits of moderate consumption and the problems of alcohol abuse.

 LO1 Describe the location and functions of body fluid.

What are fluids, and what are their functions?

You know that water, orange juice, blood, and urine are all fluids, but what makes them so? A **fluid** is a substance characterized by its ability to move freely and changeably, adapting to the shape of any container that holds it. This might not seem important, but the fluid within our cells and tissues is critical to the body's ability to function.

The main component of all fluids is water, which is made up of a precise ratio of hydrogen and oxygen (H_2O). Water is one of the six nutrient groups, and is essential to life.

Body Fluid Is the Liquid Portion of Cells and Tissues

Between 50% and 70% of a healthy adult's body weight is water. Think about it: if you weigh 150 pounds, then about 75 to 105 pounds of your body isn't solid, but fluid! When we cut a finger, we can see some of this fluid dripping out as blood, but blood alone certainly can't account for 105 pounds! So where is all this fluid hiding?

About two-thirds of our body fluid, known as *intracellular fluid*, is held within our cells (**FIGURE 8.1a**). Every cell in the body contains fluid. When cells lose their fluid, they shrink and die. On the other hand, when cells take in too much fluid, they swell and burst apart. This is why appropriate fluid balance—which we'll discuss throughout this chapter—is so critical to life.

The remaining third of our body fluid is known as *extracellular fluid* because it flows outside the cells. There are two types of extracellular fluid: tissue fluid (also known as interstitial fluid) flows between the cells that make up a particular tissue or organ (Figure 8.1b). The rest of the body's extracellular fluid flows within blood vessels or lymphatic vessels. The fluid portion of blood is called *plasma*. It transports blood cells within the body's arteries, veins, and capillaries (Figure 8.1c). The fluid in lymphatic vessels is simply called lymph (see Figure 2.12).

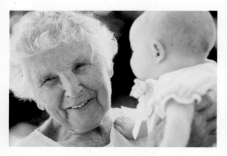

⬆ As we age, our body water content decreases: approximately 75% of an infant's body weight is composed of water, whereas an elderly adult's is only 50%, or less.

fluid A substance composed of molecules that move past one another freely. Fluids are characterized by their ability to conform to the shape of whatever container holds them.

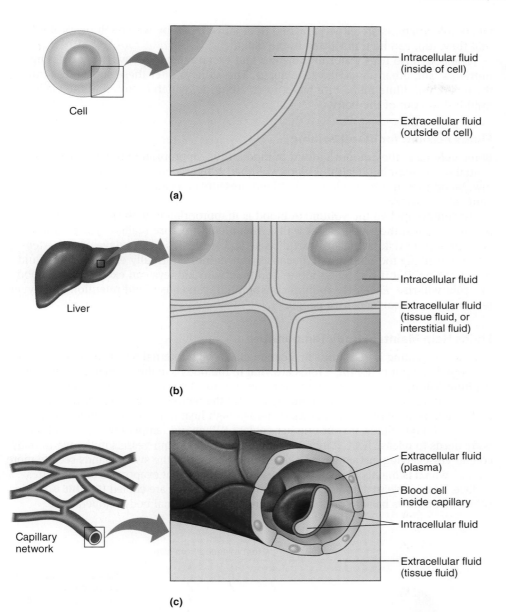

(a)

(b)

(c)

◀ FIGURE 8.1 The components of body fluid. **(a)** Intracellular fluid is contained within the cells that make up our body tissues. Extracellular fluid is external to cells. **(b)** Interstitial fluid is external to tissue cells, and **(c)** plasma is external to blood cells.

Not every tissue in the body contains the same amount of fluid. Lean tissues, such as muscle, are more than 70% fluid by weight, whereas fat tissue is between 10% and 20% fluid. Body fluid also varies according to gender. Men have more lean tissue and thus a higher percentage of total weight as body fluid than women. Our percentage of weight as body fluid also decreases as we age, from about 75% in infants to generally less than 50% in older adults. This decrease is related to the loss of lean tissue that typically occurs as we age.

Body Fluids Serve Many Critical Functions

Body fluids perform a number of functions that are critical to life.

Fluids Dissolve and Transport Substances

Water is an excellent **solvent**, which means it is capable of dissolving a variety of substances. Water-soluble substances, such as glucose, amino acids, minerals, and water-soluble vitamins, are easily transported in the bloodstream. In contrast, lipids do not dissolve in water. To overcome this chemical incompatibility, fats, cholesterol, and

solvent A substance that is capable of mixing with and breaking apart a variety of compounds. Water is an excellent solvent.

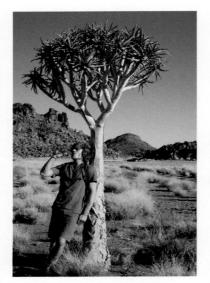

◆ A hiker needs to consume adequate amounts of water to prevent heat illness under hot and dry conditions.

fat-soluble vitamins are either attached to or surrounded by water-soluble proteins so that they, too, can be transported in the blood.

The body also uses water to transport and excrete metabolic wastes, excess micronutrients, and other unwanted substances. The kidneys filter these substances from the blood and dilute them with water to create urine, which is stored in the bladder until it flows out of the body.

Fluids Account for Blood Volume

Blood volume is the amount of fluid in blood; thus, appropriate fluid levels are essential to maintaining healthful blood volume. When blood volume is inappropriately low, blood pressure is also low. Low blood pressure can cause people to feel tired, confused, or dizzy.

In contrast, when the volume of blood is inappropriately high, it exerts greater pressure against the blood vessel walls. High blood pressure (called *hypertension*) is an important risk factor for heart disease and stroke. You can't develop hypertension by drinking too much fluid, because your kidneys normally excrete excess fluid in your urine. But if you retain more fluid than your kidneys can excrete, your blood pressure will rise. Excessive sodium consumption can cause fluid retention and hypertension in some salt-sensitive people.

Fluids Help Maintain Body Temperature

Just as overheating is disastrous to a car engine, a high internal temperature can cause the body to stop functioning. Fluids are vital to the body's ability to maintain its temperature within a safe range. Two factors account for the cooling power of fluids.

First, it takes a lot of external energy to raise the temperature of water. Because our body contains a lot of water, it takes sustained high heat to increase body temperature.

Second, body fluids are our primary coolant. When our temperature rises and our body needs to release heat, it increases the flow of blood from vessels in the warm body core to vessels lying just under the skin. At the same time, the sweat glands secrete more sweat—which is mainly water—from the skin. As this sweat evaporates off the skin's surface, heat is released and our skin and underlying blood are cooled (**FIGURE 8.2**). This cooler blood flows back to our body core and reduces internal body temperature.

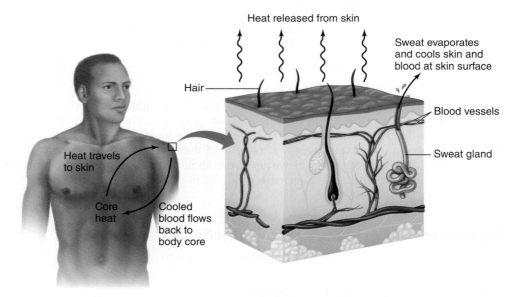

◆ **FIGURE 8.2** Evaporative cooling occurs when heat is transported from the body core through the bloodstream to the surface of the skin. When a person sweats, water evaporates into the air and carries away heat. This cools the skin and underlying blood, which then circulates back to the body core, reducing body temperature.

blood volume The amount of fluid in blood.

Fluids Protect and Lubricate Body Tissues

Water is a major part of the fluids that protect tissues. The cerebrospinal fluid that surrounds the brain and spinal column acts as a shock absorber, protecting them from damage, and amniotic fluid protects a fetus in a mother's womb.

Body fluids also act as lubricants. Fluid within our joints facilitates smooth joint motion. Fluid covering the lungs allows for their friction-free expansion and retraction within the chest cavity. Tears cleanse and lubricate the eyes. Saliva moistens the food we eat, and the mucus lining the digestive tract facilitates the smooth movement of nutrients.

recap Water is an essential nutrient. Between about 50% and 70% of a healthy adult's body weight is water. About two-thirds of our body fluid is held within the walls of our cells (intracellular fluid), and the remaining third flows outside cells (extracellular fluid). Body fluids serve many important functions, including dissolving and transporting substances, accounting for blood volume, regulating body temperature, and protecting and lubricating body tissues.

How does our body maintain fluid balance?

LO2 Identify two mechanisms by which our body gains fluid.

LO3 Identify five mechanisms by which our body loses fluid.

LO4 Discuss three potentially fatal consequences of fluid imbalance.

Our body maintains a healthy balance of fluid by a series of actions and reactions that prompt us to drink and retain fluid when we are dehydrated and to excrete excess fluid as urine when we consume more than we need.

Our Thirst Mechanism Prompts Us to Drink Fluids

Imagine that, at lunch, you ate a ham sandwich and a bag of salted potato chips. As you're leaving your afternoon class, you suddenly notice you're very thirsty and dash to the nearest drinking fountain. What made you feel so thirsty?

The body's command center for fluid intake is a cluster of nerve cells in the same part of the brain that regulates food intake—the *hypothalamus*. Within the hypothalamus is a group of cells, known as the **thirst mechanism**, that causes you to consciously desire fluids. The thirst mechanism prompts us to feel thirsty when it detects either of two conditions:

- *An increased concentration of sodium and other dissolved substances in the blood.* Remember that ham sandwich and those potato chips? Both these foods are salty and eating them temporarily increases the concentration of sodium in the blood.
- *A decrease in blood volume and blood pressure.* This can occur when we lose fluid because of excessive sweating, heavy blood loss, severe diarrhea, or simply when our fluid intake is too low.

Once the hypothalamus detects such changes, it stimulates the release of a hormone that signals the kidneys to reduce urine flow and return more water to the bloodstream. Water is drawn out of the salivary glands in the mouth in an attempt to further dilute the concentration of substances in the blood; this leaves less water available to make saliva and causes the mouth and throat to become dry. Together, these mechanisms help us retain fluid, prevent a further loss of fluid, and avoid dehydration.

Although you might think you can rely on the thirst mechanism to accurately signal when you need to drink more fluids, there are times when thirst is actually not the best predictor of fluid imbalance. Most people tend to drink only until they are no longer thirsty, but the amount of fluid they consume may not be enough to achieve fluid balance. This is particularly true when body water is rapidly lost, such as during intense exercise in the heat. Also, in older adults, the thirst mechanism is not as accurate as in younger adults. Because the thirst mechanism has these limitations, it is important that you drink regularly throughout the day, even if you don't feel particularly thirsty.

thirst mechanism A cluster of nerve cells in the hypothalamus that stimulate our conscious desire to drink fluids in response to an increase in the concentration of salt in our blood or a decrease in blood pressure and volume.

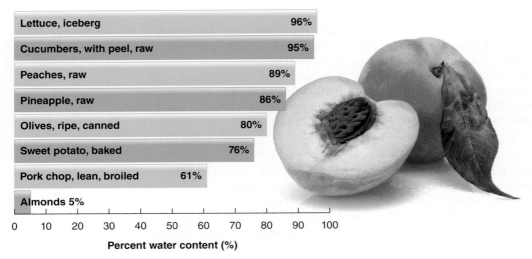

FIGURE 8.3 Water content of different foods. Much of your daily water intake comes from the foods you eat.

Data from U.S. Department of Agriculture, Agricultural Research Service. 2009. USDA National Nutrient Database for Standard Reference, Release 22. Nutrient Data Laboratory Home Page. www.ars.usda.gov/ba/bhnrc/ndl

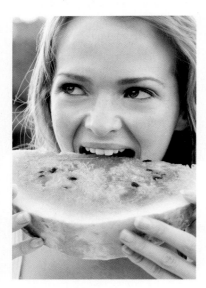

Fruits and vegetables are delicious sources of water.

metabolic water The water formed as a by-product of our body's metabolic reactions.

diuretic A substance that increases fluid loss via the urine. Common diuretics include alcohol and some prescription medications for high blood pressure and other disorders.

We Gain Fluids Through Intake and Metabolism

The fluid we need each day comes from two sources: dietary intake from the beverages and foods we consume and the body's production of metabolic water. Of course, you know that beverages are mostly water, but it isn't as easy to see the water content of foods. For example, iceberg lettuce is about 96% water, and even almonds contain a small amount of water **(FIGURE 8.3)**.

Metabolic water is the water formed as a by-product of the body's breakdown of fat, carbohydrate, and protein. This water contributes about 10% to 14% of the water our body needs each day.

We Lose Fluids Through Urine and Feces, Sweat, Evaporation, and Exhalation

Our kidneys absorb from the bloodstream any water that the body does not need. They then send the fluid, in the form of dilute urine, to the bladder for storage until we urinate. A small amount of water is also lost each day in the feces. However, when someone experiences severe diarrhea, water loss in the feces can be as high as several quarts per day.

We also lose fluid via sweat. Fluid loss in sweat is much higher during physical labor or exercise and when we are in a hot environment. In fact, some large football players can lose more than 8 quarts of fluid per day as sweat!

Water is also continuously evaporated from our skin, even when we are not obviously sweating. Finally, water is continuously exhaled from the lungs as we breathe.

FIGURE 8.4 shows the estimated amounts and types of water intake and losses for a woman expending 2,500 kcal of energy per day. It shows that her fluid losses of 3,000 mL (3 L, or just over 12 cups) per day are matched by:

- An intake of 2,200 mL (2.2 L, or about 9 cups) of fluid in beverages,
- The consumption of 500 mL (about 2 cups) of fluid in foods, and
- The production of 300 mL (about 1.3 cups) of metabolic water.

The consumption of **diuretics**—substances that increase fluid loss via the urine—can result in dangerously excessive fluid loss. Some prescription medications have a diuretic effect, and many over-the-counter weight-loss products are really just diuretics. Alcohol also has a strong diuretic effect. In the past, it was believed that caffeine-containing beverages, such as coffee, tea, and cola, acted as diuretics, but more recent research suggests that caffeinated drinks do not in fact have a significant impact on

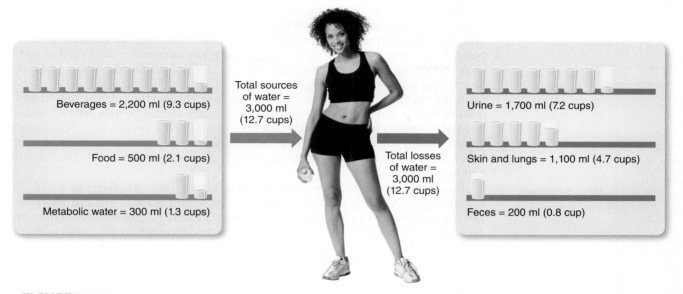

Total sources
of water =
3,000 ml
(12.7 cups)

Total losses
of water =
3,000 ml
(12.7 cups)

Beverages = 2,200 ml (9.3 cups)

Food = 500 ml (2.1 cups)

Metabolic water = 300 ml (1.3 cups)

Urine = 1,700 ml (7.2 cups)

Skin and lungs = 1,100 ml (4.7 cups)

Feces = 200 ml (0.8 cup)

▲ **FIGURE 8.4**   Amounts and categories of water sources and losses for a woman expending 2,500 kcal per day.

the hydration status of adults.[3] Although more research on this aspect needs to be done, it's probably safe to count caffeinated beverages toward your daily fluid requirements. Later in this chapter, we identify ways to determine whether or not you are adequately hydrated.

recap   The thirst mechanism prompts us to feel thirsty when it detects an increased concentration of sodium and other dissolved substances in the blood. It is also triggered by low blood volume or blood pressure. A healthy fluid level is maintained in the body by balancing intake with excretion. Primary sources of fluids include intake through beverages and foods and the production of metabolic water in the body. Fluid losses occur through urine, feces, sweating, evaporation from the skin, and exhalation from the lungs.

Fluid Imbalance Can Be Deadly

Fluid imbalances can be serious, even fatal. Dehydration, heatstroke, and water intoxication are fluid imbalances explained in this section.

Dehydration Is Common with Exercise in Hot Weather

Dehydration is a serious health problem that results when fluid losses exceed fluid intake. It occurs most often as a result of heavy exercise and/or exposure to high environmental temperatures, when loss of body water via sweating and breathing is increased.

Both the elderly and the very young are at a higher risk for dehydration. The thirst mechanism becomes less sensitive with age, so elderly people can fail to drink adequate fluid. Older adults also have less body water than younger adults, so fluid imbalances can occur more quickly. Infants are at increased risk because a larger proportion of their body weight is water; thus, they need to drink a relatively large amount of fluid for their body size. Infants also lose fluid at a higher rate and cannot tell us when they are thirsty. Fluid losses from diarrhea or vomiting must be closely monitored in infants.

In all people, relatively small losses in body water, equal to a 1% to 2% change in body weight, result in symptoms that include thirst, discomfort, and loss of appetite. More severe water losses can cause nausea, flushed skin, and mental confusion. Losses of body water greater than 8% of body weight can result in delirium, coma, and death.

dehydration A serious condition of depleted body fluid that results when fluid excretion exceeds fluid intake.

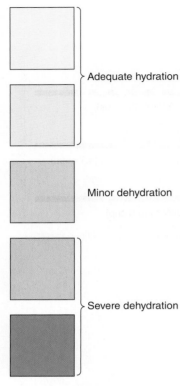

Adequate hydration

Minor dehydration

Severe dehydration

FIGURE 8.5 Urine color chart. Color variations indicate levels of hydration.

Watch a slideshow of causes and symptoms of dehydration and tips to stay hydrated at http://www.medicinenet.com and type "dehydration" in the search bar and click on "Dehydration Slideshow."

heatstroke A potentially fatal response to high temperature characterized by failure of the body's heat-regulating mechanisms commonly called *sunstroke*.

water intoxication Dilution of body fluid that results when water intake or retention is excessive; it can lead to hyponatremia; also called *overhydration*.

Earlier we discussed the importance of fluid replacement when you are physically active. How can you tell whether you're drinking enough fluid before, during, and after athletic competitions or exercise sessions? First, you can measure your body weight before and after each session, using the same scale, unclothed or just in your underwear. Whether you've lost 2 ounces or 2 pounds during your session, that weight loss is lost fluid.

A second way to monitor your fluid levels is to observe the color of your urine (**FIGURE 8.5**). If you are properly hydrated, your urine should be pale yellow, similar in color to diluted lemonade. Urine that is medium to dark yellow, like apple juice, indicates inadequate fluid intake. Very dark or brown urine, such as the color of a cola beverage, is a sign of severe dehydration and indicates potential muscle breakdown and kidney damage.

How can you minimize fluid loss related to physical activity? Begin in a well-hydrated state by slowly drinking water or, for prolonged bouts of exercise, sport beverages, at least 4 hours before the activity. During an activity, prevent dehydration by drinking water or sports beverages as needed. A marathon runner may need to drink 400 to 800 mL (1½ to 3 cups) of a sports beverage per hour during the race; however, a player in a casual tennis match may require much less. After activity, most people can restore fluid balance through normal meals, snacks, and beverages. But if your weight or the color of your urine indicates that you are significantly dehydrated, one guideline is to drink about 1,500 mL (about 6 cups) for each kilogram of body weight lost.

Heatstroke

People who work outdoors in the heat, such as farm workers, highway or construction workers, and soldiers, are particularly vulnerable to dangerous fluid loss. So are athletes who train or compete in hot weather. In 2011, five high school football players died from heatstroke.[4]

Heatstroke is a failure of the body's heat-regulating mechanism. Environment, clothing, and body size can all play a role:

- Sweating is an effective means of cooling the body only if the sweat is able to evaporate. Thus, it is less effective in a humid environment.
- Heavy or tight fitting clothing, such as a military or football uniform, padding, and helmet, significantly reduces the body's ability to dissipate heat.
- Larger individuals with a lot of muscle mass produce more body heat. In addition, people with high levels of body fat have an extra layer of insulation that makes it difficult to dissipate body heat both at rest and during exercise.

Symptoms of heatstroke include a rapid pulse, rapid shallow breathing, hot and dry skin, high body temperature, and disorientation or loss of consciousness. Heatstroke is a medical emergency: to prevent death, immediate care is essential. If you're working, training, or competing in the heat and someone collapses, call 911. Immediately remove tight, heavy clothing and immerse the victim in an ice bath if she or he is conscious and can be constantly supervised. Otherwise, apply ice packs to the victim's armpits and groin area, and sponge or continuously spray the person's body with cold water until help arrives.

You can reduce your own risk for heatstroke by maintaining a healthy fluid balance before, during, and after exercise or manual labor. If you're training, competing, or working in a hot environment and begin to feel dizzy, light-headed, disoriented, or nauseated, stop immediately. Find a cool place to rest, consume cool beverages (such as water or a sports beverage), and tell someone to notify your trainer, coach, or employer that you need assistance.

Water Intoxication

Is it possible to drink too much water? **Water intoxication**, also called *overhydration*, can occur, but it is rare. In non-athletes, it generally occurs only in people with health problems that cause the kidneys to retain too much water or during dangerous activities, such as hazing rituals and the use of certain illegal drugs. It is more common in endurance athletes, such as long-distance runners and triathletes, because kidney function is reduced during intense exercise. When athletes drink too much water and do not replace adequate sodium during a long event, their body can retain too much fluid, resulting in a potentially fatal dilution of blood sodium called *hyponatremia.* Warning signs of hyponatremia include continuing thirst despite fluid intake, nausea, headache, inability to concentrate, confusion, and possible convulsions. These symptoms indicate the need for immediate medical assistance.

recap Dehydration, heatstroke, and water intoxication can occur when water and electrolyte losses are not balanced with water and electrolyte replacement. These conditions can occur in manual laborers, soldiers, athletes, and anyone engaging in vigorous physical activity in hot weather and can be fatal.

How much fluid do we need—and what kinds?

 Compare and contrast sources of drinking water.

 Debate the health benefits and potential concerns of at least four popular beverages.

We need to drink enough fluid every day so that our body can sweat, breathe, and produce urine and feces without drawing water out of cells. But how much is "enough"? The DRI guidelines from the Institute of Medicine recommend that men consume approximately 3,000 mL (about 13 cups) of fluids daily from water and other beverages, with an additional 700 mL of water from food. Women should consume about 2,200 mL (9 cups) of fluid, as well as 500 mL of water from food.[3] Still, fluid requirements are highly individualized. For example, a male athlete training in a hot environment may need to drink up to 10 liters (about 42 cups) of fluid per day, whereas a petite, sedentary woman who works in a temperature-controlled office building may require only about 2 liters (8 cups) per day.

Public Tap Water Is Safe to Drink

Millions of Americans routinely consume tap water, which generally comes from two sources: surface water and groundwater. *Surface water* comes from lakes, rivers, and reservoirs. *Groundwater* comes from underground rock formations called *aquifers.* Many people who live in rural areas depend on groundwater pumped from a well as their water source.

The Environmental Protection Agency (EPA) sets and monitors the standards for public water systems. Water treatment plants most commonly use chlorine, a chemical effective in killing many harmful microbes, to purify water supplies. They also routinely check water supplies for hazardous chemicals, minerals, and other contaminants. Because of these efforts, the United States has one of the safest water systems in the world. The EPA does not monitor water from private wells, but it publishes recommendations for well owners to help them maintain a safe water supply. For more information on drinking water safety, go to the EPA website (see **Web Links** at the end of this chapter).

Over the past 20 years, there has been a major shift away from the use of tap water to the consumption of bottled water. Americans now spend nearly $12 billion on bottled water per year, representing about 30 billion bottles![5] The sharp rise in bottled water production and consumption is most likely due to the convenience of drinking bottled water, the health messages related to drinking more water, and the public's fears related to the safety of tap water. However, environmental concerns related to the disposal of billions of water bottles in landfills, and the burning of fossil fuels required to manufacture and transport bottled water, has begun to limit the growth of the bottled water industry. The industry has responded by using smaller bottle caps, thinner bottles, and a higher proportion of recyclable materials. Still, many universities now ban the sale of bottled water on campus, and several U.S. cities, including San Francisco, prohibit the sale of bottled water on public property.

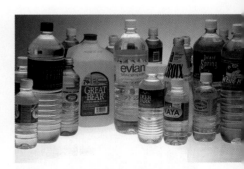

Numerous varieties of drinking water are available to consumers.

nutrition myth or fact?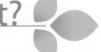

Is Bottled Water Safer Than Tap Water?

Bottled water has become increasingly popular during the past 20 years. It is estimated that Americans drink almost 9 billion gallons of bottled water each year. Many people prefer the taste of bottled water to that of tap water. They also feel that bottled water is safer than tap water. Is this true?

The Food and Drug Administration (FDA), which regulates bottled water, does not require that it meet higher quality standards than public water. Despite many people's assumptions, bottled water is taken from either surface water or groundwater sources, the same as tap water. In fact, up to 40% of bottled water sold in the United States and Canada is actually sourced from municipal tap water.[1] Look closely at the label of your favorite bottled water. If the label states "From a public water source," it has come directly from the tap!

Although many labels lack information about how the water is treated, a little research on the company's website should help you find the answer. There are several ways of treating water, but what you're looking for is either *micron filtration* or *reverse osmosis*, which have proven to be most effective against

the most common waterborne disease–causing microbes. Purification of bottled water by other types of filtration, or by treatment with ultraviolet light, ozone, or ion exchange may be less effective.

Should you spend money on bottled water? Probably not, unless you live in an area where you don't have reliable access to safe drinking water. Instead, purchase a reusable water bottle made of stainless steel, glass, or BPA-free plastic. Some of the newer bottles contain a filtration device that removes chlorine as you sip, improving the tap water's taste.

If you do choose to purchase bottled water, look for brands that carry the trademark of the International Bottled Water Association (IBWA). This association follows the regulations of the FDA. Avoid waters with added sugars, because their empty Calories can contribute significantly to your day's energy intake. Although these products may be promoted with healthful-sounding names, they're essentially "liquid candy."

For more information on bottled water, search the FDA website at www.fda.gov.

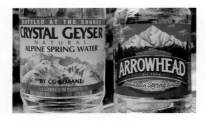

Bottled water is very popular, but how does it really compare to tap water?

The Food and Drug Administration (FDA) is responsible for the regulation of bottled water. As with tap water, bottled water is taken from either surface water or groundwater sources, but it is often treated and filtered differently. For example, carbonated water (seltzer water) contains carbon dioxide gas that either occurs naturally or is added to the water. Mineral waters contain various levels of minerals and offer a unique taste. Some brands, however, contain high amounts of sodium and should be avoided by people who are trying to reduce their sodium intake. Distilled water is mineral-free but has a "flat" taste.

Is bottled water better than tap water? Review the ***Nutrition Myth or Fact?*** feature box to find out!

All Beverages Are Not Created Equal

Many beverages contain important nutrients in addition to their water content, whereas others provide water and refined sugar but very little else. Let's review the health benefits and potential concerns of some of the most popular beverages on the market.

Milk and Milk Substitutes

Low-fat and skim milk are healthful beverage choices, because they provide protein, calcium, phosphorus, vitamin D, and usually vitamin A. Many brands of fluid milk are now "specialized" and provide additional calcium, vitamin E, essential fatty acids, and/or plant sterols (to lower serum cholesterol). Kefir, a blended yogurt drink, is also a good source of most of these nutrients. Calcium-fortified soymilk provides protein and calcium, and many brands provide vitamin D. In contrast, almond and rice milks are low in protein, with only 1 gram per cup. When purchasing flavored milk, kefir, or milk substitutes, check the Nutrition Facts panel for the sugar content. Some brands of chocolate milk, for example, can contain 6 or more teaspoons of refined sugar in a single cup!

Hot Beverages Containing Caffeine

Coffee without cream or non-dairy creamer can be a healthful choice if consumed in moderation. Research suggests that its caffeine content does not significantly decrease the body's hydration status, and the calcium in coffee drinks made with milk, such as café con leche and café latte, can be significant. Also, coffee is known to provide several types of phytochemicals that may lower the risk for certain chronic diseases. Although some people are sensitive to the caffeine in coffee, in moderation it is a safe and potentially healthful source of fluid.

Tea is second only to water as the most commonly consumed beverage in the world. With the exception of caffeine-free red tea and herbal teas, all forms of tea come from the same plant, *Camellia sinesis* and all contain caffeine. Black tea is the most highly processed (the tea leaves are fully fermented) and contains the highest level of caffeine, about half the amount in brewed coffee. Green and white teas are lower in caffeine and higher in phytochemicals thought to decrease the risk of certain chronic diseases and cancers.[6] Some research suggests that green and white teas may have antibacterial and antiviral effects.[7]

Chocolate- and cocoa-based beverages also provide caffeine, although the levels are much lower than those found in coffee, tea, or colas. Dark chocolate is rich in antioxidants known as flavanols, which may lower risk for heart attacks and stroke. Hot chocolate made with dark cocoa powder and skim or low-fat milk is a nutritious and satisfying drink.

Energy Drinks

Colas and several other soft drinks contain caffeine—typically about 35–60 mg in a 12-ounce serving. In contrast, energy drinks typically contain more than twice this amount of caffeine per serving, and a few contain up to ten times this amount. Also, many energy drinks contain guarana seed extract: guarana seeds contain more caffeine than coffee beans, so their "extract" is simply a potent source of additional caffeine. Some also contain taurine, an amino acid associated with muscle contraction.

Energy drinks represent a highly popular and rapidly growing beverage option, with over $12 billion in sales in 2012 and a predicted increase to $22 billion in sales by 2017.[8] About 30% of teenagers drink them on a regular basis, even though physicians, nutrition experts, consumer groups, and the FDA have raised significant concerns.[9]

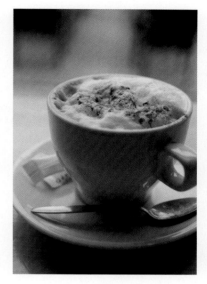

Consuming coffee drinks in moderation can be a healthful choice for adults, and the calcium content in caffeinated drinks made with milk can be significant. Avoid using cream or nonfat creamers and opt for low- or nonfat milk.

foods you don't know you love YET

Rooibos Tea

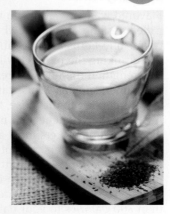

Also called red tea, rooibos (pronounced ROY-bos) is a ruddy tea with a naturally sweet, nutty flavor. The plant it comes from, *Aspalathus linearis*, is grown only in a small region of South Africa, but over the past decade rooibos has become increasingly available in markets throughout the United States. Sold both loose and in tea bags, it's prepared like black tea, and many people drink it with lemon. The increasing popularity of rooibos is due in part to its health benefits: it contains no caffeine and is rich in antioxidant phytochemicals. Traditionally, South Africans have used rooibos tea as a treatment for allergies, asthma, and skin inflammation.

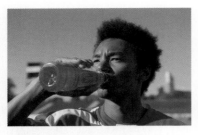

⬆ "Energy drinks" are a popular segment of the beverage market, but many contain caffeine and other substances that can cause harmful effects.

Energy drinks are uniquely dangerous not only because they contain such high levels of caffeine, but also because—unlike hot coffee and tea, which are sipped slowly—they're typically downed in a few minutes. Some are even packaged as a "shot." For example, a product called 5-Hour Energy delivers more than 200 mg of caffeine in a 2-ounce "shot." This flood of caffeine can cause blood pressure and heart rate to surge. As we noted at the beginning of this chapter, seizures, cardiac arrests, miscarriages, over 20,000 emergency room visits, and at least 18 deaths between 2009 and 2012 have been linked to consumption of energy drinks. Although the FDA limits the amount of caffeine in soft drinks, it has no legal authority to regulate the ingredients, including caffeine, in energy drinks because they are classified as dietary supplements, not food. In contrast, Canada now caps caffeine levels in energy drinks, and Mexico is proposing to ban their sale to adolescents. In addition to caffeine, energy drinks are also a source of significant added sugar. For example, a 16-ounce bottle of Rockstar Original contains 62 grams—more than 15 teaspoons—of sugar and 248 empty Calories.

A disturbing trend is the practice among adolescents of mixing energy drinks with alcoholic beverages.[10] Research has shown that when adolescents drink alcohol-laced energy drinks, they drink more alcohol and show more signs of intoxication compared to teens who consume alcohol in the absence of energy drinks. Unfortunately, caffeine seems to blunt the perception of intoxication; in other words, those who combine energy drinks with alcoholic beverages don't even realize how drunk they are. Because the combination of energy drinks and alcohol leads to a "wide awake drunk," these adolescents are also more likely to suffer physical and sexual assaults, falls, burn injuries, drownings, and traffic accidents or fatalities.

Beverages with Added Sugars

Sugar is added to many juice drinks, sweetened teas, flavored waters, and sodas. The current debate about the potential health consequences of increased use of high-fructose corn syrup (HFCS) has led many beverage companies to sweeten their products with honey, "pure cane sugar," or so-called fruit-juice concentrate. Although these sound like more healthful options, they are still simple sugars. Fruit-juice concentrate, for example, is mostly pure fructose, with none of the fiber or other nutrients that make fruit a nutritious food.

As package sizes increase, the Calorie count for sugary drinks can be unexpectedly high. Even 100% fruit juice, with no added sugar, can provide more than 100 to 150 Calories per 8-ounce glass. Recently, most large manufacturers of nonalcoholic beverages have committed to the "Clear on Calories" campaign, which requires that they list Calorie content on the front of the product. Now, when consumers buy a 20 oz bottle of sweetened tea, they'll know they're getting, for example, 250 Calories if they drink the whole bottle.

Specialty Waters

Flavored waters, made with or without added sugars, are widely available, as are so-called designer or enhanced waters. Many of these drinks are made with added nutrients and herbs and are labeled with structure–function claims stating, for example, that drinking the product will enhance memory, delay aging, boost energy levels, or strengthen the immune response. Notice, however, that the label also includes a disclaimer, such as "This statement has not been evaluated by the FDA. This product is not intended to diagnose, treat, cure, or prevent any disease." The FDA requires this disclaimer whenever a manufacturer makes a structure–function claim. In other words, manufacturers must acknowledge that the statements made on the labels of these fortified waters are not, in fact, based on research or reliable sources.

Actually, the level of nutrients is typically so much lower than what can be obtained from foods that such beverages rarely have much of an impact on health or well-being. And waters made with HFCS, honey, or other sweeteners can add more than 300 Calories to your daily diet.

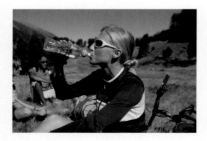

⬆ Vigorous exercise causes significant losses of water and electrolytes, which must be replenished to optimize performance and health.

One enhanced water being marketed through online sites and "health" stores is alkaline water. Promoted as a way to counteract the buildup of free radicals in the body, alkaline water supposedly delays the aging process, improves digestion, and minimizes bone loss. Typically produced through the use of an ionizer, a device that modifies its chemical profile, alkaline water has a slightly higher pH (more alkaline) than most forms of tap or bottled water. However, as soon as alkaline water is swallowed and moves into the stomach, the highly acidic gastric fluid immediately reduces the water's pH, defeating its entire purpose! Moreover, our kidneys and lungs, along with blood-based proteins, immediately respond to fluctuations in our body's pH, maintaining a healthy balance even when we drink black coffee or other acidic beverages. A product called "black water" is also being marketed to balance the body's pH level, as well as to "detoxify" the body. Black water is enriched with fulvic and humic acids; both are found in nature but neither is required to maintain health in humans. In short, no scientific evidence supports the health claims made for either alkaline water or black water.

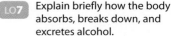

Athletes who train or compete in hot weather are vulnerable to dangerous fluid loss.

Sports Beverages and Coconut Water

A final fluid option is that of a traditional sports beverage, which provides water, electrolytes, and a source of carbohydrate, although some products now offer low-/no-sugar options. Because of the potential for fluid and electrolyte imbalances during vigorous exercise, many athletes drink sports beverages instead of plain water before, during, and after workouts. Recently, sports beverages have also become popular with recreationally active people and non-athletes. Is it really necessary or helpful for people to consume these beverages? See the *Highlight* feature on sports beverages to find out.

In addition to traditional sports beverages, coconut water is often marketed as a superior fluid for athletes, particularly for rehydration and the prevention of dehydration. However, a recent study of athletes performing 60 minutes of vigorous exercise found that coconut water was no better than a sport beverage or plain water at promoting hydration or exercise performance.[11] Moreover, subjects reported feeling more bloated and experienced greater stomach upset when drinking the coconut water. There are also claims that coconut water can delay aging, enhance the immune system, and prevent cancer, but no well-designed human studies support these claims.

As you can see, American consumers have a wide range of beverage choices available to them. Poor choices can increase your total caloric intake and lower your daily intake of nutrients. Over the past 40 years, the caloric contribution of beverages to our total energy intake has almost doubled. Plain drinking water is available free of charge, contributes no Calories, contains no additives, is highly effective in quenching thirst and maintaining hydration status, and poses no health threat. For most of us, most of the time, water really is the perfect beverage choice.

recap Fluid requirements are highly individualized and depend on body size, age, physical activity, health status, and environmental factors. All beverages provide water, and some—such as milk and calcium-fortified drinks—provide other important nutrients as well. Some beverages contain excessive amounts of caffeine, added sugars, or other potentially harmful ingredients and should be consumed in limited amounts. Pure water remains the best beverage choice for most people.

alcohol A beverage made from fermented fruits, vegetables, or grains.

drink The amount of an alcoholic beverage that provides approximately ½ fl. oz of pure ethanol.

How much alcohol is safe to drink?

Alcohol is the common name for a beverage made from fermented fruits, vegetables, and grains. Alcoholic beverages include beer, wine, and distilled spirits, such as whiskey. Although alcohol is an energy-rich compound providing 7 kcal per gram, it is not considered a nutrient because, instead of being essential to our body's functioning, it can significantly impair functioning.

Alcohol Consumption Is Described as Drinks per Day

Alcohol consumption is typically described in terms of *drinks per day*. A **drink** is defined as the amount of a beverage that provides ½ fl. oz of alcohol. Typically, that's equivalent to 1½ oz of distilled spirits (80-proof vodka, gin, whiskey, rum, scotch), 5 oz

LO7 Explain briefly how the body absorbs, breaks down, and excretes alcohol.

LO8 Discuss the health effects of moderate alcohol intake.

LO9 Describe how excessive alcohol use increases the risks of illness, injury, and death.

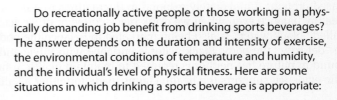

highlight

Sports Beverages: Help or Hype?

Once considered specialty products used exclusively by elite athletes, sports beverages have become popular everyday choices for both active and nonactive people. The market for these drinks has become so lucrative that many of the large soft drink companies now produce them. This surge in popularity leads us to ask three important questions:

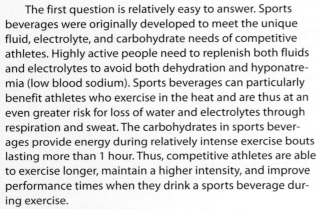

- Do sports beverages benefit highly active athletes?
- Do sports beverages benefit recreationally active people?
- Do nonactive people benefit from consuming sports beverages?

The first question is relatively easy to answer. Sports beverages were originally developed to meet the unique fluid, electrolyte, and carbohydrate needs of competitive athletes. Highly active people need to replenish both fluids and electrolytes to avoid both dehydration and hyponatremia (low blood sodium). Sports beverages can particularly benefit athletes who exercise in the heat and are thus at an even greater risk for loss of water and electrolytes through respiration and sweat. The carbohydrates in sports beverages provide energy during relatively intense exercise bouts lasting more than 1 hour. Thus, competitive athletes are able to exercise longer, maintain a higher intensity, and improve performance times when they drink a sports beverage during exercise.

In addition, sports beverages may help athletes consume more energy than they could by eating solid foods and water alone. Some competitive athletes train or compete for 6 to 8 hours each day on a regular basis. It is virtually impossible for them to consume enough solid foods to support this intense level of exercise.

Do recreationally active people or those working in a physically demanding job benefit from drinking sports beverages? The answer depends on the duration and intensity of exercise, the environmental conditions of temperature and humidity, and the individual's level of physical fitness. Here are some situations in which drinking a sports beverage is appropriate:

- before exercise or manual labor if you're concerned that dehydration might occur, especially if you are already feeling dehydrated
- during exercise or manual labor if you have recently had diarrhea or vomiting
- during exercise or manual labor in high heat and/or high humidity
- during exercise or manual labor at high altitude and in cold environments; these conditions increase fluid and electrolyte losses
- during continuous, vigorous exercise or labor lasting longer than 60 minutes in any climate
- between exercise bouts when it is difficult to consume food, such as between multiple soccer matches during a tournament

Recently, sports beverages have become very popular with people who do little or no regular exercise or manual labor. However, there's no evidence that people who do not exercise get any benefits from consuming sports beverages. Even if they live in a hot climate, they should be able to replenish the fluid and electrolytes they lose during sweating by drinking water and other beverages and eating a normal diet.

When inactive people drink sports beverages, a common consequence is inappropriate weight gain. Drinking 12 fl. oz (1.5 cups) of Gatorade adds 90 Calories to a person's daily energy intake. Many inactive people consume two to three times this amount each day, increasing their risk for overweight or obesity—with no benefit to their health.

---

of wine, or 12 oz of beer or a wine cooler (**FIGURE 8.6**). The alcohol content of distilled spirits is directly related to its **proof**: 100-proof liquor is 50% alcohol, whereas 80-proof liquor is 40% alcohol. **TABLE 8.1** compares the alcohol content of different beverages.

The 2010 *Dietary Guidelines for Americans* advise, "If alcohol is consumed, it should be consumed in moderation—up to one drink per day for women and two drinks per day for men—and only by adults of legal drinking age."[12] It's important to understand that these are *daily* guidelines; a person who drinks no alcohol Sunday through Thursday but routinely downs a six-pack on Friday and Saturday nights would not be classified as a moderate drinker! The 2010 Guidelines also identify specific groups who should not consume any alcohol at all:

- women who are or may become pregnant
- anyone younger than the legal drinking age
- people who cannot control their alcohol intake or keep it within moderate levels

proof A measure of the alcohol content of a liquid. For example, 100-proof liquor is 50% alcohol by volume, whereas 80-proof liquor is 40% alcohol by volume.

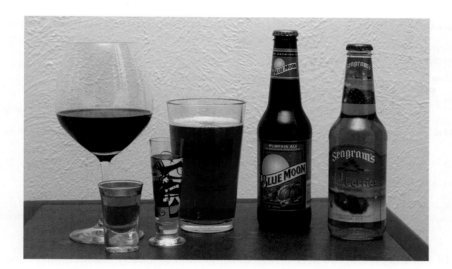

FIGURE 8.6 What does one drink look like? The National Institute on Alcohol Abuse and Alcoholism lists "one drink" as 5 oz of wine, 12 oz of beer or wine cooler, or 1½ oz of distilled spirits.

- people taking medications that can interact with alcohol
- people who drive, operate machinery, or engage in other tasks requiring attention and coordination

In the United States, fewer than half of all adults regularly consume alcohol. About 40% of Americans are lifetime or current abstainers (defined as having no alcoholic drinks within the previous 12 months); women are twice as likely as men to be lifetime abstainers.

Alcohol Absorption Rates Vary

Alcohol, which does not require digestion, is absorbed from both the stomach and the small intestine. From there, it's transported to the liver, where it is subsequently metabolized or, if consumed in excess, released into the bloodstream and rapidly distributed throughout the body.

The rate at which we absorb alcohol varies. If consumed without food, alcohol is absorbed from the stomach almost immediately. Eating a meal or snack with some fat, protein, and fiber before or with alcohol intake will slow gastric emptying and delay the intestinal absorption of alcohol. Carbonated alcoholic beverages are absorbed more rapidly than noncarbonated, resulting in the infamous intoxicating effect of champagne and sparkling wines. Women often absorb 30–35% more of a given amount of alcohol than do men of the same size, which may explain why women are often more susceptible to its effects.

TABLE 8.1   Alcohol Content of Common Alcoholic Beverages

Beverage Type	% Alcohol by Volume
Light beer, pilsner	3–4%
Regular beer, lager	5–6%
Stout beer, malt liquor	7–10%
Sparkling wine	8–12%
Table wine	9–14%
Fortified wine (sherry, port, vermouth, marsala)	16–22%
Wine cooler, fruit-flavored drinks (alcopops)	3–7%
Whiskey, vodka, rum, and other "spirits"	40–60%

TABLE 8.2 **Effects of Blood Alcohol Concentration (BAC) on Brain Activity**

Blood Alcohol Concentration (%)	Typical Response
0.02–0.05	Feeling of relaxation; euphoria; relief
0.06–0.10	Impaired judgment, fine motor control, and coordination; loss of normal emotional control; legally drunk in many states (at the upper end of the range)
0.11–0.15	Impaired reflexes and gross motor control; staggered gait; legally drunk in all states; slurred speech
0.16–0.20	Impaired vision; unpredictable behavior; further loss of muscle control
0.21–0.35	Total loss of coordination; in a stupor
0.40 and above	Loss of consciousness; coma; suppression of respiratory response; death

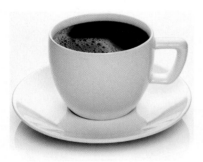

◀ Contrary to popular notions, coffee will not speed the breakdown of alcohol.

For a list of DUI/DWI laws and penalties in all fifty states, go to the Insurance Institute for Highway Safety's web page at www.iihs.org. Type "dui laws" into the Search bar, then select DUI/DWI Laws from the list.

In a healthy adult, the liver breaks down alcohol at a fairly constant rate, equal to about one drink per hour. If someone drinks more than that, such as three drinks in an hour, the excess alcohol is released back into the bloodstream, where it is distributed to all body tissues and fluids, including the brain and liver.

Despite popular notions, there is no effective way to speed up the breakdown of alcohol: it doesn't help to walk around, consume coffee or energy drinks, or use herbal or nutrient supplements. The keys to avoiding intoxication are to consume alcohol slowly, to have no more than one drink per hour, and to drink alcoholic beverages only after or while eating a meal or large snack.

As a person's alcohol intake increases over time, the liver metabolizes alcohol more efficiently and blood alcohol levels rise more slowly. This metabolic tolerance to alcohol explains why people who chronically abuse alcohol must consume larger and larger amounts before becoming intoxicated. Over time, some may need to consume twice as much alcohol as when they first started to drink to reach the same state of intoxication.

Of the alcohol we consume, a small amount, typically less than 10%, is excreted through the urine, breath, and sweat. As the blood alcohol concentration increases, so does the level of alcohol in breath vapor; this relationship forms the basis of the common Breathalyzer testing done by law enforcement agencies. It may surprise you to learn that your driving ability becomes impaired at quite low levels of alcohol consumption. For example, certain driving skills are reduced by blood alcohol concentrations (BAC) as low as 0.02%, despite the fact that most states in the United States do not charge drivers with a DUI/DWI offense if their BAC is below 0.08%. **TABLE 8.2** identifies typical responses of individuals at varying BAC levels.

recap Alcohol provides 7 kcal per gram but is not a nutrient because it is not essential to body functioning. Alcohol intake is classified in terms of "drinks per day." A drink is defined as the amount of a beverage that provides ½ fl. oz of alcohol. Fewer than half of Americans regularly consume alcohol. Alcohol absorption can be slowed by the consumption of a meal or large snack. The liver breaks down absorbed alcohol at a steady rate of approximately one drink per hour; there is no effective way to speed up this process.

Moderate Alcohol Consumption Has Health Benefits and Risks

The psychological benefits of moderate alcohol consumption are well known: it can relieve tension and anxiety while increasing a sense of relaxation and self-confidence. But moderate alcohol consumption has health benefits as well. It has been linked to a reduced risk for cardiovascular disease and certain types of strokes. Moderate alcohol intake increases levels of protective HDL-cholesterol, lowers harmful LDL-cholesterol concentrations, and reduces the risk for clot formation in the arteries. Although many people believe these benefits come only from red wines, recent studies suggest that intakes of white wine, distilled spirits, or even beer have similar effects.[13]

In the elderly, moderate alcohol consumption may stimulate appetite and improve dietary intake. Some, but not all, research suggests that moderate alcohol consumption may lower risk for cognitive impairment and other forms of dementia.[14] As research in this area continues, healthcare providers will develop a clearer picture of which groups of people might benefit from moderate alcohol intake.

Despite such benefits, moderate drinking can also be risky. A person's genetic background, state of health, use of medicines, and age all influence the short- and long-term responses to alcohol intake, even at moderate levels. For example, some studies have reported an increased risk for breast cancer among women consuming even low to moderate levels of alcohol, and others have reported an increased risk of developing high blood pressure (hypertension) among men consuming as little as two drinks per day. In addition, alcohol consumption interferes with the absorption and utilization of thiamin, folate, and vitamin B_6, increasing the risk for nutrient deficiency.

Another concern is the effect of alcohol on our waistlines. At 7 kcal/g, alcohol has a relatively high Calorie content. Only fat (9 kcal/g) has more Calories per gram. Let's take a look at the Calorie counts of some common alcoholic beverages:

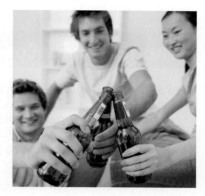

▲ Drinking beverages that contain alcohol causes an increase in water loss, because alcohol is a diuretic.

- A shot of whiskey, rum, vodka, or gin contains about 100 Calories.
- A 12-ounce can of beer and a 6-ounce glass of wine have the same Calorie count—about 150.
- A 12-ounce bottle of a wine cooler will cost you about 250 Calories.
- Many mixed drinks are loaded with Calories: a 6-ounce white Russian has about 320 Calories, and a pineapple daiquiri packs 670 Calories into just 4 ounces!

As you can see, if you're watching your weight, it makes sense to strictly limit your consumption of alcohol to stay within your daily energy needs. Alcohol intake may also increase your food intake, because alcoholic beverages enhance appetite, particularly during social events, leading some people to overeat. Both current and lifelong intakes of alcohol increase risk of obesity in males and females.

Drinking alcohol while taking any one of dozens of medications can also cause problems.[15] For example, if you are taking antihistamines for an allergy, alcohol will increase their sedative effect, making you extremely drowsy. And you can develop serious liver and kidney disease if you are regularly taking the painkiller acetaminophen (sold in many over-the-counter remedies, such as Tylenol), even if you drink only moderately.

Trace the flow of alcohol through the body and see how it affects your organs and body systems. Go to www .collegedrinkingprevention.gov and click on College Students. Then click the link "Interactive Body" to see how alcohol interacts with your body.

recap Moderate alcohol consumption is associated with health benefits as well as potential risks. Every person will have a unique metabolic and behavioral response to a given alcohol exposure and must carefully weigh the pros and cons of alcohol consumption.

Excessive Alcohol Consumption Leads to Serious Health Problems

Alcohol is a drug. It exerts a narcotic effect on virtually every part of the brain, acting as a sedative and depressant. Alcohol suppresses the area of the brain that controls reasoning and judgment, causes blurred vision and slurred speech, and impairs fine and gross motor skills (see Table 8.2). It also interferes with normal sleep patterns and reduces sexual function.

Excessive alcohol consumption negatively affects not only the drinker's physiology but also his or her mood and behavior. Many people who drink to excess experience mood swings, irritability, or intense anger, whereas others experience sadness or lethargy. In addition, alcohol impairs judgment, making a person more likely to perform or become the victim of vandalism, physical or sexual assault, and other crimes.

WHAT ABOUT **YOU?** (?)

Should You Be Concerned About How Much Alcohol You Drink?

As discussed in this chapter, alcohol contributes to societal violence as well as personal illness, disability, and death.

Answer the following questions, provided by the National Institute on Alcohol Abuse and Alcoholism (NIAAA), to help you find out if you have a drinking problem. For each question, circle Yes or No.

- Have you ever felt you should cut down on your drinking?
    YES or NO
- Have people annoyed you by criticizing your drinking?
    YES or NO
- Have you ever felt bad or guilty about your drinking?
    YES or NO
- Do you drink alone when you feel angry or sad?
    YES or NO
- Has your drinking ever made you late for school or work?
    YES or NO
- Have you ever had a drink first thing in the morning to steady your nerves or to get rid of a hangover?
    YES or NO
- Do you ever drink after promising yourself you won't?
    YES or NO

One "yes" answer suggests a possible alcohol problem. More than one "yes" answer means it is highly likely that a problem exists.

If you think you might have an alcohol problem, it's important to see a doctor or other healthcare provider right away.

She or he can help you determine if a drinking problem exists and plan the best course of action. If your doctor tells you to cut down on or stop drinking, these steps from the NIAAA can help you:

1. Write down your reasons for cutting down or stopping, such as complying with drinking-age laws or campus zero-tolerance policies, improving your health or grades, or getting along better with friends.
2. Also write down your goal (for example, *I will stop drinking alcohol as of today, May 18, 2015*).
3. To help you achieve your goal, keep a diary listing every time you have a drink, the amount and type, and what circumstances (such as peer pressure, loneliness) prompted you to drink.
4. Make sure there is no alcohol in your house, dorm room, apartment, car, locker, and so forth. Instead, keep non-alcoholic beverages that you enjoy well stocked wherever you go.
5. Learn how to say NO. You don't have to drink when other people drink. Practice ways to say no politely. For instance, you can tell people that you feel better when you drink less, or that you are watching your weight. Stay away from people who harass you about not drinking.
6. Get support. Tell your family and trusted friends about your plan to cut down or stop drinking and ask them for support in reaching your goal. Or contact your local chapter of Alcoholics Anonymous.

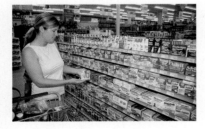

⬆ Alcohol can interfere with and increase the risks of using various over-the-counter and prescription medications.

binge drinking The consumption of 5 or more alcoholic drinks on one occasion.

Intoxication significantly increases the likelihood that a person will engage in unprotected sex, which in turn puts them at risk for sexually transmitted infections and unplanned pregnancy. And, like many drugs, it can be highly addictive.

In the absence of addiction, excessive alcohol consumption is often called as *alcohol abuse* or "problem drinking." It is characterized by drinking too *much*, too *often* or *inappropriately* (such as when pregnant, prior to driving a motor vehicle, between classes, or to deal with negative emotions). Although the legal drinking age in the United States is 21 years, nearly 20% of college students between 18 and 24 years of age can be categorized as experiencing alcohol abuse and/or dependence.[16]

How much alcohol do you drink, and should you be concerned about it? Check out the ***What About You?*** feature box to help you decide.

Binge Drinking and Alcohol Poisoning

Binge drinking, defined as consuming 5 or more alcoholic drinks on one occasion by a man (4 or more drinks for a woman), is a common type of alcohol abuse, especially on college campuses. The rate of binge drinking is highest (51%) among those 18 to 20 years of age; twice as many men report binge drinking as women. About

90% of the alcohol consumed by those under age 21 is in the form of bingeing.[17] In other words, among those too young to legally consume alcohol, it is typically an "all or nothing" situation. Many rituals associated with student life, including acceptance into a fraternity or sorority, sports events, and 21st-birthday rituals, involve binge drinking.

The negative effects of binge drinking range from being debilitating to life threatening. They include impaired motor control, disorientation, impaired judgment, memory loss, dehydration, nausea, vomiting, loss of bowel control, and accidental and intentional injuries. Potentially fatal falls, drowning, automobile accidents, and acts of physical violence often result from binge drinking. When alcohol intake is so high that it overwhelms the liver's ability to clear the alcohol from the blood, alcohol poisoning, a potentially fatal consequence of binge drinking, can occur. **Alcohol poisoning** depresses the areas of the brain that regulate breathing and cardiac function, resulting in respiratory and heart failure, then death.

Most binge drinkers lose consciousness before alcohol poisoning becomes fatal, but immediate medical care is still essential. That's because any alcohol in the stomach and intestines will continue to seep into the bloodstream, further elevating the person's BAC. As this toxic level of alcohol circulates throughout the body, it can cause brain damage or death. In addition, extremely intoxicated people can vomit while they're unconscious. If the vomit blocks their breathing passages, they can choke to death. If it is inhaled into their lungs, they can develop a life-threatening form of pneumonia. Someone who passes out after binge drinking should *never* be left alone to "sleep it off," but should be turned on his or her side and carefully watched for vomiting; cold, clammy, or bluish skin; and slow or irregular breathing patterns. If any of these signs become evident, seek emergency medical care immediately.

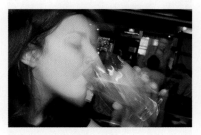

◄ Drinking too much, too often, and inappropriately are signs of alcohol abuse.

Chronic Alcohol Abuse

Chronic alcohol abuse, defined as excessive intake over a period of several months to years, impairs brain function in a number of ways. In adolescence and young adulthood, the brain is still developing, and alcohol abuse during these years can actually change brain structure and function. This may impair the development of intellect and abstract reasoning, diminish memory, and interfere with behavioral and emotional regulation. Even after becoming sober, many people who have chronically abused alcohol often continue to experience ongoing memory and learning problems.

Chronic alcohol abuse can also lead to *alcoholism* (also known as *alcohol dependence*), a disease characterized by the following four symptoms, described by the National Institute on Alcohol Abuse and Alcoholism (NIAAA):

- *Craving:* a strong need, or urge, to drink alcoholic beverages
- *Loss of control:* not being able to stop drinking once drinking has begun
- *Physical dependence:* the development of withdrawal symptoms, such as nausea, sweating, shakiness, and anxiety after stopping alcohol intake
- *Tolerance:* the need to drink larger and larger amounts of alcohol to get the same "high" or pleasurable sensations associated with alcohol intake

In addition, chronic alcohol abuse severely damages the liver. As the primary site of alcohol metabolism, the liver is extremely vulnerable to the toxic effects of alcohol. Liver cells are damaged or destroyed during excessive and binge-drinking episodes. If alcohol abuse persists, liver function continues to decline. *Fatty liver* is an early and reversible sign of damage. If drinking continues, the person may develop alcohol-related **hepatitis**, which causes loss of appetite, nausea and vomiting, abdominal pain, jaundice, and, on occasion, mental confusion. **Cirrhosis** of the liver is a chronic condition that develops after many years of alcohol abuse. It is characterized by scarring of liver tissue, impaired blood flow through the liver, and a life-threatening decline in liver function (**FIGURE 8.7**). In addition,

alcohol poisoning A potentially fatal condition in which an overdose of alcohol results in cardiac or respiratory failure.

hepatitis Inflammation of the liver; can be caused by a virus or a toxic agent, such as alcohol.

cirrhosis End-stage liver disease characterized by significant abnormalities in liver structure and function; may lead to complete liver failure.

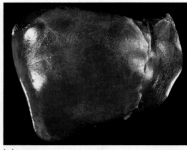

(a)

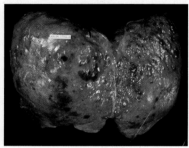

(b)

◆ **FIGURE 8.7** Cirrhosis of the liver, caused by chronic alcohol abuse. **(a)** A healthy liver. **(b)** A liver damaged by cirrhosis.

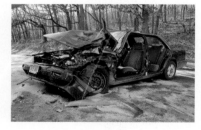

◆ Excessive alcohol consumption greatly increases the risks for car accidents and other traumatic injuries.

chronic alcohol abuse is associated with an increased risk for diabetes, bone disease, and several cancers, including cancer of the mouth, esophagus, stomach, and bladder.

Alcohol Consumption Greatly Increases the Risk for Accidental Death

Although the rate of alcohol-related traffic deaths has decreased by almost 25% over the past decade, the number remains unacceptably high. In 2012, more than 10,000 people died in automobile crashes involving a drunk driver, nearly one-third of all automotive fatalities.[18]

It is estimated that as many as 6,000 young Americans die each year from alcohol-related accidents, homicides, and suicides. Alcohol has also been implicated in 40% of all suicide attempts and fatal falls, 50% of sexual assaults, and 60% of drowning and homicides.[19]

Reading about these problems of alcohol consumption may prompt you to think about someone you know who abuses or is addicted to alcohol. If so, the *Game Plan* feature box has guidelines for helping someone with an alcohol problem get treatment.

Strategies for Limiting Alcohol Intake

As you can see, drinking too much alcohol is dangerous for many reasons. So, if you sometimes or often drink "to get drunk," a reasonable question to ask yourself is, *Why*? How does binge drinking fit in with your goals for yourself, your academic career, your professional future? If you decide that you want to drink socially, but avoid intoxication, here are some tips for staying in control:

- Take steps ahead of time to keep within your limits. For example:
  - If you're going to a bar, take only enough money to buy two beers and two sodas.
  - Have a meal or snack containing protein before you leave home.
  - Have a "No thanks" line ready. Something as simple as "No thanks, I'm good"—can help you side-step peer pressure.
- Make your first beverage a large glass of sparkling water, iced tea, diet soda, juice, or non-alcoholic beer. After that, rotate between alcoholic and non-alcoholic drinks.
- If you're mixing a drink for yourself, use less liquor and dilute it with large amounts of diet soda, water, or juice. If you're in a bar, ask the bartender to make it weak.
- Whether or not your drink is diluted, sip slowly to allow your liver time to keep up with your alcohol intake.
- Stay occupied by dancing, sampling the food, watching the game, or talking with friends.

The best strategy is to volunteer to be the designated driver. You'll have a "free pass" for the night in terms of saying no to alcohol.

recap Alcohol abuse (also called problem drinking) occurs when a person drinks too much, too often, or inappropriately. Binge drinking is the consumption of five or more drinks on one occasion. It can cause alcohol poisoning, which can be fatal. Chronic alcohol abuse can result in significant cognitive, emotional, and behavioral deficits and can lead to alcoholism. It can also severely damage the liver and increase the risk for certain cancers. Alcohol consumption, particularly in underage drinkers, is strongly associated with traumatic death.

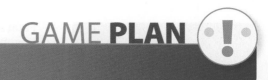

GAME **PLAN**

Strategies for Helping Someone with an Alcohol Problem Get Treatment

If you know someone who abuses alcohol by drinking too much, too often, or inappropriately or who experiences symptoms of alcoholism, what should you do? Some people respond well when confronted by a single person, whereas others benefit more from a group intervention. There should be no blaming or shaming; alcohol use disorders are medical conditions with a genetic component. The National Institute on Alcoholism and Alcohol Abuse (NIAAA) suggests the following steps to help someone with an alcohol problem get treatment:

 Stop covering up and making excuses. Many times, family and friends will make excuses to others to protect the person from the results of his or her drinking. It is important, however, to stop covering for that person so he or she can experience the full consequences of inappropriate alcohol consumption.

☐ ***Intervene at a vulnerable time.*** The best time to talk to someone about problem drinking is shortly after an alcohol-related incident such as a DUI arrest, an alcohol-related traffic accident, or a public scene. Wait until the person is sober and everyone is relatively calm.

☐ ***Be specific.*** Tell the person exactly why you are concerned; use examples of specific problems associated with his or her drinking habits (e.g., poor school or work performance; legal problems; inappropriate behaviors). Explain what will happen if the person chooses not to get help—for example, no longer going out with the person if alcohol will be available, no longer riding with him or her in motor vehicles, moving out of a shared home, and so on.

☐ ***Get help.*** Professional help is available from community agencies, healthcare providers, online sites, school or worksite wellness centers, and some religious organizations. Several contacts and websites are listed shortly. If the person indicates a willingness to get help, call immediately for an appointment and/or immediately bring him or her to a treatment center. The longer the delay, the more likely it is that the person will experience a change of heart.

 Enlist the support of others. Whether or not the person agrees to get help, calling on other friends and relatives can often be effective, especially if one of these people has battled alcohol abuse. Formal support groups such as Al-Anon and Alateen can provide additional information and guidance.

Treatment for alcohol use disorders works for many, but not all, individuals. "Success" is measured in small steps, and relapses are common. Most scientists agree that people who abuse alcohol cannot just "cut down." Complete avoidance of all alcoholic beverages is the only way for most people who abuse alcohol to achieve full and ongoing recovery.

✛ HEALTHWATCH

Can pregnant women safely consume alcohol?

LO10 Explain how alcohol intake during pregnancy can affect the fetus.

Alcohol is a known *teratogen* (a substance capable of causing birth defects). When a pregnant woman consumes alcohol, it quickly crosses the placenta into the fetal bloodstream. Since the immature fetal liver cannot effectively metabolize alcohol, it builds up in the fetal blood and tissues, increasing the risk for a variety of birth defects. The effects of maternal alcohol intake are dose-dependent: the more the mother drinks, the greater the potential harm to the fetus.

The term **fetal alcohol spectrum disorders (FASD)** is an umbrella term used to describe the range of complications that can develop when a pregnant woman consumes alcohol. It is not known how many infants are born with FASD each year, although one estimate is that there are 6 cases of FASD out of every 1,000 live births in the United States.[20]

fetal alcohol spectrum disorders (FASD) An umbrella term describing the range of effects that can occur in the child of a woman who drinks during pregnancy.

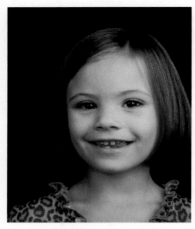

FIGURE 8.8 The facial features characteristic of children with fetal alcohol syndrome (FAS) include a short nose with a low, wide bridge; drooping eyes with an extra skinfold; and a flat, thin upper lip. Behavioral problems and learning disorders are also characteristic. The effects of FAS are irreversible.

fetal alcohol syndrome (FAS) A cluster of birth defects in the children of a mother who consumed alcohol during pregnancy, including facial deformities, impaired growth, and a spectrum of mild to severe cognitive, emotional, and physical problems.

Fetal alcohol syndrome (FAS) is the most severe form of FASD and is characterized by malformations of the face, limbs, heart, and nervous system **(FIGURE 8.8)**. Newborn and infant death rates are high, and those who survive typically have emotional, behavioral, social, learning, and developmental problems throughout life. FAS is one of the most common causes of mental retardation in the United States and is the only one that is completely preventable. FAS is usually recognized at birth, due in large part to the characteristic facial features of affected infants. However, maternal alcohol consumption can also result in various other physical, developmental, and behavioral problems that are recognized later in infancy and childhood, such as hearing and vision problems, hyperactivity, attention deficit disorder, and impaired learning.[20]

Can pregnant women safely consume small amounts of alcohol? Although some pregnant women do have an occasional alcoholic drink with no apparent ill effects, the fact is there is no amount of alcohol that is known to be safe. The 2010 *Dietary Guidelines for Americans* specifically state that "women who are pregnant or who may be pregnant" should not drink alcohol. The Guidelines confirm that "no safe level of alcohol consumption during pregnancy has been established."[12]

Breastfeeding women should also be very cautious about their use of alcohol, which rapidly enters breast milk at levels similar to those in the mother's bloodstream. In addition to inhibiting the mother's milk supply, alcohol that passes into breast milk can make the baby sleepy, depress its central nervous system, and, over time, slow the child's motor development. During the initial stages of breastfeeding, when the infant nurses nearly around the clock, alcohol consumption should be completely avoided. When feedings become less frequent, after about 3 months of age, an occasional glass of wine or beer is considered safe, as long as there is sufficient time (approximately 4 hours) before the next feeding. This will allow time for the alcohol to be metabolized by the mother and will lower maternal blood levels, thus limiting alcohol from entering the breast milk. Another option is for the mother to express breast milk before consuming alcohol and save it for a later feeding.

recap Alcohol is a known teratogen (substance capable of causing birth defects). Fetal alcohol syndrome is a condition characterized by malformations of the face, limbs, heart, and nervous system in infants born to mothers who abuse alcohol during pregnancy. A variety of other physical, developmental, and behavioral disorders can also occur if a woman drinks during her pregnancy. No amount of alcohol during pregnancy is considered safe.

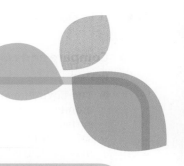

STUDY **PLAN** | MasteringNutrition™

Customize your study plan—and master your nutrition!—
in the Study Area of **MasteringNutrition**.

what can I do **today?**

Now that you've read this chapter, try making these three changes.

1 Track your fluid intake. Are you drinking enough to stay optimally hydrated?

2 Choose healthful beverages! For one full day, try avoiding all sweetened drinks and stick to plain water, coffee, tea, nonfat milk, calcium-fortified soy milk, rice milk, or almond milk, or, in limited amounts (4–6 fl. oz per day) 100% fruit or vegetable juice. Then see if you can make it a habit to limit the amount of sweetened drinks you consume on average.

3 If you drink alcohol, keep your intake moderate: no more than one standard-size drink for women, and two for men, per day.

test yourself | *answers*

1. **True.** Between approximately 50% and 70% of our body weight consists of water.

2. **False.** Persistent vomiting can lead to serious health consequences and even death.

3. **True.** Carbonated alcoholic beverages, such as champagne, are absorbed more rapidly than noncarbonated varieties of alcohol.

summary

Scan to hear an MP3 Chapter Review in **MasteringNutrition**.

LO 1 Describe the location and functions of body fluid

- Water is an essential nutrient. Between approximately 50% and 70% of a healthy adult's body weight is water.

- Body fluid held within cells is known as intracellular fluid. It accounts for about two-thirds of body water. Extracellular fluid is outside the cells. There are two types of extracellular fluid: tissue fluid, or interstitial fluid, flows between the cells; plasma and lymph are fluids that flow within blood and lymphatic vessels.

- Water acts as a solvent in our bodies, helps transport nutrients and wastes, provides protection and lubrication for our organs and tissues, and acts to maintain blood volume and pressure and body temperature.

LO 2 Identify two mechanisms by which our body gains fluid

- The primary sources of fluid intake are beverages and foods, and metabolic water produced during metabolism.

LO 3 Identify five mechanisms by which our body loses fluid

- Fluid is lost through urine, feces, sweat, evaporation, and exhalation.

LO 4 Discuss three potentially fatal consequences of fluid imbalance

- Fluid intake needs are highly variable and depend on body size, age, physical activity, health status, and environmental conditions. Dehydration occurs when water excretion exceeds water intake. Individuals at risk include the elderly, infants, people exercising heavily for prolonged periods in the heat, and individuals suffering from prolonged vomiting and/or diarrhea.

- Heat stroke is a potentially fatal condition that occurs when the body cannot release enough heat through sweat to control temperatures within a safe range. If left untreated, heat stroke can lead to death.

- Water intoxication is caused by consuming too much water. Hyponatremia, or diluted blood sodium levels, can result from water intoxication and is more common in marathon runners and other athletes who compete in long events.

LO 5 Compare and contrast sources of drinking water

- The Environmental Protection Agency (EPA) monitors public tap water, which comes from surface or ground water and ensures that it is safe to drink. Bottled water is convenient but may be derived from a public tap, and its production depletes natural resources and produces waste.

LO 6 Debate the health benefits and potential concerns of at least four popular beverages

- Milk and milk substitutes are healthful beverages, as are coffee and tea in moderation. Energy drinks typically contain more caffeine than coffee or tea and are consumed more quickly, triggering a surge of caffeine in the bloodstream that can result in cardiac arrest, seizures, and other medical emergencies. They are also high in sugar. Specialty waters are of questionable benefit and may also contain significant added sugars.

- Sports drinks can be helpful especially when dehydration is a possibility, such as working in high heat and humidity, being at high altitudes, or when exercising in heat and humidity for more than 60 minutes.

LO 7 Explain briefly how the body absorbs, breaks down, and excretes alcohol

- Alcohol is a narcotic drug. Although it provides 7 kcal/gram, it impairs, rather than promotes, human functioning and is not considered a nutrient.

- Alcohol, which does not require digestion, is absorbed from both the stomach and the small intestine. From there, it's transported to the liver, where it is subsequently metabolized or, if consumed in excess, released into the bloodstream and rapidly distributed throughout the body. Of the alcohol we consume, a small amount, typically less than 10%, is excreted through the urine, breath, and sweat.

- Alcohol absorption can be slowed by the consumption of a meal or large snack that provides some protein, fat, and fiber.

- The liver breaks down alcohol at a steady rate of approximately one drink per hour. There is no effective way to speed up this process.

LO 8 Discuss the health effects of moderate alcohol intake

- Moderate alcohol intake is associated with benefits to the cardiovascular system. It also appears to stimulate appetite and possibly reduce the risk of dementia in older adults. Other health benefits have been suggested by research. However, risk of breast cancer increases for women who drink alcohol even in moderate amounts, as does risk of hypertension in men.

LO 9 Describe how excessive alcohol use increases the risks of illness, injury, and death

- About 51% of young people between the ages of 18 and 21 report binge drinking, which is defined as having 5 or more alcoholic drinks on one occasion. Negative effects include impaired motor control, disorientation, impaired judgment, memory loss, dehydration, nausea, vomiting, loss of bowel control, and accidental and intentional injuries. Alcohol poisoning is associated with binge drinking and can be fatal.

- Chronic alcohol intake can lead to diminished memory and learning disabilities, as well as hepatitis and cirrhosis of the liver. It is also associated with an increased risk of certain cancers.

LO 10 Explain how alcohol intake during pregnancy can affect the fetus

- Fetal alcohol spectrum disorders (FASD) is a term used to describe the range of complications that can develop in the child of a woman who consumes alcohol during pregnancy. It includes fetal alcohol syndrome, which is characterized by malformations of the face, limbs, heart, and nervous system, and cognitive, emotional, and other deficits and delays throughout life. No amount of alcohol intake during pregnancy is considered safe.

review questions

LO 1 Describe the location and functions of body fluid

1. Plasma is one example of
   a. fluid outside our cells.
   b. fluid inside our cells.
   c. pure water.
   d. metabolic water.

LO 2 Identify two mechanisms by which our body gains fluid

2. Our body gains fluid by
   a. absorption and inhalation.
   b. intake and metabolism.
   c. hunger and thirst.
   d. all of the above.

LO 3 Identify five mechanisms by which our body loses fluid

3. Our body loses fluid through
   a. urine and feces.
   b. sweat.
   c. evaporation and exhalation.
   d. all of the above.

LO 4 Discuss three potentially fatal consequences of fluid imbalance

4. Pale yellow urine typically indicates
   a. adequate hydration.
   b. dehydration.
   c. heatstroke.
   d. water intoxication.

LO 5 Compare and contrast sources of drinking water

5. Water from a reservoir is
   a. distilled water.
   b. seltzer water.
   c. surface water.
   d. groundwater.

LO 6 Debate the health benefits and potential concerns of at least four popular beverages

6. Which of the following beverages contains added sugars?
   a. Mineral water
   b. Fresh-squeezed orange juice
   c. Chocolate milk
   d. All of the above

LO 7 Explain briefly how the body absorbs, breaks down, and excretes alcohol

7. Alcohol is absorbed from
   a. the stomach.
   b. the small intestine.
   c. the liver.
   d. both a and b.

LO 8 Discuss the health effects of moderate alcohol intake

8. Moderate alcohol consumption
   a. is defined as no more than two drinks per day for women and three per day for men.
   b. interferes with the absorption of some B-vitamins.
   c. decreases appetite in older adults.
   d. increases the risk for cardiovascular disease.

LO 9 Describe how excessive alcohol use increases the risks of illness, injury, and death

9. Excessive alcohol consumption
   a. is implicated in almost 10% of all traffic fatalities.
   b. increases sexual function.
   c. can cause brain damage.
   d. All of the above are true.

LO 10 Explain how alcohol intake during pregnancy can affect the fetus

10. Fetal alcohol syndrome
    a. is a range of complications that develop in an estimated 20% of pregnant women who drink alcohol.
    b. is a rare cause of mental retardation in the United States.
    c. is entirely treatable.
    d. is entirely preventable.

Answers to Review Questions are located at the back of this text.

web links

The following websites and apps explore further topics and issues related to personal health.
Visit **MasteringNutrition** for links to the websites and RSS feeds.

www.aa.org
Alcoholics Anonymous, Inc. (AA)

www.al-anon.alateen.org
Al-Anon Family Group Headquarters, Inc.

www.collegedrinkingprevention.gov
College Drinking: Changing the Culture

www.epa.gov
U.S. Environmental Protection Agency (EPA)

www.fda.gov
U.S. Food and Drug Administration (FDA)

9

Achieving and Maintaining a Healthful Body Weight

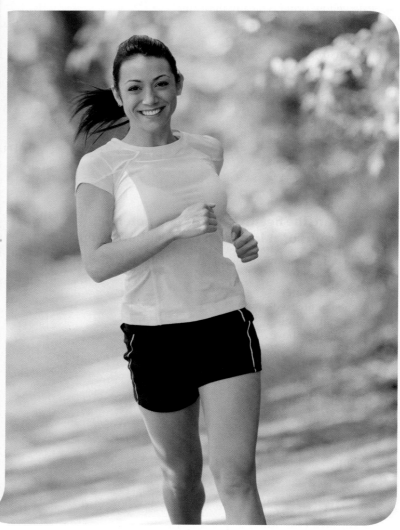

learning outcomes

After studying this chapter, you should be able to:

1 Define what is meant by a healthful weight, pp. 251–255.

2 Determine your BMI and fat distribution pattern and identify any health risks associated with these assessments, pp. 251–255.

3 State the energy balance equation and estimate your basal metabolic rate, pp. 255–266.

4 Explain how to calculate how many Calories you need to consume on average each day, pp. 255–266.

5 Discuss a range of factors thought to contribute to differences in body weight, pp. 255–266.

6 Identify three key strategies for healthful weight loss, pp. 266–276.

7 Discuss health risks associated with obesity, pp. 276–281.

8 Discuss three treatment options for obesity, pp. 276–281.

9 Identify several factors thought to contribute to the development of eating disorders, pp. 281–288.

10 Compare and contrast anorexia nervosa, bulimia nervosa, binge-eating disorder, night-eating syndrome, and the female athlete triad, pp. 281–288.

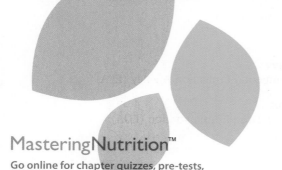

MasteringNutrition™

Go online for chapter quizzes, pre-tests, Interactive Activities, and more!

test yourself

Are these statements true or false? Circle your guess.

1. **T F** People who are physically active but overweight should not be considered healthy.

2. **T F** Although a majority of Americans are overweight, only about 10% of Americans are obese.

3. **T F** Only females get eating disorders.

Test Yourself answers can be found at the end of the chapter.

In February of 2012, at age 23, British pop singer Adele became only the second woman in history to win six Grammy Awards in one night. She has won critical acclaim from musicians of various genres and the adoration of millions of fans worldwide. Still, some critics—including fashion designer Karl Lagerfeld and comedian Joan Rivers—focus not on her big, soulful voice, but on her weight. Is Adele overweight? A size "14 to 16," she exudes supreme confidence in her tall, curvy body and insists she's not interested in losing weight just because someone else thinks she should. Rather than worry about something as "petty" as what you look like, Adele suggests that, "The first thing to do is be happy with yourself and appreciate your body."[1]

Are you happy with your weight, shape, body composition, and fitness? If not, what needs to change—your diet, your level of physical activity, or maybe just your attitude? What role do diet and physical activity play in maintaining a healthful body weight? How much of your body size and shape is due to genetics? What influence does society—including food advertising—have on your weight? And if you decide that you do need to lose weight, what's the best way to do it? In this chapter, we will explore these questions and provide some answers.

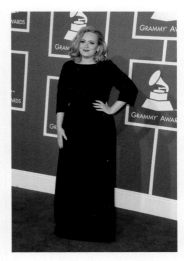

British pop singer Adele, who came under some media scrutiny for her weight, states that she is comfortable with who she is and how she looks.

Is your body weight healthful?

As you begin to think about achieving and maintaining a healthful weight, it's important to make sure you understand what a healthful body weight actually is and the various methods you can use to figure out if your own weight is healthful.

LO1 Define what is meant by a healthful weight.

LO2 Determine your BMI and fat distribution pattern and identify any health risks associated with these assessments.

Understand What a Healthful Body Weight Really Is

We can define a healthful weight as all of the following:[2]

- A weight that is appropriate for your age and physical development
- A weight that is based on your genetic background and family history of body shape and weight
- A weight that you can achieve and sustain without severely curtailing your food intake or constantly dieting
- A weight that is compatible with normal blood pressure, lipid levels, and glucose tolerance
- A weight that promotes good eating habits and allows you to participate in regular physical activity
- A weight that is acceptable to you

As you can see, a healthful weight is not one at which a person must be extremely thin or overly muscular. In addition, there is no one body type that can be defined as healthful. Thus, achieving a healthful body weight should not be dictated by the latest fad or society's expectations of what is acceptable.

Various methods are available to help you determine whether you're maintaining a healthful body weight. Let's review a few of these methods.

Determine Your Body Mass Index

Body mass index (BMI) is a commonly used comparison of a person's body weight to his or her height. You can calculate your BMI using the following equation:

$$\text{BMI (kg/m}^2\text{)} = \text{weight (kg)/height (m)}^2$$

If you're not comfortable using the metric system, there is an equation to calculate BMI using weight in pounds and height in inches:

$$\text{BMI (kg/m}^2\text{)} = [\text{weight (lb)/height (in.)}^2] \times 703$$

body mass index (BMI) A measurement representing the ratio of a person's body weight to his or her height.

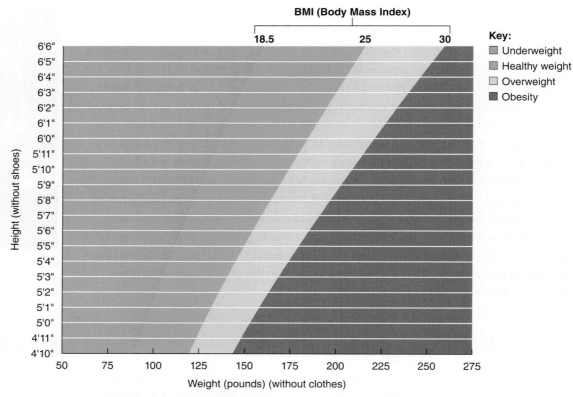

↞ FIGURE 9.1 Estimate your body mass index (BMI) using this graph. To determine your BMI, find the value for your height on the left and follow this line to the right until it intersects with the value for your weight on the bottom axis. The area on the graph where these two points intersect is your BMI.

underweight Having too little body fat to maintain health, causing a person to have a weight for a given height that is below an acceptably defined standard.

normal weight Having an adequate but not excessive level of body fat for health.

overweight Having a moderate amount of excess body fat, resulting in a person having a weight for a given height that is greater than an accepted standard but is not considered obese.

obesity Having an excess of body fat that adversely affects health, resulting in a person having a weight for a given height that is substantially greater than an accepted standard.

morbid obesity A condition in which a person's body weight exceeds 100% of normal, putting him or her at very high risk for serious health consequences.

A less exact but practical method is to use the graph in **FIGURE 9.1**, which shows approximate BMI values for your height and weight and whether your BMI is in a healthful range.

Your body mass index provides an important clue to your overall health. Physicians, nutritionists, and other scientists classify BMI accordingly:

- **Underweight** is defined as having too little body fat to maintain health, causing a person to have a weight that is below an acceptably defined standard for a given height. A person having a BMI less than 18.5 kg/m² is considered underweight.
- **Normal weight** is defined as having an adequate but not excessive level of body fat for health. It ranges from 18.5 to 24.9 kg/m².
- **Overweight** is defined as having a moderate amount of excess body fat, resulting in a person having a weight that is greater than some accepted standard for a given height but is not considered obese. Having a BMI between 25.1 and 29.9 kg/m² indicates that a person is overweight.
- **Obesity** is defined as having an excess of body fat that adversely affects health, resulting in a person having a weight that is substantially greater than some accepted standard for a given height. A BMI value between 30 and 39.9 kg/m² is consistent with obesity.
- **Morbid obesity** is defined as a BMI greater than or equal to 40 kg/m²; in this case, the person's body weight exceeds 100% of normal, putting him or her at very high risk for serious health consequences.

In addition to the effect of body weight on disease risk, researchers study the relationship between body weight and risk for premature death. Until recently, data from national surveys have indicated that having a BMI value within the healthful range means that your risk of dying prematurely is within the expected average. Thus, if your BMI value fell outside this range, either higher or lower, your risk of dying prematurely was considered greater than the average risk. However, recent evidence suggests that having a BMI in the overweight category may actually be protective against dying prematurely.[3] This study found that people who are overweight (BMI of 25 to 29.99 kg/m^2) but not obese have a 6% *lower* risk of dying prematurely than those with a normal BMI. In contrast, having a BMI in the obese category increases a person's risk of dying prematurely 18% above that of people with a BMI value in the normal-weight range.

Although calculating BMI can be very helpful in estimating these risks for young and middle-aged adults, it is limited when used with children, teens, and adults over age 65. It is also of limited value for people who have a disproportionately higher muscle mass for a given height. Let's take the example of a male weight lifter who is 5'7" tall and weighs 200 lb. Using Figure 9.1, you can see that his BMI is over 30, placing him in the high-risk category for many diseases. But is he really overweight? To answer that question, an assessment of body composition is necessary.

Measure Your Body Composition

There are many methods available to assess your **body composition**, or the amount of body fat (*adipose tissue*) and lean body mass (*lean tissue*) you have. **FIGURE 9.2** lists and describes some of the more common, but it's important to bear in mind that they can only estimate your body fat and lean body mass. Because the range of error of these methods can be 3% to more than 20%, you shouldn't use them as the sole indicator of how healthy you are.

Let's return to our weight lifter, whose BMI is over 30. Is he obese? He trains with weights 4 days per week, rides an exercise bike for about 30 minutes per session three times per week, and eats a nourishing diet. A skinfold assessment of his body composition shows that his body fat is 9%. This value is within the healthful range for men. He is an example of a person whose BMI appears to be very high but who is not actually obese.

Assess Your Fat Distribution Patterns

To complete your evaluation of your current body weight, it's important to consider the way fat is distributed throughout your body. This is because your fat distribution pattern is known to affect your risk for various diseases. **FIGURE 9.3** shows two types of fat patterning:

- In *apple-shaped fat patterning*, fat is stored mainly around the waist. Apple-shaped patterning is known to significantly increase a person's risk for many chronic diseases, such as type 2 diabetes, heart disease, and high blood pressure. It is thought that this patterning causes problems with the metabolism of fat and carbohydrate, leading to unhealthful changes in blood cholesterol, insulin, glucose, and blood pressure. Men tend to store fat in the apple-shaped pattern.
- In *pear-shaped fat patterning*, fat is stored mainly around the hips and thighs. This pattern does not seem to significantly increase a person's risk for chronic diseases. Premenopausal women tend to store fat in the pear-shaped pattern; postmenopausal women tend to store fat in the apple-shaped pattern.

You can use the following three-step method to determine your type of fat patterning:

1. Ask a friend to measure the circumference of your natural waist—that is, the narrowest part of your torso as observed from the front (**FIGURE 9.4a**).
2. Then have that friend measure your hip circumference at the maximal width of the buttocks as observed from the side (Figure 9.4b).
3. Then divide the waist value by the hip value. This measurement is called your *waist-to-hip ratio*. For example, if your natural waist is 30 inches and your hips are 40 inches, then your waist-to-hip ratio is 30 divided by 40, which equals 0.75.

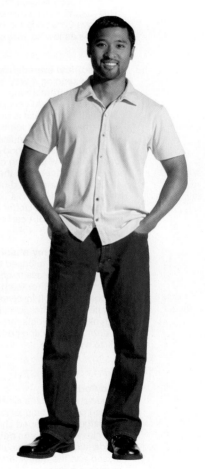

A healthful body weight is one that is appropriate for your age, your physical development, your heredity, and other factors.

body composition The ratio of a person's body fat to lean body mass.

Method		Limitations

Underwater weighing:
Considered the most accurate method. Estimates body fat within a 2–3% margin of error. This means that if your underwater weighing test shows you have 20% body fat, this value could be no lower than 17% and no higher than 23%. Used primarily for research purposes.

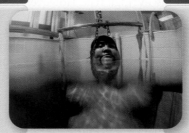

- Subject must be comfortable in water.
- Requires trained technician and specialized equipment.
- May not work well with extremely obese people.
- Must abstain from food for at least 8 hours and from exercise for at least 12 hours prior to testing.

Skinfolds:
Involves "pinching" a person's fold of skin (with its underlying layer of fat) at various locations of the body. The fold is measured using a specially designed caliper. When performed by a skilled technician, it can estimate body fat with an error of 3–4%. This means that if your skinfold test shows you have 20% body fat, your actual value could be as low as 16% or as high as 24%.

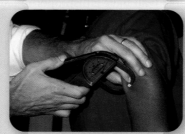

- Less accurate unless technician is well trained.
- Proper prediction equation must be used to improve accuracy.
- Person being measured may not want to be touched or to expose their skin.
- Cannot be used to measure obese people, as their skinfolds are too large for the caliper.

Bioelectrical impedance analysis (BIA):
Involves sending a very low level of electrical current through a person's body. As water is a good conductor of electricity and lean body mass is made up of mostly water, the rate at which the electricity is conducted gives an indication of a person's lean body mass and body fat. This method can be done while lying down, with electrodes attached to the feet, hands, and the BIA machine. Hand-held and standing models (which look like bathroom scales) are now available. Under the best of circumstances, BIA can estimate body fat with an error of 3–4%.

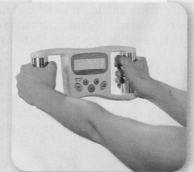

- Less accurate.
- Body fluid levels must be normal.
- Proper prediction equation must be used to improve accuracy.
- Should not eat for 4 hours and should not exercise for 12 hours prior to the test.
- No alcohol should be consumed within 48 hours of the test.
- Females should not be measured if they are retaining water due to menstrual cycle changes.

Dual-energy x-ray absorptiometry (DXA):
The technology is based on using very-low-level x-rays to differentiate among bone tissue, soft (or lean) tissue, and fat (or adipose) tissue. It involves lying for about 30 minutes on a specialized bed fully clothed, with all metal objects removed. The margin of error for predicting body fat ranges from 2% to 4%.

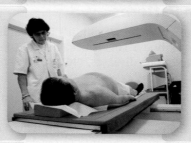

- Expensive; requires trained technician with specialized equipment.
- Cannot be used to measure extremely tall, short, or obese people, as they do not fit properly within the scanning area.

Bod Pod:
A machine that uses air displacement to measure body composition. This machine is a large, egg-shaped chamber made from fiberglass. The person being measured sits inside, wearing a swimsuit. The door is closed and the machine measures how much air is displaced. This value is used to calculate body composition. It appears promising as an easier and equally accurate alternative to underwater weighing in many populations, but it may overestimate body fat in some African American men.

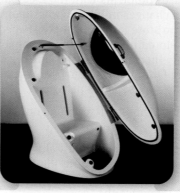

- Expensive.
- Less accurate in some populations.

FIGURE 9.2 Overview of various body composition assessment methods.

Once you figure out your ratio, how do you interpret it? An increased risk for chronic disease is associated with the following waist-to-hip ratios:

- In men, a ratio higher than 0.90
- In women, a ratio higher than 0.80

These ratios suggest an apple-shaped fat distribution pattern. In addition, waist circumference alone can indicate your risk for chronic disease. For males, your risk of chronic disease is increased if your waist circumference is above 40 inches (102 cm). For females, your risk is increased at measurements above 35 inches (88 cm).

> **recap** Body mass index, body composition, the waist-to-hip ratio, and waist circumference are tools that can help you evaluate the health of your current body weight. None of these methods is completely accurate, but most may be used appropriately as general health indicators.

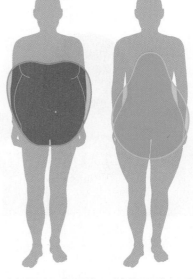

(a) Apple-shaped fat patterning   **(b) Pear-shaped fat patterning**

FIGURE 9.3 Fat distribution patterns. **(a)** An apple-shaped fat distribution pattern increases an individual's risk for many chronic diseases. **(b)** A pear-shaped distribution pattern does not seem to be associated with an increased risk for chronic disease.

What makes us gain and lose weight?

Have you ever wondered why some people are thin and others are overweight, even though they seem to eat about the same diet? If so, you're not alone. For hundreds of years, researchers have puzzled over what makes us gain and lose weight. In this section, we explore some information and current theories that may shed light on this question.

We Gain or Lose Weight When Our Energy Intake and Expenditure Are Out of Balance

Fluctuations in body weight are a result of changes in our **energy intake**, or the food we eat, and our **energy expenditure**, or the amount of energy we expend at rest, as a result of eating, and as a result of the physical activity we do. This relationship between what we eat and what we do is defined by the energy balance equation:

Energy balance occurs when energy intake = energy expenditure

Although the concept of energy balance appears simple, it is a dynamic process.[4] This means that, over time, factors that impact the energy intake side of the equation (including how many Calories we eat and the macronutrient composition of the food) need to balance with the factors that impact the energy expenditure side of the equation. **FIGURE 9.5** shows how our weight changes when either side of this equation is altered. From this figure, you can see that, to lose weight, we must expend more

LO3 State the energy balance equation and estimate your basal metabolic rate.

LO4 Explain how to calculate how many Calories you need to consume on average each day.

LO5 Discuss a range of factors thought to contribute to differences in body weight.

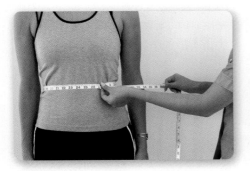

(a)   **(b)**

FIGURE 9.4 Determining your type of fat patterning. **(a)** Measure the circumference of your natural waist. **(b)** Measure the circumference of your hips at the maximal width of the buttocks as observed from the side. Dividing the waist value by the hip value gives you your waist-to-hip ratio.

energy intake The amount of food a person eats; in other words, it is the number of kilocalories consumed.

energy expenditure The energy the body expends to maintain its basic functions and to perform all levels of movement and activity.

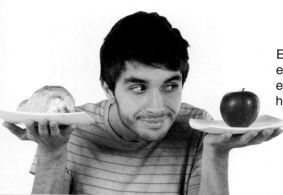

Energy balance is the relationship between the food we eat and the energy we expend each day. Finding the proper balance between energy intake and energy expenditure allows us to maintain a healthy body weight.

ENERGY DEFICIT

When you consume fewer Calories than you expend, your body will draw upon your stored energy to meet its needs. You will lose weight.

ENERGY INTAKE < ENERGY EXPENDITURE = WEIGHT LOSS

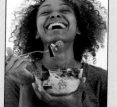

Calories in   Calories out

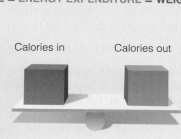

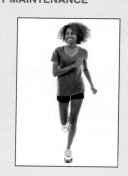

ENERGY BALANCE

When the Calories you consume meet your needs, you are in energy balance. Your weight will be stable.

ENERGY INTAKE = ENERGY EXPENDITURE = WEIGHT MAINTENANCE

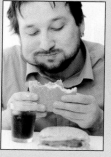

Calories in   Calories out

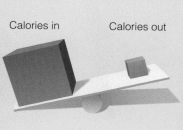

ENERGY EXCESS

When you take in more Calories than you need, the surplus Calories will be stored as fat. You will gain weight.

ENERGY INTAKE > ENERGY EXPENDITURE = WEIGHT GAIN

Calories in   Calories out

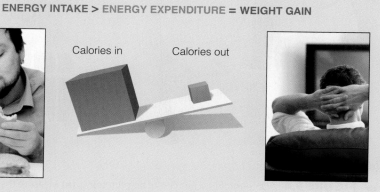

energy than we consume. In contrast, to gain weight, we must consume more energy than we expend. People who balance energy intake and expenditure maintain a consistent body weight.

Energy Intake Is the Food We Eat Each Day

Energy intake is the amount of energy in the food and beverages we consume each day. This value includes the carbohydrate, fat, protein, and alcohol that each contains; vitamins, minerals, and water contribute no kilocalories. Our daily energy intake is expressed as *kilocalories per day (kcal/day)*.

You have several options for determining how much energy you consume. For packaged foods and drinks, read the "Calories" line on the Nutrition Facts panel and make sure you adjust the value to the serving size you consume. For instance, if a serving is listed as half a cup but you routinely have a full cup, you need to double the value. To locate specific nutrient values for numerous fresh foods, including fruits, vegetables, meats, and many other foods, see the detailed Food Composition Table supplement that accompanies this text.

When our total daily energy intake exceeds the amount of energy we expend, we gain weight. An excess intake of approximately 3,500 kilocalories will result in a gain of 1 lb. Without exercise or other increased physical activity, this gain will likely be fat.

Energy Expenditure Includes More Than Just Physical Activity

Energy expenditure (also known as *energy output*) is the energy the body expends to maintain its basic functions and to perform all levels of movement and activity. We can calculate how much energy we expend in a typical 24-hour period by adding together estimates of the energy expended at rest, to process food, and to engage in physical activity. These three factors are referred to as our *basal metabolic rate (BMR)*, the *thermic effect of food (TEF)*, and the *energy cost of physical activity* (**FIGURE 9.6**).

Basal Metabolic Rate   You probably don't think about it, but your body expends a lot of energy just to maintain your functioning, even while you're sleeping. Your **basal metabolic rate (BMR)** is the energy you expend for *basal*, or *resting*, functions, including breathing, circulation, maintaining body temperature, synthesizing new cells and tissues, and so on. These basal functions require so much energy that the *majority* of your energy output each day (about 60–75%) is a result of your BMR. This means that 60% to 75% of your energy output goes to keeping you alive, aside from any physical activity.

BMR varies widely among people. The primary influence on BMR is the amount of lean body mass: people with a higher lean body mass have a higher BMR, because it takes more energy to support lean tissue. Age is another factor: BMR decreases approximately 3% to 5% per decade after age 30. Much of this change is due to a decline in lean body mass resulting from inactivity. Thus, you can prevent much of this decrease with regular physical activity. Several other factors that can affect a person's BMR are listed in **TABLE 9.1**.

How can you estimate your BMR? Begin by converting your current body weight in pounds to kilograms, by dividing pounds by 2.2. For instance, if you weigh 175 lb, your weight in kilograms is 79.5:

$$175 \text{ lb}/2.2 = 79.5 \text{ kg}$$

If you're a male, you can assume that your weight in kilograms roughly matches the kilocalories (kcal) you expend per hour: that is, 79.5 kcal per hour. Thus, your BMR for a 24-hour day is:

$$79.5 \text{ kcal per hour} \times 24 \text{ hours} = 1,908$$

Females have less lean body mass on average than males, so their BMR is considered about 90% of the BMR for males of the same weight. Thus, if you're a woman who weighs 175 lb, you'll need to multiply the 1,908 BMR for males by 0.9 to get your final value. Here's the full equation for women:

$$175 \text{ lb}/2.2 = 79.5 \text{ kg}$$
$$1,908 \times 0.9 = 1,717 \text{ BMR for women}$$

To determine how much energy you consumed in one meal or on 1 day, log on to ChooseMyPlate SuperTracker at www.choosemyplate.gov. Click on the tab for SuperTracker, then get started!

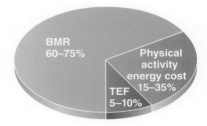

Components of energy expenditure

FIGURE 9.6   The components of energy expenditure include basal metabolic rate (BMR), the thermic effect of food (TEF), and the energy cost of physical activity. BMR accounts for 60% to 75% of our total energy output, whereas TEF and physical activity together account for 25% to 40%.

basal metabolic rate (BMR)   The energy the body expends to maintain its fundamental physiologic functions.

TABLE 9.1 Factors Affecting Basal Metabolic Rate (BMR)

Factors That Increase BMR	Factors That Decrease BMR
Higher lean body mass	Lower lean body mass
Greater height (more surface area)	Lower height
Younger age	Older age
Elevated levels of thyroid hormone	Depressed levels of thyroid hormone
Stress, fever, illness	Starvation or fasting
Male gender	Female gender
Pregnancy and lactation	
Certain drugs, such as stimulants, caffeine, and tobacco	

Thermic Effect of Food   The **thermic effect of food** is the energy we expend to digest food and to absorb, transport, metabolize, and store the nutrients. The thermic effect of food is equal to about 5% to 10% of the energy content of a meal. Thus, if a meal contains 500 kcal, the thermic effect of processing that meal is about 25 to 50 kcal. Interestingly, our body uses less energy to process fat and relatively more to process protein and carbohydrate.

Energy Cost of Physical Activity   The **energy cost of physical activity** represents about 15% to 35% of our total energy output each day. This is the energy that we expend due to any movement or work above basal levels. This includes low-intensity activities such as sitting, standing, fidgeting, and walking and higher-intensity activities such as running, skiing, and bicycling. One of the most obvious ways to increase how much energy we expend as a result of physical activity is to do more activities for a longer period of time.

TABLE 9.2 lists the energy cost of certain activities. As you can see, activities that involve moving our larger muscle groups (or more parts of the body) require more energy. The amount of energy we expend during activities is also affected by our body size. This is why the kilocalories of energy in the third column of Table 9.2 are expressed per pound of body weight.

How Many Kilocalories Do You Need?

Given everything we've discussed so far, you're probably asking yourself, "How much should I eat?" This question is not always easy to answer, because our energy needs fluctuate from day to day according to our activity level, the environmental conditions, and other factors, such as the amount and type of food we eat and our intake of caffeine. So how can you make a general estimate of how many kilocalories your body needs per day?

A simple way to estimate your total daily kilocalorie needs is to multiply your BMR by a varying amount according to how active you are. The following formula is a simplified version of one developed during a 1919 study of basal metabolism, and still in use today.[5] As with the formula for BMR, it does not account for wide variations in body composition. People who are very muscular typically need more kilocalories than the formula suggests, and the elderly and the obese need fewer. The formula is as follows:

- If you do little or no exercise or physical labor, multiply your BMR by 1.2.
- If you participate in moderate exercise or labor three to five times a week, multiply your BMR by 1.5.
- If you participate in intense exercise or labor six to seven times a week, multiply your BMR by 1.75.

thermic effect of food The energy expended as a result of processing food consumed.

energy cost of physical activity The energy expended on body movement and muscular work above basal levels.

TABLE 9.2 Energy Costs of Various Physical Activities

Activity	Intensity	Kilocalories Used per Pound per Hour
Sitting, studying (including reading or writing)	Light	0.6
Cooking or food preparation (standing or sitting)	Light	0.9
Walking (e.g., to neighbor's house)	Light	1.14
Stretching—Hatha yoga	Moderate	1.14
Cleaning (dusting, straightening up, vacuuming, changing linen, carrying out trash)	Moderate	1.58
Weight lifting (free weights, Nautilus, or universal type)	Light or moderate	1.36
Bicycling, 10 mph	Leisure (work or pleasure)	1.83
Walking, 4 mph (brisk pace)	Moderate	2.26
Aerobics	Low impact	2.26
Weight lifting (free weights, Nautilus, or universal type)	Vigorous	2.72
Bicycling 12 to 13.9 mph	Moderate	3.63
Running, 5 mph (12 minutes per mile)	Moderate	3.76
Running, 6 mph (10 minutes per mile)	Moderate	4.44
Running, 8.6 mph (7 minutes per mile)	Vigorous	5.59

Data from: The Compendium of Physical Activities Tracking Guide. Healthy Lifestyles Research Center, College of Nursing & Health Innovation, Arizona State University.

For example, let's say that a male student weighs 160 lb. To calculate his BMR, he divides his weight in pounds by 2.2 to determine his weight in kilograms, then multiplies that number by 24 hours:

$$160 \text{ lb}/2.2 = 72.72 \text{ kg} \times 24 = 1,745$$

Our student's BMR is 1,745. He does no regular exercise and spends his waking hours pretty much sitting in classes, studying, working at a computer, and so forth. Let's see how many kilocalories he needs per day to maintain his current weight and level of activity:

$$\text{BMR of } 1,745 \times 1.2 = 2,094 \text{ kcal per day}$$

If he wants to lose weight, he needs to increase his level of physical activity or consume fewer than 2,094 kcal a day. Even if he doesn't want to lose weight, he should begin a program of physical activity, at least 30 minutes a day most days of the week, to promote his wellness.

For a more precise estimate of your kilocalorie needs, you can use Table 9.2 to calculate the actual kilocalories you expend in physical activity on any given day. Then add that to your BMR. Precise calculations of energy expenditure are nearly impossible in real life, however. That's because we don't really spend long stretches of time sitting completely still or performing exactly the same activity at exactly the same pace. For instance, while you were quietly studying for an hour, did you fidget, or get up and stretch, or rush downstairs to answer the door? Despite its limitations, estimating the number of kilocalories you expend on an average day might provide you with an incentive to increase your physical activity.

Limitations of the Energy Balance Equation

As researchers have learned more about the factors that regulate body weight, the accuracy and usefulness of the classic energy balance equation illustrated in Figure 9.5

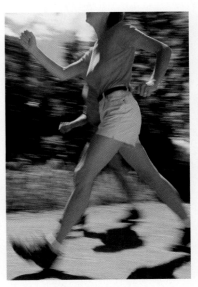

Brisk walking is a great way to expend energy.

have been called into question. Many researchers point out that the equation fails to account for many factors that can alter energy intake and expenditure or to help explain why people gain and lose weight differently.

For example, if an individual were to consume an additional 100 kcal each day above the energy needed to maintain weight (the energy content of 8 fl. oz of a cola beverage) for 10 years, he or she would consume an extra intake of 365,000 kcal! Assuming that no other changes occurred in energy expenditure, the energy balance equation tells us that this individual should gain 104 pounds. However, the equation doesn't take into account the increased BMR and cost of moving a larger body as weight increases. In a real person, that increase in energy expenditure would eventually balance the increased energy intake. The individual would then achieve energy balance and become weight stable at a higher body weight. Thus, the extra 100 kcal/day would actually result in a more realistic weight gain of a few pounds.

The inadequacy of the classic energy balance equation has prompted experts to propose a dynamic equation of energy balance that takes into account the rates of energy intake and expenditure and their effect on rate of change of fat and lean tissues in the body, not simply on body weight overall.[4]

As you can see, the energy balance equation is just the beginning of the story. Next, let's look at how genetic and physiologic factors contribute to variations in weight change.

Predict a more realistic time course for weight loss or weight gain for yourself based on a dynamic simulation model of human metabolism by going to http://bwsimulator.niddk.nih.gov.

recap The energy balance equation relates food intake to energy expenditure. Eating more energy than you expend causes weight gain, whereas eating less energy than you expend causes weight loss. The three components of this equation are basal metabolic rate, the thermic effect of food, and the energy cost of physical activity. A simple way to estimate daily energy needs is to calculate your BMR and then multiply it by a number reflecting your daily activity level.

Genetic Factors Affect Body Weight

Our genetic background influences our height, weight, body shape, basal metabolic rate, and other aspects of our physiology (how the body functions). A classic study shows that the body weights of adults who were adopted as children are similar to the weights of their biological parents, not their adoptive parents.[6] How much of our BMI can be accounted for by genetic influences remains controversial, however, with proposed values ranging from 50% to 90%.[7] This means that 10% to 50% of our BMI is accounted for by nongenetic, environmental factors and lifestyle choices such as exposure to cheap, high-energy food and low levels of physical activity. Unfortunately, this message that a relatively large proportion of our BMI is accounted for by genetic influences could discourage people who want to lose weight from making helpful lifestyle changes. One study found that individuals who were tested and found to have a higher genetic risk for obesity were more likely to report a higher fat intake and lower levels of physical activity 6 months after they received these results.[8]

Exactly how do genetic factors influence body weight? We discuss here some theories attempting to explain this link.

The FTO Gene

The existing evidence on genetics and obesity indicates that there is no one single "obesity gene." Instead, more than 120 genes currently are thought to be associated with an increased risk for obesity.[9] Nevertheless, one gene that has received a great deal of attention is the FTO (fat mass and obesity-associated) gene. This relatively common gene appears to stimulate excessive food intake and may diminish feelings of satiety; thus, it's not surprising that people who carry the gene weigh more, on average, than people who do not. A recent study indicates that physical activity can reduce the influence of the FTO gene on obesity risk in adults and children by 27%. These results highlight the importance of regular physical activity in reducing risk for obesity in people who are genetically predisposed.[10]

The Thrifty Gene Theory

The **thrifty gene theory** suggests that some people possess a gene (or genes) that causes them to be energetically thrifty. This means that, both at rest and during activity, these people expend less energy than those who do not possess this gene. The proposed purpose of this gene is to protect a person from starving to death during times of extreme food shortages. This theory has been applied to some Native American tribes, because these societies were exposed to centuries of feast and famine. Those with a thrifty metabolism survived when little food was available, and this trait was passed on to future generations. Although an actual thrifty gene (or genes) has not yet been identified, think about how people with such a gene might respond to today's food-focused environment. They would likely experience more weight gain than people without the gene, and their body would be more resistant to weight loss.

The Set-Point Theory

The **set-point theory** suggests that our body is designed to maintain our weight within a narrow range, or at a "set point." In many cases, our body appears to respond in such a way as to maintain our current weight. When we dramatically reduce energy intake (such as with fasting or strict diets), our body responds with physiologic changes that cause our BMR to drop. This reduces our energy output. At the same time, we reduce our activity because we just don't have the energy for it. These two mechanisms of energy conservation may contribute to some of the rebound weight gain many dieters experience after they quit dieting.

Conversely, overeating in some people may cause an increase in BMR and is thought to be associated with an increased thermic effect of food, as well as an increase in spontaneous movements, or fidgeting. This in turn increases energy output and may explain why some people fail to gain as much weight as might be expected from eating excess food. We don't eat exactly the same amount of food each day; some days we overeat, and other days we eat less. When you think about how much our daily energy intake fluctuates (about 20% above and below our average monthly intake), our ability to maintain a certain weight over long periods of time suggests that there is some evidence to support the set-point theory.

Can we change our set point? Many people do successfully lose weight and maintain that weight loss over long periods of time. Thus, it seems clear that we can and that the set-point theory doesn't entirely account for our body's resistance to weight loss.

recap Many factors affect our ability to gain and lose weight. Our genetic background influences our height, weight, body shape, and metabolic rate. The FTO gene variant appears to prompt overeating and weight gain. The thrifty gene theory suggests that some people possess a thrifty gene, or set of genes, that causes them to expend less energy than people who do not have this gene. The set-point theory suggests that our body is designed to maintain weight within a narrow range.

Composition of the Diet Affects Fat Storage

Scientists used to think that people would gain the same amount of weight if they ate too much food of any type, but now there is evidence to support the theory that, when we overeat high-fat foods, we're likely to gain more weight than when we overeat high-carbohydrate or high-protein foods. This may be due to the fact that eating fat doesn't cause much of an increase in metabolic rate and that the body stores fat in the form of adipose tissue quite easily. In contrast, when we eat too much protein or carbohydrate, the body's initial response is to use the energy from these macronutrients to fuel the body, with a smaller amount of the excess stored as fat. This does not mean, however, that you can eat as many low-fat foods as you want and not gain weight! Consistently overeating protein or carbohydrate will also lead to weight gain. Instead, maintain a balanced diet combining fat, carbohydrate, and protein and reduce dietary fat to less than 35% of total energy. This strategy may help reduce your storage of fat energy as adipose tissue.

thrifty gene theory A theory that suggests that some people possess a gene (or genes) that causes them to be energetically thrifty, resulting in their expending less energy at rest and during physical activity.

set-point theory A theory that suggests that the body raises or lowers energy expenditure in response to increased and decreased food intake and physical activity. This action maintains an individual's body weight within a narrow range.

Metabolic Factors Influence Weight Loss and Gain

Four metabolic factors are thought to increase a person's risk for weight gain and resistance to weight loss.[4] These factors include:

- Relatively low metabolic rate. Obese individuals weigh more and have a higher amount of lean tissue than people of normal weight, and thus will have a higher absolute BMR. However, at any given size, people vary in their relative BMR—it can be high, normal, or low. People who have a relatively low BMR are more at risk for weight gain and are resistant to weight loss.
- Low level of spontaneous physical activity (fidgeting). People who exhibit less spontaneous physical activity are at increased risk for weight gain.
- Low sympathetic nervous system (SNS) activity. The SNS plays an important role in regulating all components of energy expenditure, and people with lower SNS activity are more prone to obesity and more resistant to weight loss.
- Low fat metabolism. Some people use relatively more carbohydrate for energy, which means that less fat is used. Instead, it's stored in adipose tissue. Thus, these people are at higher risk for gaining weight.

Physiologic Factors Influence Body Weight

Recall that the hypothalamus plays an important role in regulating hunger and satiety. Researchers theorize that some people may have an insufficient satiety mechanism, which prevents them from feeling full after a meal, allowing them to overeat.

Many hormones and functional proteins play a role in food intake, energy metabolism, and body weight. For instance, two hormones produced in the gastrointestinal tract, cholecystokinin (CCK) and peptide YY (PYY), promote satiety and thus decrease food intake. *Leptin*, a protein hormone produced by adipose cells, also acts to reduce food intake and cause a decrease in body weight and body fat. People who are obese tend to have very high amounts of leptin in their body, but unfortunately they appear to be insensitive to its effects. Researchers are currently studying the role of leptin in starvation and overeating, and it appears it might play a role in cardiovascular and kidney complications that result from obesity.

Factors that can decrease satiety (or increase food intake) include *ghrelin*, a protein synthesized in the stomach, neuropeptide Y, an amino acid–containing compound produced in the hypothalamus, and the decreased blood glucose level that occurs when we haven't eaten for a while.

Uncoupling proteins have recently become the focus of research into body weight. These proteins play a role in energy metabolism in the mitochondria of our cells; mitochondria work to generate energy and are found in skeletal muscle cells and adipose cells. Some research suggests that a person with more uncoupling proteins or a higher activity of these proteins would be more resistant to weight gain and obesity. One type of uncoupling protein is found exclusively in **brown adipose tissue**, a type of adipose tissue that has more mitochondria than white adipose tissue. It is found in significant amounts in people of normal weight,[11] whereas people who are obese have lower amounts.[12] These findings suggest a possible role of brown adipose tissue in obesity.

Cultural and Economic Factors Affect Food Choices and Body Weight

Cultural factors (including religious beliefs, learned food preferences, and food-related values) affect our food choices, eating patterns, and body weight. In addition, because both parents work outside the home in most American families, more people are embracing the "fast-food culture," in which eating out, ordering take-out meals, and grabbing prepared foods from grocery stores is the norm.

Coinciding with these cultural influences on food intake are cultural factors that promote inactivity. These include the shift from manual labor to more sedentary jobs and increased access to labor-saving devices in all areas of our lives. Even seemingly minor changes—such as walking through an automated door instead of pushing a door open—add up to a lower expenditure of energy by the end of the day. Other

↟ Behaviors learned as a child can affect adulthood weight and physical activity patterns.

brown adipose tissue A type of adipose tissue that has more mitochondria than white adipose tissue, and which can increase energy expenditure by uncoupling certain steps in the energy production process.

nutrition myth or fact?

Does It Cost More to Eat Right?

The shelves of American supermarkets are filled with an abundance of healthful food options: organic meats and produce, exotic fish, out-of-season fresh fruits and vegetables that are flown in from warmer climates, whole-grain breads and cereals, and low-fat and low-sodium options of traditional foods. With all of this choice, it would seem easy for anyone to consume healthful foods throughout the year. But a closer look at the prices of these foods suggests that, for many, they simply are not affordable. This raises the question "Does eating right have to be expensive?"

It is a fact that organic foods are more expensive than non-organic options. However, there is little evidence indicating that organic foods are richer in nutrients than non-organic foods. In addition, some of the lowest cost foods currently available in stores are also some of the most nutritious: these include beans, lentils, and other legumes, seasonal fruits, root vegetables (such as potatoes and winter squashes), cooking oils high in mono- and polyunsaturated fats, and frozen as well as canned fruits and vegetables, which are generally just as nutritious as fresh options. A recent study that did a cost comparison of more and less nutrition foods in U.S. supermarkets found that it is possible to choose more nutritious foods from various common food categories without spending more money.[1] Thus, people can still eat healthfully on a tight budget.

Here are some more tips to help you save money when shopping for healthful foods:

- Buy whole grains, such as cereals, brown rice, and pastas in bulk—they store well for longer periods and provide a good base for meals and snacks.
- Buy frozen vegetables on sale and stock up—these are just as healthful as fresh vegetables, require less preparation, and are typically cheaper.

- If lower-sodium options of canned beans and other vegetables are more expensive, buy the less expensive regular option and drain the juice from the vegetables before cooking.
- Consume leaner meats and in smaller amounts—by eating less, you'll not only save money but reduce your total intake of energy and fat while still obtaining the nutrients that support good health.
- Choose frozen fish or canned salmon or tuna packed in water as an alternative to fresh fish.
- Avoid frozen or dehydrated prepared meals. They are usually expensive; high in sodium, saturated fats, and energy; and low in fiber and other important nutrients.
- Buy generic or store brands of foods—be careful to check the labels to ensure that the foods are similar in nutrient value to the higher priced options.
- Cut coupons from local newspapers and magazines and watch the sale circulars, so that you can stock up on healthful foods you can store.
- Consider cooking more meals at home; you'll have more control over what goes into your meals, and you'll be able to cook larger amounts and freeze leftovers for future meals.

As you can see, eating healthfully does not have to be expensive. However, it helps to become a savvy consumer by reading food labels, comparing prices, and gaining the skills and confidence to cook at home. The information shared throughout this text should help you acquire these skills, so that you can eat healthfully even on a limited budget!

---

cultural barriers to being physically active include lack of physically active role models to emulate, acceptance of larger body size, cultural prohibitions against exercise in some ethnic minority groups, and fear for personal safety, particularly among women.

Economic status is related to health status, particularly in developed countries such as the United States: people of lower economic status have reduced access to healthcare and higher rates of obesity and related chronic diseases than people with higher incomes.[13] In addition, economic factors strongly impact our food choices and eating behaviors. It is a common belief that healthful foods are expensive and that only wealthy people can afford to purchase them. While it is true that certain foods considered more healthful, such as organic foods, produce out-of-season, and certain meats and fish, can be costly, does healthful eating always have to be expensive? Refer to the **Nutrition Myth or Fact?** feature to learn more about whether a healthful diet can also be an affordable one.

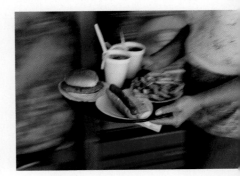

▲ Fast foods may be inexpensive and filling, but most are high in saturated fat, salt, and sugar.

Social Factors Influence Behavior and Body Weight

As you know, appetite can be experienced in the absence of hunger. It's commonly stimulated by social situations and cues that promote eating—and overeating. Social factors also influence our level of physical activity.

To test your understanding of a serving size, take an interactive quiz from the National Institutes of Health. Just enter "NIH Portion Distortion" into your Internet browser and select Portion Distortion, WeCan®. This will take you to the Portion Distortion home page; then click on the Portion Distortion I and II links, and explore the other resources located there.

Some Social Factors Promote Overeating

Encouragement from family and friends to eat the way they do can induce people to overeat. For example, the pressure to overeat on holidays is high as family members or friends offer extra servings of favorite holiday foods and follow a large meal with a rich dessert.

A key social factor in the tendency of Americans to overeat is our easy access to food throughout the day. Vending machines selling junk foods are everywhere, shopping malls are filled with fast-food restaurants, and serving sizes have become so large that many Americans are suffering from "portion distortion" **(FIGURE 9.7)**. This easy access to high-energy meals and snacks leads many people to overeat.

The more often we eat out, the less control we have over the energy and nutrient content of our meals. This makes it easy to overeat. The National Restaurant Association reports restaurant industry sales for 2010 at $587 billion, with projections for 2014 at $683 billion.[14] When was the last time you ate a home-cooked meal? Although typically inexpensive, the meals served at many of the diners, fast-food restaurants, and cafeterias favored by students offer large serving sizes high in empty Calories. Whether or not you know the precise Calorie count for the foods you select, you can eat out healthfully—if you're smart about it! The *Game Plan* box identifies some tactics for eating smart when eating out.

20 Years Ago   Today

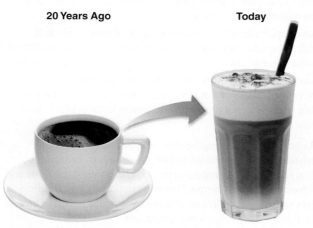

8 fluid ounces, 42 Calories   16 fluid ounces, 350 Calories

FIGURE 9.7 A cup of coffee has increased from 8 fl. oz to 16 fl. oz over the past 20 years and now commonly contains Calorie-dense flavored syrup as well as steamed whole milk.

Some Social Factors Promote Inactivity

Social factors can also cause people to be less physically active. For instance, we don't even have to spend time or energy preparing food anymore, because everything either is ready to serve or requires just a few minutes to cook in a microwave oven. Other social factors promoting inactivity include living in an unsafe community or an area with harsh weather and coping with family, community, and work responsibilities that don't involve physical activity. Among children, decreased activity often results from lack of recreational facilities and a reduction in physical education in schools.

Another social factor promoting inactivity in both children and adults is the increasing dominance of technology in our choices of entertainment. Instead of participating in sports or gathering for a dance at the community hall, we go to the movies or stay at home watching television, surfing the Internet, and playing video games. By reducing energy expenditure, these behaviors contribute to weight gain. For instance, a study of 11- to 13-year-old schoolchildren found that children who watched more than 2 hours of television per night were more likely to be overweight or obese than children who watched less than 2 hours per night. Similarly, television watching in adults has been shown to be associated with weight gain over a four-year period.[15]

Social Pressures Can Promote Underweight

On the other hand, social pressures to maintain a lean body are great enough to encourage some people to undereat, or to avoid foods they perceive as "bad," especially fats. Our society ridicules, and often ostracizes, overweight people, many of whom face discrimination in employment and other areas of their lives. A recent study found that children who are obese are 60% more likely to experience bullying than children of normal weight.[16] Moreover, media images of waiflike fashion models and men in tight jeans with muscular chests and abdomens encourage many people—especially adolescents and young adults—to skip meals, resort to crash diets, and exercise obsessively. Even some people of normal body weight push themselves to achieve an unrealistic and unattainable weight goal, in the process threatening their health and even their lives (see the *Healthwatch* section later in this chapter for the consequences of disordered eating).

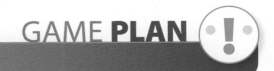

GAME **PLAN**

Tactics for Eating Smart When Eating Out

During the past 20 years, there has been phenomenal growth in the restaurant industry, particularly in the fast-food market. During this period, rates of obesity have increased dramatically. The lunches in **FIGURE 9.8** are both from popular fast-food restaurants, McDonald's and Subway. The lunch on the left, a Big Mac hamburger with extra-large french fries and an apple pie, provides 1,429 Calories and contains 47% of its total energy as fat. In contrast, the Subway cold-cut trio sandwich, granola bar, and a medium apple provides 610 Calories and contains 31% of its total energy as fat. So as you can see, eating out can be a part of a healthful diet—as long as you make smart choices.

Try these tactics the next time you eat out:

- ☐ Avoid all-you-can-eat buffet-style restaurants.
- ☐ Choose lower-fat or "lite" versions of your favorite meals.
- ☐ Order a healthful appetizer as your entreé.
- ☐ If a child-size portion is available for your menu choice, order it.
- ☐ Share your meal with a friend. Many restaurant meals are large enough for two people.
- ☐ Order any meat item grilled or broiled. Avoid fried foods.
- ☐ Instead of a hamburger, choose a chicken burger, fish burger, or veggie burger.
- ☐ Order a meatless dish filled with vegetables and whole grains.

- ☐ Avoid dishes with a lot of cheese or a cream sauce. Also avoid cream-based soups.
- ☐ Instead of french fries, order a salad and choose low-fat or nonfat dressing.
- ☐ To drink, choose water, tea, diet drinks, or skim milk. Also, request skim milk in lattés and other coffee drinks. Beware of milkshakes! A large McDonald's chocolate milkshake comes in at 500 Calories!
- ☐ Watch out for "yogurt parfaits" offered at several fast-food restaurants. Many are loaded with empty Calories.
- ☐ Skip dessert or share one with friends! Another healthful alternative is to order fresh fruit for dessert.
- ☐ Don't feel you have to eat everything you are served. If you're full, stop!

About 1,430 Calories (kcal)

McDonald's Big Mac hamburger
French fries, extra large
3 tbsp. ketchup
Apple pie

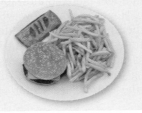

About 610 Calories (kcal)

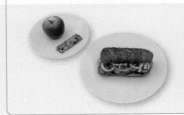

Subway cold-cut trio 6"sandwich
Granola bar, hard, with
    chocolate chips, 1 bar (24 g)
1 fresh medium apple

▲ **FIGURE 9.8** The energy density of two fast-food meals. The meal on the left is higher in total Calories and fat; the one on the right is the preferred choice for someone trying to eat a healthful diet.

By now it should be clear that how a person gains, loses, and maintains body weight is a complex matter. Most people who are overweight have tried several weight-loss programs unsuccessfully and have therefore given up all weight-loss attempts. Some even suffer from severe depression related to their body weight. Should we condemn these people as failures and continue to pressure them to lose weight? Should people who are overweight but otherwise healthy (for example, with normal blood pressure, lipids, and glucose levels) be advised to lose weight? As we continue to search for ways to help people achieve and maintain a healthful body weight, our society must take measures to reduce the social pressures facing people who are overweight or obese.

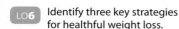 When we overeat, the body stores the extra energy from dietary fat more readily than the energy from carbohydrate or protein. Metabolic and physiologic factors, such as various energy-regulating hormones, influence body weight by their effects on energy expenditure, satiety, and appetite. Cultural, economic, and social factors can significantly influence the amounts and types of food we eat and our level of physical activity. Social pressures on those who are overweight can drive people to use harmful methods to achieve an unrealistic body weight.

LO6 Identify three key strategies for healthful weight loss.

How can you achieve and maintain a healthful body weight?

Now that you understand what constitutes a healthful body weight, how are you feeling about yours? You might decide that you'd like to lose weight, but are you really committed to making the changes required? To find out, check out the ***What About You?*** box. If your results suggest that you are, then take heart. Losing weight and maintaining that loss are goals well within your reach using three primary strategies:

- Gradual reduction in energy intake
- Incorporation of regular and appropriate physical activity
- Application of behavior modification techniques

In this section, we first discuss popular diet plans, which may or may not incorporate these strategies. We then explain how to design a personalized weight-loss program that includes all three of them.

If You Decide to Follow a Popular Weight-Loss Plan, Choose One Based on the Three Strategies

If you'd like to lose weight, the information ahead will help you design your own personalized diet plan. If you'd feel more comfortable following an established plan, however, many are available. How can you know whether or not it is based on sound dietary principles, and whether its promise of long-term weight loss will prove true for *you*? Look to the three strategies just identified: Does the plan promote gradual reductions in energy intake? Does it advocate increased physical activity? Does it include strategies for modifying your eating and activity-related behaviors? Reputable diet plans incorporate all of these strategies. Unfortunately, many dieters are drawn to fad diets, which do not.

Avoid Fad Diets

Beware of fad diets! They are simply what their name implies—fads that do not result in long-term, healthful weight changes. Although fad diets enjoy short-term popularity, most will "die" within a year, only to be born again as a "new and improved" fad diet. The goal of the person or company designing and marketing a fad diet is to make money. How can you tell if the program you are interested in qualifies as a fad diet? Check out the ***Highlight*** feature box on fad diets for some telltale signs.

Diets Focusing on Macronutrient Composition May or May Not Work for You

Many weight-loss diets encourage increased consumption of certain macronutrients and restrict the consumption of others. Provided here is a brief review of three such diets and their general effects on weight loss and health.[17]

Diets High in Carbohydrate and Moderate in Fat and Protein   Nutritionally balanced high-carbohydrate, moderate-fat and protein diets typically contain 55–60% of total energy intake as carbohydrate, 20–30% of total energy intake as fat, and 15–20% of energy intake as protein. These diets include Weight Watchers, Jenny Craig, and

WHAT ABOUT **YOU** ?

Are You Ready to Jump Start Your Weight Loss?

If you are overweight or obese, complete each of the following questions by circling the response(s) that best represents your situation or attitudes, then total your points for each section. Section 1 indicates the factors that may predispose you to excess weight and make weight loss more challenging. Section 2 assesses how ready you are to begin losing weight right now.

Section 1 Family, Weight, and Diet History

1. How many people in your immediate family (parents or siblings) are overweight or obese?
   a. No one is overweight or obese (0 points)
   b. One person (1 point)
   c. Two people (2 points)
   d. Three or more people (3 points)

2. During which periods of your life were you overweight or obese? (Circle all that apply.)
   a. Birth through age 5 (1 point)
   b. Ages 6 to 11 (1 point)
   c. Ages 12 to 13 (1 point)
   d. Ages 14 to 18 (2 points)
   e. Ages 19 to present (2 points)

3. How many times in the last year have you made an effort to lose weight but have had little or no success?
   a. None. I've never thought about it. (0 points)
   b. I've thought about it, but I've never tried hard to lose weight. (1 point)
   c. I have tried 2 to 3 times. (1 point)
   d. I have tried at least once a month. (2 points)
   e. I have tried so many times, I can't remember the number. (3 points)

                                      Total points: _____

Scoring

A score higher than 3 suggests that you may have several challenges ahead as you begin a weight loss program. The higher you score, the greater the likelihood of challenges.

Your own weight problems may be related, at least in part to the eating habits and preferences you learned at home, and it may take a conscious effort to change them. If in the past you tried repeatedly to lose weight but returned to your old behaviors, you may have to reframe your thinking.

Section 2 Readiness to Change
Attitudes and Beliefs About Weight loss

1. What is/are your main reason(s) for wanting to lose weight? (Circle all that apply.)
   a. I want to please someone I know or attract a new person. (0 points)
   b. I want to look great and/or fit into smaller size clothes for an upcoming event (wedding, vacation, date, etc.). (1 point)
   c. Someone I know has had major health problems because of being overweight/obese. (1 point)
   d. I want to improve my health and/or have more energy. (2 points)
   e. I was diagnosed with a health problem (prediabetes, diabetes, high blood pressure, etc.) because of being overweight/obese. (2 points)

2. What do you think about your weight and body shape? (Circle all that apply.)
   a. I'm fine with being overweight, and if others don't like it, tough! (0 points)
   b. My weight hurts my energy levels and my performance and holds me back. (1 point)
   c. I feel good about myself, but think I will be happier if I lose some of my weight. (1 point)
   d. I'm self-conscious about my weight and uncomfortable in my skin. (1 point)
   e. I'm really worried that I will have a major health problem if I don't change my behaviors now. (2 points)

Daily Eating Patterns

3. Which of the following statements describes you? (Circle all that apply.)
   a. I think about food several times a day, even when I'm not hungry. (0 points)
   b. There are some foods or snacks that I can't stay away from, and I eat them even when I'm not hungry. (0 points)
   c. I tend to eat more meat and fatty foods and never get enough fruits and veggies. (0 points)
   d. I've thought about the weaknesses in my diet and have some ideas about what I need to do. (1 point)
   e. I haven't really tried to eat a "balanced" diet, but I know that I need to start now. (1 point)

—Continued next page

Continued—

4. When you binge or eat things you shouldn't or too much at one sitting, what are you likely to do? (Circle all that apply.)

   a. Not care and go off of my diet. (0 points)

   b. Feel guilty for a while, but then do it again the next time I am out. (0 points)

   c. Fast for the next day or two to help balance the high consumption day. (0 points)

   d. Plan ahead for next time and have options in mind so that I do not continue to overeat. (1 point)

   e. Acknowledge that I have made a slip and get back on my program the next day. (1 point)

5. On a typical day, what are your eating patterns? (Circle all that apply.)

   a. I skip breakfast and save my Calories for lunch and dinner. (0 points)

   b. I never really sit down for a meal. I am a "grazer" and eat whatever I find that is readily available. (0 points)

   c. I try to eat at least five servings of fruits and veggies and restrict saturated fats in my diet. (1 point)

   d. I eat several small meals, trying to be balanced in my portions and getting foods from different food groups. (1 point)

Commitment to Weight Loss and Exercise

6. How would you describe your current support system for helping you lose weight? (Circle all that apply.)

   a. I believe I can do this best by doing it on my own. (0 points)

   b. I am not aware of any sources that can help me. (0 points)

   c. I have two to three friends or family members I can count on to help me. (1 point)

   d. There are counselors on campus with whom I can meet to plan a successful approach to weight loss. (1 point)

   e. I have the resources to join Weight Watchers or other community or online weight loss programs. (1 point)

7. How committed are you to exercising? (Circle all that apply.)

   a. Exercise is uncomfortable, embarrassing, and/or I don't enjoy it. (0 points)

   b. I don't have time to exercise. (0 points)

   c. I'd like to exercise, but I'm not sure how to get started. (1 point)

   d. I've visited my campus recreation center or local gym to explore my options for exercise. (2 points)

   e. There are specific sports or physical activities I do already, and I can plan to do more of them. (2 points)

8. What statement best describes your motivation to start a weight loss/lifestyle change program?

   a. I don't want to start losing weight. (0 points)

   b. I am thinking about it sometime in the distant future. (0 points)

   c. I am considering starting within the next few weeks; I just need to make a plan. (1 point)

   d. I'd like to start in the next few weeks, and I'm working on a plan. (2 points)

   e. I already have a plan in place, and I'm ready to begin tomorrow. (3 points)

   Total points: _____

others that follow the general guidelines of the DASH Diet and the USDA Food Guide. All of these diet plans emphasize that weight loss occurs when energy intake is lower than energy expenditure. The goal is gradual weight loss, or about 1 to 2 lb of body weight per week. Typical suggested energy deficits are between 500 and 1,000 kcal per day. It is recommended that women eat no less than 1,000 to 1,200 kcal per day and that men consume no less than 1,200 to 1,400 kcal per day. Regular physical activity is encouraged.

To date, these types of low-energy diets have been researched more than any others. A substantial amount of high-quality scientific evidence (from randomized controlled trials) indicates that they may be effective in decreasing body weight—at least initially. In addition, the people who lose weight on these diets may improve their blood lipid levels and decrease their blood pressure. However, recently published results from a randomized controlled trial following almost 50,000 U.S. women for 7 years indicate that, contrary to established beliefs, this type of diet does not result in significant long-term weight loss or reduce the risks for breast and colorectal cancers or cardiovascular disease.[17–20] Many limitations affected the study findings, however,

Scoring

A score higher than 8 indicates that you may be ready to change; the higher your score above 8, the more successful you may be. If you scored lower than 8, consider the following:

In order to lose weight, you will need to change your daily eating habits. Overeating (or eating poorly) may be a response to your food attitudes rather than to physical hunger. Poor eating may also reflect your emotional responses toward food, and/or unhealthy dietary choices. To increase your commitment to weight loss and exercise, think of friends or family who can support your efforts to stick to your plan. Also consider the wealth of available resources and where you can go for help. Having a plan and sticking to it will be crucial as you begin your weight loss journey!

Your Plan for Chance

The Assess Yourself identifies six areas of importance in determining your readiness for weight loss. If you wish to lose weight to improve your health, understanding your attitudes about food and exercise will help you succeed in your plan.

Today, you can: Set "SMART" goals for weight loss and give them a reality check. Are they specific, measurable, achievable, relevant, and time-oriented? For example rather than aiming to lose 15 pounds this month (which probably wouldn't be healthy or achievable), set a comfortable goal to lose 5 pounds. Realistic goals will encourage weight-loss success by boosting your confidence in your ability to make lifelong healthy changes.

Begin keeping a food log and identifying the triggers that influence your eating habits. Think about what you can do to eliminate or reduce the influence of your most common food triggers.

Within the next 2 weeks, you can: Get in the habit of incorporating more fruits, vegetables, and whole grains in your diet and eating less fat. The next time you make dinner, look at the proportions on your plate. If vegetables and whole grains do not take up most of the space, substitute 1 cup of the meat, pasta, or cheese in your meal with 1 cup of legumes, salad greens, or a favorite vegetable. You'll reduce the number of calories while eating the same amount of food!

Aim to incorporate more exercise into your daily routine. Visit your campus rec center or a local gym, and familiarize yourself with the equipment and facilities that are available. Try a new machine or sports activity, and experiment until you find a form of exercise you really enjoy.

By the end of the semester, you can: Get in the habit of grocery shopping every week and buying healthy, nutritious foods while avoiding high-fat, high-sugar, or overly processed foods. As you make healthy foods more available and unhealthy foods less available, you'll find it easier to eat better.

Chart your progress and reward yourself as you meet your goals. If your goal is to lose weight and you successfully take off 10 pounds, reward yourself with a new pair of jeans or other article of clothing (which will likely fit better than before!).

and more research needs to be done before we are able to determine the long-term effectiveness of higher carbohydrate diets on weight loss and disease risks.

Diets Low in Carbohydrate and High in Fat and Protein Low-carbohydrate, high-fat and -protein diets cycle in and out of popularity on a regular basis. By definition, these types of diets generally contain about 55% to 65% of total energy intake as fat and most of the remaining balance of daily energy intake as protein. Examples include Dr. Atkins' Diet Revolution, the Carbohydrate Addict's Diet, and Protein Power. These diets minimize the role of restricting total energy intake on weight loss. They instead advise participants to restrict carbohydrate intake, proposing that carbohydrates are addictive and that they cause significant overeating, insulin surges leading to excessive fat storage, and an overall metabolic imbalance that leads to obesity. The goal is to reduce carbohydrates enough to cause ketosis, which will decrease blood glucose and insulin levels and can reduce appetite.

Countless people claim to have lost substantial weight on these types of diets. Although quality scientific studies are just beginning to be conducted, the current

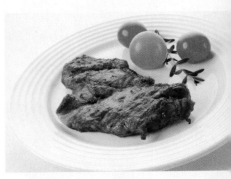

"Low-carb" diets may lead to weight loss but are nutritionally inadequate and can have negative side effects.

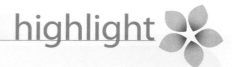

highlight

The Anatomy of Fad Diets

Fad diets are weight-loss programs that enjoy short-term popularity and are sold based on a marketing gimmick that appeals to the public's desires and fears. In addition, the goal of the person or company designing and marketing the diet is not to improve public health but to make money. How can you tell if the program you are interested in is a fad diet? Here are some telltale signs:

- The promoters of the diet claim that the program is new, improved, or based on some new discovery; however, no scientific data are available to support these claims.

- The program is touted for its ability to result in rapid weight loss or body-fat loss, usually more than 2 lb per week, and may claim that weight loss can be achieved with little or no physical exercise.

- The diet includes special foods and supplements, many of which are expensive and/or difficult to find or can be purchased only from the diet promoter. Common recommendations for these diets include avoiding certain foods, eating only a special combination of certain foods, and including magic foods in the diet that "burn" fat and speed up metabolism.

- The diet includes a rigid menu that must be followed daily or allows only a few, select foods each day. Alternatively, the diet focuses on one macronutrient group (such as protein) and severely restricts the others (such as carbohydrate and fat). Variety and balance are discouraged, and certain foods (such as all dairy products or all foods made with refined flour) are entirely forbidden.

- Many fad diets identify certain foods and/or supplements as critical to the success of the diet and usually claim that these substances can cure or prevent a variety of health ailments or that the diet can stop the aging process.

In a world in which many of us feel we have to meet a certain physical standard to be attractive and "good enough," fad diets flourish, with millions of people trying one each year.[2] Unfortunately, the only people who usually benefit from them are their marketers, who can become very wealthy promoting programs that don't work.

---

limited evidence suggests that individuals following them, in both free-living and experimental conditions, do lose weight. In addition, it appears that those people who lose weight may also experience positive metabolic changes similar to those seen with higher carbohydrate diets.

So are low-carb diets effective? A recent review of all the published studies of these diets resulted in the conclusion that low-carb diets are just as effective, and possibly more effective, in promoting weight loss and reducing cardiovascular disease risk for a period of up to 1 year.[21] However, the authors conclude that long-term health benefits of this type of a diet are unknown at this time, and more research is needed.

Low-Fat and Very-Low-Fat Diets Low-fat diets contain 11–19% of total energy as fat, whereas very-low-fat diets contain less than 10% of total energy as fat. Both of these types of diets are high in carbohydrate and moderate in protein. Examples include Dr. Dean Ornish's Program for Reversing Heart Disease and the New Pritikin Program. These diets do not focus on total energy intake but emphasize eating foods higher in complex carbohydrates and fiber. Consumption of sugar and white flour is very limited. The Ornish diet is vegetarian, whereas the Pritikin diet allows 3.5 oz of lean meat per day. Regular physical activity is a key component of these diets.

Data are limited on the effectiveness of these programs for two reasons. First, they were not originally designed for weight loss but to decrease or reverse heart disease. Second, they are not popular with consumers, who view them as too restrictive and difficult to follow. However, high-quality evidence suggests that people following these diets do lose weight, and some data suggest that the diets may also decrease blood pressure and blood levels of LDL-cholesterol, triglycerides, glucose, and insulin. Low-fat diets are low in vitamin B_{12}, and very-low-fat diets are low in essential fatty acids, vitamins B_{12} and E, and zinc. Thus, supplementation is needed. These types of diets are not considered safe for people with diabetes who are insulin dependent (either type 1 or type 2) or for people with carbohydrate-malabsorption illnesses.

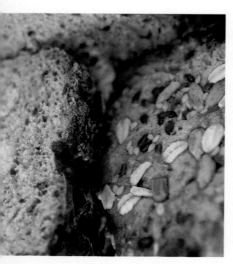

Low-fat and very-low-fat diets emphasize eating foods higher in complex carbohydrates and fiber.

If You Decide to Design Your Own Weight-Loss Plan, Include the Three Strategies

As we noted earlier, a healthful and effective weight-loss plan involves a modest reduction in energy intake, incorporating physical activity into each day, and practicing changes in behavior that can help you reduce your energy intake and increase your energy expenditure. To further assist you, guidelines for a sound weight-loss plan are identified in the *Game Plan* box. Following are some guidelines for designing your own personalized diet plan that incorporates these strategies.

Set Realistic Goals

The first key to safe and effective weight loss is setting realistic goals related to how much weight to lose and how quickly (or slowly) to lose it. Although gradual weight loss is frustrating for most people, it is much more likely to be maintained over time. A realistic goal is to lose about 0.5 to 2 pounds per week. A weight-loss plan should never provide less than a total of 1,200 kcal per day unless you are under a physician's supervision. Your weight-loss goals should also take into consideration any health-related concerns you have. After checking with your physician, you may decide initially to set a goal of simply maintaining your current weight and preventing additional weight gain. After your weight has remained stable for several weeks, you might then write down realistic goals for weight loss.

Goals that are more likely to be realistic and achievable share the following characteristics:

- *They are specific:* Telling yourself "I will eat less this week" is not helpful, because the goal is not specific. An example of a specific goal is "I will eat only half of my restaurant entrée tonight and take the rest home and eat it tomorrow for lunch."
- *They are reasonable:* If you are not presently physically active, it would be unreasonable to set a goal of exercising for 30 minutes every day. A more reasonable goal would be to exercise for 15 minutes per day, 3 days per week. Once you've achieved that goal, you can increase the frequency, intensity, and time of exercise according to the improvements in fitness that you have experienced.
- *They are measurable:* Effective goals are ones you can measure. An example is "I will lose at least half a pound by May 1." Recording your specific, measurable goals will help you better determine whether you are achieving them.

By monitoring your progress regularly, you can determine whether you are meeting your goals or whether you need to revise them based on accomplishments or challenges that arise.

Eat Smaller Portions of Lower-Calorie Foods

Two of the biggest weight-loss challenges are understanding what a healthful portion size is and then reducing the portion sizes of the foods and beverages we consume. It has been suggested that effective weight-loss strategies include reducing both the portion size and the energy density of foods.[22] To help you get started, here are some specific suggestions from the Weight-Control Information Network:[23]

- Follow the amounts recommended in the USDA Food Patterns (Chapter 1). Making this change involves understanding what constitutes a portion and measuring foods to determine whether they meet or exceed the recommended amounts.
- To help increase your understanding of the portion sizes of packaged foods, measure out the amount of food that is identified as 1 serving on the Nutrition Facts panel and eat it from a plate or bowl instead of straight out of the box or bag.
- Try using smaller dishes, bowls, and glasses. This will make your portion appear larger, and you'll be eating or drinking less.
- When cooking at home, put a serving of the entrée on your plate; then freeze any leftovers in single-serving containers. This way, you won't be tempted to eat the whole batch before the food goes bad, and you'll have ready-made servings for future meals.

Steps Toward Sustained Weight Loss

Now that you know how to spot a fad diet, you may be wondering what makes a weight-loss plan sound. That is, what should you do to lose weight and keep it off while staying well nourished and healthy? An expert panel from the National Institutes of Health recommends the following steps toward weight loss that lasts.[3]

Dietary Recommendations

☐ Aim for a weight loss of 0.5 to 2 lb per week. Remember that 1 lb of fat is equal to about 3,500 kilocalories.

☐ To achieve this rate of weight loss, reduce your current energy intake by approximately 250 to 1,000 kilocalories a day. A weight-loss plan should never provide less than a total of 1,200 kilocalories a day.

☐ Aim for a total fat intake of 15% to 25% of total energy intake and choose unsaturated rather than saturated or *trans* fats.

☐ Limit your intake of simple sugars.

☐ Consume 25 to 35 grams of fiber a day.

☐ Consume 1,000 to 1,500 mg of calcium a day.

☐ Select leaner cuts of meat (such as the white meat of poultry and extra-lean ground beef) and reduced-fat or skim dairy products.

☐ Select lower-fat food-preparation methods (baking, broiling, and grilling instead of frying).

☐ Save high-fat, high-Calorie snack foods for occasional special treats.

Steps for Increasing Your Physical Activity

☐ Try to do a minimum of 30 minutes of moderate physical activity most, preferably all, days of the week. Moderate physical activity includes walking, jogging, riding a bike, roller blading, and so forth.

☐ Ideally, do 45 minutes or more of moderate physical activity at least 5 days per week.

☐ Keep clothes and equipment for physical activity in convenient places.

☐ Move throughout the day, such as by taking stairs, pacing while talking on the phone, or doing sit-ups while watching television.

☐ Join an exercise class, mall-walking group, running club, yoga group, or any other group of people who are physically active.

☐ Use the "buddy" system by exercising with a friend or relative and calling this support person when you need an extra boost to stay motivated.

☐ Prioritize exercise by writing it down, along with your classes and other engagements, in your daily planner.

■ To help you fill up, take second helpings of plain vegetables. That way, dessert may not seem so tempting!

■ When buying snacks, go for single-serving, prepackaged items. If you buy larger bags or boxes, divide the snack into single-serving bags.

■ When you have a treat, such as ice cream, measure out ½ cup, eat it slowly, and enjoy it!

Additional strategies you can incorporate include eliminating extra foods high in saturated fats, such as butter, cheese sauces, doughnuts, and cakes. Select lower-fat versions of the foods listed in the USDA Food Patterns (ChooseMyPlate.gov). This means selecting leaner cuts of meat (such as the white meat of poultry and extra-lean ground beef) and reduced-fat or skim dairy products and using lower-fat preparation methods (such as baking and broiling instead of frying). In addition, switch from sugary drinks to low-Calorie or non-Calorie drinks throughout the day.

Increase the number of times each day that you choose foods that are relatively low in energy density. This includes salads (with low- or non-Calorie dressings), fruits, vegetables, and soups (broth-based). These foods are low in energy, but because they contain relatively more water and fiber than more energy-dense foods, they can help you feel satiated without having to consume large amounts of energy.

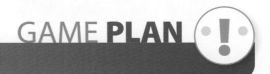

GAME **PLAN**

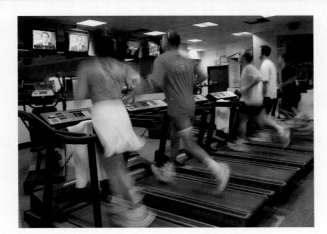

⬅ Joining an exercise class can help you increase your physical activity.

Steps for Modifying Your Food-Related Behavior

☐ Eat only at set times in one location. Do not eat while studying, working, driving, watching television, and so forth.

☐ Keep a log of what you eat, when, and why. Note any triggers you discover and list ways to avoid them.

☐ Avoid shopping when you are hungry.

☐ Avoid buying problem foods—that is, foods you have difficulty eating in moderate amounts.

☐ Avoid purchasing high-fat, high-sugar food from vending machines and convenience stores.

☐ At fast-food restaurants, choose small portions of foods lower in fat and simple sugars.

☐ Follow the serving sizes indicated as part of the USDA Food Patterns at MyPlate.gov.

☐ Serve your food portions on smaller dishes, so that they appear larger.

☐ Avoid feelings of deprivation by eating small, regular meals throughout the day.

☐ Whether at home or dining out, share food with others.

☐ Prepare healthful snacks to take with you, so that you won't be tempted by foods from vending machines, fast-food restaurants, and so forth.

☐ Chew food slowly, taking at least 20 minutes to eat a full meal and stopping at once if you begin to feel full.

☐ Reward yourself for positive behaviors by getting a massage, buying new clothes, or going to a movie or concert.

☐ Set reasonable goals and don't punish yourself if you deviate from your plan (and you will—everyone does). Ask others to avoid responding to any slips you make.

Data from National Heart, Lung, and Blood Institute Expert Panel, National Institutes of Health. 1998. *Clinical Guidelines on the Identification, Evaluation, and Treatment of Overweight and Obesity in Adults.* Washington, DC: Government Printing Office.

FIGURE 9.9 illustrates two sets of meals, one higher in energy and one lower in energy. You can see from this figure that simple changes to a meal, such as choosing lower-fat dairy products, smaller portion sizes, and foods that are relatively less dense in energy, can reduce energy intake without sacrificing taste, pleasure, or nutritional quality!

Participate in Regular Physical Activity

The *Dietary Guidelines for Americans* emphasize the role of physical activity in maintaining a healthful weight. Why is being physically active so important? Of course, we expend extra energy during physical activity, but there's more to it than that, because exercise alone (without a reduction of energy intake) does not result in dramatic weight loss. Instead, one of the most important reasons for being regularly active is that it helps us maintain or increase our lean body mass and our BMR. In contrast, energy restriction alone causes us to lose lean body mass. As you've learned, the more lean body mass we have, the more energy we expend over the long term.

While very few weight-loss studies have documented long-term maintenance of weight loss, those that have find that only people who are regularly active are able to maintain most of their weight loss. The National Weight Control Registry is an

a day of meals

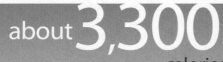

about 3,300 calories (kcal)

about 1,700 calories (kcal)

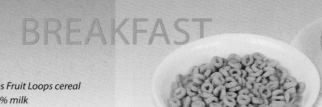

BREAKFAST

1½ cups Fruit Loops cereal
1 cup 2% milk
1 cup orange juice
2 slices white toast
1 tbsp. butter (on toast)

1½ cups Cheerios cereal
1 cup skim milk
½ fresh pink grapefruit

LUNCH

McDonald's Big Mac hamburger
French fries, extra large
3 tbsp. ketchup
Apple pie

Subway cold-cut trio 6" sandwich
Granola bar, hard, with chocolate chips, 1 bar (24 g)
1 fresh medium apple

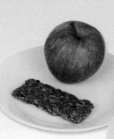

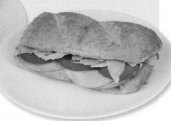

DINNER

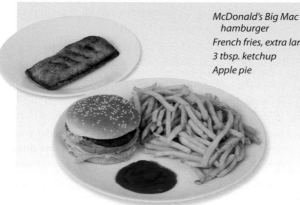

4.5 oz ground beef (80% lean, crumbled), cooked
2 medium taco shells
2 oz cheddar cheese
2 tbsp. sour cream
4 tbsp. store-bought salsa
1 cup shredded lettuce
½ cup refried beans
6 Oreos

5 oz ground turkey, cooked
2 soft corn tortillas
1 oz low-fat cheddar cheese
4 tbsp. store-bought salsa
1 cup shredded lettuce
1 cup cooked mixed veggies

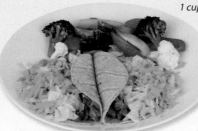

nutrient analysis

3,319 kcal
44.1% of energy from carbohydrates
44.2% of energy from fat
15.6% of energy from saturated fat
12.5% of energy from protein
31.4 grams of dietary fiber
4,752 milligrams of sodium

Saves 1,600 kcals!

nutrient analysis

1,753 kcal
44.6% of energy from carbohydrates
31.5% of energy from fat
10.6% of energy from saturated fat
21% of energy from protein
24.9 grams of dietary fiber
3,161 milligrams of sodium

foods you don't know you love YET

Air-Popped Popcorn

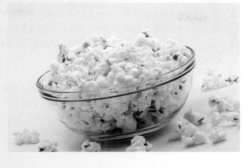

Popcorn is one of the most popular snacks in the United States. What would a night at the movies be without it? Unfortunately, the versions sold in movie theaters typically contain alarmingly high levels of fat, salt, and Calories. A quick Internet search reveals that even a small size at the nation's largest movie theater chains can pack between 400 and 700 Calories! Even microwave popcorns can contain excessive fat and salt, and many of the lower-fat brands contain *trans* fats. But have you ever tried popcorn in its natural state? Without all the additives, popcorn is naturally low in fat and high in fiber, and contains no salt or sugar.

You can make a healthy popcorn snack by air-popping it—no fancy gadget required! Just put 1/8 cup (2 tablespoons) of popcorn kernels into a brown paper lunch bag. Fold the bag two or three times at the top, about an inch per fold, and set it upright on your microwave turntable. Pop for about 2 minutes, but watch and listen closely: as soon as the popping slows down, stop the microwave. Otherwise, you risk burned popcorn and a smoky kitchen! Many options are also available today from manufacturers who offer fat- and salt-free air-popped popcorn in premeasured amounts. Always be sure to tilt the bag away from you when you open it, because hot steam will escape. If you wish, add a small amount of melted butter (100 Calories per tablespoon) and a pinch of salt for flavoring. For more zest, try instead adding a little parmesan cheese, or even garlic or chili powder. Air-popped popcorn can be a delicious, low-Calorie, healthful snack!

ongoing project documenting the habits of people who have lost at least 30 pounds and kept their weight off for at least 1 year. Of the more than 4,000 people studied thus far, the average weight loss was 73 pounds over 5.7 years.[24] Almost all the people (89%) reported changing both physical activity and dietary intake to lose weight and maintain weight loss. No one form of exercise seems to be most effective, but many people report doing some form of aerobic exercise (walking is the most commonly reported form of activity) for approximately 1 hour per day most days of the week. In fact, on average, this group expended more than 2,600 kcal each week through physical activity!

In addition to expending energy and maintaining lean body mass and BMR, regular physical activity improves our mood, results in a higher quality of sleep, increases self-esteem, and gives us a sense of accomplishment. All of these changes enhance our ability to engage in long-term healthful lifestyle behaviors.

Incorporate Appropriate Behavior Modifications into Daily Life

Successful weight loss and long-term maintenance of a healthful weight require people to modify their behaviors. Some of the behavior modifications related to food and physical activity have been discussed in the previous sections. Here are a few more practical changes you can make to help you lose weight and keep it off:

- Shop for food only when you are not hungry.
- Avoid buying problem foods—that is, foods that you may have difficulty eating in moderate amounts.
- Avoid feelings of deprivation by eating small, regular meals throughout the day.
- Eat only at set times in one location. Do not eat while studying, working, driving, watching television, and so forth.

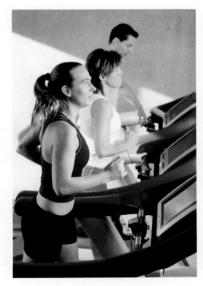

◄ Participating in regular and appropriate physical activity is one of the main components of a weight-change plan.

- Keep a log of what you eat, when, and why. Try to identify social or emotional cues that cause you to overeat, such as getting a poor grade on an exam or feeling lonely. Then strategize about other ways to cope, such as calling a friend.
- Whether at home or dining out, share food with others.
- Prepare healthful snacks to take with you, so that you won't be tempted by foods from vending machines, fast-food kiosks, and so forth.
- Chew food slowly, taking at least 20 minutes to eat a full meal and stopping at once if you begin to feel full.
- Always use appropriate utensils.
- Leave food on your plate or store it for the next meal.
- Don't punish yourself for deviating from your plan (and you probably will—almost everyone does). Ask your friends and family to be supportive and not dwell on the occasional slip-up.

recap Achieving and maintaining a healthful body weight involves gradual reductions in energy intake, such as by eating smaller portions and limiting dietary fat; incorporating regular physical activity; and applying appropriate behavior modification techniques. Fad diets do not incorporate these strategies and do not result in long-term, healthful weight change. A variety of diets based on macronutrient composition may promote weight loss but may or may not result in long-term maintenance of the lower body weight.

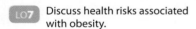 HEALTHWATCH

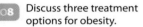 **LO7** Discuss health risks associated with obesity.

LO8 Discuss three treatment options for obesity.

How can you avoid obesity?

At the beginning of this chapter, we defined obesity as having an amount of excess body fat that adversely affects health, resulting in a person having a weight for a given height that is substantially greater than some accepted standard. People with a BMI between 30 and 39.9 are considered obese. Morbid obesity occurs when a person's body weight exceeds 100% of normal. People who are morbidly obese have a BMI greater than or equal to 40.

Why Is Obesity Harmful?

Obesity rates in the United States have increased more than 50% during the past 20 years, and it is now estimated that about 35.7% of adults 20 years and older are obese.[25] The alarming rise in obesity is a major health concern, because it is linked to many chronic diseases and complications:

- Hypertension
- Dyslipidemia, including elevated total cholesterol, triglycerides, and LDL-cholesterol and decreased HDL-cholesterol
- Type 2 diabetes
- Heart disease
- Stroke
- Gallbladder disease
- Osteoarthritis
- Sleep apnea
- Certain cancers, such as colon, breast, endometrial, and gallbladder
- Menstrual irregularities and infertility
- Gestational diabetes, premature fetal deaths, neural tube defects, and complications during labor and delivery
- Depression
- Alzheimer's disease, dementia, and cognitive decline

Abdominal obesity, specifically a large amount of visceral fat that is stored deep within the abdomen (**FIGURE 9.10**), is one of five risk factors collectively referred to as *metabolic syndrome*. As we discussed earlier in this text (see Chapters 3 and 4), a diagnosis of metabolic syndrome increases a person's risk for heart disease, type 2 diabetes, and stroke. It is typically made if a person has three or more of the following risk factors:

- abdominal obesity (defined as a waist circumference greater than or equal to 40 inches for men and 35 inches for women),
- higher-than-normal triglyceride levels (greater than or equal to 150 mg/dL),
- lower-than-normal HDL-cholesterol levels (less than 40 mg/dL in men and 50 mg/dL in women),
- elevated blood pressure (greater than or equal to 130/85 mm Hg), and
- fasting blood glucose levels greater than or equal to 100 mg/dL, including people with diabetes.

People with metabolic syndrome are twice as likely to develop heart disease and five times as likely to develop type 2 diabetes than people without metabolic syndrome. About 34% of adults in the United States have metabolic syndrome, and rising obesity rates are contributing to increased rates.[26]

Obesity is also associated with an increased risk of premature death: as discussed previously, having a BMI equal to or greater than 30 kg/m^2 increases a person's risk of dying prematurely 18% above that of people with a BMI value in the range of 18.5–24.99 kg/m^2. Several of the obesity-related diseases just listed are leading causes of death in the United States.

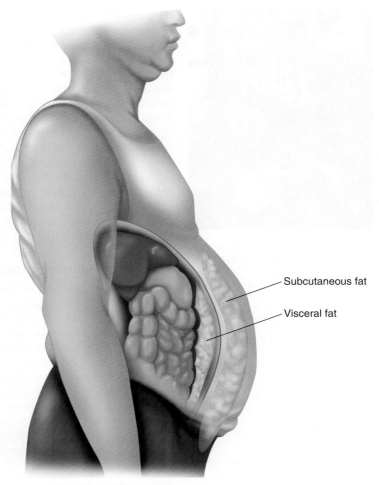

Subcutaneous fat

Visceral fat

▲ **FIGURE 9.10**   Abdominal obesity, specifically a high amount of visceral fat stored deep within the abdomen, is one of the risk factors for metabolic syndrome.

Why Do People Become Obese?

Obesity is known as a **multifactorial disease**, meaning that there are many things that cause it. Although it is certainly true that overeating plays a role, it is also true that some people are more susceptible to becoming obese than others, and some are more resistant to weight loss and maintaining weight loss. Research on the causes of obesity is ongoing, but let's explore some current theories.

Genetic and Physiologic Factors Influence Obesity Risk

The same genetic, metabolic, and physiologic factors that influence energy metabolism, food intake, and satiety also, of course, influence a person's risk of developing obesity. Additional hormonal factors include an abnormally low level of thyroid hormone and an abnormally high level of the stress-hormone cortisol, both of which can lead to weight gain and obesity. A physician can check your blood for levels of these hormones. Certain prescription medications, including steroids used for asthma and other disorders, seizure medications, and some antidepressants, can slow basal metabolic rate or stimulate appetite, leading to weight gain and obesity.[27]

Childhood Obesity Is Linked to Adult Obesity

The prevalence of obesity in children and adolescents increased at an alarming rate in the United States over the last fifty years, and approximately 17% of this age group are now estimated to be obese.[28] Health data demonstrate that these children are

multifactorial disease Any disease that may be attributable to one or more of a variety of causes.

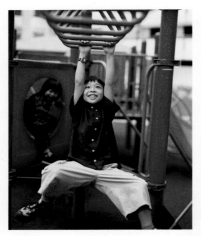

◆ Adequate physical activity is instrumental in preventing childhood obesity.

already showing signs of chronic disease while they are young, including elevated blood pressure, high LDL-cholesterol levels, and changes in insulin and glucose metabolism that may increase their risk for type 2 diabetes (formerly known as *adult onset diabetes*). In some instances, children as young as 5 years of age have been diagnosed with type 2 diabetes. Unfortunately, many of these children are likely to maintain these disease risk factors into adulthood. Moreover, although some children who are obese grow up to have a normal body weight, it has been estimated that about 70% of children who are obese maintain their higher weight as adults.[29]

Having either one or two overweight parents increases the risk for obesity by two to four times. This may be explained in part by genetics and in part by unhealthful eating patterns or lack of physical activity within the family. We know that children who eat healthful diets that do not contain a lot of empty Calories and are very physically active are unlikely to become obese. In contrast, children who eat a lot of empty Calories and spend most of their time on the computer or in front of the television are more likely to be obese. When these patterns are carried into adolescence and adulthood, the obesity is likely to persist.

Social Factors Appear to Influence Obesity Risk

Poverty has been linked to obesity. One reason for this may be that high-Calorie processed foods cost less and are easier to find and prepare than more healthful foods, such as fresh fruits and vegetables. Other reasons may include reduced access to safe places to walk, hike, or engage in other forms of physical activity, not to mention the cost of membership in a health club, gym, or commercial weight-loss program. Poverty also typically reduces access to high-quality healthcare, including health education and other types of preventive care.

Our social ties may also have a subtle influence on our risk for obesity. Although their data have been challenged, researchers from Harvard Medical School evaluated a social network of more than 12,000 people and concluded that an individual's risk of becoming obese increases significantly—by 37% to 57%—if the person has a spouse, sibling, or friend who has become obese.[30]

Does Obesity Respond to Treatment?

Ironically, up to 40% of women and 25% of men are dieting at any given time. How can obesity rates be so high when there are so many people dieting? Although relatively few studies have tracked weight-loss maintenance, evidence from one study suggests that only about 20% of obese people are successful at long-term weight loss.[24] In this study, success was defined as losing at least 10% of initial body weight and maintaining the loss for at least 1 year. The results suggest that about 80% of obese people who are dieting fail to lose weight or to keep it off. Although these statistics might suggest that obesity somehow resists intervention, that's not the case. Bearing in mind that 20% of people do succeed in long-term weight loss, the question becomes "How do they do it?"

Lifestyle Changes Can Help

The first line of defense in treating obesity in adults is a diet with a deficit of 500 to 1,000 Calories a day, along with physical activity at least 30 minutes a day, five days a week. Up to 60 minutes a day may be necessary to lose weight and maintain a healthful weight over time. Psychotherapy can be helpful in challenging patients to examine the thought patterns, situations, and stressors that may be undermining their efforts at weight loss. Support groups such as Overeaters Anonymous (OA) also help many people maintain their dietary and activity changes.

Weight Loss Can Be Enhanced with Prescribed Medications

The biggest complaint about the lifestyle recommendations for healthful weight loss is that they are difficult to maintain. In response to this challenge, prescription drugs have been developed to assist people with weight loss. These drugs typically act as appetite suppressants and may also increase satiety.

To learn more about the complex factors contributing to the rise in obesity in the United States, watch a video from CDC-TV, the video channel of the U.S. Centers for Disease Control and Prevention, at http://www.cdc.gov/. Type in "Obesity CDC-TV" into the search box to get started.

Weight-loss medications should be used only with proper supervision from a physician. Physician involvement is so critical because many drugs developed for weight loss have serious side effects. Some have even proven deadly. These life-threatening drugs have been banned, yet they still serve as examples illustrating that the treatment of obesity through pharmacologic means is neither simple nor risk-free.

Seven prescription weight-loss drugs are currently available.[31] The long-term safety of many of these drugs is still being explored:

- Diethylpropion (brand name Tenuate), phentermine (brand name Adipex), benzphetamine (brand name Didrex), phendimetrazine (brand name Bontril), and lorcaserin (brand name Belviq) are drugs that decrease appetite and increase feelings of fullness. Side effects include increased blood pressure and heart rate, nervousness, insomnia, dry mouth, and constipation.
- Combination phentermine-topiramate (brand name Qsymia) also works by decreasing appetite and increasing feelings of fullness. Side effects include increased heart rate, tingling of hands and feet, dry mouth, constipation, anxiety, and birth defects. Because of this increased risk for birth defects, women of child-bearing years must avoid getting pregnant while taking this medication.
- Orlistat (brand name Xenical) is a drug that acts to inhibit the absorption of dietary fat from the intestinal tract. Orlistat is also available in a reduced-strength form (brand name Alli) that is available without a prescription. Side effects include intestinal cramps, gas, diarrhea, and oily spotting. Although rare, liver damage can occur.

Although the use of prescribed weight-loss medications is associated with side effects and a certain level of risk, they are justified for people who are obese. That's because the health risks of obesity override the risks of the medications. They are also advised for people who have a BMI greater than or equal to 27 kg/m² who also have other significant health risk factors such as heart disease, high blood pressure, and type 2 diabetes.

Surgery Can Be Used to Treat Morbid Obesity

Generally, bariatric surgery is advised in people with a BMI greater than or equal to 40 kg/m² or in people with a BMI greater than or equal to 35 kg/m² who have other life-threatening conditions such as diabetes, hypertension, or elevated cholesterol levels. The three most common types of weight-loss surgery performed are sleeve gastrectomy, gastric bypass, and gastric banding **(FIGURE 9.11)**.

Surgery is considered a last resort for morbidly obese people who have not been able to lose weight with energy restriction, exercise, and medications. This is because

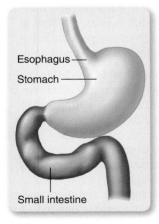

(a) Normal anatomy

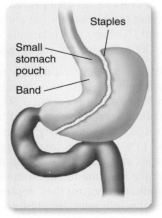

(b) Sleeve gastrectomy

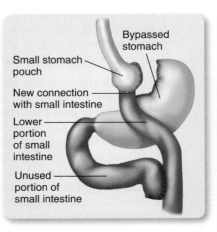

(c) Gastric bypass

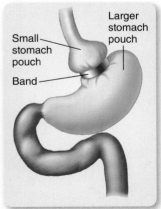

(d) Gastric banding

FIGURE 9.11 Various forms of surgery alter the normal anatomy **(a)** of the gastrointestinal tract to promote weight loss. Sleeve gastrectomy **(b)**, gastric bypass, **(c)** and gastric banding **(d)** are three surgical procedures used to reduce morbid obesity.

the risks of surgery in people with morbid obesity are extremely high. They include an increased rate of infections, formation of blood clots, and adverse reactions to anesthesia. After the surgery, many recipients face a lifetime of problems with chronic diarrhea, vomiting, intolerance to dairy products and other foods, dehydration, and nutritional deficiencies resulting from alterations in nutrient digestion and absorption that occur with bypass procedures. Thus, the potential benefits of the procedure must outweigh the risks. If the immediate threat of serious disease and death is more dangerous than the risks associated with surgery, then the procedure is justified.

Liposuction is a cosmetic surgical procedure that removes fat cells from localized areas in the body. It is not recommended or typically used to treat obesity or morbid obesity. Instead, it is often used by normal or mildly overweight people to "spot reduce" fat from various areas of the body. This procedure is not without risks; blood clots, skin and nerve damage, adverse drug reactions, and perforation injuries can and do occur as a result of liposuction. It can also cause deformations in the area where the fat is removed. This procedure is not the solution to long-term weight loss, because the millions of fat cells that remain in the body after liposuction enlarge if the person continues to overeat. In addition, although liposuction may reduce the fat content of a localized area, it does not reduce a person's risk for the diseases that are more common among overweight or obese people. Only traditional weight loss with diet and exercise can reduce body fat and the risks for chronic diseases.

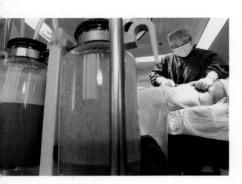

▲ Liposuction removes fat cells from specific areas of the body.

recap Obesity is caused by genetic, metabolic, and physiologic factors, a history of childhood obesity, overeating, and lack of adequate physical activity. Treatments for obesity and morbid obesity include a low-energy diet in combination with regular physical activity; weight-loss prescription medications; and weight-loss surgery.

What if you are underweight?

With so much emphasis in the United States on obesity and weight loss, some find it surprising that many people are trying to gain weight. These include people who are clinically underweight—that is, people with a BMI less than 18.5. Being underweight can be just as unhealthful as being obese, because underweight increases the risk for infections, osteoporosis, and other diseases and can even be fatal. In addition, many athletes want to gain weight in order to increase their strength and power for competition.

To gain weight, people must eat more energy than they expend. Although overeating large amounts of high-saturated-fat foods (such as bacon, sausage, and cheese) can cause weight gain, doing this without exercising is not considered healthful because most of the weight gained is fat, and high-fat diets increase our risks for cardiovascular and other diseases. Unless there are medical reasons to eat a high-fat diet, it is recommended that people trying to gain weight eat a diet that is relatively low in dietary fat (less than 35% of total Calories) and relatively high in complex carbohydrates (55% of total Calories). The following are recommendations for weight gain:

- Eat a diet that includes about 500 to 1,000 kcal per day more than is needed to maintain current body weight. Although we don't know precisely how much extra energy is needed to gain 1 lb, a common estimate is about 3,500 kcal. Thus, eating 500 to 1,000 kcal per day in excess should result in a gain of 1 to 2 lb of weight each week.
- Eat a diet that contains about 55% of total energy from carbohydrate, 25% to 35% of total energy from fat, and 10% to 20% of total energy from protein.
- Eat frequently, including meals and numerous snacks throughout the day. Many underweight people do not take the time to eat often enough.
- Avoid the use of tobacco products, because they depress appetite and increase metabolic rate, which prevent weight gain. In addition, they increase our risks for lung, mouth, esophageal, and other cancers.

■ Exercise regularly and incorporate weight lifting or some other form of resistance training into your exercise routine. This form of exercise is most effective in increasing muscle mass. Performing aerobic exercise (such as walking, running, bicycling, or swimming) at least 30 minutes a day for 3 days per week will help maintain a healthy cardiovascular system.

The key to gaining weight is to eat frequent meals throughout the day and to select energy-dense foods. When selecting foods that are higher in fat, make sure you select foods higher in polyunsaturated and monounsaturated fats (such as peanut butter, olive and canola oils, and avocados). Smoothies and milkshakes made with low-fat milk or yogurt are another great way to take in a lot of energy. Eating fruit or raw vegetables with peanut butter, hummus, guacamole, or cream cheese and including salad dressings on your salad are other ways to increase the energy density of foods. The biggest challenge to weight gain is setting aside time to eat; by packing a lot of foods to take with you throughout the day, you can increase your opportunities to eat more.

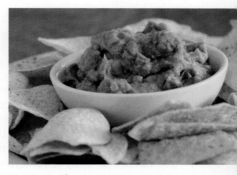

⬆ Eating frequent nutrient- and energy-dense snacks can help promote weight gain.

recap Weight gain can be achieved by eating about 500 to 1,000 kcal per day more than is needed to maintain present weight and by performing weight lifting and aerobic exercise. Eating frequent, healthy meals and snacks throughout the day and avoiding the use of tobacco products are important strategies.

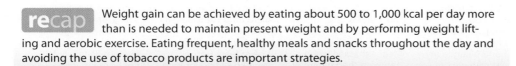

✚ HEALTHWATCH

Disordered eating: are you at risk?

Disordered eating is a general term used to describe a variety of atypical eating behaviors that people use to achieve or maintain a lower body weight. These behaviors may be as simple as going on and off diets or as extreme as refusing to eat any fat. Such behaviors don't usually continue for long enough to make the person seriously ill, nor do they significantly disrupt the person's normal routine.

In contrast, some people restrict their eating so much or for so long that they become dangerously ill. These people have an **eating disorder**, a psychiatric condition that involves extreme body dissatisfaction and long-term eating patterns that negatively affect body functioning. Three clinically diagnosed eating disorders are anorexia nervosa, bulimia nervosa, and binge-eating disorder. Whereas anorexia nervosa is characterized by extreme food restriction, bulimia nervosa and binge-eating disorder are characterized by extreme intake of food. These disorders will be discussed in more detail shortly.

LO9 Identify several factors thought to contribute to the development of eating disorders.

LO10 Compare and contrast anorexia nervosa, bulimia nervosa, binge-eating disorder, night-eating syndrome, and the female athlete triad.

Eating Behaviors Occur on a Continuum

When does normal dieting cross the line into disordered eating? Eating behaviors occur on a *continuum,* a spectrum that can't be divided neatly into parts. An example is a rainbow—where exactly does the red end and the orange begin? Thinking about eating behaviors as a continuum makes it easier to understand how a person can progress from relatively normal eating behaviors to a pattern that is disordered. For instance, let's say that for several years you've skipped breakfast in favor of a mid-morning snack, but now you find yourself avoiding the cafeteria until early afternoon. Is this normal? To answer that question, you'd need to consider your feelings about food and your **body image**—the way you perceive your body.

Take a moment to consider the statements in the ***What About You?*** feature box. It will help clarify how you feel about your body and whether or not you're at risk for an eating disorder.

disordered eating A general term used to describe a variety of abnormal or atypical eating behaviors that are used to keep or maintain a lower body weight.

eating disorder A clinically diagnosed psychiatric disorder characterized by severe disturbances in body image and eating behaviors.

body image A person's perception of his or her body's appearance and functioning.

WHAT ABOUT **YOU** (?)

Are You at Risk for an Eating Disorder?

Take a look at the Eating Issues and Body Image Continuum (**FIGURE 9.12**). Which of the five columns best describes your feelings about food and your body? If you identify with the statements on the left side of the continuum, you probably have few issues with food or body image. Most likely, you accept your body size and view food as a normal part of maintaining your health and fueling your daily physical activity.

As you progress to the right side of the continuum, food and body image become bigger issues, with food restriction becoming the norm. If you identify with the statements on the far right, you are probably afraid of eating and dislike your body. If so, you should consult a healthcare professional as soon as possible. The earlier you seek treatment, the more likely you can take ownership of your body and develop a healthful approach to food.

• I am not concerned about what others think regarding what and how much I eat. • When I am upset or depressed I eat whatever I am hungry for without any guilt or shame. • I feel no guilt or shame no matter how much I eat or what I eat. • Food is an important part of my life but only occupies a small part of my time. • I trust my body to tell me what and how much to eat.	• I pay attention to what I eat in order to maintain a healthy body. • I may weigh more than what I like, but I enjoy eating and balance my pleasure with eating with my concern for a healthy body. • I am moderate and flexible in goals for eating well. • I try to follow Dietary Guidelines for healthy eating.	• I think about food a lot. • I feel I don't eat well most of the time. • It's hard for me to enjoy eating with others. • I feel ashamed when I eat more than others or more than what I feel I should be eating. • I am afraid of getting fat. • I wish I could change how much I want to eat and what I am hungry for.	• I have tried diet pills, laxatives, vomiting, or extra time exercising in order to lose or maintain my weight. • I have fasted or avoided eating for long periods of time in order to lose or maintain my weight. • I feel strong when I can restrict how much I eat. • Eating more than I wanted to makes me feel out of control.	• I regularly stuff myself and then exercise, vomit, or use diet pills or laxatives to get rid of the food or calories. • My friends/family tell me I am too thin. • I am terrified of eating fat. • When I let myself eat, I have a hard time controlling the amount of food I eat. • I am afraid to eat in front of others.
FOOD IS NOT AN ISSUE	**CONCERNED/WELL**	**FOOD PREOCCUPIED/ OBSESSED**	**DISRUPTIVE EATING PATTERNS**	**EATING DISORDERED**
BODY OWNERSHIP	**BODY ACCEPTANCE**	**BODY PREOCCUPIED/ OBSESSED**	**DISTORTED BODY IMAGE**	**BODY HATE/ DISASSOCIATION**
• Body image is not an issue for me. • My body is beautiful to me. • My feelings about my body are not influenced by society's concept of an ideal body shape. • I know that the significant others in my life will always find me attractive. • I trust my body to find the weight it needs to be at so I can move and feel confident about my physical body.	• I base my body image equally on social norms and my own self-concept. • I pay attention to my body and my appearance because it is important to me, but it only occupies a small part of my day. • I nourish my body so it has the strength and energy to achieve my physical goals. • I am able to assert myself and maintain a healthy body without losing my self-esteem.	• I spend a significant amount time viewing my body in the mirror. • I spend a significant amount time comparing my body to others. • I have days when I feel fat. • I am preoccupied with my body. • I accept society's ideal body shape and size as the best body shape and size. • I believe that I'd be more attractive if I were thinner, more muscular, etc.	• I spend a significant amount of time exercising and dieting to change my body. • My body shape and size keep me from dating or finding someone who will treat me the way I want to be treated. • I have considered changing or have changed my body shape and size through surgical means so I can accept myself. • I wish I could change the way I look in the mirror.	• I often feel separated and distant from my body—as if it belongs to someone else. • I hate my body and I often isolate myself from others. • I don't see anything positive or even neutral about my body shape and size. • I don't believe others when they tell me I look OK. • I hate the way I look in the mirror.

FIGURE 9.12 The Eating Issues and Body Image Continuum. The progression from normal eating (far left) to eating disorders (far right) occurs on a continuum.

From Smiley, King, and Avey. University of Arizona Campus Health Service. Original Continuum by C. Shisslak. Preventive Medicine and Public Health. Copyright ©1997 Arizona Board of Regents. Reprinted by permission.

Many Factors Contribute to Disordered Eating Behaviors

The factors that result in the development of disordered eating are very complex, but research indicates that a number of genetic, social, and psychological factors may contribute in any particular individual.

Influence of Genetics

Overall, the diagnosis of anorexia nervosa or bulimia nervosa is several times more common in people with a sibling or parent who also has an eating disorder.[32,33] Although molecular research has identified a vast array of potential genetic factors in eating disorders, no specific gene or genes has been identified conclusively; moreover, researchers agree that both genetic and environmental factors play a role.[34]

Influence of Social Factors

Every day, we are confronted with advertisements in which computer-enhanced images of lean men and women promote everything from beer to cars. As this media saturation has increased over the last century, so has the incidence of eating disorders. However, research specifically linking eating disorders to the influence of media has shown mixed results.

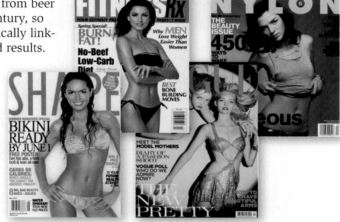

On the other hand, research does suggest that family dynamics can influence the development of an eating disorder. The risk for anorexia nervosa, for example, is increased in people who have a family member with an eating disorder, an anxiety disorder, clinical depression, or a substance use disorder.[33] Some studies have found that a mother's concern about a child's weight is significant in predicting an eating disorder.[35]

A history of childhood sexual abuse has been reported in from 20–50% of patients with anorexia nervosa or bulimia nervosa. A history of trauma in adulthood is also more common, including rape or aggravated assault.[36] Peer relationships also appear to strongly influence body image and risk of developing an eating disorder.[37] For example, one study found that the risk of anorexia nervosa decreased as the BMI of one's peers increased.[38] Intriguingly, another study found that peer feedback interacts with media images of "thin-ideal" models to affect an adolescent's body image either positively or negatively.[39]

▲ Photos of celebrities and models are often airbrushed, or altered to "enhance" physical appearance. Unfortunately, many people believe that these are accurate portrayals and strive to reach unrealistic levels of physical beauty.

Influence of Psychological Factors

Patients in treatment for eating disorders are much more likely to also be experiencing another psychiatric disorder—such as clinical depression, an anxiety disorder, or a substance abuse disorder—than the general population.[36] Personality might also play a role: A number of studies suggest that people with anorexia nervosa tend to be perfectionistic, socially inhibited, and compliant.[40] Unfortunately, many studies observe these behaviors only in individuals who are very ill and in a state of starvation, which may affect personality. Thus, it is difficult to determine if personality is the cause or the effect of the disorder. In contrast to people with anorexia, people with bulimia tend to be more impulsive, have low self-esteem, and demonstrate an extroverted, erratic personality style that seeks attention and admiration. In these people, negative moods are more likely to cause overeating than food restriction.[40]

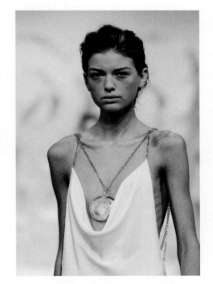

recap Eating behaviors occur along a continuum. *Disordered eating* is a general term that describes a variety of atypical eating behaviors people use to achieve or maintain a lower body weight; whereas an *eating disorder* is a recognized psychiatric condition that involves extreme body dissatisfaction and long-term eating patterns that negatively affect body functioning. The development of disordered eating behaviors and eating disorders may be influenced by genetics, social factors, and personality.

▲ The preferred look among runway models can require extreme emaciation, often achieved by self-starvation and/or drug abuse.

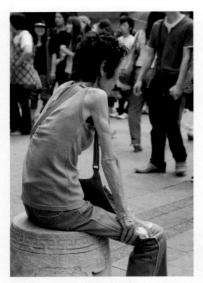

⬅ People with *anorexia nervosa* experience an extreme drive for thinness, resulting in potentially fatal weight loss.

anorexia nervosa A serious, potentially life-threatening eating disorder that is characterized by self-starvation, which eventually leads to a deficiency in the energy and essential nutrients the body requires to function normally.

amenorrhea The absence of menstruation. In females who had previously been menstruating, the absence of menstrual periods for 3 or more months.

bulimia nervosa A serious eating disorder characterized by recurrent episodes of binge eating and compensatory behaviors in order to prevent weight gain, such as self-induced vomiting.

binge eating Consumption of a large amount of food in a short period of time, usually accompanied by a feeling of loss of self-control.

purging An attempt to rid the body of unwanted food by vomiting or other compensatory means, such as excessive exercise, fasting, or laxative abuse.

Anorexia Nervosa Is a Potentially Deadly Eating Disorder

Anorexia nervosa is an eating disorder characterized by an extremely low body weight achieved through self-starvation, which eventually leads to a severe nutrient deficiency. According to the American Psychiatric Association, depending on how narrowly or broadly the condition is defined, between 0.3% to 3.7% of American females develops anorexia.[36] Although estimates vary widely, at least 4% of people with anorexia nervosa die prematurely from complications of the disorder, making it the most common and deadly psychiatric disorder diagnosed in women.[41] Anorexia also occurs in males, but the prevalence is much lower than in females.[36]

The classic sign of anorexia nervosa is an extremely restrictive eating pattern that leads to self-starvation. These individuals may fast completely, restrict energy intake to only a few Calories per day, or eliminate all but one or two food groups from their diet. They also have an intense fear of weight gain, and even small amounts (for example, 1–2 lb) trigger high stress and anxiety.

In women, **amenorrhea** (experiencing no menstrual periods for at least 3 months) is a common feature of anorexia. It occurs when a young woman consumes insufficient energy to maintain normal body functions. The signs of an eating disorder such as anorexia may be somewhat different in men. For more information, see the *Highlight* feature box on eating disorders in men.

Treatment brings full recovery in 50–70% of adolescents diagnosed with anorexia nervosa, and another 20% experience significant improvement.[36] However, left untreated, anorexia eventually leads to a deficiency in energy and other nutrients that are required by the body to function normally. The body will then use stored fat and lean tissue (such as organ and muscle tissue) as an energy source to maintain brain tissue and vital body functions. The body will also shut down or reduce nonvital body functions to conserve energy. Electrolyte imbalances can lead to heart failure and death. **FIGURE 9.13** highlights many of the health problems that occur in people with anorexia nervosa.

Bulimia Nervosa Is Characterized by Bingeing and Purging

Bulimia nervosa (commonly referred to as just *bulimia*) is an eating disorder characterized by repeated episodes of binge eating and purging. **Binge eating** is usually defined as a quantity of food that is large for the person and for the amount of time in which it is eaten. For example, a person may eat a dozen brownies with 2 quarts of ice cream in 30 minutes. While eating, the person may experience a sense of euphoria similar to a drug-induced high. **Purging** is an action taken to prevent weight gain, such as vomiting, laxative use, or excessive exercise.

The prevalence of bulimia is higher than that of anorexia, but the mortality rate is somewhat lower—an estimated 1%, although unintentional drug overdose and suicide are not uncommon in this group.[36] Although the prevalence of bulimia nervosa is higher in women, rates for men are significant in some predominately "thin-build" sports in which participants are encouraged or required to maintain a low body weight (such as horse racing, wrestling, crew, and gymnastics). Individuals in these sports typically do not have all the characteristics of bulimia nervosa, however, and the purging behaviors they practice typically stop once the sport is discontinued.

In addition to the recurrent and frequent binge-eating and purging episodes, the signs and symptoms of bulimia nervosa may include a chronically inflamed and sore throat, tooth decay and staining, gastroesophageal reflux, swelling in the neck and below the jaw, and dehydration. These problems are due to the use of vomiting as a method of purging. Chronic irregular bowel movements and constipation may result in people with bulimia who chronically abuse laxatives. Also, although a person with bulimia typically purges after most episodes, many do not do so on every occasion, or the purging method may be ineffective. Therefore, the weight gained as a result of binge eating can be significant.

highlight

Eating Disorders in Men: Are They Different?

Like many people, you might find it hard to believe that men develop eating disorders or, if they do, their disorders must be somehow "different," right? To explore this question, let's take a look at what research has revealed about similarities and differences between men and women with eating disorders.

Until about a decade ago, little research was conducted on eating disorders in males. Recently, however, eating disorder experts have begun to examine the gender-differences debate in detail and have discovered that eating disorders in males are largely similar to eating disorders in females. But some differences *do* exist. For instance, men with disordered eating are less concerned about actual body weight (scale weight) than females but are more concerned about body composition (percentage of muscle mass compared with fat mass). Also, males are commonly driven by a desire to improve athletic performance, to avoid being teased for being fat, to avoid obesity-related illnesses observed in male family members, and to improve a homosexual relationship. Similar factors are rarely reported by women.

The methods that men and women use to achieve weight loss also appear to differ. Males are more likely to use excessive exercise as a means of weight control, whereas females are more likely to use severe energy restriction, vomiting, and laxative abuse. These weight-control differences may stem from the societal biases surrounding dieting and male behavior; that is, dieting is considered to be more "acceptable" for women, whereas the overwhelming sociocultural belief is that "real men don't diet."

Recently, some psychologists who work with men have identified a disorder called *muscle dysmorphia (MD),* which has been classified variously as an eating disorder or as a body-image disorder.[4] Men with MD are distressed by the idea that they are not sufficiently lean and muscular, spend long hours lifting weights, and follow an extremely specialized diet. The disorder has also been called *reverse anorexia nervosa,* and indeed, men with MD perceive themselves as small and frail even though they are actually quite large and muscular. Frequently, men with MD abuse anabolic steroids, but no matter how "buff" or "chiseled" they become, their anatomy cannot match their ideal. Additionally, whereas people with anorexia eat little of anything, men with MD tend to consume excessive amounts of high-protein foods and dietary supplements, such as protein powders.

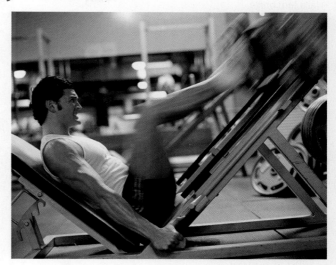

Men are more likely than women to exercise excessively in an effort to control their weight.

Men with MD do share some characteristics with men and women with true anorexia nervosa. For instance, they tend to have low self-esteem and a perfectionistic personality.[4] They also report "feeling fat" and engage in behaviors indicating an obsession with appearance (such as looking in the mirror).[5] They express significant discomfort with the idea of having to expose their body to others (for example, take off their clothes in the locker room), and they have increased rates of mental illness.[6]

The following are outward signs that someone may be struggling with MD:

- A rigid and excessive schedule of weight training
- Strict adherence to a high-protein, muscle-enhancing diet
- Use of anabolic steroids, protein powders, or other muscle-enhancing drugs or supplements
- Poor attendance at work, school, social, or sports activities because of interference with training schedule or dietary restrictions
- Frequent and critical self-evaluation of body composition

Although muscle dysmorphia isn't typically life-threatening, it can certainly cause distress and despair. Therapy—especially participation in an all-male support group—can help.

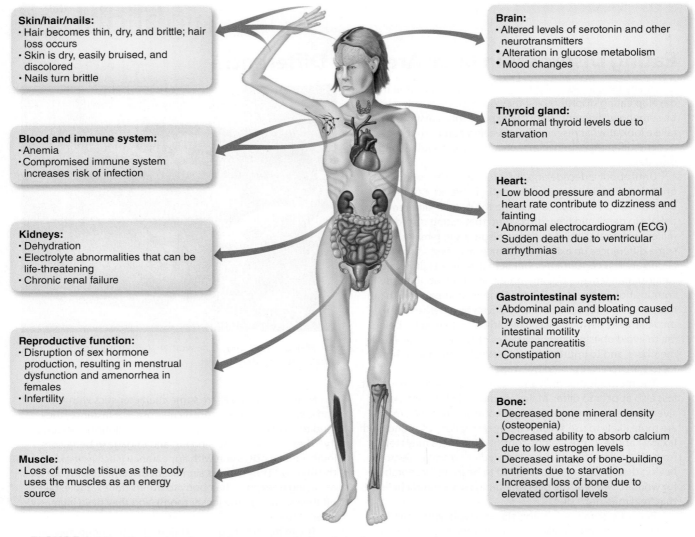

Skin/hair/nails:
- Hair becomes thin, dry, and brittle; hair loss occurs
- Skin is dry, easily bruised, and discolored
- Nails turn brittle

Blood and immune system:
- Anemia
- Compromised immune system increases risk of infection

Kidneys:
- Dehydration
- Electrolyte abnormalities that can be life-threatening
- Chronic renal failure

Reproductive function:
- Disruption of sex hormone production, resulting in menstrual dysfunction and amenorrhea in females
- Infertility

Muscle:
- Loss of muscle tissue as the body uses the muscles as an energy source

Brain:
- Altered levels of serotonin and other neurotransmitters
- Alteration in glucose metabolism
- Mood changes

Thyroid gland:
- Abnormal thyroid levels due to starvation

Heart:
- Low blood pressure and abnormal heart rate contribute to dizziness and fainting
- Abnormal electrocardiogram (ECG)
- Sudden death due to ventricular arrhythmias

Gastrointestinal system:
- Abdominal pain and bloating caused by slowed gastric emptying and intestinal motility
- Acute pancreatitis
- Constipation

Bone:
- Decreased bone mineral density (osteopenia)
- Decreased ability to absorb calcium due to low estrogen levels
- Decreased intake of bone-building nutrients due to starvation
- Increased loss of bone due to elevated cortisol levels

FIGURE 9.13 The impact of *anorexia nervosa* on the female body.

The following are the most dangerous health consequences associated with bulimia:

- Electrolyte imbalance typically caused by dehydration and the loss of potassium and sodium from the body with frequent vomiting. This can lead to irregular heartbeat and even heart failure and death.
- Gastrointestinal problems: inflammation, ulceration, and possible rupture of the esophagus and stomach from frequent bingeing and vomiting.

Binge-Eating Disorder Can Cause Significant Weight Gain

When was the last time a friend or relative confessed to you about "going on an eating binge"? Most likely, they explained that the behavior followed some sort of stressful event, such as a problem at work, the breakup of a relationship, or a poor grade on an exam. Many people have one or two binge episodes every year or so, in response to stress. But in people with **binge-eating disorder**, the behavior occurs frequently and is not usually followed by purging. This lack of compensation for the

To learn more about eating disorders, visit the website of the National Institute of Mental Health at www.nimh.nih.gov. From the index at right, choose "Eating Disorders." Then scroll down the page, where, on the right, you can click on "Publication About Eating Disorders." You can access it as a PDF or order a hard copy for free.

binge-eating disorder An eating disorder characterized by binge eating an average of twice a week or more, typically without compensatory purging.

binge distinguishes binge-eating disorder from bulimia nervosa and explains why the person tends to gain a lot of weight.

The prevalence of binge-eating disorder is estimated to be 2% of the adult population, but it is much higher—perhaps as high as 30%—among the obese.[36] About one-third of patients are men. Our current food environment, which offers an abundance of good-tasting, cheap food any time of the day, makes it difficult for people with binge-eating disorder to avoid food triggers.

Disordered Eating Can Be Part of a Syndrome

A *syndrome* is a type of disorder characterized by the presence of two or more distinct health problems that tend to occur together. Two syndromes involving disordered eating behaviors are night-eating syndrome and the female athlete triad.

Night-eating syndrome was first described in a group of patients who were not hungry in the morning but spent the evening and night eating and reported having insomnia. It is associated with obesity because, although night eaters don't binge, they do consume significant energy, and they don't compensate for the excess energy intake. The distinguishing characteristic of night-eating syndrome is time: at least 25% of the day's energy intake occurs between the evening meal and breakfast the following morning. Night eating is also characterized by insomnia and a depressed mood. In short, night eaters appear to have a unique combination of three disorders: an eating disorder, a sleep disorder, and a mood disorder.[42]

The **female athlete triad** is a serious syndrome that consists of three clinical conditions in some physically active females: low energy availability (inadequate energy intake to maintain menstrual function—with or without eating disorders), menstrual dysfunction (such as amenorrhea), and low bone density **(FIGURE 9.14)**.[43] Sports that emphasize leanness or a thin body build may place a young girl or a woman at risk for the female athlete triad. These include figure skating, gymnastics, and diving. Classical ballet dancers are also at increased risk for the disorder.

Active women experience the general social and cultural demands placed on women to be thin, as well as pressure from their coach, teammates, judges, and/or spectators to meet weight standards or body-size expectations for their sport. As the pressure to be thin mounts, they may engage in disordered eating behaviors.

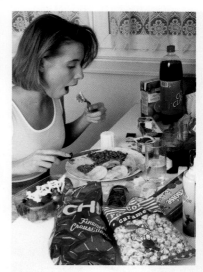

People with *bulimia nervosa* consume relatively large amounts of food in very brief periods of time.

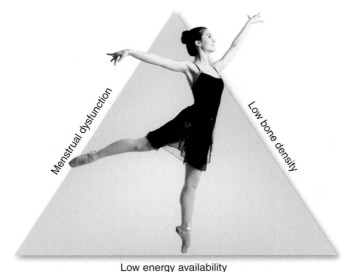

Menstrual dysfunction

Low bone density

Low energy availability

FIGURE 9.14 The female athlete triad is a syndrome consisting of three coexisting disorders: low energy availability (with or without eating disorders), menstrual dysfunction (such as amenorrhea), and low bone density. Energy availability is defined as *dietary energy intake* (how much energy you take in through foods) minus *exercise energy expenditure* (how much energy you expend through exercise).

night-eating syndrome A disorder characterized by intake of more than 25% of the day's energy late at night. Individuals with this disorder also experience mood and sleep disorders.

female athlete triad A syndrome combining three clinical conditions in some physically active females: low energy availability (with or without eating disorders), menstrual dysfunction, and low bone density.

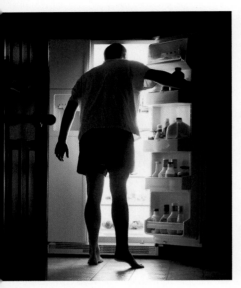

People with night-eating syndrome consume most of their daily energy between 8 PM and 6 AM.

Low energy availability combined with high levels of physical activity can disrupt the menstrual cycle and reduce levels of the reproductive hormones estrogen and progesterone. When estrogen levels in the body are low, it is difficult for bone to retain calcium, and gradual loss of bone mass occurs. Thus, many female athletes are at increased risk for fractures.

Treatment for Disordered Eating Requires a Multidisciplinary Approach

As with any health problem, prevention is the best treatment for disordered eating. People having trouble with eating and body image issues need help to deal with these issues before they develop into something more serious.

Treating anyone with disordered eating requires a multidisciplinary approach. In addition to a physician and psychologist, a nutritionist, the person's coach (if an athlete), and family members and friends all must work together. Patients who are severely underweight, display signs of malnutrition, are medically unstable, or are suicidal may require immediate hospitalization. Conversely, patients who are underweight but are still medically stable may enter an outpatient program designed to meet their specific needs. Some outpatient programs are extremely intensive, requiring patients to come in each day for treatment, whereas others are less rigorous, requiring only weekly visits for meetings with a psychiatrist or eating disorder specialist.

recap Anorexia nervosa is a potentially life-threatening disorder in which a person refuses to maintain a minimally normal body weight. Bulimia nervosa is characterized by binge eating followed by purging. In contrast, in binge-eating disorder, no purging typically occurs, and significant weight gain is likely. Night-eating syndrome is a combination of an eating disorder, a sleep disorder, and a mood disorder. The female athlete triad is a syndrome consisting of low energy availability, menstrual dysfunction, and low bone density. Treatment of eating disorders requires a multidisciplinary approach. Severely malnourished patients require hospitalization as a life-saving measure.

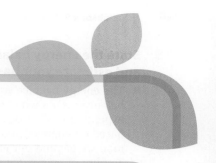

Customize your study plan—and master your nutrition!—in the Study Area of **MasteringNutrition**.

what can I do **today?**

Now that you've read this chapter, try making these three changes.

1 Calculate your body mass index from your current height and weight, and measure your waist-to-hip ratio to determine if your body weight and shape are in the healthy range.

2 If you need to lose weight, list three realistic, measurable goals you can begin to work toward today to help you achieve a healthy weight.

3 If you eat out today, whether in the campus cafeteria or at your favorite fast-food restaurant, consciously choose a healthier alternative to your usual meal and skip the sugary drink.

test yourself | *answers*

1. **False.** Health can be defined in many ways. A person who is overweight but exercises regularly and has no additional risk factors for various diseases (such as unhealthful blood lipid levels or smoking) is considered healthy.

2. **False.** According to the Centers for Disease Control and Prevention, the United States has an overall obesity rate of 35.7% for adults.

3. **False.** Males also are diagnosed with eating disorders, but the incidence is much lower than for females.

summary

Scan to hear an MP3 Chapter Review in **MasteringNutrition**.

LO **1** **Define what is meant by a healthful weight**

■ A healthful body weight is one that is appropriate for your age and physical development; is consistent with your genetic background and family history; can be achieved and sustained without constant dieting; is consistent with normal blood pressure, lipid levels, and glucose tolerance; promotes good eating habits and allows for regular physical activity; and is acceptable to you.

LO **2** **Determine your BMI and fat distribution pattern and identify any health risks associated with these assessments**

■ Body mass index (BMI) is a measurement that compares weight to height. It is useful as an indication of disease risks associated with overweight and obesity in groups of people. A BMI less than 18.5 places a person in the underweight category. Underweight is defined as having too little body fat to maintain health. A BMI of 18.5 to 25 is considered normal. A BMI between 25.1 and 29.9 is defined as overweight, which is defined as having a moderate amount of excess body fat, resulting in a person having a weight for a given height that is greater than some accepted standards but is not considered obese. A BMI greater than or equal to 30 is obesity, a state in which excess body fat adversely affects health, resulting in a person having a weight for a given height that is substantially greater than some accepted standards. Morbid obesity, a BMI greater than or equal to 40, occurs when a person's body weight exceeds 100% of normal, which puts him or her at very high risk for serious health consequences.

■ In addition to BMI, a person's fat distribution pattern affects risk for various diseases. In apple-shaped fat patterning, fat is stored mainly around the waist. In pear-shaped fat patterning, fat is stored mainly around the hips and thighs. Apple-shaped patterning is known to significantly increase a person's risk for many chronic diseases, such as type 2 diabetes, heart disease, and high blood pressure.

LO 3 **State the energy balance equation and estimate your basal metabolic rate**

- The energy balance equation states that energy balance occurs when energy intake equals energy expenditure. That is, we lose or gain weight based on changes in our energy intake or the food we eat and our energy expenditure or the amount of energy we expend at rest, as a result of eating and physical activity.

- Basal metabolic rate, or BMR, is the energy needed to maintain the body's resting functions. BMR accounts for 60% to 75% of total daily energy needs. To estimate your BMR, divide your weight in pounds by 2.2 to derive your weight in kilograms. Males can then multiply this number by 24 hours per day to derive the number of Calories they expend in basal metabolism per day. Females expend somewhat fewer Calories on average; thus, they need to multiply their 24-hour total by 0.9.

LO 4 **Explain how to calculate how many Calories you need to consume on average each day**

- The number of Calories you expend each day includes the energy cost of physical activity (the energy that we expend for physical movement above basal levels) plus basal metabolism. To estimate your needs, multiply your BMR by 1.2 if you are inactive; by 1.5 if you are moderately active; and by 1.75 if you participate in intense activity more than five days a week.

- Unfortunately, the energy balance equation fails to account for many factors that can alter energy intake and expenditure or to help explain why people gain and lose weight differently.

LO 5 **Discuss a range of factors thought to contribute to differences in body weight**

- Our genetic heritage influences our risk for obesity. Factors such as the FTO gene variant, possessing a thrifty gene (or genes), or maintaining a weight set point may affect a person's risk for obesity. Overeating high-fat foods may promote weight gain more readily than overeating protein or carbohydrate. Four metabolic factors thought to influence body weight are a relatively low BMR, a low level of spontaneous physical activity, low sympathetic nervous system (SNS) activity, and low fat metabolism. Also, a variety of hormones and functional proteins play a role in food intake, energy metabolism, and body weight.

- Cultural, economic, and social factors can influence the types and amounts of foods that are eaten, as well as the level of physical activity. For example, financial limitations may lead people to choose less healthful but more satiating foods and reduce access to parks, fitness centers, and other places where they could engage in physical activity.

LO 6 **Identify three key strategies for healthful weight loss**

- A sound weight-change plan involves a gradual reduction in energy intake by eating smaller portions of lower-fat foods; incorporating physical activity into each day; and practicing changes in behavior that can assist someone in meeting realistic weight-change goals.

LO 7 **Discuss health risks associated with obesity**

- Obesity and morbid obesity are associated with significantly increased risks for many diseases, including cardiovascular disease, type 2 diabetes, gallbladder disease, osteoarthritis, infertility, dementia, and sleep apnea. They also increase the risk of premature death. Abdominal obesity is a risk factor for the metabolic syndrome.

LO 8 **Discuss three treatment options for obesity**

- Obesity can be treated with low-energy diets and regular physical activity. Prescription medications and surgery can assist with weight loss but should be considered only when the risks of obesity override the risks associated with these therapies.

LO 9 **Identify several factors thought to contribute to the development of eating disorders**

- Disordered eating is a general term used to describe a variety of abnormal or atypical eating behaviors that are used to achieve or maintain a lower body weight. In contrast, an eating disorder is a psychiatric disorder characterized by extreme body dissatisfaction and long-term eating patterns that negatively affect body functioning.

- A number of factors are thought to contribute to the development of eating disorders, including genetics, family and other social factors, the presence of another psychiatric disorder, and possibly personality traits.

LO 10 **Compare and contrast anorexia nervosa, bulimia nervosa, binge-eating disorder, night-eating syndrome, and the female athlete triad**

- Clinically diagnosed psychiatric eating disorders include the following: Anorexia nervosa is a medical disorder in which an individual uses severe food restriction and other practices to maintain a body weight that interferes with normal functions. Bulimia nervosa is an eating disorder characterized by recurrent episodes of binge eating, followed by some form of purging. Binge-eating disorder is the consumption of a large amount of food in a short period of time (such as within 2 hours) without compensatory behaviors.

■ In contrast to the three psychiatric eating disorders are two syndromes involving disordered eating behaviors: Night-eating syndrome involves consumption of at least 25% of the day's Calories at night; insomnia; and a depressed mood. The female athlete triad is characterized by the presence of three coexisting disorders: low energy availability (for example, because of inadequate intake), menstrual dysfunction such as amenorrhea, and low bone density.

review questions

LO 1 Define what is meant by a healthful weight

1. A healthful body weight is
   a. a weight that is compatible with normal blood pressure, lipid levels, and glucose tolerance.
   b. a weight that you can achieve and sustain as long as you're constantly dieting.
   c. a weight characterized by pear-shaped fat patterning.
   d. all of the above.

LO 2 Determine your BMI and fat distribution pattern and identify any health risks associated with these assessments

2. The ratio of a person's body weight to height is represented as his or her
   a. body composition.
   b. basal metabolic rate.
   c. bioelectrical impedance.
   d. body mass index.

LO 3 State the energy balance equation and estimate your basal metabolic rate

3. Energy balance occurs when
   a. energy expended via the basal metabolic rate, thermal effect of food, and effect of physical activity equals energy intake.
   b. energy expended via the basal metabolic rate, temperature regulation, and exercise is greater than energy intake.
   c. energy expended via the body mass index, basal metabolic rate, and effect of physical activity equals energy intake.
   d. energy expended via the body mass index, thermal effect of food, and effect of physical activity is greater than energy intake.

LO 4 Explain how to calculate how many Calories you need to consume on average each day

4. To calculate how many Calories you need each day,
   a. multiply your BMI by 1.2.
   b. multiply your BMI by a varying amount according to how active you are.
   c. multiply your BMR by a varying amount according to how active you are.
   d. divide your weight in pounds by 2.2, then multiply by 24.

LO 5 Discuss a range of factors thought to contribute to differences in body weight

5. The set-point theory proposes that
   a. obese people have a gene not found in slender people that regulates their weight, so that it always hovers near a given set point.
   b. obese people have a gene that causes them to be energetically thrifty.
   c. all people have a genetic set point for their body weight.
   d. all people of a given height, build, and gender should be able to maintain about the same body weight.

LO 6 Identify three key strategies for healthful weight loss

6. Three key strategies for healthful weight loss are
   a. dramatic reduction in energy intake; vigorous aerobic exercise daily; and behavior modification.
   b. gradual reduction in energy intake; regular and appropriate physical activity; and behavior modification.
   c. consumption of fewer than 1,200 Calories a day; 60 minutes of exercise daily; and psychological counseling.
   d. gradual reduction in energy intake; 30–60 minutes of aerobic exercise daily; and participation in a support group.

LO 7 Discuss health risks associated with obesity

7. Obesity increases the risk for
   a. heart disease.
   b. type 2 diabetes.
   c. premature death.
   d. all of the above.

LO 8 Discuss three treatment options for obesity

8. Which of the following statements about obesity treatment is true?
   a. A low-Calorie diet and exercise are the first line of defense.
   b. Most prescription weight loss medications work by speeding up peristalsis and thereby reducing nutrient absorption.
   c. Weight-loss surgery is recommended only for people who are overweight or moderately obese, because it is too dangerous for the morbidly obese.
   d. Liposuction is a recommended and effective obesity treatment.

LO **9** **Identify several factors thought to contribute to the development of eating disorders**

9. Factors thought to contribute to eating disorders include
   a. genetic inheritance.
   b. history of sexual abuse.
   c. presence of another psychiatric disorder.
   d. all of the above.

LO **10** **Compare and contrast anorexia nervosa, bulimia nervosa, binge-eating disorder, night-eating syndrome, and the female athlete triad**

10. The eating disorder most likely to result in significant weight gain is
    a. anorexia nervosa.
    b. bulimia nervosa.
    c. binge-eating disorder.
    d. the female athlete triad.

Answers to Review Questions are located at the back of this text.

web links

The following websites and apps explore further topics and issues related to personal health.
Visit **MasteringNutrition** for links to the websites and RSS feeds.

www.anad.org
National Association of Anorexia Nervosa and Associated Disorders

www.eatright.org
Academy of Nutrition and Dietetics

www.ftc.gov
Federal Trade Commission

www.nationaleatingdisorders.org
National Eating Disorders Association

www.niddk.nih.gov
National Institute of Diabetes and Digestive and Kidney Diseases

www.nih.gov
National Institutes of Health

www.nimh.nih.gov
National Institute of Mental Health (NIMH)

www.oa.org
Overeaters Anonymous

www.obesity.org
The Obesity Society

www.sneb.org
Society for Nutrition Education and Behavior

Nutrition and Physical Activity
Keys to Good Health

10

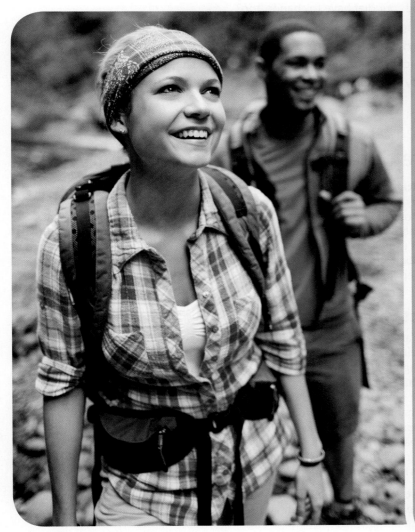

learning outcomes

After studying this chapter, you should be able to:

1 Compare and contrast the concepts of physical activity, leisure-time physical activity, exercise, and physical fitness, pp. 294–296.

2 Identify the four components of physical fitness, pp. 294–296.

3 List at least four health benefits of being physically active on a regular basis, pp. 294–296.

4 Explain how to identify and achieve your personal fitness goals, pp. 296–303.

5 Describe the FITT principle and calculate your maximal and training heart rate range, pp. 296–303.

6 List and describe at least three processes by which the body breaks down fuels to support physical activity, pp. 303–307.

7 Discuss at least three changes in nutrient needs that can occur in response to an increase in physical activity or vigorous exercise training, pp. 307–316.

8 Describe the concept of carbohydrate loading, and discuss situations in which this practice may be beneficial to athletic performance, pp. 307–316.

9 Discuss several deceptive tactics companies use to market ergogenic aids, pp. 317–321.

10 Identify the claims for, research evidence on, and potential health risks of at least three ergogenic aids, pp. 317–321.

test yourself

Are these statements true or false? Circle your guess.

1. **T F** Only about half of all Americans perform adequate levels of physical activity.

2. **T F** Eating extra protein helps us build muscle.

3. **T F** During exercise, our desire to drink is enough to prompt us to consume enough water or fluids.

Test Yourself answers can be found at the end of the chapter.

MasteringNutrition™

Go online for chapter quizzes, pre-tests, Interactive Activities, and more!

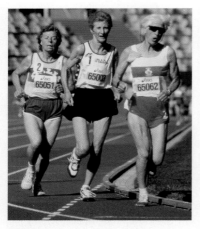

⬆ With the help of a nutritious diet, many people are able to remain physically active—and even competitive—throughout adult life.

In the summer of 2013, Lillian Web of Florida and Harold Bach of North Dakota each won a gold medal for the 100-meter dash in track and field at the National Senior Games. Web did it in just over 38 seconds, and Bach's time was less than 22 seconds. If these performance times don't amaze you, perhaps they will when you consider these athletes' ages: Web was 99 years old, and Bach was 93!

There's no doubt about it: regular physical activity dramatically improves our strength, stamina, health, and longevity. But what qualifies as "regular physical activity"? In other words, how much do we need to do to reap the benefits? And if we do become more active, does our diet have to change, too?

A nourishing diet and regular physical activity are like teammates, interacting in a variety of ways to improve our strength and stamina and increase our resistance to many chronic diseases and acute illnesses. In this chapter, we define physical activity, identify its many benefits, and discuss the nutrients needed to maintain an active life.

LO1 Compare and contrast the concepts of physical activity, leisure-time physical activity, exercise, and physical fitness.

LO2 Identify the four components of physical fitness.

LO3 List at least four health benefits of being physically active on a regular basis.

What are the benefits of physical activity?

The term **physical activity** describes any movement produced by muscles that increases energy expenditure. Different categories of physical activity include occupational, household, leisure-time, and transportation.[1] **Leisure-time physical activity** is any activity not related to a person's occupation that includes competitive sports, planned exercise training, and recreational activities, such as hiking, walking, and bicycling. **Exercise** is therefore considered a subcategory of leisure-time physical activity and refers to activity that is purposeful, planned, and structured.[2]

Physical Activity Increases Our Fitness

A lot of people are looking for a "magic pill" that will help them maintain weight loss, reduce their risk for diseases, make them feel better, and improve their quality of sleep. Although many people are not aware of it, regular physical activity is this "magic pill." That's because it promotes **physical fitness**: the ability to carry out daily tasks with vigor and alertness, without undue fatigue, and with ample energy to enjoy leisure-time pursuits and meet unforeseen emergencies.[1]

The four components of physical fitness are cardiorespiratory fitness, which is the ability of the heart, lungs, and blood vessels to supply working muscles; musculoskeletal fitness, which is fitness of the muscles and bones; flexibility; and body composition (**TABLE 10.1**).[3] These are achieved through three types of exercise:

■ **Aerobic exercise** involves the repetitive movement of large muscle groups, which increases the body's use of oxygen and promotes cardiovascular health. In your

physical activity Any movement produced by muscles that increases energy expenditure; includes occupational, household, leisure-time, and transportation activities.

leisure-time physical activity Any activity not related to a person's occupation; includes competitive sports, recreational activities, and planned exercise training.

exercise A subcategory of leisure-time physical activity; any activity that is purposeful, planned, and structured.

physical fitness The ability to carry out daily tasks with vigor and alertness, without undue fatigue, and with ample energy to enjoy leisure-time pursuits and meet unforeseen emergencies.

aerobic exercise Exercise that involves the repetitive movement of large muscle groups, increasing the body's use of oxygen and promoting cardiovascular health.

TABLE 10.1 The Components of Fitness

Fitness Component	Examples of Activities One Can Do to Achieve Fitness in Each Component
Cardiorespiratory	Aerobic-type activities, such as walking, running, swimming, cross-country skiing
Musculoskeletal fitness:	Resistance training, weight lifting, calisthenics, sit-ups, push-ups
Muscular strength	Weight lifting or related activities using heavier weights with few repetitions
Muscular endurance	Weight lifting or related activities using lighter weights with more repetitions
Flexibility	Stretching exercises, yoga
Body composition	Aerobic exercise, resistance training

daily life, you get aerobic exercise when you walk to school, work, or a bus stop or take the stairs to a third-floor classroom.

- **Resistance training** is a form of exercise in which our muscles work against resistance, such as against handheld weights. Carrying grocery bags or books and moving heavy objects are everyday activities that make our muscles work against resistance.
- **Stretching** exercises are those that increase flexibility, because they involve lengthening muscles using slow, controlled movements. You can perform stretching exercises even while you're sitting in a classroom by flexing, extending, and rotating your neck and limbs.

Physical Activity Reduces Our Risk for Chronic Disease

In addition to contributing to our fitness, physical activity can reduce our risk for certain diseases. Specifically, the health benefits of physical activity include (FIGURE 10.1):

- *Reduces our risks for, and complications of, heart disease, stroke, and high blood pressure:* Regular physical activity increases high-density lipoprotein (HDL) cholesterol (the "good" cholesterol) and lowers triglycerides in the blood, improves the strength of the heart, helps maintain healthy blood pressure, and limits the progression of atherosclerosis ("hardening of the arteries").
- *Reduces our risk for obesity:* Regular physical activity maintains lean body mass and promotes more healthful levels of body fat, may help in appetite control, and increases energy expenditure and the use of fat as an energy source.
- *Reduces our risk for type 2 diabetes:* Regular physical activity enhances the action of insulin, which improves the cells' uptake of glucose from the blood. In addition, it can improve blood glucose control in people with diabetes, which in turn reduces the risk for, or delays the onset of, diabetes-related complications.

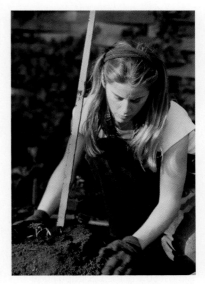

Moderate physical activity, such as gardening, helps maintain overall health.

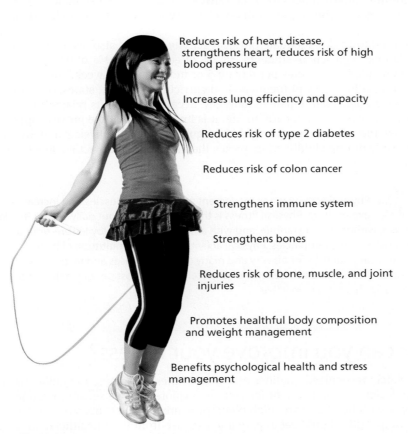

Reduces risk of heart disease, strengthens heart, reduces risk of high blood pressure

Increases lung efficiency and capacity

Reduces risk of type 2 diabetes

Reduces risk of colon cancer

Strengthens immune system

Strengthens bones

Reduces risk of bone, muscle, and joint injuries

Promotes healthful body composition and weight management

Benefits psychological health and stress management

FIGURE 10.1 Health benefits of regular physical activity.

resistance training Exercise in which our muscles act against resistance.

stretching Exercise in which muscles are gently lengthened using slow, controlled movements.

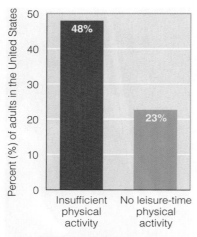

← FIGURE 10.2 Rates of physical inactivity in the United States. Almost 50% of the U.S. population does not do enough physical activity to meet national health recommendations, and 23% report doing no leisure-time physical activity.

Data from Centers for Disease Control and Prevention. 2014. Facts About Physical Activity. Available at http://www.cdc.gov/physicalactivity/data/facts.html; and Centers for Disease Control and Prevention, Office of Surveillance, Epidemiology. and Laboratory Services. Behavioral Risk Factor Surveillance System. 2012. Prevalence and Trend Data. Exercise – 2012. Available at http://apps.nccd.cdc.gov/brfss/list.asp?cat=EX&yr=2012&qkey=8041&state=All

Sitting too long, studying for tomorrow's exam? Stretching can help! Learn some simple stretches by watching the how-to video collection at www.mayoclinic.org and typing in "desk stretches."

■ *May reduce our risk for colon cancer:* Although the exact role that physical activity may play in reducing the risk of colon cancer is still unknown, we do know that regular physical activity enhances gastric motility, which reduces the transit time of potentially cancer-causing agents through the gut.

■ *Reduces our risk for osteoporosis:* Regular physical activity, especially weight-bearing exercise, increases bone density and enhances muscular strength and flexibility, thereby reducing the likelihood of falls and the incidence of fractures and other injuries when falls occur.

Regular physical activity is also known to improve our sleep patterns, reduce our risk for upper respiratory infections by improving immune function, and reduce anxiety and mental stress. It can also be effective in treating mild and moderate depression.

Many Americans Are Inactive

For most of our history, humans were very physically active. This was not by choice but because their survival depended on it. They expended a considerable amount of energy each day foraging and hunting for food, planting and harvesting food, preparing food once it was acquired, and securing shelter. In addition, their diet was composed primarily of small amounts of lean meats and naturally grown vegetables and fruits. This lifestyle pattern contrasts considerably with today's, which is characterized by sedentary jobs, easy access to an overabundance of energy-dense foods, and few opportunities for, or little interest in, expending energy through occupational or recreational activities.

Given these changes, it isn't surprising that most people find the "magic pill" of regular physical activity difficult to swallow. The Centers for Disease Control and Prevention report that almost 50% of people in the United States do not do enough physical activity to meet national health recommendations, and 23% admit to doing no leisure-time physical activity at all **(FIGURE 10.2)**.[4,5] These statistics are reflected in the high rates of obesity, heart disease, and type 2 diabetes in industrialized countries.

This trend toward inadequate physical activity levels is also occurring in young people. Among high school students, 38.5% of girls and 59.9% of boys are meeting the recommended 60 minutes per day on 5 or more days per week.[6] Although physical education (PE) is part of the mandated curriculum in most states, only 31.5% of high school students participate in daily PE. Because our habits related to eating and physical activity are formed early in life, it is imperative that we provide opportunities for children and adolescents to engage in regular, enjoyable physical activity. An active lifestyle during childhood increases the likelihood of an active, healthier life as an adult.

recap Physical activity is any movement produced by muscles that increases energy expenditure. Physical fitness is the ability to carry out daily tasks with vigor and alertness, without undue fatigue, and with ample energy to enjoy leisure-time pursuits and meet unforeseen emergencies. Physical activity provides a multitude of health benefits, including reducing our risks for obesity and many chronic diseases and relieving anxiety and stress. Despite the many health benefits of physical activity, most people in the United States, including many children, are inactive.

LO4 Explain how to identify and achieve your personal fitness goals.

LO5 Describe the FITT principle and calculate your maximal and training heart rate range.

How can you improve your fitness?

Several widely recognized qualities of a sound fitness program, and guidelines to help you design one that is right for you, are explored in this section. Keep in mind that people with heart disease, high blood pressure, diabetes, obesity, osteoporosis, asthma, or arthritis should get approval to exercise from their healthcare practitioner prior to starting a fitness program. In addition, a medical evaluation should be

WHAT ABOUT **YOU?**

Taking the President's Challenge Adult Fitness Test

The President's Challenge Adult Fitness test is designed for adults 18 years of age and older who are in good general health. The tests assess aerobic fitness, muscle strength and endurance, flexibility, and body composition. Detailed instructions for completing each test can be found at http://www.adultfitnesstest.org/. Below is a form for recording your test results. It is suggested that you do these tests with a partner to assist you with keeping track of your time and scores on each test.

Before getting started, make sure you're healthy enough to take the test. Go to http://www.adultfitnesstest.org and search under "risk questionnaire," to complete the American Heart Association Physical Activity Readiness Questionnaire.

1. **Aerobic Fitness** – you must enter either a 1-mile walk time and heart rate or enter a 1.5-mile run time

   Mile walk time: _____ minutes _____ seconds

   Heart rate (after walk): _____ beats per minute

Weight: _____ lb (required for result calculation)

OR

1.5-mile run time: _____ minutes _____ seconds

2. **Muscular Strength and Endurance**

   Half sit-ups: _____ (in 1 minute)

   Push-ups: _____

3. **Flexibility**

   Sit and Reach _____ inches

4. **Body Composition**

   Body mass index: Height _____ feet _____ inches

   Weight _____ lb

   Waist measurement _____ inches

Once you complete the form, enter your data online to get your fitness score at http://www.adultfitnesstest.org and search under "data entry."

conducted before starting an exercise program for an apparently healthy but currently inactive man 40 years or older or woman 50 years or older.

Assess Your Current Level of Fitness

Before beginning any fitness program, it is important to know your initial level of fitness. This information can then be used to help you design a fitness program that meets your goals and is appropriate for you. How can you go about estimating your current fitness level? The President's Council on Fitness, Sports and Nutrition can help! Check out the **What About You?** box to take The President's Challenge Adult Fitness Test.

Identify Your Personal Fitness Goals

A fitness program that is ideal for you is not necessarily right for everyone. Before designing or evaluating any program, it is important to define your personal fitness goals. Do you want to prevent osteoporosis, diabetes, or another chronic disease that runs in your family? Do you simply want to increase your energy and stamina? Or do you intend to compete in athletic events? Each of these scenarios requires a unique fitness program. This concept is referred to as the *specificity principle*: specific actions yield specific results.

Training is generally defined as activity leading to skilled behavior. Training is very specific to any activity or goal. For example, if you wanted to train for athletic competition, a traditional approach that includes planned, purposive exercise sessions under the guidance of a trainer or coach would be beneficial. If you wanted to achieve cardiorespiratory fitness, you would likely be advised to participate in an aerobics class at least three times a week or jog for at least 20 minutes three times a week.

In contrast, if your goal is to transition from doing no regular physical activity to doing enough physical activity to maintain your overall health, you could follow the minimum recommendations put forth in the 2008 Physical Activity Guidelines for Americans.[7] To gain significant health benefits, including reducing the risk for chronic diseases, you can participate in at least 30 minutes per day of moderate intensity aerobic physical activity (such as gardening, brisk walking, or basketball). The activity need not be completed in one session. You can divide the amount of physical activity into two or more shorter sessions throughout the day as long as the total cumulative time is achieved (for example, brisk walking for 10 minutes three times per day). Although these minimum guidelines are appropriate for achieving health benefits, performing physical activities at a higher intensity and for longer duration will confer even greater health benefits and more significant improvements in physical fitness.

Make Your Program Consistent, Varied, and Fun!

A number of factors motivate us to be active. Some are *intrinsic* factors, which are those done for the satisfaction a person gains from engaging in the activity. Examples include the desire to gain competence, the desire to be challenged by the activity and enhance our skills, and enjoyment. In contrast, *extrinsic* motivators are rewards or outcomes separate from the behavior itself.[8] Some of the most common extrinsic factors are desires to improve appearance and to increase fitness. Recently, some employers have been offering financial incentives to log in time at the company's fitness center. This would be another example of an extrinsic factor.

If we're going to reap the benefits of physical activity, we need to do it consistently. People who are regularly active tend to be more motivated by intrinsic factors, including enjoyment, whereas extrinsic factors appear to be more important to people who are not regularly active or are trying to engage in activity for the first time.[9]

Thus an important motivator in maintaining regular physical activity is enjoyment—or fun! What activities do you consider fun? If you enjoy the outdoors, hiking, camping, fishing, and rock climbing are potential activities for you. If you would rather exercise with friends between classes, walking, climbing stairs, jogging, roller-blading, or bicycle riding may be more appropriate. Or you may prefer to use the programs and equipment at your campus or community fitness center or purchase your own treadmill and free weights.

Variety is also important to maintaining your fitness and your interest in being regularly active. Although some people enjoy doing similar activities day after day, many get bored with the same fitness routine. Incorporating a variety of activities into your fitness program will help maintain your interest and increase your enjoyment while promoting different types of fitness identified in Table 10.1. Variety can be achieved by:

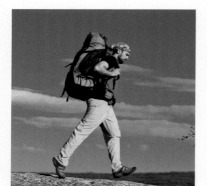

◆ Hiking is a leisure-time activity that can contribute to your physical fitness. An important component for any activity is how much you enjoy doing it.

- combining aerobic exercise, resistance training, and stretching;
- combining indoor and outdoor activities throughout the week;
- taking different routes when you walk or jog each day;
- watching a movie, reading a book, or listening to music while you ride a stationary bicycle or walk on a treadmill; and
- participating in different activities each week, such as walking, dancing, bicycling, yoga, weight lifting, swimming, hiking, and gardening.

This "smorgasbord" of activities can increase your fitness without leading to monotony and boredom.

recap A sound fitness program must meet your personal fitness goals, such as reducing your risks for disease or preparing for competition in athletic events. It should also be fun and include activities you enjoy. Variety and consistency are important to help you maintain interest and achieve physical fitness in all components.

Appropriately Overload Your Body

In order to improve your fitness, you must place an extra physical demand on your body. This is referred to as the **overload principle**. A word of caution is in order here: *the overload principle does not advocate subjecting your body to inappropriately high stress,* because this can lead to exhaustion and injuries. In contrast, an appropriate overload on various body systems will result in healthy improvements in fitness.

overload principle The principle of placing an extra physical demand on your body to improve your fitness level.

	Frequency	Intensity	Time and Type
Cardiorespiratory fitness 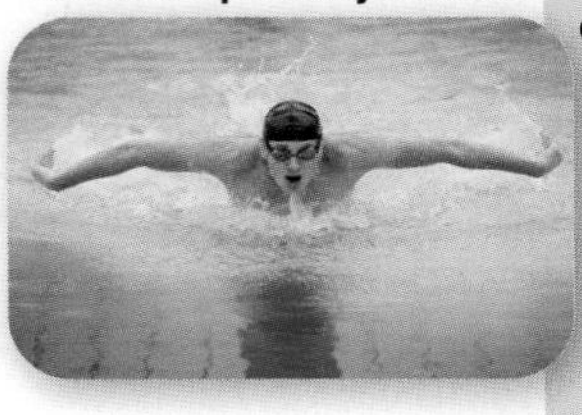	At least 30 minutes most days of the week	50–70% maximal heart rate for moderate intensity; 70–85% maximal heart rate for vigorous intensity	At least 30 consecutive minutes Choose swimming, walking, running, cycling, dancing, or other aerobic activities
Muscular fitness 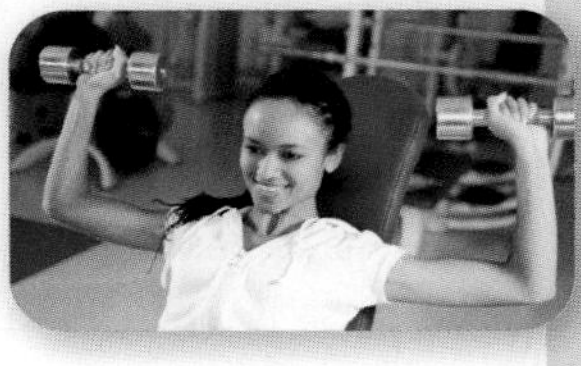	2–3 days per week	70–85% maximal weight you can lift	1–3 sets of 8–12 lifts for each set A minimum of 8–10 exercises involving the major muscle groups such as arms, shoulders, chest, abdomen, back, hips, and legs, is recommended.
Flexibility 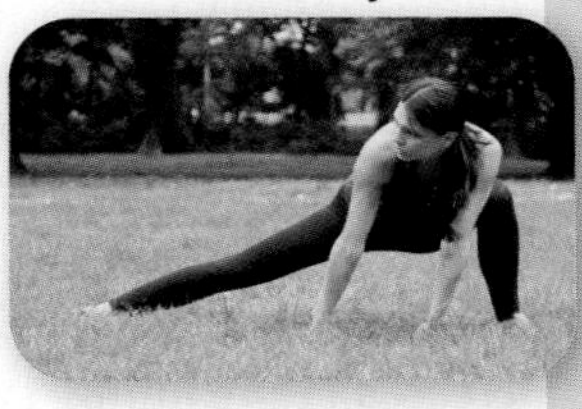	2–4 days per week	Stretching through full range of motion	For stretching, perform 2–4 repetitions per stretch. Hold each stretch for 15–30 seconds. Or try yoga, tai chi, or other flexibility programs.

FIGURE 10.3 Using the FITT principle to achieve cardiorespiratory and musculoskeletal fitness and flexibility. The recommendations in this figure follow the 2008 Physical Activity Guidelines for Americans (still in effect today).

To achieve an appropriate overload, four factors should be considered, collectively known as the FITT principle: *f*requency, *i*ntensity, *t*ime, and *t*ype of activity. You can use the FITT principle to design either a general physical fitness program or a performance-based exercise program. **FIGURE 10.3** shows how the FITT principle applies to a cardiorespiratory and muscular fitness program. Let's consider each of the FITT principle's four factors in more detail.

Frequency

Frequency refers to the number of activity sessions per week. Depending on your goals for fitness, the frequency of your activities will vary. The Physical Activity Guidelines for Americans recommend engaging in aerobic (cardiorespiratory) activities for at least 150 minutes a week. To achieve cardiorespiratory fitness, training should be at least 3 to 5 days per week. On the other hand, training more than 6 days per week does not cause significant gains in fitness but can substantially increase the risks for injury. Training 3 to 6 days per week appears optimal to achieve and maintain cardiorespiratory fitness. In contrast, only 2 to 3 days of training are needed to achieve muscular fitness.

Intensity

Intensity refers to the amount of effort expended or to how difficult the activity is to perform. We can describe the intensity of activity as low, moderate, or vigorous:

- **Low-intensity activities** are those that cause very mild increases in breathing, sweating, and heart rate. Examples include walking at a leisurely pace, fishing, and light housecleaning.

frequency The number of activity sessions per week you perform.

intensity The amount of effort expended during the activity, or how difficult the activity is to perform.

low-intensity activities Activities that cause very mild increases in breathing, sweating, and heart rate.

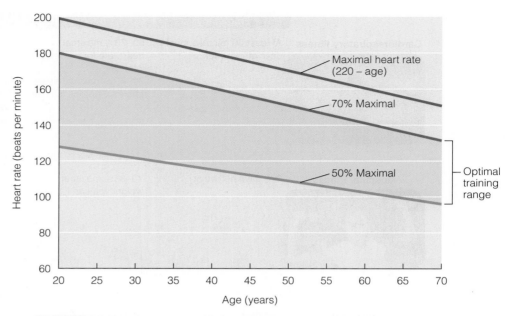

⬆ FIGURE 10.4 This heart rate training chart can be used to estimate aerobic exercise intensity. The top line indicates the predicted maximal heart rate value for a person's age (220 – age). The shaded area represents the heart rate values that fall between 50% and 70% of maximal heart rate, which is the range generally recommended to achieve aerobic fitness.

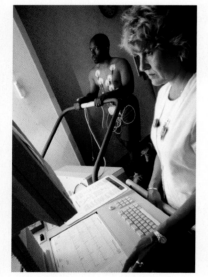

⬆ Testing in a fitness lab is the most accurate way to determine maximal heart rate.

moderate-intensity activities Activities that cause noticeable increases in breathing, sweating, and heart rate.

vigorous-intensity activities Activities that produce significant increases in breathing, sweating, and heart rate; talking is difficult when exercising at a vigorous intensity.

maximal heart rate The rate at which your heart beats during maximal-intensity exercise.

- **Moderate-intensity activities** cause moderate increases in breathing, sweating, and heart rate. For instance, you can carry on a conversation, but not continuously. Examples include brisk walking, water aerobics, doubles tennis, ballroom dancing, and bicycling slower than 10 miles per hour.
- **Vigorous-intensity activities** produce significant increases in breathing, sweating, and heart rate, so that talking is difficult when exercising. Examples include jogging, running, racewalking, singles tennis, aerobics, bicycling 10 miles per hour or faster, jumping rope, and hiking uphill with a heavy backpack.

Traditionally, heart rate has been used to indicate level of intensity during aerobic activities. You can calculate the range of exercise intensity that is appropriate for you by estimating your **maximal heart rate**, which is the rate at which your heart beats during maximal-intensity exercise. Maximal heart rate is estimated by subtracting your age from 220.

FIGURE 10.4 shows an example of a heart rate training chart, which you can use to estimate the intensity of your own workout. The Centers for Disease Control and Prevention makes the following recommendations:[10]

- To achieve moderate-intensity physical activity, your target heart rate should be 50–70% of your estimated maximal heart rate. Older adults and anyone who has been inactive for a long time may want to exercise at the lower end of the moderate-intensity range.
- To achieve vigorous-intensity physical activity, your target heart rate should be 70–85% of your estimated heart rate. Those who are physically fit or are striving for a more rapid improvement in fitness may want to exercise at the higher end of the vigorous-intensity range.
- Competitive athletes generally train at a higher intensity, around 80–95% of their maximal heart rate.

Although the calculation of *220 minus age* has been used extensively for years to predict maximal heart rate, it was never intended to accurately represent everyone's true maximal heart rate or to be used as the standard of aerobic training intensity. The most accurate way to determine your own maximal heart rate is to complete a

WHAT ABOUT **YOU?**

What's Your Maximal Heart Rate and Training Range?

You can estimate your maximal heart rate by using the following easy calculation:

your maximal heart rate = 220 minus your age

Let's say you are 20 years old:

your maximal heart rate = 220 – 20
= 200 beats per minute (bpm)

Now let's calculate your training range. As we said in the text, for non-athletes this number is 50% to 70% of your maximal heart rate. If you want to work out at the lower end of your range, you should multiply your maximal heart rate by 50%. If your maximal heart rate is 200, your equation is

lower end of your training range
= 200 bpm × 0.50 = 100 bpm

If you want to work out at the higher end of your range, you should multiply your maximal heart rate by 70%:

higher end of your training range
= 200 bpm × 0.70 = 140 bpm

Thus, your training range is between 100 and 140 bpm.

maximal exercise test in a fitness laboratory; however, this test is not commonly conducted with the general public and can be very expensive. Although not completely accurate, the estimated maximal heart rate method can still be used to give you a general idea of your aerobic training range.

So what is your maximal heart rate and training range? To find out, try the easy calculation in the *What About You?* feature box.

Time of Activity

Time of activity refers to how long each session lasts. To achieve general health, you can do multiple short bouts of activity that add up to 30 minutes each day. However, to achieve higher levels of fitness, it is important that the activities be done for at least 20 to 30 consecutive minutes.

For example, let's say you want to compete in triathlons. To be successful during the running segment of the triathlon, you will need to be able to run at least 5 miles. Thus, it is appropriate for you to train so that you can complete 5 miles during one session and still have enough energy to swim and bicycle during the race. You will need to consistently train at a distance of 5 miles; you will also benefit from running longer distances.

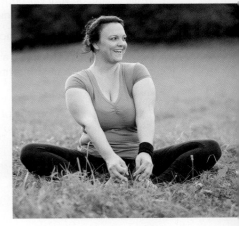

Stretching should be included in the warm-up before, and the cool-down after, exercise.

Type of Activity

Type of activity refers to the range of physical activities a person can engage in to promote health and physical fitness. Many examples are illustrated in Table 10.1 and Figure 10.3. The types of activity you choose to engage in will depend on your goals for health and physical fitness, your personal preferences, and the range of activities available to you.

Include a Warm-Up and a Cool-Down Period

To properly prepare for and recover from an exercise session, warm-up and cool-down activities should be performed. **Warm-up**, also called preliminary exercise, includes general activities, such as gentle aerobics, calisthenics, and then stretching followed by specific activities that prepare you for the actual activity, such as jogging or swinging a golf club. Your warm-up should be brief (5 to 10 minutes), gradual, and sufficient to increase muscle and body temperature but should not cause fatigue or deplete energy stores.

Warming up prior to exercise is important, because it properly prepares your muscles for exertion by increasing blood flow and body temperature. It enhances the body's flexibility and may also help prepare you psychologically for the exercise session or athletic event.

time of activity The amount of time that a given exercise session lasts, not including warm-up and cool-down periods.

type of activity The range of physical activities a person can engage in to promote health and physical fitness.

warm-up Activities that prepare you for an exercise session, including stretching, calisthenics, and movements specific to the exercise you are about to engage in; also called preliminary exercise.

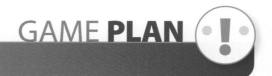

GAME **PLAN**

Tips for Increasing Your Physical Activity

There are 1,440 minutes in every day. Spend just 30 of those minutes in physical activity, and you'll be taking an important step toward improving your health. Here are some tips for working activity into your daily life:

☐ Walk as often and as far as possible: park your car farther away from your dorm, a lecture hall, or shops; walk to school or work; go for a brisk walk between classes; get on or off the bus one stop away from your destination. And don't be in such a rush to reach your destination—take the long way and burn a few more Calories.

☐ Take the stairs instead of the elevator.

☐ Exercise while watching television—for example by doing sit-ups, stretching, or using a treadmill or stationary bike.

☐ While talking on your cell phone, memorizing vocabulary terms, or practicing your choral part, don't stand still—pace!

☐ Turn on some music and dance!

☐ Get an exercise partner: join a friend for walks, hikes, cycling, skating, tennis, or a fitness class.

☐ Take up a group sport.

☐ Register for a class from the physical education department in an activity you've never tried before, maybe yoga or fencing.

☐ Register for a dance class, such as jazz, tap, or ballroom.

☐ Use the pool, rock-climbing wall, or other facilities at your campus fitness center, or join a health club, gym, or YMCA/YWCA in your community.

☐ Join an activity-based club, such as a skating, tennis, or hiking club.

☐ Play golf without using a golf cart—choose to walk and carry your clubs instead.

☐ Choose a physically active vacation that provides daily activities combined with exploring new surroundings.

If you have been inactive for a while, use a sensible approach by starting out slowly. Gradually build up the time you spend doing the activity by adding a few minutes every few days until you reach 30 minutes a day. As this 30-minute minimum becomes easier, gradually increase the length of time you spend in activity, the intensity of the activities you choose, or both.

Cool-down activities are done after the exercise session. The cool-down should be gradual and allow your body to slowly recover. Your cool-down should include some of the same activities you performed during the exercise session, but at a low intensity, and you should allow ample time for stretching. Cooling down after exercise assists in the prevention of injury and may help reduce muscle soreness.

Map your walking, running, or cycling route and share it with friends—or check out dozens of fitness loops right in your neighborhood by going to www.livestrong.com and clicking "Loops" under the Fitness tab.

Keep It Simple, Take It Slow

There are 1,440 minutes in every day. Spend just 30 of those minutes in physical activity, and you'll be taking an important step toward improving your health. See the *Game Plan* feature box for working daily activity into your life.

If you have been inactive for a while, use a sensible approach by starting out slowly. The first month is an initiation phase, which is the time to start to incorporate relatively brief bouts of physical activity into your daily life and reduce the time you spend in sedentary activities. Gradually build up the time you spend doing the activity by adding a few minutes every few days until you reach 30 minutes a day.

The next 4 to 6 months is the improvement phase, in which you can increase the intensity and duration of the activities you engage in. As you become more fit, the 30-minute minimum becomes easier, and you'll need to gradually increase either the length of time you spend in activity, the intensity of the activities you choose, or both to continue to progress toward your fitness goals. Once you've reached your goals and a plateau in your fitness gains, you've entered into the maintenance phase. At this point you can either maintain your current activity levels, or you may choose to reevaluate your goals and alter your training accordingly.

cool-down Activities done after an exercise session is completed; they should be gradual and allow your body to slowly recover from exercise.

To improve fitness, you must place an appropriate overload on your body. Follow the FITT principle: *FITT* stands for frequency, intensity, time, and type of activity. Frequency is the number of activity sessions per week. Intensity is how difficult the activity is to perform. Time of activity is how long each activity session lasts. Type refers to the range of physical activities one can engage in. Warm-up exercises prepare the muscles for exertion by increasing blood flow and temperature. Low-intensity cool-down activities help prevent injury and may help reduce muscle soreness.

What fuels our activities?

To perform exercise, or muscular work, we must be able to generate energy. The common currency of energy for virtually all cells in the body is **adenosine triphosphate (ATP)**. As you might guess from its name, a molecule of ATP includes an organic compound called adenosine and three phosphate groups (**FIGURE 10.5**). When one of the phosphates is cleaved, or broken away, from ATP, energy is released. The products remaining after this reaction are adenosine diphosphate (ADP) and an independent inorganic phosphate group (P_i). In a mirror image of this reaction, the body regenerates ATP by adding a phosphate group back to ADP. In this way, we continually provide energy to our cells.

The amount of ATP stored in a muscle cell is very limited; it can keep the muscle active for only about 1 to 3 seconds. When more energy is needed, a high-energy compound called **creatine phosphate (CP)** can be broken down to support the regeneration of ATP. Because this reaction can occur in the absence of oxygen, it is referred to as **anaerobic** (meaning "without oxygen").

Muscle tissue contains about four to six times as much CP as ATP, but that is still not enough to fuel long-term activities. CP is used the most during very intense, short bouts of activity, such as lifting, jumping, and sprinting. Together, our stores of ATP and CP can support a *maximal* physical effort for only about 3 to 15 seconds. As a result, we rely on other energy sources, such as carbohydrate and fat, to support activities of longer duration (**FIGURE 10.6**).

The Breakdown of Carbohydrates Provides Energy for Exercise

During activities lasting about 30 seconds to 3 minutes, our body needs an energy source that can be used quickly to produce ATP. The breakdown of carbohydrates, specifically glucose, provides this quick energy in a process called **glycolysis**. The

LO6 List and describe at least three processes by which the body breaks down fuels to support physical activity.

adenosine triphosphate (ATP) The common currency of energy for virtually all cells of the body.

creatine phosphate (CP) A high-energy compound that can be broken down for energy and used to regenerate ATP.

anaerobic Means "without oxygen"; refers to metabolic reactions that occur in the absence of oxygen.

glycolysis The breakdown of glucose; yields two ATP molecules and two pyruvic acid molecules for each molecule of glucose.

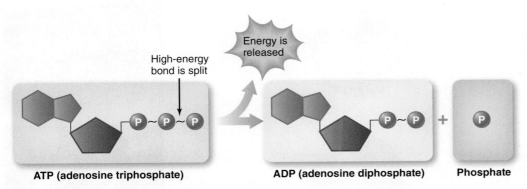

FIGURE 10.5 Structure of adenosine triphosphate (ATP). Energy is produced when ATP is split into adenosine diphosphate (ADP) and inorganic phosphate (P_i).

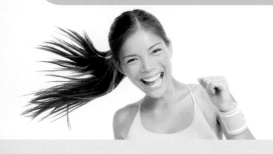

focus figure 10.6 | What Fuels Our Activities?

Depending on the duration and intensity of the activity, our bodies may use ATP-CP, carbohydrate, or fat in various combinations to fuel muscular work. Keep in mind that the amounts and sources shown below can vary based on the person's fitness level and health, how well fed the person is before the activity, and environmental temperatures and conditions.

SPRINT START (0–3 seconds)
A short, intense burst of activity like sprinting is fueled by ATP and creatine phosphate (CP) under anaerobic conditions.

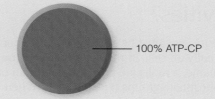
100% ATP-CP

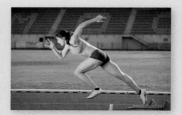

100-M DASH (10–12 seconds)
ATP and CP provide energy for about 10 seconds of quick, intense activity, after which energy is provided as ATP from the breakdown of carbohydrates.

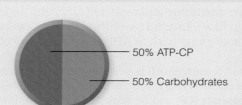
50% ATP-CP
50% Carbohydrates

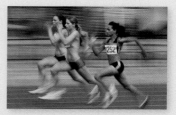

1500-M RACE (4–6 minutes)
Energy derived from ATP and CP is small and would be exhausted after about 10 seconds of the race. At this point, most of the energy is derived from aerobic metabolism of primarily carbohydrates.

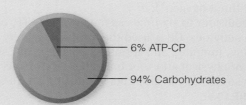
6% ATP-CP
94% Carbohydrates

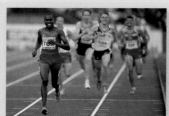

10-KM RACE (30–40 minutes)
During moderately intense activities such as a 10-kilometer race, ATP is provided by fat and carbohydrate metabolism. As the intensity increases, so does the utilization of carbohydrates for energy.

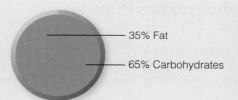
35% Fat
65% Carbohydrates

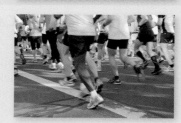

MARATHON (2.5–3 hours)
During endurance events such as marathons, ATP is primarily derived from carbohydrates, and to a lesser extent, fat. A very small amount of energy is provided by the breakdown of amino acids to form glucose.

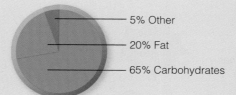
5% Other
20% Fat
65% Carbohydrates

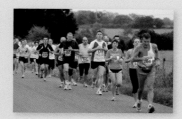

DAY-LONG HIKE (5.5–7 hours)
The primary energy source for events lasting several hours at low intensity is fat (free fatty acids in the bloodstream) which derive from triglycerides stored in fat cells. Carbohydrates contribute a relatively smaller percentage of energy needs.

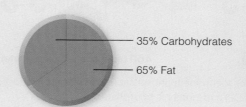
35% Carbohydrates
65% Fat

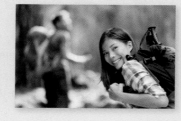

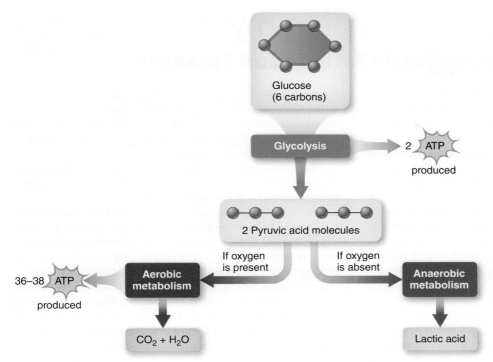

FIGURE 10.7 The breakdown of one molecule of glucose, or the process of glycolysis, yields two molecules of pyruvic acid and two ATP molecules. The further metabolism of pyruvic acid in the presence of insufficient oxygen (anaerobic process) results in the production of lactic acid. The metabolism of pyruvic acid in the presence of adequate oxygen (aerobic process) yields thirty-six to thirty-eight molecules of ATP.

most common source of glucose during exercise comes from glycogen stored in our muscles and glucose found in our blood. As shown in **FIGURE 10.7**, for every glucose molecule that goes through glycolysis, two ATP molecules are produced. The primary end product of glycolysis is **pyruvic acid**.

When oxygen availability is limited in the cell, pyruvic acid is converted to **lactic acid** (see the blue section of Figure 10.7). For years, it was assumed that lactic acid was a useless, even potentially toxic by-product of high-intensity exercise. We now know that lactic acid is an important intermediate of glucose breakdown and that it plays a critical role in supplying fuel for working muscles, the heart, and resting tissues. But does it cause muscle fatigue and soreness? See the *Nutrition Myth or Fact?* box.

The major advantage of glycolysis is that it is the fastest way that we can regenerate ATP for exercise, other than the ATP–CP system. However, this high rate of ATP production can be sustained for only a brief period of time, generally less than 3 minutes. To continue to exercise, we must rely on the aerobic energy system to provide adequate ATP.

In the presence of oxygen, pyruvic acid can go through additional metabolic pathways. Although this process is slower than glycolysis, the breakdown of one glucose molecule going through aerobic metabolism yields thirty-six to thirty-eight ATP molecules for energy (recall that glycolysis yields only two). Thus, this aerobic process supplies eighteen times more energy! Another advantage of the aerobic process is that it does not result in significant production of metabolic by-products that contribute to muscle fatigue, which means that a low-intensity activity can be performed for hours. Aerobic metabolism of glucose is the primary source of fuel for our muscles during activities lasting from 3 minutes to 4 hours (see Figure 10.6).

We can store only a limited amount of glycogen in our body. An average, well-nourished man who weighs about 154 lb (70 kg) can store about 200 to 500 grams of muscle glycogen, which is equal to 800 to 2,000 kilocalories of energy. Although

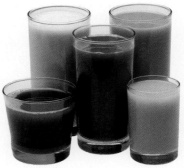

Fruit and vegetable juices can be good sources of carbohydrates.

pyruvic acid The primary end product of glycolysis.

lactic acid A compound that results when pyruvic acid is metabolized.

nutrition myth or fact?

Does Lactic Acid Cause Muscle Fatigue and Soreness?

Lactic acid is a by-product of glycolysis. For many years, both scientists and athletes believed that lactic acid caused both muscle fatigue and soreness. Does recent scientific evidence support this belief?

The exact causes of muscle fatigue are not known, and there appear to be many contributing factors. Recent evidence suggests that fatigue may be due not only to the accumulation of many acids and other metabolic by-products, such as inorganic phosphate,[1] but also to the depletion of creatine phosphate and changes in calcium in the cells that affect muscle contraction. Depletion of muscle glycogen, liver glycogen, and blood glucose, as well as psychological factors, can all contribute to fatigue.[2] Thus, it appears that lactic acid contributes to fatigue but does not cause it independently.

So what causes muscle soreness? As with fatigue, there are probably many factors. It is hypothesized that soreness usually results from microscopic tears in the muscle fibers as a result of strenuous exercise. This damage triggers an inflammatory reaction, which causes an influx of fluid and various chemicals to the damaged area. These substances work to remove damaged tissue and initiate tissue repair, but they may also stimulate pain. However, it appears highly unlikely that lactic acid is an independent cause of muscle soreness.

Recent studies indicate that lactic acid is produced even under aerobic conditions! This means it is produced at rest as well as during exercise at any intensity. The reasons for this constant production of lactic acid are still being studied. What we do know is that lactic acid is an important fuel for resting tissues, for working cardiac and skeletal muscles, and even for the brain both at rest and during exercise.[3-4] That's right—skeletal muscles not only *produce* lactic acid but also *use* it for energy, both directly and after it is converted into glucose and glycogen in the liver. We also know that endurance training improves the muscles' ability to use lactic acid for energy. Thus, contrary to being a waste product of glucose metabolism, lactic acid is actually an important energy source for muscle cells during rest and exercise.

---

trained athletes can store more muscle glycogen than the average person, even their body does not store enough glycogen to provide an unlimited energy supply for long-term activities. Thus, we also need a fuel source that is very abundant and can be broken down under aerobic conditions, so that it can support activities of lower intensity and longer duration. This fuel source is fat.

Aerobic Breakdown of Fats Supports Exercise of Low Intensity and Long Duration

The triglyceride molecule is the primary storage form of fat in our cells. Its three fatty acid molecules provide much of the energy we need to support long-term activity.

There are two major advantages of using fatty acids as a fuel. First, fat is a very abundant energy source, even in lean people. For example, a man who weighs 154 lb (70 kg) who has a body fat level of 10% has approximately 15 lb of body fat, which is equivalent to more than 50,000 kcal of energy! This is significantly more energy than can be provided by muscle glycogen (800 to 2,000 kcal). Second, fat provides 9 kcal of energy per gram, whereas carbohydrate provides only 4 kcal per gram, which means that fat supplies more than twice as much energy per gram as carbohydrate. The primary disadvantage of using fat as a fuel is that the breakdown process is relatively slow; thus, fat is used predominantly as a fuel source during activities of lower intensity and longer duration. Fat is also our primary energy source during rest, sitting, and standing in place.

What specific activities are primarily fueled by fat? Walking long distances uses fat stores, as do other low- to moderate-intensity forms of exercise. Fat is also an important fuel source during endurance events such as marathons (26.2 miles) and ultramarathons (49.9 or more miles). Endurance exercise training improves our ability to use fat for energy, which may be one reason that endurance athletes tend to have lower body fat levels than people who do not exercise.

Our body is continually using some combination of carbohydrate and fat for energy. At rest, we use very little carbohydrate, relying mostly on fat. However, this does not mean that we can reduce our body fat by resting and doing very little activity!

To lose weight and reduce body fat, a person needs to exercise regularly and reduce energy intake, so that a negative energy balance results. During maximal exercise (at 90% to 100% effort), we are using virtually all carbohydrate. However, most activities we do each day involve some use of both fuels.

When it comes to eating properly to support regular physical activity or exercise training, the nutrient to focus on is carbohydrate. This is because most people store more than enough fat to support exercise, whereas our storage of carbohydrate is limited. It is especially important that we maintain adequate stores of glycogen for moderate to intense exercise.

Amino Acids Are Not Major Sources of Fuel During Exercise

Proteins, or more specifically amino acids, are not major energy sources during exercise. Amino acids can be used directly for energy if necessary, but they are more often used to make glucose to maintain our blood glucose levels during exercise. Amino acids also help build and repair tissues after exercise. Depending on the intensity and duration of the activity, amino acids may contribute about 1% to 6% of the energy needed.[11]

Given this, why are so many people concerned about their protein intake? Our muscles are not stimulated to grow when we eat extra dietary protein. Only appropriate physical training can stimulate our muscles to grow and strengthen. Thus, although we need enough dietary protein to support activity and recovery, consuming very high amounts does not provide an added benefit. The protein needs of athletes are only slightly higher than the needs of non-athletes, and most of us eat more than enough protein to support even the highest requirements for competitive athletes! Thus, there is generally no need for recreationally active people or even competitive athletes to consume protein or amino acid supplements.

recap Adenosine triphosphate, or ATP, is the common energy source for all cells of the body. ATP and creatine phosphate stored in our muscle cells can fuel only brief spurts of activity. To support activities that last longer, energy is produced from the breakdown of glucose. Fat is broken down slowly to support activities of low intensity and long duration. Amino acids help build and repair tissues after exercise but contribute only 1% to 6% of the energy needed during exercise. We generally consume more than enough protein in our diet to support regular exercise and do not need protein or amino acid supplements.

What kind of diet supports physical activity?

Lots of people wonder, "Do my nutrient needs change if I become more physically active?" The answer to this question depends on the type, intensity, and duration of the activity in which you participate. It is not necessarily true that our requirement for every nutrient is greater if we are physically active.

People who are performing moderate-intensity daily activities for health can follow the dietary guidelines put forth in the USDA Food Patterns. For smaller or less active people, the lower end of the range of recommendations for each food group may be appropriate. For larger or more active people, the higher end of the range is suggested. Modifications may be necessary for people who exercise vigorously every day, particularly for athletes training for competition. TABLE 10.2 provides an overview of the nutrients that can be affected by regular, vigorous exercise training. Each of these nutrients is described in more detail in the following section.

LO7 Discuss at least three changes in nutrient needs that can occur in response to an increase in physical activity or vigorous exercise training.

LO8 Describe the concept of carbohydrate loading, and discuss situations in which this practice may be beneficial to athletic performance.

Vigorous Exercise Increases Energy Needs

Athletes generally have higher energy needs than moderately physically active or sedentary people. The amount of extra energy needed to support regular training is

TABLE 10.2   Suggested Intakes of Nutrients to Support Vigorous Exercise

Nutrient	Functions	Suggested Intake
Energy	Supports exercise, activities of daily living, and basic body functions	Depends on body size and the type, intensity, and duration of activity For many female athletes: 1,800 to 3,500 kcal/day For many male athletes: 2,500 to 7,500 kcal/day
Carbohydrate	Provides energy, maintains adequate muscle glycogen and blood glucose; high-complex-carbohydrate foods provide vitamins and minerals	45% to 65% of total energy intake Depending on sport and gender, should consume 6–10 grams of carbohydrate per kg of body weight per day
Fat	Provides energy, fat-soluble vitamins, and essential fatty acids; supports production of hormones and transport of nutrients	20% to 35% of total energy intake
Protein	Helps build and maintain muscle; provides building material for glucose; is an energy source during endurance exercise; aids recovery from exercise	10% to 35% of total energy intake Endurance athletes: 1.2–1.5 grams per kg body weight Strength athletes: 1.3–1.8 grams per kg body weight
Water	Maintains temperature regulation (adequate cooling); maintains blood volume and blood pressure; supports all cell functions	Consume fluid before, during, and after exercise Consume enough to maintain body weight Consume at least 8 cups (64 fl. oz) of water daily to maintain regular health and activity Athletes may need up to 10 liters (170 fl. oz) every day; more is required if exercising in a hot environment
B-vitamins	Critical for energy production from carbohydrate, fat, and protein	May need slightly more (one to two times the RDA) for thiamin, riboflavin, and vitamin B_6
Calcium	Builds and maintains bone mass; assists with nervous system function, muscle contraction, hormone function, and transport of nutrients across cell membrane	Meet the current RDA: 14–18 years: 1,300 mg/day 19–50 years: 1,000 mg/day 51–70 years: 1,000 mg/day (males); 1,200 mg/day (females) 71 and older: 1,200 mg/day
Iron	Primarily responsible for the transport of oxygen in blood to cells; assists with energy production	Consume at least the RDA: Males: 14–18 years: 11 mg/day 19 years and older: 8 mg/day Females: 14–18 years: 15 mg/day 19–50 years: 18 mg/day 51 and older: 8 mg/day

determined by the type, intensity, and duration of the activity. In addition, the energy needs of male athletes are higher than those of female athletes, because male athletes weigh more, have more muscle mass, and expend more energy during activity. This is relative, of course: a large woman who trains 3 to 5 hours each day will probably need more energy than a small man who trains 1 hour each day. The energy needs of athletes can range from only 1,500 to 1,800 kcal/day for a small female gymnast to more than 7,500 kcal/day for a male cyclist competing in the Tour de France cross-country cycling race.

FIGURE 10.8 shows an example of 1 day's meals that total about 1,800 kcal and 4,000 kcal, with the carbohydrate content of these foods meeting more than 60% of total energy intake. As you can see, athletes who need 4,000 kcal per day need to consume very large quantities of food. However, the heavy demands of daily physical training, work, school, and family responsibilities often leave these athletes with little time to eat adequately. Thus, many athletes meet their energy demands by planning regular meals and snacks and **grazing** (eating small meals throughout the day) consistently. They may also take advantage of the energy-dense snack foods and meal replacements specifically designed for athletes participating in vigorous training. These steps help athletes maintain their blood glucose levels and energy stores.

grazing The practice of consistently eating small meals throughout the day; done by many athletes to meet their high-energy demands.

a day of meals

about **1,800** calories (kcal)

about **4,000** calories (kcal)

BREAKFAST

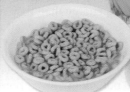
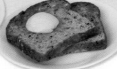
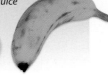

1 cup Cheerios
4 oz skim milk
1 medium banana
6 fl. oz orange juice

1-½ cups Cheerios
8 fl. oz skim milk
1 medium banana
2 slices whole-wheat toast
1 tbsp. butter
6 fl. oz orange juice

LUNCH

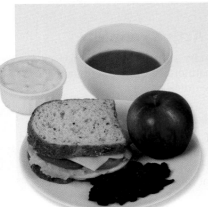
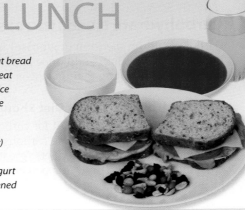

Turkey sandwich:
2 slices whole-wheat bread
3 oz turkey lunch meat
1 oz Swiss cheese slice
1 leaf iceberg lettuce
2 slices tomato
1 cup tomato soup
   (made with water)
1 large apple
8 oz nonfat fruit yogurt
¼ cup dried, sweetened
   cranberries

2 turkey sandwiches, each with:
2 slices whole-wheat bread
3 oz turkey lunch meat
1 oz Swiss cheese slice
1 leaf iceberg lettuce
2 slices tomato
2 cups tomato soup
   (made with water)
Two 8 oz containers of low-fat
   fruit yogurt
¼ cup trail mix
12 fl. oz Gatorade

DINNER

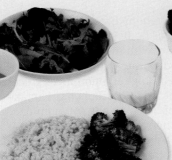
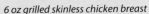
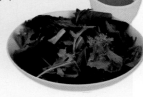
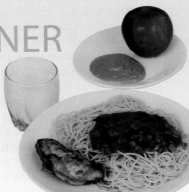

4 oz grilled skinless chicken breast
1-½ cups mixed salad greens
1 tbsp. French salad dressing
1 cup steamed broccoli
½ cup cooked brown rice
4 fl. oz skim milk
1 cup fresh blackberries

6 oz grilled skinless chicken breast
3 cups mixed salad greens
3 tbsp. French salad dressing
2 cups cooked spaghetti noodles
1 cup spaghetti sauce with meat
8 fl. oz skim milk
1 large apple
2 tbsp. peanut butter

nutrient analysis

1,797 kcal
60.8% of energy from carbohydrates
15.7% of energy from fat
4.7% of energy from saturated fat
23.5% of energy from protein
35 grams of dietary fiber
2,097 milligrams of sodium

More energy for activity!

nutrient analysis

3,984 kcal
59.4% of energy from carbohydrates
22.6% of energy from fat
7.0% of energy from saturated fat
18.0% of energy from protein
45.4 grams of dietary fiber
6019 milligrams of sodium

If an athlete is losing body weight, his or her energy intake is inadequate. Conversely, weight gain may indicate that energy intake is too high. Weight maintenance is generally recommended to maximize performance. If weight loss is warranted, food intake should be lowered no more than 200 to 500 kcal/day, and athletes should try to lose weight prior to the competitive season, if at all possible. Weight gain may be necessary for some athletes and can usually be accomplished by consuming 500 to 700 kcal/day more than needed for weight maintenance. The extra energy should come from a healthy balance of carbohydrate (45% to 60% of total energy intake), fat (20% to 35% of total energy intake), and protein (10% to 35% of total energy intake).

Many athletes are concerned about their weight. Jockeys, boxers, wrestlers, judo athletes, and others are required to "make weight"—to meet a predefined weight category. Others, such as distance runners, gymnasts, figure skaters, and dancers, are required to maintain a very lean figure for performance and aesthetic reasons. These athletes tend to eat less energy than they need to support vigorous training, which puts them at risk for inadequate intakes of all nutrients. These athletes are also at a higher risk of suffering from health consequences resulting from poor energy and nutrient intake, including eating disorders, osteoporosis, menstrual disturbances (in women), dehydration, heat and physical injuries, and even death. It is also important to understand that athletes should not adopt low-carbohydrate diets in an attempt to lose weight. As we discuss next, carbohydrates are a critical energy source for maintaining exercise performance.

Carbohydrate Needs Increase for Many Active People

Carbohydrate (in the form of glucose) is one of the primary sources of energy for a body in training. Both endurance athletes and strength athletes require adequate carbohydrate to maintain their glycogen stores and provide quick energy.

How Much of an Athlete's Diet Should Be Carbohydrates?

You may recall that the AMDR for carbohydrates is 45% to 65% of total energy intake. Athletes should consume carbohydrate intakes within this recommended range. Although high-carbohydrate diets (greater than 60% of total energy intake) have been recommended in the past, this percentage value may not be appropriate or achievable for many athletes.

When Should Carbohydrates Be Consumed?

It is important for athletes not only to consume enough carbohydrate to maintain glycogen stores but also to time their intake optimally. Our body stores glycogen very rapidly during the first 24 hours of recovery from exercise, with the highest storage rates occurring during the first few hours.[12] Higher carbohydrate intakes during the first 24 hours of recovery from exercise are associated with higher amounts of glucose being stored as muscle glycogen. It is recommended that a daily carbohydrate intake of approximately 6 to 10 grams of carbohydrate per kg of body weight will optimize muscle glycogen stores in many athletes. However, this need may be much greater in athletes who are training heavily daily, because they have less time to recover and require more carbohydrate to support both training and storage needs.

If an athlete has to perform or participate in training bouts that are scheduled less than 8 hours apart, he or she should try to consume enough carbohydrate in the few hours following training to allow for ample glycogen storage. However, with a longer recovery time (generally 12 hours or more), the athlete can eat when he or she chooses, and glycogen levels should be restored as long as the total carbohydrate eaten is sufficient.

Interestingly, studies have shown that muscle glycogen can be restored to adequate levels in the muscle whether the food is eaten in small, multiple snacks or in larger meals.[12] There is also evidence that consuming high glycemic-index foods during the immediate postrecovery period results in higher glycogen storage than is achieved as a result of eating low glycemic-index foods. This may be due to a greater malabsorption of the carbohydrate in low glycemic-index foods, because these foods contain more indigestible forms of carbohydrate.[12]

What Food Sources of Carbohydrate Support Are Good for Athletes?

What are good carbohydrate sources to support vigorous training? In general, fiber-rich, less-processed carbohydrate foods, such as whole grains and cereals, fruits, vegetables, and juices, are excellent sources that also supply fiber, vitamins, and minerals. Guidelines recommend that intake of simple sugars be less than 10% of total energy intake, but some athletes who need very large energy intakes to support training may need to consume more. In addition, as previously mentioned, glycogen storage can be enhanced by consuming foods with a high glycemic index immediately postrecovery. Thus, there are advantages to consuming a wide variety of carbohydrate sources.

As a result of time constraints, many athletes have difficulties consuming enough food to meet carbohydrate demands. Sports drinks and energy bars have been designed to help athletes increase their carbohydrate intake. TABLE 10.3 identifies some energy bars and other simple, inexpensive snacks and meals that provide 50 to 100 grams of carbohydrate.

Carbohydrate loading may benefit endurance athletes, such as cross-country skiers.

When Does Carbohydrate Loading Make Sense?

As you know, carbohydrate is a critical energy source to support exercise—particularly endurance-type activities—yet we have a limited capacity to store them. So it's not surprising that discovering ways to maximize our storage of carbohydrates has been at the forefront of sports nutrition research for many years. The practice of **carbohydrate loading**, also called *glycogen loading,* involves altering both exercise duration and carbohydrate intake to maximize the amount of muscle glycogen. TABLE 10.4 provides a schedule for carbohydrate loading for an endurance athlete.

Athletes who may benefit from carbohydrate loading are those competing in marathons, ultramarathons, long-distance swimming, cross-country skiing, and triathlons.

carbohydrate loading The practice of altering training and carbohydrate intake so that muscle glycogen storage is maximized; also known as *glycogen loading.*

TABLE 10.3   Carbohydrate and Total Energy in Various Foods

Food	Amount	Carbohydrate (grams)	Energy from Carbohydrate (%)	Total Energy (kcal)
Sweetened applesauce	1 cup	50	97	207
Large apple	1 each	50	82	248
with saltine crackers	8 each			
Whole-wheat bread	1-oz. slice	50	71	282
with jelly	4 tsp			
and skim milk	12 fl. oz			
Spaghetti (cooked)	1 cup	50	75	268
with tomato sauce	¼ cup			
Brown rice (cooked)	1 cup	100	88	450
with mixed vegetables	½ cup			
and apple juice	12 fl. oz			
Grape Nuts cereal	½ cup	100	84	473
with raisins	⅜ cup			
and skim milk	8 fl. oz			
Clif Bar (chocolate chip)	2.4 oz	43	72	230
Meta-Rx (fudge brownie)	100 g	41	41	400
Power Bar (chocolate)	1 bar	45	75	240
PR Bar Ironman	50 g	22	44	200

Source: Data adapted from: Manore, M. M., N. Meyer, and J. L. Thompson. 2009. *Sport Nutrition for Health and Performance,* 2nd edn. Champaign, IL: Human Kinetics.

TABLE 10.4 Recommended Carbohydrate Loading Guidelines for Endurance Athletes

Days Prior to Event	Exercise Duration (in minutes)	Carbohydrate Content of Diet (g per kg body weight)
6	90 (at 70% max effort)	5 (moderate)
5	40 (at 70% max effort)	5 (moderate)
4	40 (at 70% max effort)	5 (moderate)
3	20 (light training)	10 (high)
2	20 (light training)	10 (high)
1	Rest	10 (high)
Day of race	Competition	Precompetition food and fluid

Source: Data adapted from *Current Trends in Performance Nutrition,* by Marie Dunford. Champaign, IL: Human Kinetics, 2005.

Athletes who compete in baseball, American football, 10K runs, walking, hiking, weight lifting, and most swimming events will not gain any performance benefits from this practice, nor will people who regularly participate in moderately intense physical activities to maintain fitness.

It is important to emphasize that, even in endurance events, carbohydrate loading does not always improve performance. There are many adverse side effects of this practice, including extreme gastrointestinal distress, particularly diarrhea. We store water along with the extra glycogen in our muscles, which leaves many athletes feeling heavy and sluggish. Athletes who want to try carbohydrate loading should experiment prior to competition to determine whether it is a helpful approach for them.

recap The type, intensity, and duration of activities we participate in determine our nutrient needs. Men generally need more energy than women because of their greater muscle mass and higher body weight. In general, athletes should consume at least 45% to 60% of their total energy as carbohydrate. Consuming carbohydrate sources within the first few hours of recovery can maximize carbohydrate storage rates. Carbohydrate loading involves altering physical training and the diet so that the storage of muscle glycogen is maximized in an attempt to enhance endurance performance.

Moderate Fat Consumption Is Enough to Support Most Activities

Fat is an important energy source for both moderate physical activity and vigorous endurance training. When athletes reach a physically trained state, they are able to use more fat for energy; in other words, they become better "fat burners." This can also occur in people who are not athletes but who regularly participate in aerobic-type fitness activities. This training effect occurs for a number of reasons, including an increase in the number and activity of various enzymes involved in fat metabolism, an improved ability of the muscles to store fat, and an improved ability to extract fat from the blood for use during exercise. By using fat as a fuel, athletes can spare carbohydrate, so that they can use it during prolonged, intense training or competition.

Many athletes concerned with body weight and physical appearance believe they should eat less than 15% of their total energy intake as fat, but this is inadequate to support vigorous activity. Moreover, if fat consumption is too low, levels of the fat-soluble vitamins and essential fatty acids may be too low to maintain health and performance. Instead, a fat intake of 20% to 35% of total energy intake is recommended for most athletes, with less than 10% of total energy intake as saturated fat. Notice that these are the same recommendations as for non-athletes. Athletes who have

foods you don't know you love YET

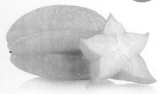

Star Fruit

There's a new "star" in the fruit galaxy—the star fruit! Also known as carambola, the star fruit is native to the Philippines, Indonesia, India, and Sri Lanka. Because it thrives in warm, humid conditions, star fruit are now grown in the United States in Florida and Hawaii. Its name reflects its unique shape, with ridges running down its sides, which cause it to look like a star when cut in cross section. There are both tart and sweet types of star fruit, and they taste like a combination of lemons, pineapples, and plums. Star fruit are an excellent source of water and vitamin C, and they are naturally low in fat and sodium. To enjoy star fruit, no peeling is necessary—simply wash them, remove any damaged areas, slice crosswise to get the star shape, and enjoy!

chronic disease risk factors, such as high blood lipids, high blood pressure, or unhealthful blood glucose levels, should work with their physician to adjust their intake of fat and carbohydrate according to their health risks.

Many Athletes Have Increased Protein Needs

The protein intakes suggested for active people range from 1.0 to 1.8 grams per kg body weight. At the lower end of this range are people who exercise four to five times a week for 30 minutes or less. At the upper end are athletes who train five to seven times a week for more than an hour a day. Protein intakes as high as 1.8 to 2.0 grams per kg per day may help to prevent the loss of lean body mass during periods when an athlete may be restricting energy to promote fat loss.[13]

Most inactive people and many athletes in the United States consume more than enough protein to support their needs.[14] However, some athletes do not consume enough protein, including those with very low energy intakes, vegetarians or vegans who do not consume high-protein food sources, and young athletes who are growing and are not aware of their higher protein needs.

In 1995, Dr. Barry Sears published *The Zone: A Dietary Road Map*, a book that claims numerous benefits of a high-protein, low-carbohydrate diet for competitive athletes.[15] Since that time, Sears has published more than a dozen spin-offs, all of which recommend the consumption of a 40-30-30 diet, or one composed of 40% carbohydrate, 30% fat, and 30% protein. Dr. Sears claims that high-carbohydrate diets impair athletic performance because of the unhealthful effects of insulin. These claims have not been supported by research, and in fact, many of Dr. Sears's claims are not consistent with human physiology. The primary problem with the Zone Diet for athletes is that it is too low in both energy and carbohydrate to support training and performance.

High-quality protein sources include lean meats, poultry, fish, eggs, low-fat dairy products, legumes, and soy products. By following their personalized MyPlate food patterns, people of all fitness levels can consume more than enough protein without the use of supplements or specially formulated foods.

recap Athletes and other physically active people use more fat for energy. A dietary fat intake of 20% to 35% is generally recommended, with less than 10% of total energy intake as saturated fat. Protein needs can be somewhat higher for athletes, but most people in the United States already consume more than twice their daily needs. Although low-carbohydrate, high-protein diets have been marketed to athletes, they are generally too low in carbohydrate and total energy to support training and competition.

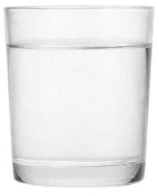

▲ Water is essential for maintaining fluid balance and preventing dehydration.

Regular Exercise Increases Our Need for Fluids

In this chapter, we will provide a brief overview on the role of water during exercise. A detailed discussion of fluid and electrolyte balance is provided in Chapter 8.

Heat production can increase by fifteen to twenty times during heavy exercise! As explained in Chapter 8, the primary way in which we dissipate this heat is through sweating, which is also called **evaporative cooling**. When body temperature rises, more blood (which contains water) flows to the surface of the skin. In this way, heat is carried from the core of our body to the surface of our skin. By sweating, the water (and body heat) leaves our body, and the air around us picks up the evaporating water from our skin, cooling our body.

Heat illnesses occur because, when we exercise in the heat, our muscles and skin constantly compete for blood flow. When there is no longer enough blood flow to simultaneously provide adequate blood to our muscles and our skin, muscle blood flow takes priority and evaporative cooling is inhibited. Dehydration significantly increases the risk for heat illnesses. **FIGURE 10.9** identifies the symptoms of dehydration during heavy exercise. As discussed in Chapter 8, *heatstroke* occurs when the body cannot release enough heat in the form of sweat to keep the body temperature within a safe range.

How can we prevent dehydration and heat illnesses such as heatstroke? Obviously, adequate fluid intake is critical before, during, and after exercise. Unfortunately, our thirst mechanism cannot be relied on to signal when we need to drink. If we rely only on our feelings of thirst, we will not consume enough fluid to support exercise.

General fluid replacement recommendations are based on maintaining body weight. Athletes who are training and competing in hot environments should weigh themselves before and after the training session or event and should regain the weight lost over the subsequent 24-hour period. They should avoid losing more than 2–3% of body weight during exercise, because performance can be impaired with fluid losses as small as 1% of body weight.

TABLE 10.5 identifies the guidelines for proper fluid replacement. For activities lasting less than 1 hour, plain water is generally adequate to replace fluid losses. However, for training and competition lasting longer than 1 hour in any weather, sports beverages containing carbohydrate and electrolytes are recommended. These beverages are also recommended for people who will not drink enough water because they don't like the taste. If drinking these beverages will promote adequate hydration, they are appropriate to use.

evaporative cooling Another term for sweating, which is the primary way in which we dissipate heat.

Inadequate Intakes of Some Vitamins and Minerals Can Diminish Health and Performance

When people train vigorously for athletic events, their requirements for certain vitamins and minerals may be altered. Many highly active people do not eat enough food

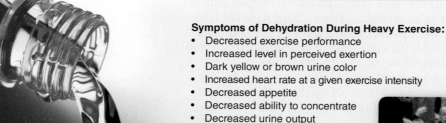

Symptoms of Dehydration During Heavy Exercise:
- Decreased exercise performance
- Increased level in perceived exertion
- Dark yellow or brown urine color
- Increased heart rate at a given exercise intensity
- Decreased appetite
- Decreased ability to concentrate
- Decreased urine output
- Fatigue and weakness
- Headache and dizziness

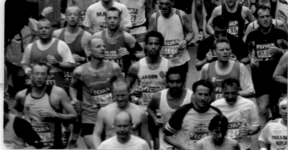

▲ **FIGURE 10.9** Symptoms of dehydration during heavy exercise.

TABLE 10.5   Guidelines for Fluid Replacement

Activity Level	Environment	Fluid Requirements (liters per day)
Sedentary	Cool	2–3
Active	Cool	3–6
Sedentary	Warm	3–5
Active	Warm	5–10

Before Exercise or Competition

- Drink adequate fluids during 24 hours before the event; should be able to maintain body weight.
- Slowly drink about 0.17 to 0.24 fl. oz per kg body weight of water or a sports drink at least 4 hours before exercise or an event to allow time for excretion of excess fluid prior to the event.
- Slowly drink another 0.10 to 0.17 fl. oz per kg body weight about 2 hours before the event.
- Consuming beverages with sodium and/or small amounts of salted snacks at a meal will help stimulate thirst and retain fluids consumed.

During Exercise or Competition

- Drink early and regularly throughout the event to sufficiently replace all water lost through sweating.
- The amount and rate of fluid replacement depend on a person's rate of sweating and the exercise duration, weather conditions, and opportunities to drink.
- Fluids should be cooler than the environmental temperature and flavored to enhance taste and promote fluid replacement.

During Exercise or Competition That Lasts More Than 1 Hour

- Fluid replacement beverage should contain 5–10% carbohydrate to maintain blood glucose levels; sodium and other electrolytes should be included in the beverage in amounts of 0.5–0.7 gram of sodium per liter of water to replace the sodium lost by sweating.

Following Exercise or Competition

- Consume about 3 cups of fluid for each pound of body weight lost.
- Fluids after exercise should contain water to restore hydration status, carbohydrates to replenish glycogen stores, and electrolytes (for example, sodium and potassium) to speed rehydration.
- Consume enough fluid to permit regular urination and to ensure the urine color is very light or light yellow in color; drinking about 125–150% of fluid loss is usually sufficient to ensure complete rehydration.

In General

- Products that contain fructose should be limited, because these may cause gastrointestinal distress.
- Caffeine and alcohol should be avoided, because these products increase urine output and reduce fluid retention.
- Carbonated beverages should be avoided, because they reduce the desire for fluid intake due to stomach fullness.

Source: Data adapted from Murray, R. 1997. Drink more! Advice from a world class expert. *ACSM's Health Fitness J.* 1:19–23; American College of Sports Medicine. 2007. Position stand, exercise and fluid replacement. *Med. Sci. Sports Exerc.* 39(2): 377–390; and Casa, D. J., L. E. Armstrong, S. K. Hillman, S. J. Montain, R. V. Reiff, B. S. E. Rich, W. O. Roberts, and J. A. Stone. 2000. National Athletic Trainers' Association position statement: fluid replacement for athletes. *J. Athletic Training.* 35:212–224.

or a variety of foods that allows them to consume enough of these nutrients, yet it is imperative that active people do their very best to eat an adequate, varied, and balanced diet to try to meet their increased needs.

B-Vitamins

The B-vitamins are directly involved in energy metabolism. There is reliable evidence that—as a population—active people may require slightly more thiamin, riboflavin, and vitamin B_6 than the current RDA because of increased production of energy and inadequate dietary intake in some active people.[14] However, these increased needs are easily met by consuming adequate energy and plentiful fiber-rich carbohydrates. Active people at risk for poor B-vitamin status are those who consume inadequate energy or who consume mostly refined-carbohydrate foods, such as soda pop and sugary snacks. Vegan athletes and active people may be at risk for inadequate intake of vitamin B_{12}; food sources enriched with this nutrient include soy and cereal products.

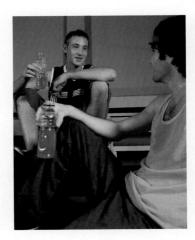

Drinking sports beverages during training and competition lasting more than 1 hour replaces fluid, carbohydrates, and electrolytes.

Calcium

Calcium supports proper muscle contraction and ensures bone health. Calcium intakes are inadequate for most women in the United States, including both sedentary and active women. This is most likely due to the failure to consume foods that are high in calcium, particularly dairy products. Although vigorous training does not appear to increase our need for calcium, we need to consume enough calcium to support bone health. If we do not, stress fractures and severe loss of bone can result.

Some female athletes suffer from a syndrome known as the female athlete triad (see Chapter 9). In the female athlete triad, nutritional inadequacies cause irregularities in the menstrual cycle and hormonal disturbances that can lead to a significant loss of bone mass. Thus, for female athletes, consuming the recommended amounts of calcium is critical. For female athletes who are physically small and have lower energy intakes, calcium supplementation may be needed to meet current recommendations.

Iron

Iron, a part of the hemoglobin molecule, is critical for the transport of oxygen in our blood to our cells and working muscles. Iron is also involved in energy production. Research has shown that active people lose more iron in the sweat, feces, and urine than do inactive people and that endurance runners lose iron when their red blood cells break down in their feet due to the high impact of running. Female athletes and non-athletes lose more iron than male athletes because of menstrual blood losses, and females in general tend to eat less iron in their diet. Vegetarian athletes and active people may also consume less iron. Thus, many athletes and active people are at higher risk for iron deficiency. Depending on its severity, poor iron status can impair athletic performance and our ability to maintain regular physical activity.

A phenomenon known as *sports anemia* was identified in the 1960s. Sports anemia is not true anemia, but a transient decrease in iron stores that occurs at the start of an exercise program for some people, as well as in some athletes who increase their training intensity. Exercise training increases the amount of water in our blood (called *plasma volume*); however, the amount of hemoglobin does not increase until later into the training period. Thus, the iron content in the blood appears to be low but instead is falsely depressed due to increases in plasma volume. Sports anemia, because it is not true anemia, does not affect performance.

In general, it appears that physically active females are at relatively high risk of suffering from the first stage of iron depletion, in which iron stores are low.[16] Because of this, it is suggested that blood tests of iron stores and monitoring of dietary iron intakes be routinely done for active females.[16] In some cases, iron needs cannot be met through the diet, and supplementation is necessary. Iron supplementation should be done with a physician's approval and proper medical supervision.

recap Regular exercise increases fluid needs. Fluid is critical to cool our internal body temperature and prevent heat illnesses such as heatstroke. Dehydration is a serious threat during exercise in extreme heat and high humidity. Active people may need more thiamin, riboflavin, and vitamin B_6 than inactive people. Exercise itself does not increase our calcium needs, but many women, including active women, do not consume enough calcium. Some female athletes suffer from the female athlete triad, a condition that involves the interaction of low energy availability, menstrual dysfunction, and bone loss. Many active people require more iron, particularly female athletes and vegetarian athletes.

Are ergogenic aids necessary for active people?

Many competitive athletes and even some recreationally active people search continually for that something extra that will enhance their performance. **Ergogenic aids** are substances used to improve exercise and athletic performance. For example, nutrition supplements can be classified as ergogenic aids, as can anabolic steroids and other pharmaceuticals. Interestingly, people report using ergogenic aids not only to enhance athletic performance but also to improve their physical appearance, prevent or treat injuries and diseases, and help them cope with stress. Some people even report using them because of peer pressure!

As you have learned in this chapter, adequate nutrition is critical to athletic performance and to regular physical activity, and products such as sports bars and beverages can help athletes maintain their competitive edge. However, as we will explore shortly, many ergogenic aids are not effective, some are dangerous, and most are very expensive. For the average consumer, it is virtually impossible to track the latest research findings for these products. In addition, many have not been adequately studied, and unsubstantiated claims surrounding them are rampant. So how can you become a more educated consumer about ergogenic aids?

Early in the text (in Chapter 1) we explained how to determine if a website is reliable and how to evaluate research and claims made by companies promoting their products. The sale of ergogenic aids is a multibillion-dollar industry, and some companies resort to misleading claims to boost their share of the market. Beware of the following deceptive tactics used to market ergogenic aids:

- Taking published research out of context, applying the findings in an unproven manner, or having inappropriate control over study results. Some companies claim that research has been done or is currently being done but fail to provide specific information.
- Paying celebrities to endorse products—remember that testimonials can be faked, bought, and exaggerated.
- Stating that the product is patented and that this proves its effectiveness. Patents are granted to indicate differences among products; they do not indicate effectiveness.
- Advertising through infomercials and mass-media marketing videos. Although the Federal Trade Commission (FTC) regulates false claims in advertising, products are generally investigated only if they pose significant public danger.
- Offering mail-order fitness evaluations or anabolic measurements. Most of these evaluations are inappropriate and inaccurate.

A recent review of the evidence underpinning sports performance products, which includes drinks, supplements, clothing, and footwear, found that there was inadequate information available to perform a critical appraisal of approximately half the products.[17] In addition, when studies were conducted to assess a product's effectiveness, only 2.7% of the studies were judged to be of high quality and at low risk of bias. Thus, the authors of this review concluded that the currently available evidence is not of sufficient quality to inform the public about the benefits and risks of these products.

New ergogenic aids are introduced virtually every month. It is therefore not possible to discuss every available product here. However, a brief review of a number of currently popular ergogenic aids is provided.

Anabolic Products Are Promoted as Muscle and Strength Enhancers

Many ergogenic aids are said to be **anabolic**, meaning that they build muscle and increase strength. Most anabolic substances promise to increase testosterone, which is the hormone associated with male sex characteristics that increases muscle size and

LO9 Discuss several deceptive tactics companies use to market ergogenic aids.

LO10 Identify the claims for, research evidence on, and potential health risks of at least three ergogenic aids.

Want to learn what the U.S. Food and Drug Administration is doing to crack down on fraudulent health claims and the companies that make them? Click on www.fda.gov and click on the "Drugs" tab. Under "Emergency Preparedness," click on the "Bioterrorism and Drug Preparedness" link to read more.

ergogenic aids Substances used to improve exercise and athletic performance.

anabolic The term used for a substance that builds muscle and increases strength.

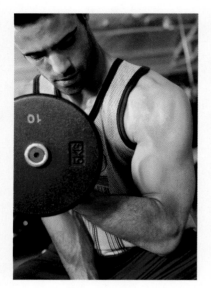

Anabolic substances are often marketed to people trying to increase muscle size, but they carry risks for harmful side effects.

strength. Although some anabolic substances are effective, they are generally associated with harmful side effects.

Anabolic Steroids

Anabolic steroids are testosterone-based drugs known to be effective in increasing muscle size, strength, power, and speed. They have been used extensively by strength and power athletes; however, they are illegal in the United States, and their use is banned by all major collegiate and professional sports organizations, in addition to both the U.S. and the International Olympic Committees. Proven long-term and irreversible effects of steroid use include infertility; early closure of the plates of the long bones, resulting in permanently shortened stature; shriveled testicles, enlarged breast tissue (that can be removed only surgically), and other signs of "feminization" in men; enlarged clitoris, facial hair growth, and other signs of "masculinization" in women; increased risk for certain forms of cancer; liver damage; unhealthful changes in blood lipids; hypertension; severe acne; hair thinning or baldness; and depression, delusions, sleep disturbances, and extreme anger (so-called roid rage).

Androstenedione and Dehydroepiandrosterone

Androstenedione ("andro") and dehydroepiandrosterone (DHEA) are precursors of testosterone. Manufacturers of these products claim that taking them will increase testosterone levels and muscle strength. Androstenedione became very popular after baseball player Mark McGwire claimed he used it during the time he was breaking home run records. Contrary to popular claims, studies have found that neither androstenedione nor DHEA increases testosterone levels, and androstenedione has been shown to lead to unhealthy changes in blood lipids and increase a person's risk for heart disease.[18] There are no studies that support claims that these products improve strength or increase muscle mass.

Gamma-Hydroxybutyric Acid

Gamma-hydroxybutyric acid, or GHB, is a central nervous system depressant. It was once promoted as an alternative to anabolic steroids for building muscle. The production and sale of GHB were never approved in the United States; however, it was illegally produced and sold on the black market as a dietary supplement. For many users, GHB caused only dizziness, tremors, or vomiting, but others experienced severe side effects, including seizures, respiratory depression, sedation, and coma. Many people were hospitalized, and some died.

In 2001, the federal government placed GHB on the Controlled Substances list, making its manufacture, sale, and possession illegal. A form of GHB is available by prescription for the treatment of narcolepsy, a rare sleep disorder, but extra paperwork is required by the prescribing physician, and prescriptions are closely monitored. After the ban, a similar product (gamma-butyrolactone, or GBL) was marketed in its place. This product was also found to be dangerous and was removed from the market by the FDA. Recently, another replacement product called BD (also known as 1,4-butanediol) was also banned by the FDA, because it has caused at least seventy-one deaths, with forty more under investigation. BD is an industrial solvent and is listed on ingredient labels as tetramethylene glycol, butylene glycol, or sucol-B. Side effects include wild, aggressive behavior; nausea; incontinence; and sudden loss of consciousness.

Creatine

Creatine is a supplement that has become wildly popular with strength and power athletes. Creatine, or creatine phosphate, is found in meat and fish and stored in our muscles. As described earlier, our body uses creatine phosphate (CP) to regenerate ATP. It is theorized that creatine supplements make more CP available to replenish ATP, which prolongs a person's ability to train and perform in short-term, explosive activities, such as weight lifting and sprinting. Between 1994 and 2014, almost

6,000 research articles related to creatine and exercise in humans were published. Creatine does not seem to enhance performance in aerobic-type events, but it has been shown to increase the work performed and the amount of strength gained during resistance exercise and enhance sprint performance in swimming, running, and cycling.[19]

Although side effects such as dehydration, muscle cramps, and gastrointestinal disturbances have been reported with creatine use, there is very little information on how the long-term use of creatine affects health. Further research is needed to determine the effectiveness and safety of creatine use over prolonged periods of time.

Protein and Amino Acid Supplements and Beta-Hydroxy-Beta-Methylbutyrate (HMB)

Protein and amino acid supplements have long been popular and are widely available in health food stores and on the Internet. Examples of these products include various protein powders and individual amino acids, such as glutamine and arginine. Although manufacturers claim that these products build muscle mass and enhance strength, research indicates that they do not.[14,20–21]

As discussed in Chapter 5, recent evidence suggests that dietary protein, and particularly the amino acid leucine, are important triggers to enhance the synthesis of protein in the muscle.[13] Beta-hydroxy-beta-methylbutyrate (or HMB), is a metabolite of leucine. The evidence is mixed supporting whether HMB can build muscle mass and increase strength.[22–24] However, as noted in Chapter 5, you can derive the benefits of leucine by consuming a glass of milk after exercise, with no need to purchase expensive supplements that may be ineffective.

Some Products Are Said to Optimize Fuel Use During Exercise

Certain ergogenic aids are touted as increasing energy levels and improving athletic performance by optimizing our use of fat, carbohydrate, and protein. The products reviewed here include caffeine, ephedrine, carnitine, chromium, ribose, beta-alanine, and nitrate.

Caffeine

Caffeine is a stimulant that makes us feel more alert and energetic, decreasing feelings of fatigue during exercise. Although previous research found that caffeine increases the use of fat as a fuel during endurance exercise, the current consensus from sports nutrition experts is that the primary ergogenic effect of caffeine is due to its effect on the central nervous system.[25]

We noted in Chapter 8 that some energy drinks contain very high amounts of caffeine. Although these drinks have become popular with athletes, they should be avoided during exercise, because severe dehydration can result from the combination of fluid loss from exercise and caffeine consumption. Side effects of high amounts of caffeine include increased blood pressure, increased heart rate, dizziness, insomnia, headache, and gastrointestinal distress. However, recent research indicates that low doses of caffeine (2 to 3 mg per kg body weight, or the equivalent of 1 mug of coffee) are effective in enhancing performance and are associated with minimal side effects.[26]

Ephedrine

Ephedrine, also known as ephedra, Chinese ephedra, or *ma huang,* is a strong stimulant marketed as a weight-loss supplement and energy enhancer. Because it is associated with severe and dangerous side effects, including headache, nausea, anxiety, irregular heart rate, high blood pressure, and death, it is illegal to sell ephedra-containing dietary supplements in the United States.[27] However, ephedra can still be found in traditional Chinese herbal remedies and in herbal teas. The use of ephedra

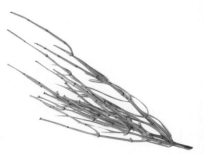

Ephedrine is made from the herb *Ephedra sinica* (Chinese ephedra).

does not appear to enhance athletic performance, but supplements containing both caffeine and ephedra have been shown to prolong the amount of exercise that can be done until exhaustion is reached. Ephedra is known to promote short-term weight loss in sedentary women, but its impact on weight loss and body fat levels in athletes is unknown.

Carnitine

Carnitine is a compound made from amino acids that is found in the membrane of mitochondria. Carnitine helps shuttle fatty acids into the mitochondria, so that they can be used for energy. It has been proposed that exercise training depletes our cells of carnitine and that supplementation should restore carnitine levels, thereby enabling us to improve our use of fat as a fuel source. Thus, carnitine is marketed not only as a performance-enhancing substance but also as a fat burner. Research studies of carnitine supplementation do not support these claims, because neither the transport of fatty acids nor their oxidation appears to be enhanced with chronic supplementation.[28] The use of carnitine supplements has not been associated with significant side effects.

Chromium

Chromium is a trace mineral that enhances insulin's action of increasing the transport of amino acids into the cell. It is found in whole-grain foods, cheese, nuts, mushrooms, and asparagus. It is theorized that many people are chromium deficient and that supplementation will enhance the uptake of amino acids into muscle cells, which will increase muscle growth and strength. Like carnitine, chromium is marketed as a fat burner, because it is speculated that its effect on insulin stimulates the brain to decrease food intake. Chromium supplements are available as chromium picolinate and chromium nicotinate. Early studies of chromium supplementation showed promise, but more recent, better-designed studies do not support any benefit of chromium supplementation for muscle mass, muscle strength, body fat, or exercise performance.[29]

Ribose

Ribose is a five-carbon sugar that is critical to the production of ATP. Ribose supplementation is claimed to improve athletic performance by increasing work output and by promoting a faster recovery time from vigorous training. Although early research on ribose suggested that it improves exercise tolerance in patients with heart disease, more recent studies have reported that ribose supplementation has no impact on athletic performance.[30-33]

Beta-Alanine

Beta-alanine is a nonessential amino acid that has been identified as the limiting factor in the production of *carnosine*, a compound synthesized in skeletal muscle that is thought to buffer acids produced during exercise and thereby enhance a person's ability to perform short-term, high-intensity activities.[34-35] Recent evidence suggests that beta-alanine supplementation can increase muscle carnosine levels and delay the onset of muscle fatigue. Additionally, beta-alanine supplementation results in improved exercise performance during single or repeated high-intensity exercise bouts or maximal muscle contractions.[34-35] It appears that several weeks of supplementation is needed to increase muscle carnosine levels and positively affect performance.[35]

Nitrate

Nitric oxide is a compound involved in numerous physiological processes, including regulating blood flow, muscle contraction, mitochondrial function, and glucose uptake. Nitric oxide can be produced by consuming a concentrate of foods high in nitrate, including beetroot, spinach, lettuce, arugula, celery, and watercress. The most commonly used and studied product to date is concentrated beetroot juice. Recent research indicates that beetroot juice supplementation improves cycling time trial performance in distances from 4 to 16.1 km, and in 5 km running performance.[36-38] However, findings from studies examining endurance exercise performance in elite athletes have not shown any benefits of beetroot supplementation.[39-40] Thus, the ergogenic effect of nitrate may be dependent on intensity, duration, and type of exercise and the training status of the person performing the activity. Dietary sources of nitrate have also been proposed to promote cardiovascular health.[41]

From this review of ergogenic aids, you can see that many are not effective and some are dangerous. It is important to be a savvy consumer when considering these products to make sure you're not wasting your money or putting your health at risk by using them.

recap Ergogenic aids are substances used to improve exercise and athletic performance. Anabolic steroids are effective in increasing muscle size, power, and strength, but they are illegal and can cause serious health problems. Androstenedione and dehydroepiandrosterone are precursors of testosterone; neither has been shown to effectively increase testosterone levels, strength, or muscle mass. GHB and its derivatives are illegal substances associated with dangerous sedation and death. Creatine supplements are popular and can enhance sprint performance in swimming, running, and cycling. Protein and amino acid supplements do not increase muscle growth or strength, and the effects of HMB on performance are unclear. Caffeine is a stimulant that decreases fatigue during exercise; in contrast, ephedrine is a stimulant that has potentially fatal side effects. Carnitine, chromium, and ribose are marketed as ergogenic aids, but studies do not support their effectiveness. Two relatively new ergogenic aids that appear to have positive impacts on performance include beta-alanine and nitrate.

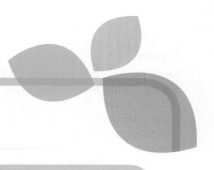

Customize your study plan—and master your nutrition!—in the Study Area of **MasteringNutrition**.

what can I do **today?**

Now that you've read this chapter, try making these three changes.

1 For 1 day, leave your car parked at home and try walking, cycling, or taking public transportation to school or work.

2 Exercise for at least 30 minutes today. Before you do, estimate your training heart rate range. During your workout, keep track of your heart rate and try to keep it within your target training range.

3 Use the information in this chapter to design an activity plan that will help you increase your daily level of physical activity.

test yourself | *answers*

1. **True.** Almost 50% of Americans do not do enough physical activity. Moreover, about half of these people—25% of the population—report doing no leisure-time physical activity at all.

2. **False.** Our muscles are not stimulated to grow when we eat extra protein, whether as food or as supplements. Weight-bearing exercise appropriately stresses the body and produces increased muscle mass and strength.

3. **False.** Unfortunately, our thirst mechanism cannot be relied on to signal when we need to drink. If we rely solely on our feelings of thirst, we might not drink enough to support vigorous exercise.

summary

Scan to hear an MP3 Chapter Review in **MasteringNutrition**.

LO 1 Compare and contrast the concepts of physical activity, leisure-time physical activity, exercise, and physical fitness

- Physical activity is any movement produced by muscles that increases energy expenditure. It includes occupational, household, leisure-time, and transportation activities. Exercise is a subcategory of leisure-time physical activity and is purposeful, planned, and structured.

- Physical fitness is defined as the ability to carry out daily tasks with vigor and alertness, without undue fatigue, and with ample energy to enjoy leisure-time pursuits and meet unforeseen emergencies.

LO 2 Identify the four components of physical fitness

- Physical fitness includes four components: cardiorespiratory fitness, which is the ability of the heart, lungs, and blood vessels to supply working

muscles; musculoskeletal fitness, which is fitness of the muscles and bones; flexibility; and body composition. These can be achieved through regular aerobic exercise, resistance training, and stretching.

LO 3 List at least four health benefits of being physically active on a regular basis

- Physical activity provides a multitude of health benefits, including reducing risks for heart disease, stroke, high blood pressure, obesity, type 2 diabetes, and osteoporosis. It can also improve our sleep patterns, reduce our risk for upper respiratory infections by improving immune function, reduce anxiety and mental stress, and relieve mild and moderate depression. Despite these benefits, almost half of all Americans are insufficiently active.

LO 4 Explain how to identify and achieve your personal fitness goals

- To identify your personal fitness goals, apply the specificity principle: specific actions yield specific results. To achieve your goals, appropriately overload your body. The overload principle states that you need to place an extra physical demand on your body to achieve improvements in fitness.

LO 5 Describe the FITT principle and calculate your maximal and training heart rate range

- Four factors are collectively known as the FITT principle: frequency, intensity, time, and type of activity. Frequency refers to the number of activity sessions per week. Intensity refers to how difficult the activity is to perform. You can calculate the range of exercise intensity that is appropriate for you by estimating your maximal heart rate, which is the rate at which your heart beats during maximal-intensity exercise. Maximal heart rate is estimated by subtracting your age from 220. Time refers to how long each activity session lasts. Type is the range of physical activities a person can engage in to promote health and physical fitness.

- Warm-up, or preliminary exercise, is important to get prepared for exercise. Warm-up exercises prepare the muscles for exertion by increasing blood flow and temperature. Cool-down activities are done after an exercise session is complete. Cool-down activities assist in the prevention of injury and may help reduce muscle soreness.

LO 6 List and describe at least three processes by which the body breaks down fuels to support physical activity

- Adenosine triphosphate, or ATP, is the common energy source for all cells of the body. The amount of ATP stored in a muscle cell is limited and can keep a muscle active for only 1 to 3 seconds.

- Creatine phosphate stored in muscles can be broken down to provide short bursts of energy.

- The body breaks down glucose from blood and muscle glycogen to fuel long-term activity.

- Fat can be broken down to support activities of low intensity and long duration. Its breakdown process is relatively slow, so it cannot support quick, high-intensity activities.

- Amino acids can be used to make glucose to maintain blood glucose levels during exercise and can contribute from 3% to 6% of the energy needed during exercise (although this is not a preferred energy source). Amino acids also help build and repair tissues after exercise.

LO 7 Discuss at least three changes in nutrient needs that can occur in response to an increase in physical activity or vigorous exercise training

- Athletes generally have higher energy needs than moderately physically active or sedentary people.

- It is generally recommended that athletes consume at least 45% to 65% of their total energy as carbohydrate. This is the AMDR for non-athletes as well. A dietary fat intake of 20% to 35% is generally recommended, with less than 10% of total energy intake as saturated fat. The protein intakes suggested for active people range from 1.0 to 1.8 grams per kg body weight, but most Americans already consume more than twice their daily needs for protein.

- Regular exercise increases our fluid needs to help cool our internal body temperature and prevent dehydration and heat illnesses, including heat syncope, heat cramps, heat exhaustion, and heatstroke.

- Athletes may need more thiamin, riboflavin, and vitamin B_6 than do inactive people. Many people do not consume enough calcium and are at risk for decreased bone density and increased risk of fractures. Many active individuals require additional iron, particularly female athletes and vegetarian athletes.

LO 8 Describe the concept of carbohydrate loading, and discuss situations in which this practice may be beneficial to athletic performance

- Carbohydrate loading alters physical training and the diet, such that the storage of muscle glycogen is maximized. It is used to enhance endurance performance, for example in marathons, ultramarathons, long-distance swimming, cross-country skiing, and triathlons.

LO 9 Discuss several deceptive tactics companies use to market ergogenic aids

- Ergogenic aids are substances used to improve exercise and athletic performance. Many ergogenic aids are not effective, and some are dangerous. Their marketing campaign may use deceptive tactics such as taking published research out of context, paying celebrities to endorse products, or stating that a patent for the product proves its effectiveness.

LO 10 Identify the claims for, research evidence on, and potential health risks of at least three ergogenic aids

- Anabolic steroids build muscle and increase strength, but have several proven and dangerous long-term effects, including increased risk for hypertension, certain forms of cancer, liver damage, depression, delusions, sleep disturbances, and extreme anger.

- Neither androstenedione nor DHEA improves strength or muscle mass.

- GHB and similar replacement products are illegal and dangerous.

- Creatine supplementation does not seem to enhance performance in aerobic-type events, but it has been shown to increase the work performed and the amount of strength gained during resistance exercise and enhance sprint performance in swimming, running, and cycling.

- Protein and amino acid supplementation does not build muscle mass or enhance strength. The evidence for the effectiveness of HMB, a metabolite of the amino acid leucine, is mixed.

- Caffeine is a stimulant that decreases fatigue during exercise; in contrast, ephedrine is a stimulant that has potentially fatal side effects. Carnitine, chromium, and ribose are marketed as ergogenic aids but studies do not support their effectiveness. Two relatively new ergogenic aids that appear to have positive impacts on performance include beta-alanine and nitrate.

review questions

LO **1** **Compare and contrast the concepts of physical activity, leisure-time physical activity, exercise, and physical fitness**

1. Exercise is
   a. a subcategory of leisure-time physical activity.
   b. activity that is purposeful, planned, and structured.
   c. not related to a person's occupation.
   d. all of the above.

LO **2** **Identify the four components of physical fitness**

2. The four components of physical fitness are
   a. cardiorespiratory fitness, musculoskeletal fitness, flexibility, and body composition.
   b. cardiorespiratory fitness, strength, stamina, and flexibility.
   c. aerobic capacity, muscular strength, chronic disease resistance, and maintenance of a healthful body weight.
   d. cardiorespiratory efficiency, musculoskeletal strength, flexibility, and chronic disease resistance.

LO **3** **List at least four health benefits of being physically active on a regular basis**

3. To support a daylong hike, the body predominantly uses which nutrient for energy?
   a. protein
   b. carbohydrate
   c. fat
   d. water

LO **4** **Explain how to identify and achieve your personal fitness goals**

4. To achieve your personal fitness goals,
   a. identify specific actions likely to yield the specific results you're seeking.
   b. design a fitness program that is consistent, varied, and fun.
   c. appropriately overload your body.
   d. all of the above.

LO **5** **Describe the FITT principle and calculate your maximal and training heart rate range**

5. For achieving and maintaining aerobic fitness, the intensity range during exercise typically recommended is
   a. 25% to 50% of your estimated maximal heart rate.
   b. 35% to 75% of your estimated maximal heart rate.
   c. 50% to 70% of your estimated maximal heart rate.
   d. 75% to 95% of your estimated maximal heart rate.

LO **6** **List and describe at least three processes by which the body breaks down fuels to support physical activity**

6. The amount of ATP stored in a muscle cell can keep a muscle active for about
   a. 1 to 3 seconds.
   b. 10 to 30 seconds.
   c. 1 to 3 minutes.
   d. 1 to 3 hours.

LO **7** **Discuss at least three changes in nutrient needs that can occur in response to an increase in physical activity or vigorous exercise training**

7. Athletes participating in an intense athletic competition lasting more than 1 hour should drink
   a. beverages containing caffeine.
   b. beverages containing carbohydrates and electrolytes.
   c. plain, room-temperature water.
   d. nothing.

LO **8** **Describe the concept of carbohydrate loading, and discuss situations in which this practice may be beneficial to athletic performance**

8. Which of the following statements about carbohydrate loading is true?
   a. Carbohydrate loading involves altering the duration and intensity of exercise and intake of carbohydrate such that the storage of fat is minimized.
   b. Carbohydrate loading results in increased storage of glycogen in muscles and the liver.
   c. Carbohydrate loading is beneficial for most athletes prior to most competitive events.
   d. All of the above are true.

LO **9** **Discuss several deceptive tactics companies use to market ergogenic aids**

9. An advertisement in which a former Olympic gold medalist endorses an ergogenic aid
   a. is an example of an illegal scam.
   b. is an example of a deceptive marketing tactic.

   c. is trustworthy if the athlete mentions that studies have shown it is effective.
   d. is probably trustworthy because the athlete has an Olympic medal.

LO **10** **Identify the claims for, research evidence on, and potential health risks of at least three ergogenic aids**

10. Creatine
    a. seems to enhance performance in aerobic-type events.
    b. appears to increase a person's risk for bladder cancer.
    c. seems to increase strength gained in resistance exercise.
    d. is stored in the liver.

Answers to Review Questions are located at the back of this text.

web links

The following websites and apps explore further topics and issues related to personal health. Visit **MasteringNutrition** for links to the websites and RSS feeds.

www.acsm.org
American College of Sports Medicine

www.heart.org/HEARTORG/
American Heart Association

http://ods.od.nih.gov
NIH Office of Dietary Supplements

www.webmd.com
WebMD Health

http://www.win.niddk.nih.gov
Weight-control Information

11

Nutrition Throughout the Life Cycle

learning outcomes

After studying this chapter, you should be able to:

1 Explain why a nourishing diet is important even before conception, pp. 327–338.

2 Identify the range of optimal weight gain during the three trimesters of pregnancy, pp. 327–338.

3 Discuss nutrient needs and some common nutrition-related concerns of pregnant women, pp. 327–338.

4 Discuss the advantages and challenges of breastfeeding, pp. 339–346.

5 Discuss nutrient needs, timing of introduction to and type of solid foods, and common nutrition-related concerns of infants, pp. 339–346.

6 Discuss nutrient needs and some common nutrition-related concerns of toddlers, pp. 346–348.

7 Identify changes in nutrient needs for school-age children, as well as the effect of school attendance on children's nutrition, pp. 348–352.

8 Explain how adolescents' rapid growth affects their nutritional status, pp. 353–355.

9 Discuss changes in an older adult's body, functions, and nutrient needs, pp. 356–363.

10 Identify some common nutrition-related concerns of older adults, pp. 356–363.

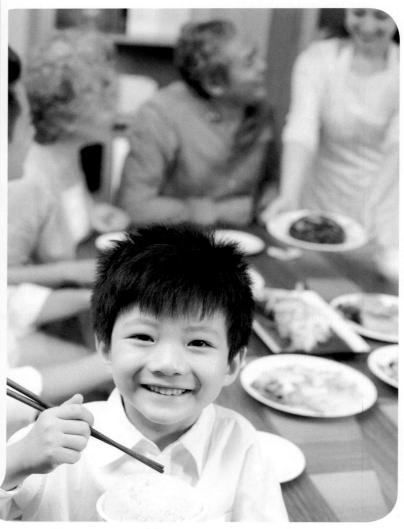

MasteringNutrition™

Go online for chapter quizzes, pre-tests, Interactive Activities, and more!

test yourself

Are these statements true or false? Circle your guess.

1. **T F** Despite popular belief, very few pregnant women actually experience morning sickness, food cravings, or food aversions.

2. **T F** Most infants begin to require solid foods by about 3 months (12 weeks) of age.

3. **T F** More than 10% of Americans age 65 and older experience food insecurity.

Test Yourself answers can be found at the end of the chapter.

On Sunday afternoons, the Harris family gathers for dinner at the Long Beach apartment of their 88-year-old great-great-grandmother, Anabelle. Anabelle is as thin as a rail, as are her 70-year-old daughter and 67-year-old son. But when her granddaughters, who are cooking the family meal, send everyone to the table, a change becomes evident. Almost all of Anabelle's grandchildren and their spouses are overweight, as are most of her great-grandchildren. Even her "darling" 2-year-old great-great-granddaughter, Tina-Marie, is chubby. Anabelle worries about everyone's weight. One of her grandsons had a heart attack last year. During her pregnancy with Tina-Marie, Anabelle's great-granddaughter developed gestational diabetes, and several other family members have been diagnosed with type 2 diabetes. Anabelle's family isn't alone in their weight problems: approximately 32% of American children and adolescents (age 2 to 19 years) are overweight or obese, along with more than 68% of American adults.[1] In addition, type 2 diabetes occurs in about 10% of all American adults and is on the rise.[2]

Why have rates of obesity and its associated chronic diseases skyrocketed in the past 10 years, and what can be done to promote weight management across the life span? How do our nutrient needs change as we grow and age, and what other nutrition-related concerns develop in each life stage? This chapter will help you answer these questions.

Starting out right: healthful nutrition in pregnancy

From conception through infancy, adequate nutrition is essential for tissue formation and growth, including neurologic development. Our ability to reach peak physical and intellectual potential as adults is in part determined by the nutrition we receive during fetal development and the first year of life.

LO1 Explain why a nourishing diet is important even before conception.

LO2 Identify the range of optimal weight gain during the three trimesters of pregnancy.

LO3 Discuss nutrient needs and some common nutrition-related concerns of pregnant women.

Why Is Nutrition Important Before Conception?

Several factors make nutrition important even before **conception**—the point at which a woman's ovum (egg) is fertilized with a man's sperm. First, an adequate and varied preconception diet reduces the risk for nutrient-deficiency problems, providing "insurance" during those first few weeks of life. For example, low folate intake by a pregnant woman during the first 28 days after conception—typically before the woman even realizes she is pregnant—may cause the fetal spinal cord tissues to fail to close, resulting in problems ranging from paralysis to an absence of brain tissue. For this reason, all women capable of becoming pregnant are encouraged to consume 400 µg of folic acid daily from fortified foods, such as cereals, or supplements, in addition to natural sources of folate from a varied, healthful diet. Note that consuming adequate folate should be a health habit that is established *before* a woman attempts to conceive.

Also prior to conception, women must avoid alcohol, illegal drugs, and other known **teratogens** (substances that cause birth defects). Women should also consult their healthcare provider about their consumption of caffeine, prescription medications, and herbs and other dietary supplements. Smoking increases the risk for a low-birth-weight baby and infant mortality, so women should quit smoking before getting pregnant.

Third, the mother's health prior to conception greatly influences the future health of her child. The offspring of women who are obese at the time of conception are at much higher risk for obesity and birth defects, such as congenital heart defects.[3]

conception The uniting of an ovum (egg) and sperm to create a fertilized egg.

teratogen Any substance that can cause a birth defect.

Children of diabetic women are much more likely to develop type 2 diabetes, high blood pressure, and unhealthful blood lipid levels as adults compared with the offspring of non-diabetic women. Women with a healthy pre-pregnancy weight have the best chance of an uncomplicated pregnancy and delivery, with low risk for negative outcomes, such as prolonged labor and cesarean section. Women who are underweight or overweight prior to conception are at greater risk for pregnancy-related complications. Additionally, certain nutrient deficiencies in a pregnant woman may alter the genetic profile of her child.

Finally, maintaining a balanced and nourishing diet before conception reduces a woman's risk of developing a health problem during her pregnancy. Although some problems are beyond the woman's control, others, from iron-deficiency anemia to high blood pressure, are less likely in women following a healthful diet.

The man's nutrition and lifestyle prior to pregnancy are important as well, because malnutrition contributes to abnormalities in sperm.[4,5] Here are some findings:

- Obesity is associated with increased male infertility, including lower sperm counts, quality, and motility.
- Omega 3 fatty acids are higher in the sperm of fertile men versus those of infertile men.
- Men with high folate intake have fewer sperm defects compared with those with lower intakes.
- Antioxidants, such as vitamins C and E and lycopene, have been linked to improved sperm quality and fertility.
- Men who abuse alcohol, smoke, or use illegal drugs are more likely to produce defective sperm than men who avoid such practices.

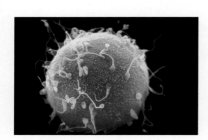

▲ During conception, a sperm fertilizes an egg.

Why Is Nutrition Important During Pregnancy?

A balanced, nourishing diet throughout pregnancy provides the nutrients needed to support fetal growth and development without depriving the mother of the nutrients she needs to maintain her own health. It also minimizes the risks of excessive weight gain.

In clinical practice, the calculation of weeks in a pregnancy begins with the date of the first day of a woman's last menstrual period. A full-term pregnancy lasts 38 to 42 weeks and is divided into three **trimesters**, with each trimester lasting about 13 to 14 weeks.

The first trimester (approximately weeks 1 to 13) begins when the ovum and sperm unite to form a single, fertilized cell. Over the next few weeks, layers of cells develop into the distinct tissues of the developing **embryo**.

By about week 8, the embryo's skeleton and muscles have begun to develop. A primitive heart has begun to beat, and digestive organs are forming. During the next few weeks, the embryo continues to grow and change dramatically into a recognizable human **fetus**.

Not surprisingly, the embryo is most vulnerable to teratogens during the first trimester (**FIGURE 11.1**). Alcohol, illegal drugs, certain medications, high potency supplements, and other environmental factors can interfere with embryonic development and cause birth defects. Deficiencies of nutrients such as folate can also harm the embryo. In some cases, the damage is so severe that the pregnancy is naturally terminated in a **spontaneous abortion** (also called a *miscarriage*), most commonly in the first trimester.

It is also during the first trimester that the **placenta** forms, which provides nutrients to the fetus and removes wastes. The placenta is connected to the fetus via the **umbilical cord**, emerging from the fetus's navel (see the top photo in Figure 11.1).

During the second trimester (approximately weeks 14 to 27 of pregnancy), the fetus grows to approximately 10 inches and gains about 2 lb. Bones become harder and organ systems continue to mature.

During the third trimester (approximately week 28 to birth), the fetus gains nearly half its body length and three-quarters of its body weight! At the time of birth, an average baby is about 18 to 22 inches long and weighs 7.5 lb. Brain growth is rapid throughout this trimester and for the first 2 years of life.

trimester Any one of three stages of pregnancy, each lasting 13 to 14 weeks.

embryo The human growth and developmental stage lasting from the third week to the end of the eighth week after conception.

fetus The human growth and developmental stage lasting from the beginning of the ninth week after conception to birth.

spontaneous abortion The natural termination of a pregnancy and expulsion of the fetus and pregnancy tissues because of a genetic, developmental, or physiologic abnormality that is so severe that the pregnancy cannot be maintained; also known as *miscarriage*.

placenta A pregnancy-specific organ formed from both maternal and embryonic tissues. It is responsible for oxygen, nutrient, and waste exchange between mother and fetus.

umbilical cord The cord containing arteries and veins that connects the baby (from the navel) to the mother via the placenta.

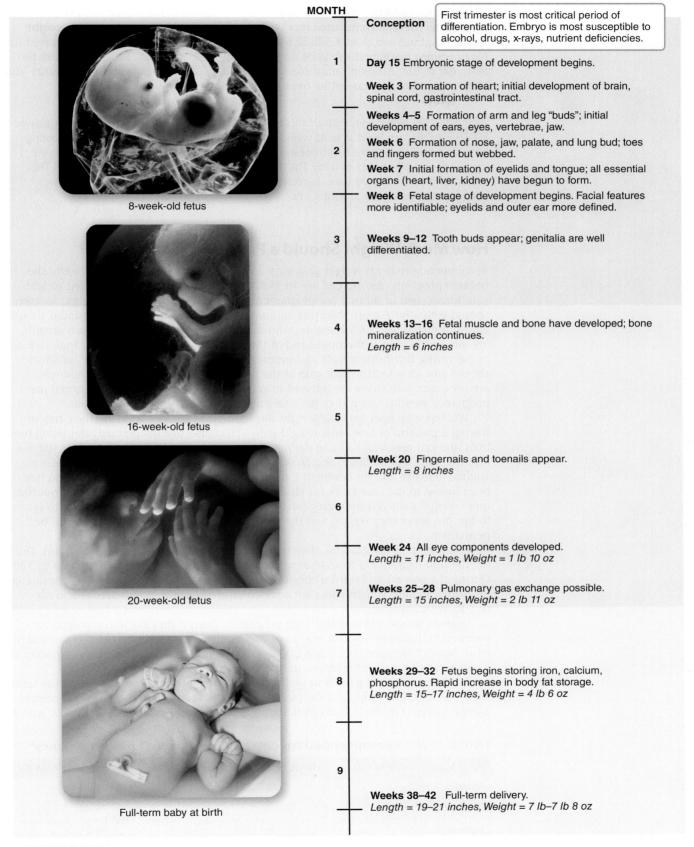

MONTH

Conception

> First trimester is most critical period of differentiation. Embryo is most susceptible to alcohol, drugs, x-rays, nutrient deficiencies.

1

Day 15 Embryonic stage of development begins.

Week 3 Formation of heart; initial development of brain, spinal cord, gastrointestinal tract.

Weeks 4–5 Formation of arm and leg "buds"; initial development of ears, eyes, vertebrae, jaw.

2

Week 6 Formation of nose, jaw, palate, and lung bud; toes and fingers formed but webbed.

Week 7 Initial formation of eyelids and tongue; all essential organs (heart, liver, kidney) have begun to form.

Week 8 Fetal stage of development begins. Facial features more identifiable; eyelids and outer ear more defined.

8-week-old fetus

3

Weeks 9–12 Tooth buds appear; genitalia are well differentiated.

4

Weeks 13–16 Fetal muscle and bone have developed; bone mineralization continues.
Length = 6 inches

5

16-week-old fetus

Week 20 Fingernails and toenails appear.
Length = 8 inches

6

Week 24 All eye components developed.
Length = 11 inches, Weight = 1 lb 10 oz

7

Weeks 25–28 Pulmonary gas exchange possible.
Length = 15 inches, Weight = 2 lb 11 oz

20-week-old fetus

8

Weeks 29–32 Fetus begins storing iron, calcium, phosphorus. Rapid increase in body fat storage.
Length = 15–17 inches, Weight = 4 lb 6 oz

9

Full-term baby at birth

Weeks 38–42 Full-term delivery.
Length = 19–21 inches, Weight = 7 lb–7 lb 8 oz

FIGURE 11.1 A timeline of embryonic and fetal development.

Generally, a birth weight of at least 5.5 lb is considered a marker of a successful pregnancy. An undernourished mother is likely to give birth to a **low-birth-weight** infant weighing less than 5.5 lb at birth. Low-birth-weight infants are at increased risk for infection, learning disabilities, impaired physical development, and death in the first year of life. Although nutrition is not the only factor contributing to maturity and birth weight, its role cannot be overstated.

recap Nutrition is critical both before and during pregnancy. A full-term pregnancy lasts from 38 to 42 weeks and is traditionally divided into trimesters lasting 13 to 14 weeks. During the first trimester, cells differentiate and divide rapidly to form the various tissues of the human body. The fetus is especially vulnerable during this time. The second and third trimesters are characterized by profound growth and maturation. An adequate birth weight is at least 5.5 lb.

How Much Weight Should a Pregnant Woman Gain?

Recommendations for weight gain vary according to a woman's weight *before* she became pregnant. As you can see in **TABLE 11.1**, the average recommended weight gain for women of normal pre-pregnancy weight is 25 to 35 lb; underweight women should gain a little more than this amount, and overweight and obese women should gain somewhat less.[6] Adolescents, who may not have completed their own growth, are advised to gain at the upper end of these ranges, because they are at high risk of delivering low-birth-weight and premature infants. Small women, 5'2" or shorter, should aim for a total weight gain at the lower end of these ranges. Women who are pregnant with twins are advised to gain 37 to 54 lb if they were of normal pre-pregnancy weight, less if they became pregnant while overweight or obese.

Women who gain *too little* weight during their pregnancy increase their risk of having a preterm or low-birth-weight baby. They also risk dangerously depleting their own nutrient reserves. Gaining *too much* weight during pregnancy increases the risk that the fetus will be large, and large babies have increased risks for trauma during vaginal delivery and for cesarean birth. Also, increased pregnancy weight gain has been linked to increased risk for childhood and adolescent obesity.[7] In addition, the more weight gained during pregnancy, the more difficult it is for the mother to return to her pre-pregnancy weight and the more likely it is that her weight gain will be permanent.

In addition to the amount of weight, the *pattern* of weight gain is important. During the first trimester, a woman of normal weight should gain no more than 3 to 5 lb. During the second and third trimesters, an average of about 1 lb a week is considered healthful. Smaller weight gains are advised for overweight (0.6 lb/week) and obese (0.5 lb/week) women.[6]

Women should never diet during pregnancy, even if they begin the pregnancy overweight, because this can lead to nutrient deficiencies for both the mother and the fetus. Instead, women concerned about their weight should consult their physician or a registered dietitian experienced in working with prenatal populations.

Of the total weight gained in pregnancy, 10 to 12 lb are accounted for by the fetus itself, the amniotic fluid, and the placenta (**FIGURE 11.2**). Another 3 to 8 lb represent a natural increase in the volume of the mother's blood and extracellular fluid. A woman

TABLE 11.1 Recommended Weight Gain for Women During Pregnancy[6]

Pre-Pregnancy Weight Status	Body Mass Index (kg/m²)	Recommended Weight Gain (lb)
Normal	18.5–25.0	25–35
Underweight	<18.5	28–40
Overweight	25.1–29.9	15–25
Obese	≥30.0	11–20

low birth weight A weight of less than 5.5 lb at birth.

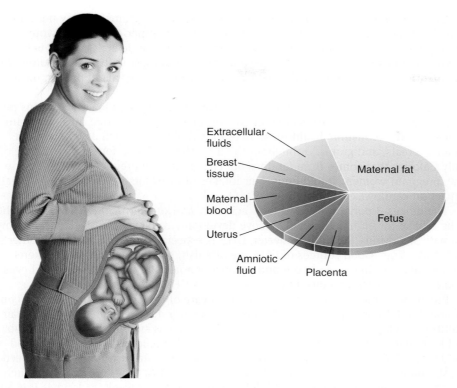

Extracellular fluids

Breast tissue

Maternal blood

Uterus

Amniotic fluid

Placenta

Maternal fat

Fetus

◄ **FIGURE 11.2** The weight gained during pregnancy is distributed between the mother's own tissues and the pregnancy-specific tissues.

can expect to be about 10 to 12 lb lighter immediately after the birth and, within about 2 weeks, another 5 to 8 lb lighter because of fluid loss.

After the first 2 weeks, losing the remainder of the pregnancy weight depends on more energy being expended than is taken in. Appropriate physical activity can help women lose those extra pounds. Also, because the production of breast milk requires significant energy, breastfeeding helps many new mothers lose the remaining weight.

What Are a Pregnant Woman's Nutrient Needs?

The requirements for nearly all nutrients increase during pregnancy to accommodate the growth and development of the fetus without depriving the mother of the nutrients she needs to maintain her own health. The DRI tables located in the end pages of this textbook identify the DRIs for pregnant women in three age groups.

Macronutrient Needs of Pregnant Women

During the first trimester, a woman should maintain approximately the same Calorie intake as during her nonpregnant days. Instead of eating more, she should attempt to maximize the nutrient density of what she eats. For example, she should drink low-fat milk; calcium-fortified soy, almond, or rice milk; or orange juice rather than soft drinks.

During the last two trimesters of pregnancy, energy needs increase by about 350 to 450 kcal/day. For a woman normally consuming 2,000 kcal/day, an extra 400 kcal represents only a 20% increase in energy intake, a goal that can be met more easily than many pregnant women realize. For example, 1 cup of low-fat yogurt and two pieces of whole-wheat toast spread with a tablespoon of peanut butter is about 400 kcal. At the same time, some vitamin and mineral needs increase by 50% or more. The key for getting adequate micronutrients while not consuming too many extra Calories is choosing nutrient-dense foods.

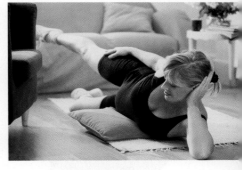

◄ Following a physician-approved exercise program helps pregnant women maintain a positive body image and prevent excess weight gain.

During pregnancy, protein needs increase to about 1.1 grams per day per kilogram of body weight, an increase of about 25 grams of protein per day.[8] Many women already eat this much protein every day. If not, however, it does not take much food to add 25 grams of protein. Remember that yogurt and toast with peanut butter we just mentioned? This light meal provides the additional 25 grams of protein most women need.

Pregnant women should aim for a carbohydrate intake of at least 175 grams per day.[8] Glucose is the primary metabolic fuel of the developing fetus; thus, pregnant women need to consume healthful sources of carbohydrate, such as whole-grain breads, cereals, and grains, throughout the day. The guideline for the percentage of daily Calories that comes from fat does not change during pregnancy. Like anyone else, pregnant women should limit their intakes of *trans* fats because of their negative impact on cardiovascular health.

The omega-3 polyunsaturated fatty acid *docosahexaenoic acid (DHA)* is thought to be critical for both neurologic and eye development. Because the fetal brain grows dramatically during the third trimester, DHA is especially important in the mother's diet at this time. Good sources of DHA are oily fish, such as anchovies, mackerel, salmon, and sardines. It is also found in lower amounts in tuna, chicken, and eggs (some eggs are DHA-enhanced by feeding hens a DHA-rich diet).

Pregnant women who eat fish should be aware of the potential for mercury contamination, because even a limited intake of mercury during pregnancy can impair a fetus's developing nervous system. Large fish, such as swordfish, shark, tile fish, and king mackerel, have high levels of mercury and should be avoided. The Food and Drug Administration recommends that women who are pregnant or breastfeeding should eat at least 8 to 12 oz (2 to 3 servings) of most other types of fish, such as salmon, shrimp, tilapia, cod, and light canned tuna, per week, as long as it is adequately cooked.[9]

Micronutrient Needs of Pregnant Women

The needs for certain micronutrients increase during pregnancy. See **TABLE 11.2** for an overview of these changes. The key micronutrients are discussed in this section.

Folate As noted earlier, adequate folate is critical during the first 28 days after conception, when it is required for the formation and closure of the **neural tube**—an embryonic structure that eventually becomes the brain and spinal cord. Folate deficiency is associated with neural tube defects such as **spina bifida** (**FIGURE 11.3**) and **anencephaly**, a fatal defect in which there is a partial absence of brain tissue.[10] To reduce the risk for a neural tube defect, all women capable of becoming pregnant are encouraged to consume 400 μg of folic acid per day from supplements, fortified foods, or both in addition to a variety of foods naturally high in folate. Adequate folate intake does not guarantee normal neural tube development, because the precise cause of neural tube defects is unknown, and in some cases there is a genetic component.

Folate deficiency can also result in macrocytic anemia (a condition in which blood cells do not mature properly) and has been associated with low birth weight and preterm delivery. The RDA for folate for pregnant women is 600 μg/day, a full 50% increase over the RDA for a nonpregnant female.[10]

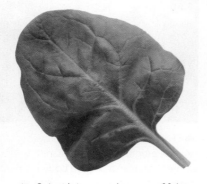

⬆ Spinach is a good source of folate.

neural tube Embryonic tissue that forms a tube, which eventually becomes the brain and spinal cord.

spina bifida An embryonic neural tube defect that occurs when the spinal vertebrae fail to completely enclose the spinal cord, allowing it to protrude.

anencephaly A fatal neural tube defect in which there is a partial absence of brain tissue, most likely caused by failure of the neural tube to close.

TABLE 11.2 **Nutrient Recommendations for Pregnant Adult Women**

Micronutrient	Pre-Pregnancy	Pregnancy	% Increase
Folate	400 μg/day	600 μg/day	50
Vitamin B$_{12}$	2.4 μg/day	2.6 μg/day	8
Vitamin C	75 mg/day	85 mg/day	13
Vitamin A	700 μg/day	770 μg/day	10
Iron	18 mg/day	27 mg/day	50
Zinc	8 mg/day	11 mg/day	38

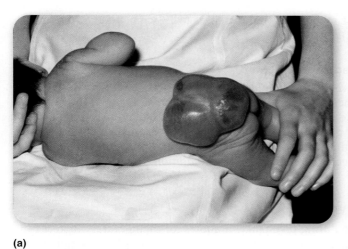

(a)

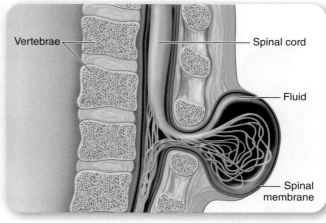

Vertebrae — Spinal cord

— Fluid

— Spinal membrane

(b)

👉 **FIGURE 11.3** Spina bifida, a common neural tube defect. **(a)** An external view of an infant with spina bifida. **(b)** An internal view of the protruding spinal cord tissue and fluid-filled sac.

Vitamin B₁₂ Vitamin B_{12} (cobalamin) is vital during pregnancy, because it regenerates the active form of folate.[10] The RDA for vitamin B_{12} for pregnant women is shown in Table 11.2. It can easily be obtained from animal food sources; however, deficiencies have been observed in women following a vegan diet. Fortified foods and supplementation provide these women with the necessary B_{12}.

Vitamin A As seen in Table 11.2, vitamin A needs increase during pregnancy, and deficiency has been linked to low birth weight and preterm delivery. However, the consumption of excessive amounts of vitamin A, particularly during the first trimester, increases the risk for the birth of an infant with cleft lip or palate, heart defects, and abnormalities of the central nervous system.[11] A well-balanced diet supplies sufficient vitamin A, so supplementation even at low levels is not recommended.

Vitamin D Despite the role of vitamin D in calcium absorption, the RDA for this nutrient does not increase during pregnancy. However, pregnant women with darkly pigmented skin and/or limited sun exposure who do not regularly drink milk will benefit from vitamin D supplementation. Vitamin D can be highly toxic, however, so excessive intakes must be avoided.[12]

Calcium Growth of the fetal skeleton requires calcium. However, the RDA for calcium does not change during pregnancy; it remains at 1,300 mg/day for pregnant adolescents and 1,000 mg/day for adult pregnant women, in part because pregnant women absorb calcium from their diet more efficiently than nonpregnant women.[12]

Iron During pregnancy, the demand for red blood cells increases to accommodate the needs of the expanded maternal blood volume, growing uterus, placenta, and fetus.[11] Thus, more iron is needed (see Table 11.2). Fetal demand for iron increases even further during the last trimester, when the fetus stores iron in the liver for use during the first few months of life. This iron storage is protective for the infant because breast milk is low in iron.

Severely inadequate iron intake certainly has the potential to harm the fetus; however, in most cases, the fetus builds adequate stores by "robbing" maternal iron, prompting iron-deficiency anemia in the mother. During pregnancy, maternal iron deficiency causes pallor and exhaustion, but at birth it endangers her life: anemic women are more likely to die during or shortly after childbirth, because they are less able to tolerate blood loss and fight infection. To ensure adequate iron during pregnancy, an iron supplement (as part of, or separate from, a full-spectrum prenatal supplement) is routinely prescribed during the last two trimesters.

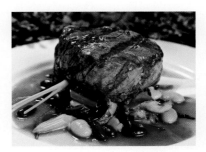

👉 Meats provide protein and heme iron, which are important for both maternal and fetal nutrition.

Zinc Because zinc has critical roles in DNA and protein synthesis, it is very important that adequate zinc status be maintained during pregnancy. The RDA for zinc for

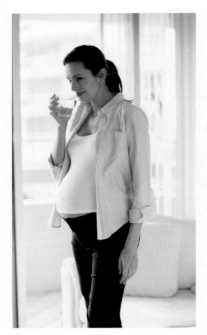

It's important that pregnant women drink about 10 cups of fluid a day.

adult pregnant women is 11 mg per day and increases to 12 mg per day for pregnant adolescents (see Table 11.2).[11]

Do Pregnant Women Need Supplements?

Prenatal multivitamin and mineral supplements are not strictly necessary during pregnancy, but most healthcare providers recommend them. Meeting all the nutrient needs would otherwise take careful and somewhat complex dietary planning. Prenatal supplements are especially good insurance for vegans, adolescents, and others whose diet is low in one or more micronutrients. It is important that pregnant women understand, however, that supplements are to be taken *in addition to*, not as a substitute for, a nutrient-rich diet.

Fluid Needs of Pregnant Women

Fluid plays many vital roles during pregnancy. It allows for the necessary increase in the mother's blood volume, acts as a lubricant, and helps regulate body temperature. Fluid that the mother consumes also helps maintain the **amniotic fluid** that surrounds, cushions, and protects the fetus in the uterus. The AI for fluid intake is approximately 2.3 liters (10 cups) of fluid as beverages, including drinking water.[13]

recap During the last two trimesters of pregnancy, energy needs increase by about 350 to 450 kcal/day. Pregnant women should consume enough energy from nutrient-dense foods to support an appropriate weight gain, typically 25 to 35 lb. Folate deficiency has been associated with neural tube defects. Most healthcare providers recommend prenatal supplements as well as an iron supplement for pregnant women. More fluid is needed during pregnancy to provide for increased maternal blood volume and amniotic fluid.

Nutrition-Related Concerns for Pregnant Women

Conditions involving a particular nutrient, such as neural tube defects and iron-deficiency anemia, have already been discussed. The following are some of the most common discomforts and disorders of pregnant women that are related to their general nutrition.

Morning Sickness

More than half of all pregnant women experience **morning sickness**, or *nausea and vomiting of pregnancy (NVP)*. It is thought to be related at least in part to the effect of pregnancy-related hormones on the brain and gastrointestinal (GI) tract. The symptoms vary from occasional mild queasiness to constant nausea with bouts of vomiting. In truth, "morning sickness" is not an appropriate name because about 80% of pregnant women report that their symptoms last all day. Except in severe cases, the mother and fetus do not suffer lasting harm. However, some women experience such frequent vomiting that they require hospitalization.

There is no cure for morning sickness. However, some women find it helpful to snack lightly throughout the day rather than consuming three larger meals. Greasy and high-fat foods should be avoided, as should strong cooking odors. Some women find that cold or room-temperature foods are less likely to cause nausea. Alternative therapies such as meditation, biofeedback, and acupressure wrist bands may also help.

Food Cravings

It seems as if nothing is more stereotypical about pregnancy than the image of a frazzled husband getting up in the middle of the night to run to the convenience store to get his pregnant wife some pickles and ice cream. This image, although humorous, is far from reality. Although some women have specific cravings, most crave a type of food (such as "something sweet" or "something salty") rather than a particular food.

amniotic fluid The watery fluid contained in the innermost membrane of the sac containing the fetus. It cushions and protects the growing fetus.

morning sickness Varying degrees of nausea and vomiting associated with pregnancy, most commonly in the first trimester.

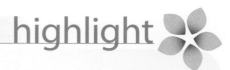

highlight

The Danger of Nonfood Cravings

A few weeks after her nurse told her she was pregnant, Darlene started feeling "funny." She'd experience bouts of nausea lasting several hours every day, and her appetite seemed to disappear. At the grocery store, she'd wander through the aisles with an empty cart, confused about what foods she should be choosing for her growing baby and unable to find anything that appealed to her. Eventually, she'd return home with a few things: frozen macaroni and cheese dinners, cereal bars, orange and grape soda—and a large bag of ice. She took cupfuls of ice from the soda machine at the assembly plant where she worked and ate it throughout the day. Each weekend, she went through more than a boxful of popsicles to "settle her stomach." Even her favorite strawberry ice cream no longer appealed to her.

At Darlene's next checkup, her nurse became concerned because she had lost weight. "I want to eat the stuff like in those pictures you gave me," Darlene confessed, "but I don't like it very much." She was too embarrassed to admit to anyone, even the nurse, that the only thing she really wanted to eat was ice.

Some people contend that a pregnant woman with unusual food cravings is intuitively seeking needed nutrients. Arguing against this theory is the phenomenon of *pica*—the craving and consumption of nonfood material, which often occurs during pregnancy. A woman with pica may crave ice, clay, dirt, chalk, coffee grounds, baking soda, laundry starch, or any other substance. The cause of these nonfood cravings is not known; however, people with developmental disabilities are at increased risk. Lower socioeconomic status and

family stress have also been implicated, as have cultural factors. For example, in the United States, pica is more common among pregnant African American women than women from other racial or ethnic groups. The practice of eating clay has been traced to central Africa, and researchers theorize that people taken from central Africa and sent as slaves to the United States brought the practice with them. In addition, nutrient deficiencies have been associated with pica, although it is not at all clear that nutrient deficiencies cause it. In fact, the inhibition of nutrient absorption caused by the ingestion of clay and other substances may produce nutrient deficiency.

No matter the cause, pica is dangerous. Consuming ice can lead to inadequate weight gain if, as with Darlene, the ice substitutes for food. The ingestion of clay, starch, and other substances can not only inhibit absorption of nutrients but also cause constipation, intestinal blockage, and even excessive weight gain. Women with pica are known to be at risk for high lead exposure, which may impair the neurodevelopment of the fetus and increase the risk for pregnancy-related complications. The ingestion of certain substances, such as dish-washing liquid, can lead to such severe vomiting and diarrhea that the individual experiences electrolyte disturbances that lead to seizures or death.

Some pregnant women with pica find food items they can substitute for the craved nonfood—for instance, peanut butter for clay or nonfat powdered milk for starch. If a woman experiences pica, she should talk with her healthcare provider immediately.

Most cravings are, of course, for edible substances. But a surprising number of pregnant women crave nonfoods, such as laundry starch, chalk, and clay. This craving, called **pica**, is the subject of the *Highlight* box.

Gestational Diabetes

Gestational diabetes is defined as impaired glucose tolerance identified during pregnancy. New diagnostic standards will nearly double the frequency of diagnosed gestational diabetes, to a level as high as 18% of pregnant women.[14] It is usually a temporary condition in which a pregnant woman is unable to produce enough insulin or becomes insulin resistant, resulting in elevated levels of blood glucose. Obesity is a common risk factor. Because of the high rate of obesity among young women and the new diagnostic criteria, it is expected that the number of women diagnosed with gestational diabetes will greatly increase in the next few years.

As many as 10% of women with gestational diabetes develop type 2 diabetes shortly after the birth, and 40% to 60% will become diabetic over the next 10 to 20 years. Fortunately, gestational diabetes has no short-term ill effects on the fetus if blood glucose levels are strictly controlled through diet, physical activity, and/or medication. Over the long term, however, the offspring of women with gestational diabetes may remain at higher risk for type 2 diabetes and other disorders. If blood glucose

pica An abnormal craving to eat something not fit for food, such as clay, chalk, paint, or other nonfood substances.

gestational diabetes In a pregnant woman, insufficient insulin production or insulin resistance that results in consistently high blood glucose levels; the condition typically resolves after birth occurs.

is not adequately controlled, gestational diabetes can result in a type of maternal high blood pressure, discussed in the next section. It can also result in a baby that is too large as a result of receiving too much glucose across the placenta during fetal life. Infants who are overly large are at risk for early birth and trauma during vaginal birth and may need to be delivered by cesarean section.

Hypertensive Disorders of Pregnancy

About 7% to 8% of U.S. pregnant women develop some form of hypertension, or high blood pressure, yet it accounts for almost 16% of pregnancy-related deaths. A woman who develops high blood pressure during pregnancy, with no other complications, is diagnosed with *gestational hypertension.* A more complex and severe hypertensive disorder during pregnancy is *preeclampsia,* in which the elevated blood pressure is accompanied by sudden weight gain and loss of protein in the urine. If left untreated, hypertensive disorders during pregnancy can lead to seizures and kidney failure that are life-threatening for both the mother and the fetus.

No one knows exactly what causes hypertensive disorders during pregnancy, but deficiencies in dietary protein, vitamin C, vitamin E, calcium, and magnesium seem to increase the risk. Pregnant adolescents and women who are pregnant for the first time are at higher risk, as are African American and low-income women. Management focuses mainly on blood pressure control. Typical treatment includes medication and close medical oversight. In nearly all women without a history of hypertension, blood pressure returns to normal within about a day after childbirth.

⬆ Pregnant women should have their blood pressure measured to test for gestational hypertension.

Adolescent Pregnancy

The adolescent birthrate in the United States has fallen to its lowest level in the past 60 years: 29.4 births for every 1,000 women aged 15 to 19 years. Nevertheless, this rate is among the highest of all industrialized nations.[15] Adolescents who become pregnant face greater nutritional challenges than adult women for several reasons:

- An adolescent's body is still changing and growing: peak bone mass has not yet been reached, and full stature may not have been attained. This demand for tissue growth keeps calorie and nutrient needs during adolescence very high. Iron-deficiency anemia is common among pregnant adolescents, increasing the risk for preterm birth and other complications.
- Many adolescents have not yet established healthful eating patterns, yet as shown in **TABLE 11.3**, pregnant adolescents have increased nutrient needs compared to non-pregnant adolescents.
- Pregnant adolescents are less likely than older women to receive early and regular prenatal care.
- Pregnant adolescents are more likely to smoke and less likely to understand the consequences of prenatal smoking, alcohol consumption, and drug abuse.
- Pregnant adolescents with excessive prenatal weight gain are more likely to retain the excess weight after delivery than are adult women, increasing their risk for adult obesity.

TABLE 11.3   Differences in Nutrient Recommendations Between Nonpregnant and Pregnant Adolescents

Nutrient	Nonpregnant Adolescent	Pregnant Adolescent	% Increase
Folate	400 µg/day	600 µg/day	50
Vitamin B$_{12}$	2.4 µg/day	2.6 µg/day	8
Vitamin C	65 mg/day	80 mg/day	23
Vitamin A	700 µg/day	750 µg/day	7
Iron	15 mg/day	27 mg/day	80
Zinc	9 mg/day	12 mg/day	33
Iodine	150 µg/day	220 µg/day	47

With regular prenatal care and close attention to proper nutrition and other healthful behaviors, both the adolescent mother and her infant are as likely to have positive outcomes as are older mothers and their infants.

Vegetarianism

With the possible exception of iron and zinc, vegetarian women who consume dairy products and eggs (lacto-ovo-vegetarians) have no nutritional concerns beyond those encountered by every pregnant woman. In contrast, women who are vegan need to pay more attention than usual to their intake of nutrients that are derived primarily or wholly from animal products. These include vitamin D (unless regularly exposed to sunlight throughout the pregnancy), vitamin B_6, vitamin B_{12}, calcium, iron, and zinc. Supplements and/or fortified foods containing these nutrients are usually necessary.

Consumption of Caffeine

Caffeine readily crosses the placenta and thus quickly reaches the fetus, but at what dose and to what extent it causes fetal harm is still a subject of controversy and study. There is general agreement that women who consume less than about 200 mg of caffeine per day (the equivalent of one to two small cups of coffee) are not harming the fetus. Evidence suggests that consuming higher daily doses of caffeine (the higher the dose, the stronger the evidence) may slightly increase the risk for miscarriage, stillbirth, and other problems for the fetus. It is sensible, then, for pregnant women to limit daily caffeine intake to no more than the equivalent of one 12-ounce cup of coffee.[16]

Consumption of Alcohol

Alcohol is a known teratogen that readily crosses the placenta and accumulates in the fetal bloodstream. The immature fetal liver cannot readily metabolize alcohol, and its presence in fetal blood and tissues is associated with a variety of birth defects, including *fetal alcohol syndrome* (see Chapter 8). According to the CDC, approximately 8 percent of U.S. pregnant women report drinking alcohol, and 2 percent admit to binge drinking, consuming 4 or more drinks at one sitting.[17]

Heavy drinking during the first trimester typically results in fetal malformations such as heart defects and facial abnormalities. Because many women do not even realize they are pregnant until several weeks after conception, public health officials recommend not only that pregnant women abstain from all alcoholic beverages, but also women who are trying to become pregnant or suspect they may be pregnant should abstain.

Smoking

Several components and metabolites of tobacco are toxic to the fetus, including lead, cyanide, nicotine, and carbon monoxide. Fetal nourishment, growth, and development may be impaired by reduced oxygen levels in fetal blood and reduced placental blood flow.

Maternal smoking greatly increases the risk for miscarriage, stillbirth, placental abnormalities, poor fetal growth, preterm delivery, and low birth weight.[18] The effects of maternal smoking continue after birth: sudden infant death syndrome (SIDS) and respiratory illnesses occur with greater frequency in the children of smokers than the children of nonsmokers.

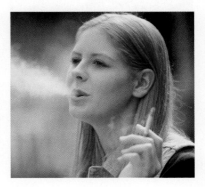

Cigarette smoking may interfere with nutrient metabolism.

Legal and Illegal Drugs

The U.S. Food and Drug Administration (FDA) rigorously tests prescription and over-the-counter medications for safety and effectiveness; however, little is known about the effects of many of these drugs on fetal development. In general, pregnant women should consult their healthcare provider about continuing to use any medication, especially in the first trimester.

In 2011, 5% of pregnant women in the United States used illicit drugs. Many street drugs decrease oxygen and nutrient delivery to the fetus by reducing placental blood flow.[19] As a result, the child may suffer from developmental disabilities. All women are strongly advised to stop taking illegal drugs *before* becoming pregnant. If a woman using illegal drugs discovers she is pregnant, she should seek healthcare immediately.

Herbal Supplements

Many pregnant women feel that, as "natural" products, herbals are safe. This is a dangerous assumption. Herbal supplements typically are not tested for purity, safety, or effectiveness. Pregnant women should always consult with their healthcare provider before using any type of herbal product.

Food Safety

Because of the risk for foodborne illness, pregnant women should avoid a few specific foods. These include unpasteurized milk; raw or partially cooked eggs; raw or undercooked meat, fish, or poultry; unpasteurized juices; and raw sprouts. Soft cheeses, such as Brie, feta, Camembert, Roquefort, and Mexican-style cheeses, also called *queso blanco* or *queso fresco,* should be avoided unless they are clearly labeled as made with pasteurized milk.

As discussed earlier, fish is an excellent source of the omega-3 essential fatty acid DHA and, in appropriate amounts, is a healthful addition to a balanced prenatal diet. However, certain types of fish should be avoided because of their high mercury content.[9] All fish should be thoroughly cooked to kill any disease-causing bacteria or parasites. Pregnant women should avoid sushi and other raw fish, as well as raw oysters and clams.

To view a slide show on exercise during and after pregnancy, go to www.webmd.com. Enter "pregnancy fitness moves slideshow" in the search bar, then click on the first link.

Maintaining Fitness

Exercise can help keep a woman physically fit during pregnancy. Other benefits of exercise during pregnancy include the following:[20]

- Exercise improves mood, helping women feel more in control of their changing body, increasing self confidence and reducing postpartum depression.
- Expending additional energy through exercise compensates for extra energy consumed when a ravenous appetite kicks in.
- Regular moderate exercise reduces the risk for pregnancy-related complications such as gestational diabetes, helps keep blood pressure down, and offers all the cardiovascular benefits seen in nonpregnant individuals.
- Regular exercise can shorten the duration of active labor.
- A woman who exercises throughout pregnancy will have an easier time resuming a fitness routine and losing weight after the birth.

If a woman was not active prior to pregnancy, she should begin an exercise program slowly and progress gradually under the guidance of her healthcare provider. Federal guidelines recommend that pregnant women get at least 150 minutes of moderate-intensity aerobic activity per week. Brisk walking, hiking, swimming, and water aerobics are excellent choices. Healthy women who already do vigorous-intensity aerobic activity, such as running, or more than 150 minutes of activity can continue doing so during and after their pregnancy provided they stay healthy and discuss with their healthcare provider how and when activity should be adjusted over time.[21]

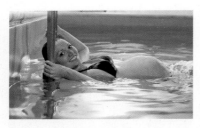

⬆ During pregnancy, women should adjust their physical activity to comfortable, low-impact exercises.

recap Pregnant women may experience a variety of nutrition-related concerns during pregnancy, from morning sickness to gestational diabetes. These can seriously affect maternal and fetal health. Because adolescents' bodies are still growing and developing, their nutrient needs during pregnancy become so high that adequate nourishment for the mother and baby becomes difficult. Women who follow a vegan diet usually need to consume multivitamin and mineral supplements during pregnancy. Any use of alcohol, illegal drugs, and tobacco can be dangerous to the woman and her fetus. Pregnant women should avoid certain foods associated with foodborne illness. Exercise (provided the mother has no contraindications) can enhance the health of a pregnant woman.

Nutrition in infancy

In the first year of life, infants generally grow about 10 inches and triple their weight—a growth rate more rapid than will ever occur again. At the same time, their limited physical activity means that the majority of their energy expenditure is to support growth.

LO4 Discuss the advantages and challenges of breastfeeding.

LO5 Discuss nutrient needs, timing of introduction to and type of solid foods, and common nutrition-related concerns of infants.

What Are the Benefits of Breastfeeding?

Throughout most of human history, infants have thrived on only one food: breast milk. Breastfeeding is universally recognized as the ideal method of infant feeding because of the nutritional quality and health benefits of breast milk.[22] La Leche League International is an advocacy group for breastfeeding: its publications, website, and local meetings are all valuable resources for breastfeeding mothers and their families. Many hospitals and HMOs also offer breastfeeding classes.

Nutritional Quality of Breast Milk

During pregnancy, the woman's body is prepared to produce breast milk by the development of the milk-producing glands, called *alveoli* (**FIGURE 11.4**). At birth, changing hormone levels stimulate milk production. In the first few days after birth, the breast milk is called **colostrum**. This yellowish fluid is rich in protein, vitamins A and E, and antibodies that help protect the newborn from infection.

Within 2 to 4 days, colostrum is replaced by mature breast milk. The amount and types of proteins in breast milk are ideally suited to the human infant: they are easily digested in the infant's immature GI tract, reducing the risk for gastric distress; they prevent the growth of harmful bacteria; and they include antibodies that help prevent infection while the infant's immune system is still immature.

The primary carbohydrate in breast milk is lactose. Lactose provides energy and promotes the growth of beneficial gut bacteria. It also aids in the absorption of calcium. Breast milk has more lactose than cow's milk does.

As with protein, the amount and types of fat in breast milk are ideally suited to the human infant, especially omega-3 DHA and omega-6 arachidonic acid (ARA), which have been shown to be essential for the growth and development of the infant's nervous system and the retina of the eyes. Many people are surprised to learn that the fat content of breast milk is higher than that of whole cow's milk. The energy provided by these fats, however, supports the rapid rate of growth during the first year of life.

The fat content of breast milk actually changes during the course of every feeding: the milk that is first released is watery and is thought to satisfy the infant's initial thirst. As the feeding continues, the fat content increases, until the very last 5% or so of the milk produced is similar to cream. This milk is thought to trigger a sense of fullness, prompting the infant to stop nursing. Breast milk is also relatively high in cholesterol, which supports the rapid growth and development of the brain and nervous system.

Breast milk is a good source of readily absorbed calcium and magnesium. It is low in iron, but the iron it does contain is easily absorbed (recall that the fetus stores iron in preparation for the first few months of life). Most experts agree that breast milk can meet the iron needs of full-term healthy infants for the first 6 months, after which iron-rich foods are needed.

Breast milk alone is entirely sufficient to sustain an infant for the first 6 months of life. Throughout the next 6 months of infancy, as solid foods are gradually introduced, breast milk remains the baby's primary source of superior-quality nutrition. The

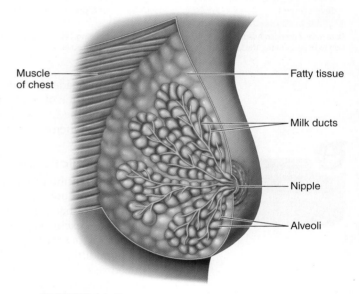

Muscle of chest · Fatty tissue · Milk ducts · Nipple · Alveoli

FIGURE 11.4 Anatomy of the breast. During pregnancy, hormones secreted by the placenta prepare the breast for lactation.

colostrum The first fluid made and secreted by the breasts from late in pregnancy to about a week after birth. It is rich in immune factors and protein.

TABLE 11.4 Benefits of Breastfeeding

Benefits to Infant	Benefits to Mother	Benefits to Family/Society
Provides superior level and balance of nutrients for infant growth, health, and development	Increases level of oxytocin, resulting in less postpartum bleeding and more rapid return of uterus to pre-pregnant state	Reduces healthcare costs and employee absenteeism for care attributable to infant/child illness
Decreases incidence and severity of a wide range of infectious diseases, including diarrhea, bacterial meningitis, and respiratory infections	Delays resumption of menstrual periods, causing reduced menstrual blood loss over the months after the birth and preserving maternal iron	Decreases family food expenditures: cost of purchasing extra food for lactating mother is less than half the cost of purchasing infant formula
Is associated with decreased risk for both type 1 and type 2 diabetes	Delays resumption of ovulation and thereby increases spacing between pregnancies	Decreases environmental burden for production and transport of formula, bottles, artificial nipples, and so on
Has possible protective effect against sudden infant death syndrome (SIDS), several chronic digestive diseases, leukemia, lymphoma, Hodgkin disease, asthma, and allergies	Promotes an earlier return to pre-pregnancy weight	Reduces caregiver time away from infant/siblings to prepare infant food: breast milk requires no preparation and is always the perfect temperature
Is associated with reduced risk for childhood and adulthood overweight and obesity	Improves bone remineralization in months after birth	
Is associated with enhanced cognitive development	Reduces the woman's risk for ovarian cancer and premenopausal breast cancer	

Data from: American Academy of Pediatrics, Section on Breastfeeding. February 2005. Policy Statement: Breastfeeding and the use of human milk. *Ped.* 115(2):496–506. In addition to these benefits, the La Leche League and other breastfeeding advocacy organizations identify emotional and psychological benefits of skin-to-skin suckling.

American Academy of Pediatrics (AAP) encourages exclusive breastfeeding (no food or other source of nourishment) for the first 6 months of life, continuing breastfeeding for at least the first year of life and, if acceptable within the family unit, into the second year of life or longer.[22]

Immunologic Benefits for Breastfed Infants

Protective antibodies and immune cells are passed directly from the mother to the newborn through breast milk. It has been shown that breastfed infants have a lower incidence of bacterial infections. In fact, it has been estimated that, if 90% of U.S. infants were exclusively breastfed for 6 months, medical expenses would be decreased by $13 billion per year and over 900 infant deaths would be prevented.[23]

In addition, breast milk is nonallergenic, and breastfeeding is associated with a reduced risk for wheezing, asthma, and cow's milk allergies during infancy, childhood, and adulthood. Breastfed babies also die less frequently from **sudden infant death syndrome (SIDS)** and have a decreased chance of developing diabetes, overweight and obesity, hypercholesterolemia, and chronic digestive disorders in later life.

Physiologic Benefits for the Mother

Breastfeeding causes uterine contractions that speed the return of the uterus to prepregnancy size and reduce bleeding. Many women also find that breastfeeding helps them lose the weight they gained during pregnancy, particularly if they breastfeed for more than 6 months.

Breastfeeding also suppresses **ovulation**, lengthening the time between pregnancies and giving a mother's body the chance to recover before she conceives again. Ovulation may not cease completely, however, so it is still possible to become pregnant while breastfeeding. The benefits of breastfeeding are summarized in **TABLE 11.4**.

Effects of Drugs and Other Substances on Breast Milk

Many substances make their way into breast milk, including illegal and prescription drugs, over-the-counter drugs, and even substances from foods the mother eats. All illegal drugs should be assumed to pass into breast milk and should be avoided by breastfeeding mothers. Prescription drugs vary in the degree to which they pass into breast milk. Breastfeeding mothers should inform their healthcare provider that they

Visit the La Leche League home page, where you'll find answer pages, podcasts, and links to breastfeeding families, at www.llli.org.

sudden infant death syndrome (SIDS) A condition marked by the sudden death of a previously healthy infant; the most common cause of death in infants more than 1 month of age.

ovulation The release of an ovum (egg) from a woman's ovary.

are breastfeeding. In some cases, a woman may be advised to switch to formula feeding while she is taking a certain medication.

Caffeine, alcohol, and nicotine all rapidly enter breast milk. Caffeine can make the baby agitated and fussy, whereas alcohol can make the baby sleepy and, over time, slow motor development, in addition to inhibiting the mother's milk supply. Nicotine interferes with infant sleep patterns, and maternal smoking increases the risk for respiratory illness in the infant.

Some substances that the mother eats, such as compounds found in garlic, onions, peppers, broccoli, and cabbage, are distasteful enough to the infant to prevent proper feeding. Although some high-risk babies may have allergic reactions to foods the mother has eaten, such as wheat, cow's milk, or eggs, there is no strong evidence that limiting maternal food choices during lactation provides additional protection against infant allergies.

Although environmental contaminants can enter the breast milk, the benefits of breastfeeding almost always outweigh potential risks. Fresh fruits and vegetables eaten by lactating women should be thoroughly washed and peeled to minimize exposure to pesticide and fertilizer residues. The mother's exposure to solvents, paints, gasoline fumes, furniture strippers, and similar products should also be limited.

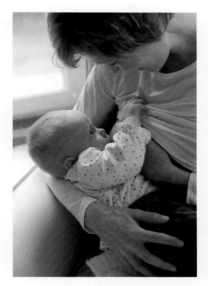

Breastfeeding has important benefits for both the mother and the infant.

What Are a Breastfeeding Woman's Nutrient Needs?

You might be surprised to learn that breastfeeding requires even more energy and nutrients than pregnancy! This is because breast milk has to supply an adequate amount of all the nutrients an infant needs to grow and develop. The current DRIs during breastfeeding (also called *lactation*) are listed in tables at the back of this textbook.

Nutrient Recommendations for Breastfeeding Women

It's estimated that milk production requires about 700 to 800 kcal/day. It is generally recommended that breastfeeding women aged 19 years and above consume 330 kcal/day above their pre-pregnancy energy needs during the first 6 months of breastfeeding and 400 additional kcal/day during the second 6 months.[8] This additional energy is sufficient to support milk production while allowing for an energy deficit that helps women gradually lose any excess weight gained during pregnancy. It is very important that breastfeeding women avoid severe energy restriction, because this practice can decrease milk production.

Of the macronutrients, carbohydrate and protein needs are increased. An additional 15 to 25 grams of protein/day and 80 grams of carbohydrate/day above pre-pregnancy requirements are recommended.[8]

Although the needs for several vitamins and minerals increase over the requirements of pregnancy, the DRI for iron decreases significantly—to just 9 mg/day.[11] This is because iron is not a significant component of breast milk, and breastfeeding usually suppresses menstruation for at least a few months, reducing iron losses. The recommended calcium intake for a lactating woman is the same as for all women between the ages of 19 and 50 years—that is, 1,000 mg/day. Because of their own continuing growth, however, teen mothers who are breastfeeding should continue to consume 1,300 mg/day.[12]

Do Breastfeeding Women Need Supplements?

If a breastfeeding woman appropriately increases her energy intake and does so with nutrient-dense foods, her nutrient needs can usually be met without supplements. However, there is nothing wrong with taking a basic multivitamin for insurance, as long as it is not considered a substitute for proper nutrition. Breastfeeding women should consume omega-3 fatty acids either in fish or supplements to support the infant's developing nervous system, and women who don't consume dairy products should monitor their calcium and vitamin D intakes carefully. Women following a vegan diet should consume a vitamin B_{12} supplement or include B_{12}–fortified foods in their diets.

Fluid Recommendations for Breastfeeding Women

Because fluid is lost with every feeding, lactating women need to consume about an extra quart (about 1 liter) of fluid per day. The AI for fluid recommends about 13 cups of beverages each day to facilitate milk production and prevent dehydration.[13]

What Is the Nutritional Quality of Infant Formula?

Women with certain infectious diseases are advised not to breastfeed, as are women using certain prescription medications and women who abuse drugs.[22] Other women choose not to breastfeed for other reasons. If breastfeeding is not feasible, several types of commercial formulas provide nutritious alternatives. Most formulas are based on cow's milk that is modified to make it more appropriate for human infants. Soy-based formulas are a good alternative for infants who are lactose intolerant (although this is rare in infants) or who cannot tolerate the proteins in cow's milk–based formulas. Soy formulas may also satisfy the requirements of families who are strict vegans. However, soy-based formulas are not without controversy. Because soy contains isoflavones, or plant forms of estrogens, there is some concern over the effects these compounds have on growing infants. In addition, soy itself is a common allergen.

Cow's milk should *not* be introduced to infants under 1 year of age. Cow's milk is too high in protein, and the protein is difficult to digest, leading to gastrointestinal bleeding. In addition, cow's milk has too much sodium, too little iron, and a poor balance of other vitamins and minerals for infants. Goat's milk, soy milk, almond milk, and rice milk are also inappropriate for infants.

When bottle-feeding an infant, parents and caretakers need to pay close attention to their infant's cues for hunger and fullness. Although most parents instinctively recognize when their baby needs to eat, it is often harder for them to know when to stop. Some infants turn their head away from the nipple or tightly close their lips; others simply nod off or fall asleep. Older infants may actually push away the bottle or initiate playlike behaviors.

Once the baby's teeth start coming in, he or she should not be allowed to fall asleep while sucking on the bottle. This practice allows the formula to pool around the teeth and, without the normal release of saliva that occurs when the baby is awake, can lead to a form of severe dental decay known as *baby bottle syndrome* **(FIGURE 11.5)**.

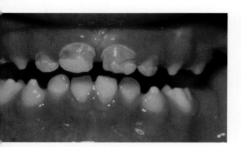

FIGURE 11.5 Leaving a baby alone with a bottle can result in the tooth decay of baby bottle syndrome.

What Are an Infant's Nutrient Needs?

Three characteristics of infants combine to make their nutritional needs unique. These are (1) their high energy needs compared with their body weight, (2) their immature digestive tracts and kidneys, and (3) their small body size. The DRIs for infants are based on the nutrient values of breast milk and are listed in the tables at the back of this textbook.

Macronutrient Needs of Infants

Infants grow rapidly and need to consume about 40 to 50 kcal/pound of body weight per day. About 40% to 50% of an infant's caloric intake should come from fat. Intakes below this level can be harmful before the age of 2 years. Omega-6 and omega-3 fatty acids are essential for the rapid brain growth, retinal maturation, and nervous system development that happen in the first 1 to 2 years of life.

Although carbohydrate and protein are also essential for infant growth and development, no more than 20% of an infant's daily energy requirement should come from protein. Immature kidneys are not able to process and excrete the excess nitrogen from higher protein diets.

Micronutrient Needs of Infants

Breast milk and commercial formulas provide most of the vitamins and minerals infants need. However, several micronutrients may warrant supplementation.

All infants are routinely given an injection of vitamin K shortly after birth. This provides vitamin K until the infant's intestines can develop their own healthful bacteria, which then provide the needed vitamin K.

Breast milk is low in vitamin D, and deficiencies of this nutrient are common, especially in breastfed infants with darkly pigmented skin and those with limited sunlight exposure. Thus, breastfed infants are commonly prescribed a vitamin D supplement, even in sunny climates.[22] Vitamin D deficiency is also becoming more common in formula-fed infants, particularly dark-skinned infants, those with low sun exposure, and those consuming less than 1 liter (32 ounces) of infant formula per day.

Breastfed infants also require additional iron beginning no later than 6 months of age, because the infant's iron stores become depleted and breast milk is a poor source of iron. Iron is extremely important for mental and physical development and the prevention of iron-deficiency anemia. Infant rice cereal fortified with iron, an excellent choice as a first food, can serve as an additional iron source, as can puréed meats. Many infant formulas are already fortified with iron, thus formula-fed infants rarely need an iron supplement.

Depending on the fluoride content of the household water supply, breastfed infants over the age of 6 months may need a fluoride supplement. Most brands of bottled water have low levels of fluoride, and many home water treatment systems remove fluoride. On the other hand, fluoride toxicity may be a risk for infants simultaneously exposed to fluoridated toothpaste and rinses, fluoridated water, and fluoride supplements.

There are special conditions in which additional supplements may be needed for breastfed infants. For example, a vegan mother's breast milk may be low in vitamin B_{12}, and a supplement of this vitamin should be given to the baby.

Fluid Recommendations for Infants

Fluid is critical for everyone, but for infants the balance is more delicate for two reasons. First, infants have a relatively large body surface area, so they proportionally lose more water through evaporation than adults do. Second, their kidneys are immature and unable to concentrate urine. As a result, they are at increased risk for dehydration. An infant needs about 2 fl. oz of fluid per pound of body weight, and either breast milk or formula is almost always adequate in providing this amount. Experts have confirmed that "infants exclusively fed human milk do not require supplemental water."[13] To save money, some families dilute infant formula with extra water. This practice is extremely dangerous. Overhydration can cause nutrient imbalances, such as hyponatremia (low blood sodium), as well as inadequate weight gain and failure to thrive.

recap Breast milk provides superior nutrition and heightened immunity for infants. Mothers who breastfeed experience the benefit of increased post-pregnancy weight loss and suppressed ovulation. If breastfeeding is not feasible, several types of commercial formulas provide nutritious alternatives. Vitamin D supplements may be recommended for exclusively breastfed infants; iron and fluoride supplements may be prescribed for infants older than 6 months of age.

When Do Infants Begin to Need Solid Foods?

Despite recommendations from the American Academy of Pediatrics that infants not be given solid foods before the age of 4 months, nearly 40% of mothers report doing just that.[24] Before 4 to 6 months of age, however, most infants are not physically or developmentally able to consume solid food. The suckling response, present at birth, depends on a particular movement of the tongue that draws liquid out of a breast or bottle. When very young infants are spoon-fed solid food, the *extrusion reflex* causes most of the food to be pushed back out of the mouth. This reflex action must begin to subside before solid foods can be successfully introduced, typically after 4 to 6 months of age.

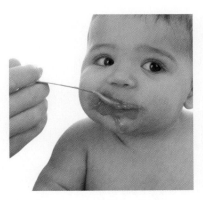

The extrusion reflex will push solid food out of an infant's mouth.

In addition, to minimize the risk of choking or gagging, the infant must have gained muscular control of the head and neck. The infant must also be able to sit up (with or without support).

An infant is also not ready for solid foods until the digestive system has matured. Infants are able to digest and absorb lactose from the time of their birth; however, they lack adequate levels of the enzyme amylase, for the digestion of starch, until the age of 3 to 4 months. If an infant is fed solid foods too soon, starches remain undigested, contributing to diarrhea and bloating, and proteins can be absorbed intact and undigested, setting the stage for allergies. In addition, the kidneys must have matured so that they are better able to process electrolytes and nitrogen waste products, as well as properly concentrate urine.

When deciding which foods to introduce first, parents must consider their infant's nutrient needs and the risk for an allergic reaction. At about 6 months of age, infant iron stores become depleted; thus, the first food introduced is often iron-fortified infant cereal. Rice cereal rarely triggers an allergic response and is easy to digest. Cereal and other solid foods should always be fed to the infant from a spoon, not placed into a bottle.

Parents should not introduce another new food for at least 4 to 5 days to carefully watch for signs of a food allergy or intolerance, including a rash, unexplained diarrhea, runny nose, or wheezing. If all goes well with the rice cereal, another single-grain cereal (other than wheat, which is highly allergenic) can be introduced, or the family may choose to introduce a different single-item food, such as a strained vegetable or meat. Some nutritionists recommend pureed meats or poultry because they are good sources of iron and zinc, whereas others encourage the introduction of vitamin C–rich vegetables. It is wise to introduce strained vegetables before fruits because, once a child becomes accustomed to the sweetness of bananas, peaches, and other fruits, the relative blandness of most vegetables may be less appealing.

Commercial baby foods are convenient and are typically made without added salt or sugar; however, homemade baby foods are usually cheaper and reflect the food patterns of the family. Gradually, a variety of foods should be introduced to the infant by the end of the first year. Throughout the first year, solid foods should only be a supplement to, not a substitute for, breast milk or formula.

What Not to Feed an Infant

The following foods should *never* be offered to an infant:

- *Foods that could cause choking:* Foods such as grapes, chunks of hot dogs or cheese, nuts, popcorn, raw carrots, raisins, and hard candies cannot be chewed adequately by infants and can cause choking.
- *Corn syrup and honey:* These may contain spores of the bacterium *Clostridium botulinum*. These spores can produce a toxin that can be fatal. Children older than 1 year can safely consume these substances because their digestive tract is mature enough to kill any *C. botulinum* spores.
- *Alternatives to breast milk or infant formula*, including cow's milk, goat's milk, soy milk, almond milk, and rice milk. These beverages are too high in certain nutrients and too low in others for infant nutrition. Children can begin to consume these milks after their first birthday.
- *Large quantities of fruit juices:* Fruit juices are poorly absorbed in the infant digestive tract, causing diarrhea if consumed in excess. There is no nutritional reason to feed fruit juice to infants younger than 6 months of age; infants 6 to 12 months should be limited to 4 to 6 oz of 100% pasteurized fruit juice (no sweeteners added) per day, with no more than 2 to 4 oz given at a time.
- *Too much salt and sugar:* Infant foods should not be prepared with added salt or other seasonings. Cookies, cakes, and other excessively sweet, processed foods should be avoided.
- *Too much breast milk or formula:* As nutritious as breast milk and formula are, once infants reach the age of 6 months, solid foods should be introduced gradually. Six months of age is a critical time; it is when a baby's iron stores begin to be depleted. Overreliance on breast milk or formula can result in a condition known as *milk anemia*.

For a list of foods that increase a child's risk for choking, go to www.choosemyplate.gov and type "choking hazards" into the search bar. Click on the first link.

recap In the absence of breastfeeding, commercial formulas provide adequate nutrition for infants. Solid foods can gradually be introduced into an infant's diet at 4 to 6 months of age, beginning with rice cereal, then moving to single-item vegetables or meats. Parents should avoid foods that represent a choking hazard, foods containing honey or corn syrup, alternatives to breast milk or formula, and foods and beverages high in salt and sugar.

Nutrition-Related Concerns for Infants

Nutrition is one of the biggest concerns of new parents. Infants cannot speak, and their cries are sometimes indecipherable. Feeding time can be frustrating for parents, especially if the child is not eating, not growing appropriately, or has problems such as diarrhea, vomiting, or persistent skin rashes. Following are some nutrition-related concerns for infants.

Allergies

As noted earlier, breastfeeding minimizes the risk for allergy development, as does delaying the introduction of solid foods until 4 to 6 months of age. One of the most common allergies in infants is to the proteins in cow's milk–based formulas. Egg whites, peanuts and other nuts, wheat, soy, and citrus are other common allergens.

Each new food should be introduced in isolation, so that any allergic reaction can be identified and the particular food avoided. If there is a strong family history of food allergies, parents should be especially watchful when introducing new foods to their infant and should examine food and beverage labels closely for offending ingredients.

Colic

Perhaps nothing is more frustrating to new parents than the relentless crying spells of some infants, typically referred to as **colic**. In this condition, infants who appear happy, healthy, and well nourished suddenly begin to cry or even shriek and continue for hours, no matter what their caregiver does to console them. The spells tend to occur at the same time of day, typically late in the afternoon or early in the evening, and often occur daily for a period of several weeks. Overstimulation of the nervous system, feeding too rapidly, swallowing of air, and intestinal gas pain are considered possible culprits, but the precise cause is unknown. For breastfed infants, colic spells are sometimes reduced when the mother switches to a bland diet. For formula-fed infants, a change in the type of formula sometimes helps.

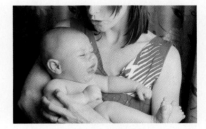

Colicky babies will begin crying for no apparent reason, even if they otherwise appear well nourished and happy.

Gastroesophageal Reflux

Particularly common in preterm infants, gastroesophageal reflux occurs in about 3% of newborns. Typically, as the gastrointestinal tract matures within the first 12 months of life, this condition resolves. Caretakers should avoid overfeeding the infant, keep the infant upright after each feeding, and watch for choking or gagging. Some infants improve when fed whey-enriched formulas.

Iron-Deficiency Anemia

As stated earlier, full-term infants are born with sufficient iron stores to last for approximately the first 6 months of life. In older infants and toddlers, however, iron is the mineral most likely to be deficient. Iron-deficiency anemia causes pallor, lethargy, and impaired growth. Iron-fortified formula and cereals are good sources of this mineral. Overconsumption of cow's milk remains a common cause of anemia among U.S. infants and children.

Dehydration

Whether the cause is diarrhea, vomiting, prolonged fever, or inadequate fluid intake, dehydration is extremely dangerous to infants and if left untreated can quickly result

colic A condition in infants marked by inconsolable crying for unknown reasons that lasts for hours at a time.

in death. Treatment includes providing fluids, a task that is difficult if vomiting is occurring. In some cases, the physician may recommend that a pediatric electrolyte solution, readily available at most grocery and drug stores, be administered on a temporary basis. In more severe cases, hospitalization and the administration of intravenous fluids may be necessary.

 recap The risk for food allergies can be reduced by breastfeeding and delaying the introduction of solid foods until the infant is at least 4 to 6 months of age. Infants with colic or gastroesophageal reflux present special challenges, but both conditions generally improve over time. Iron-deficiency anemia is easily prevented through the use of iron-fortified cereals. Dehydration is extremely dangerous to infants, and prompt fluid/electrolyte replacement is essential.

LO6 Discuss nutrient needs and some common nutrition-related concerns of toddlers.

Nutrition for toddlers

The rapid growth rate of infancy begins to slow during toddlerhood—the period from 12 to 36 months of age. During the second and third years of life, a toddler will grow a total of about 5.5 to 7.5 inches and gain an average of 9 to 11 lb. However, toddlers expend significant energy to fuel their increasing levels of activity. **TABLE 11.5** identifies the nutrient recommendations for toddlers, children, and adolescents.

What Are a Toddler's Nutrient Needs?

A healthy toddler generally requires about 1,000 kcal per day. Toddlers need more fat than adults, up to 40% of total Calories, and should not be given low-fat or skim milk, yogurt, or cheese until at least age 2. Toddlers' protein and carbohydrate needs increase modestly; most of the carbohydrates they eat should be complex, and refined carbohydrates should be kept to a minimum. As toddlers grow, their micronutrient needs increase.

Toddlers sometimes become so busy playing that they ignore or fail to recognize the thirst sensation, so caregivers need to make sure an active toddler is drinking adequately. The recommended total fluid intake for toddlers is about 4 cups of beverages.[13] Suggested beverages include plain water, milk and soy milk, and limited amounts of diluted fruit juices.

Given their typically erratic eating habits, toddlers can develop nutrient deficiencies. That's why many pediatricians recommend a multivitamin and mineral supplement formulated especially for toddlers.

Encouraging Nutritious Food Choices with Toddlers

Toddlers tend to be choosy about what they eat. Some avoid entire food groups, such as all meats or vegetables. Others will suddenly refuse all but one or two favorite foods (such as peanut butter on crackers) for several days or longer. Still others eat in extremely small amounts, seemingly satisfied by a single slice of apple or two bites of toast. These behaviors concern many parents, but as long as healthful food is abundant and choices are varied, toddlers have the ability to match their intake with their needs. Parents who offer only foods of high nutritional quality can usually feel confident that their toddlers are getting the nutrition they need, even if their choices seem odd or erratic on any particular day. Food should never be "forced" on a child; doing so sets the stage for eating and control issues later in life.

Toddlers' stomachs are still very small, and they cannot consume all the Calories they need in three meals. They need several small meals and snacks and should eat every 2 to 3 hours. One successful feeding technique is to create a snack tray filled with small portions of nutritious food choices and leave it within reach of the child's play area. The child can then "graze" while he or she plays. A snack tray plus a spill-proof cup of water is particularly useful on car trips.

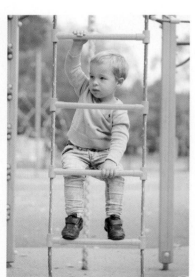

Toddlers expend significant amounts of energy actively exploring their world.

TABLE 11.5   **Nutrient Recommendations for Children and Adolescents**

Nutrient	Toddlers (1 to 2 years)	Children (3 to 8 years)	Children (9 to 13 years)	Adolescents (14 to 18 years)
Carbohydrate	130 grams/day	130 grams/day	130 grams/day	130 grams/day
Fat	No DRI	No DRI	No DRI	No DRI
Protein	1.10 grams/kg body weight per day	0.95 gram/kg body weight per day	0.95 gram/kg body weight per day	0.85 gram/kg body weight per day
Vitamin A	300 µg/day	400 µg/day	600 µg/day	Boys = 900 µg/day Girls = 700 µg/day
Vitamin C	15 mg/day	25 mg/day	45 mg/day	Boys = 75 mg/day Girls = 65 mg/day
Vitamin E	6 mg/day	7 mg/day	11 mg/day	15 mg/day
Calcium	500 mg/day	800 mg/day	1,300 mg/day	1,300 mg/day
Iron	7 mg/day	10 mg/day	8 mg/day	Boys = 11 mg/day Girls = 15 mg/day
Zinc	3 mg/day	5 mg/day	8 mg/day	Boys = 11 mg/day Girls = 9 mg/day
Fluid	1.3 liters/day	1.7 liters/day	Boys = 2.4 liters/day Girls = 2.1 liters/day	Boys = 3.3 liters/day Girls = 2.3 liters/day

Firm foods pose a choking hazard. Never feed a toddler nuts, carrots, grapes, raisins, cherry tomatoes, hard candies, hot dogs, or cheese sticks. Foods should be soft and sliced into strips or wedges that are easy for children to grasp. As the child develops more teeth and becomes more coordinated, food choices can become more varied.

Foods prepared for toddlers should also be fun. Parents can use cookie-cutters to turn a peanut butter sandwich into a pumpkin face or arrange cooked peas or carrot slices to look like a smiling face on top of mashed potatoes. Diluted fruit juice and low-fat yogurt can be frozen into "popsicles" or blended into "milkshakes."

Even at mealtime, portion sizes should be small. One tablespoon of a food for each year of age constitutes a serving throughout the preschool years (**FIGURE 11.6**). Realistic portion sizes can give toddlers a sense of accomplishment when they "eat it all up" and lessen parents' fears that their child is not eating enough.

Introduce new foods gradually. Most toddlers are leery of new foods, spicy foods, hot (temperature) foods, mixed foods (such as casseroles), and foods with strange textures. A helpful rule is to require the child to eat at least one bite of a new food: if the child does not want the rest, nothing negative should be said and the child should be praised just for the willingness to try. Although it may take as many as 12–15 attempts, parents should reintroduce the new food a few weeks later because, over time, toddlers will often accept foods they once rejected.[25]

Nutrition-Related Concerns for Toddlers

As during infancy, new foods should be presented one at a time, and the toddler should be monitored for allergic reactions for 4 to 5 days before introducing additional new foods. Although many food allergies subside as a child ages, toddlers remain at risk.

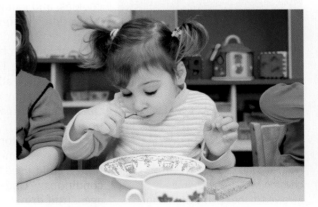

FIGURE 11.6   Portion sizes for preschoolers should be much smaller than those for older children. Use the following guideline: 1 tablespoon of food for each year of age equals 1 serving. For example, 2 tbsp. of rice, 2 tbsp. of black beans, and 2 tbsp. of chopped tomatoes is appropriate for a 2-year-old toddler.

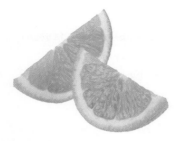

 Foods that may cause allergies, such as peanut butter and citrus fruits, should be introduced to toddlers one at a time.

For toddlers, a lacto-ovo-vegetarian diet in which dairy foods and eggs are included can be as wholesome as a diet including meats and fish. However, because meat is an excellent source of zinc and heme iron, the most readily absorbed form of iron, families who do not serve meat must be careful to include enough zinc and iron from other sources in their child's diet, such as fortified cereals. In contrast, a vegan diet, in which no foods of animal origin are consumed, poses several potential nutritional risks for toddlers. For this reason, families that wish to feed their toddler a vegan diet are advised to consult their pediatrician or a registered dietitian.

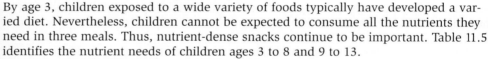 Toddlers are highly active and need to consume enough energy to fuel their growth and activity. Total energy, fat, and protein requirements are higher for toddlers than for infants. Until age 2, healthy toddlers of appropriate weight should drink whole milk to meet calcium requirements and sustain adequate fat intake. Toddlers require small, frequent, nutritious meals and snacks, and food should be cut in small pieces, so that it is easy to handle, chew, and swallow. Because toddlers are becoming more independent and can self-feed, parents need to be alert for choking and should watch for allergies and monitor weight gain. Feeding vegan diets to toddlers is controversial, because it poses potential deficiencies for several nutrients.

LO7 Identify changes in nutrient needs for school-age children, as well as the effect of school attendance on children's nutrition.

Nutrition throughout childhood

Children experience an average growth of 2 to 4 inches per year throughout childhood. Between the ages of 3 and 13, children begin to make some of their own food choices. The impact of these decisions on children's health can be profound, so age-appropriate nutrition education is critical.

What Are a Child's Nutrient Needs?

By age 3, children exposed to a wide variety of foods typically have developed a varied diet. Nevertheless, children cannot be expected to consume all the nutrients they need in three meals. Thus, nutrient-dense snacks continue to be important. Table 11.5 identifies the nutrient needs of children ages 3 to 8 and 9 to 13.

As compared with toddlers, children need more protein but a lower percentage of fat—about 25% to 35% of total energy.[8] The need for carbohydrate remains the same as for toddlers.[8] Fiber-rich carbohydrates are important, and simple sugars should come from fruits and fruit juices, with refined-carbohydrate items (such as cakes, cookies, and candies) saved for occasional treats.

Children who fail to consume the recommended 5 or more servings of fruits and vegetables each day may become deficient in vitamins A, C, and E. Minerals of concern continue to be calcium, iron, and zinc, which come primarily from animal-based foods (see Table 11.5). Notice that calcium needs increase dramatically in children age 9 to 13 years to allow for increased bone growth and density.

If there is any doubt that a child's nutrient needs are not being met for any reason (for instance, breakfasts are skipped, lunches are traded, or parents lack money for nourishing food), a vitamin/mineral supplement that provides no more than 100% of the daily value for the micronutrients may help correct any existing deficit.

Fluid recommendations for children are shown in Table 11.5. The exact amount of fluid a child needs varies according to their level of physical activity and the weather conditions.[13] Under most circumstances, water is the beverage of choice; sports beverages, fruit drinks, and sodas provide excess Calories that can, over time, contribute to inappropriate weight gain.

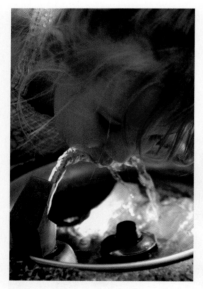

 Fluid intake is important for children, who may become so involved in their play that they ignore the sensation of thirst.

Encouraging Nutritious Food Choices with Children

Most children can understand that some foods will "help them grow up healthy and strong" and that other foods will not. Because children want to grow as quickly as possible, parents can capitalize on this natural desire and, using age-appropriate language, encourage children to eat foods high in fiber-rich carbohydrates, protein, and micronutrients.

However, peer pressure can be extremely difficult for both parents and their children to deal with during this life stage. If a popular child is snacking on chips and soda, it may be hard for a child to have an apple and milk without embarrassment. Nevertheless, parents are powerful role models and should "set the tone" with their own healthful eating and activity patterns. Families can also choose restaurants where "children's meals" reflect the standards of the National Restaurant Association's Kids LiveWell program, which defines goals for total calories, fat, and sodium or help their children select healthful menu choices.[26]

Families can also take advantage of online tools, such as the MyPlate.gov/KIDS/ site, where a child can print out activity sheets and play interactive games and parents can learn how to improve children's food choices (**FIGURE 11.7**). As their children mature, parents can continue to involve children in meal planning and food purchasing decisions. For instance, children can grow foods in small container gardens, develop their own shopping list with nutritious favorites, and help with age-appropriate food-preparation activities. If children have input into what is going into their body, they are more likely to take an active role in their health.

To download a free booklet containing 40 kid-tested healthy meals, go to http://www.nhlbi.nih.gov and click on the "Public" tab. Then click on the link for *Deliciously Healthy Family Meals* on the right-hand side.

What Is the Effect of School Attendance on Nutrition?

Children's school attendance can affect their nutrition in several ways. First, in the hectic time between waking and getting out the door, many children minimize or skip breakfast completely. Students who eat breakfast perform better on schoolwork, have improved attention spans, and demonstrate fewer behavioral problems than their peers who skip breakfast.[27-32] Many schools offer free or low-cost school breakfasts to help children avoid hunger in the classroom.[27] You've probably heard someone claim that breakfast is the most important meal of the day. Is it true? See the **Nutrition Myth or Fact?** box.

Another consequence of attending school is that, with no one monitoring what they eat, children do not always consume adequate amounts of food. They may spend their lunchtime talking or playing with friends rather than eating. Some schools schedule playground breaks before, rather than after, lunch, allowing children time to burn off their pent-up energy as well as build their hunger and thirst.

The impact of the National School Breakfast and Lunch Programs on children's diets is enormous: 99% of public schools participate in at least one of the programs, serving nearly 32 million children. On the surface, it would appear that school breakfasts and lunches would be expected to improve children's diets, because they must meet certain nutritional standards. For example:

- Students must be offered fruits, vegetables, and whole grains every day.
- Milk must be fat-free or low fat.
- Calories, averaged over a week, and portion sizes must be appropriate for the age of the children being served.
- Sodium, saturated fats, and *trans* fats must be reduced to specified levels.

In addition, vending machines and other sources of food on school campuses must meet specific nutrient guidelines.

Despite these regulations, some caution remains. The actual amount of nutrients a student *gets* depends on what the student actually *eats*. So, a child might eat the slice of whole-wheat cheese pizza and the low fat milk, but skip the apple and carrot sticks. Also keep in mind that children can still bring high-fat and high-sugar snacks and beverages from home or trade with classmates who bring them.

The good news is that many schools are working to ensure a more healthful food environment. Many now offer salad bars, fresh fruit bowls, baked potato bars, and soup stations to entice students into more healthful choices. Some schools now cultivate a garden where children help to grow the vegetables that will be used in their lunches. Moreover, the U.S. Department of Agriculture has developed several programs to improve children's nutrition, for example, by providing children with less common fruits and vegetables they might not otherwise have had the chance to try.

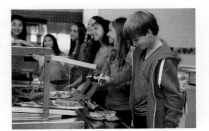

School-age children may receive a standard school lunch, but many choose less healthful foods when given the opportunity.

Healthy Eating for Preschoolers Daily Food Plan

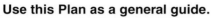
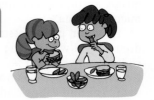

Use this Plan as a general guide.

● These food plans are based on average needs. Do not be concerned if your child does not eat the exact amounts suggested. Your child may need more or less than average. For example, food needs increase during growth spurts.

● Children's appetites vary from day to day. Some days they may eat less than these amounts; other days they may want more. Offer these amounts and let your child decide how much to eat.

Food group	2 year olds	3 year olds	4 and 5 year olds	What counts as:
Fruits	1 cup	1 - 1½ cups	1 - 1½ cups	½ cup of fruit? ½ cup mashed, sliced, or chopped fruit ½ cup 100% fruit juice ½ medium banana 4-5 large strawberries
Vegetables	1 cup	1½ cups	1½ - 2 cups	½ cup of veggies? ½ cup mashed, sliced, or chopped vegetables 1 cup raw leafy greens ½ cup vegetable juice 1 small ear of corn
Grains Make half your grains whole	3 ounces	4 - 5 ounces	4 - 5 ounces	1 ounce of grains? 1 slice bread 1 cup ready-to-eat cereal flakes ½ cup cooked rice or pasta 1 tortilla (6" across)
Protein Foods	2 ounces	3 - 4 ounces	3 - 5 ounces	1 ounce of protein foods? 1 ounce cooked meat, poultry, or seafood 1 egg 1 Tablespoon peanut butter ¼ cup cooked beans or peas (kidney, pinto, lentils)
Dairy Choose low-fat or fat-free	2 cups	2 cups	2½ cups	½ cup of dairy? ½ cup milk 4 ounces yogurt ¾ ounce cheese 1 string cheese

Some foods are easy for your child to choke on while eating. Skip hard, small, whole foods, such as popcorn, nuts, seeds, and hard candy. Cut up foods such as hot dogs, grapes, and raw carrots into pieces smaller than the size of your child's throat—about the size of a nickel.

There are many ways to divide the Daily Food Plan into meals and snacks. View the "Meal and Snack Patterns and Ideas" to see how these amounts might look on your preschooler's plate at www.choosemyplate.gov/preschoolers.html.

FIGURE 11.7 MyPlate Healthy Eating for Preschoolers: Daily Food Plan.

Data adapted from *MyPlate Healthy Eating for Preschoolers: Daily Food Plan. USDA Food and Nutrition Service.*

nutrition myth or fact?

Is Breakfast the Most Important Meal of the Day?

What did you eat for breakfast this morning? Whole-grain cereal with low-fat milk? A strawberry toaster pastry? Nothing? What does it matter, anyway? Sure, you've heard the saying that breakfast is the most important meal of the day, but that's just a myth—isn't it? As long as you eat a nutritious meal at lunch and dinner, why should skipping breakfast matter?

Over the past two decades, dozens of published studies have pointed to the importance of a healthful breakfast.[1-6] Most of these studies cite two key health benefits: First, breakfast supports our physical and mental functioning. Second, it helps us maintain a healthful weight. Let's examine the evidence for each of these claims.

The word *breakfast* was initially used as a verb meaning "to break the fast"—that is, to end the hours of fasting that naturally occur during a night of sleep. When we fast, our body breaks down stored nutrients to provide energy to fuel the resting

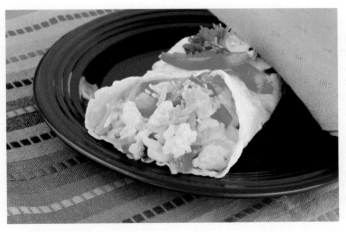

◀ Breakfast doesn't have to be boring! A breakfast burrito with scrambled eggs, low-fat cheese, and vegetables served in a whole-grain tortilla provides energy and nutrients to start your day off right.

body. First, cells break down glycogen stores in the muscle tissues and liver, using the "freed" glucose for energy. These stores last about 12 hours. But people who skip breakfast fast much longer than that: if they finish dinner around 7:00 PM and don't eat again until noon the next day, they're going without fuel for 17 hours! Long before this point, essentially all the stored glycogen is used up, and the body turns to fatty acids and amino acids for fuel.

If you're like many people, when your blood glucose is low, you experience not only hunger but also weakness, shakiness, irritability, and poor concentration. So it's not surprising that children and teens who skip breakfast don't function as well—either physically or academically—as their breakfast-eating peers. What exactly are the benefits of eating breakfast?

- Eating breakfast improves children's ability to learn.[3-5] Children who eat breakfast exhibit improved memory recall, score higher on cognitive tests, have fewer behavioral and emotional problems, and are less likely to have to repeat a grade than children who arrive at school hungry and unfed.

- Eating a complete breakfast helps children perform better on demanding mental tasks and improves their attention and memory. Children make fewer mistakes and work faster in math and vocabulary.[3]

- Breakfast improves students' behavior, including improving their reaction to frustration, reducing disciplinary office referrals, decreasing tardiness, and increasing school attendance rates.[3]

- Children who skip breakfast "up-regulate" their appetites, leading to overeating later in the day. Teens who eat breakfast are more likely to experience longer periods of fullness and have reduced night time snacking compared with those who tend to skip breakfast.[6]

What do you think? Is breakfast the most important meal of the day? And what—if anything—will you be having for breakfast tomorrow?

Nutrition-Related Concerns for Children

Two significant nutrition-related concerns for children are food insecurity and overweight. Surprisingly, these can occur simultaneously.

Childhood Food Insecurity

Although most children in the United States grow up with an abundant and healthful supply of food, approximately 21% of U.S. households with children are faced with *food insecurity*, a term used to describe a household's inability to ensure a consistent, dependable supply of safe and nutritious food.[33] This statistic is definitely at odds with America's image as "the land of plenty."

The effects of food insecurity can be very harmful to children.[33] Without an adequate breakfast, they will not be able to concentrate or pay attention to their parents and teachers. Impaired nutrient status can blunt children's immune responses, making them more susceptible to common childhood illnesses. Increased rates of hospitalizations have been linked to food insecurity. Children's rates of anxiety and suicide are also increased with food insecurity. Finally, maternal depression is more common within food-insecure households, creating an environment that often leads to poor mental health outcomes in the child.

Options for families facing food insecurity include a number of government and privately funded programs, including school breakfast and lunch programs, WIC (Special Supplemental Nutrition Program for Women, Infants and Children) and the Supplemental Nutrition Assistance Program (SNAP), previously termed the Food Stamp program. Private, church-based, and community food pantries and kitchens can provide a narrow range of foods for a limited period of time.

Obesity Watch: Encouraging an Active and Healthful Lifestyle

The CDC (U.S. Centers for Disease Control and Prevention) classifies children as overweight when their BMI is at or above the 85th percentile and lower than the 95th percentile; that is, the child's body mass index is higher than that of 85% of U.S. children of the same age and gender. The CDC considers a child to be obese if his or her BMI is at or above the 95th percentile. During the past 30 years, the rate of obesity has doubled or even tripled for U.S children. Currently, about 12% of preschoolers, 17% of children 6 to 11 years old, and 18% of youth 12 to 19 years old are classified as obese.[1]

There are some recent encouraging signs, however, including a 43% decrease in the obesity rate among 2- to 5-year-olds over the past 7 years.[1] A slight decrease in calorie intake, along with national campaigns to decrease "screen time" (television, video games, computer usage), improve school meals, and increase physical activity in children may be responsible for these improvements.

Obese and overweight children are at higher risk for several health problems including asthma, sleep apnea, impaired mobility, and emotional problems due to intense teasing, low self-esteem, and social isolation. Among children who are overweight, rates of type 2 diabetes have increased tenfold over the past 20 years. Increasing numbers of obese children are also experiencing high blood lipids and high blood pressure.

Experts agree that the main culprits in childhood obesity are similar to those involved in adult obesity: eating too much and moving around too little. Thus, they recommend a two-pronged approach: establishing healthful eating practices that work for the whole family and increasing physical activity. Parents should work to consistently provide nutritious food choices, encourage children to eat a healthful breakfast every morning, and sit down to a shared family meal each evening or as often as possible.[34] The television should be off throughout mealtimes to encourage attentive eating and true enjoyment of the food. Children should engage in physical activity for at least an hour each day.[35] For younger children, this can be divided into two or three shorter sessions. Parents should encourage children to replace sedentary activities with shared activities, such as ball games, bike rides, and hikes, or one of the newly developed electronic game systems that offer virtual tennis, dancing, and other simulations.

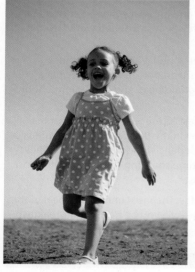

▲ Active, healthy-weight children are less likely to become overweight adults.

recap Children experience an average growth of 2 to 4 inches per year. They need a lower percentage of fat Calories than toddlers but slightly more than adults (25% to 35% of energy). Micronutrient needs increase because of growth and maturation. Children can become easily dehydrated, especially during vigorous activity in warm weather. Peer pressure influences children's nutritional choices. Involving children in food growing, purchasing, and preparation can help. School meals must meet federal nutrition guidelines, but the foods that children actually choose to eat can be high in saturated fat, sugar, and energy and low in nutrients. Food insecurity and obesity are significant nutritional concerns for U.S. children.

Nutrition for adolescents

Explain how adolescents' rapid growth affects their nutritional status.

The adolescent years begin with the onset of **puberty**, the period in life in which secondary sexual characteristics develop and there is the capacity for reproducing. Adolescence is characterized by increasing independence and self-reliance. All teens deal with their emerging sexuality, and some experiment with behaviors, such as smoking and drinking, that lie outside their traditional cultural or social boundaries. During this stage, they may ignore their parents' attempts to improve their diet, or they may adopt a diet that is much more healthful than that of their parents.

Adolescent Growth and Activity Patterns

The nutritional needs of adolescents are influenced by their rapid growth in height, increased weight, changes in body composition, and individual levels of physical activity. Both boys and girls experience *growth spurts,* or periods of accelerated growth, during which their height increases by an average of 20% to 25%. Growth spurts for girls tend to begin around 10 to 11 years of age, and they typically grow a total of 2 to 8 inches. Growth spurts for boys begin around 12 to 13 years of age, and they tend to grow 4 to 12 inches.

The average weight gained by girls and boys during this time is 35 and 45 lb, respectively. The weight gained by girls and boys is dramatically different in terms of its composition. Girls tend to gain significantly more body fat than boys, who tend to gain more muscle mass.

The physical activity levels of adolescents are highly variable. Many are physically active in sports or other organized physical activities, whereas others become less interested in sports and more interested in intellectual or artistic pursuits. This variability results in highly individual energy needs.

What Are an Adolescent's Nutrient Needs?

Adolescents need a significant amount of energy to maintain their health, support their dramatic growth and maturation, and fuel their physical activity. Still, adolescence is often a time in which overweight begins. Dieting to lose weight should be undertaken only under the guidance of a physician or registered dietitian.

The AMDR for carbohydrate for adolescents is the same as for adults. The AMDR for fat is slightly higher: 25% to 35% of total energy.[8] The RDA for protein for adolescents is similar to that of adults, at 0.85 gram of protein per kilogram of body weight per day.[8] This amount is assumed to be sufficient to support health and to cover the additional needs of growth and development during the adolescent stage.

Adequate calcium intake is critical to achieve peak bone density. The RDA for calcium remains high throughout adolescence and can be difficult to consume for teens who do not drink milk or calcium-fortified beverages.[12]

As shown in Table 11.5, the iron needs of adolescents are relatively high to replace the blood lost during menstruation in girls and to support the growth of muscle mass in boys.[11] If energy intake is adequate and adolescents consume animal products each day, they should be able to meet their iron needs. However, adolescents who limit their food intake or follow a vegetarian diet can have difficulty meeting the RDA for iron.

Vitamin A is critical to support the rapid growth and development that occurs during adolescence. Consuming at least 5 servings of fruits and vegetables each day can help teens meet their RDA (see Table 11.5).[11]

If an adolescent is unable or unwilling to eat adequate amounts of nutrient-dense foods, a multivitamin and mineral supplement that provides no more than 100% of the Daily Value for the micronutrients can be beneficial. As with younger children and adults, a supplement should not be considered a substitute for a healthful diet.

The AI for total fluid for adolescent boys is about 11 cups as beverages, including water. The AI for girls is about 8 cups as beverages. Boys are generally more active than girls and have more lean tissue, so they require a higher fluid intake. Highly

puberty The period of life in which secondary sexual characteristics develop and people are biologically capable of reproducing.

active adolescents who are exercising in the heat may have higher fluid needs than the AI and should drink often to avoid dehydration.[13] Adolescents should be cautioned against excessive consumption of energy drinks, sports beverages, and high sugar/high fat drinks from coffee shops and encouraged to drink more water, low-fat or skim milk, soy milk, unsweetened tea or coffee, and 100% fruit juices.

Encouraging Nutritious Food Choices with Adolescents

Adolescents make most of their own food choices, and many are buying and preparing a significant amount of the foods they consume. Although parents can still be effective role models,[34] adolescents are generally strongly influenced by their peers, the mass media, the environments in which they spend most of their time, and their own developing sense of what foods compose a healthful diet.

Many adolescent diets lack adequate amounts of vegetables, fruits, low-fat dairy, and whole grains. Many teens eat on the run at fast-food restaurants, convenience stores, and vending machines, where these healthful foods may not be available. In addition, many teens skip meals. For instance, adolescent girls often skip breakfast, because they believe it might make them fat. In reality, teens who start their day with breakfast have a higher diet quality and are at lower risk for overweight or obesity compared with those who skip breakfast.[34]

Parents and school food service programs can capitalize on adolescents' preferences for pizza, burgers, spaghetti, and sandwiches by providing more healthful versions of these foods, as well as appealing vegetable-based sides. In addition, stocking the refrigerator with raw fruits and vegetables that are already cleaned and sliced may encourage adolescents to eat more of these foods as between-meal snacks. Teens should also be encouraged to consume adequate milk and other calcium-enriched beverages.

Nutrition-Related Concerns for Adolescents

Obesity prevention continues to be a concern during adolescence. Additional concerns are disordered eating, low bone density, acne, and the use of alcohol and tobacco products.

Obesity Watch: Balancing Food and Physical Activity

Although expected and healthful, weight gain during adolescence can become excessive, increasing the risk for the early onset of type 2 diabetes, hypertension, and high blood lipid levels. A teen's energy intake must be balanced with adequate physical activity. Like younger children, adolescents should participate in at least 60 minutes of physical activity each day; however, fewer than 30% of high school students actually meet this guideline.[35] Daily physical education in school can help reduce the prevalence of overweight and obesity among adolescents; however, rates of participation now fall below 40%, with only 24% of high school seniors attending physical education classes on a daily basis. Community-based sports leagues or clubs are options for some adolescents and an increasing number of teenagers are joining commercial gyms as a social outlet.

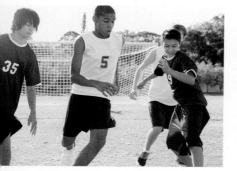

◆ The nutrient needs of adolescents are affected by their activity levels.

Disordered Eating and Eating Disorders

An initially appropriate concern about body image and weight can turn into a dangerous obsession during this emotionally challenging life stage. Clinical eating disorders frequently begin during adolescence and occur in boys *and* girls. Parents, teachers, and friends should be aware of the warning signs, which include rapid and excessive weight loss, a preoccupation with weight and body image, going to the bathroom regularly after meals, and signs of frequent vomiting or laxative use (see Chapter 9).

Bone-Density Watch

Early adolescence, 13 to 15 years of age, is a crucial time for ensuring adequate dietary calcium in order to maximize bone mineral density and reduce the risk for osteoporosis. Meeting the adolescent RDA for calcium (1,300 mg/day) requires a daily consumption of at least 4 servings (4 cups) of milk or other dairy foods,

foods you don't know you love YET

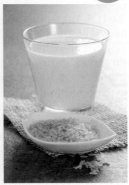

Milk Alternatives

You know you need to replenish your body's stores of calcium every day, throughout the day, but what if you don't like milk? Milk alternatives to the rescue! Soy milk, almond milk, and rice milk—all of which are available in most larger grocery stores nationwide—are plant-based beverages that typically are enriched with as much calcium (not to mention vitamin D) as a glass of cow's milk. Many brands are also enriched with vitamin B$_{12}$, making them ideal for people following a vegan diet. They're also low in saturated fat and cholesterol free, and they come in a variety of flavors, from vanilla to coffee.

calcium-fortified foods and beverages, or supplements. Unfortunately, many adolescents fail to meet this recommendation. Although not the only factor, milk consumption during adolescence is strongly linked to higher bone mineral content and lower risk for adult bone fractures.[36]

Adolescent Acne and Diet

The hormonal changes that occur during puberty are largely responsible for the acne flare-ups that plague 80% to 90% of adolescents. Emotional stress, genetic factors, and personal hygiene are most likely secondary contributors. But what about foods? Current research does not support a link between acne and consumption of chocolate, salt, or total fat intake. There is some evidence that high glycemic index diets may be associated with an increase in acne prevalence, severity, or duration.[37] On the other hand, a healthful diet, rich in fruits, vegetables, whole grains, fish, and lean meats, provides nutrients to optimize skin health and maintain an effective immune system.

Prescription medications, including a vitamin A derivative called Accutane, effectively control severe forms of acne. Neither Accutane nor any other prescription vitamin A derivative should be used by women who are pregnant or who may become pregnant. Accutane is a known teratogen, causing severe fetal malformations, and has been associated with depression, suicidal thoughts or actions, inflammatory bowel disease, and other disorders. For these reasons, the drug is typically prescribed only for teens who have severe, disfiguring acne, and regular medical monitoring is essential.

Use of Alcohol and Tobacco

Many adolescents experiment with alcohol and tobacco. (The risks of alcohol consumption are discussed in Chapter 8.) Cigarette smoking diminishes appetite, interferes with nutrient metabolism, reduces physical fitness, damages the lungs, increases the incidence of respiratory illness, and promotes addiction to nicotine. Most people who begin smoking during adolescence continue to smoke in adulthood, increasing their risks for lung cancer, heart disease, osteoporosis, and emphysema.

recap Adolescents experience rapid increases in height, weight, and lean body mass and fat mass, so their energy needs can be very high. Because many adolescents fail to eat a variety of nutrient-dense foods, their intakes of some nutrients may be deficient. Calcium is needed to optimize bone growth and to achieve peak bone density, and iron needs are increased because of increased muscle mass in boys and the onset of menstruation in girls. Obesity can occur during adolescence as a result of increased appetite and food intake and decreased physical activity. Disordered eating behaviors typically develop in adolescence. Consumption of alcohol and cigarette smoking are additional risks.

Discuss changes in an older adult's body, functions, and nutrient needs.

 Identify some common nutrition-related concerns of older adults.

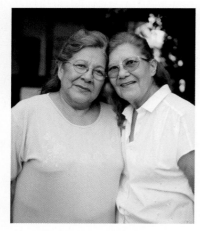

⬆ Older adults have unique nutritional needs.

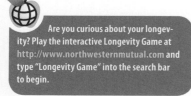

Are you curious about your longevity? Play the interactive Longevity Game at http://www.northwesternmutual.com and type "Longevity Game" into the search bar to begin.

life expectancy The expected number of years remaining in one's life, typically stated from the time of birth.

life span The highest age reached by any member of a species; currently, the human life span is 122 years.

Nutrition for older adults

The U.S. population is getting older each year. It is estimated that, by the year 2050, there will be nearly 89 million Americans age 65 and older, about twice as many as are currently alive.[38] In addition, the number of *centenarians*, persons over the age of 100 years, and *super centenarians*, over 110 years, continues to grow.

In 2011, **life expectancy**, which is the average number of years that a person can be expected to live, was 78.7 years in the United States.[39] Whereas some researchers have argued that the growing rate of obesity and its medical consequences will drive down U.S. life expectancy over the next several decades, others refute this claim, saying that future advances in healthcare will balance this factor.

Life span is the age to which the longest-living member of the species has lived. Madame Jeanne Calment, born in 1875, survived to the age of 122 and is generally acknowledged as having lived longer than anyone else in the world. Researchers have made great progress toward understanding the aging of humans, but much remains unknown. Scientists can't even agree on why we age or when the aging process begins. Some believe aging is programmed into our genes, whereas others view aging as the consequence of progressive cellular damage. As the debate continues, however, gerontologists agree that humans can positively influence the aging process through personal lifestyle choices, such as eating a nourishing diet, participating in regular physical activity, and avoiding smoking and substance abuse.

Physiologic Changes That Accompany Aging

With age comes the decline of taste, odor, and tactile and visual perception: the more each of these functions becomes impaired, the greater is the potential impact on the person's food intake. For example, the loss of visual acuity may result in difficulty reading food labels, including nutrient information and "pull dates" for perishable foods. Driving skills decline, limiting the ability of some older Americans to get to markets that sell healthful, affordable foods. Older adults may no longer be able to read their favorite recipes or distinguish the small markings on temperature knobs on ovens and stoves. Their diet may thus consist of a few foods that are easy to prepare, such as cereal with milk and sandwiches with cold cuts, and may lack the variety necessary to prevent nutrient deficiencies.

With increasing age, salivary production declines. As a result, teeth are more susceptible to decay, chewing and swallowing become more difficult, and the risk for choking increases. Reduced gastric acid production limits the absorption of minerals such as calcium, iron, and zinc and food sources of folic acid and vitamin B_{12}. Lack of intrinsic factor reduces the absorption of vitamin B_{12}, whether from food or supplements. Older adults may also experience a delay in gastric emptying, resulting in a prolonged sense of fullness and a reduced appetite. Because only about 30% of older adults retain an "adequate" level of lactase activity, many restrict their milk intake and fail to consume adequate calcium.

Age-Related Changes in Body Composition

With aging, muscle mass declines, leading to impaired physical functioning in the elderly. It has been estimated that women and men lose 20% to 25% of their lean body mass, respectively, as they age from 35 to 70 years. Decreased production of certain hormones, chronic diseases, and an increasingly sedentary lifestyle contribute to this loss of muscle, as does a poor diet. Along with adequate dietary intake of Calories as well as protein and other nutrients, regular physical activity, including strength or resistance training, can help adults maintain or enhance their muscle mass and strength as they age.

Body fat increases from young adulthood through middle age, peaking at approximately 55 to 65 years of age. With aging, body fat shifts from subcutaneous stores, just below the skin, to internal or visceral fat stores. Maintaining an appropriate energy intake and remaining physically active can help keep body fat at a healthy level.

Bone mineral density declines with age, increasing the risk for fracture. Among older women, the onset of menopause leads to a sudden and dramatic loss of bone due to the lack of estrogen. Although less dramatic, bone loss in elderly males also occurs, due in part to decreasing levels of testosterone. A nourishing diet with adequate protein, calcium, phosphorus, and vitamin D and regular weight-bearing activity can reduce these losses.

Age-Related Changes in Organ Function

With increasing age, the kidneys lose their ability to concentrate waste products, leading to an increase in urine output and greater risk for dehydration. Bladder control also often declines. The aged liver is less efficient at breaking down drugs and alcohol, and the aged heart lacks the endurance to sustain a sudden increase in physical activity. In most instances, older adults can adapt to these age-related changes through minor lifestyle adjustments, such as reducing their alcohol consumption and gradually increasing their physical activity.

The number of neurons in the brain decreases with age, impairing memory, reflexes, coordination, and learning ability. Although many people believe that dementia is an inevitable part of the aging process, this is not true: diet, physical activity, intellectual stimulation, social contact, and other factors can help preserve the health of the brain as well as the body.

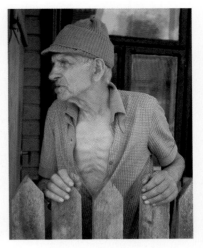

▲ A variety of gastrointestinal and other physiologic changes can lead to weight loss in older adults.

Factors That Accelerate the Aging Process

There is no doubt that genes exert tremendous influence on the aging process. Siblings of centenarians, those who live to be at least 100 years old, are four times more likely to live into their nineties than others. The brother of Madame Calment, previously mentioned as the world's oldest human, survived to the age of 97. A number of studies currently under way suggest that our genetic makeup influences our cellular aging and life span.

As cells age, they undergo many changes in structure and function. Some cells, such as skeletal and cardiac muscle, atrophy (decrease in size), whereas others, including fat cells, enlarge. Many gerontologists have linked the aging process to a progressive accumulation of free radicals, known to damage DNA and various cell proteins. Others cite a progressive failure in DNA repair. Still others point to an abnormal attachment of glucose to proteins in our tissues. Cell membrane function declines with age, allowing waste products to accumulate within the cell and preventing the normal uptake of nutrients and oxygen.

The way we live greatly influences the way we age. Whereas **chronological age** can never change, **biological age** is largely due to our personal lifestyle choices. Accelerated or unsuccessful aging is marked by premature loss of function, high rates of disability, and multiple disease complications. Lifestyle factors that accelerate aging include smoking, sun exposure, alcohol consumption, overeating and poor food choices, and low levels of physical activity.

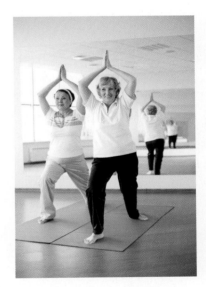

▲ A less physically active lifestyle will lead to lower total energy requirements in older adults.

recap The physiologic changes that occur with aging include sensory declines, loss of muscle mass and lean tissue, increased fat mass, decreased bone density, and impaired ability to absorb and metabolize various nutrients. Body organs lose functional capacity and are less tolerant of stressors. Many of these changes influence the nutritional needs of older adults and their ability to consume a healthful diet; however, diet and other lifestyle choices can greatly influence the rate and extent of these changes.

What Are an Older Adult's Nutrient Needs?

The requirements for many nutrients are the same for older adults as for young and middle-aged adults. A few nutrient requirements increase, and a few are actually lower.

chronologic age Age as defined by calendar years, from date of birth.

biologic age Physiologic age as determined by health and functional status; often estimated by scored questionnaires.

Energy and Macronutrient Recommendations for Older Adults

The energy needs of older adults are lower than those of younger adults. This decrease is primarily due to a loss of muscle mass and lean tissue, which results in a lower basal metabolic rate, and a more sedentary lifestyle, which lowers total energy requirements. Some of this decrease in energy expenditure is an inevitable response to aging, but part of the decrease can be delayed or minimized by staying physically active. Because their energy needs are lower, older adults need to pay particularly close attention to consuming a diet high in nutrient-dense foods but not too high in energy in order to avoid weight gain. Refer to the nearby **Highlight** feature box to learn more about the theory of caloric restriction, which proposes that energy-restricted diets may significantly prolong our life span.

The DRIs for total fat, protein, and carbohydrate for older adults are the same as those for adults of all ages.[8] Some researchers have argued in favor of increasing the RDA for protein for older adults; however, the issue remains unresolved.

After age 50, fiber needs decrease slightly along with decreased energy needs. Approximately 30 grams of fiber per day for men and 21 grams per day for women is assumed sufficient to reduce the risks for constipation and diverticular disease, to maintain healthful blood levels of glucose and lipids, and to provide good sources of nutrient-dense, low-energy foods.

Micronutrient Recommendations for Older Adults

Although zinc recommendations are the same for adults of all ages, and iron recommendations are the same for males of all ages and actually decreased for older females, these micronutrients are critical for immune defense, wound healing, and many other functions. Intakes of both zinc and iron can be inadequate in older adults who eat less red meat, poultry, and fish.

Vitamin A requirements are also the same for adults of all ages; however, older adults should be careful not to consume more than the RDA, because absorption of vitamin A is actually greater in older adults. Thus, this group is at greater risk for vitamin A toxicity, which can cause liver damage, neurologic problems, and increased risk for bone fracture.[11]

The micronutrient recommendations that change with age are identified in **TABLE 11.6**. Notice that the need for Vitamin D increases for adults over the age of 70 years, due in part to the decreased ability to synthesize vitamin D when exposed to sunlight.[12] Calcium requirements are increased for women over the age of 51 years and men over the age of 70 years; the need for calcium increases at an earlier age for women because of the hormonal changes that occur with menopause and their negative effects on bone health.[12]

Older adults need to pay close attention to consuming adequate amounts of the B-vitamins, particularly vitamin B_{12}, vitamin B_6, and folate. Inadequate intakes of

TABLE 11.6   Nutrient Recommendations That Change with Increased Age

Key Nutrient Recommendations	Rationale
Vitamin D *Increased need* for vitamin D from 600 IU/day for adults age 18 to 70 years to 800 IU/day for adults over age 70 years	Decreased bone density Decreased ability to synthesize vitamin D in our skin Decreased absorption of dietary calcium
Calcium *Increased need* for calcium from 1,000 mg/day for adults 19–50 years to 1,200 mg/day for women 51 years of age and older and men 71 years and older	Decreased bone density Decreased absorption of dietary calcium
B-Vitamins *Increased need* for vitamin B_6 and need for vitamin B_{12} *as a supplement or from fortified foods*	Lower levels of gastric juice Decreased absorption of food B_{12} from gastrointestinal tract Increased need to reduce homocysteine levels and to optimize immune function

highlight

Can We Live Longer by Eating a Low-Energy Diet?

How old do you want to live to be—80 years, 90, 100? World-wide, throughout human history, legends have told of a "fountain of youth" which reverses decades of aging in any-one who drinks its waters. Of course no one believes such tales any longer, but pick up a fashion or fitness magazine and you're likely to find modern equivalents: anti-aging diets, supplements, cosmetics, spa treatments, and other therapies. If you were to read that you could live to celebrate your 100th birthday in good health by eating less, would you do it?

A practice known as *Calorie restriction* (CR) has been getting a great deal of press lately. The practice typically involves eating 20 to 30 percent fewer Calories than your body needs to maintain your normal weight—while still getting enough vitamins and other nutrients to keep your body functioning in good health.

Research has shown that CR can significantly extend the life span of rats, mice, fish, flies, and yeast cells as well as non-human primates such as monkeys. But only in the past few years have researchers begun to design and conduct studies of CR in humans. Some of the beneficial metabolic effects of CR reported in several, but not all, human studies include:

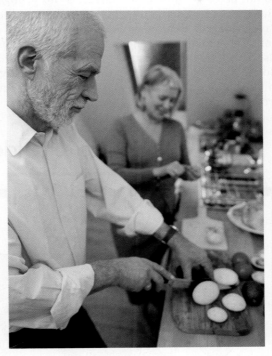

⬆ Maintaining a calorically restricted diet that is also highly nutritious requires significant meal planning and preparation.

- Decreased fat mass
- Decreased blood glucose levels, serum LDL and total cholesterol; increased serum HDL cholesterol
- Decreased blood pressure
- Decreased oxidative stress, chronic inflammation, and DNA damage
- Protective changes in various hormone levels

In contrast, there are other metabolic effects that are potentially harmful:

- Decreased energy expenditure, beyond that expected for the weight loss that occurred, which suggests a generalized slowing of metabolic rate (may increase tendency for rapid weight gain if person resumes normal calorie intake)
- Decreased lean body mass
- Decreased core body temperature

Based on animal research, the benefits of CR for humans are predicted to correlate to the age at which the program begins. The later in life the CR protocol is started, the lower the expected benefit. For example, if a person did not start CR until the age of 55 years, he or she would be expected to gain only 4 months of extended life! It has been estimated that humans would need to restrict their typical energy intake by at least 20% for 40 years or more to gain an addition 4–5 years of healthy living. If you normally eat about 2,000 kcal/day, a 20% reduction would result in an energy intake of about 1,600 kcal/day. Although this might not seem excessive, it would be very difficult to maintain every day for a lifetime.

In the absence of high-quality human studies, several CR groups, including the "CRONies" (Caloric Restriction with Optimal Nutrition), have provided researchers with some data. Most of the CRONies are males in their late 30s to mid-50s. One report indicated that most CRONies had followed the CR diet for about 10 years and reduced their caloric intake by about 30%. Overall, members report improved blood lipids and the other health benefits listed earlier.

Those who follow the CR lifestyle spend many hours planning their meals, face limited options for eating meals outside their home, and the challenge of following the CR restrictions while dining with family members and friends.

Also, those who follow the CR program report several side effects. The top three complaints are constant hunger, frequently feeling cold, and a loss of libido (sex drive). Finally, the long-term effects of the diet are not known. There is concern that, if initiated in early adulthood, CR might reduce bone density or lead to inappropriate loss of muscle mass. And because the production of female reproductive hormones is linked to a certain level of body fat, CR could impair a woman's fertility. Interestingly, as noted earlier, most of the members of the CRONies are males.

Considering the possible benefits and known risks of CR, do you feel it is a good option for those hoping to live a very long and healthy life? Would you commit to such a lifestyle? Scientists will continue to study the CR diet to determine if, in fact, it is a safe and effective approach.

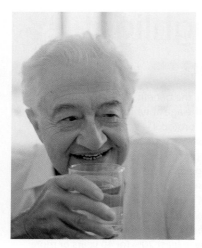

these vitamins increases blood levels of homocysteine, an amino acid that some researchers have linked to increased risk for heart disease and dementia. Older adults need larger amounts of vitamin B_6 in their diet, and they should get most of their vitamin B_{12} from supplements or fortified foods.[10]

Fluid Recommendations for Older Adults

The AI for fluid is the same for older and younger adults.[13] Many elderly people do not perceive thirst as effectively as do younger adults and can develop dehydration. Some older adults intentionally limit their beverage intake, because they have urinary incontinence or do not want to be awakened for nighttime urination. This practice can endanger their health, so it is important for these individuals to seek treatment for the incontinence and continue to drink plenty of fluids. Notice that fluids are part of the Tufts University MyPlate for Older Adults, shown in **FIGURE 11.8**. At least eight 1-cup (8 oz) servings of water or other fluid are recommended.

Older adults need the same amount of fluids as other adults.

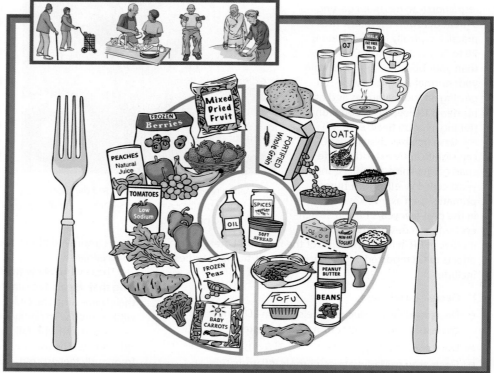

©2011 Tufts University

Source: Tufts University School of Nutrition

FIGURE 11.8 The Tufts University MyPlate for Older Adults illustrates healthful food and fluid choices appropriate for older adults.

Copyright 2011 Tufts University. For details about the MyPlate for Older Adults, please see http://nutrition.tufts.edu/research/myplate-older-adults

recap Older adults have lower energy needs because of their loss of lean tissue and lower physical activity levels. Fat, protein, and carbohydrate recommendations are the same as for younger adults, but their fiber needs decrease slightly. Micronutrients of concern for older adults include zinc and iron, calcium, vitamin D, vitamin B_{12}, vitamin B_6, and folate. Older adults are at increased risk for dehydration, so ample fluid intake should be encouraged.

Healthy Eating Tips for Older Adults

For older adults struggling with illness, chronic pain, or limited financial resources, planning healthy meals can be a challenge. Here are a few suggestions on how to improve the diet of your grandparents or other older adults:

- Encourage them to stock up on healthful ready-to-eat foods, such as pre-packaged salads, frozen low-fat entrées, ready-made grilled chicken, pre-cut fruits and vegetables, and low-sodium soups.
- Suggest that they eat their main meal when their appetite is strongest. For many, that means a substantial breakfast or lunch, with a smaller dinner.
- Provide visual cues to a healthy diet, such as a healthy foods shopping list print-out from http://nutrition.about.com. Type in "Healthy Foods Grocery" for a complete shopping list.
- Collect examples of simple but healthful menus and recipes from consumer magazines and put them into a binder. Use highlighters to emphasize the meals that include their favorite foods.
- Encourage them to share meals with others as often as possible. Most older adults eat better when there is someone to socialize with during meals.

Nutrition-Related Concerns for Older Adults

Older adults have a number of unique medical, social, and nutritional concerns that are closely interrelated.

Overweight and Underweight: A Delicate Balancing Act

Not surprisingly, overweight and obesity are of concern to older adults. The elderly population as a whole has a high risk for heart disease, hypertension, type 2 diabetes, and cancer, and these diseases are more prevalent in people who are overweight or obese. It is estimated that older adults who were overweight or obese at age 65 incur up to 17% higher medical expenses over their lifetime compared with those of normal weight at age 65.

Although some healthcare providers question the value of attempting obesity treatment among older adults, even moderate weight loss in obese elderly people can improve their physical functioning. The preferred interventions are the same as for younger adults: the use of dietary modifications to achieve an energy deficit while retaining adequate nutrient intakes, gradual and medically appropriate initiation of physical activity, and culturally appropriate behavior modification. The use of more aggressive interventions such as weight-loss drugs and bariatric surgery in the elderly remains relatively rare and not well researched.

Underweight may actually be more risky for older adults than overweight, because mortality rates are higher in underweight elderly. Many older adults lose weight as a result of illness, medication, loss of ability to perform self-care, tooth loss or mouth pain, alcoholism, smoking, or economic hardship. In addition, depression and reduced social contact, which can develop after the death of family members and friends or when adult children move out of the area, can cause older adults to lose the desire to prepare nourishing meals for themselves. Dementia can cause older adults to forget to eat, to eat only an extremely limited diet, or to store foods inappropriately (for example, meats or milk in a cabinet rather than in the refrigerator). Any of these factors can result in underweight and frailty, significantly increasing the person's risk for serious illness, injuries (such as fractures), and death.

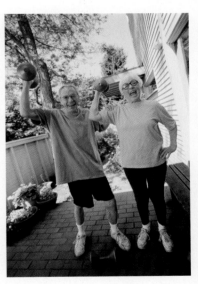

Older adults should participate in regular physical activity to maintain a healthful weight and reduce the risk for low bone mass.

Osteoporosis

Osteoporosis is a complex disease that develops over an extended period of time and manifests in the elderly in fractures of the hip, wrist, and spine. It is estimated that 55% of Americans over the age of 50 will have an osteoporosis-related bone fracture in their lifetime. By the year 2020, more than 61 million older Americans will suffer from osteoporosis. As many as 38% of elderly male hip fracture patients will die of complications related to the fracture within 1 year of the incident.

Age-Related Eye Disorders

Cataracts, a cloudiness of the eye lens that impairs vision, develop in almost 70% of adults in their eighties. *Macular degeneration,* deterioration of the retina of the eye that causes a loss or distortion of vision, is the most common cause of blindness in elderly Americans. Sunlight exposure and smoking increase the risk for each condition.

Recent research suggests, but does not prove, that dietary choices may slow the progress of these degenerative eye diseases. For example, vitamins C and E, zinc, and two phytochemicals, lutein and zeaxanthin, may provide protection against these diseases. Although the research is not yet conclusive, older adults can benefit by eating foods rich in these nutrients, primarily richly colored fruits and vegetables, nuts, and whole grains. In contrast, there is no evidence that vision-enhancing supplements are effective in preventing these age-related disorders.

Use of Medications and Supplements

Although persons 65 years of age and above account for only 13% of the U.S. population, they are prescribed about 35% of all medications, and they experience almost 40% of all adverse drug effects, in part because of **polypharmacy**, or the use of five or more prescription drugs at any given time. A small but significant number of older adults use ten or more medications, a practice known as *excessive polypharmacy*. It should come as no surprise, then, that older adults make more than 175,000 emergency room visits annually for medication-related problems.

Drugs can also interact adversely with nutrients. Some medications affect appetite, either increasing or decreasing food intake, and others alter nutrient digestion and absorption. Several drugs negatively impact the activation or metabolism of nutrients such as vitamin D, folate, and vitamin B_6, whereas others increase the kidneys' excretion of nutrients. Conversely, nutrient intake can affect the action of certain drugs. For example, excessive vitamin K can block the action of anticoagulant drugs. A compound in grapefruit juice inhibits the breakdown of as many as 85 different drugs, leading to as much as a tenfold increase in blood drug levels and potential overdose. TABLE 11.7 summarizes a few of the more common drug–nutrient interactions that place older adults at risk.

Supplement usage continues to grow among all segments of the U.S. population, including the elderly. The Institute of Medicine, in establishing the DRI for vitamin B_{12}, specifically stated that adults over the age of 50 years should obtain most of their B_{12} "by consuming foods fortified with B_{12} or a B_{12}-containing supplement."[10] Older adults

TABLE 11.7 Examples of Common Drug–Nutrient Interactions

Category of Drug	Common Nutrient/Food Interactions
Antacids	May decrease the absorption of iron, calcium, folate, and vitamin B_{12}
Antibiotics	May reduce the absorption of calcium, fat-soluble vitamins; reduce the production of vitamin K by gut bacteria
Anticonvulsants	Interfere with activation of vitamin D
Anticoagulants ("blood thinners")	Oppose the clotting activity of vitamin K
Antidepressants	May cause weight gain as a result of increased appetite; may inappropriately lower serum sodium levels
Antiretroviral agents (treatment of HIV/AIDS)	Reduce the absorption of most nutrients
Aspirin	Lowers blood folate levels; increases loss of iron due to GI bleeding
Diuretics	Some types may increase urinary loss of potassium, sodium, calcium, and magnesium; some cause retention of potassium and other electrolytes
Laxatives	Increase fecal excretion of dietary fat, fat-soluble vitamins, calcium, and other minerals

polypharmacy The concurrent use of five or more medications.

should consult their healthcare provider about the need for other single-nutrient or multivitamin/mineral supplements.

What Social Programs Provide Food to Older Adults in Need?

Approximately 14% of older adults experience hunger or food insecurity at some point during any given year.[40] The most common cause of food insecurity and hunger among older adults is lack of income and poverty. Poverty levels are highest for those 85 years of age and older, primarily because of medical expenses. Older adults in poverty may live in areas with few or no supermarkets, may not be able to afford transportation to buy healthful food, and may fear leaving their home to shop for groceries. Low-income elderly households may also lack working refrigerators and/or stoves, limiting the types of foods they can buy, store, and prepare.

The federal government has developed an extensive network of food and nutrition services for older Americans. Many of them are coordinated with state and local governments, as well as nonprofit or community organizations. They include the following:

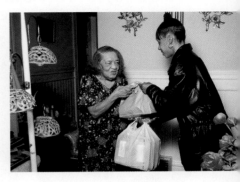

For homebound disabled and older adults, community programs provide nourishing, balanced meals as well as vital social contact.

- *Supplemental Nutrition Assistance Program (SNAP):* Older adults account for about 17% of all household recipients. Participants are provided with a monthly allotment, typically in the form of a prepaid debit card. Food-insecure seniors participating in SNAP are less likely to suffer from depression compared with nonparticipants who are food insecure. Unfortunately, older Americans who are eligible for SNAP are far less likely to participate compared with younger groups.[41]
- *Child and Adult Care Program:* This program provides healthful meals and snacks to older and functionally impaired adults in qualified adult day-care settings.
- *Commodity Supplemental Food Program:* Unlike SNAP benefits, this program is not intended to provide a complete array of foods. Instead, specific commodity foods are distributed, including cereals, peanut butter, dry beans, rice or pasta, and canned juice, fruits, vegetables, meat, poultry, and tuna. These foods are rich in nutrients typically lacking in the diets of older adults.
- *Seniors' Farmers' Market Nutrition Program:* This program, sponsored by the U.S. Department of Agriculture, provides coupons to low-income seniors, so that they can buy eligible foods at farmers' markets, roadside stands, and community-supported agriculture (CSA) programs. Seniors benefit from the nutritional advantages of fresh local produce and are often able to increase the variety of the foods they eat.
- *Nutrition Services Incentive Program:* The Department of Health and Human Services, through the Administration on Aging, provides funds and USDA commodity foods to individual state agencies for meals for senior citizens. There are no income criteria; any person 60 years or above (and spouse, even if younger) can take part in this program. Meals are served at senior centers and other locations in the community. This program also provides nutrition and health education and usually offers transportation to and from the meal site. For qualified homebound elders, meals can be delivered to their homes.

Participation in nutrition programs for the elderly improves the dietary quality and nutrient intakes of older adults. Unfortunately, many of these programs have long waiting lists and are unable to meet the current demands of their communities. With the ever-increasing number of elderly people, legislators must continue to commit adequate funding for these essential services.

recap Both overweight and underweight can contribute to poor health in older adults. Osteoporosis is increasingly common in both men and women in this age group, as are fracture-related deaths. Risk for eye disorders may be reduced by intakes of foods rich in antioxidants and phytochemicals. An older adult's nutrition can influence the effectiveness of certain medications, and some drugs affect nutrient status. A number of social services are available to older adults who are unable to secure a healthful diet.

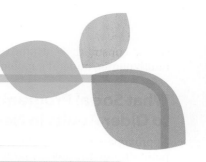

STUDY **PLAN** | MasteringNutrition™

Customize your study plan—and master your nutrition!—
in the Study Area of **MasteringNutrition**.

what can I do **today?**

Now that you've read this chapter, try making these three changes.

1 If you're a woman of childbearing age, whether or not you intend to become pregnant, make sure you consume at least 400 µg of folic acid daily.

2 Male or female, if you smoke, stop. Visit your healthcare provider or campus health services center for help in quitting, or join a smoking cessation program in your community.

3 Commit to regular physical activity. It can help you maintain your muscle mass and strength as you age.

test yourself | *answers*

1. **False.** More than half of all pregnant women experience morning sickness, and food cravings or aversions are also common.

2. **False.** Most infants do not have a physiologic need for solid food until about 6 months of age.

3. **True.** About 14% of older adults in the United States are unable to acquire adequate, nutritious food throughout the year.

summary

Scan to hear an MP3 Chapter Review in **MasteringNutrition**.

LO **1** Explain why a nourishing diet is important even before conception

- Nutrition is important before conception because critical stages of cell division, tissue differentiation, and organ development occur in the early weeks of pregnancy, often before a woman even knows she is pregnant. For example, 400 mg of folic acid daily is recommended for all women of childbearing age.

LO **2** Identify the range of optimal weight gain during the three trimesters of pregnancy

- A plentiful, nourishing diet is important throughout pregnancy to provide the energy and nutrients needed to support fetal development without depriving the mother of nutrients she needs to maintain her own health. Pregnant women of normal weight should consume adequate energy to gain 25 to 35 lb during pregnancy. Women who are underweight should gain slightly more, and women who are overweight or obese should gain less.

LO **3** Discuss nutrient needs and some common nutrition-related concerns of pregnant women

- Pregnant women need to be especially careful to consume adequate amounts of folate, vitamin B_{12}, vitamin C, vitamin D, calcium, iron, and other nutrients. Adolescents' bodies are still growing and developing; thus, their nutrient needs during pregnancy are higher than those of older pregnant women.

- A majority of pregnant women experience nausea and/or vomiting during pregnancy, called morning sickness, and some crave specific types of foods and nonfood substances (pica).

- Gestational diabetes and hypertension are nutrition-related disorders that can seriously affect maternal and fetal health.

- Alcohol is a teratogen and should not be consumed in any amount during pregnancy. Cigarette smoking reduces placental transfer of oxygen and nutrients, limiting fetal growth and development.

LO **4** **Discuss the advantages and challenges of breastfeeding**

- Breastfeeding women require more energy than is needed during pregnancy. Protein needs increase, and an overall nutritious diet with plentiful fluids is important in maintaining milk quality and quantity, as well as preserving the mother's health.

- Breast milk offers superior nutrition and protects the infant from infections and allergies. It also provides health benefits to the mother: Mothers who breastfeed experience the benefit of increased postpregnancy weight loss and suppressed ovulation.

- The American Academy of Pediatrics encourages exclusive breastfeeding (no food or other source of nourishment) for the first 6 months of life, continuing breastfeeding for at least the first year of life and, if acceptable within the family unit, into the second year of life or longer.

LO **5** **Discuss nutrient needs, timing of introduction to and type of solid foods, and common nutrition-related concerns of infants**

- Because infant stores of iron become depleted after about 6 months, a supplement or iron-fortified cereal is recommended for older breastfeeding infants. Breastfeeding infants also require a vitamin D supplement.

- Breast milk or formula is entirely sufficient for the first 6 months of life. Solid foods can be introduced one at a time after 4 to 6 months of age, with breast milk or formula remaining very important throughout the first year. Choking foods, honey, and excessive amounts of fruit juice, salty foods, and sweet foods must be avoided.

- Nutrition-related concerns for infants include the potential for allergies, colic, gastroesophageal reflux, dehydration, and anemia.

LO **6** **Discuss nutrient needs and some common nutrition-related concerns of toddlers**

- Toddlers grow more slowly than infants but are far more active. To provide adequate energy, toddlers should drink whole milk rather than low- or nonfat milk until they reach the age of 2 years. They require small, frequent, nutritious snacks and meals to consume adequate levels of nutrients.

- Feeding vegan diets to toddlers is controversial and poses potential deficiencies for protein, iron, calcium, zinc, vitamin D, and vitamin B_{12}.

LO **7** **Identify changes in nutrient needs for school-age children, as well as the effect of school attendance on children's nutrition**

- They need a lower percentage of fat Calories than toddlers but slightly more than adults (25% to 35% of energy). Micronutrient needs increase because of growth and maturation. Children can become easily dehydrated, especially during vigorous activity in warm weather. Peer pressure influences children's nutritional choices. Involving children in food growing, purchasing, and preparation can help.

- Many school-aged children skip breakfast and do not choose healthful foods during school lunch periods. School lunches are nutritious as planned and meet federal guidelines, but the foods that children choose to eat at school can be high in fat, sugar, and energy and low in nutrients.

- Food insecurity and obesity are significant nutritional concerns for U.S. children.

LO **8** **Explain how adolescents' rapid growth affects their nutritional status**

- Adolescents experience rapid increases in height, weight, and lean body mass and fat mass, so their energy needs can be very high. Because many adolescents fail to eat a variety of nutrient-dense foods, their intakes of some nutrients may be deficient.

- Many adolescents replace whole grains, fruits, and vegetables with fast foods and snack foods, placing them at risk for nutrient deficiencies. Calcium is needed to optimize bone growth and to achieve peak bone density, and iron needs are increased because of increased muscle mass in boys and menstruation in girls.

LO **9** **Discuss changes in an older adult's body, functions, and nutrient needs**

- Some of the physiologic changes that occur with aging, including decreased bone mass, muscle mass, and strength, can be lessened with a nutritious diet and regular physical activity.

- Recommendations for total fat, protein, and carbohydrate intake are unchanged throughout adulthood; however, fiber needs decrease slightly for older adults.

- Micronutrients of concern for older adults include calcium, iron, zinc, vitamin D, vitamin B_{12}, vitamin B_6, and folate. Older adults are at increased risk for dehydration, so ample fluid intake is important.

LO **10** **Identify some common nutrition-related concerns of older adults**

- Being overweight or underweight are concerns in older adulthood, because both increase the risk for illness and premature mortality. Some studies have shown links between dietary patterns and risk of age-related conditions, such as cataracts and dementia.

- Medications can interfere with nutrient absorption and metabolism, and nutrients can also interfere with the actions of medications. Polypharmacy can present a challenge to the older adults when medications interact or interfere with each other.

- Food-assistance programs for low-income older adults, such as the Supplemental Nutrition Assistance Program and Nutrition Services Incentive Program, can provide important nourishment to this vulnerable population.

review questions

LO **1** **Explain why a nourishing diet is important even before conception**

1. Folate deficiency in the first weeks after conception has been linked with which of the following problems in newborns?
   a. High blood pressure
   b. Neural tube defects
   c. Abnormally high birth weight
   d. Poor bone mineralization

LO **2** **Identify the range of optimal weight gain during the three trimesters of pregnancy**

2. A total pregnancy weight gain of 25–35 pounds is recommended for women who
   a. were of normal weight prior to pregnancy.
   b. were underweight prior to pregnancy.
   c. were overweight prior to pregnancy.
   d. were underweight prior to pregnancy and are carrying twins.

LO **3** **Discuss nutrient needs and some common nutrition-related concerns of pregnant women**

3. During pregnancy,
   a. women need a higher percentage of Calories from fat.
   b. women have a higher RDA for protein.
   c. Calorie needs increase by about 550–600 kcal/day.
   d. all of the above are true.

LO **4** **Discuss the advantages and challenges of breastfeeding**

4. Which of the following statements about breast milk is true?
   a. Both antibodies and immune cells are passed from mother to infant in breast milk.
   b. Breast milk is especially high in glucose.
   c. Breast milk alone is entirely sufficient to sustain an infant for the first 12 months of life.
   d. All of the above are true.

LO **5** **Discuss nutrient needs, timing of introduction to and type of solid foods, and common nutrition-related concerns of infants**

5. Which of the following nutrients should be added to the diet of breastfed infants when they are around 6 months of age?
   a. Fiber
   b. Fat
   c. Iron
   d. Vitamin C

LO **6** **Discuss nutrient needs and some common nutrition-related concerns of toddlers**

6. Of the following foods, which would be the most appropriate choice to serve a toddler?
   a. Grapes
   b. Grape juice
   c. A whole-grain cracker with smooth peanut butter
   d. A yogurt parfait made with ⅓ cup nonfat yogurt topped with ¼ cup chopped walnuts and ¼ cup chopped grapes

LO **7** **Identify changes in nutrient needs for school-age children, as well as the effect of school attendance on children's nutrition**

7. Which of the following is a common nutrition-related consequence of attending school?
   a. Schoolchildren may feel too rushed in the morning to eat breakfast.
   b. Schoolchildren do not always eat adequate amounts of food.
   c. Schoolchildren do not always eat the most nutritious parts of their school lunch.
   d. all of the above

LO 8 Explain how adolescents' rapid growth affects their nutritional status

8. The RDA for calcium for adolescents is
   a. less than that for young children.
   b. less than that for adults.
   c. less than that for pregnant adults.
   d. greater than that for children, adults, and pregnant adults.

LO 9 Discuss changes in an older adult's body, functions, and nutrient needs

9. Which of the following is needed in increased amounts in older adulthood?
   a. Fiber
   b. Vitamin D
   c. Carbohydrate
   d. Energy (kcal/day)

LO 10 Identify some common nutrition-related concerns of older adults

10. Why are older adults often at risk for inappropriate weight loss?
    a. Certain drugs interfere with normal appetite.
    b. Depression and social isolation decrease food intake.
    c. Many elderly people have limited incomes and have no transportation to shop for healthful foods.
    d. All of the above are correct.

Answers to Review Questions are located at the back of this text.

web links

The following websites and apps explore further topics and issues related to personal health.
Visit **MasteringNutrition** for links to the websites and RSS feeds.

www.aap.org
American Academy of Pediatrics

www.aarp.org
American Association for Retired Persons

www.aoa.gov
The Department of Health and Human Services, Administration on Aging

www.diabetes.org
American Diabetes Association

www.livingto100.com
The Living to 100 Life Expectancy Calculator

www.llli.org
La Leche League

www.marchofdimes.com
March of Dimes

www.nihseniorhealth.gov
The National Institutes of Health, SeniorHealth

www.nofas.org
National Organization on Fetal Alcohol Syndrome

www.teamnutrition.usda.gov
MyPlate for Kids

Food Safety, Technology, and the New Food Movement

learning outcomes

After reading this chapter, you will be able to:

1 Summarize the two main reasons that foodborne illness is a critical concern in the United States, pp. 369–372.

2 Identify the types of microorganisms most commonly involved in foodborne illness, pp. 372–377.

3 Describe strategies for preventing foodborne illness at home, while eating out, and when traveling to other countries, pp. 377–382.

4 Compare and contrast the different methods manufacturers use to preserve foods, pp. 382–383.

5 Debate the safety of food additives, including the role of the GRAS list, pp. 383–385.

6 Describe the process of genetic modification and discuss the potential risks and benefits associated with genetically modified organisms, pp. 385–387.

7 Describe the process by which persistent organic pollutants accumulate in foods, pp. 388–393.

8 Discuss the regulation, labeling, benefits, and limitations of organic foods, pp. 388–393.

9 Explain how corporate agricultural practices have threatened sustainability and reduced food diversity, and identify several initiatives embraced by the food movement to reverse these trends, pp. 393–398.

10 Discuss two issues of food equity: food insecurity and unfair trade practices, pp. 393–398.

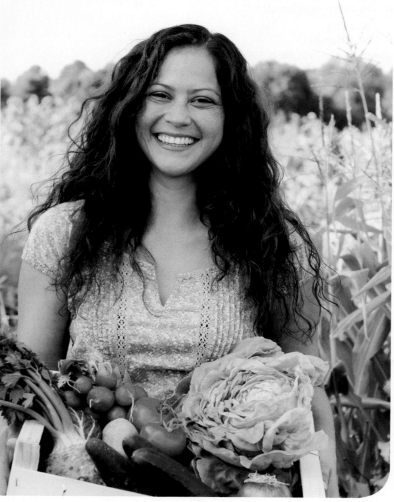

MasteringNutrition™

Go online for chapter quizzes, pre-tests, Interactive Activities, and more!

test yourself

Are these statements true or false? Circle your guess.

1. **T** **F** Mold is the most common cause of food poisoning.

2. **T** **F** Freezing destroys any microorganisms that might be lurking in your food.

3. **T** **F** More than 10% of Americans are unable to obtain enough food to meet their needs every day.

Test Yourself answers can be found at the end of the chapter.

A cruise. The epitome of luxury. The ads promise panoramic views of romantic landscapes, comfort, fun, and great-tasting food. . . . So why do healthcare professionals sometimes refer to a cruise ship as a "floating petri dish"?

The answer, in a word, is norovirus. Infection with this highly contagious virus typically causes 1–3 days of forceful vomiting and diarrhea, but it can be more severe and even fatal. In any given year, over 90% of diarrheal disease outbreaks on cruise ships are caused by norovirus. During the same week in January, 2014, for example, it sickened 700 people on one Caribbean cruise, and 170 on another. Norovirus doesn't hit only cruise lines, but also hospitals and nursing homes, restaurants, workplaces, and college campuses.

Norovirus is spread by direct person-to-person contact as well as in food or water. Food can become contaminated while it is being grown, shipped, handled, or prepared, most commonly when workers with virus particles on their hands touch the food. Although a variety of foods have been associated with outbreaks, foods that are eaten raw, such as leafy vegetables, fruit, and shellfish, are most commonly involved.[1]

But norovirus is not the only microbe contaminating our food supply. In just the first few weeks of 2014, *Salmonella* bacteria, which cause severe abdominal cramps and diarrhea, were found in eggs, parsley, tomatoes, cheese, and even cat and dog food.[2] And *Listeria monocytogenes*, a type of bacteria that can cause pregnant women to miscarry, showed up in hummus, smoked salmon, and a variety of cheeses during the same brief period.[2] What's worse, these are just two of several bacteria that cause foodborne illness.

How do disease-causing agents enter our food and water supplies, and how can we protect ourselves from them? What makes food spoil, and what keeps it fresh? Which aspects of industrial food production help consumers, and which put us at risk? We explore these and other questions in this chapter.

Why is foodborne illness a critical concern?

 Summarize the two main reasons that foodborne illness is a critical concern in the United States.

Foodborne illness is a term used to encompass any symptom or disorder that arises from ingesting food or water contaminated with disease-causing (*pathogenic*) microscopic organisms (called *microorganisms*), their toxic secretions, or chemicals (such as mercury or pesticides). You probably refer to foodborne illness as *food poisoning*.

Foodborne Illness Affects Millions of Americans Annually

According to the Centers for Disease Control and Prevention (CDC), approximately 48 million Americans—1 out of every 6—report experiencing foodborne illness each year. Of these, 128,000 are hospitalized and 3,000 die.[3] The people most at risk for serious foodborne illness include

- developing fetuses, infants, and young children, because their immune system is immature;
- people who are very old or have a chronic illness, because their immune system may be compromised;
- people with acquired immunodeficiency syndrome (AIDS); and
- people who are receiving immune-system-suppressing drugs, such as transplant recipients and cancer patients.

Although the statistics may seem frightening, most experts consider our food supply safe. That's partly because not all cases of food contamination make all people

foodborne illness An illness transmitted by food or water contaminated by a pathogenic microorganism, its toxic secretions, or a toxic chemical.

TABLE 12.1 Government Agencies That Regulate Food Safety

Name of Agency	Year Established	Role in Food Regulations	Website
U.S. Department of Agriculture (USDA)	1785	Oversees safety of meat, poultry, and eggs sold across state lines; also regulates which drugs can be used to treat sick cattle and poultry	www.usda.gov
U.S. Food and Drug Administration (FDA)	1862	Regulates food standards of food products (except meat, poultry, and eggs) and bottled water; regulates food labeling and enforces pesticide use as established by EPA	www.fda.gov
Centers for Disease Control and Prevention (CDC)	1946	Works with public health officials to promote and educate the public about health and safety; able to track information needed in identifying foodborne illness outbreaks	www.cdc.gov
Environmental Protection Agency (EPA)	1970	Regulates use of pesticides and which crops they can be applied to; establishes standards for water quality	www.epa.gov

sick; in fact, even virulent strains cause illness in only a small percentage of people who consume the tainted food. Moreover, modern technology has given us an array of techniques to preserve foods. We discuss these later in this chapter.

Moreover, food safety in the United States is monitored by several government agencies. In addition to the CDC, mentioned earlier, the United States Department of Agriculture (USDA), Food and Drug Administration (FDA), and Environmental Protection Agency (EPA) monitor and regulate food safety, production, and preservation. Information about these agencies and how to access them appear in **TABLE 12.1**.

Food Production Is Increasingly Complex

Despite safeguards, foodborne illness has emerged as a major public health threat in recent years. One reason is that more foods are mass-produced than ever before, with a combination of ingredients from a much greater number of sources, including fields, feedlots, and a variety of processing facilities all over the world. These various sources can remain hidden not only to consumers but even to food companies using the ingredients. Contamination can occur at any point from farm to table (**FIGURE 12.1**), and when it does, it can be difficult to trace.

Moreover, oversight of food safety, according to the government's own descriptions, is both fragmented and underfunded.[4] Over the last few decades, for example, government inspection of food-production facilities has declined just as the number of facilities, both here and overseas, has skyrocketed. Farms and production facilities are often inspected by private auditors who have a financial interest in completing the job quickly and perfunctorily.

New food safety legislation, the FDA Food Safety Modernization Act (FSMA), which was signed into law in January 2011, is beginning to strengthen our food safety system.[4] Among its provisions are the following:

- New requirements for food processors to prevent contamination
- New requirements for food importers to verify the safety of food from their suppliers
- New FDA enforcement tools, including mandatory recall authority
- A new, more rigorous inspection schedule

Moreover, in January 2013, the FDA proposed two new rulings requiring farmers and food processors, whether foreign or domestic, to develop a formal plan for preventing contamination and for correcting any problems that arise. Additional rules are expected to follow.[5]

Although it is too soon to judge the effectiveness of these provisions, the most recent data from the CDC are not encouraging. As compared with 2006–2008, the 2012 incidence of foodborne infection with two common bacterial culprits had increased, and infections with another five had neither increased nor decreased significantly.[6]

For information—including posters, podcasts, and videos—on a variety of food safety topics, go to http://www.cdc.gov, type in "food safety" in the search bar, and click on "For Consumers."

Farms

Animals raised for meat can harbor harmful microorganisms, and crops can be contaminated with pollutants from irrigation, runoff from streams, microorganisms or toxins in soil, or pesticides. Contamination can also occur during animal slaughter or from harvesting, sorting, washing, packing, and/or storage of crops.

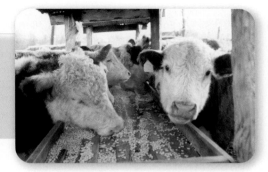

▲ **FIGURE 12.1**   Food is at risk for contamination at any of the five stages from farm to table, but following food safety guidelines can reduce the risks.

Processing

Some foods, such as produce, may go from the farm directly to the market, but most foods are processed. Processed foods may go through several steps at different facilities. At each site, people, equipment, or environments may contaminate foods. Federal safeguards, such as cleaning protocols, testing, and training, can help prevent contamination.

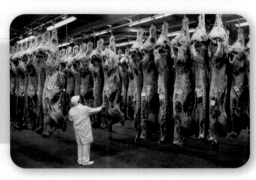

Transportation

Foods must be transported in clean, refrigerated vehicles and containers to prevent multiplication of microorganisms and microbial toxins.

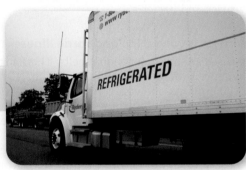

Retail

Employees of food markets and restaurants may contaminate food during storage, preparation, or service. Conditions such as inadequate refrigeration or heating may promote multiplication of microorganisms or microbial toxins. Establishments must follow FDA guidelines for food safety and pass local health inspections.

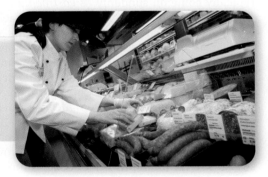

Table

Consumers may contaminate foods with unclean hands, utensils, or surfaces. They can allow the multiplication of microorganisms and microbial toxins by failing to follow the food-safety guidelines for storing, preparing, cooking, and serving foods discussed in this chapter.

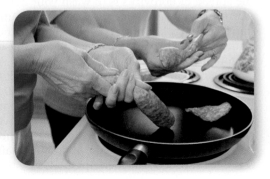

Foodborne illness affects 48 million Americans a year. Contamination can occur at any point from farm to table. The Centers for Disease Control and Prevention, the Food and Drug Administration, the United States Department of Agriculture, and the Environmental Protection Agency monitor and regulate food production and preservation. The Food Safety Modernization Act of 2011 increased the oversight of food production by federal agencies and authorized the FDA to swiftly recall contaminated foods from the market, and new rules are under development.

LO2 Identify the types of microorganisms most commonly involved in foodborne illness.

What causes most foodborne illness?

A *pathogen* is any agent capable of generating disease. The consumption of food containing pathogenic microorganisms results in *food infections*. *Food intoxications* result from consuming food tainted with harmful substances called *toxins*. Chemical residues in foods, such as pesticides and pollutants, can also cause illness. Residues are discussed later in this chapter.

Several Types of Microorganisms Contaminate Foods

The two types of microorganisms that most commonly cause food infections are viruses and bacteria.

Viruses Involved in Foodborne Illness

Viruses are not independent cells. Their survival depends on their ability to infect the living cells of humans and other animals, plants, and even other microorganisms.

Norovirus, the virus introduced at the beginning of this chapter, is responsible for 49% of all foodborne illness annually in the United States (**FIGURE 12.2**). In fact, it causes more foodborne illness than all other microbial culprits put together, about 19 to 21 million cases annually.[7]

Norovirus is so common and contagious that many people refer to it simply as "the stomach flu"; however, it is not a strain of influenza. Symptoms of infection typically come on suddenly as *gastroenteritis*, inflammation of the lining of the stomach and intestines. This causes stomach cramps as well as both vomiting and diarrhea. Because the vomiting begins abruptly, the person is likely to be in a social setting. Because it is forceful, anyone nearby is likely to become contaminated. Another characteristic that makes norovirus so contagious is that, whereas most viruses perish quickly in a dry environment, norovirus is able to survive on dry surfaces and objects, from countertops to utensils, for days or even weeks. Also, ingestion of even a few "particles" of norovirus can result in full-blown illness.[7]

College campuses commonly report outbreaks. In 2013, for instance, several campuses in the Northeast experienced norovirus outbreaks, sending hundreds of students to their campus health center or to the hospital. The best way to prevent the spread of norovirus is to wash your hands, kitchen surfaces, and utensils with warm, soapy water. Alcohol-based hand sanitizers may be used in addition to hand washing, but not as a substitute.[7] If you experience vomiting or diarrhea, immediately clean and disinfect all nearby surfaces and remove and wash laundry thoroughly.

Whereas norovirus is estimated to infect up to 21 million Americans annually, hepatitis A virus (HAV) causes about 17,000 infections.[8] Like norovirus, HAV can be transmitted person-to-person or via contaminated foods and water supplies. The term *hepatitis* means inflammation of the liver. This causes jaundice (a yellowish skin tone), the most common sign of HAV infection.[8] Typically, the symptoms of HAV infection include a mild fever, abdominal pain, and nausea and vomiting that lasts a few weeks. Rarely, in elderly patients and those with preexisting liver disease, HAV infection can lead to liver failure and even death.

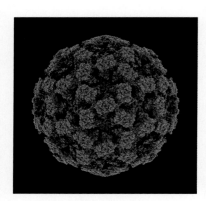

▲ **FIGURE 12.2** Norovirus is the leading cause of foodborne infection in the United States. It is responsible for more foodborne illness from known agents than all other viruses, bacteria, and parasites combined.

viruses A group of noncellular infectious agents that are usually smaller than bacteria, lack independent metabolism, and are incapable of growth or reproduction outside living cells.

bacteria Microorganisms that lack a true nucleus and reproduce by division or by forming spores.

parasite A microorganism that simultaneously derives benefit from and harms its host.

helminth A multicellular microscopic worm.

TABLE 12.2   Six Most Common Bacterial Causes of Foodborne Illness

Bacteria	Incubation Period	Duration	Symptoms	Foods Most Commonly Affected	Steps for Prevention
Salmonella (more than 2,300 types)	12–24 hours	4–7 days	Nausea Diarrhea Abdominal pain Chills Fever Headache	Raw or undercooked eggs, poultry, and meat Raw milk and dairy products Seafood Fruits and vegetables	Cook foods thoroughly. Avoid cross-contamination. Only drink pasteurized milk. Practice proper hand washing and sanitizing.
Clostridium perfringens	8–22 hours	24 hours	Abdominal cramps Diarrhea Dehydration	Beef Poultry Gravies Leftovers	Cook foods thoroughly and serve hot. Refrigerate leftovers promptly. Reheat leftovers thoroughly before serving.
Escherichia coli (O157:H7 and other strains that can cause human illness)	2–4 days	3–7 days or longer	Diarrhea (may be bloody) Abdominal cramps Nausea Can lead to kidney failure	Contaminated water Unpasteurized milk Raw or rare ground beef, sausages Unpasteurized juices Uncooked fruits and vegetables Prepackaged raw cookie dough	Only drink pasteurized milk. Cook foods properly. Avoid cross-contamination.
Shigella (several species)	12–50 hours	1–2 days	Abdominal cramps Diarrhea Fever Vomiting Blood and pus	Poultry Salad and other raw vegetables Dairy products	Practice proper hand washing and sanitizing.
Campylobacter (several species)	1–7 days	2–10 days	Headache Diarrhea Nausea Abdominal cramps	Raw and undercooked meat, poultry, eggs Cake icing Untreated water Unpasteurized milk	Only drink pasteurized milk. Cook foods properly. Avoid cross-contamination.
Staphylococcus aureus (which produces an enterotoxin)	1–6 hours	1–2 days	Severe vomiting Abdominal cramps Diarrhea	Custard- or cream-filled baked goods Ham Poultry Dressings, sauces, and gravies Eggs Potato salad	Refrigerate foods. Practice proper hand washing and sanitizing.

Source: Data from Iowa State University Extension, Food Safety. Updated June 22, 2010. *Common Foodborne Pathogens.* http://www.extension.iastate.edu/foodsafety/pathogens/index.cfm? parent=37; U.S. Food and Drug Administration, Foodborne Illnesses: What You Need to Know, Updated October 31, 2013, from http://www.fda.gov/Food/FoodborneIllnessContaminants/ FoodborneIllnessesNeedToKnow/default.htm; and L. H. Gould, et al., Surveillance for Foodborne Disease Outbreaks—United States, 1998–2008, *MMWR*, June 28, 2013 / 62(SS02);1–34.

Bacteria Involved in Foodborne Illness

In contrast to viruses, **bacteria** are cellular microorganisms; however, they lack the true cell nucleus common to plant and animal cells, and they reproduce either by dividing in two or by forming reproductive spores. Many thrive in the intestines of birds and mammals, including humans; in fact, as we explained in Chapter 2, our gastrointestinal tract contains trillions of probiotic bacteria that contribute to our health and functioning.

In contrast, pathogenic bacteria are capable of causing disease. Foodborne bacterial illness commonly occurs when we ingest pathogenic bacteria living in or on undercooked or raw foods or fluids. These bacteria, which often come from human or animal feces, can damage our cells and tissues either directly or by secreting a destructive toxin. The six bacterial pathogens responsible for the greatest number of foodborne illnesses among Americans are identified in **TABLE 12.2**. Of these, the most deadly is *Salmonella* (**FIGURE 12.3**).

Other Microorganisms Involved in Foodborne Illness

Parasites are microorganisms that simultaneously derive benefit from and harm their host. They are responsible for only about 1% of foodborne illnesses. The following are the most common culprits:

■ **Helminths** are multicellular worms, such as tapeworms (**FIGURE 12.4**), flukes, and roundworms. They reproduce by releasing their eggs into vegetation or water.

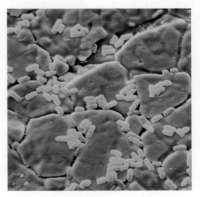

▲ **FIGURE 12.3** *Salmonella* is the leading cause of bacterial foodborne illness, causing more than a million infections annually. Infection can cause fever, diarrhea, and abdominal cramps, and cells of some strains of *Salmonella* can perforate the intestines and invade the blood, causing systemic infection and death.

Hooks   Sucker

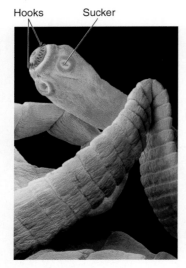

FIGURE 12.4 Tapeworms have long, wormlike bodies and hooks and suckers, which help them attach to human tissues.

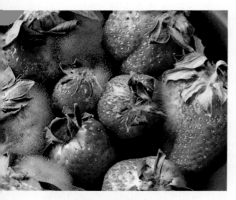

FIGURE 12.5 Molds rarely cause foodborne illness, in part because they look so unappealing that we throw the food away.

protozoa Single-celled, mobile microorganisms.

fungi Plantlike, spore-forming organisms that can grow as either single cells or multicellular colonies.

prion A protein that misfolds and becomes infectious; prions are not living cellular organisms or viruses.

toxin Any harmful substance; in microbiology, a chemical produced by a microorganism that harms tissues or causes harmful immune responses.

Animals, including fish, then consume the contaminated matter. The eggs hatch inside their host, and larvae develop in the host's flesh, where they can survive long after the host is killed for food. Thoroughly cooking beef, pork, or fish destroys the larvae. In contrast, people who eat contaminated foods either raw or undercooked consume living larvae, which then mature into adult worms in their small intestine. Some worms cause only mild nausea and diarrhea, but others can grow large enough to cause intestinal obstruction or travel through the bloodstream to invade muscle tissue. Undercooked pork, for example, can harbor the larvae of a helminth called *Trichinella*. Consumption results in trichinellosis, which can cause months of diarrhea, fatigue, and muscle pain or even, with heavy doses, result in death.[9]

- **Protozoa** are single-celled parasites implicated in food- and waterborne illness. One of these, *Toxoplasma gondii*, is the last of our top culprits in foodborne illness, and is second only to *Salmonella* as a cause of death.[3] Another common agent is *Giardia*, various species of which cause a diarrheal illness called *giardiasis*. Both *T. gondii* and *Giardia* live in the intestines of infected animals and humans and pass into food and water from stools. People typically ingest these parasites by swallowing contaminated water or by eating undercooked or raw contaminated food. Many people infected with these parasites never develop symptoms, or experience only a mild, flu-like illness; however, in vulnerable populations, *T. gondii* can lead to organ damage, and infection during pregnancy can cause a miscarriage, stillbirth, or eye or brain damage in the newborn.[10,11]

Fungi are plantlike, spore-forming organisms that can grow as either single cells or multicellular colonies. Three common types are yeasts, which are globular, molds, which are long and thin, and the familiar mushrooms. Foodborne illnesses are rarely caused by microscopic fungi, in part because very few species are capable of causing serious disease in people with healthy immune systems, and these few are not typically foodborne. The CDC lists only one foodborne fungus, *Cryptococcus*, which almost exclusively affects patients with compromised immunity.[12] In addition, unlike bacterial growth, which is invisible and often tasteless, fungal growth typically makes food look and taste so unappealing that we immediately discard it **(FIGURE 12.5)**.

A foodborne illness in beef cattle that has had front-page exposure in recent years is mad cow disease, or *bovine spongiform encephalopathy* (*BSE*). This neurological disorder is caused by a **prion**, a proteinaceous infectious particle that is self-replicating. Prions start out as normal proteins of animal tissues, then misfold and become infectious. When they do, they can transform other normal proteins into abnormally shaped prions until they eventually cause illness.

The human form of BSE can develop in people who consume contaminated meat or tissue. If you eat beef, are you at risk? See the ***Nutrition Myth or Fact?*** box and find out.

Some Foodborne Illness Is Due to Toxins

Some species of bacteria and fungi secrete chemicals, called **toxins**, that are responsible for serious and even life-threatening illnesses. These toxins bind to body cells and can cause a variety of symptoms, such as diarrhea, vomiting, organ damage, convulsions, and paralysis. Toxins can be categorized depending on the type of cell they bind to; the two primary types of toxins associated with foodborne illness are neurotoxins, which damage the nervous system and can cause paralysis, and enterotoxins, which target the gastrointestinal system and generally cause severe diarrhea and vomiting.

Bacterial Toxins

One of the most common and deadly neurotoxins is produced by the bacterium *Clostridium botulinum*. The botulism toxin blocks nerve transmission to muscle cells and causes paralysis, including paralysis of the muscles required for breathing. A common source of contamination is food in a damaged (split, pierced, or bulging) can. If you spot damaged canned goods while shopping, notify the store manager.

nutrition myth or fact?

Mad Cow Disease: Is It Safe to Eat Beef?

Mad cow disease is a fatal neurological disorder in cattle caused by a *prion*, which is an abnormally folded, infectious protein. Prions influence other proteins to take on their abnormal shape, and these abnormal proteins damage nerve tissue, notably in the brain and spinal cord. The disease can occur in sheep and other animals as well as cows.

Mad cow disease is technically known as *bovine spongiform* (spongelike) *encephalopathy (BSE)* because the disease eats away at a cow's brain, leaving it full of holes. Eventually, the brain can no longer control vital functions and the cow literally "goes mad" and dies. Unfortunately, people who eat contaminated meat from infected cattle will also be infected. Symptoms may take years to appear, but eventually the person may develop the human form of mad cow disease, called *variant Creutzfeldt-Jakob disease (vCJD)*. As of 2013, this disease had killed 177 people in Great Britain, and another 51 in other nations.[1]

Scientists are not certain how the prions are introduced to cattle. They think that cattle become infected by eating feed containing tissue from the brains and spinal cords of other infected cattle. Decades ago in Great Britain and Europe, it was common practice to feed livestock with meal made from other animals. This practice has ceased, and the number of deaths attributed to vCJD has declined steadily from its peak of 28 in the year 2000.[1]

For many years, experts in North America believed BSE to be a problem limited to Europe. But then, eight cases of BSE were found in cows in Canada from 2003 to 2006. And in December 2003, the first case of mad cow disease

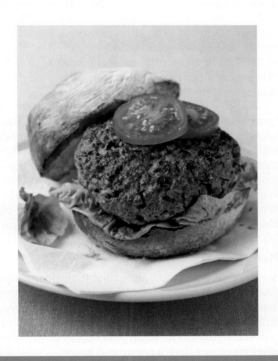

was reported in the United States. Since then, three additional cases have been confirmed, the most recent in April of 2012.[2] So if you eat beef, are you at risk?

To date, only one case of vCJD has been confirmed in Canada and one in the United States, and these individuals are thought to have acquired the disease while in the United Kingdom. The low incidence of vCJD in North America may reflect longstanding preventive practices. For instance, the United States has a system of three interlocking safeguards against BSE. The first and most important of these is the practice of removing, prior to slaughter, the parts of an animal that would contain BSE should an animal have the disease. The second is rigorous control of the quality of animal feed. The third safeguard—which led to the April 2012 detection in a cow culled for lameness—is an ongoing BSE surveillance program in which carcasses are routinely sampled for BSE.[2]

So is it safe for Americans to eat beef? The USDA is working together with other government agencies and the U.S. beef industry to eliminate the use of unapproved animal feed and to improve technologies and procedures to detect BSE before an animal is approved for consumption. The beef industry is highly motivated to maintain food safety, because reduced beef consumption would translate into millions of dollars in lost income. In May, 2013, the intergovernmental World Organization for Animal Health upgraded the United States' risk classification for BSE to "negligible."[3] Thus, although it may not be possible to guarantee the safety of U.S. beef, adherence to strict safety standards has minimized the risk of an outbreak of vCJD.

If you inadvertently purchase food in a damaged can, or find that the container spurts liquid when you open it, throw it out immediately. *Never* taste the food, because even a microscopic amount of botulism toxin can be deadly.[13] Other common sources of *C. botulinum* are foods improperly canned at home and raw honey.

Some strains of *E. coli* are particularly dangerous, because they produce a toxin called *Shiga toxin*. These types are referred to as Shiga toxin-producing *E. coli* or STEC. The most common STEC is *E. coli* O157. This species alone is responsible for more than 2,000 hospitalizations each year.[3] In vulnerable populations, infection with one of the STECs can result in kidney failure and, in some cases, death.

Eating spoiled fish, commonly tuna or mackerel, is unwise because bacteria responsible for the spoilage release toxins into the fish. The result is *scombrotoxic fish poisoning*, which causes headache, vomiting, a rash, sweating, and flushing within

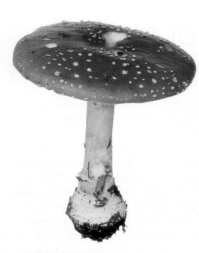

⬆ **FIGURE 12.6** Some mushrooms, such as this fly agaric, contain toxins that can cause illness or even death.

a few minutes to 2 hours after consumption. Symptoms are usually mild and resolve within a few hours in healthy people.[14]

Fungal Toxins

Some fungi produce poisonous chemicals called *mycotoxins*. (The prefix *myco* means "fungus.") These toxins are typically found in grains stored in moist environments. In some instances, moist conditions in the field encourage fungi to reproduce and release their toxins on the surface of growing crops. Long-term consumption of mycotoxins can cause organ damage or cancer.

A highly visible fungus that causes food intoxication is the poisonous mushroom. Most mushrooms are not toxic, but a few, such as the death cap mushroom (*Amanita phalloides*), can be fatal. Some poisonous mushrooms are quite colorful **(FIGURE 12.6)**, a fact that helps explain why the victims of mushroom poisoning are often children.[15]

Toxic Algae

Have you ever walked a beach and noticed a red sign warning that the area was closed to all shellfishing? Almost certainly the cause was a harmful algal bloom (HAB), commonly known as a "red tide," during which certain species of toxic algae reach dangerous levels in the ocean waters, sometimes even turning them purple, pink, or red. Mussels, clams, and other shellfish consume these toxic algae as they filter seawater for food. Humans who then eat the seafood, which typically looks, smells, and tastes normal, develop *paralytic shellfish poisoning* (PSP). The effects of PSP can be limited to nausea, vomiting, diarrhea, dizziness, and disorientation. However, as its name suggests, PSP can also cause paralysis and sometimes results in death.[16]

Finfish can also be contaminated with toxic algae. Ciguatoxins are marine toxins commonly found in fresh fish caught off the coasts of Hawaii, Puerto Rico, the Virgin Islands, and other tropical regions. They are produced by algae called *dinoflagellates*, which are consumed by small fish. The toxins become progressively more concentrated as larger fish eat these small fish, and high concentrations can be present in grouper, sea bass, snapper, and a number of other large fish from tropical regions. Symptoms of ciguatoxin poisoning include nausea, vomiting, diarrhea, headache, itching, a "pins-and-needles" feeling, and even nightmares or hallucinations, but the illness is rarely fatal and typically resolves within a few weeks.[14]

Plant Toxins

A variety of plants contain toxins that, if consumed, can cause illness. As humans evolved, we learned to avoid such plants. However, one plant toxin is still commonly found in kitchens. Potatoes that have turned green contain the toxin solanine, which forms along with chlorophyll—a harmless green pigment—when the potatoes are exposed to light. The toxin also occurs in the sprouts that form on stored potatoes, whether or not they have turned green.

Solanine is very toxic even in small amounts. Potatoes that appear green beneath the skin should be thrown away, and any sprouts forming on a stored potato should be removed. Toxicity causes vomiting, diarrhea, fever, headache, and other symptoms, and can progress to shock. Very rarely, the poisoning can be fatal.[17] You can avoid the greening and sprouting of potatoes by storing them for only short periods in a dark cupboard or brown paper bag in a cool area.

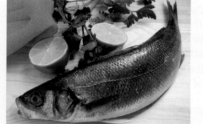

⬆ Sea bass may look appealing, but like several other large predatory tropical fish, it can be contaminated with a high concentration of marine toxins.

The Body Responds to Contaminants with Acute Illness

Many contaminants are killed in the mouth by antimicrobial enzymes in saliva or in the stomach by hydrochloric acid. Any that survive these chemical assaults usually trigger vomiting and/or diarrhea as the gastrointestinal tract attempts to expel them. Simultaneously, the white blood cells of the immune system are activated, and a generalized inflammatory response causes the person to experience nausea, fatigue, fever, and muscle aches. Depending on the state of one's health, the precise microorganism or toxin involved, and the "dose" ingested, the symptoms can range from mild to severe.

To diagnose a foodborne illness, a specimen—usually blood or stool—must be analyzed. Treatment usually involves keeping the person hydrated and comfortable, because most foodborne illness tends to be self-limiting; the person's vomiting and/ or diarrhea, though unpleasant, rid the body of the offending agent. In more severe cases, hospitalization may be necessary.

In the United States, all confirmed cases of foodborne illness must be reported to the state health department, which in turn reports these illnesses to the CDC in Atlanta, Georgia. The CDC monitors its reports for indications of epidemics of food-borne illness and assists local and state agencies in controlling such outbreaks.

Certain Conditions Help Microorganisms Multiply in Foods

Given the correct environmental conditions, microorganisms can thrive in many types of food. Four factors affect the survival and reproduction of food microorganisms:

- *Temperature:* Many microorganisms capable of causing human illness thrive at moderately cool to warm temperatures, from about 40°F to 140°F (4°C to 60°C) as stated by the USDA. You can think of this range of temperatures as the **danger zone** (FIGURE 12.7). These microorganisms can be destroyed by thoroughly heating or cooking foods, and their reproduction can be slowed by refrigeration and freezing. We identify safe cooking and food-storage temperatures later in this chapter.
- *Humidity:* Many microorganisms require a high level of moisture; thus, foods such as boxed dried pasta do not make suitable microbial homes, although cooked pasta left at room temperature would prove hospitable.
- *Acidity:* Most microorganisms have a preferred pH range in which they thrive. For instance, *Clostridium botulinum* loves alkaline environments. It cannot grow or produce its toxin in acidic environments, so the risk for botulism is decreased in citrus fruits, pickles, and tomato-based foods. In contrast, alkaline foods, such as fish and most vegetables are a magnet for *C. botulinum.*
- *Oxygen content:* Many microorganisms require oxygen to function; thus, food-preservation techniques that remove oxygen, such as industrial canning and bottling, keep foods safe for consumption. In contrast, *C. botulinum* thrives in an oxygen-free environment. For this reason, the canning process heats foods to an extremely high temperature to destroy this organism. It is not uncommon for food producers to voluntarily recall canned goods because of concerns that the food had not been heated high enough to destroy *C. botulinum.*

In addition, microorganisms need an entryway into a food. Just as our skin protects our body from microbial invasion, the peels, rinds, and shells of many foods seal off access to the nutrients within. Eggshells are a good example of a natural food barrier. Once such a barrier is removed, however, the food loses its primary defense against contamination.

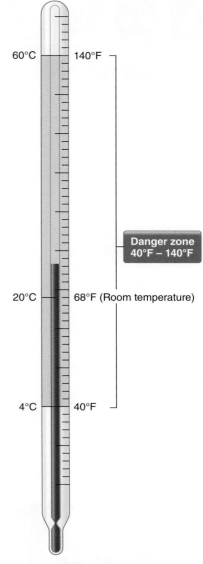

▲ **FIGURE 12.7** The danger zone is a range of temperature at which many pathogenic microorganisms thrive. Notice that "room temperature" (about 68°F) is within the danger zone!

recap Food infections result from the consumption of food containing pathogenic microorganisms, such as viruses and bacteria, whereas food intoxications result from consuming food containing toxins. The body has several defense mechanisms that help rid us of offending microorganisms or their toxins. To reproduce in foods, microorganisms require a precise range of temperature, humidity, acidity, and oxygen content.

danger zone Range of temperature (about 40°F to 140°F [4°C to 60°C]) at which many microorganisms capable of causing human disease thrive.

How can you prevent foodborne illness?

The U.S. Department of Health and Human Services' food safety website, called foodsafety.gov, identifies four basic steps for reducing your risk of foodborne illness (FIGURE 12.8).

 Describe strategies for preventing foodborne illness at home, while eating out, and when traveling to other countries.

CLEAN   SEPARATE   COOK   CHILL

▲ **FIGURE 12.8** This food safety logo from foodsafety.gov helps you remember the four steps for reducing your risk of foodborne illness.

Clean: Wash Your Hands and Kitchen Surfaces Often

One of the easiest and most effective ways to prevent foodborne illness is to wash your hands before and after handling food. Remove any rings or bracelets before you begin, because jewelry can harbor bacteria. Scrub hands with warm, soapy water for at least 20 seconds, being sure to wash underneath your fingernails and between your fingers.[18] Although you should wash dishes in hot water, it's too harsh for hand washing: it causes the surface layer of the skin to break down, increasing the risk that microorganisms will be able to penetrate your skin. Dry your hands on a clean towel or fresh paper towel.

Thoroughly wash utensils, containers, cutting boards, and countertops with soap and hot water. Rinse. You may sanitize them with a solution of 1 tablespoon (or more) of chlorine bleach to 1 gallon of water. Flood the surface with the bleach solution and allow it to air dry. Wash fruits and vegetables thoroughly under running water just before eating, cutting, or cooking them. Washing fruits and vegetables with soap or detergent or using commercial produce washes is not recommended.[18]

Separate: Don't Cross-Contaminate

Cross-contamination is the spread of microorganisms from one food to another. This commonly occurs when raw foods, such as chicken and vegetables, are cut using the same knife, prepared on the same cutting board, or stored on the same plate. Keep raw meat, poultry, eggs, and seafood and their juices away from ready-to-eat food. Use separate cutting boards, utensils, and plates. When preparing meals with a marinade, reserve some of the fresh marinade in a clean container; then add the raw ingredients to the remainder. In this way, some uncontaminated marinade will be available if needed later in the cooking process. Raw food should always be marinated in the refrigerator.

Beware of cross-contamination while food shopping. For example, the displaying of food products such as cooked shrimp on the same bed of ice as raw seafood is not safe, nor is slicing cold cuts with the same knife used to trim raw meat. Report such practices to your local health authorities.

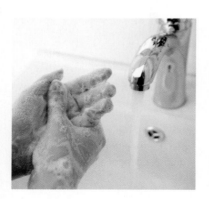

▲ One of the most effective strategies for preventing foodborne illness is simply to wash your hands thoroughly.

cross-contamination Contamination of one food by another via the unintended transfer of microorganisms through physical contact.

Chill: Store Foods in the Refrigerator or Freezer

The third rule for keeping food safe from bacteria is to promptly refrigerate or freeze it. Remember the danger zone: microorganisms that cause foodborne illness can reproduce rapidly in foods left at room temperature. Refrigeration (at or below 40°F) and freezing (at or below 0°F)[18] do not kill all microorganisms, but cold temperatures diminish their ability to reproduce in quantities large enough to cause illness. Also, many naturally occurring enzymes that cause food spoilage are deactivated at cold temperatures.

Shopping for Perishable Foods

When shopping for food, purchase refrigerated and frozen foods last. Put packaged meat, poultry, or fish into a plastic bag before placing it in your shopping cart. This prevents drippings from those foods from coming into contact with others in your cart.

Don't purchase foods that have passed their "sell by," "best used by," or other expiration date on the label.[18] The "sell by" date indicates the last day a product can be sold and still maintain its quality during normal home storage and consumption. The "best used by" date tells you how long a product will maintain optimum quality before eating. If the stamped date has passed, notify the store manager. These foods should be promptly removed from the shelves.

After you purchase perishable foods, get them home and into the refrigerator or freezer within 1 hour. If your trip home will be longer than an hour, take along a cooler to transport them in.

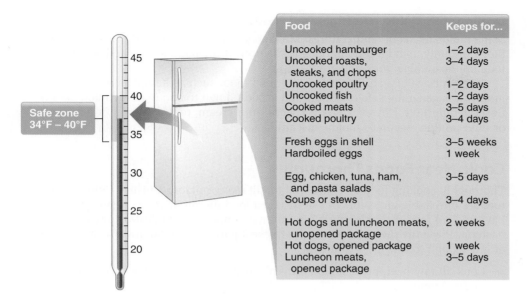

Food	Keeps for...
Uncooked hamburger	1–2 days
Uncooked roasts, steaks, and chops	3–4 days
Uncooked poultry	1–2 days
Uncooked fish	1–2 days
Cooked meats	3–5 days
Cooked poultry	3–4 days
Fresh eggs in shell	3–5 weeks
Hardboiled eggs	1 week
Egg, chicken, tuna, ham, and pasta salads	3–5 days
Soups or stews	3–4 days
Hot dogs and luncheon meats, unopened package	2 weeks
Hot dogs, opened package	1 week
Luncheon meats, opened package	3–5 days

Safe zone 34°F – 40°F

▲ **FIGURE 12.9**   While it's important to keep a well-stocked refrigerator, it's also important to know how long foods will keep.

Data from U.S. Department of Agriculture, Food Safety and Inspection Services. May 11, 2010. Fact Sheets. Safe Food Handling. Refrigeration and Food Safety. www.fsis.usda.gov/Fact_Sheets/Refrigeration_&_Food_Safety/index.asp#4

Refrigerating Foods at Home

As soon as you get home from shopping, put meats, eggs, cheeses, milk, and any other perishable foods in the refrigerator. Store meat, poultry, and seafood in the back of the refrigerator away from the door, so that they stay cold, and on the lowest shelf, so that their juices do not drip onto any other foods. If you are not going to use raw poultry, fish, or ground beef within 2 days of purchase, store it in the freezer. A guide for refrigerating foods is provided in **FIGURE 12.9**.

After a meal, refrigerate leftovers promptly—even if still hot—to discourage microbial growth. The standard rule is to refrigerate leftovers within *2 hours* of serving.[18] If the temperature is above 90°F, such as at a picnic, then foods should be refrigerated within 1 hour. A larger quantity of food takes longer to cool, so divide and conquer: separate leftovers into shallow containers for quicker cooling. Finally, avoid keeping leftovers for more than a few days. If you don't plan to finish a dish within the recommended time frame, freeze it.

Freezing and Thawing Foods

The temperature in your freezer should be set at 0°F. Use a thermometer and check it periodically. If your electricity goes out, avoid opening the freezer until the power is restored. When the power does come back on, check the temperature on the top shelf. If it is at or below 40°F, the food should still be safe to eat, or refreeze.

As with refrigeration, smaller packages will freeze more quickly. So rather than attempting to freeze an entire casserole, divide the food into multiple small portions in freezer-safe containers; then freeze.

Sufficient thawing will ensure adequate cooking throughout, which is essential to preventing foodborne illness. Thaw poultry on the bottom shelf of the refrigerator, in a large bowl to catch its juices. Never thaw frozen meat, poultry, or seafood on a kitchen counter or in a basin of warm water. Room temperatures allow growth of bacteria on the surface of food. You can also thaw foods in your microwave, following the manufacturer's instructions.

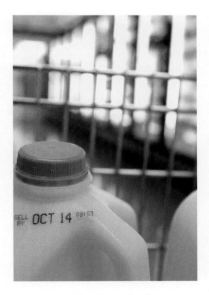

▲ The "sell by" date tells the store how long to display the product for sale.

🌐 For more information about thawing foods safely, check out www.fsis.usda.gov. Type "big thaw" in the Search box, then click on "The Big Thaw."

Dealing with Molds in Refrigerated Foods

Some molds like cool temperatures. Mold spores are common in the atmosphere, and they randomly land on food in open containers. If the temperature and acidity of the food are hospitable, they will grow.

If the surface of a small portion of a solid food, such as hard cheese, becomes moldy, it is generally safe to cut off that section down to about an inch and eat the unspoiled portion. However, if soft cheese, sour cream, tomato sauce, or another soft or fluid product becomes moldy, discard it.

Cook: Heat Foods Thoroughly

Thoroughly cooking food is a sure way to kill many microorganisms. Color and texture are unreliable indicators of safety. Use a food thermometer to ensure that you have cooked food to a safe minimum internal temperature to destroy any harmful bacteria. Place the thermometer in the thickest part of the food, away from bone, fat, or gristle, and follow these guidelines:[18]

- Cook all raw beef, pork, lamb and veal steaks, chops, and roasts to a minimum internal temperature of 145°F (62.8°C).
- Cook all raw ground beef, pork, lamb, and veal to an internal temperature of 160°F (71.1°C).
- Cook all poultry to an internal temperature of 165°F (73.9°C).

If you barbecue, checking the food's temperature with a food thermometer should be part of your routine. See the **Game Plan** feature box for more advice on grilling and barbecuing foods.

Microwave cooking is convenient, but you need to be sure your food is thoroughly and evenly cooked and that there are no cold spots in the food where bacteria can thrive. For best results, cover food, stir often, and rotate for even cooking. Raw and semi-raw (such as marinated or partly cooked) fish delicacies, including sushi and sashimi, may be tempting, but their safety cannot be guaranteed. Always cook fish thoroughly. When done, fish should be opaque and flake easily with a fork. If you're wondering how sushi restaurants can guarantee the safety of their food, the short answer is they can't. All fish to be used for sushi must be flash frozen in a process that effectively kills any parasites that are in the fish, but does not necessarily kill bacteria or viruses. In April of 2012, 316 people in 26 states experienced foodborne illness after consuming sushi made with tuna contaminated with *Salmonella* bacteria.[19] Thus, eating raw seafood remains risky.

Protect Yourself from Toxins in Foods

Killing microorganisms with heat is an important step in keeping food safe, but it won't protect you against their toxins. That's because many toxins are unaffected by heat and are capable of causing severe illness even when the microorganisms that produced them have been destroyed. For example, let's say you prepare a casserole for a team picnic. Too bad you forget to wash your hands before serving it to your teammates, because you contaminate the casserole with the bacterium *Staphylococcus aureus*, which is commonly found on skin. You and your friends go off and play soccer, leaving the food in the sun, and a few hours later you take the rest of the casserole home. At supper, you heat the leftovers thoroughly, thinking that this will kill any bacteria that multiplied while it was left out. That night you experience nausea, severe vomiting, and abdominal pain. What happened? While your food was left out, *Staphylococcus* multiplied in the casserole and produced a toxin (**FIGURE 12.10**). When you reheated the food, you killed the microorganisms, but their toxin was unaffected by the heat. When you then ate the food, the toxin made you sick.

Be Choosy When Eating Out—Close to Home or Far Away

When choosing a place to eat out, avoid restaurants that don't look clean. Grimy tabletops and dirty restrooms indicate indifference to hygiene. On the other hand,

GAME **PLAN** !

Staying Food-Safe at Your Next Barbecue

It's the end of the term and you and your friends are planning a lakeside barbecue to celebrate! Here are some tips from the U.S. Food and Drug Administration for preventing foodborne illness at any outdoor gathering.[4]

☐ *Wash your hands, utensils, and food-preparation surfaces.* Even in outdoor settings, food safety begins with hand washing. Take along a water jug, some soap, and paper towels or a box of moist disposable towelettes. Keep all utensils and platters clean when preparing foods.

☐ *Keep foods cold during transport.* Use coolers with ice or frozen gel packs to keep food at or below 40°F. It's

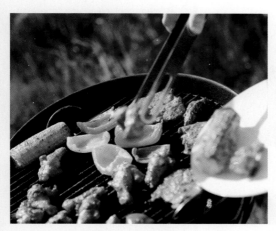

⬆ At a barbecue, it's essential to heat foods to the proper temperature.

easier to maintain a cold temperature in small coolers. Consider packing three: put beverages in one cooler, washed fruits and vegetables and containers of potato salad in another, and wrapped, frozen meat, poultry, and seafood in another. Keep coolers in the air-conditioned passenger compartment of your car, rather than in a hot trunk.

☐ *Grill foods thoroughly.* Use a food thermometer to be sure the food has reached an adequate internal temperature before serving.

☐ *Avoid cross-contamination.* When taking food from the grill to the table, never use the same platter or utensils that previously held raw meat or seafood!

☐ *Keep hot foods hot.* Keep grilled food hot until it is served by moving it to the side of the grill, just away from the coals, so that it stays hot but doesn't overcook. If grilled food isn't going to be eaten right away, wrap it well and place it in an insulated container.

☐ *Keep cold foods cold.* Cold foods, such as chicken salad, should be kept in a bowl of ice during your barbecue. Drain off water as the ice melts and replace the ice frequently. Don't let any perishable food sit out longer than 2 hours. In temperatures above 90°F, don't let food sit out for more than 1 hour.

cleanliness of areas used by the public doesn't guarantee that the kitchen is clean. That is why health inspections are important. Public health inspectors randomly visit and inspect the food-preparation areas of all businesses that serve food, whether eaten in or taken out. When in doubt, check the inspection results posted in the restaurant.

Another way to protect yourself when dining out is by ordering foods to be cooked thoroughly. If you order a hamburger and it arrives pink in the middle, or scrambled eggs and they arrive runny, send the food back to be cooked thoroughly.

When planning a trip, tell your physician your travel plans and ask about vaccinations needed or any medications that you should take along in case you get sick. Pack a waterless antibacterial hand cleanser and, once you arrive in your destination, keep it with you and use it frequently. When dining, select foods and beverages carefully. All raw food has the potential for contamination. (See Chapter 2.)

recap Foodborne illness can be prevented at home by following four tips: *Clean*: wash your hands and kitchen surfaces often. *Separate*: isolate foods to prevent cross-contamination. *Chill*: store foods in the refrigerator or freezer. *Cook*: heat foods long enough and at the correct temperatures to ensure proper cooking. When eating out, avoid restaurants that don't look clean and ask that all food be cooked thoroughly.

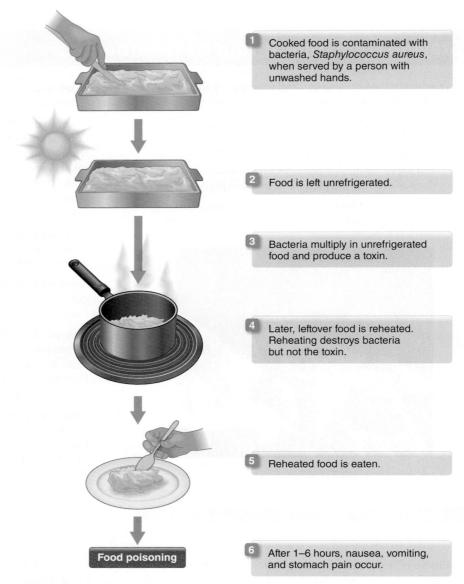

1   Cooked food is contaminated with bacteria, *Staphylococcus aureus*, when served by a person with unwashed hands.

2   Food is left unrefrigerated.

3   Bacteria multiply in unrefrigerated food and produce a toxin.

4   Later, leftover food is reheated. Reheating destroys bacteria but not the toxin.

5   Reheated food is eaten.

Food poisoning

6   After 1–6 hours, nausea, vomiting, and stomach pain occur.

FIGURE 12.10   Food contamination can occur long after the microorganism itself has been destroyed.

LO4   Compare and contrast the different methods manufacturers use to preserve foods.

How is food spoilage prevented?

Any food that has been harvested and that people aren't ready to eat must be preserved in some way or, before long, it will degrade enzymatically and become home to a variety of microorganisms. Even processed foods have the potential to spoil.

The most ancient methods of preserving foods include salting, sugaring, drying, and smoking, all of which draw the water out of the plant or animal cells. By dehydrating the food, these methods make it inhospitable to microorganisms and dramatically slow the action of enzymes that would otherwise degrade the food. Natural methods of cooling also have been used for centuries, including storing foods in underground cellars, caves, running streams, and even "cold pantries"— north-facing rooms of the house that were kept dark and unheated and often were stocked with ice.

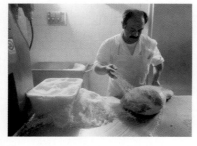

A worker salting a Parma ham.

More recently, technological advances have helped food producers preserve the integrity of their products for months and even years between harvesting and consumption:

- *Canning:* Developed in the late 1700s, canning involves washing and blanching the food, placing it in cans, siphoning out the air, sealing the cans, and then heating them to a very high temperature. Canned food has an average shelf life of at least 2 years from the date of purchase.
- *Pasteurization:* The technique called **pasteurization** exposes a beverage or other food to heat high enough to destroy microorganisms but for a short enough period of time that the taste and quality of the food are not affected. For example, in *flash pasteurization*, milk or other liquids are heated to 162°F (72°C) for 15 seconds. Although some people claim that unpasteurized milk, juices, and ciders taste better, drinking these products puts you at risk for foodborne illness.
- **Irradiation** is a process that exposes foods to gamma rays from radioactive metals. Energy from the rays penetrates food and its packaging, killing or disabling microorganisms in the food. The process does not cause foods to become radioactive! A few nutrients, including thiamin and vitamins A, E, and K, are lost, but these losses are also incurred in conventional processing and preparation. Although irradiated food has been shown to be safe, the FDA requires that all irradiated foods be labeled with a "radura" symbol and a caution against irradiating the food again **(FIGURE 12.11)**.
- *Aseptic packaging:* You probably know aseptic packaging best as "juice boxes." Food and beverages are first heated, then cooled, then placed in sterile containers. The process uses less energy and materials than traditional canning, and the average shelf life is about 6 months.
- *Modified atmosphere packaging:* In this process, the oxygen in a package of food is replaced with an inert gas, such as nitrogen or carbon dioxide. This prevents a number of chemical reactions that spoil food, and it slows the growth of bacteria that require oxygen. The process can be used with a variety of foods, including meats, fish, vegetables, and fruits.
- *High-pressure processing* is a technique in which the food to be preserved is subjected to an extremely high pressure. This inactivates most bacteria while retaining the food's quality and freshness.

> **recap** Salting, sugaring, drying, smoking, and cooling have been used for centuries to preserve food. Canning, pasteurization, irradiation, and several packaging techniques are used to preserve a variety of foods during shipping, as well as on grocer and consumer shelves.

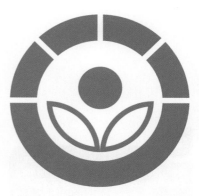

▲ **FIGURE 12.11** The U.S. Food and Drug Administration requires the Radura—the international symbol of irradiated food—to be displayed on all irradiated food sold in the United States.

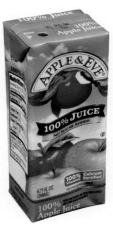

 Aseptic packaging allows foods to be stored unrefrigerated for several months without spoilage.

What are food additives, and are they safe?

Have you ever picked up a loaf of bread and started reading its ingredients? You'd expect to see flour, yeast, water, and some sugar, but what are all those other items? They are collectively called *food additives*, and they are in almost every processed food. **Food additives** are chemicals that don't occur naturally in the food, but are added to enhance the food in some way. More than 3,000 different food additives are currently used in the United States. **TABLE 12.3** identifies only a few of the most common.

Food Additives Include Nutrients and Preservatives

Vitamins and minerals are added to foods as nutrients and as preservatives. Vitamin E is usually added to fat-based products to keep them from going rancid, and vitamin C is used as an antioxidant in many foods. Iodine is added to table salt to help decrease the incidence of goiter, a condition that causes the thyroid gland to enlarge. Vitamin D

LO5 Debate the safety of food additives, including the role of the GRAS list.

pasteurization A form of sterilization using high temperatures for short periods of time.

irradiation A sterilization process in which food is exposed to gamma rays or high-energy electron beams to kill microorganisms. Irradiation does not impart any radiation to the food being treated.

food additive A substance or mixture of substances intentionally put into food to enhance its appearance, safety, palatability, and quality.

TABLE 12.3   Examples of Common Food Additives

Food Additive	Foods Found In
Coloring Agents	
Beet extract	Beverages, candies, ice cream
Beta-carotene	Beverages, sauces, soups, baked goods, candies, macaroni and cheese mixes
Caramel	Beverages, sauces, soups, baked goods
Tartrazine	Beverages, cakes and cookies, ice cream
Preservatives	
Alpha-tocopherol (vitamin E)	Vegetable oils
Ascorbic acid (vitamin C)	Breakfast cereals, cured meats, fruit drinks
BHA	Breakfast cereals, chewing gum, oils, potato chips
BHT	Breakfast cereals, chewing gum, oils, potato chips
Calcium proprionate/sodium proprionate	Bread, cakes, pies, rolls
EDTA	Beverages, canned shellfish, margarine, mayonnaise, processed fruits and vegetables, sandwich spreads
Propyl gallate	Mayonnaise, chewing gum, chicken soup base, vegetable oils, meat products, potato products, fruits, ice cream
Sodium benzoate	Carbonated beverages, fruit juice, pickles, preserves
Sodium chloride (salt)	Most processed foods
Sodium nitrate/sodium nitrite	Bacon, corned beef, lunch meats, smoked fish
Sorbic acid/potassium sorbate	Cakes, cheese, dried fruits, jellies, syrups, wine
Sulfites (sodium bisulfite, sulfur dioxide)	Dried fruits, processed potatoes, wine
Texturizers, Emulsifiers, and Stabilizers	
Calcium chloride	Canned fruits and vegetables
Carageenan/pectin	Ice cream, chocolate milk, soy milk, frostings, jams, jellies, cheese, salad dressings, sour cream, puddings, syrups
Cellulose gum/guar gum/gum arabic/locust gum/xanthan gum	Soups and sauces, gravies, sour cream, ricotta cheese, ice cream, syrups
Gelatin	Desserts, canned meats
Lecithin	Mayonnaise, ice cream
Humectants	
Glycerin	Chewing gum, marshmallows, shredded coconut
Propylene glycol	Chewing gum, gummy candies

Want to look up the unfamiliar ingredients listed on the packages of your favorite foods? Check out the FDA database at www.fda.gov. Type "GRAS database" into the search bar to get started.

is added to milk, and calcium is added to soy milk, rice milk, almond milk, and some juices to promote bone health. Folate is added to cereals, breads, and other foods to help prevent certain types of birth defects.

The following two preservatives have raised health concerns:

- *Sulfites:* A small segment of the population is sensitive to sulfites, preservatives used in many beers and wines and some other processed foods. These people can experience asthma, headaches, or other symptoms after eating food containing the offending preservatives.
- *Nitrites:* Commonly used to preserve processed meats, nitrites can be converted to *nitrosamines* during the cooking process. Nitrosamines have been found to be carcinogenic in animals, so the FDA has required all foods with nitrites to contain additional antioxidants to decrease the formation of nitrosamines.

Other Food Additives Include Flavorings, Colorings, and Other Agents

Flavoring agents are used to replace the natural flavors lost during food processing. In contrast, *flavor enhancers* have little or no flavor of their own but accentuate the natural flavor of foods. One of the most common flavor enhancers used is monosodium glutamate (MSG). In some people, MSG causes symptoms such as headaches, difficulty breathing, and heart palpitations.

Common food colorings include beet juice, which imparts a red color; beta-carotene, which gives a yellow color; and caramel, which adds brown color. The coloring tartrazine (FD&C Yellow #5) causes an allergic reaction in some people, and its use must be indicated on the product packaging.

Texturizers are added to foods to improve their texture. Emulsifiers help keep fats evenly dispersed within foods. Stabilizers give foods "body" and help them maintain a desired texture or color. Humectants keep foods such as marshmallows, chewing gum, and shredded coconut moist and stretchy. Desiccants prevent moisture absorption from the air; for example, they are used to prevent table salt from forming clumps.[20]

Are Food Additives Safe?

Federal legislation was passed in 1958 to regulate food additives. The Delaney Clause, also enacted in 1958, states, "No additive may be permitted in any amount if tests show that it produces cancer when fed to man or animals or by other appropriate tests." Before a new additive can be used in food, the producer of the additive must demonstrate its safety to the FDA by submitting data on its reasonable safety. The FDA determines the additive's safety based on these data.

Also in 1958, the U.S. Congress recognized that many substances added to foods would not require this type of formal review by the FDA prior to marketing and use, because their safety had already been established through long-term use or because their safety had been recognized by qualified experts through scientific studies. These substances are exempt from the more stringent testing criteria for new food additives and are referred to as substances that are **Generally Recognized as Safe (GRAS)**. The GRAS list identifies substances that have either been tested and determined by the FDA to be safe and approved for use in the food industry or are deemed safe as a result of consensus among experts qualified by scientific training and experience. The GRAS list is updated as needed. In 2013, for example, the FDA proposed removing partially hydrogenated oils (PHOs), the major dietary source of *trans* fatty acids, from the GRAS list.[21]

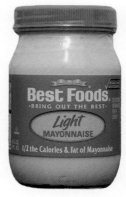

◄ Mayonnaise contains emulsifiers to prevent separation of fats.

recap Food additives are chemicals intentionally added to foods to enhance their color, flavor, texture, nutrient density, moisture level, or shelf life. Although there is continuing controversy over food additives in the United States, the FDA regulates additives used in our food supply and considers safe those it approves.

How is genetic modification used in food production?

In **genetic modification**, also referred to as *genetic engineering*, the genetic material, or DNA, of an organism is altered to bring about specific changes in its seeds or offspring. Selective breeding is one example of genetic modification; for example, Brahman cattle, which have poor-quality meat but high resistance to heat and humidity, are bred with English shorthorn cattle, which have good meat but low resistance to heat and humidity. The outcome of this selective breeding process is Santa Gertrudis cattle, which have the desired characteristics of higher-quality meat and resistance to heat and humidity. Although selective breeding is effective and has helped increase crop yields and improve the quality and quantity of our food supply, it is a relatively slow and imprecise process, because a great deal of trial and error typically occurs before the desired characteristics are achieved.

Recently, advances in biotechnology have moved genetic modification beyond selective breeding. These advances include the manipulation of the DNA of living

LO6 Describe the process of genetic modification and discuss the potential risks and benefits associated with genetically modified organisms.

Generally Recognized as Safe (GRAS) List established by Congress to identify substances used in foods that are generally recognized as safe based on a history of long-term use or on the consensus of qualified research experts.

genetic modification The process of changing an organism by manipulating its genetic material.

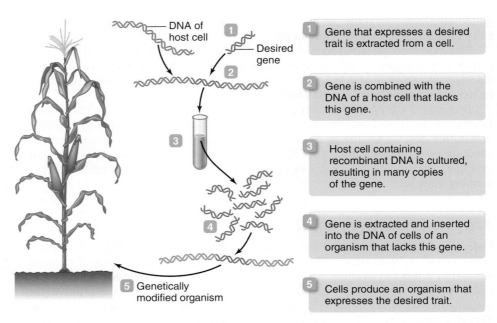

1. Gene that expresses a desired trait is extracted from a cell.

2. Gene is combined with the DNA of a host cell that lacks this gene.

3. Host cell containing recombinant DNA is cultured, resulting in many copies of the gene.

4. Gene is extracted and inserted into the DNA of cells of an organism that lacks this gene.

5. Cells produce an organism that expresses the desired trait.

FIGURE 12.12 Recombinant DNA technology involves producing plants and other organisms that contain modified DNA, which enables them to express desirable traits that are not present in the original organism.

cells of one organism to produce the desired characteristics of a different organism. Called **recombinant DNA technology**, the process commonly begins when scientists isolate from an animal, a plant, or a microbial cell a particular segment of DNA—one or more genes—that codes for a protein conferring a desirable trait, such as salt tolerance in tomato plants **(FIGURE 12.12)**. Scientists then splice the DNA into a "host cell," usually a microorganism. The cell is cultured to produce many copies—a *gene library*—of the beneficial gene. Then, many scientists can readily obtain the gene to modify other organisms that lack the desired trait—for example, traditional tomato plants. The modified DNA causes the plant's cells to build the protein of interest, and the plant expresses the desired trait. The term *genetically modified organism* (*GMO*) refers to any organism in which the DNA has been altered using recombinant DNA technology.

Cultivation of GMO food crops began in 1996. Typically, they have been used to induce resistance to pesticides. This means that genetically modified crops can be sprayed more liberally with chemicals that kill weeds and insects—in theory, without harming the crops or the surrounding ecology. Genetic modification can also increase a plant's resistance to disease or make crops more tolerant of environmental conditions, such as drought or poor soil. Another use is to increase the nutritional value of a crop. Researchers have modified soybeans and canola, for instance, to increase their content of monounsaturated fatty acids.

Since 1996, an increasing number and quantity of food crops have been genetically modified. The most common are corn and soybeans. The USDA reports that, in 2013, 80% of all corn crops and 93% of all soybean crops grown in the United States were genetically engineered varieties.[22] As the use of genetic modification increases, however, critics point to research indicating significant risks, not only to the environment but also to human health. For more information on this controversy, see the *Highlight* feature box.

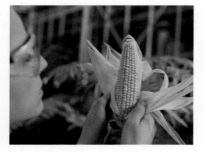

Corn is one of the most widely cultivated genetically modified crops.

recombinant DNA technology A type of genetic modification in which scientists combine DNA from different sources to produce a transgenic organism that expresses a desired trait.

recap In genetic modification, the genetic material, or DNA, of an organism is altered to enhance certain qualities. In agriculture, genetic modification is often used to improve crop protection or to increase nutrients in the resulting food. Genetic modification is also used in animals and microorganisms.

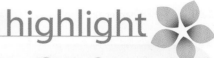

Genetically Modified Organisms: A Blessing or a Curse?

Many genetically modified organisms (GMOs) are animal and plant foods. The terms for these foods—biotech foods, gene foods, and "frankenfoods"—suggest divergent views of their potential benefits and risks to the environment and to human health.

Supporters envision an ever-expanding role for genetic engineering in food production. They identify numerous potential benefits resulting from the application of this technology, including:[5]

- enhanced taste and nutritional quality of food;
- crops that grow faster, have higher yields, can be grown in inhospitable soils, and have increased resistance to pests, diseases, droughts, herbicides, and spoilage;
- increased production of high-quality meat, eggs, and milk;
- improved animal health as a result of increased disease resistance and overall hardiness;
- environmentally responsible outcomes such as a reduction in use of an insecticide called Bt; use of less harmful pesticides; reduced water use by drought-tolerant species; reduced use of energy and emmission of greenhouse gases because of reduced need for ploughing and pesticide spraying; and conservation of soil due to higher productivity; and
- increased food security worldwide by increasing the income of small farmers, improving crop yields, and producing food crops with greater resistance to drought.

Despite these benefits, there is significant opposition to GMOs. Detractors cite a wide range of environmental and human health risks, including the following:

- Genes have been transferred to nontarget species through cross-pollination, resulting in the spread of undesirable plants, including superweeds that are tolerant to conventional herbicides. Indeed, from 1996–2011, despite the decline in the use of the insecticide Bt, the rapid spread of herbicide-resistant superweeds in the United States led to an overall 7% increase in pesticide use.[6] While the increased use of herbicides fosters the evolution of superweeds, it destroys native weeds on which insects and other organisms may depend for their survival. For example, the loss of milkweed near GMO crops has contributed to a dramatic decline in the population of monarch butterflies.[7]
- There is a potential for significant loss of biodiversity. GM crops use the same seeds—and thus the same

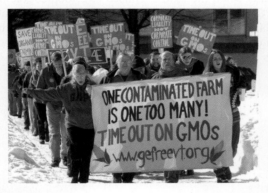

⬥ Many people oppose the genetic engineering of foods for environmental, health, or economic reasons.

genes—over and over again throughout a region. The resulting loss in genetic diversity increases the vulnerability of the crops to climatic events, pests, and plant diseases. This loss of diversity can also affect other species that share the local ecology.[8]

- Genes have been transferred from GM crops to other crops intended for food, tainting them with potential allergens and nonfood-grade ingredients. Although crops are rigorously screened for known allergens, we have no way of screening for the transfer of new, unknown allergens.[8,9]
- Undesirable genes could be transferred from GM foods to cells of the body or to the GI flora, adversely affecting human health. For example, if antibiotic-resistant genes were transferred, susceptibility to infectious disease could increase.[8]

Despite these concerns, the World Health Organization (WHO) points out that no effects on human health have been demonstrated as a result of the consumption of GM foods in countries where they have been approved.[8] Moreover, the FDA has the same standards of testing for GMO foods as for foods from traditionally bred plants, and has not found evidence that GMO foods are less safe, lower in nutrients, more toxic, or more likely to cause an allergic reaction.[10]

In addition to environmental and human health concerns, detractors assert that GMOs have reduced economic opportunity. For example, the seed industry has become increasingly controlled by just three large bioengineering firms that have bought up small, local seed companies, then increased prices to farmers for their genetically engineered seed. At the same time, the firms require farmers to sign contracts promising that they will not save and use the seeds from their GM crops. Critics say that this monopoly has had tragic consequences. By one estimate, a quarter million farmers have taken their lives because of debt induced by the high cost of nonrenewable genetically engineered seed.[11]

Many argue that, at the very least, all GM foods should be labeled so that consumers know what they're purchasing. Although the FDA supports voluntary labeling of GMO foods, as of 2014, there was no requirement that all genetically engineered foods be identified as such.[10] However, nationwide polls over the past several years have continually shown that more than 90% of Americans support labeling of GMO foods.[12]

As GMOs and genetically modified foods have been available only since 1996, it may be many years before we have any long-term studies of their impact on the world.

Describe the process by which persistent organic pollutants accumulate in foods.

 Discuss the regulation, labeling, benefits, and limitations of organic foods.

How do residues harm our food supply?

Food **residues** are chemicals that remain in foods despite cleaning and processing. Three types of residues of global concern are persistent organic pollutants, pesticides, and the hormones and antibiotics used in animals. The health concerns related to residues include skin rashes, nerve damage, cancer, and the development of antibiotic-resistant pathogenic bacteria.

Persistent Organic Pollutants Can Cause Illness

Some chemicals released into the atmosphere as a result of industry, agriculture, automobile emissions, and improper waste disposal can persist in soil or water for years or even decades. These chemicals, collectively referred to as **persistent organic pollutants (POPs)**, can travel thousands of miles in gases or as airborne particles, in rain, snow, rivers, and oceans, eventually entering the food supply through the soil or water.[23] If a pollutant gets into the soil, a plant can absorb the chemical into its structure and pass it on as part of the food chain. Animals can also absorb the pollutant into their tissues or consume it when feeding on plants growing in the polluted soil. Fat-soluble pollutants are especially problematic, because they tend to accumulate in the animal's body tissues in ever-greater concentrations as they move up the food chain. This process is called **biomagnification**. The POPs are then absorbed by humans when the animal is used as a food source (**FIGURE 12.13**).

POP residues have been found in virtually all categories of foods, including baked goods, fruit, vegetables, meat, poultry, fish, and dairy products. Significant levels have been detected all over the Earth, even in pristine regions of the Arctic thousands of miles from any known source.[23]

residues Chemicals that remain in the foods we eat despite cleaning and processing.

persistent organic pollutants (POPs) Chemicals released into the environment as a result of industry, agriculture, or improper waste disposal; automobile emissions also are considered POPs.

biomagnification Process by which persistent organic pollutants become more concentrated in animal tissues as they move from one creature to another through the food chain.

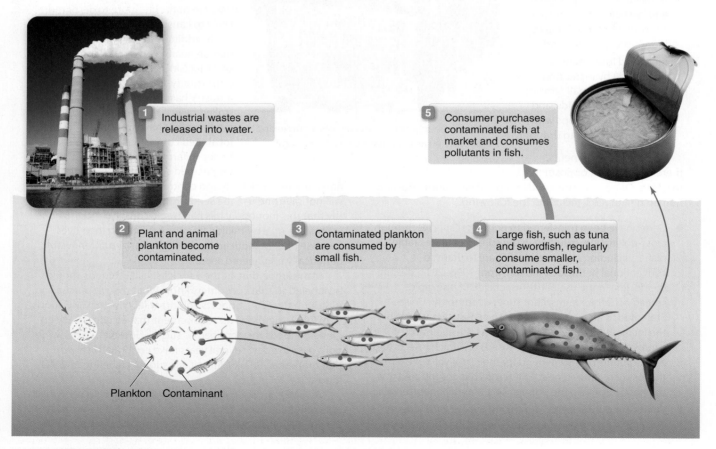

FIGURE 12.13 Biomagnification of persistent organic pollutants in the food supply.

Mercury and Lead Are Nerve Toxins

Mercury, a naturally occurring element, is found in soil, rocks, and water. It is also released into the air by pulp and paper processing and the burning of garbage and fossil fuels. As mercury falls from the air, it finds its way to streams, rivers, lakes, and the ocean, where it accumulates. Fish absorb mercury as they feed on aquatic organisms, and this mercury is passed on to us when we consume the fish. As mercury accumulates in the body, it has a toxic effect on the nervous system.

Large predatory fish, such as swordfish, shark, king mackerel, and tilefish, tend to contain the highest levels of mercury.[24] Because mercury is especially toxic to the developing nervous system of fetuses and growing children, pregnant and breastfeeding women and young children are advised to avoid eating these types of fish. Canned tuna, salmon, cod, pollock, sole, shrimp, mussels, and scallops do not contain high levels of mercury and are safe to consume; however, the FDA recommends that pregnant women and young children eat no more than two servings (12 oz) per week of any type of fish.[24]

Lead is another POP of concern. It can be found naturally in the soil, water, and air, but also occurs as industrial waste from leaded gasoline, lead-based paints, and lead-soldered cans, now outlawed but decomposing in landfills. Older homes may have high levels of lead paint dust, or the lead paint may be peeling in chips, which young children may put it their mouths. Some ceramic mugs and other dishes are fired with lead-based glaze, allowing residues to build up in foods. Excessive lead exposure can cause serious learning and behavioral disorders in children and cardiovascular and kidney disease in adults.

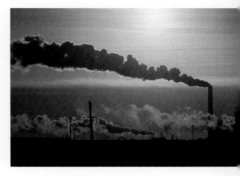

One of the ways mercury is released into the environment is by burning fossil fuels.

Endocrine Disruptors Disturb Hormonal Functions

Endocrine disruptors are chemicals thought to interfere with our body's endocrine system, which includes a variety of organs that release hormones. Hormones play a role in a vast number of body processes, but endocrine disruptors are particularly associated with reproductive problems, nerve disorders, and adverse effects on our immune system.[25]

Two types of endocrine disruptors found in plastic food containers can leach into foods. A chemical called *bisphenol A (BPA)* is routinely used in the linings of canned foods and in some plastic food packaging with the recycling code 3 or 7. BPA is a form of synthetic estrogen, a female reproductive hormone, and some research has linked it to genital abnormalities, breast and prostate cancer, miscarriage, reduced sperm count, and even heart disease and diabetes. *Phthalates*, a large group of plasticizers present in plastic food packaging with the recycling code 3, have been linked to a variety of reproductive-system disorders, especially in males; for example, a recent study found a 20% reduction in fertility among men whose urine tested high in phthalates.[26]

Here are some recommendations for consumers who want to limit their exposure to BPA and phthalates:[27]

- Reduce your consumption of canned foods.
- Avoid purchasing food in plastic containers with the recycling codes 3 or 7.
- Never put hot beverages or foods (coffee, soups, etc.) in these containers and do not microwave foods in these containers. They are more likely to leach endocrine disruptors when they become heated.
- Whenever possible, choose glass, porcelain, or stainless steel containers for beverages and foods.

Dioxins are another category of endocrine disruptors. These are industrial pollutants typically formed as a result of combustion processes, such as waste incineration or the burning of wood, coal, or oil. Dioxins enter the soil and can persist in the environment for many years. There is concern that long-term exposure to dioxins can result in an increased risk for reproductive system disorders, liver damage, cancer, and other disorders.[28] Because dioxins easily accumulate in the fatty tissues of animals, most dioxin exposure in humans occurs through dietary intake of animal fats.[29] Whereas the EPA has been working to reduce dioxin emissions into the

For a guide to safe seafood consumption, go to www.nrdc.org, type in "Mercury" and click to download the Natural Resources Defense Council's wallet card.

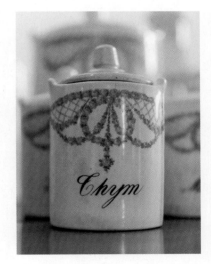

Antique porcelain is often coated with lead-based glaze.

endocrine disruptors Chemicals that may interfere with the body's endocrine system and produce adverse developmental, reproductive, neurological, and immune effects.

environment, the USDA and the FDA have been collaborating on efforts to monitor and reduce the dioxin levels in the U.S. food supply. To reduce your personal exposure to dioxins, eat meat less frequently, trim the fat from the meats you consume, and avoid fatty meats. Choose nonfat milk and yogurt, and low-fat cheeses, and replace butter with plant oils.

Pesticides Protect Against Crop Losses—But at a Cost

Pesticides are a family of chemicals used in both fields and farm storage areas to decrease the destruction and crop losses caused by weeds, animals, insects, and fungi and other microorganisms. They increase overall crop yield and allow for greater crop diversity. The three most common types of pesticides used in food production are

- *herbicides,* which are used to control weeds and other unwanted plant growth;
- *insecticides,* which are used to control insects that can infest crops; and
- *fungicides,* which are used to control plant-destroying fungal growth.

Some pesticides used today are naturally derived and/or have a low impact on the environment. These include **biopesticides**, which are species-specific and work to suppress a pest's population, not eliminate it. For example, pheromones are a biopesticide that disrupts insect mating by attracting males into traps. Biopesticides also do not leave residues on crops—most degrade rapidly and are easily washed away with water.

In contrast, pesticides made from petroleum-based products can leave residues on foods. The liver is responsible for detoxifying these chemicals. But if the liver is immature, as in a fetus, an infant, or a child, it may not be able to effectively detoxify the pesticides. In 2012, the American Academy of Pediatrics published a report describing the harmful effects of pesticides on children and recommending that families strictly limit their exposure.[30] Moreover, adults whose liver is already stressed by disease or alcohol abuse may suffer physical consequences from pesticide residues. These include nerve damage, cancer, and other problems. It is therefore essential to wash all produce carefully.

The EPA is responsible for regulating the labeling, sale, distribution, use, and disposal of all pesticides in the United States. Before a pesticide can be accepted by the EPA for use, it must be determined that it performs its intended function with minimal impact to the environment. Once the EPA has certified a pesticide, states can set their own regulations for its use. The EPA offers the following strategies for reducing your level of exposure to pesticides.[31]

- Wash and scrub all fresh fruits and vegetables thoroughly under running water.
- Peel fruits and vegetables whenever possible and discard the outer leaves of leafy vegetables, such as cabbage and lettuce. Trim the excess fat from meat and remove the skin from poultry and fish, because some pesticide residues collect in the fat.
- Eat a variety of foods from various sources, because this can reduce the risk of exposure to a single pesticide.
- Consume more organically grown foods.
- If you garden, avoid using fertilizers and pesticides to keep these chemicals out of your groundwater and your foods.
- Filter your tap water, whether it comes from a municipal water system or a well, to reduce your exposure to pesticides, fertilizers, and other contaminants.

Growth Hormones and Antibiotics Are Used in Animals

Introduced in the U.S. food supply in 1994, **recombinant bovine growth hormone (rBGH)** is a genetically engineered growth hormone. It is used in beef herds to induce animals to grow more muscle tissue and less fat. It is also injected into a third of U.S. dairy cows to increase milk output.

pesticides Chemicals used either in the field or in storage to decrease destruction by predators or disease.

biopesticides Primarily insecticides, these chemicals use natural methods to reduce damage to crops.

recombinant bovine growth hormone (rBGH) A genetically engineered hormone injected into dairy cows to enhance their milk output.

Although the FDA has allowed the use of rBGH in the United States, both Canada and the European Union have banned its use for two reasons:

- The available evidence shows an increased risk for mastitis (inflamed udders), in dairy cows injected with rBGH.[32] Farmers treat mastitis with antibiotics, promoting the development of strains of pathogenic bacteria that are resistant to antibiotics.
- The milk of cows receiving rBGH has higher levels of a hormone called insulin-like growth factor (IGF-1). This hormone can pass into the bloodstream of humans who drink milk from cows that receive rBGH, and some studies have shown that an elevated level of IGF-1 in humans may increase the risk for certain cancers. However, the evidence from these studies is inconclusive.[32]

The American Cancer Society suggests that more research is needed to help better appraise these health risks. In the meantime, consumer concerns about rBGH have caused a significant decline in sales of milk from cows treated with rBGH.[32]

Antibiotics are also routinely given to animals raised for food. Although the FDA has recently taken steps to phase out the use of antibiotics to enhance animal growth, they are still used to reduce the number of disease outbreaks in overcrowded production facilities. As a result, cows, pigs, and other animals treated with antibiotics have become significant reservoirs of virulent antibiotic-resistant strains of bacteria—so-called "superbugs." In 2011, federal testing of supermarket meats found that 39% of chicken products, 55% of ground beef, 69% of pork, and 81% of ground turkey harbored significant amounts of superbug bacteria.[33] Another study found a particularly dangerous superbug, methicillin-resistant *Staphylococcus aureus* (MRSA), in 100% of swine 9 to 12 weeks old on hog farms in Illinois and Iowa.[34] This superbug cannot be killed with common antibiotics, including methicillin, penicillin, and amoxicillin. Infection with MRSA can cause symptoms ranging from a mild skin rash to widespread invasion of tissues, including the bloodstream. MRSA blood infections are sometimes fatal.[35]

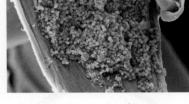

The resistant strain of bacteria responsible for methicillin-resistant *Staphylococcus aureus* (MRSA).

You can reduce your exposure to growth hormones and antibiotics by choosing organic eggs, milk, yogurt, and cheeses and by eating free-range meat from animals raised without the use of these chemicals. You can also reduce your risk by eating vegetarian and vegan meals more often.

Organic Agriculture Reduces Residues

In the population boom that followed the end of World War II, the demand for food increased dramatically. The American chemical industry helped increase agricultural production by providing a variety of new fertilizers and pesticides, including an insecticide called DDT, which began poisoning not just insects, but fish and birds, from the time it was first released for agricultural use in 1945. Then, in 1962, marine biologist Rachel Carson published *Silent Spring*, a book in which she described the harmful effects of DDT and other synthetic pesticides. The book's title, for example, referred to the effect of pesticides on songbirds, whose extinction would someday lead to a "silent spring." Scientists found Carson's research convincing, and readers flocked to her cause, creating a small but ever-growing demand for organic food.

Defining Organic

The term **organic** describes crops that are grown without the use of synthetic fertilizers, toxic and persistent pesticides, genetic engineering, or irradiation. Contrary to common belief, organic farmers can use pesticides as a final option for pest control when all other methods have proven insufficient, but they are restricted to a limited number that have been approved for use in organic production. Animals must be raised without growth hormones or antibiotics, fed with 100% organic feed, and have access to the outdoors. Also, to be certified organic, farms must employ practices that conserve resources, including soil and water, and promote ecological balance and biodiversity. Farms certified as organic must pass an inspection by a government-approved certifier who verifies that the farmer is following all USDA organic standards.[36]

A recent national survey indicates that more than 4% of all food products sold in the United States are now organic. Between 1990 and 2011, sales of organic products

organic Produced without the use of synthetic fertilizers, toxic and persistent pesticides, genetic engineering, or irradiation.

foods you don't know you love YET

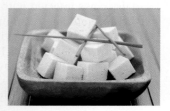

Tofu

If you're a vegetarian, you probably eat tofu several times a week. If not, you're in for a pleasant surprise. Tofu is made by causing soy milk to coagulate, forming curds, so it's 100% plant food. Yet it provides 9 grams of protein per 4-oz serving, making it a nutritious substitute for meat. What's more, tofu is free from the dioxins, hormones, and antibiotics that can be present as residues in animal-based foods. You can find tofu in almost any market, and a quick Internet search will reveal thousands of ways to prepare it. Or buy a four-pack of frozen, ready-made tofu burgers. Add veggies and a whole-grain bun for a high-protein, low-fat, residue-free meal!

in the United States skyrocketed from $1 billion to over $31 billion, and industry experts project that the market will continue to grow by at least 9% annually.[37]

Standards for Organic Labeling

In 2002, the National Organic Program (NOP) of the USDA established organic standards that provide uniform definitions for all organic products. Any product claiming to be organic must comply with the following definitions:[36]

- *100% organic:* products containing only organically produced ingredients, excluding water and salt
- *organic:* products containing 95% organically produced ingredients by weight, excluding water and salt, with the remaining ingredients consisting of those products not commercially available in organic form
- *made with organic ingredients:* a product containing more than 70% organic ingredients

If a processed product contains less than 70% organically produced ingredients, then those products cannot use the term *organic* in the principal display panel, but ingredients that are organically produced can be specified on the ingredients statement on the information panel. Products that are "100% organic" and "organic" may display the USDA organic seal (**FIGURE 12.14**).

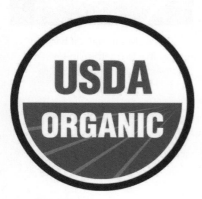

⬆ **FIGURE 12.14** The USDA organic seal identifies foods that are at least 95% organic.

Benefits and Costs of Organic Foods

Over the past few decades, hundreds of studies have attempted to compare the nutrient levels of organic foods to those of foods conventionally grown. The results have been inconclusive. For example, two large review studies published in 2011 and 2012 reached opposite conclusions on this issue, one finding consistently higher levels of nutrients in organic produce, and the other finding no nutritional advantage.[38,39] Then, in 2014, a comprehensive review study concluded that organically grown produce does indeed have a higher level of antioxidant nutrients and phytochemicals.[40]

Many people choose organic foods because of concerns about their exposure to pesticide residues, and indeed, the study just mentioned joined another recent study finding that organically produced foods were about 30% less likely to be contaminated with detectable pesticide residues or antibiotic-resistant bacteria.[39,40] In addition, as we noted earlier, the EPA advises Americans to reduce their total exposure to pesticides by consuming more organically grown foods.

Because organic foods tend to cost more than foods conventionally grown, it makes sense to spend more for organic when the alternative—the conventionally grown version—is likely to retain a high pesticide residue. **TABLE 12.4** identifies the

TABLE 12.4   The Environmental Working Group's Shopper's Guide to Pesticides in Produce

The Dirty Dozen Plus™: Buy These Organic	The Clean Fifteen™: Lowest in Pesticides
1. Apples	1. Asparagus
2. Celery	2. Avocados
3. Cherry tomatoes	3. Cabbage
4. Cucumbers	4. Cantaloupe
5. Grapes	5. Sweet corn
6. Hot peppers	6. Eggplant
7. Nectarines—imported	7. Grapefruit
8. Peaches	8. Kiwi
9. Potatoes	9. Mangoes
10. Spinach	10. Mushrooms
11. Strawberries	11. Onions
12. Sweet bell peppers	12. Papayas
PLUS:* Kale, collard greens, yellow crookneck squash, and zucchini	13. Pineapples
	14. Sweet peas—frozen
	15. Sweet potatoes

*Although they don't make the "Dirty Dozen" list, these foods are commonly contaminated with residues particularly toxic to the nervous system.
Source: Environmental Working Group. (2013). EWG's 2013 Shopper's Guide to Pesticides in Produce. http://www.ewg.org/foodnews/summary.php

foods that the Environmental Working Group advises should be your priority organic purchases. If your food budget is limited, spend your money on the organically grown versions of these foods. The table also identifies the fifteen foods that tend to be lowest in pesticide residues. You can feel confident purchasing conventional versions of these.

recap Persistent organic pollutants (POPs) of concern include mercury, lead, BPA, phthalates, and dioxins. Pesticides are used to prevent or reduce food crop losses but are potential toxins; therefore, it is essential to wash all produce carefully. Use of recombinant bovine growth hormone (rBGH) and antibiotics raises concerns about bovine and human health. The USDA organic seal identifies foods that are at least 95% organic; that is, they have been produced without the use of synthetic fertilizers, toxic and persistent pesticides, genetic engineering, irradiation, antibiotics, or growth hormones.

What's behind the rising food movement?

In 1993, four children in Washington State died after eating fast-food hamburgers contaminated with *E. coli*. Though certainly not the first food-safety incident to capture public attention, it marked a turning point, after which Americans increasingly questioned the assumption that all of our food is always entirely safe to eat. A national debate about food safety and food politics began; a series of investigative news articles, books, and films explored not only the health risks but also the environmental and social costs of contemporary methods of food production. Advocates for public health, animal welfare, farmland preservation, the rights of farmworkers, and environmental quality all came together in a common cause. The food movement was born.

 LO9 Explain how corporate agricultural practices have threatened sustainability and reduced food diversity, and identify several initiatives embraced by the food movement to reverse these trends.

 LO10 Discuss two issues of food equity: food insecurity and unfair trade practices.

Although a comprehensive discussion of the food movement isn't possible here, let's look at three of its broadest concerns: sustainability, diversity, and food equity.

Sustainability Preserves Resources

The U.S. Environmental Protection Agency (EPA) defines **sustainability** as the ability to satisfy basic economic, social, and security needs now and in the future without undermining the natural resource base and environmental quality on which life depends.[41] Whereas some people view sustainability as a lofty but impractical ideal, others point out that it's a necessary condition of human survival. That's because sustainable practices can reduce pollution of our air, soil, and water and preserve resources for future generations. To achieve these goals, experts argue that we must reduce our dependence on corporate farming. To understand the impact of corporate farming, let's review some history.

Like other modern wars, World War II led to innovations in industrial technology, engineering, and chemistry. After the war ended, these innovations were directed toward agriculture, specifically toward increasing worldwide food production to meet the food needs of a dramatically increasing postwar population. Together, the new technologies and practices became known as the **green revolution**, a massive program that led to improved seed quality, fertilizers, and pesticides, as well as new techniques for farming and irrigation, which doubled crop yields throughout the world.[42] As part of the green revolution, for example, new **high-yield varieties** of grain were produced by cross-breeding plants and selecting for the most desirable traits. It's estimated that these new varieties of rice, corn, and wheat have saved millions of people from starvation since the 1960s.

Although it has achieved higher yields at lower costs, the green revolution has also created new problems. Because it requires the use of expensive chemical fertilizers, pesticides, irrigation, and mechanical harvesters to reduce labor costs, it has mostly benefited larger, wealthier landowners rather than small, family farms. Moreover, environmental costs associated with the green revolution have included the following:

- Loss of topsoil due to erosion from heavy tilling, from extensive planting of row crops such as corn and soybeans, and from run-off due to irrigation
- Diminished biodiversity as traditional, resistant local species have been replaced with high-yield varieties that are more fragile
- Development of insecticide-resistant species of insects and herbicide-resistant varieties of weeds as use of agrochemical products has intensified
- Depletion and pollution of water supplies from irrigation techniques requiring heavy water consumption and from agrochemical run-off
- Depletion of fossil fuels and increased release of greenhouse gases[42]

In response to these drawbacks of the Green Revolution, a new global movement toward **sustainable agriculture** has evolved. The goal of the sustainable agriculture movement is to develop local, site-specific farming methods that improve soil conservation, crop yields, and food security in a sustainable manner, minimizing the adverse environmental impact. For example, soil erosion can be controlled by **crop rotation**, by terracing sloped land for the cultivation of crops, and by tillage that minimizes disturbance to the topsoil. Organic farming is one method of sustainable agriculture, because to be certified organic, farms must commit to sustainable agricultural practices, including avoiding the use of synthetic fertilizers and toxic and persistent pesticides.

Meat production is a particularly controversial issue within the sustainable agriculture movement. Research data point to the inefficiency of eating meat from grain-fed cattle instead of eating the grains themselves, both in terms of the resources required and the level of greenhouse gas emissions generated. Livestock production also leads to deforestation, further contributing to global warming. Sustainable meat production minimizes the use of antibiotics and synthetic hormones, allows for the use of otherwise unusable plants for high-quality animal feed, recycles animal wastes for fertilizers and fuel, and practices humane treatment of animals.

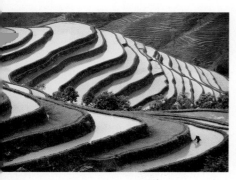

Terracing sloped land to avoid soil erosion is one practice of sustainable agriculture.

sustainability The ability to meet or satisfy basic economic, social, and security needs now and in the future without undermining the natural resource base and environmental quality on which life depends.

green revolution The tremendous increase in global productivity between 1944 and 2000 due to selective cross-breeding or hybridization to produce high-yield grains and industrial farming techniques.

high-yield varieties Semi-dwarf varieties of plants that are unlikely to fall over in wind and heavy rains and thus can carry larger amounts of seeds, greatly increasing the yield per acre.

sustainable agriculture Term referring to techniques of food production that preserve the environment indefinitely.

crop rotation The practice of alternating crops in a particular field to prevent nutrient depletion and erosion of the soil and to help with control of crop-specific pests.

Food Diversity Supports a Healthful Diet

Corporate farming has also reduced **food diversity**—that is, the variety of different species of food crops available. Beginning in the 1960s, revisions of the federal Agricultural Adjustment Act, commonly called the "farm bill," provided financial incentives for America's farmers to "get big or get out."[43] The number of small farms dwindled, and the remaining industrial operations focused on increasing their production of the few subsidized crops, such as corn. These few crops then began to monopolize the food supply. Because no subsidies were paid for production of fresh fruits and vegetables, their availability and variety plummeted, and they became more expensive.

As a result of this monopolization, the average American diet lost its variety. As you know, variety is a key component of a healthful diet: different species of fruits, vegetables, and whole grains provide different combinations of nutrients, fiber, and phytochemicals that support our health. Moreover, variety reduces the vulnerability of crops to pests and climate events. For this reason, our loss of food diversity increases our risk for widespread food shortages. And the problem is not limited to the United States. A 2014 study found that, worldwide, over the past 50 years, national food supplies have become increasingly similar, based on a dwindling number of crop plants, and as a result, global food security is threatened.[44]

Recently, experts in sustainable agriculture, public health, and nutrition have increasingly challenged this loss of food diversity. They advocate "slow food." The mission of the global Slow-Food network is to promote the cultivation and consumption of nutritious, fresh food produced in ways that preserve biodiversity, sustain the environment, and ensure animal welfare.[45] One characteristic of slow food is that, to the extent possible, it is locally grown. Although there's no precise definition of a "local food," the term typically refers to food grown within a few hundred miles of the consumer. Consuming local food limits energy use and greenhouse gas emissions from transportation (so-called "food miles"). Also, because these foods move much more quickly from farm to table, they tend to be fresher, retaining more of their micronutrients. Unfortunately, consuming foods harvested in-season from a local farm simply isn't possible year-round in many regions of the world. Even with greenhouse cultivation, the energy costs of raising and storing the food for consumption throughout a long winter can easily exceed the costs of transporting foods grown in warmer climates thousands of miles away.[46] For more information on the Slow Food movement, see the **Web Links** at the end of this chapter.

Several Initiatives Promote Sustainability and Diversity

Recently, the food movement has embraced a variety of initiatives to protect the environment and challenge the monopolization of our food supply. The following are some practical ways that individuals, communities, and corporations are promoting sustainability and food diversity:

- *Family farms:* For three decades, the number of farms in the United States has been decreasing, from 2.48 million in 1982 to 2.11 million in 2012.[47] However, since 2007, the number of small farms (1 to 9 acres) has not declined, and in some states, mainly in New England and the Southwest, they have increased. Some small farmers are taking advantage of programs offering land at reduced prices, community support, and mentoring. Many of these small farms are dedicated to organic farming, crop diversity, and other practices of sustainable agriculture.
- *Community supported agriculture (CSA):* In CSA programs, a farmer sells a certain number of "shares" to the public. Shares typically consist of a box of produce from the farm on a regular basis, such as once weekly throughout the growing season. Farmers get cash early on, as well as guaranteed buyers. Consumers get fresh, locally grown food. Together, farmers and consumers develop ongoing relationships as they share the bounty in a good year, and the losses when weather extremes or blight reduces yield. Although there is no national database on CSA programs, the organization LocalHarvest lists over 4,000.[48]

food diversity The variety of different species of plant crops or animal sources of food.

Find a farmers' market near you! Go to the USDA's Farmers' Market Search page at http://ams.usda.gov. Click on "Farmers Markets and Local Food Marketing," then choose "Find a Farmers Market."

- *Farmers' markets:* There are now more than 8,000 farmers' markets in the United States, more than four times the number when the USDA began compiling these data in 1994.[49] Along with CSAs, farmers' markets help meet the growing demand for locally grown food.
- *School gardens:* The School Garden Association of America was founded in 1910, and during World Wars I and II, school gardening became part of the war effort; however, in the postwar decades, school gardens dwindled. Recently, concerns about childhood obesity, the poor quality of children's diets, and their reduced opportunities for physical activity have renewed interest in school gardens. In partnership with the AmeriCorps Service Network, a new effort called FoodCorps is increasing school garden programs across the United States. In addition to promoting student acceptance of fruits and vegetables, school garden programs teach valuable lessons in nutrition, agriculture, and even cooking. In many schools, cafeterias incorporate the foods into the school lunch menu.[50]
- *Entrepreneurship:* A number of prominent venture capital (VC) firms in Silicon Valley are now investing in food start-ups dedicated to preserving human health and the environment. In 2012 alone, VCs poured about $350 million into organic foods, vegan versions of cheese, eggs, burgers, and other animal foods, and services that bring fresh produce from local farms directly to consumers' doors.[51]
- *Corporate involvement:* Whereas many smaller natural-food companies have long made sustainable agriculture part of their company identity, only recently has the food movement moved into corporate America. In the past few years, Walmart, Kellog, McDonald's, and several other corporations have initiated organization efforts including partnerships with local growers to promote sustainable agriculture.

Food Equity Promotes a Fair Sharing of Resources

You might think of the food movement as affluent Americans shopping at a farmers' market. However, another broad issue in the food movement is **food equity**: sharing the world's food resources fairly. Food equity is reduced when poverty limits a family's access to nutritious foods and by unfair trade practices. We explore these issues briefly here.

Food Insecurity

Despite the dramatic advances in food production brought about by the green revolution, 870 million people worldwide were hungry in 2012.[52] The World Hunger Education Service estimates that 1 in 8 people in the world is chronically undernourished, and most of these people live in developing nations.[52]

Any situation that results in inadequate food for an individual or community will prompt undernutrition. Climate events, wars, poor farming practices, crop diseases, and other factors can diminish a food supply. However, the major cause of undernutrition in the world is unequal distribution of food because of poverty. In the developing world, more than three-fourths of malnourished children live in countries with food surpluses.[53]

Unequal distribution also occurs in the United States, again largely because of poverty. As shown in **FIGURE 12.15**, the U.S. Department of Agriculture (USDA) estimates that 14.5% of U.S. households (about 17.6 million households) experienced **food insecurity** in 2012.[54] This means that the people living in these homes were unable to obtain enough food to meet their physical needs every day. More than one-third of these households, about 7 million, had *very low food security*, meaning that normal eating patterns of one or more members of the household were disrupted and food intake was reduced at times during the year because they had insufficient money or other resources for food.

Those at higher risk for food insecurity are households with income ranging from below the official U.S. poverty threshold (which was $23,850 for a family of four in 2014) to as much as 185% of the poverty threshold.[54,55] Also at increased risk are families consisting of single mothers or single fathers and their children, African American and Hispanic families, elderly people living on a fixed income, migrant laborers, and workers in minimum-wage jobs.

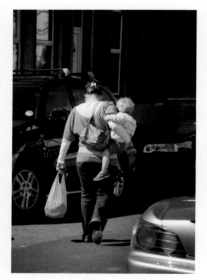

⬆ Single parents face unique economic challenges that can leave them and their children vulnerable to food insecurity.

food equity Fair distribution of the world's food resources.

food insecurity Condition in which the individual is unable to regularly obtain enough food to provide sufficient energy and nutrients to meet physical needs.

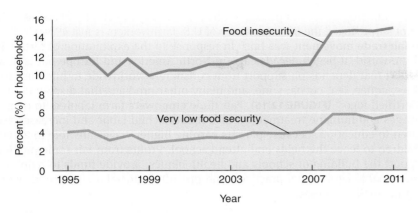

FIGURE 12.15 Prevalence of food insecurity and very low food security in U.S. households, 1995–2012.

Coleman-Jensen, A., M. Nord, and A. Singh. (2013, September). *Household Food Security in the United States in 2012.* U.S. Dept. of Agriculture, Economic Research Service. Available at http://www.ers.usda.gov.

Overall, people who are food-insecure are more likely to live in areas known as **food deserts**—geographic areas where people lack access to affordable, nutritious food. There are no reliable statistics on how many Americans live in food deserts, because there is no standard definition; however, the CDC reports that the problem does affect a small percentage of Americans, mostly those who live far from a large grocery store and do not have access to transportation.[56] Not only isolated rural regions, but also inner-city neighborhoods can be food deserts.

Increasing Access to Food

A variety of programs can increase access to nourishing food. For example, as part of a new national initiative called Healthy Corner Stores, cities from Philadelphia to Sacramento have invested in corner stores to increase city residents' access to healthy foods such as fresh produce.[57] Urban agriculture is also helping to decrease the number of food deserts. Across the United States, city governments are changing zoning codes to encourage the cultivation of vegetable gardens on rooftops, in abandoned parking lots, and even as part of the landscaping on municipal properties.

Moreover, several government programs help low-income Americans acquire food over extended periods of time. Among these programs are the Supplemental Nutrition Assistance Program (SNAP, previously called the Food Stamp Program), which helps low-income individuals of all ages; the Special Supplemental Nutrition Program for Women, Infants and Children (WIC), which helps pregnant women and children to age 5; the National School Lunch and National School Breakfast Programs, which help low-income schoolchildren; and the Summer Food Service Program, which helps low-income children in the summer. In addition, the U.S. Department of Agriculture distributes surplus foods to charitable agencies for distribution to needy families.

In the less developed nations, many international organizations help improve the nutrient status of the poor by enabling them to produce their own foods. For example, both USAID and the Peace Corps have agricultural education programs, the World Bank provides loans to fund small business ventures, and many nonprofit and nongovernmental organizations (NGOs) support community and family farms.

Fair Trade

As it has displaced small-scale farmers, corporate farming has also monopolized agricultural labor, forcing farmworkers to accept poverty-level wages and substandard and even dangerous living conditions. In the past decade, for example, the owners of seven Florida farms have been convicted of beating, chaining, and stealing from laborers in conditions that a Florida District Attorney described as "slavery." While performing backbreaking labor, America's 6 million farmworkers are continually exposed to UV radiation,

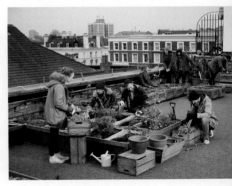

Eagle Street Rooftop Farm is a 6,000-square foot organic vegetable garden located on top of a warehouse in Brooklyn, New York.

food desert Community in which residents lack access to affordable fresh fruits and vegetables and other healthful foods.

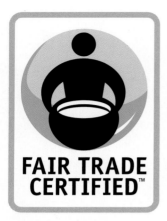

FIGURE 12.16 The Fair Trade Certified logo guarantees that the product has been produced equitably, without exploitation of workers or the environment.

pesticides, and crop dusts and pests and often lack basic sanitation and access to health-care.[43] Not surprisingly, the life expectancy of U.S. farmworkers is just 49 years.[58]

The **fair trade** movement was born in response to the exploitation of farm laborers around the world. It began decades ago in North America and Europe but is now a global effort that depends on support from consumers worldwide to purchase fruits, vegetables, coffee, tea, cocoa, wine, and many other products that display the Fair Trade Certified logo[59] (**FIGURE 12.16**). Fair trade empowers farm laborers to demand living wages and humane treatment. It also reduces child labor and increases access of children to education, because parents earning higher wages are able to allow their children to leave the fields and attend school. Profits from fair trade purchases also support the building of schools and health clinics, provide funds to help farmers adopt sustainable agricultural practices, and provide financial assistance for women to set up in small businesses.[58]

Your Actions Can Promote Sustainability, Diversity, and Food Equity

In a climate in which power over food is ever more tightly controlled, the food movement is providing ordinary citizens a means to promote change. Here are some ways that you can join them!

The choices you make when you shop can contribute to sustainability and food equity, because your purchases influence local and global markets. Within your food budget, buy organic foods to reduce the use of synthetic pesticides and fertilizers. Buy produce from a local farmers' market to encourage greater local availability of fresh foods. This reduces the costs and resources devoted to distribution, transportation, and storage of foods. And purchase Fair Trade foods to support equitable production worldwide.

The amount of meat you eat also affects the environment and the global food supply, because the production of plant-based foods uses fewer natural resources and releases fewer greenhouse gases than the production of animal-based foods. To promote reduced meat consumption on campus, talk with your food services manager about sponsoring "Meatless Mondays." See the *Web Links* for a link to the Meatless Monday website, where you can download a Meatless Monday Goes to College toolkit.

You know that physical activity is important in maintaining health, but walking, biking, and taking public transportation also limits your consumption of nonrenewable fossil fuels. When it's time to purchase a car, research your options and choose the one with the best fuel economy.

To fight food insecurity in the United States, consider joining the National Student Campaign Against Hunger and Homelessness. See the *Web Links* for their website. Alternatively, you can gather foods for local food banks, volunteer to work in a soup kitchen, help distribute food to homebound elderly, or start a community or school garden. You can also hold fund-raisers and donate cash directly.

Get the word out! If you find an organization whose goals you share, recommend them on your social networking page. Or send a short article about the organization's work to your campus news site, with suggestions about how other students can support their work.

As Francis Moore Lappe, author of the groundbreaking *Diet for a Small Planet*, explains, the food movement encourages us to think with an "eco-mind," refusing to accept scarcity and oppression for some in the name of production for many. By promoting the values of fairness, connection, and abundance, involvement in the movement encourages us to make choices in ways that can change our world.[58]

fair trade A trading partnership promoting equity in international trading relationships and contributing to sustainable development by securing the rights of marginalized producers and workers.

recap The food movement seeks to increase the sustainability of our agricultural practices to preserve natural resources for future generations. It also opposes the loss of diversity of our food supply prompted by corporate agriculture and supports the growth of smaller, local farms offering a variety of fresh produce. Poverty and unfair trade practices reduce food equity—access to a fair share in the world's food and other resources.

STUDY PLAN | MasteringNutrition™

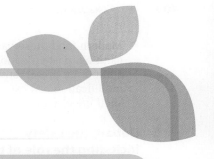

Customize your study plan—and master your nutrition!—
in the Study Area of **MasteringNutrition**.

what can I do **today?**

Now that you've read this chapter, try making these three changes.

1 Before every meal, whether you're preparing it yourself or eating out, wash your hands!

2 Buy a thermometer for your refrigerator and freezer. If you eat meat, buy a meat thermometer. Then start to use them!

3 If you purchase an apple today, pay the extra cash for organic. Apples top the list of high-pesticide foods.

test yourself | *answers*

1. **False.** A majority of cases of foodborne illness are caused by just one species of virus, called norovirus. Bacteria also commonly cause foodborne illness. Mold is not usually a culprit.

2. **False.** Freezing destroys some microorganisms but only inhibits the ability of other microorganisms to reproduce. When the food is thawed, these cold-tolerant microorganisms resume reproduction.

3. **True.** In 2008 through 2012, the last five years for which data are available, more than 14% of American households have experienced food insecurity.

chapter summary

Scan to hear an MP3 Chapter Review in **MasteringNutrition**.

LO 1 Summarize the two main reasons that foodborne illness is a critical concern in the United States

■ According to the CDC, about 48 million Americans report experiencing foodborne illness each year. Moreover, food production is increasingly complex, with more foods mass-produced than ever before, using a combination of ingredients from a much greater number of sources, including fields, feedlots, and a variety of processing facilities all over the world. Contamination can occur at any point from farm to table, and when it does, it can be difficult to trace.

LO 2 Identify the types of microorganisms most commonly involved in foodborne illness

■ Food infections result from the consumption of food containing pathogenic microorganisms, such as bacteria, whereas food intoxications result from consuming food in which microorganisms have secreted toxins. Chemical residues in food can also cause illness.

■ Food infections are most commonly caused by viruses, especially the norovirus; bacteria such as *Salmonella*; and parasites, such as helminths.

LO 3 Describe strategies for preventing foodborne illness at home, while eating out, and when traveling to other countries

■ To reproduce in foods, microorganisms require a precise range of temperature, humidity, acidity, and oxygen content. You can prevent foodborne illness at home by washing your hands and kitchen surfaces often, separating foods to prevent cross-contamination, storing foods in the refrigerator or freezer, and cooking foods to their proper temperatures.

■ When traveling, avoid raw foods and choose beverages that are boiled, bottled, or canned, without ice.

LO 4 Compare and contrast the different methods manufacturers use to preserve foods

■ Some of the oldest techniques for food preservation include salting, sugaring, drying, smoking, and cooling.

■ Modern food preservation techniques include canning, pasteurization, aseptic packaging, addition of preservatives, and irradiation. Genetic modification can extend the ripening time or shelf life of foods.

LO **5** **Debate the safety of food additives, including the role of the GRAS list**

■ Food additives are natural or synthetic ingredients added to foods during processing to enhance them in some way. They include flavorings, colorings, nutrients, texturizers, and other additives.

■ The GRAS list identifies hundreds of substances that are generally recognized as safe for use in foods.

LO **6** **Describe the process of genetic modification and discuss the potential risks and benefits associated with genetically modified organisms**

■ In genetic modification, the genetic material, or DNA, of an organism is altered to enhance certain qualities. Techniques include selective breeding and recombinant DNA technology, in which scientists isolate from an animal, a plant, or a microbial cell a particular segment of DNA—one or more genes—that codes for a protein conferring a desirable trait, then use it to modify a different organism's DNA.

■ Genetic modification can increase a plant's resistance to disease or harsh environmental conditions or improve its nutrient value or yield. Concerns include risks to the environment, including loss of native habitats, and potential threats to human health.

LO **7** **Describe the process by which persistent organic pollutants accumulate in foods**

■ Persistent organic pollutants (POPs) are chemicals released into the atmosphere as a result of industry, agriculture, automobile emissions, and improper waste disposal. Through a process called biomagnification, plants, animals, and fish absorb the chemicals from contaminated soil or water and pass them in increasingly greater concentrations up the food chain.

LO **8** **Discuss the regulation, labeling, benefits, and limitations of organic foods**

■ Organic crops are grown without the use of synthetic fertilizers, toxic and persistent pesticides, genetic engineering, or irradiation. Animals must be raised without growth hormones or antibiotics, fed with 100% organic feed, and have access to the outdoors. Although pesticides prevent or reduce crop losses, they are potential toxins, but organically grown foods are less likely to be contaminated with detectable pesticide residues. Recombinant bovine growth hormone (rBGH) is injected into conventional beef and dairy cows to increase their yield and is banned by some countries because of concerns related to human health. Indiscriminate use of antibiotics in animals has led to the development of antibiotic-resistant bacteria. The USDA regulates organic farming standards and inspects and certifies farms that follow all USDA Organic Standards.

■ A few recent research studies indicate that some organic foods may have higher levels of some nutrients and phytochemicals than nonorganic foods, but there is insufficient evidence to claim that organic foods are generally more nutritious than nonorganic foods.

LO **9** **Explain how corporate agricultural practices have threatened sustainability and reduced food diversity, and identify several initiatives embraced by the food movement to reverse these trends**

■ Although it has achieved higher yields at lower costs, corporate agriculture has led to depletion of topsoil, freshwater, and fossil fuels, and increased levels of agrochemical run-off and greenhouse gas emissions. Corporate farming has also reduced food diversity—that is, the variety of different species of food crops available. This occurred as subsidies led to the increased production of certain crops such as corn, which began to monopolize the food supply.

■ Initiatives to improve sustainability and diversity include the slow food movement, the increase in family farms, farmers' markets, community-supported agriculture, and school gardens. Entrepreneurship and corporate involvement are also important.

LO **10** **Discuss two issues of food equity: food insecurity and unfair trade practices**

■ About 14.5% of U.S. households (about 17.6 million households) experienced food insecurity in 2012. Overall, people who are food-insecure are more likely to live in areas known as food deserts—geographic areas where people lack access to affordable, nutritious food.

■ As it has displaced small-scale farmers, corporate farming has also monopolized agricultural labor, forcing farmworkers to accept poverty-level wages and substandard living conditions. The fair trade movement attempts to combat the exploitation of farm laborers around the world.

review questions

LO **1** **Summarize the two main reasons that foodborne illness is a critical concern in the United States**

1. Which of the following statements about food safety is true?
   a. Federal inspections of food production facilities have decreased over the last few decades.
   b. The United States Department of Agriculture oversees the safety of all foods produced in or imported into the United States.
   c. Foodborne illness causes 3 million hospitalizations in the United States each year.
   d. Both a and b are true.

LO **2** **Identify the types of microorganisms most commonly involved in foodborne illness**

2. The microorganism most commonly involved in foodborne illness is
   a. *E. coli*.
   b. norovirus.
   c. *Giardia*.
   d. *Cryptococcus*.

LO **3** **Describe strategies for preventing foodborne illness at home, while eating out, and when traveling to other countries**

3. The temperature in your refrigerator should be at or below
   a. 0°F.
   b. 20°F.
   c. 40°F.
   d. 60°F.

LO **4** **Compare and contrast the different methods manufacturers use to preserve foods**

4. A food preservation technique in which the oxygen in a food is replaced with an inert gas is
   a. pasteurization.
   b. irradiation.
   c. modified atmosphere packaging.
   d. high-pressure processing.

LO **5** **Debate the safety of food additives, including the role of the GRAS list**

5. Food additives that have raised health concerns include
   a. sodium chloride and potassium sorbate.
   b. sulfites and nitrites.
   c. lecithin and glycerin.
   d. all of the above.

LO **6** **Describe the process of genetic modification and discuss the potential risks and benefits associated with genetically modified organisms**

6. The process in which a gene conferring a beneficial trait is spliced into another organism is technically known as
   a. biodiversification.
   b. selective breeding.
   c. gene therapy.
   d. recombinant DNA technology.

LO **7** **Describe the process by which persistent organic pollutants accumulate in foods**

7. Which of the following best describes how biomagnification occurs?
   a. Conventional fertilizers and pesticides are sprayed onto food crops.
   b. Industrial pollutants initiate DNA mutations that lead to cancer.
   c. Animal wastes contaminate soils where food crops are grown.
   d. Industrial contaminants become more concentrated in animal tissues as they move up the food chain.

LO **8** **Discuss the regulation, labeling, benefits, and limitations of organic foods**

8. Foods that are labeled *100% organic*
   a. contain only organically produced ingredients, excluding water and salt.
   b. may display the EPA's organic seal.
   c. can include genetically modified organisms.
   d. contain foods from plant sources only.

LO **9** **Explain how corporate agricultural practices have threatened sustainability and reduced food diversity, and identify several initiatives embraced by the food movement to reverse these trends**

9. Corporate farming has
   a. increased food production and decreased global hunger.
   b. increased the use of synthetic pesticides and fertilizers and decreased crop diversity.
   c. increased the emission of greenhouse gases and depleted water supplies.
   d. all of the above.

LO **10** **Discuss two issues of food equity: food insecurity and unfair trade practices**

10. Which of the following statements about food insecurity is true?

a. Workers in minimum-wage jobs are at increased risk for food insecurity.

b. In the United States, nearly 1 million households experience very low food security.

c. Food insecurity in the United States has been declining for about the past decade.

d. None of the above is true.

Answers to Review Questions are located at the back of this text.

web links

The following websites and apps explore further topics and issues related to personal health.
Visit **MasteringNutrition** for links to the websites and RSS feeds.

http://www.cdc.gov
CDC Food Safety Homepage

This is the CDC's site for information about foodborne illness outbreaks, food safety tips, and more.

www.epa.gov
U.S. Environmental Protection Agency: Pesticides

This site provides information on safe pesticide use in your home or garden, how to reduce pesticide residues in foods, and regulation of pesticides.

www2.epa.gov
Environmental Protection Agency's Sustainability Tips

This site offers a wide variety of tips and tools to help you reduce your environmental footprint.

www.fairtradeusa.org
Fair Trade USA

Visit this website to find out why "Every Purchase Matters!"

www.foodsafety.gov
Foodsafety.gov

Use this website as a gateway to food safety information from recalls to updates, food safety tips, and more.

www.ota.com
Organic Trade Association

This website provides lots of information about the production and marketing of organic food.

www.meatlessmonday.com/
Meatless Monday

This website offers information on the environmental and health benefits of going meatless one day a week, as well as recipes for vegetarian meals and a toolkit to promote Meatless Mondays on your campus.

http://www.slowfoodusa.org/
Slow Food USA

Slow Food links the pleasure of growing, preparing, and consuming food with commitment to our communities and environment. Visit this site to learn more about the slow food movement and get involved.

www.studentsagainsthunger.org/
National Student Campaign Against Hunger and Homelessness

Visit their site to find out what they're up to and how to get involved.

appendices

appendices

appendix A

The USDA Food Guide Evolution

Early History of Food Guides

Did you know that in the United States food guides in one form or another have been around for over 125 years?

That's right. Back in 1885 a college chemistry professor named Wilber Olin (W. O.) Atwater helped bring the fledgling science of nutrition to a broader audience by introducing scientific data boxes that became the basis for the first known U.S. food guide. Those early dietary standards focused on defining the nutritional needs of an "average man" in terms of his daily consumption of proteins and calories. These became food composition tables defined in three sweeping categories; protein, fats and carbohydrate; mineral matter; and fuel values. As early as 1902, Atwater advocated for three foundational nutritional principles that we still support today; the concepts of variety, proportionality, and moderation in food choices and eating.

These ideas were adapted a few years later by a nutritionist named Caroline Hunt, who developed a food "buying" guide divided into five categories: meats and proteins; cereals and starches; vegetables and fruits; fatty foods; and sugar, based on a 2,800 calorie-per-day diet.

Starting in the 1930s and 1940s, on through the following 30 years to the early 1970s, these concepts were further developed and experimented with, evolving from 12 food groups to a "Basic Seven" group approach, to the "Basic Four," and from there to a "Hassel-Free" construct that briefly increased the number of groups up to five. While all these approaches had drawbacks and received critical scrutiny, they were nonetheless important and necessary attempts to provide Americans with reliable guidelines based on the best scientific data and practices available at the time.

The USDA Food Guide Pyramid

Beginning around the early 1980s these concepts began to assume forms we've become familiar with today. In the process, important philosophical goals became attached to the development of a comprehensive guide. These core values included the following goals for a guide:

- it must encompass a broad focus on **overall health**;
- it should emphasize the use of **current research**;
- it should be an approach that includes the **total diet**, rather than parts or pieces;
- it should be **useful**;
- it should be **realistic**;
- it should be **flexible**;
- it should be **practical**;
- and it must be **evolutionary**, in that it should be able to adapt to new information that comes to light.

Additionally, the essential steps needed to develop a modern food guide became articulated. These are readily apparent in the first USDA Food Guide Pyramid released in 1992, which attempted for the first time to create a graphic representation of the guidelines. The steps required the inclusion of:

- Nutritional Goals
- Food Groups
- Serving Sizes
- Nutrient Profiles
- Numbers of Servings, including addressing the need for adequacy and moderation.

Remarkably, W. O. Atwater's early principles of *variety, proportionality, and moderation* remain relevant and appropriate to our modern graphic guidelines. The attempts to develop a conceptual framework for selecting the types and amounts of food that can support a nutritionally sound diet continue to evolve. Nutritionists and other health professionals are still working to find better ways to communicate to a large and diverse audience how to translate recommendations for nutrient intake into recommendations on which food to eat, and in what amounts.

Let's take a look at the evolution of the modern Food Guide over the past quarter-century:

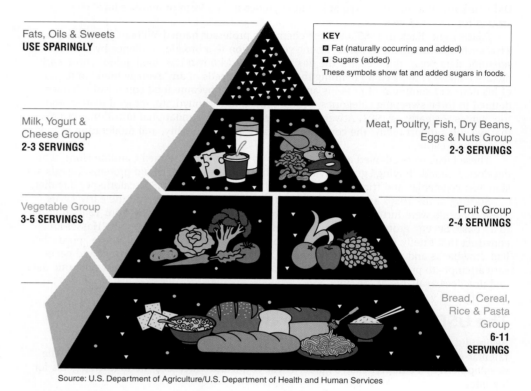

Fats, Oils & Sweets
USE SPARINGLY

KEY
◻ Fat (naturally occurring and added)
▽ Sugars (added)
These symbols show fat and added sugars in foods.

Milk, Yogurt &
Cheese Group
2-3 SERVINGS

Meat, Poultry, Fish, Dry Beans,
Eggs & Nuts Group
2-3 SERVINGS

Vegetable Group
3-5 SERVINGS

Fruit Group
2-4 SERVINGS

Bread, Cereal,
Rice & Pasta
Group
**6-11
SERVINGS**

Source: U.S. Department of Agriculture/U.S. Department of Health and Human Services

◆ FIGURE A.1   The 1992 Food Guide Pyramid. This representation of the USDA guidelines took several years to develop and attempted to convey in a single image all the key aspects of a nutritional guide.

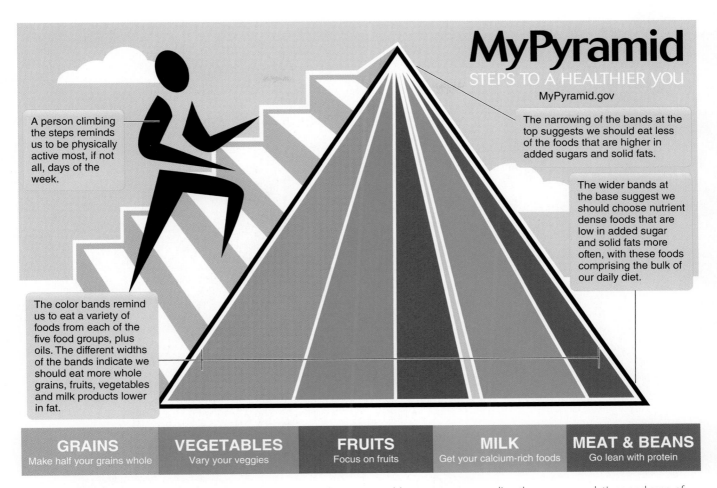

MyPyramid
STEPS TO A HEALTHIER YOU
MyPyramid.gov

A person climbing the steps reminds us to be physically active most, if not all, days of the week.

The narrowing of the bands at the top suggests we should eat less of the foods that are higher in added sugars and solid fats.

The wider bands at the base suggest we should choose nutrient dense foods that are low in added sugar and solid fats more often, with these foods comprising the bulk of our daily diet.

The color bands remind us to eat a variety of foods from each of the five food groups, plus oils. The different widths of the bands indicate we should eat more whole grains, fruits, vegetables and milk products lower in fat.

GRAINS Make half your grains whole	**VEGETABLES** Vary your veggies	**FRUITS** Focus on fruits	**MILK** Get your calcium-rich foods	**MEAT & BEANS** Go lean with protein

FIGURE A.2 The USDA revised the food guide pyramid in 2005 to address concerns regarding the recommendations and ease-of-use for a general audience. They put forth the MyPyramid Food Guidance System, which continues with the "pyramid" concept, but in a simpler presentation.

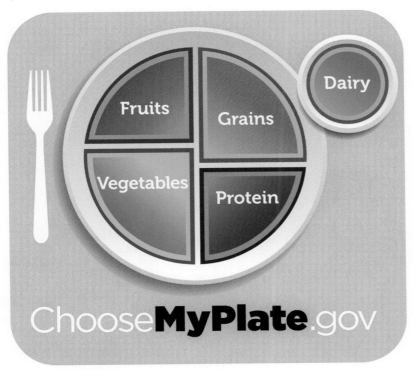

Choose**MyPlate**.gov

FIGURE A.3 In May 2011 the USDA made a dramatic change by withdrawing the pyramid concept and focusing instead on conveying core information in a simple, direct, and easy-to-follow way, as MyPlate. In MyPlate, the icons are intended as healthy eating reminders, rather than as specific messages encompassing detailed information.

Data adapted from www.nal.usda.gov/fnic/history/hist.htm and http://www.choosemyplate.gov/downloads/MyPlate/ABriefHistoryOfUSDAFoodGuides.pdf

appendix B

Calculations and Conversions

Calculation and Conversion Aids

Commonly Used Metric Units

millimeter (mm): one-thousandth of a meter (0.001)
centimeter (cm): one-hundredth of a meter (0.01)
kilometer (km): one-thousand times a meter (1,000)
kilogram (kg): one-thousand times a gram (1,000)
milligram (mg): one-thousandth of a gram (0.001)
microgram (μg): one-millionth of a gram (0.000001)
milliliter (ml): one-thousandth of a liter (0.001)

International Units

Some vitamin supplements may report vitamin content as International Units (IU).
To convert IU to

- Micrograms of vitamin D (cholecalciferol), divide the IU value by 40 or multiply by 0.025.
- Milligrams of vitamin E (alpha-tocopherol), divide the IU value by 1.5 if vitamin E is from natural sources. Divide the IU value by 2.22 if vitamin E is from synthetic sources.
- Vitamin A: 1 IU = 0.3 μg retinol or 3.6 μg beta-carotene.

Retinol Activity Equivalents

Retinol Activity Equivalents (RAE) are a standardized unit of measure for vitamin A. RAE account for the various differences in bioavailability from sources of vitamin A. Many supplements will report vitamin A content in IU, as just shown, or Retinol Equivalents (RE).

1 RAE = 1 μg retinol
12 μg beta-carotene
24 μg other vitamin A carotenoids

To calculate RAE from the RE value of vitamin carotenoids in foods, divide RE by 2.
For vitamin A supplements and foods fortified with vitamin A, 1 RE = 1 RAE.

Folate

Folate is measured as Dietary Folate Equivalents (DFE). DFE account for the different factors affecting bioavailability of folate sources.

1 DFE = 1 μg food folate
0.6 μg folate from fortified foods
0.5 μg folate supplement taken on an empty stomach
0.6 μg folate as a supplement consumed with a meal

To convert micrograms of synthetic folate, such as that found in supplements or fortified foods, to DFE:

$$\mu g \text{ synthetic} \times \text{folate } 1.7 = \mu g \text{ DFE}$$

For naturally occurring food folate, such as spinach, each microgram of folate equals 1 microgram DFE:

$$\mu g \text{ folate} = \mu g \text{ DFE}$$

Conversion Factors

Use the following table to convert U.S. measurements to metric equivalents:

Original Unit	Multiply By	To Get
ounces avdp	28.3495	grams
ounces	0.0625	pounds
pounds	0.4536	kilograms
pounds	16	ounces
grams	0.0353	ounces
grams	0.002205	pounds
kilograms	2.2046	pounds
liters	1.8162	pints (dry)
liters	2.1134	pints (liquid)
liters	0.9081	quarts (dry)
liters	1.0567	quarts (liquid)
liters	0.2642	gallons (U.S.)
pints (dry)	0.5506	liters
pints (liquid)	0.4732	liters
quarts (dry)	1.1012	liters
quarts (liquid)	0.9463	liters
gallons (U.S.)	3.7853	liters
millimeters	0.0394	inches
centimeters	0.3937	inches
centimeters	0.03281	feet
inches	25.4000	millimeters
inches	2.5400	centimeters
inches	0.0254	meters
feet	0.3048	meters
meters	3.2808	feet
meters	1.0936	yards
cubic feet	0.0283	cubic meters
cubic meters	35.3145	cubic feet
cubic meters	1.3079	cubic yards
cubic yards	0.7646	cubic meters

Length: U.S. and Metric Equivalents

¼ inch = 0.6 centimeter
1 inch = 2.5 centimeters
1 foot = 0.3048 meter
30.48 centimeters
1 yard = 0.91144 meter
1 millimeter = 0.03937 inch
1 centimeter = 0.3937 inch
1 decimeter = 3.937 inches
1 meter = 39.37 inches
1.094 yards
1 micrometer = 0.00003937 inch

Weights and Measures

Food Measurement Equivalencies from U.S. to Metric

Capacity

⅕ teaspoon	=	1 milliliter
¼ teaspoon	=	1.25 milliliters
½ teaspoon	=	2.5 milliliters
1 teaspoon	=	5 milliliters
1 tablespoon	=	15 milliliters
1 fluid ounce	=	28.4 milliliters
¼ cup	=	60 milliliters
⅓ cup	=	80 milliliters
½ cup	=	120 milliliters
1 cup	=	225 milliliters
1 pint (2 cups)	=	473 milliliters
1 quart (4 cups)	=	0.95 liter
1 liter (1.06 quarts)	=	1,000 milliliters
1 gallon (4 quarts)	=	3.84 liters

Weight

0.035 ounce	=	1 gram
1 ounce	=	28 grams
¼ pound (4 ounces)	=	114 grams
1 pound (16 ounces)	=	454 grams
2.2 pounds (35 ounces)	=	1 kilogram

U.S. Food Measurement Equivalents

3 teaspoons	=	1 tablespoon
½ tablespoon	=	1½ teaspoons
2 tablespoons	=	⅛ cup
4 tablespoons	=	¼ cup
5 tablespoons + 1 teaspoon	=	⅓ cup
8 tablespoons	=	½ cup
10 tablespoons + 2 teaspoons	=	⅔ cup
12 tablespoons	=	¾ cup
16 tablespoons	=	1 cup
2 cups	=	1 pint
4 cups	=	1 quart
2 pints	=	1 quart
4 quarts	=	1 gallon

Volumes and Capacities

1 cup	=	8 fluid ounces
		½ liquid pint
1 milliliter	=	0.061 cubic inch
1 liter	=	1.057 liquid quarts
		0.908 dry quart
		61.024 cubic inches
1 U.S. gallon	=	231 cubic inches
		3.785 liters
		0.833 British gallon
		128 U.S. fluid ounces
1 British Imperial gallon	=	277.42 cubic inches
		1.201 U.S. gallons
		4.546 liters
		160 British fluid ounces

1 U.S. ounce, liquid or fluid	=	1.805 cubic inches
		29.574 milliliters
		1.041 British fluid ounces
1 pint, dry	=	33.600 cubic inches
		0.551 liter
1 pint, liquid	=	28.875 cubic inches
		0.473 liter
1 U.S. quart, dry	=	67.201 cubic inches
		1.101 liters
1 U.S. quart, liquid	=	57.75 cubic inches
		0.946 liter
1 British quart	=	69.354 cubic inches
		1.032 U.S. quarts, dry
		1.201 U.S. quarts, liquid

Energy Units

1 kilocalorie (kcal)	=	4.2 kilojoules
1 millijoule (MJ)	=	240 kilocalories
1 kilojoule (kJ)	=	0.24 kcal
1 gram carbohydrate	=	4 kcal
1 gram fat	=	9 kcal
1 gram protein	=	4 kcal

Temperature Standards

	°Fahrenheit	°Celsius
Body temperature	98.6°	37°
Comfortable room temperature	65–75°	18–24°
Boiling point of water	212°	100°
Freezing point of water	32°	0°

Temperature Scales

To Convert Fahrenheit to Celsius:

$$[(°F - 32) \times 5]/9$$

1. Subtract 32 from °F.
2. Multiply (°F − 32) by 5; then divide by 9.

To Convert Celsius to Fahrenheit:

$$[(°C \times 9)/5] + 32$$

1. Multiply °C by 9; then divide by 5.
2. Add 32 to (°C × 9/5).

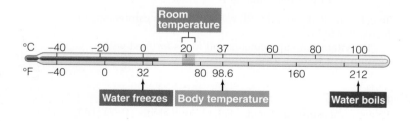

appendix C

Foods Containing Caffeine

Source: Data from USDA Nutrient Database for Standard Reference, Release 22.

Beverages

Food Name	Serving	Caffeine/Serving (mg)
Beverage mix, chocolate flavor, dry mix, prepared w/milk	1 cup (8 fl. oz)	7.98
Beverage mix, chocolate malt powder, fortified, prepared w/milk	1 cup (8 fl. oz)	5.3
Beverage mix, chocolate malted milk powder, no added nutrients, prepared w/milk	1 cup (8 fl. oz)	7.95
Beverage, chocolate syrup w/o added nutrients, prepared w/milk	1 cup (8 fl. oz)	5.64
Beverage, chocolate syrup, fortified, mixed w/milk	1 cup milk and 1 tbsp. syrup	2.63
Cocoa mix w/aspartame and calcium and phosphorus, no sodium or vitamin A, low kcal, dry, prepared	6 fl. oz water and 0.53 oz packet	5
Cocoa mix w/aspartame, dry, low kcal, prepared w/water	1 packet dry mix with 6 fl. oz water	1.92
Cocoa mix, dry mix	1 serving (3 heaping tsp. or 1 envelope)	5.04
Cocoa mix, dry, w/o added nutrients, prepared w/water	1 oz packet with 6 fl. oz water	4.12
Cocoa mix, fortified, dry, prepared w/water	6 fl. oz H_2O and 1 packet	6.27
Cocoa, dry powder, high-fat or breakfast, plain	1 piece	6.895
Cocoa, hot, homemade w/whole milk	1 cup	5
Coffee liqueur, 53 proof	1 fl. oz	9.048
Coffee liqueur, 63 proof	1 fl. oz	9.05
Coffee w/cream liqueur, 34 proof	1 fl. oz	2.488
Coffee mix w/sugar (cappuccino), dry, prepared w/water	6 fl. oz H_2O and 2 rounded tsp. mix	74.88
Coffee mix w/sugar (French), dry, prepared w/water	6 fl. oz H_2O and 2 rounded tsp. mix	51.03
Coffee mix w/sugar (mocha), dry, prepared w/water	6 fl. oz and 2 round tsp. mix	33.84
Coffee, brewed	1 cup (8 fl. oz)	94.8
Coffee, brewed, prepared with tap water, decaffeinated	1 cup (8 fl. oz)	2.37
Coffee, instant, prepared	1 cup (8 fl. oz)	61.98
Coffee, instant, regular, powder, half the caffeine	1 cup (8 fl. oz)	30.99
Coffee, instant, decaffeinated	1 cup (8 fl. oz)	1.79
Coffee and cocoa (mocha) powder, with whitener and low-calorie sweetener	1 cup	405.48
Coffee, brewed, espresso, restaurant-prepared	1 cup (8 fl. oz)	502.44
Coffee, brewed, espresso, restaurant-prepared, decaffeinated	1 cup (8 fl. oz)	2.37
Energy drink, with caffeine, niacin, pantothenic acid, vitamin B_6	1 fl. oz	9.517
Milk beverage mix, dairy drink w/aspartame, low kcal, dry, prep	6 fl. oz	4.08
Milk, lowfat, 1% fat, chocolate	1 cup	5
Milk, whole, chocolate	1 cup	5
Soft drink, cola w/caffeine	1 fl. oz	2
Soft drink, cola, w/higher caffeine	1 fl. oz	8.33
Soft drink, cola or pepper type, low kcal w/saccharin and caffeine	1 fl. oz	3.256
Soft drink, cola, low kcal w/saccharin and aspartame, w/caffeine	1 fl. oz	4.144
Soft drink, lemon-lime soda, w/caffeine	1 fl. oz	4.605
Soft drink, low kcal, not cola or pepper, with aspartame and caffeine	1 fl. oz	4.44
Soft drink, pepper type, w/caffeine	1 fl. oz	3.07
Tea mix, instant w/lemon flavor, w/saccharin, dry, prepared	1 cup (8 fl. oz)	16.59
Tea mix, instant w/lemon, unsweetened, dry, prepared	1 cup (8 fl. oz)	26.18
Tea mix, instant w/sugar and lemon, dry, no added vitamin C, prepared	1 cup (8 fl. oz)	28.49
Tea mix, instant, unsweetened, dry, prepared	1 cup (8 fl. oz)	30.81
Tea, brewed	1 cup (8 fl. oz)	47.36
Tea, brewed, prepared with tap water, decaffeinated	1 cup (8 fl. oz)	2.37
Tea, instant, unsweetened, powder, decaffeinated	1 tsp.	1.183
Tea, instant, w/o sugar, lemon-flavored, w/added vitamin C, dry prepared	1 cup (8 fl. oz)	26.05
Tea, instant, with sugar, lemon-flavored, decaffeinated, no added vitamin	1 cup	9.1

Cake, Cookies, and Desserts

Food Name	Serving	Caffeine/Serving (mg)
Brownie, square, large (2-3/4" × 7/8")	1 piece	1.12
Cake, chocolate pudding, dry mix	1 oz	1.701
Cake, chocolate, dry mix, regular	1 oz	3.118
Cake, German chocolate pudding, dry mix	1 oz	1.985
Cake, marble pudding, dry mix	1 oz	1.985
Candies, chocolate-covered, caramel with nuts	1 cup	35.34
Candies, chocolate-covered, dietetic or low-calorie	1 cup	16.74
Candy, milk chocolate w/almonds	1 bar (1.45 oz)	9.02
Candy, milk chocolate w/rice cereal	1 bar (1.4 oz)	9.2
Candy, raisins, milk-chocolate-coated	1 cup	45
Chocolate chips, semisweet, mini	1 cup chips (6 oz package)	107.12
Chocolate, baking, unsweetened, square	1 piece	22.72
Chocolate, baking, Mexican, square	1 piece	2.8
Chocolate, sweet	1 oz	18.711
Cookie Cake, Snackwell Fat Free Devil's Food, Nabisco	1 serving	1.28
Cookie, Snackwell Caramel Delights, Nabisco	1 serving	1.44
Cookie, chocolate chip, enriched, commercially prepared	1 oz	3.118
Cookie, chocolate chip, homemade w/margarine	1 oz	4.536
Cookie, chocolate chip, lower-fat, commercially prepared	3 pieces	2.1
Cookie, chocolate chip, refrigerated dough	1 portion, dough spooned from roll	2.61
Cookie, chocolate chip, soft, commercially prepared	1 oz	1.985
Cookie, chocolate wafers	1 cup, crumbs	7.84
Cookie, graham crackers, chocolate-coated	1 oz	13.041
Cookie, sandwich, chocolate, cream-filled	3 pieces	3.9
Cookie, sandwich, chocolate, cream-filled, special dietary	1 oz	0.85
Cupcake, chocolate w/frosting, low-fat	1 oz	0.86
Doughnut, cake, chocolate w/sugar or glaze	1 oz	0.284
Doughnut, cake, plain w/chocolate icing, large (3-1/2")	1 each	1.14
Fast food, ice cream sundae, hot fudge	1 sundae	1.58
Fast food, milk beverage, chocolate shake	1 cup (8 fl. oz)	1.66
Frosting, chocolate, creamy, ready-to-eat	2 tbsp. creamy	0.82
Frozen yogurt, chocolate	1 cup	5.58
Fudge, chocolate w/nuts, homemade	1 oz	1.984
Granola bar, soft, milk-chocolate-coated, peanut butter	1 oz	0.85
Granola bar, w/coconut, chocolate-coated	1 cup	5.58
Ice cream, chocolate	1 individual (3.5 fl. oz)	1.74
Ice cream, chocolate, light	1 oz	0.85
Ice cream, chocolate, rich	1 cup	5.92
M&M's Peanut Chocolate	1 cup	18.7
M&M's Plain Chocolate	1 cup	22.88
Milk chocolate	1 cup chips	33.6
Milk-chocolate-coated coffee beans	1 NLEA serving	48
Milk dessert, frozen, fat-free milk, chocolate	1 oz	0.85
Milk shake, thick, chocolate	1 fl. oz	0.568
Pastry, éclair/cream puff, homemade, custard-filled w/chocolate	1 oz	0.567
Pie crust, chocolate-wafer-cookie-type, chilled	1 crust, single 9"	11.15
Pie, chocolate mousse, no bake mix	1 oz	0.284
Pudding, chocolate, instant dry mix prepared w/reduced-fat (2%) milk	1 oz	0.283
Pudding, chocolate, regular dry mix prepared w/reduced-fat (2%) milk	1 oz	0.567
Pudding, chocolate, ready-to-eat, fat-free	4 oz can	2.27
Syrups, chocolate, genuine chocolate flavor, light, Hershey	2 tbsp.	1.05
Topping, chocolate-flavored hazelnut spread	1 oz	1.984
Yogurt, chocolate, nonfat milk	1 oz	0.567
Yogurt, frozen, chocolate, soft serve	0.5 cup (4 fl. oz)	2.16

appendix D

U.S. Exchange Lists for Meal Planning

From Choose Your Foods: Exchange Lists For Diabetes.
© Academy of Nutrition and Dietetics. Adapted and reprinted with permission.

Starch

One starch choice has 15 grams of carbohydrate, 3 grams of protein, 1 gram of fat, and 80 calories.

Icon Key

✔ = Good source of fiber
! = Extra fat
▥ = High in sodium

Food	Serving Size
Bread	
Bagel	¼ large bagel (1 oz)
! Biscuit	1 biscuit (2½ inches across)
Breads, loaf-type	
white, whole-grain, French, Italian, pumpernickel, rye, sourdough, unfrosted raisin or cinnamon	1 slice (1 oz)
✔ reduced-calorie, light	2 slices (1½ oz)
Breads, flat-type (flatbreads)	
chapatti	1 oz
ciabatta	1 oz
naan	3¼-inch square (1 oz)
pita (6 inches across)	½ pita
roti	1 oz
✔ sandwich flat buns, whole-wheat	1 bun, including top and bottom (1½ oz)
! taco shell	2 taco shells (each 5 inches across)
tortilla, corn	1 small tortilla (6 inches across)
tortilla, flour (white or whole-wheat)	1 small tortilla (6 inches across) or ⅓ large tortilla (10 inches across)
Cornbread	1¾-inch cube (1½ oz)
English muffin	½ muffin
Hot dog bun or hamburger bun	½ bun (¾ oz)
Pancake	1 pancake (4 inches across, ¼ inch thick)
Roll, plain	1 small roll (1 oz)
! Stuffing, bread	⅓ cup
Waffle	1 waffle (4-inch square or 4 inches across)
Cereals	
✔ Bran cereal (twigs, buds, or flakes)	½ cup
Cooked cereals (oats, oatmeal)	½ cup
Granola cereal	¼ cup

Food	Serving Size
Grits, cooked	½ cup
Muesli	¼ cup
Puffed cereal	1½ cups
Shredded wheat, plain	½ cup
Sugar-coated cereal	½ cup
Unsweetened, ready-to-eat cereal	¾ cup
Grains (Including Pasta and Rice)	
Unless otherwise indicated, serving sizes listed are for cooked grains.	
Barley	⅓ cup
Bran, dry	
✔ oat	¼ cup
✔ wheat	½ cup
✔ Bulgur	½ cup
Couscous	⅓ cup
Kasha	½ cup
Millet	⅓ cup
Pasta, white or whole-wheat (all shapes and sizes)	⅓ cup
Polenta	⅓ cup
Quinoa, all colors	⅓ cup
Rice, white, brown, and other colors and types	⅓ cup
Tabbouleh (tabouli), prepared	½ cup
Wheat germ, dry	3 Tbsp
Wild rice	½ cup
Starchy Vegetables	
All of the serving sizes for starchy vegetables on this list are for cooked vegetables.	
Breadfruit	¼ cup
Cassava or dasheen	⅓ cup
Corn	½ cup
on cob	4- to 4½-inch piece (½ large cob)
✔ Hominy	¾ cup
✔ Mixed vegetables with corn or peas	1 cup
Marinara, pasta, or spaghetti sauce	½ cup
✔ Parsnips	½ cup
✔ Peas, green	½ cup
Plantain	⅓ cup
Potato	
baked with skin	¼ large potato (3 oz)

Food	Serving Size
boiled, all kinds	½ cup or ½ medium potato (3 oz)
! mashed, with milk and fat	½ cup
French-fried (oven-baked)*	1 cup (2 oz)
✓ Pumpkin puree, canned, no sugar added	¾ cup
✓ Squash, winter (acorn, butternut)	1 cup
✓ Succotash	½ cup
Yam or sweet potato, plain	½ cup (3 ½ oz)

Crackers and Snacks

Note: Some snacks are high in fat. Always check food labels.

Crackers

Food	Serving Size
animal	8 crackers
✓ crispbread	2 to 5 pieces (¾ oz)
graham, 2 ½-inch square	3 squares
nut and rice	10 crackers
oyster	20 crackers
! round, butter-type	6 crackers
saltine-type	6 crackers
! sandwich-style, cheese or peanut butter filling	3 crackers
whole-wheat, baked	5 regular 1 ½-inch squares or 10 thins (¾ oz)
Granola or snack bar	1 bar (¾ oz)
Matzoh, all shapes and sizes	¾ oz
Melba toast	4 pieces (each about 2 by 4 inches)

*Note: Restaurant-style French fries are on the **Fast Foods** list, **page D-11**.

Food	Serving Size
Popcorn	
✓ no fat added	3 cups
‼ with butter added	3 cups
Pretzels	¾ oz
Rice cakes	2 cakes (4 inches across)

Snack chips

Food	Serving Size
baked (potato, pita)	about 8 chips (¾ oz)
‼ regular (tortilla, potato)	about 13 chips (1 oz)

! count as 1 starch choice + 1 fat choice (1 starch choice plus 5 grams of fat)

‼ count as 1 starch choice + 2 fat choices (1 starch choice plus 10 grams of fat)

Note: for other snacks, see the **Sweets, Desserts, and Other Carbohydrates** list, **page D-4**.

Beans, Peas, and Lentils

The choices on this list count as 1 starch choice + 1 lean protein choice.

Food	Serving Size
✓ Baked beans, canned	⅓ cup
✓ Beans (black, garbanzo, kidney, lima, navy, pinto, white), cooked or canned, drained and rinsed	½ cup
✓ Lentils (any color), cooked	½ cup
✓ Peas (black-eyed and split), cooked or canned, drained and rinsed	½ cup
🧂 ✓ Refried beans, canned	½ cup

Note: Beans, lentils, and peas are also found on the **Protein** list, **page D-6**.

Fruits

One fruit choice has 15 grams of carbohydrate and 60 calories.

Icon Key

✓ = Good source of fiber
! = Extra fat
🧂 = High in sodium

Food	Serving Size
Fruits	

The weights listed include skin, core, seeds, and rind.

Food	Serving Size
Apple, unpeeled	1 small apple (4 oz)
Apples, dried	4 rings
Applesauce, unsweetened	½ cup
Apricots	
canned	½ cup
dried	8 apricot halves
fresh	4 apricots (5 ½ oz total)
Banana	1 extra-small banana, about 4 inches long (4 oz)
✓ Blackberries	1 cup
Blueberries	¾ cup
Cantaloupe	1 cup diced
Cherries	
sweet, canned	½ cup
sweet, fresh	12 cherries (3 ½ oz)
Dates	3 small (deglet noor) dates or 1 large (medjool) date

Food	Serving Size
Dried fruits (blueberries, cherries, cranberries, mixed fruit, raisins)	2 Tbsp
Figs	
dried	3 small figs
✓ fresh	1 ½ large or 2 medium figs (3 ½ oz total)
Fruit cocktail	½ cup
Grapefruit	
fresh	½ large grapefruit (5 ½ oz)
sections, canned	¾ cup
Grapes	17 small grapes (3 oz total)
✓ Guava	2 small guava (2 ½ oz total)
Honeydew melon	1 cup diced
Kiwi	½ cup sliced
Loquat	¾ cup cubed
Mandarin oranges, canned	¾ cup

Food	Serving Size	Food	Serving Size
Mango	½ small mango (5 ½ oz) or ½ cup	dried (prunes)	3 prunes
Nectarine	1 medium nectarine (5 ½ oz)	fresh	2 small plums (5 oz total)
✓ Orange	1 medium orange (6 ½ oz)	Pomegranate seeds (arils)	½ cup
Papaya	½ papaya (8 oz) or 1 cup cubed	✓ Raspberries	1 cup
		✓ Strawberries	1 ¼ cup whole berries

Peaches

- canned . . . . ½ cup
- fresh . . . . 1 medium peach (6 oz)

Pears

- canned . . . . ½ cup
- ✓ fresh . . . . ½ large pear (4 oz)

Pineapple

- canned . . . . ½ cup
- fresh . . . . ¾ cup

Plantain, extra-ripe (black), raw . . . . ¼ plantain (2 ¼ oz)

Plums

- canned . . . . ½ cup

Tangerine . . . . 1 large tangerine (6 oz)

Watermelon . . . . 1 ¼ cups diced

Fruit Juice

Food	Serving Size
Apple juice/cider	½ cup
Fruit juice blends, 100% juice	⅓ cup
Grape juice	⅓ cup
Grapefruit juice	½ cup
Orange juice	½ cup
Pineapple juice	½ cup
Pomegranate juice	½ cup
Prune juice	⅓ cup

Milk and Milk Substitutes

One carbohydrate choice has 15 grams of carbohydrate and about 70 calories. One fat choice has 5 grams of fat and 45 calories.

Food	Serving Size	Choices per Serving
Milk and Yogurts		
Fat-Free (skim) or Low-Fat (1%)		
milk, buttermilk, acidophilus milk, lactose-free milk	1 cup	1 fat-free milk
evaporated milk	½ cup	1 fat-free milk
yogurt, plain or Greek; may be sweetened with an artificial sweetener	⅔ cup (6 oz)	1 fat-free milk
Chocolate milk	1 cup	1 fat-free milk + 1 carbohydrate
Reduced-fat (2%)		
milk, acidophilus milk, kefir, lactose-free milk	1 cup	1 reduced-fat milk
yogurt, plain	⅔ cup (6 oz)	1 reduced-fat milk
Whole		
milk, buttermilk, goat's milk	1 cup	1 whole milk
evaporated milk	½ cup	1 whole milk
yogurt, plain	1 cup (8 oz)	1 whole milk
chocolate milk	1 cup	1 whole milk + 1 carbohydrate
Other Milk Foods and Milk Substitutes		
Eggnog		
fat-free	⅓ cup	1 carbohydrate
low-fat	⅓ cup	1 carbohydrate + ½ fat
whole milk	⅓ cup	1 carbohydrate + 1 fat
Rice drink		
plain, fat-free	1 cup	1 carbohydrate
flavored, low-fat	1 cup	2 carbohydrates
Soy milk		
light or low-fat, plain	1 cup	½ carbohydrate + ½ fat
regular, plain	1 cup	½ carbohydrate + 1 fat
Yogurt with fruit, low-fat	⅔ cup (6 oz)	1 fat-free milk + 1 carbohydrate

Note: Unsweetened nut milks (such as almond milk and coconut milk) are on the **Fats** list, **page D-8**.

Nonstarchy Vegetables

One nonstarchy vegetable choice (1/2 cup cooked or 1 cup raw) has 5 grams of carbohydrate, 2 grams of protein, 0 grams of fat, and 25 calories.

Icon Key

✔ = Good source of fiber

! = Extra fat

🧂 = High in sodium

Nonstarchy Vegetables

Amaranth leaves (Chinese spinach)	Hearts of palm
Artichoke	✔ Jicama
Artichoke hearts (no oil)	Kale
Asparagus	Kohlrabi
Baby corn	Leeks
Bamboo shoots	Mixed vegetables (without starchy vegetables, legumes, or pasta)
Bean sprouts (alfalfa, mung, soybean)	Mushrooms, all kinds, fresh
Beans (green, wax, Italian, yard-long beans)	Okra
Beets	Onions
Broccoli	Pea pods
Broccoli slaw, packaged, no dressing	Peppers (all varieties)
✔ Brussels sprouts	Radishes
Cabbage (green, red, bok choy, Chinese)	Rutabaga
✔ Carrots	🧂 Sauerkraut, drained and rinsed
Cauliflower	Spinach
Celery	Squash, summer varieties (yellow, pattypan, crookneck, zucchini)
Chayote	Sugar snap peas
Coleslaw, packaged, no dressing	Swiss chard
Cucumber	Tomato
Daikon	Tomatoes, canned
Eggplant	🧂 Tomato sauce (unsweetened)
Fennel	Tomato/vegetable juice
Gourds (bitter, bottle, luffa, bitter melon)	Turnips
Green onions or scallions	Water chestnuts
Greens (collard, dandelion, mustard, purslane, turnip)	

Note: Salad greens (like arugula, chicory, endive, escarole, lettuce, radicchio, romaine, and watercress) are on the **Free Foods** list, **page D-9**.

Sweets, Desserts, and Other Carbohydrates

One carbohydrate choice has 15 grams of carbohydrate and about 70 calories. One fat choice has 5 grams of fat and 45 calories.

Icon Key

✔ = Good source of fiber

! = Extra fat

🧂 = High in sodium

Food	Serving Size	Choices per Serving
Beverages, Soda, and Sports Drinks		
Cranberry juice cocktail	½ cup	1 carbohydrate
Fruit drink or lemonade	1 cup (8 oz)	2 carbohydrates
Hot chocolate, regular	1 envelope (2 Tbsp or ¾ oz) added to 8 oz water	1 carbohydrate
Soft drink (soda), regular	1 can (12 oz)	2½ carbohydrates
Sports drink (fluid replacement type)	1 cup (8 oz)	1 carbohydrate
Brownies, Cake, Cookies, Gelatin, Pie, and Pudding		
Biscotti	1 oz	1 carbohydrate + 1 fat
Brownie, small, unfrosted	1¼-inch square, ⅞-inch high (about 1 oz)	1 carbohydrate + 1 fat

Food	Serving Size	Choices per Serving
Cake		
angel food, unfrosted	1/12 of cake (about 2 oz)	2 carbohydrates
frosted	2-inch square (about 2 oz)	2 carbohydrates + 1 fat
unfrosted	2-inch square (about 1 oz)	1 carbohydrate + 1 fat
Cookies		
100-calorie pack	1 oz	1 carbohydrate + ½ fat
chocolate chip cookies	2 cookies, 2 ¼ inches across	1 carbohydrate + 2 fats
gingersnaps	3 small cookies, 1 ½ inches across	1 carbohydrate
large cookie	1 cookie, 6 inches across (about 3 oz)	4 carbohydrates + 3 fats
sandwich cookies with crème filling	2 small cookies (about ⅔ oz)	1 carbohydrate + 1 fat
sugar-free cookies	1 large or 3 small cookies (¾ to 1 oz)	1 carbohydrate + 1 to 2 fats
vanilla wafer	5 cookies	1 carbohydrate + 1 fat
Cupcake, frosted	1 small cupcake (about 1 ¾ oz)	2 carbohydrates + 1 to 1 ½ fats
Flan	½ cup	2 ½ carbohydrates + 1 fat
Fruit cobbler	½ cup (3 ½ oz)	3 carbohydrates + 1 fat
Gelatin, regular	½ cup	1 carbohydrate
Pie		
commercially prepared fruit, 2 crusts	1/6 of 8-inch pie	3 carbohydrates + 2 fats
pumpkin or custard	1/8 of 8-inch pie	1 ½ carbohydrates + 1 ½ fats
Pudding		
regular (made with reduced-fat milk)	½ cup	2 carbohydrates
sugar-free or sugar- and fat-free (made with fat-free milk)	½ cup	1 carbohydrate

Candy, Spreads, Sweets, Sweeteners, Syrups, and Toppings

Food	Serving Size	Choices per Serving
Blended sweeteners (mixtures of artificial sweeteners and sugar)	1 ½ Tbsp	1 carbohydrate
Candy		
chocolate, dark or milk type	1 oz	1 carbohydrate + 2 fats
chocolate "kisses"	5 pieces	1 carbohydrate + 1 fat
hard	3 pieces	1 carbohydrate
Coffee creamer, nondairy type		
powdered, flavored	4 tsp	½ carbohydrate + ½ fat
liquid, flavored	2 Tbsp	1 carbohydrate
Fruit snacks, chewy (pureed fruit concentrate)	1 roll (¾ oz)	1 carbohydrate
Fruit spreads, 100% fruit	1 ½ Tbsp	1 carbohydrate
Honey	1 Tbsp	1 carbohydrate
Jam or jelly, regular	1 Tbsp	1 carbohydrate
Sugar	1 Tbsp	1 carbohydrate
Syrup		
chocolate	2 Tbsp	2 carbohydrates
light (pancake-type)	2 Tbsp	1 carbohydrate
regular (pancake-type)	1 Tbsp	1 carbohydrate

Condiments and Sauces

Food	Serving Size	Choices per Serving
Barbecue sauce	3 Tbsp	1 carbohydrate
Cranberry sauce, jellied	¼ cup	1 ½ carbohydrates
Curry sauce	1 oz	1 carbohydrate + 1 fat
Gravy, canned or bottled	½ cup	½ carbohydrate + ½ fat
Hoisin sauce	1 Tbsp	½ carbohydrate
Marinade	1 Tbsp	½ carbohydrate
Plum sauce	1 Tbsp	½ carbohydrate
Salad dressing, fat-free, cream-based	3 Tbsp	1 carbohydrate
Sweet-and-sour sauce	3 Tbsp	1 carbohydrate

Note: You can also check the **Fats** list and **Free Foods** list for other condiments.

Food	Serving Size	Choices per Serving
Doughnuts, Muffins, Pastries, and Sweet Breads		
Banana nut bread	1-inch slice (2 oz)	2 carbohydrates + 1 fat
Doughnut		
cake, plain	1 medium doughnut (1 ½ oz)	1 ½ carbohydrates + 2 fats
hole	2 holes (1 oz)	1 carbohydrate + 1 fat
yeast-type, glazed	1 doughnut, 3 ¾ inches across (2 oz)	2 carbohydrates + 2 fats
Muffin		
regular	1 muffin (4 oz)	4 carbohydrates + 2 ½ fats
lower-fat	1 muffin (4 oz)	4 carbohydrates + ½ fat
Scone	1 scone (4 oz)	4 carbohydrates + 3 fats
Sweet roll or Danish	1 pastry (2 ½ oz)	2 ½ carbohydrates + 2 fats
Frozen Bars, Frozen Dessert, Frozen Yogurt, and Ice Cream		
Frozen pops	1	½ carbohydrate
Fruit juice bars, frozen, 100% juice	1 bar (3 oz)	1 carbohydrate
Ice cream		
fat-free	½ cup	1 ½ carbohydrates
light	½ cup	1 carbohydrate + 1 fat
no-sugar-added	½ cup	1 carbohydrate + 1 fat
regular	½ cup	1 carbohydrate + 2 fats
Sherbet, sorbet	½ cup	2 carbohydrates
Yogurt, frozen		
fat-free	⅓ cup	1 carbohydrate
regular	½ cup	1 carbohydrate + 0 to 1 fat
Greek, lower-fat or fat-free	½ cup	1 ½ carbohydrates

Protein

One lean protein choice has 0 grams of carbohydrate, 7 grams of protein, 2 grams of fat, and 45 calories.

Icon Key

✔ = Good source of fiber

! = Extra fat

🧂 = High in sodium (based on the sodium content of a typical 3-oz serving of meat, unless 1 oz or 2 oz is the normal serving size)

Food	Serving Size
Lean Protein	
Note: 1 oz is usually the serving size for meat, fish, poultry, or hard cheeses.	
Beef: ground (90% or higher lean/10% or lower fat); select or choice grades trimmed of fat: roast (chuck, round, rump, sirloin),steak (cubed, flank, porterhouse,T-bone), tenderloin	1 oz
🧂 Beef jerky	½ oz
Cheeses with 3 grams of fat or less per oz	1 oz
Curd-style cheeses: cottage-type (all kinds); ricotta (fat-free or light)	¼ cup (2 oz)
Egg substitutes, plain	½ cup
Egg whites	2
Fish	
fresh or frozen, such as catfish, cod, flounder, haddock, halibut, orange roughy, tilapia, trout	1 oz
salmon, fresh or canned	1 oz

Food	Serving Size
sardines, canned	2 small sardines
tuna, fresh or canned in water or oil and drained	1 oz
🧂 smoked: herring or salmon (lox)	1 oz
Game: buffalo, ostrich, rabbit, venison	1 oz
🧂 Hot dog with 3 grams of fat or less per oz. Note: May contain carbohydrate.	1 hot dog (1 ¾ oz)
Lamb: chop, leg, or roast	1 oz
Organ meats: heart, kidney, liver Note: May be high in cholesterol.	1 oz
Oysters, fresh or frozen	6 medium oysters
Pork, lean	
🧂 Canadian bacon	1 oz
🧂 ham	1 oz
rib or loin chop/roast, tenderloin	1 oz
Poultry, without skin: chicken; Cornish hen; domestic duck or goose (well-drained of fat); turkey; lean ground turkey or chicken	1 oz

Food	Serving Size
🧂 Processed sandwich meats with 3 grams of fat.......1 oz or less per oz: chipped beef, thin-sliced deli meats, turkey ham, turkey pastrami	
🧂 Sausage with 3 grams of fat or less per oz.............1 oz	
Shellfish: clams, crab, imitation shellfish,.............1 oz lobster, scallops, shrimp	
Veal: cutlet (no breading), loin chop, roast ....1 oz	

Medium-Fat Protein

One medium-fat protein choice has 0 grams of carbohydrate, 7 grams of protein, 5 grams of fat, and 75 calories.

Note: 1 oz is usually the serving size for meat, fish, poultry, or hard cheeses.

Food	Serving Size
Beef trimmed of visible fat: ground beef..............1 oz (85% or lower lean/15% or higher fat), corned beef, meatloaf, prime cuts of beef (rib roast), short ribs, tongue	
Cheeses with 4 to 7 grams of fat per oz:..............1 oz feta, mozzarella, pasteurized processed cheese spread, reduced-fat cheeses	
Cheese, ricotta (regular or part-skim) ....¼ cup (2 oz)	
Egg ....1 egg	
Fish: any fried..1 oz	
Lamb: ground, rib roast ....1 oz	
Pork: cutlet, ground, shoulder roast ....1 oz	
Poultry with skin: chicken, dove, pheasant, ...1 oz turkey, wild duck, or goose; fried chicken	
🧂 Sausage with 4 to 7 grams of fat per oz...............1 oz	

High-Fat Protein

These foods are high in saturated fat, cholesterol, and calories and may raise blood cholesterol levels if eaten on a regular basis. Try to eat 3 or fewer choices from this group per week.

Note: 1 oz is usually the serving size for meat, fish, poultry, or hard cheeses.

Food	Serving Size
Bacon, pork..2 slices (1 oz each before cooking)	
🧂 Bacon, turkey......................................3 slices (½ oz each before cooking)	
Cheese, regular: American, blue-veined, ...1 oz brie, cheddar, hard goat, Monterey jack, Parmesan, queso, and Swiss	
! Hot dog: beef, pork, or combination.................1 hot dog (10 hot dogs per 1 lb-sized package)	
Hot dog: turkey or chicken..........................1 hot dog (10 hot dogs per 1 lb-sized package)	
Pork: sausage, spareribs...........................1 oz	
🧂 Processed sandwich meats with 8 grams of...........1 oz fat or more per oz: bologna, hard salami, pastrami	
🧂 Sausage with 8 grams fat or more per oz: ....1 oz bratwurst, chorizo, Italian, knockwurst, Polish, smoked, summer	

Protein

Icon Key

✓ = Good source of fiber

! = Extra fat

🧂 = High in sodium (based on the sodium content of a typical 3-oz serving of meat, unless 1 oz or 2 oz is the normal serving size)

Food	Serving Size	Choices per Serving

Plant-Based Protein

Because carbohydrate and fat content varies among plant-based proteins, you should read the food labels.

	Food	Serving Size	Choices per Serving
	"Bacon" strips, soy-based	2 strips (½ oz)	1 lean protein
✓	Baked beans, canned	⅓ cup	1 starch + 1 lean protein
✓	Beans (black, garbanzo, kidney, lima, navy, pinto, white), cooked or canned, drained and rinsed	½ cup	1 starch + 1 lean protein
	"Beef" or "sausage" crumbles, meatless	1 oz	1 lean protein
	"Chicken" nuggets, soy-based	2 nuggets (1½ oz)	½ carbohydrate + 1 medium-fat protein
✓	Edamame, shelled	½ cup	½ carbohydrate + 1 lean protein
	Falafel (spiced chickpea and wheat patties)	3 patties (about 2 inches across)	1 carbohydrate +1 high-fat protein
	Hot dog, meatless, soy-based	1 hot dog (1½ oz)	1 lean protein
✓	Hummus	⅓ cup	1 carbohydrate + 1 medium-fat protein
✓	Lentils, any color, cooked or canned, drained and rinsed	½ cup	1 starch + 1 lean protein
	Meatless burger, soy-based	3 oz	½ carbohydrate + 2 lean proteins
✓	Meatless burger, vegetable and starch-based	1 patty (about 2½ oz)	½ carbohydrate + 1 lean protein
	Meatless deli slices	1 oz	1 lean protein
	Mycoprotein ("chicken" tenders or crumbles), meatless	2 oz	½ carbohydrate + 1 lean protein
	Nut spreads: almond butter, cashew butter, peanut butter, soy nut butter	1 Tbsp	1 high-fat protein
✓	Peas (black-eyed and split peas), cooked or canned, drained and rinsed	½ cup	1 starch + 1 lean protein
🧂 ✓	Refried beans, canned	½ cup	1 starch + 1 lean protein
	"Sausage" breakfast-type patties, meatless	1 (1½ oz)	1 medium-fat protein
	Soy nuts, unsalted	¾ oz	½ carbohydrate + 1 medium-fat protein
	Tempeh, plain, unflavored	¼ cup (1½ oz)	1 medium-fat protein
	Tofu	½ cup (4 oz)	1 medium-fat protein
	Tofu, light	½ cup (4 oz)	1 lean protein

Fat

One fat choice has 5 grams of fat and 45 calories.

Food	Serving Size	Food	Serving Size

Unsaturated Fats—Monounsaturated Fats

Almond milk (unsweetened) ....1 cup

Avocado, medium ....2 Tbsp (1 oz)

Nut butters (trans fat-free): almond butter, ...1½ tsp
cashew butter, peanut butter (smooth
or crunchy)

Nuts

almonds...6 nuts

Brazil ....2 nuts

cashews...6 nuts

filberts (hazelnuts) ....5 nuts

macadamia......................................3 nuts

mixed (50% peanuts) ....6 nuts

peanuts ....10 nuts

pecans ....4 halves

pistachios ....16 nuts

Oil: canola, olive, peanut ....1 tsp

Olives

black (ripe) 8

green, stuffed....................................10 large

Spread, plant stanol ester-type

light...1 Tbsp

regular ....2 tsp

Unsaturated Fats—Polyunsaturated Fats

Margarine

lower-fat spread (30 to 50% vegetable............1 Tbsp
oil, *trans* fat-free)

stick, tub (*trans* fat-free), or squeeze ....1 tsp
(*trans* fat-free)

Mayonnaise

reduced-fat......................................1 Tbsp

regular ....1 tsp

Mayonnaise-style salad dressing

reduced-fat......................................1 Tbsp

regular ....2 tsp

Nuts

pignolia (pine nuts) ....1 Tbsp

walnuts, English ....4 halves

Oil: corn, cottonseed, flaxseed, grapeseed, ...1 tsp
safflower, soybean, sunflower

Salad dressing

reduced-fat (Note: May contain carbohydrate.)....2 Tbsp

regular ....1 Tbsp

Seeds

flaxseed, ground.................................1½ Tbsp

pumpkin, sesame, sunflower ....1 Tbsp

Tahini or sesame paste..............................2 tsp

Saturated Fats

Bacon, cooked, regular or turkey ....1 slice

Butter

reduced-fat......................................1 Tbsp

stick..1 tsp

whipped...2 tsp

Butter blends made with oil

reduced-fat or light ....1 Tbsp

regular ....1½ tsp

Chitterlings, boiled ....2 Tbsp (½ oz)

Coconut, sweetened, shredded ....2 Tbsp

Coconut milk, canned, thick

light..⅓ cup

regular ....1½ Tbsp

Coconut milk beverage (thin), unsweetened..........1 cup

Cream

half-and-half.....................................2 Tbsp

heavy ....1 Tbsp

light..1½ Tbsp

whipped...2 Tbsp

Cream cheese

reduced-fat......................................1½ Tbsp (¾ oz)

regular ....1 Tbsp (½ oz)

Lard..1 tsp

Oil: coconut, palm, palm kernel ....1 tsp

Salt pork ....¼ oz

Shortening, solid ....1 tsp

Sour cream

reduced-fat or light ....3 Tbsp

regular ....2 Tbsp

Free Foods

A "free" food is any food or drink choice that has less than 20 calories and 5 grams or less of carbohydrate per serving.

Icon Key

✔ = Good source of fiber
! = Extra fat
🧂 = High in sodium

Food	Serving Size	Food	Serving Size
Low Carbohydrate Foods		*Salad dressing*	
Candy, hard (regular or sugar-free)	1 piece	fat-free	1 Tbsp
Fruits		fat-free, Italian	2 Tbsp
Cranberries or rhubarb, sweetened with sugar substitute	½ cup	Sour cream, fat-free or reduced-fat	1 Tbsp
Gelatin dessert, sugar-free, any flavor		*Whipped topping*	
Gum, sugar-free		light or fat-free	2 Tbsp
Jam or jelly, light or no-sugar-added	2 tsp	regular	1 Tbsp
Salad greens (such as arugula, chicory, endive, escarole, leaf or iceberg lettuce, purslane, romaine, radicchio, spinach, watercress)		**Condiments**	
		Barbecue sauce	2 tsp
		Catsup (ketchup)	1 Tbsp
Sugar substitutes (artificial sweeteners)		Chili sauce, sweet, tomato-type	2 tsp
Syrup, sugar-free	2 Tbsp	Horseradish	
Vegetables: any **raw** nonstarchy vegetables (such as broccoli, cabbage, carrots, cucumber, tomato)	½ cup	Hot pepper sauce	
		Lemon juice	
		Miso	1½ tsp
Vegetables: any **cooked** nonstarchy vegetables (such as carrots, cauliflower, green beans)	¼ cup	*Mustard*	
		honey	1 Tbsp
Reduced-Fat or Fat-Free Foods		brown, Dijon, horseradish-flavored, wasabi-flavored, or yellow	
Cream cheese, fat-free	1 Tbsp (½ oz)	Parmesan cheese, grated	1 Tbsp
Coffee creamers, nondairy		Pickle relish (dill or sweet)	1 Tbsp
liquid, flavored	1½ tsp	*Pickles*	
liquid, sugar-free, flavored	4 tsp	🧂 dill	1½ medium pickles
powdered, flavored	1 tsp		
powdered, sugar-free, flavored	2 tsp	sweet, bread and butter	2 slices
Margarine spread		sweet, gherkin	¾ oz
fat-free	1 Tbsp	Pimento	
reduced-fat	1 tsp	Salsa	¼ cup
Mayonnaise		🧂 Soy sauce, light or regular	1 Tbsp
fat-free	1 Tbsp	Sweet-and-sour sauce	2 tsp
reduced-fat	1 tsp	Taco sauce	1 Tbsp
Mayonnaise-style salad dressing		Vinegar	
fat-free	1 Tbsp	Worcestershire sauce	
reduced-fat	2 tsp	Yogurt, any type	2 Tbsp

Free Foods

Icon Key

✔ = Good source of fiber
! = Extra fat
🧂 = High in sodium

Drinks/Mixes

🧂 Bouillon, broth, consommé
Bouillon or broth, low sodium
Carbonated or mineral water
Club soda
Cocoa powder, unsweetened (1 Tbsp)
Coffee, unsweetened or with sugar substitute
Diet soft drinks, sugar-free
Drink mixes (powder or liquid drops), sugar-free
Tea, unsweetened or with sugar substitute
Tonic water, sugar-free

Water
Water, flavored, sugar-free

Seasonings

Flavoring extracts (for example, vanilla, almond, or peppermint)
Garlic, fresh or powder
Herbs, fresh or dried
Kelp
Nonstick cooking spray
Spices
Wine, used in cooking

Combination Foods

One carbohydrate choice has 15 grams of carbohydrate and about 70 calories.

Icon Key

√ = Good source of fiber

! = Extra fat

🧂 = High in sodium

Food	Serving Size	Choices per Serving
Entrees		
🧂 Casserole-type entrees (tuna noodle, lasagna, spaghetti with meatballs, chili with beans, macaroni and cheese)	1 cup (8 oz)	2 carbohydrates + 2 medium-fat proteins
🧂 Stews (beef/other meats and vegetables)	1 cup (8 oz)	1 carbohydrate + 1 medium-fat protein + 0 to 3 fats
Frozen Meals/Entrees		
🧂 Burrito (beef and bean)	1 burrito (5 oz)	3 carbohydrates + 1 lean protein + 2 fats
Dinner-type healthy meal (includes dessert and is usually less than 400 calories)	about 9–12 oz	2 to 3 carbohydrates + 1 to 2 lean proteins + 1 fat
"Healthy"-type entree (usually less than 300 calories)	about 7–10 oz	2 carbohydrates + 2 lean proteins
Pizza		
🧂 cheese/vegetarian, thin crust	¼ of a 12–inch pizza (4½–5 oz)	2 carbohydrates + 2 medium-fat proteins
🧂 meat topping, thin crust	¼ of a 12–inch pizza (5 oz)	2 carbohydrates + 2 medium-fat proteins + 1½ fats
🧂 cheese/vegetarian or meat topping, rising crust	⅙ of 12–inch pizza (4 oz)	2½ carbohydrates + 2 medium-fat proteins
🧂 Pocket sandwich	1 sandwich (4½ oz)	3 carbohydrates + 1 lean protein + 1 to 2 fats
🧂 Pot pie	1 pot pie (7 oz)	3 carbohydrates + 1 medium-fat protein + 3 fats
Salads (Deli-Style)		
Coleslaw	½ cup	1 carbohydrate + 1½ fats
Macaroni/pasta salad	½ cup	2 carbohydrates + 3 fats
🧂 Potato salad	½ cup	1½ to 2 carbohydrates + 1 to 2 fats
Tuna salad or chicken salad	½ cup (3½ oz)	½ carbohydrate + 2 lean proteins + 1 fat
Soups		
🧂 √ Bean, lentil, or split pea soup	1 cup (8 oz)	1½ carbohydrates + 1 lean protein
🧂 Chowder (made with milk)	1 cup (8 oz)	1 carbohydrate + 1 lean protein + 1½ fats
🧂 Cream soup (made with water)	1 cup (8 oz)	1 carbohydrate + 1 fat
🧂 Miso soup	1 cup (8 oz)	½ carbohydrate + 1 lean protein
🧂 Ramen noodle soup	1 cup (8 oz)	2 carbohydrates + 2 fats
🧂 Rice soup/porridge (congee)	1 cup (8 oz)	1 carbohydrate
🧂 Tomato soup (made with water), borscht	1 cup (8 oz)	1 carbohydrate
🧂 Vegetable beef, chicken noodle, or other broth-type soup (including "healthy"-type soups, such as those lower in sodium and/or fat)	1 cup (8 oz)	1 carbohydrate + 1 lean protein

Fast Foods

One carbohydrate choice has 15 grams of carbohydrate and about 70 calories.

Icon Key

✓ = Good source of fiber

! = Extra fat

🧂 = High in sodium

Food	Serving Size	Choices per Serving
Main Dishes/Entrees		
Chicken		
🧂 breast, breaded and fried*.	1 (about 7 oz)	1 carbohydrate + 6 medium-fat proteins
breast, meat only**	1	4 lean proteins
drumstick, breaded and fried*.	1 (about 2½ oz)	½ carbohydrate + 2 medium-fat proteins
drumstick, meat only**.	1	1 lean protein + ½ fat
🧂 nuggets or tenders.	6 (about 3½ oz)	1 carbohydrate + 2 medium-fat proteins + 1 fat
thigh, breaded and fried*	1 (about 5 oz)	1 carbohydrate + 3 medium-fat proteins + 2 fats
thigh, meat only**.	1	2 lean proteins + ½ fat
wing, breaded and fried*.	1 wing (about 2 oz).	½ carbohydrate + 2 medium-fat proteins
wing, meat only**.	1 wing	1 lean protein
🧂 ✓ Main dish salad (grilled chicken type, no dressing or croutons)	1 salad (about 11½ oz)	1 carbohydrate + 4 lean proteins
Pizza		
🧂 cheese, pepperoni, or sausage, regular or thick crust	⅛ of a 14-inch pizza (about 4 oz)	2½ carbohydrates + 1 high-fat protein + 1 fat
🧂 cheese, pepperoni, or sausage, thin crust	⅛ of a 14-inch pizza (about 2¾ oz)	1½ carbohydrates + 1 high-fat protein + 1 fat
🧂 cheese, meat, and vegetable, regular crust	⅛ of a 14-inch pizza (about 5 oz)	2½ carbohydrates + 2 high-fat proteins
Asian		
🧂 Beef/chicken/shrimp with vegetables in sauce	1 cup (about 6 oz)	1 carbohydrate + 2 lean proteins + 1 fat
Egg roll, meat.	1 egg roll (about 3 oz)	1½ carbohydrates + 1 lean protein + 1½ fats
Fried rice, meatless.	1 cup	2½ carbohydrates + 2 fats
Fortune cookie	1 cookie.	½ carbohydrate
🧂 Hot-and-sour soup.	1 cup	½ carbohydrate + ½ fat
🧂 Meat with sweet sauce.	1 cup (about 6 oz)	3½ carbohydrates + 3 medium-fat proteins + 3 fats
🧂 Noodles and vegetables in sauce (chow mein, lo mein).	1 cup	2 carbohydrates + 2 fats
Mexican		
🧂 ✓ Burrito with beans and cheese	1 small burrito (about 6 oz)	3½ carbohydrates + 1 medium-fat protein + 1 fat
🧂 Nachos with cheese.	1 small order (about 8 nachos)	2½ carbohydrates + 1 high-fat protein + 2 fats
🧂 Quesadilla, cheese only	1 small order (about 5 oz)	2½ carbohydrates + 3 high-fat proteins
Taco, crisp, with meat and cheese	1 small taco (about 3 oz)	1 carbohydrate + 1 medium-fat protein + ½ fat
🧂 ✓ Taco salad with chicken and tortilla bowl	1 salad (1 lb, including tortilla bowl)	3½ carbohydrates + 4 medium-fat proteins + 3 fats
🧂 Tostada with beans and cheese	1 small tostada (about 5 oz)	2 carbohydrates + 1 high-fat protein
Sandwiches		
Breakfast Sandwiches		
🧂 Breakfast burrito with sausage, egg, cheese	1 burrito (about 4 oz)	1½ carbohydrates + 2 high-fat proteins
🧂 Egg, cheese, meat on an English muffin	1 sandwich.	2 carbohydrates + 3 medium-fat proteins + ½ fat

*Definition and weight refer to food **with** bone, skin, and breading.

Definition refers to above food **without bone, skin, and breading.

Food	Serving Size	Count As
Egg, cheese, meat on a biscuit	1 sandwich	2 carbohydrates + 3 medium-fat proteins + 2 fats
Sausage biscuit sandwich	1 sandwich	2 carbohydrates + 1 high-fat protein + 4 fats
Chicken Sandwiches		
grilled with bun, lettuce, tomatoes, spread	1 sandwich (about 7½ oz)	3 carbohydrates + 4 lean proteins
crispy, with bun, lettuce, tomatoes, spread	1 sandwich (about 6 oz)	3 carbohydrates + 2 lean proteins + 3½ fats
Fish sandwich with tartar sauce and cheese	1 sandwich (5 oz)	2½ carbohydrates + 2 medium-fat proteins + 1½ fats
Hamburger		
regular with bun and condiments (catsup, mustard, onion, pickle)	1 burger (about 3½ oz)	2 carbohydrates + 1 medium-fat protein + 1 fat
4 oz meat with cheese, bun, and condiments (catsup, mustard, onion, pickle)	1 burger (about 8½ oz)	3 carbohydrates + 4 medium-fat protein + 2½ fats
Hot dog with bun, plain	1 hot dog (about 3½ oz)	1½ carbohydrates + 1 high-fat protein + 2 fats
Submarine sandwich (no cheese or sauce)		
less than 6 grams fat	1 6-inch sub	3 carbohydrates + 2 lean proteins
regular	1 6-inch sub	3 carbohydrates + 2 lean proteins + 1 fat
Wrap, grilled chicken, vegetables, cheese, and spread	1 small wrap (about 4 to 5 oz)	2 carbohydrates + 2 lean proteins + 1½ fats

Sides/Appetizers

Food	Serving Size	Count As
French fries	1 small order (about 3½ oz)	2½ carbohydrates + 2 fats
	1 medium order (about 5 oz)	3½ carbohydrates + 3 fats
	1 large order (about 6 oz)	4½ carbohydrates + 4 fats
Hashbrowns	1 cup/medium order (about 5 oz)	3 carbohydrates + 6 fats
Onion rings	1 serving (8 to 9 rings, about 4 oz)	3½ carbohydrates + 4 fats
Salad, side (no dressing, croutons or cheese)	1 small salad	1 nonstarchy vegetable

Beverages and Desserts

Food	Serving Size	Count As
Coffee, latte (fat-free milk)	1 small order (about 12 oz)	1 fat-free milk
Coffee, mocha (fat-free milk, no whipped cream)	1 small order (about 12 oz)	1 fat-free milk + 1 carbohydrate
Milkshake, any flavor	1 small shake (about 12 oz)	5½ carbohydrates + 3 fats
	1 medium shake (about 16 oz)	7 carbohydrates + 4 fats
	1 large shake (about 22 oz)	10 carbohydrates + 5 fats
Soft-serve ice cream cone	1 small	2 carbohydrates + ½ fat

Alcohol

One alcohol equivalent or choice (½ oz absolute alcohol) has about 100 calories. One carbohydrate choice has 15 grams of carbohydrate and about 70 calories.

Alcoholic Beverage	Serving Size	Choices per Serving
Beer		
light (less than 4.5% abv)	12 fl oz	1 alcohol equivalent + ½ carbohydrate
regular (about 5% abv)	12 fl oz	1 alcohol equivalent + 1 carbohydrate
dark (more than 5.7% abv)	12 fl oz	1 alcohol equivalent + 1 to 1½ carbohydrates
Distilled spirits: (80 or 86 proof): vodka, rum, gin, whiskey, tequila	1½ fl oz	1 alcohol equivalent
Liqueur, coffee (53 proof)	1 fl oz	1 alcohol equivalent + 1 carbohydrate
Sake	1 fl oz	½ alcohol equivalent
Wine		
champagne/sparkling	5 fl oz	1 alcohol equivalent
dessert (sherry)	3½ fl oz	1 alcohol equivalent + 1 carbohydrate
dry, red or white (10% abv)	5 fl oz	1 alcohol equivalent

Note: The abbreviation "% abv" refers to the percentage of alcohol by volume.

appendix E

Stature-for-Age Charts

CDC Growth Charts: United States
Stature-for-age percentiles: Boys, 2 to 20 years

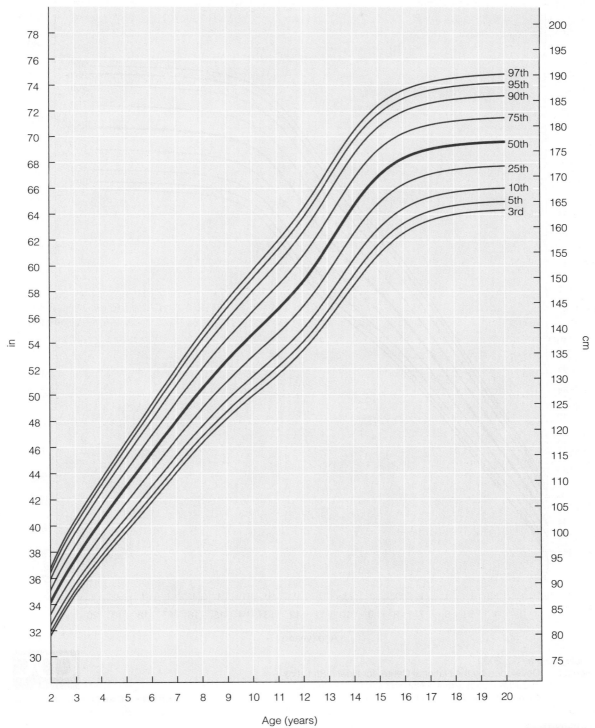

in

cm

Age (years)

Published May 30, 2000.
Source: Developed by the National Center for Health Statistics
in collaboration with the National Center for Chronic
Disease Prevention and Health Promotion (2000).

SAFER · HEALTHIER · PEOPLE™

E-1

CDC Growth Charts: United States
Stature-for-age percentiles: Girls, 2 to 20 years

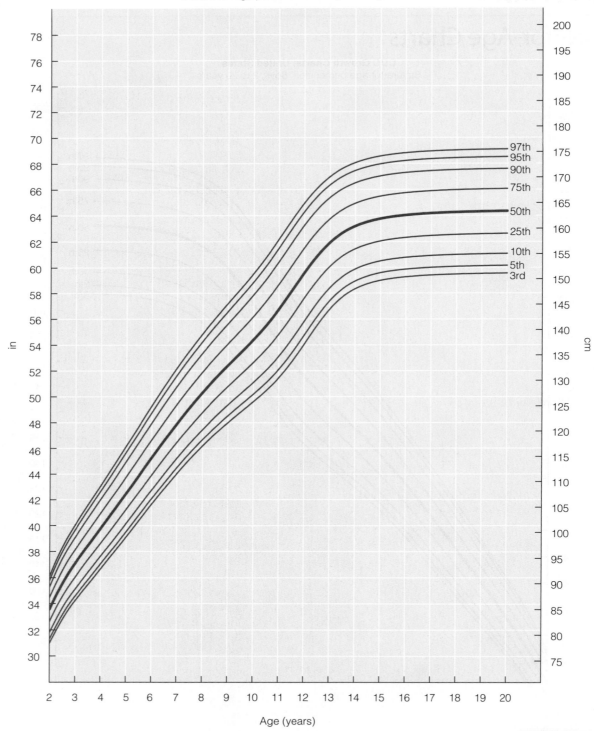

Age (years)

Published May 30, 2000.
Source: Developed by the National Center for Health Statistics in collaboration with the National Center for Chronic Disease Prevention and Health Promotion (2000).

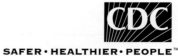

SAFER · HEALTHIER · PEOPLE™

appendix F

Organizations and Resources

Academic Journals

International Journal of Sport Nutrition and Exercise Metabolism
Human Kinetics
P.O. Box 5076
Champaign, IL 61825-5076
(800) 747-4457
www.humankinetics.com/IJSNEM

Journal of Nutrition
Department of Nutrition
Pennsylvania State University
126-S Henderson Building
University Park, PA 16802-6504
(814) 865-4721
www.nutrition.org

Nutrition Research
Elsevier: Journals Customer Service
6277 Sea Harbor Drive
Orlando, FL 32887
(877) 839-7126
www.journals.elsevierhealth.com/periodicals/NTR

Nutrition
Elsevier: Journals Customer Service
6277 Sea Harbor Drive
Orlando, FL 32887
(877) 839-7126
www.journals.elsevierhealth.com/periodicals/NUT

Nutrition Reviews
International Life Sciences Institute
Subscription Office
P.O. Box 830430
Birmingham, AL 35283
(800) 633-4931
www.ingentaconnect.com/content/ilsi/nure

Obesity Research
North American Association for the Study
of Obesity (NAASO)
8630 Fenton Street, Suite 918
Silver Spring, MD 20910
(301) 563-6526
www.nature.com/oby/index.html

International Journal of Obesity
Journal of the International Association for
the Study of Obesity
Nature Publishing Group
The Macmillan Building
4 Crinan Street
London N1 9XW
United Kingdom
www.nature.com/ijo

Journal of the American Medical Association
American Medical Association
P.O. Box 10946
Chicago, IL 60610-0946
(800) 262-2350
www.jama.ama-assn.org

New England Journal of Medicine
10 Shattuck Street
Boston, MA 02115-6094
(617) 734-9800
www.nejm.org

American Journal of Clinical Nutrition
The American Journal of Clinical Nutrition
9650 Rockville Pike
Bethesda, MD 20814-3998
(301) 634-7038
www.ajcn.org

Journal of the American Dietetic Association
Elsevier, Health Sciences Division
Subscription Customer Service
6277 Sea Harbor Drive
Orlando, FL 32887
(800) 654-2452
www.adajournal.org

Aging

Administration on Aging
U.S. Health & Human Services
200 Independence Avenue, SW
Washington, DC 20201
(877) 696-6775
www.aoa.gov

American Association of Retired Persons (AARP)
601 E. Street, NW
Washington, DC 20049
(888) 687-2277
www.aarp.org

Health and Age
Sponsored by the Novartis Foundation for Gerontology &
The Web-Based Health Education Foundation
Robert Griffith, MD
Executive Director
573 Vista de la Ciudad
Santa Fe, NM 87501
www.healthandage.com

National Council on the Aging
300 D Street, SW, Suite 801
Washington, DC 20024
(202) 479-1200
www.ncoa.org

International Osteoporosis Foundation
5 Rue Perdtemps
1260 Nyon
Switzerland
41 22 994 01 00
www.iofbonehealth.org

National Institute on Aging
Building 31, Room 5C27
31 Center Drive, MSC 2292
Bethesda, MD 20892
(301) 496-1752
www.nia.nih.gov

Osteoporosis and Related Bone Diseases National Resource Center
2 AMS Circle
Bethesda, MD 20892-3676
(800) 624-BONE
www.hiams.nih.gov/health_info/bone/

American Geriatrics Society
The Empire State Building
350 Fifth Avenue, Suite 801
New York, NY 10118
(212) 308-1414
www.americangeriatrics.org

National Osteoporosis Foundation
1232 22nd Street, NW
Washington, DC 20037-1292
(202) 223-2226
www.nof.org

Alcohol and Drug Abuse

National Institute on Drug Abuse
6001 Executive Boulevard, Room 5213
Bethesda, MD 20892-9561
(301) 443-1124
www.nida.nih.gov/nidahome.html

National Institute on Alcohol Abuse and Alcoholism
5635 Fishers Lane, MSC 9304
Bethesda, MD 20892-9304
www.niaaa.nih.gov

Alcoholics Anonymous
Grand Central Station
P.O. Box 459
New York, NY 10163
www.aa.org

Narcotics Anonymous
P.O. Box 9999
Van Nuys, CA 91409
(818) 773-9999
www.na.org

National Council on Alcoholism and Drug Dependence
20 Exchange Place, Suite 2902
New York, NY 10005
(212) 269-7797
www.ncadd.org

National Clearinghouse for Alcohol and Drug Information
11420 Rockville Pike
Rockville, MD 20852
(800) 729-6686
www.store.samhsa.gov/home

Canadian Government

Health Canada
A.L. 0900C2
Ottawa, ON K1A 0K9
(613) 957-2991
www.hc-sc.gc.ca/english

National Institute of Nutrition
408 Queen Street, 3rd Floor
Ottawa, ON K1R 5A7
(613) 235-3355
www.nin.ca/public_html

Agricultural and Agri-Food Canada
Public Information Request Service
Sir John Carling Building
930 Carling Avenue
Ottawa, ON K1A 0C5
(613) 759-1000
www.agr.gc.ca

Bureau of Nutritional Sciences
Sir Frederick G. Banting Research Centre
Tunney's Pasture (2203A)
Ottawa, ON K1A 0L2
(613) 957-0352
www.hc-sc.gc.ca/food-aliment/ns-sc/e_nutrition.html

Canadian Food Inspection Agency
59 Camelot Drive
Ottawa, ON K1A 0Y9
(613) 225-2342
www.inspection.gc.ca/english/toce.shtml

Canadian Institute for Health Information
CIHI Ottawa
377 Dalhousie Street, Suite 200
Ottawa, ON K1N 9N8
(613) 241-7860
www.cihi.ca

Canadian Public Health Association
1565 Carling Avenue, Suite 400
Ottawa, ON K1Z 8R1
(613) 725-3769
www.cpha.ca

Canadian Nutrition and Professional Organizations

Dietitians of Canada
480 University Avenue, Suite 604
Toronto, ON M5G 1V2
(416) 596-0857
www.dietitians.ca

Canadian Diabetes Association
National Life Building
1400-522 University Avenue
Toronto, ON M5G 2R5
(800) 226-8464
www.diabetes.ca

National Eating Disorder Information Centre
CW 1-211, 200 Elizabeth Street
Toronto, ON M5G 2C4
(866) NEDIC-20
www.nedic.ca

Canadian Pediatric Society
100-2204 Walkley Road
Ottawa, ON K1G 4G8
(613) 526-9397
www.cps.ca

Canadian Dietetic Association
480 University Avenue, Suite 604
Toronto, ON M5G 1V2
(416) 596-0857
www.dietitians.ca

Disordered Eating

American Psychiatric Association
1000 Wilson Boulevard, Suite 1825
Arlington, VA 22209
(703) 907-7300
www.psych.org

National Institute of Mental Health
Office of Communications
6001 Executive Boulevard, Room 8184, MSC 9663
Bethesda, MD 20892
(866) 615-6464
www.nimh.nih.gov

National Association of Anorexia Nervosa and Associated Disorders (ANAD)
Box 7
Highland Park, IL 60035
(847) 831-3438
www.anad.org

National Eating Disorders Association
603 Stewart Street, Suite 803
Seattle, WA 98101
(206) 382-3587
www.nationaleatingdisorders.org

Eating Disorder Referral and Information Center
2923 Sandy Pointe, Suite 6
Del Mar, CA 92014
(858) 792-7463
www.edreferral.com

Anorexia Nervosa and Related Eating Disorders, Inc. (ANRED)
E-mail: jarinor@rio.com
www.anred.com

Overeaters Anonymous
P.O. Box 44020
Rio Rancho, NM 87174
(505) 891-2664
www.oa.org

Exercise, Physical Activity, and Sports

American College of Sports Medicine (ACSM)
P.O. Box 1440
Indianapolis, IN 46206-1440
(317) 637-9200
www.acsm.org

American Physical Therapy Association (ASNA)
1111 North Fairfax Street
Alexandria, VA 22314
(800) 999-APTA
www.apta.org

Gatorade Sports Science Institute (GSSI)
617 West Main Street
Barrington, IL 60010
(800) 616-GSSI
www.gssiweb.com

National Coalition for Promoting Physical Activity (NCPPA)
1010 Massachusetts Avenue, Suite 350
Washington, DC 20001
(202) 454-7518
www.ncppa.org

Sports, Wellness, Eating Disorder and Cardiovascular Nutritionists (SCAN)
P.O. Box 60820
Colorado Springs, CO 80960
(719) 635-6005
www.scandpg.org

President's Council on Physical Fitness and Sports
Department W
200 Independence Avenue, SW
Room 738-H
Washington, DC 20201-0004
(202) 690-9000
www.fitness.gov

American Council on Exercise
4851 Paramount Drive
San Diego, CA 92123
(858) 279-8227
www.acefitness.org

The International Association for Fitness Professionals (IDEA)
10455 Pacific Center Court
San Diego, CA 92121
(800) 999-4332, ext. 7
www.ideafit.com

Food Safety

Food Marketing Institute
655 15th Street, NW
Washington, DC 20005
(202) 452-8444
www.fmi.org

Agency for Toxic Substances and Disease Registry (ATSDR)
ORO Washington Office
Ariel Rios Building
1200 Pennsylvania Avenue, NW
M/C 5204G
Washington, DC 20460
(888) 422-8737
www.atsdr.cdc.gov

Food Allergy and Anaphylaxis Network
11781 Lee Jackson Highway, Suite 160
Fairfax, VA 22033-3309
(800) 929-4040
www.foodallergy.org

Foodsafety.gov
www.foodsafety.gov

The USDA Food Safety and Inspection Service
Food Safety and Inspection Service
United States Department of Agriculture
Washington, DC 20250
www.fsis.usda.gov

Consumer Reports
Web Site Customer Relations Department
101 Truman Avenue
Yonkers, NY 10703
www.consumerreports.org

Center for Science in the Public Interest: Food Safety
1875 Connecticut Avenue, NW
Washington, DC 20009
(202) 332-9110
www.cspinet.org/foodsafety

Center for Food Safety and Applied Nutrition
5100 Paint Branch Parkway
College Park, MD 20740
(888) SAFEFOOD
www.cfsan.fda.gov

Food Safety Project
Dan Henroid, MS, RD, CFSP
HRIM Extension Specialist and Website Coordinator
Hotel, Restaurant and Institution Management
9e MacKay Hall
Iowa State University
Ames, IA 50011
(515) 294-3527
www.extension.iastate.edu/foodsafety

Organic Consumers Association
6101 Cliff Estate Road
Little Marais, MN 55614
(218) 226-4164
www.organicconsumers.org

Infancy and Childhood

Administration for Children and Families
370 L'Enfant Promenade, SW
Washington, DC 20447
www.acf.hhs.gov

The American Academy of Pediatrics
141 Northwest Point Boulevard
Elk Grove Village, IL 60007
(847) 434-4000
www.aap.org

Kidnetic.com
E-mail: contactus@kidnetic.com
www.kidnetic.com

Kidshealth: The Nemours Foundation
12735 West Gran Bay Parkway
Jacksonville, FL 32258
(866) 390-3610
www.kidshealth.org

National Center for Education in Maternal and Child Health
Georgetown University
Box 571272
Washington, DC 20057
(202) 784-9770
www.ncemch.org

Birth Defects Research for Children, Inc.
930 Woodcock Road, Suite 225
Orlando, FL 32803
(407) 895-0802
www.birthdefects.org

USDA/ARS Children's Nutrition Research Center at Baylor College of Medicine
1100 Bates Street
Houston, TX 77030
www.bcm.edu

Keep Kids Healthy.com
www.keepkidshealthy.com

International Agencies

UNICEF
3 United Nations Plaza
New York, NY 10017
(212) 326-7000
www.unicef.org

World Health Organization
Avenue Appia 20
1211 Geneva 27
Switzerland
41 22 791 21 11
www.who.int/en

The Stockholm Convention on Persistent Organic Pollutants
11–13 Chemin des Anémones
1219 Châtelaine
Geneva, Switzerland
41 22 917 8191
www.chm.pops.int

Food and Agricultural Organization of the United Nations
Viale delle Terme di Caracalla
00100 Rome, Italy
39 06 57051
www.fao.org

International Food Information Council Foundation
1100 Connecticut Avenue, NW
Suite 430
Washington, DC 20036
(202) 296-6540

Pregnancy and Lactation

San Diego County Breastfeeding Coalition
c/o Children's Hospital and Health Center
3020 Children's Way, MC 5073
San Diego, CA 92123
(800) 371-MILK
www.breastfeeding.org

National Alliance for Breastfeeding Advocacy
Barbara Heiser, Executive Director
9684 Oak Hill Drive
Ellicott City, MD 21042-6321
OR
Marsha Walker, Executive Director
254 Conant Road
Weston, MA 02493-1756
www.naba-breastfeeding.org

American College of Obstetricians and Gynecologists
409 12th Street, SW,
P.O. Box 96920
Washington, DC 20090
www.acog.org

La Leche League
1400 N. Meacham Road
Schaumburg, IL 60173
(847) 519-7730
www.lalecheleague.org

National Organization on Fetal Alcohol Syndrome
900 17th Street, NW
Suite 910
Washington, DC 20006
(800) 66 NOFAS
www.nofas.org

March of Dimes Birth Defects Foundation
1275 Mamaroneck Avenue
White Plains, NY 10605
(888) 663-4637
www.marchofdimes.org

Professional Nutrition Organizations

Association of Departments and Programs of Nutrition (ANDP)
Dr. Marilynn Schnepf, ANDP Chair
316 Ruth Leverton Hall
Nutrition and Health Sciences
University of Nebraska–Lincoln
Lincoln, NE 68583-0806
www.fshn.hs.iastate.edu/andp

North American Association for the Study of Obesity (NAASO)
8630 Fenton Street, Suite 918
Silver Spring, MD 20910
(301) 563-6526
www.obesity.org

American Dental Association
211 East Chicago Avenue
Chicago, IL 60611-2678
(312) 440-2500
www.ada.org

American Heart Association
National Center
7272 Greenville Avenue
Dallas, TX 75231
(800) 242-8721
www.heart.org/HEARTORG

American Dietetic Association (ADA)
120 South Riverside Plaza, Suite 2000
Chicago, IL 60606-6995
(800) 877-1600
www.eatright.org

The American Society for Nutrition (ASN)
9650 Rockville Pike, Suite L-4500
Bethesda, MD 20814-3998
(301) 634-7050
www.nutrition.org

The Society for Nutrition Education
7150 Winton Drive, Suite 300
Indianapolis, IN 46268
(800) 235-6690
www.sne.org

American College of Nutrition
300 S. Duncan Avenue, Suite 225
Clearwater, FL 33755
(727) 446-6086
www.americancollegeofnutrition.org

American Obesity Association
1250 24th Street, NW, Suite 300
Washington, DC 20037
(800) 98-OBESE

American Council on Health and Science
1995 Broadway
Second Floor
New York, NY 10023
(212) 362-7044
www.acsh.org

American Diabetes Association
ATTN: National Call Center
1701 North Beauregard Street
Alexandria, VA 22311
(800) 342-2383
www.diabetes.org

Institute of Food Technologies
525 W. Van Buren, Suite 1000
Chicago, IL 60607
(312) 782-8424
www.ift.org

ILSI Human Nutrition Institute
One Thomas Circle, Ninth Floor
Washington, DC 20005
(202) 659-0524
www.ilsi.org

Trade Organizations

American Meat Institute
1700 North Moore Street
Suite 1600
Arlington, VA 22209
(703) 841-2400
www.meatami.com

National Dairy Council
10255 W. Higgins Road, Suite 900
Rosemont, IL 60018
(312) 240-2880
www.nationaldairycouncil.org

United Fresh Fruit and Vegetable Association
1901 Pennsylvania Ave. NW, Suite 1100
Washington, DC 20006
(202) 303-3400
www.unitedfresh.org

U.S.A. Rice Federation
Washington, DC
4301 North Fairfax Drive, Suite 425
Arlington, VA 22203
(703) 236-2300
www.usarice.com

U.S. Government

The USDA National Organic Program
Agricultural Marketing Service
USDA-AMS-TMP-NOP
Room 4008-South Building
1400 Independence Avenue, SW
Washington, DC 20250-0020
(202) 720-3252
www.ams.usda.gov

U.S. Department of Health and Human Services
200 Independence Avenue, SW
Washington, DC 20201
(877) 696-6775
www.hhs.gov

Food and Drug Administration (FDA)
5600 Fishers Lane
Rockville, MD 20857
(888) 463-6332
www.fda.gov

Environmental Protection Agency
Ariel Rios Building
1200 Pennsylvania Avenue, NW
Washington, DC 20460
(202) 272-0167
www.epa.gov

Federal Trade Commission
600 Pennsylvania Avenue, NW
Washington, DC 20580
(202) 326-2222
www.ftc.gov

Office of Dietary Supplements
National Institutes of Health
6100 Executive Boulevard, Room 3B01, MSC 7517
Bethesda, MD 20892
(301) 435-2920
www.ods.od.nih.gov

Nutrient Data Laboratory Homepage
Beltsville Human Nutrition Center
10300 Baltimore Avenue
Building 307-C, Room 117
BARC-East
Beltsville, MD 20705
(301) 504-8157
www.nal.usda.gov/fnic/foodcomp

National Digestive Disease Clearinghouse
2 Information Way
Bethesda, MD 20892-3570
(800) 891-5389
www.digestive.niddk.nih.gov

The National Cancer Institute
NCI Public Inquiries Office
Suite 3036A
6116 Executive Boulevard, MSC 8322
Bethesda, MD 20892-8322
(800) 4-CANCER
www.cancer.gov

The National Eye Institute
31 Center Drive, MSC 2510
Bethesda, MD 20892-2510
(301) 496-5248
www.nei.nih.gov

The National Heart, Lung, and Blood Institute
Building 31, Room 5A52
31 Center Drive, MSC 2486
Bethesda, MD 20892
(301) 592-8573
www.nhlbi.nih.gov

Institute of Diabetes and Digestive and Kidney Diseases
Office of Communications and Public Liaison
NIDDK, NIH, Building 31, Room 9A04
Center Drive, MSC 2560
Bethesda, MD 20892
(301) 496-4000
www.niddk.nih.gov

National Center for Complementary and Alternative Medicine
NCCAM Clearinghouse
P.O. Box 7923
Gaithersburg, MD 20898
(888) 644-6226
www.nccam.nih.gov

U.S. Department of Agriculture (USDA)
14th Street, SW
Washington, DC 20250
(202) 720-2791
www.usda.gov

Centers for Disease Control and Prevention (CDC)
1600 Clifton Road
Atlanta, GA 30333
(404) 639-3311/Public Inquiries: (800) 311-3435
www.cdc.gov

National Institutes of Health (NIH)
9000 Rockville Pike
Bethesda, MD 20892
(301) 496-4000
www.nih.gov

Food and Nutrition Information Center
Agricultural Research Service, USDA
National Agricultural Library, Room 105
10301 Baltimore Avenue
Beltsville, MD 20705-2351
(301) 504-5719
www.nal.usda.gov/fnic

National Institute of Allergy and Infectious Diseases
NIAID Office of Communications and Public Liaison
6610 Rockledge Drive, MSC 6612
Bethesda, MD 20892
(301) 496-5717
www.niaid.nih.gov

Weight and Health Management

The Vegetarian Resource Group
P.O. Box 1463, Dept. IN
Baltimore, MD 21203
(410) 366-VEGE
www.vrg.org

American Obesity Association
1250 24th Street, NW
Suite 300
Washington, DC 20037
(202) 776-7711
www.obesity.org

Anemia Lifeline
(888) 722-4407
www.anemia.com

The Arc
(301) 565-3842
E-mail: info@thearc.org
www.thearc.org

Bottled Water Web
P.O. Box 5658
Santa Barbara, CA 93150
(805) 879-1564
www.bottledwaterweb.com

The Food and Nutrition Board
Institute of Medicine
500 Fifth Street, NW
Washington, DC 20001
(202) 334-2352
www.iom.edu

The Calorie Control Council
www.caloriecontrol.org

TOPS (Take Off Pounds Sensibly)
4575 South Fifth Street
P.O. Box 07360
Milwaukee, WI 53207
(800) 932-8677
www.tops.org

Shape Up America!
15009 Native Dancer Road
N. Potomac, MD 20878
(240) 631-6533
www.shapeup.org

World Hunger

Center on Hunger, Poverty, and Nutrition Policy
Tufts University
Medford, MA 02155
(617) 627-3020
www.tufts.edu/nutrition

Freedom from Hunger
1644 DaVinci Court
Davis, CA 95616
(800) 708-2555
www.freedomfromhunger.org

Oxfam International
1112 16th Street, NW, Suite 600
Washington, DC 20036
(202) 496-1170
www.oxfam.org

WorldWatch Institute
1776 Massachusetts Avenue, NW
Washington, DC 20036
(202) 452-1999
www.worldwatch.org

Food First
398 60th Street
Oakland, CA 94618
(510) 654-4400
www.foodfirst.org

The Hunger Project
15 East 26th Street
New York, NY 10010
(212) 251-9100
www.thp.org

U.S. Agency for International Development
Information Center
Ronald Reagan Building
Washington, DC 20523
(202) 712-0000
www.usaid.gov

references

Chapter 1

1. US Burden of Disease Collaborators. 2013. The state of US Health, 1990–2010. Burden of diseases, injuries, and risk factors. *JAMA.* 310(6):591–606.
2. Institute of Medicine, Food and Nutrition Board. 2003. *Dietary Reference Intakes: Applications in Dietary Planning.* Washington, DC: National Academies Press.
3. U.S. Department of Agriculture and U.S. Department of Health and Human Services. 2010. *Dietary Guidelines for Americans, 2010.* 7th edn. Washington, DC: U.S. Government Printing Office.
4. Young, L. R., and M. Nestle. 1998. Variations in perceptions of a "medium" food portion: implications for dietary guidance. *J. Am. Diet. Assoc.* 98:458–459.
5. Young, L. R., and M. Nestle. 2002. The contribution of expanding portion sizes to the U.S. obesity epidemic. *American Journal of Public Health.* 92(2):246–249.
6. U.S. Department of Health and Human Services. 2014. U.S. Food and Drug Administration. Nutrition Facts Label: Proposed Changes Aim to Better Inform Food Choices. www.fda.gov/ForConsumers/ConsumerUpdates/ucm387114.htm.
7. Winterfelt, E. A., M. L. Bogle, and L. L. Ebro. 2005. *Dietetics Practice and Future Trends.* 2nd edn. Sudbury, MA: Jones and Bartlett.
8. Agricultural Research Service. June 6, 2008. Founding American Nutrition Science. ARS Timeline. www.ars.usda.gov/is/timeline/nutrition.htm.
9. Rising, K., P. Bacchetti, and L. Bero. 2008. Reporting bias in drug trials submitted to the Food and Drug Administration: review of publication and presentation. *PLoS Medicine.* 5(11):e217. Doi:10.1371/journal.pmed.0050217.
10. Schott, G., H. Pachl, U. Limbach, U. Gundert-Remy, W. Ludwig, and K. Lieb. 2010. The financing of drug trials by pharmaceutical companies and its consequences: Part 1. A qualitative, systematic review of the literature on possible influences on the findings, protocols, and quality of drug trials. *Deutsch Aerzteblatt International.* 107(16):279–285.

Feature Box Reference

1. Fogel, J., and S. B. S. Shlivko. 2010. Weight problems and spam e-mail for weight loss products. *South. Med. J.* 103(1):31–36.

Chapter 2

1. Abou-Samra, R., et al. 2011. Effect of different protein sources on satiation and short-term satiety when consumed as a starter. *Nutrition Journal 2011,* December 23(10):139.
2. Bianconi, E., et al. 2013. An estimation of the number of cells in the human body. *Ann Hum Biol.* Nov–Dec; 40(6):463–471.
3. National Digestive Diseases Information Clearinghouse (NDDIC). April 30, 2012. Heartburn, gastroesophageal reflux (GER), and gastroesophageal reflux disease (GERD). NIH Publication No. 07-0882.
4. National Digestive Diseases Information Clearinghouse (NDDIC). October 30, 2013. H. pylori and peptic ulcers. NIH Publication No. 10-4225.
5. National Digestive Diseases Information Clearinghouse (NDDIC). November 27, 2013. NSAIDs and peptic ulcers. NIH Publication No. 10-4644.
6. U.S. Food and Drug Administration (FDA). April 17, 2013. Food allergies: what you need to know. www.fda.gov/Food/ResourcesForYou/Consumers/ucm079311.htm.

7. National Institutes of Allergy and Infectious Disease. (NIAID). July 2012. Food allergy: an overview. NIH Publication No. 12-5518.
8. National Institute of Diabetes and Digestive and Kidney Diseases (NIDDK). January 8, 2014. Celiac Disease Awareness Campaign.
9. Ludvigsson, J. F., et al. 2013. The Oslo definitions for coeliac disease and related terms. *Gut* 2013;62:43–52. doi:10.1136/gutjnl-2011-301346.
10. Rubio-Tapia, A., J. F. Ludvigsson, T. L. Brantner, J. A. Murray, and J. E. Everhart. 2012. The prevalence of celiac disease in the United States. *American Journal of Gastroenterology.* 2012;107:1538–1544.
11. National Digestive Diseases Information Clearinghouse (NDDIC). November 25, 2013. Diarrhea. NIH Publication No. 11-2749.
12. Grundmann, O., and S. L. Yoon. 2010. Irritable bowel syndrome: Epidemiology, diagnosis, and treatment: an update for health-care practitioners. *Journal of Gastroenterology and Hepatology.* 25:691–699.
13. National Digestive Diseases Information Clearinghouse (NDDIC). October 7, 2013. Irritable bowel syndrome. NIH Publication No. 13-693.

Feature Box References

1. Corella D., and J. M. Ordovas. 2009. Nutrigenomics in cardiovascular medicine. *Circ. Cardiovasc. Genet.* 2:637–651.
2. Barker, D. J. P., M. Lampl, T. Roseboom, and N. Winder. 2012. Resource allocation in utero and health in later life. *Placenta* 33:e30–e34.
3. Meadows, G. G. 2012. Diet, nutrients, phytochemicals, and cancer metastasis suppressor genes. *Cancer Metastasis Rev.* Dec; 31(3–4):441–454.
4. Zeisel, S. H. 2010. A grand challenge for nutrigenomics. *Front Gene.* 2010 December 13;1(2). doi: 10.3389/fgene.2010.00002. Available at http://www.uncnri.org/pdf/A%20grand%20challenge%20for%20nutrigenomics.pdf.
5. National Human Genome Research Institute. 2012. NIH Human Microbiome Project defines normal bacterial makeup of the body. *NIH News.* http://www.genome.gov/27549144.
6. Hemarajata, P., and J. Versalovic. 2013. Effects of probiotics on gut microbiota: mechanisms of intestinal immunomodulation and neuromodulation. *Therap Adv Gastroenterol.* January; 6(1):39–51. Available at http://www.ncbi.nlm.nih.gov/pmc/articles/PMC3539293/.
7. Stanghellini, V., et al. 2010. Gut microbiota and related diseases: clinical features. *Intern Emerg Med.* Oct;5 Suppl 1:S57–S63.
8. Draganov, P. V. 2009. Recent advances and remaining gaps in our knowledge of associations between gut microbiota and human health. *World J Gastroenterol.* 15(1):81–85.
9. Krajmalnik-Brown, R., Z. E. Ilhan, D. W. Kang, and J. K. DiBaise. 2012. Effects of gut microbes on nutrient absorption and energy regulation. *Nutr Clin Pract.* Apr; 27(2): 201–214.
10. Dinan, T. G., C. Stanton, and J. F. Cryan. 2013. Psychobiotics: a novel class of psychotropic. *Biological Psychiatry.* 74 (10):720.
11. United States Food and Drug Administration. 2012, April 6. Regulatory information: complementary and alternative medicine products and their regulation by the Food and Drug Administration. Available at http://www.fda.gov/RegulatoryInformation/Guidances/ucm144657.htm#iv.
12. National Digestive Diseases Information Clearinghouse (NDDIC). November 27, 2013. NSAIDs and peptic ulcers. NIH Publication No. 10-4644.
13. National Digestive Diseases Information Clearinghouse (NDDIC). November 25, 2013. Diarrhea. NIH Publication No. 11-2749.

Chapter 3

1. Sears, B. 2011. *The Zone Diet.* London: Thorsons.
2. Atkins, R. C. 2003. *Dr. Atkins' New Diet Revolution.* London: Vermilion.
3. U.S. Department of Agriculture and U.S. Department of Health and Human Services. 2010. *Dietary Guidelines for Americans, 2010,* 7th edn. Washington, DC: U.S. Government Printing Office.
4. Denova-Gutiérrez, E., G. Huitrón-Bravo, J. O. Talavera, S. Castañon, K. Gallegos-Carrillo, Y. Flores, and J. Salmerón. 2010. Dietary glycemic index, dietary glycemic load, blood lipids, and coronary heart disease. *J. Nutr. Metab.* Doi:10.1155/2010/170680.
5. Hu, J., C. La Vecchia, L. S. Augustin, E. Negri, M. de Groh, H. Morrison, L. Mery, Canadian Cancer Registries Epidemiology Research Group. 2013. Glycemic index, glycemic load and cancer risk. *Ann. Oncol.* 24(1): 245–251.
6. Institute of Medicine, Food and Nutrition Board. 2002. *Dietary Reference Intakes for Energy, Carbohydrates, Fiber, Fat, Protein and Amino Acids (Macronutrients).* Washington, DC: The National Academy of Sciences.
7. Welsh J. A., A. Sharma, J. L. Abramson, V. Vaccarino, C. Gillespie, and M. B. Vos. 2010. Caloric sweetener consumption and dyslipidemia among US adults. *JAMA* 303:1490–1497.
8. Huang, C., J. Huang, Y. Tian, X. Yang, and D. Gu. 2014. Sugar sweetened beverages consumption and risk of coronary heart disease: a meta-analysis of prospective studies. *Atherosclerosis* 234(1):11–16.
9. De Koning L., V. S. Malik, M. D. Kellogg, E. B. Rimm, W. C. Willett, and F. B. Hu. 2012. Sweetened beverage consumption, incident coronary heart disease, and biomarkers of risk in men. *Circulation* 125:1735–1741.
10. Johnson R. K., L. J. Appel, M. Brands, B. V. Howard, M. Lefevre, R. H. Lustig, F. Sacks, L. M. Steffen, and J. Wylie-Rosett. 2009. Dietary sugars intake and cardiovascular health: a scientific statement from the American Heart Association. *Circulation* 120:1011–1020.
11. Hu, F. B., and V. S. Malik. 2010. Sugar-sweetened beverages and risk of obesity and type 2 diabetes: epidemiologic evidence. *Physiol. Behav.* 100(1):47–54.
12. Fagherazzi, G., A. Vilier, D. S. Sartorelli, M. Lajous, B. Balkau, and F. Clavel-Chapelon. 2013. Consumption of artificially and sugar-sweetened beverages and incident type 2 diabetes in the Etude Epidémiologique auprès des femmes de la Mutuelle Générale de l'Education Nationale-European Investigation into Cancer and Nutrition cohort. *Am. J. Clin. Nutr.* Epub ahead of print, doi:10.3945/ajcn.112.050997.
13. Basu S., P. Yoffee, N. Hills, and R. H. Lustig. 2013. The relationship of sugar to population-level diabetes prevalence: an econometric analysis of repeated cross-sectional data. *PLoS ONE* 8(2): e57873. doi:10.1371/journal.pone.0057873.
14. Malik V. S., B. M. Popkin, G. A. Gray, J.-P. Després, and F. B. Hu. 2010. Sugar-sweetened beverages, obesity, type 2 diabetes mellitus, and cardiovascular disease risk. *Circulation* 121:1356–1364.
15. Te Moranga L., S. Mallard, and J. Mann. 2013. Dietary sugars and body weight: systematic review and meta-analyses of randomised controlled trials and cohort studies. *BMJ* 346:e7492.
16. International Food Information Council Foundation. 2013, August. Facts About Low-Calorie Sweeteners. http://www.foodinsight.org/Content/5438/LCS%20Fact%20Sheet_rev%202.pdf
17. International Food Information Council Foundation. 2011. Everything You Need to Know About Aspartame. Available at: http://www.foodinsight.org/Content/3848/FINAL_Aspartame%20Brochure_Web%20Version_11-2011.pdf
18. Gardner, C., J. Wylie-Rosett, S. S. Gidding, L. M. Steffen, R. K. Johnson, D. Reader, and A. H. Lichtenstein. 2012. Nonnutritive sweeteners: current use and health perspectives. A scientific statement from the American Heart Association and the American Diabetes Association. *Diab. Care,* 35:1798–1808.
19. National Diabetes Information Clearinghouse (NDIC). 2011. National Diabetes Statistics 2011. Diagnosed Diabetes. National Institutes of Health Publication No. 11-3892. http://diabetes.niddk.nih.gov/dm/pubs/statistics/index.htm.
20. Dalleck, L. C., and E. M. Kjelland. 2012. The prevalence of metabolic syndrome and metabolic syndrome risk factors in college-aged students. *American Journal of Health Promotion* 270(1), 37–42.

Chapter 4

1. Food and Drug Administration (FDA). US Dept of Health and Human Services. FDA Facts: Questions and Answers Regarding trans Fat. January 2014. Available at: http://www.fda.gov/downloads/food/popularTopics/ucm385846.pdf
2. United States Department of Agriculture (USDA) and Department of Health and Human Services (DHHS). 2010. Dietary Guidelines for Americans, 2010. Available at: http://www.cnpp.usda.gov/Publications/DietaryGuidelines/2010/PolicyDoc/PolicyDoc.pdf
3. Institute of Medicine (IOM), Food and Nutrition Board. 2005. *Dietary Reference Intakes for Energy, Carbohydrate, Fiber, Fat, Fatty Acids, Cholesterol, Protein, and Amino Acids (Macronutrients).* Washington, DC: National Academies Press.
4. Baum S. J., P. M. Kris-Etherton, W. C. Willett, A. H. Lichtenstein, L. L. Rudel, K. C. Maki, et al. 2012. Fatty acids in cardiovascular health and disease: a comprehensive update. *Journal of Clinical Lipidology* 6(3):216–234.
5. Mozaffarian D., and J. H. Wu. 2011. Omega-3 fatty acids and cardiovascular disease: effects on risk factors, molecular pathways, and clinical events. *Journal of the American College of Cardiology* 58(20):2047–2067.
6. Manore M. M., N. L. Meyer, and J. Thompson. 2009. *Sport Nutrition for Health and Performance,* 2nd edn. Champaign, IL: Human Kinetics.
7. Ormrod D. J., C. C. Holmes, and T. E. Miller. 1998. Dietary chitosan inhibits hypercholesterolaemia and atherogenesis in the apolipoprotein E-deficient mouse model of atherosclerosis. *Atherosclerosis.* 138(2):329–334.
8. Mhurchu C. N., C. A. Dunshea-Mooij, D. Bennett, and A. Rodgers. 2005b. Chitosan for overweight or obesity. Cochrane database of systematic reviews (Online) (Cochrane Database Syst Rev) 2005(3): CD003892. 2005b.
9. Mhurchu C. N., C. Dunshea-Mooij, D. Bennet, and A. Rodgers. 2005a. Effect of chitosan on weight loss in overweight and obese individuals: a systemic review of randomized control trials. *Obesity Rev.* 6:35–42.
10. Jull A. B., C. Ni Mhurchu, D. A. Bennett, C. A. Dunshea-Mooij, and A. Rodgers. 2008. Chitosan for overweight or obesity. Cochrane database of systematic reviews (Online) (Cochrane Database Syst Rev) (3): CD003892. 2008;3.
11. Manore, M. M. 2012. Dietary Supplements for Improving Body Composition and Reducing Body Weight: Where is the evidence? *Int J Sport Nutr Exerc Metab* 22(2):139–154.
12. Mayo Clinic. 2010. Alli Weight-Loss Pill: Does It Work? MayoClinic.com. www.mayoclinic.com/health/alli/WT00030
13. Rodriguez N. R., N. M. DiMarco, and S. Langley. 2009. Position of the American Dietetic Association, Dietitians of Canada, and the American College of Sports Medicine: Nutrition and Athletic Performance. *J. Am. Diet. Assoc.* 109:509–527.
14. Lichtenstein, A. H., and L. Van Horn. 1998. Very low fat diets. *Circulation* 98:935–939.
15. Kris-Etherton, P. M., W. S. Harris, L. J. Appel, and the Nutrition Committee of the American Heart Association. 2002. Fish consumption, fish oil, omega-3 fatty acids and cardiovascular disease. *Circulation* 106:2747–2757.
16. Flock, M. R., W. S. Harris, & P. M. Kris-Etherton. 2013. Long-chain omega-3 fatty acids: time to establish a dietary reference intake. *Nutr. Rev.* 71(10):692–707. doi:10.1111/nure.12071.

17. Eckel, R. H., J. M. Jakicic, J. D. Ard, N. H. Miller, V. S. Hubbard, C. A. Nonas, . . . S. Z. Yanovski. (2013). 2013 AHA/ACC Guideline on Lifestyle Management to Reduce Cardiovascular Risk: A Report of the American College of Cardiology/American Heart Association Task Force on Practice Guidelines. *J. Am. Coll. Cardiol.* doi:10.1016/j.jacc.2013.11.003.

18. Burillo, E., P. Martín-Fuentes, R. Mateo-Gallego, L. Baila-Rueda, A. Cenarro, E. Ros, and F. Civeira. 2012. Omega-3 fatty acids and HDL. How do they work in the prevention of cardiovascular disease? *Current vascular pharmacology, 10*(4):432–441.

19. Mozaffarian, D., M. B. Katan, A. Ascherio, M. J. Stampher, and W. C. Willet. 2006. Trans fatty acids and cardiovascular disease. *N. Engl. J. Med.* 354(15):1601–1613.

20. Centers for Disease Control and Prevention (CDC). 2013. Heart Disease Prevention: What Can You Do? Available at: http://www.cdc.gov/heartdisease/what_you_can_do.htm.

21. Expert Panel on Detection, Evaluation, and Treatment of High Blood Cholesterol in Adults, National Institutes of Health. 2001. Executive summary of the Third Report of the National Cholesterol Education Program (NCEP) Expert Panel on Detection, Evaluation, and Treatment of High Blood Cholesterol in Adults (Adult Treatment Panel III). *JAMA* 285(19):2486–2509.

22. American Cancer Society (ACS). 2013. Cancer Prevention and Early Detection Facts and Figures, 2013. Atlanta: American Cancer Society, 2013. Available at: http://www.cancer.org/acs/groups/content/@epidemiologysurveilance/documents/document/acspc-037535.pdf.

23. Alexander, D. D., L. M. Morimoto, P. J. Mink, and K. A. Lowe. 2010. Summary and meta-analysis of prospective studies of animal fat intake and breast cancer. *Nutr. Res. Rev.* 23(1):169–179.

24. Makarem, N., U. Chandran, E. V. Bandera, and N. Parekh. 2013. Dietary fat in breast cancer survival. *Annu. Rev. Nutr.* 33:319–348.

25. Magalhães, B., B. Peleteiro, and N. Lunet. 2012. Dietary patterns and colorectal cancer: systematic review and meta-analysis. *European J. Cancer Prevention, 21*(1):15–23.

26. Hori, S., E. Butler, and J. McLoughlin. 2011. Prostate cancer and diet: food for thought? *Brit. J. Urology International, 107*(9):1348–1359.

27. Crowe, F. L., T. J. Key, P. N. Appleby, R. C. Travis, K. Overvad, M. U. Jakobsen, . . . E. Riboli. 2008. Dietary fat intake and risk of prostate cancer in the European Prospective Investigation into Cancer and Nutrition. *Am. J. Clin. Nutr.* 87(5):1405–1413.

Feature Box References

1. Eckel, R. H., J. M. Jakicic, J. D. Ard, N. H. Miller, V. S. Hubbard, C. A. Nonas, . . . S. Z. Yanovski. 2013. 2013 AHA/ACC Guideline on Lifestyle Management to Reduce Cardiovascular Risk: A Report of the American College of Cardiology/American Heart Association Task Force on Practice Guidelines. *J. Am. Coll. Cardiol.* doi:10.1016/j.jacc.2013.11.003.

2. Almario, R. U., and S. E. Karakas. 2013. Lignan content of the flaxseed influences its biological effects in healthy men and women. *J. Am. Coll. Nutr. 32*(3), 194–199.

Chapter 5

1. Stahler, C. 2009. How many vegetarians are there? *Vegetarian Journal.* Issue 4. http://www.vrg.org/journal/vj2009issue4/2009_issue4_2009_poll.php.

2. Smith, M. I., T. Yatsunenko, M. J. Manary, I. Trehan, R. Mkakosya, J. Cheng, . . . J. I. Gordon. 2013. Gut microbiomes of Malawian twin pairs discordant for kwashiorkor. *Science* 339:548–554.

3. Chowdhury, R., S. Warnakula, S. Kunutsor, F. Crowe, H. A. Ward, L. Johnson, . . . Di Angelantonio. 2014. Association of dietary, circulating, and supplement fatty acids with coronary risk: a systematic review and meta-analysis. *Ann. Intern. Med.* 160(6):398–406.

4. American Dietetic Association. 2009. Position of the American Dietetic Association: vegetarian diets. *J. Am. Diet. Assoc.* 109:1266–1282.

5. Calvez, J., N. Poupin, C. Chesneau, C. Lassale, and D. Tomé. 2012. Protein intake, calcium balance and health consequences. *Eur. J. Clin. Nutr.* 66:281–295.

6. Martin, W. F., L. E. Armstrong, and N. R. Rodriguez. 2005. Dietary protein intake and renal function. *Nutr. Metabol.* 2:25. www.nutritionandmetabolism.com/content/2/1/25.

7. Ha, V., J. L. Sievenpiper, R. J. de Souza, V. H. Jayalath, A. Mirrahimi, A. Agarwal, . . . D. A. Jenkins. 2014. Effect of dietary pulse intake on established therapeutic lipid targets for cardiovascular risk reduction: a systematic review and meta-analysis of randomized controlled trials. CMAJ, e-pub ahead of print, doi: 10.1503/cmaj.131727.

8. Sabaté, J. M., and Y. Ang. 2009. Nuts and health outcomes: new epidemiological evidence. *Am. J. Clin. Nutr.* 89(suppl): 1643S–1648S.

9. Li, T. Y., A. M. Brennan, N. M. Wedick, C. Mantzoros, N. Rifai, and F. B. Hu. 2009. Regular consumption of nuts is associated with a lower risk of cardiovascular disease in women with type 2 diabetes. *J. Nutr.* 139(7):1333–1338.

10. Pan, A., Q. Sun, J. E. Manson, W. C. Willett, and F. B. Hu. 2013. Walnut consumption is associated with lower risk of type 2 diabetes in women. *J. Nutr.* 143:512–518.

11. Phillips, S. M., and L. J. C. van Loon. 2011. Dietary protein for athletes: from requirements to optimum adaptation. *J. Sports Sci.* 29(suppl. 1):S29–S38.

12. American Dietetic Association. 2009. Position of the American Dietetic Association: Vegetarian Diet. *J. Am. Diet. Assoc.* 109:1266–1282.

13. Institute of Medicine, Food and Nutrition Board. 2002. *Dietary Reference Intakes for Energy, Carbohydrate, Fiber, Fat, Fatty Acids, Cholesterol, Protein, and Amino Acids (Macronutrients).* Washington, DC: National Academies Press.

Feature Box References

1. American College of Sports Medicine, American Dietetic Association, and Dietitians of Canada. 2009. Joint position statement. Nutrition and athletic performance. *Med. Sci. Sports Exerc.* 41(3):709–731.

2. Phillips, S. M., and L. J. C. van Loon. 2011. Dietary protein for athletes: from requirements to optimum adaptation. *J. Sports Sci.* 29(suppl. 1):S29–S38.

3. Brehm, B. J., and D. A. D'Alessio. 2008. Benefits of high-protein weight loss diets: enough evidence for practice? *Curr. Opin. Endocrinol. Diabetes Obes.* 15:416–421.

4. McConnon, A., G. W. Horgan, C. Lawton, J. Stubbs, R. Shepherd, A. Astrup, . . . M. M. Raats. 2013. Experience and acceptability of diets of varying protein content and glycemic index in an obese cohort: results from the Diogenes trial. *Eur. J. Clin. Nutr.* 67(9):990–995.

5. Chowdhury, R., S. Warnakula, S. Kunutsor, F. Crowe, H. A. Ward, L. Johnson, . . . E. Di Angelantonio. 2014. Association of dietary, circulating, and supplement fatty acids with coronary risk: a systematic review and meta-analysis. *Ann. Intern. Med.* 160(6):398–406.

6. Clifton, P. M., K. Bastiaans, and J. B. Keogh. 2009. High protein diets decrease total and abdominal fat and improve CVD risk profile in overweight and obese men and women with elevated triacylglycerol. *Nutr. Metab. Cardiovas. Dis.* 19:548–554.

7. Russell, W. R., S. W. Gratz, S. H. Duncan, G. Holtrop, J. Ince, L. Scobbie, . . . H. J. Flint. 2011. High-protein, reduced-carbohydrate weight-loss diets promote metabolite profiles likely to be detrimental to colonic health. *Am. J. Clin. Nutr.* 93(5):1062–1072.

8. U.S. Department of Health and Human Services. U.S. Food and Drug Administration. 2013. Food. Guidance for

Industry: A Food Labeling Guide (11. Appendix C: Health Claims). http://www.fda.gov/food/guidanceregulation/guidancedocumentsregulatoryinformation/labelingnutrition/ucm064919.htm.

9. American Heart Association. 2014. Getting Healthy. Nutrition Center. Try These Tips for Heart-health Grocery Shopping. http://www.heart.org/HEARTORG/GettingHealthy/NutritionCenter/HeartSmartShopping/Try-These-Tips-for-Heart-Healthy-Grocery-Shopping_UCM_001884_Article.jsp.

10. Centers for Disease Control and Prevention. 2013. Cancer Prevention and Control. Cancer Among Men. http://www.cdc.gov/cancer/dcpc/data/men.htm.

11. American Cancer Society. 2013. Soybean. http://www.cancer.org/treatment/treatmentsandsideeffects/complementaryand alternativemedicine/dietandnutrition/soybean.

12. Shedd-Wise, K. M., D. Lee Alekel, H. Hofmann, K. B. Hanson, D. J. Schiferl, L. N. Hanson, and M. D. van Loan. 2011. The Soy Isoflavones for Reducing Bone Loss (SIRBL) study: three year effects on pQCT bone mineral density and strength measures in postmenopausal women. *J. Clin. Densitom.* 14(1):47–57.

Chapter 6

1. Bernstein, L. 2000. Dementia without a cause: lack of vitamin B_{12} can cause dementia. *Discover*, February 21.

2. Druesne-Pecollo, N., P. Latino-Martel, T. Norat, E. Barrandon, S. Bertrais, P. Galan, and S. Hercberg. 2010. Beta-carotene supplementation and cancer risk: a systematic review and meta-analysis of randomized controlled trials. *Int. J. Cancer.* 127(1):172–184.

3. World Health Organization (WHO). 2013. Micronutrient deficiencies. Vitamin A deficiency. http://www.who.int/nutrition/topics/vad/en/index.html.

4. Institute of Medicine, Food and Nutrition Board. 2010. *Dietary Reference Intakes for Calcium and Vitamin D.* Washington, DC: National Academy Press.

5. Adams, J. S., and M. Hewison. 2010. Update on vitamin D. *J. Clin. Endocrinol. Metab.* 95:471–478.

6. Holick, M. F., N. C. Binkley, H. A. Bischoff-Ferrari, C. M. Gordon, D. A. Hanley, R. P. Heaney, M. Hassan Murad, and C. M. Weaver. 2011. Evaluation, treatment, and prevention of vitamin D deficiency: an Endocrine Society Clinical Practice Guideline. *J. Clin. Endocrinol. Metab.* 96:1911–1930.

7. Yetley, E. A., et al. 2009. Dietary Reference Intakes for vitamin D: Justification for a review of the 1997 values. *Am. J. Clin. Nutr.* 89:719–727.

8. Holick, M. F. 2006. Resurrection of vitamin D deficiency and rickets. *J. Clin. Invest.* 116:2062–2072.

9. Weisberg, P., K. S. Scanlon, R. Li, and M. E. Cogswell. 2004. Nutritional rickets among children in the United States: review of cases reported between 1986 and 2003. *Am. J. Clin. Nutr.* 80(suppl.):1697S–1705S.

10. Institute of Medicine, Food and Nutrition Board. 2002. *Dietary Reference Intakes for Vitamin A, Vitamin K, Arsenic, Boron, Chromium, Copper, Iodine, Iron, Manganese, Molybdenum, Nickel, Silicon, Vanadium, and Zinc.* Washington, DC: National Academies Press.

11. National Institutes of Health. Office of Dietary Supplements (ODS). 2011. Vitamin B6. Dietary Supplement Fact Sheet. http://ods.od.nih.gov/factsheets/VitaminB6-HealthProfessional/

12. Weck, M. N., and H. Brenner. 2006. Prevalence of chronic atrophic gastritis in different parts of the world. *Cancer Epidemiol Biomarkders Prev* 15:1083–1094.

13. Adamu, M. A., M. N. Weck, D. Rothenbacher, and H. Brenner. 2011. Incidence and risk factors for the development of chronic atrophic gastritis: five year follow-up of a population-based cohort study. *Int. J. Cancer* 128:1652–1658.

14. Tang, W., H. Wilson, Z. Whang, B. S. Levison, R. A. Koeth, E. B. Britt, X. Fu, Y. Wu, and S. L. Hazen. 2013. Intestinal microbial

metabolism of phosphatidylcholine and cardiovascular risk. *New Eng. J. Med.* 368:1575–1584.

15. Gahche, J., R. Bailey, V. Burt, J. Hughes, E. Yetley, J. Dwyer, M. F. Picciano, M. McDowell, and C. Sempos. 2011. Dietary supplement use among U.S. adults has increased since NHANES III (1988–1994). NCHS Data Brief. Number 61. www.cdc.gov/nchs/data/databriefs/db61.htm.

16. American Dietetic Association. 2009. Position of the American Dietetic Association: Nutrient Supplementation. *J. Am. Diet. Assoc.* 109:2073–2085.

17. American Cancer Society. 2014. Cancer Facts & Figures 2014. http://www.cancer.org/research/cancerfactsstatistics/cancerfactsfigures2014/index

18. Durko, L., and E. Malecka-Panas. 2014. Lifestyle modifications and colorectal cancer. *Curr Colorectal Cancer Rep.* 2014; 10: 45–54.

19. Deschasaux, M., C. Pouchieu, M. His, S. Hercberg, P. Latino-Martel, and M. Touvier. 2014. Dietary total and insoluble fiber intakes are inversely associated with prostate cancer risk. *J. Nutr.* 144(4):504–510.

20. Aune, D., D. S. Chan, D. C. Greenwood, A. R. Vieira, D. A. Rosenblatt, R. Vieira, and T. Norat. 2012. Dietary fiber and breast cancer risk: a systematic review and meta-analysis of prospective studies. *Ann. Oncol.* 23(6):1394–1402.

21. Shukla, S., and S. Gupta. 2010. Apigenin: a promising molecule for cancer prevention. *Pharm. Res.* 27(6):962–978.

22. Ohio State University. 2013, May 20. Compound in Mediterranean diet makes cancer cells 'mortal'. *ScienceDaily.*

23. Abdull Razis, A. F., and N. M. Noor. 2013. Cruciferous vegetables: dietary phytochemicals for cancer prevention. *Asian Pac. J. Cancer Prev.* 14(3): 1565–1570.

24. American Cancer Society. 2012. American Cancer Society Guidelines on Nutrition and Physical Activity for Cancer Prevention. http://www.cancer.org/healthy/eathealthygetactive/acsguidelinesonnutritionphysicalactivityforcancerprevention/acs-guidelines-on-nutrition-and-physical-activity-for-cancer-prevention-intro.

Feature Box References

1. Institute of Medicine, Food and Nutrition Board. 2010. *Dietary Reference Intakes for Calcium and Vitamin D.* Washington, DC: National Academy Press.

2. Allan, G. M., and B. Arroll. 2014. Prevention and treatment of the common cold: making sense of the evidence. *CMAJ.* 186(3):190–199.

3. National Institute of Allergy and Infectious Diseases. April 13, 2011. Common Cold. http://www.niaid.nih.gov/topics/commonCold/Pages/prevention.aspx.

4. National Center for Complementary and Alternative Medicine. 2013. Dietary and Herbal Supplements. http://nccam.nih.gov/health/supplements/.

5. Bailey, R. L., J. J. Gahche, C. V. Lentino, J. T. Dwyer, J. S. Engel, P. R. Thomas, et al. 2011. Dietary supplement use in the United States, 2003–2006. *J. Nutr.* 141(2):261–266.

6. U.S. Government Accountability Office. 2010. Herbal Dietary Supplements: Examples of Deceptive or Questionable Marketing Practices and Potentially Dangerous Advice. GAO-10-662T. www.gao.gov/new.items/d10662t.pdf.

Chapter 7

1. Gropper, S. S., and J. L. Smith. 2013. *Advanced Nutrition and Human Metabolism*, 6th edn. Belmont, CA: Wadsworth Cengage Learning.

2. Institute of Medicine (IOM), Food and Nutrition Board. 2001. *Dietary Reference Intakes for Vitamin A, Vitamin K, Arsenic, Boron, Chromium, Copper, Iodine, Iron, Manganese, Molybdenum, Nickel, Silicon, Vanadium, and Zinc.* Washington, DC: National Academies Press.

3. Eckhert, C. D. 2014. Trace elements. In: Ross A. C., B. Caballero, R. J. Cousins, K. L. Tucker, and T. R. Ziegler, eds. *Modern Nutrition in Health and Disease*, 11th edn, pp. 245–259. Philadelphia: Lippincott Williams & Wilkins.

4. United States Department of Agriculture (USDA) and Department of Health and Human Services (DHHS). 2010. Dietary Guidelines for Americans, 2010. Available at http://www.cnpp.usda.gov/Publications/DietaryGuidelines/2010/PolicyDoc/PolicyDoc.pdf.

5. Institute of Medicine (IOM), Food and Nutrition Board. 2004. *Dietary Reference Intakes for Water, Potassium, Sodium, Chloride and Sulfate.* Washington, DC: National Academies Press.

6. Sacks, F. M., L. P. Svetkey, W. M. Vollmer, L. J. Appel, G. A. Bray, D. Harsha, . . . P.-H. Lin. 2001. Effects on blood pressure of reduced dietary sodium and the Dietary Approaches to Stop Hypertension (DASH) diet. *N. Engl. J. Med.* 344:3–10.

7. National Institutes of Health (NIH), Office of Dietary Supplements. 2013. Selenium QuickFacts. http://ods.od.nih.gov/factsheets/Selenium-QuickFacts/

8. Centers for Disease Control and Prevention (CDC). 2002. Iron Deficiency—United States, 1999–2000. *Morbidity and Mortality Weekly Report.* 51(40):871–920. www.cdc.gov/mmwr/PDF/wk/mm5140.pdf.

9. Spanierman, C. S. 2013. Iron toxicity. Medscape Emedicine. http://emedicine.medscape.com/article/815213-overview#a0101.

10. Institute of Medicine, Food and Nutrition Board. 2011. *Dietary Reference Intakes for Calcium, Phosphorus, Magnesium, Vitamin D, and Fluoride.* Washington, DC: National Academies Press.

11. Heaney, R. P., and K. Rafferty. 2001. Carbonated beverages and urinary calcium excretion. *Am. J. Clin. Nutr.* 74:343–347.

12. Wu, C. H., Y. C. Yang, W. J. Yao, F. H. Lu, J. S. Wu, and C. J. Chang. 2002. Epidemiological evidence of increased bone mineral density in habitual tea drinkers. *Arch. Intern. Med.* 162:1001–1006.

13. Dew, T. P., A. J. Day, and M. R. Morgan. 2007. Bone mineral density, polyphenols and caffeine: a reassessment. *Nutr Res. Rev.* 20(1):89–105 doi: http://dx.doi.org/10.1017/S0954422407738805.

14. WebMD. (2013). Causes of Osteoporosis. http://www.webmd.com/osteoporosis/guide/strong-bones.

15. National Osteoporosis Foundation (NOF). 2012. What Women Need to Know. http://nof.org/articles/235. Accessed May 2014.

16. National Institutes of Health. 2013. The Surgeon General's Report on Bone Health and Osteoporosis: What It Means to You. http://www.niams.nih.gov/health_Info/Bone/SGR/surgeon_generals_report.asp.

17. Levis, S., and V. S. Lagari. 2012. The role of diet in osteoporosis prevention and management. *Current osteoporosis reports.* 10(4):296–302. doi: http://dx.doi.org/10.1007/s11914-012-0119-y.

Feature Box References

1. Evans, G. W. 1989. The effect of chromium picolinate on insulin controlled parameters in humans. *Int. J. Biosoc. Med. Res.* 11:163–180.

2. Hasten, D. L., E. P. Rome, D. B. Franks, and M. Hegsted. 1992. Effects of chromium picolinate on beginning weight training students. *Int. J. Sports Nutr.* 2:343–350.

3. Lukaski, H. C., W. W. Bolonchuk, W. A. Siders, and D. B. Milne. 1996. Chromium supplementation and resistance training: effects on body composition, strength, and trace element status of men. *Am. J. Clin. Nutr.* 63:954–965.

4. Hallmark, M. A., T. H. Reynolds, C. A. DeSouza, C. O. Dotson, R. A. Anderson, and M. A. Rogers. 1996. Effects of chromium and resistive training on muscle strength and body composition. *Med. Sci. Sports Exerc.* 28:139–144.

5. Walker, L. S., M. G. Bemben, D. A. Bemben, and A. W. Knehans. 1998. Chromium picolinate effects on body composition and muscular performance in wrestlers. *Med. Sci. Sports Exerc.* 30:1730–1737.

6. Campbell, W. W., L. J. Joseph, S. L. Davey, D. Cyr-Campbell, R. A. Anderson, and W. J. Evans. 1999. Effects of resistance training and chromium picolinate on body composition and skeletal muscle in older men. *J. Appl. Physiol.* 86:29–39.

7. Volpe, S. L., H. W. Huang, K. Larpadisorn, and I. I. Lesser. 2001. Effect of chromium supplementation and exercise on body composition, resting metabolic rate and selected biochemical parameters in moderately obese women following an exercise program. *J. Am. Coll. Nutr.* 20:293–306.

8. Campbell, W. W., L. J. O. Joseph, R. A. Anderson, S. L. Davey, J. Hinton, and W. J. Evans. 2002. Effects of resistive training and chromium picolinate on body composition and skeletal muscle size in older women. *Int. J. Sports Nutr. Exerc. Metab.* 12:125–135.

9. Lukaski H. C., W. A. Siders, and J. G. Penland. 2007. Chromium picolinate supplementation in women: effects on body weight, composition and iron status. *Nutr.* 23:187–185.

10. Tian, H., X. Guo, X. Wang, X. He, R. Sun, S. Ge, and Z. Zhang. 2013. Chromium picolinate supplementation for overweight or obese adults. *The Cochrane database of systematic reviews.* 11.

11. Onakpoya, I., P. Posadzki, and E. Ernst. 2013. Chromium supplementation in overweight and obesity: a systematic review and meta-analysis of randomized clinical trials. *Obes. Rev.* 14(6):496–507.

12. Centers for Disease Control and Prevention (CDC). 2013. Common Colds: Protect Yourself and Others. http://www.cdc.gov/Features/Rhinoviruses/. Accessed March 2013.

13. National Institute of Allergy and Infectious Diseases (NIAID), National Institutes of Health. 2012. The Common Cold. www3.niaid.nih.gov/topics/commonCold/Pages/overview.aspx. Accessed May 2014.

14. Prasad, A. 1996. Zinc: the biology and therapeutics of an ion. *Ann. Intern. Med.* 125:142–143.

15. Jackson, J. L., E. Lesho, and C. Peterson. 2000. Zinc and the common cold: A meta-analysis revisited. *J. Nutr.* 130:1512S–1515S.

16. Sigh, M., and R. R. Das. 2011. Zinc for the common cold. *Cochrane Database of Systemic Reviews.* Issue 2. Art. No. Cd001364, doi:10.1002/14651858.

17. Hemila, H. 2011. Zinc lozenges may shorten the duration of colds: a systemic review. *Open Respiratory Medicine Journal.* 5:51–58.

18. Das, R. R., and M. Singh. 2014. Oral zinc for the common cold. *JAMA.* 311(14):1440–1441.

19. Keller, J. L., A. J. Lanou, and N. D. Barnard. 2002. The consumer cost of calcium from food supplements. *J. Am. Diet. Assoc.* 102:1669–1671.

Chapter 8

1. Center for Food Safety and Applied Nutrition Adverse Event Reporting System. 2012. Voluntary and Mandatory Reports on 5-Hour Energy, Monster Energy, and Rockstar Energy Drink. Available at http://www.fda.gov/downloads/AboutFDA/CentersOffices/OfficeofFoods/CFSAN/CFSANFOIAElectronicReadingRoom/UCM328270.pdf. (Accessed March 2014).

2. National Institute on Alcohol Abuse and Alcoholism. 2014. Alcohol Facts and Statistics. Available at http://www.niaaa.nih.gov/alcohol-health/overview-alcohol-consumption/alcohol-facts-and-statistics. (Accessed March 2014).

3. Institute of Medicine, Food and Nutrition Board. 2004. *Dietary Reference Intakes: Water, Potassium, Sodium, Chloride, and Sulfate.* Washington, DC: National Academies Press.

4. Mueller, F. O., and R. C. Cantu. 2012. *Annual Survey of Catastrophic Football Injuries, 1977–2012.* National Center for Catastrophic Sports Injury Research. Available at http://nccsir.unc.edu/. (Accessed March 2014).

5. International Bottled Water Association. 2013. U.S. Consumption of Bottled Water Shows Continued Growth, Increasing 6.2 Percent in 2012; Sales up 6.7 Percent. Available at http://www.bottledwater.org/us-consumption-bottled-water-shows-continued-growth-increasing-62-percent-2012-sales-67-percent. (Accessed March 2014).

6. da Silva Pinto, M. 2013. Tea: a new perspective on health benefits. *Food Res Intl.* http://dx.doi.org/10.1016/j.foodres.2013.01.038 (Accessed March 2014)

7. Laine, M. L., and W. Crielaard. 2012. Functional foods/ingredients and periodontal diseases. *Eur J Nutr* 51(Suppl 2):S27–S30.

8. Knowles, D. Marketed to teens, energy drink sales poised to nearly double over the next five years, despite health warnings from pediatricians. *The New York Daily News,* February 13, 2013.

9. Pomeranz, J. L., C. R. Munsell, and J. L. Harris. 2013. Energy drinks: an emerging public health hazard for youth. *J Public Health Policy.* Doi:10.1057/jphp.2013.6.

10. Patrick, M. E., and J. L. Maggs. 2013. Energy drinks and alcohol: Links to alcohol behaviors and consequences across 56 days. *J Adolescent Health.* Doi.org/10.1016/j.jadohealth.2013.09.013.

11. Kalman, D. S., S. Feldman, D. R. Krieger, and R. J. Bloomer. 2012. Comparison of coconut water and a carbohydrate-electrolyte sport drink on measures of hydration and physical performance in exercise-trained men. *J Int Soc Sports Nutr,* 2012 Jan 18;9(1):1. doi: 10.1186/1550-2783-9-1.

12. U.S. Department of Agriculture and U.S. Department of Health and Human Services. 2010. *Dietary Guidelines for Americans, 2010,* 7th ed. Washington, DC: U.S. Government Printing Office.

13. Poli, A., F. Marangoni, F. A. Avogaro, et al. 2013. Moderate alcohol use and health: A consensus document. *Nutrition, Metabolism & Cardiovascular Diseases.* 23:487–504.

14. Hogenkamp, P. S., C. Benedict, P. Sjögren, L. Kilander, L. Lind, and H. B. Schiöth. 2014. Late-life alcohol consumption and cognitive function in elderly men. *Age.* 36:243–249.

15. National Institute on Alcohol Abuse and Alcoholism. 2014. Harmful Interactions: Mixing alcohol with medicines. NIH Publication No. 13-5329. Available at http://pubs.niaaa.nih.gov/publications/Medicine/medicine.htm. (Accessed March 2014).

16. National Institute on Alcohol Abuse and Alcoholism. 2013. College Drinking. Available at http://pubs.niaaa.nih.gov/publications/CollegeFactSheet/CollegeFactSheet.pdf. (Accessed March 2014).

17. Centers for Disease Control and Prevention. 2012. Alcohol and Public Health: Fact Sheets – Binge Drinking. Available at www.cdc.gov/alcohol/fact-sheets/binge-drinking.htm (Accessed March 2014).

18. National Highway Traffic Safety Administration. 2013. Impaired Driving. Available at http://www.nhtsa.gov/Impaired. (Accessed March 2014).

19. National Institute on Alcohol Abuse and Alcoholism. Rethinking Drinking: Alcohol and your health. Available at http://rethinkingdrinking.niaaa.nih.gov/WhatsTheHarm/WhatAreTheRisks.asp. (Accessed March 2014).

20. Centers for Disease Control and Prevention. 2012. Fetal Alcohol Spectrum Disorders (FASDs): Facts about FASD. Available at www.cdc.gov/fasd (Accessed March 2014).

Feature Box Reference

1. Corporate Accountability International. n.d. Think Outside the Bottle. Available at http://www.stopcorporateabuse.org/think-outside-bottle (Accessed March 2014).

Chapter 9

1. 60 Minutes Overtime Staff. 2012, February 12. Adele talks about her body image and weight. *CBS News.* Available at http://www.cbsnews.com/news/adele-talks-about-her-body-image-and-weight/.

2. Manore, M. M, N. L. Meyer, and J. Thompson. 2009. *Sport Nutrition for Health and Performance,* 2nd edn. Champaign, IL: Human Kinetics.

3. Flegal, K. M., B. K. Kit, H. Orpana, and B. I. Graubard. 2013. Association of all-cause mortality with overweight and obesity using standard body mass index categories. A systematic review and meta-analysis. *JAMA* 309(1):71–82.

4. Galgani, J., and E. Ravussin. 2008. Energy metabolism, fuel selection and body weight regulation. *Int. J. Obes.* 32:S109–S119.

5. Harris, J., and F. Benedict. 1919. *A Biometric Study of Basal Metabolism in Man.* Washington, DC: Carnegie Institute of Washington.

6. Stunkard, A. J., T. I. A. Sørensen, C. Hanis, T. W. Teasdale, R. Chakraborty, W. J. Schull, and F. Schulsinger. 1986. An adoption study of human obesity. *N. Engl. J. Med.* 314:193–198.

7. Bouchard, C. 2010. Defining the genetic architecture of the predisposition to obesity: a challenging but not insurmountable task. *Am. J. Clin. Nutr.* 91:5–6.

8. Bloss, C. S., N. J. Stork, and E. J. Topol. 2011. Effect of direct-to-consumer genomewide profiling to assess disease risk. *N. Engl. J. Med.* 364(6):524–534.

9. Razquin, C., A. Marti, and J. A. Martinez. 2011. Evidences on three relevant obesogenes: MC4R, FTO, and PPARY. *Mol. Nutr. Food Res.* 55(1):136–149.

10. Kilpeläinen, T. O., L. Qi, S. Brage, S. J. Sharp, E. Sonestedt, E. Demerath, T. Ahmad, et al. 2011. Physical activity attenuates the influence of FTO variants on obesity risk: a meta-analysis of 218,166 adults and 19,268 children. *PLoS Med.* 8(11)e1001116, Epub 2011 Nov 1.

11. Lee, P., M. M. Swarbrick, and K. K. Ho. 2013. Brown adipose tissue in adult humans: a metabolic renaissance. *Endocr. Rev.* 34(3):413–438.

12. Cypess, A. M., S. Lehman, G. Williams, I. Tal, D. Rodman, A. B. Goldfine, . . . C. R. Kahn. 2009. Identification and importance of brown adipose tissue in adult humans. *N. Engl. J. Med.* 360(15):1509–1517.

13. Levine, J. A. 2011. Poverty and obesity in the U.S. *Diabetes,* 60(11):2667–2668.

14. National Restaurant Association. 2014. Restaurant.org/Forecast. Available at http://www.restaurant.org/News-Research/Research/Facts-at-a-Glance.

15. Ding D., T. Sugiyama, and N. Owen. 2012. Habitual active transport, TV viewing and weight gain: a four-year follow-up study. *Prev Med* 54: 201–204.

16. Lumeng, J. C., P. Forrest, D. P. Appugliese, N. Kaciroti, R. F. Corwyn, and R. H. Bradley. 2010. Weight status as a predictor of being bullied in third through sixth grades. *Pediatrics.* 125(6):e1301–e1307.

17. Prentice, R. L., B. Caan, R. T. Chlebowski, et al. 2006. Low-fat dietary pattern and risk of invasive breast cancer: the Women's Health Initiative Randomized Controlled Dietary Modification Trial. *JAMA* 295:629–642.

18. Beresford, S. A., K. C. Johnson, C. Ritenbaugh, et al. 2006. Low-fat dietary pattern and risk of colorectal cancer: the Women's Health Initiative Randomized Controlled Dietary Modification Trial. *JAMA* 295:643–654.

19. Howard, B. V., L. Van Horn, J. Hsia, et al. 2006. Low-fat dietary pattern and risk of cardiovascular disease: the Women's Health Initiative Randomized Controlled Dietary Modification Trial. *JAMA* 295:655–666.

20. Howard B. V., J. E. Manson, M. L. Stefanick, et al. 2006. Low-fat dietary pattern and weight change over 7 years: the Women's Health Initiative Dietary Modification Trial. *JAMA* 295:39–49.

21. Hession, M., C. Rolland, U. Kulkarni, A. Wise, and J. Broom. 2009. Systematic review of randomized controlled trials of low-carbohydrate vs. low-fat/low-calorie diets in the management of obesity and its co-morbidities. *Obes. Rev.* 10(1):36–50.

22. Raynor, H. A., S. M. Looney, E. A. Steeves, M. Spence, and A.A. Gorin. 2012. The effects of an energy density prescription on diet quality and weight loss: a pilot randomized controlled trial. *J. Acad. Nutr. Diet.* 112(9):1397–1402.

23. National Institute of Diabetes and Digestive and Kidney Diseases. Weight-control Information Network. 2012. Just Enough for You. About Food Portions. NIH Publication No. 09-5287. Available at: http://win.niddk.nih.gov/publications/just_enough.htm.

24. Wing, R. R., and S. Phelan. 2005. Long-term weight loss maintenance. *Am. J. Clin. Nutr.* 82(suppl):222S–225S.

25. Ogden, C. L., M. D. Carroll, B. K. Kitt, and K. M. Flegal. 2012. Prevalence of obesity in the United States, 2009–2010. NCHS data brief no 82. Available at http://www.cdc.gov/nchs/data/databriefs/db82.pdf.

26. Ervin, R. B. 2009. Prevalence of metabolic syndrome among adults 20 years of age and over, by sex, age, race and ethnicity, and body mass index: United States, 2003–2006. *Nat. Health Stat. Rep.* 13:1–4. Available at http://www.cdc.gov/nchs/data/nhsr/nhsr013.pdf.

27. National Institute of Diabetes and Digestive and Kidney Diseases. Weight-control Information Network. 2012. Understanding Adult Obesity. NIH Publication No. 06-3680 Available at http://www.win.niddk.nih.gov/publications/understanding.htm.

28. Centers for Disease Control and Prevention. 2014. Overweight and Obesity. Childhood Obesity Facts. Available at http://www.cdc.gov/obesity/data/childhood.html.

29. Centers for Disease Control and Prevention. 2014. Adolescent and School Health. Childhood Obesity Facts. Available at http://www.cdc.gov/healthyyouth/obesity/facts.htm.

30. Christakis, N. A., and J. H. Fowler. 2007. The spread of obesity in a large social network over 32 years. *N. Engl. J. Med.* 357(4):370–379.

31. Mayo Clinic. 2013. Weight Loss. Prescription Drugs: Can They Help You? Available at www.mayoclinic.org/healthy-living/weight-loss/in-depth/weight-loss-drugs/art-20044832?pg = 2.

32. American Psychiatric Association. 2013. *Diagnostic and Statistical Manual of Mental Disorders, 5th Edition, DSM-5.* Washington, D.C.: American Psychiatric Association.

33. Steinhausen, H.-C., H. Jakobsen, D. Helenius, P. Munk-Jørgensen, and M. Strober. 2014. A nation-wide study of the family aggregation and risk factors in anorexia nervosa over three generations. *Int. J. Eating Disorders*, Apr 28 (Epub ahead of print), doi: 10.1002/eat.22293.

34. Boraska, V., C. S. Franklin, J. A. Floyd, et al. 2014. A genome-wide association study of anorexia nervosa. *Molecular Psychiatry.* Feb 11 (Epub ahead of print), doi: 10.1038/mp.2013.187.

35. Allen, K. L., L. Y. Gibson, N. J. McLean, E. A. Davis, and S. M. Byrne. 2014. Maternal and family factors and child eating pathology: risk and protective relationships. *Int. J. Eating Disorders*, 2:11, http://www.jeatdisord.com/content/2/1/11.

36. American Psychiatric Association. 2013. Eating Disorders: Epidemiology. *APA Practice Guidelines.* Available at http://psychiatryonline.org/content.aspx?bookid = 28&sectionid = 1671672.

37. Keel, P. K., and K. J. Forney. 2013. Psychosocial Risk Factors for Eating Disorders. *Int. J. Eating Disorders*, 46(5):433–439.

38. Costa-Font, J., and M. Jofre-Bonet. 2011, Anorexia, body image, and peer effects: evidence from a sample of European women. *Centre for Economic Performance*: CEP Discussion Paper No. 1098. Available at http://cep.lse.ac.uk/pubs/download/dp1098.pdf.

39. Veldhuis, J., E. A. Konijn, and J. C. Seidel. 2014. Negotiated media effects. Peer feedback modifies effects of media's thin-body ideal on adolescent girls. *Appetite*, 73:172–182.

40. Keel, P. K., T. A. Brown, L. A. Holland, and L. D. Bodell. 2012. Empirical Classification of Eating Disorders. *Annual Rev. Clin. Psychol.*, 8:381–404.

41. National Association of Anorexia Nervosa and Associated Disorders. 2014. Eating Disorder Statistics. Available at http://www.anad.org/get-information/about-eating-disorders/eating-disorders-statistics/.

42. Vander Wal, J. S. 2012. Night eating syndrome: a critical review of the literature. *Clin. Psychol. Rev.*, 32:49–59.

43. Nattiv, A., A. B. Loucks, M. M. Manore, C. F. Sanborn, J. Sundgot-Borgen, and M. P. Warren. 2007. The female athlete triad. *Med. Sci. Sports Exerc.* 39(10):1867–1882.

Feature Box References

1. Katz D. L., K. Doughty, V. Njike, J. A. Treu, J. Reynolds, J. Walker, E. Smith, and C. Katz. 2011. A cost comparison of more and less nutritious food choices in US supermarkets. *Pub. Health Nutr.* 14(9):1693–1699.

2. Academy of Nutrition and Dietetics. 2012. Tip of the Day. Say No to the Dangers of Fad Diets. Available at http://www.eatright.org/Public/content.aspx?id = 6851&terms = fad%20diets.

3. Lumeng, J. C., P. Forrest, D. P. Appugliese, N. Kaciroti, R. F. Corwyn, and R. H. Bradley. 2010. Weight status as a predictor of being bullied in third through sixth grades. *Pediatrics.* 125(6):e1301–e1307.

4. Murray, S. B., E. Rieger, L. Karlov, and S.W. Touyz. 2013. An investigation of the transdiagnostic model of eating disorders in the context of muscle dysmorphia. *Eur. Eat. Disord. Rev.*, 21(2):160–164.

5. Murray, S. B., E. Rieger, S. W. Touyz, and Y. de la Garza Garcia. 2010. Muscle dysmorphia and the DSM-V conundrum: where does it belong? A Review Paper. *Int. J. Eating Disorders* 43(6):483–491.

6. Weltzin, T. E. 2013. A Silent Problem: Males with Eating Disorders in the Workplace. National Association of Anorexia Nervosa and Associated Disorders. Available at www.anad.org/get-information/males-eating-disorders/medical-director-on-males-with-eds-in-the-workplace/.

Chapter 10

1. U.S. Department of Health and Human Services. 2008. *Physical Activity Guidelines for Americans.* Available at http://www.health.gov/paguidelines/guidelines/.

2. Caspersen, C. J., K. E. Powell, and G. M. Christensen. 1985. Physical activity, exercise, and physical fitness: definitions and distinctions for health-related research. *Public Health Rep.* 100:126–131.

3. Heyward, V., and A. Gibson. 2014. *Advanced Fitness Assessment and Exercise Prescription,* 7th edn. Champaign, IL: Human Kinetics.

4. Centers for Disease Control and Prevention. 2014. Facts About Physical Activity. Available at http://www.cdc.gov/physicalactivity/data/facts.html.

5. Centers for Disease Control and Prevention, Office of Surveillance, Epidemiology, and Laboratory Services. Behavioral Risk Factor Surveillance System. 2012. Prevalence and Trend Data. Exercise – 2012. Available at http://apps.nccd.cdc.gov/brfss/list.asp?cat = EX&yr = 2012&qkey = 8041&state = All.

6. Centers for Disease Control and Prevention. 2012. Youth risk behavior surveillance—United States, 2011. *MMWR.* 61(SS-4):1–168.

7. United States Department of Health and Human Services. 2009. *2008 Physical Activity Guidelines for Americans.* Available at http://health.gov/paguidelines/guidelines/default.aspx#toc

8. Ryan, R. M., C. M. Frederick, D. Lepes, N. Rubio, and K. M. Sheldon. 1997. Intrinsic motivation and exercise adherence. *Int. J. Sport Psychol.* 28:335–354.

9. Buckworth, J., R. E. Lee, G. Regan, L. K. Schneider, and C. C. DeClemente. 2007. Decomposing intrinsic and extrinsic motivation for exercise: application to stages of motivational readiness. *Psychol. Sport Exerc.* 8(4):441–461.

10. Centers for Disease Control and Prevention. 2011. Physical Activity for Everyone. Target Heart Rate and Estimated Maximum Heart Rate. Available at www.cdc.gov/physicalactivity/everyone/measuring/heartrate.html.

11. American College of Sports Medicine, American Dietetic Association, and Dietitians of Canada. 2009. Nutrition and athletic performance. Joint position statement. *Med. Sci. Sports Exerc.* 41:709–731.

12. Burke, L. 2010. Nutrition for recovery after training and competition. In: Burke, L., and V. Deakin, eds. *Clinical Sports Nutrition,* 4th edn, pp. 358–392. New York: McGraw-Hill.

13. Phillips, S. M., and L. J. C. van Loon. 2011. Dietary protein for athletes: from requirements to optimum adaptation. *J. Sports Sci.* 29(S1):S29–S38.

14. Manore, M., N. L. Meyer, and J. Thompson. 2009. *Sports Nutrition for Health and Performance.* 2nd edn. Champaign, IL: Human Kinetics.

15. Sears, B. 1995. *The Zone: A Dietary Road Map.* New York: HarperCollins.

16. Sinclair, L. M., and P. S. Hinton. 2005. Prevalence of iron deficiency with and without anemia in recreationally active men and women. *J. Am. Diet. Assoc.* 105(6):975–978.

17. Heneghan, C., J. Howick, B. O'Neill, P. J. Gill, D. S. Lasserson, D. Cohen, . . . M. Thompson. 2012. The evidence underpinning sports performance products: a systematic assessment. *BMJ Open*, 2:e001702. Doi:10.1136/bmjopen-2012-001702.

18. Calfee, R., and P. Fadale. 2006. Popular ergogenic drugs and supplements in young athletes. *Pediatrics* 117(3):e577–e589.

19. Tarnopolsky, M. A. 2010. Caffeine and creatine use in sport. *Ann. Nutr. Metab.* 57(Suppl 2):1–8.

20. Finn, K. J., R. Lund, and M. Rosene-Treadwell. 2003. Glutamine supplementation did not benefit athletes during short-term weight reduction. *J. Sports Sci. Med.* 2:163–168.

21. Campbell, B. I., P. M. La Bounty, and M. Roberts. 2004. The ergogenic potential of arginine. *J. Int. Soc. Sports Nutr.* 1(2):35–38.

22. Zanchi, N. E., F. Gerlinger-Romero, L. Guimarães-Ferreira, M. Alves de Siqueira Filho, V. Felitti, F. Santos Lira, M. Seelaender, and A. H. Lancha, Jr. 2011. HMB supplementation: clinical and athletic performance effects and mechanisms of action. *Amino Acids.* 40:1015–1025.

23. Ransone, J., K. Neighbors, R. Lefavi, and J. Chromiak. 2003. The effect of [beta]-hydroxy [beta]-methylbutryrate on muscular strength and body composition in collegiate football players. *J. Strength Conditioning Res.* 17(1):34–39.

24. Williams, M. 2006. Dietary supplements and sports performance: metabolites, constituents, and extracts. *J. Int. Soc. Sports Nutr.* 3(2):1–5.

25. Burke, L. M. 2008. Caffeine and sports performance. *Appl. Physiol. Nutr. Metab.* 33:1319–1334.

26. Skinner T. L., D. G. Jenkins, D. R. Taaffe, M. D. Leveritt, and J. S. Coombes. 2013. Coinciding exercise with peak serum caffeine does not improve cycling performance. *J. Sci. Med. Sport.* 16(1):54–59.

27. National Institutes of Health, National Center for Complementary and Alternative Medicine (NCCAM). 2013. Herbs at a glance. Ephedra. NCCAM Publication No. D336. Available at http://nccam.nih.gov/health/ephedra.

28. Burke, L., E. Broad, G. Cox, B. Desbrow, C. Dziedzic, S. Gurr, . . . G. Slater. 2010. Supplements and sports foods. In: Burke, L., and V. Deakin, eds. *Clinical Sports Nutrition*, 4th edn, pp. 419–500. Sydney: McGraw Hill.

29. Kreider, R. B., N. A. Schwarz, and B. Leutholtz. 2012. Optimizing nutrition for exercise and sports. In: Temple, N. J., T. Wilson, and D. R. Jacobs, Jr, eds. *Nutritional Health*, 3rd edn, pp. 391–434. New York: Humana Press.

30. Pliml, W., T. von Arnim, A. Stablein, H. Hofmann, H. G. Zimmer, and E. Erdmann. 1992. Effects of ribose on exercise-induced ischaemia in stable coronary artery disease. *Lancet* 340(8818): 507–510.

31. Earnest, C. P., G. M. Morss, F. Wyatt, A. N. Jordan, S. Colson, T. S. Church, . . . A. Lucia. 2004. Effects of a commercial herbal-based formula on exercise performance in cyclists. *Med. Sci. Sports Exerc.* 36(3):504–509.

32. Hellsten, Y., L. Skadhauge, and J. Bangsbo. 2004. Effect of ribose supplementation on resynthesis of adenine nucleotides after intense intermittent training in humans. *Am. J. Physiol. Regul. Integr. Comp. Physiol.* 286:R182–R188.

33. Kreider, R. B., C. Melton, M. Greenwood, C. Rasmussen, J. Lundberg, C. Earnest, and A. Almada. 2003. Effects of oral D-ribose supplementation on anaerobic capacity and selected metabolic markers in healthy males. *Int. J. Sport Nutr. Exerc. Metab.* 13(1):76–86.

34. Artioli, G. G., B. Gualano, A. Smith, J. Stout, and A. H. Lancha, Jr. 2010. Role of ß-alanine supplementation on muscle carnosine and exercise performance. *Med. Sci. Sports Exerc.* 42(6):1162–1173.

35. Derave, W., I. Everaert, S. Beeckman, and A. Baguet. 2010. Muscle carnosine metabolism and ß-alanine supplementation in relation to exercise and training. *Sports Med.* 40(3):247–263.

36. Lansley, K. E., P. G. Winyard, S. J. Bailey, A. Vanhatalo, D. P. Wilkerson, J. R. Blackwell, . . . A. M. Jones. 2011. Acute dietary nitrate supplementation improves cycling time trial performance. *Med. Sci. Sports Exerc.* 43:1125–1131.

37. Cermak, N. M., M. J. Gibala, and L. J. van Loon. 2012. Nitrate supplementation's improvement of 10-km time-trial performance in trained cyclists. *Int. J. Sport Nutr. Exerc. Metab.* 22:64–71.

38. Murphy, M., K. Eliot, R. M. Heuertz, and E. Weiss. 2012. Whole beetroot consumption acutely improves running performance. *J. Acad. Nutr. Diet.* 112:548–552.

39. Cermak, N. M., P. Res, R. Stinkens, J. O. Lundberg, M. J. Gibala, and L. J. C. van Loon. 2012. No improvement in endurance performance after a single dose of beetroot juice. *Int. J. Sport Nutr. Exerc. Metab.* 22(6):470–478.

40. Bescós, R., V. Ferrer-Roca, P. A. Galilea, A. Roig, F. Drobnic, A. Sureda, . . . A. Pons. 2012. Sodium nitrate supplementation does not enhance performance of endurance athletes. *Med. Sci. Sports Exerc.* 44(12):2400–2409.

41. Lundberg, J. O., M. Carlström, F. J. Larsen, and E. Weitzberg. 2011. Roles of dietary inorganic nitrate in cardiovascular health and disease. *Cardiovasc. Res.* 89:525–532.

Feature Box References

1. Westerblad, H., D. G. Allen, and J. Lännergren. 2002. Muscle fatigue: lactic acid or inorganic phosphate the major cause? *News Physiol. Sci.* 17(1):17–21.

2. Brooks, G., T. Fahey, and K. Baldwin. 2005. *Exercise Physiology: Human Bioenergetics and Its Applications*. New York: McGraw-Hill.

3. Brooks, G. A. 2009. Cell-cell and intracellular lactate shuttles. *J. Physiol.* 587(23):5591–5600.

4. van Hall G., M. Stromstad, P. Rasmussen, O. Jans, M. Zaar, C. Gam, . . . and H. B. Nielsen. 2009. Blood lactate is an important energy source for the human brain. *J. Cerebral Blood Flow & Metab.* 29(6):1121–1129.

Chapter 11

1. Ogden, C. L., M. D. Carroll, B. K. Kitt, and K. M. Flegal. 2014. Prevalence of childhood and adult obesity in the United States, 2011-2012. *JAMA* 311:806–814.

2. American Diabetes Association. 2013. Fast Facts: Data and Statistics about Diabetes. Available at http://professional.diabetes.org/admin/UserFiles/0%20-%20Sean/FastFacts%20March%202013.pdf. (Accessed March 2014).

3. Brite, J., S. K. Laughon, J. Troendle, and J. Mills. 2013. Maternal overweight and obesity and risk of congenital heart defects in offspring. *International J Obesity* doi:10.1038/ijo.2013.244.

4. Delimaris, I., and S. M. Piperakis. 2014. The importance of nutritional factors on human male fertility: a toxicological approach. *J Transl Toxicol* 1:52–59.

5. Spitz, A. Male Fertility and Nutrition. Available from www.theafa.org/article/male-fertility-and-nutrition/. (Accessed March 2014).

6. Rasmussen, K. M., and A. L. Yaktine, eds., Committee to Reexamine IOM Pregnancy Weight Guidelines; Institute of Medicine; National Research Council. 2009. *Weight Gain During Pregnancy: Reexamining the Guidelines*. Washington, DC: National Academies Press.

7. Ludwig, D. S., H. L. Rouse, and J. Currie. 2013. Pregnancy weight gain and childhood body weight: a within-family comparison. *PLOS Medicine* 10(10):e1001521. Doi:10.137/journal.pmed.1001521.

8. Institute of Medicine, Food and Nutrition Board. 2002. *Dietary Reference Intakes for Energy, Carbohydrate, Fiber, Fat, Fatty Acids, Cholesterol, Protein, and Amino Acids*. Washington, DC: National Academies Press.

9. U.S. Food and Drug Administration. 2014.–Fish: What Pregnant Women and Parents Should Know: Draft updated advice by FDA and EPA. Available at http://www.fda.gov/Food/FoodborneIllness Contaminants/Metals/ucm393070.htm#Advice. (Accessed June 2014).

10. Institute of Medicine, Food and Nutrition Board. 1998. *Dietary Reference Intakes for Thiamin, Riboflavin, Niacin, Vitamin B$_6$, Folate, Vitamin B$_{12}$, Pantothenic Acid, Biotin, and Choline*. Washington, DC: National Academies Press.

11. Institute of Medicine, Food and Nutrition Board. 2001. *Dietary Reference Intakes for Vitamin A, Vitamin K, Arsenic, Boron, Chromium, Copper, Iodine, Iron, Manganese, Molybdenum, Nickel, Silicon, Vanadium, and Zinc*. Washington, DC: National Academies Press.

12. Institute of Medicine, Food and Nutrition Board. 2011. *Dietary Reference Intakes for Calcium and Vitamin D*. Washington, DC: National Academies Press.

13. Institute of Medicine, Food and Nutrition Board. 2004. *Dietary Reference Intakes for Water, Potassium, Sodium, Chloride, and Sulfate*. Washington, DC: National Academies Press.

14. American Diabetes Association. 2013. Standards of Medical Care in Diabetes—2013. *Diabetes Care*. 36:S11–S66.

15. U.S. Department of Health & Human Services. Office of Adolescent Health. 2013. Trends in Teen Pregnancy and Childbearing. Available at www.dhhs.gov/ash/oah/adolescent-health-topics/reproductive-health/teen-pregnancy/trends.html (Accessed April 2014)

16. March of Dimes. 2014. Caffeine in Pregnancy. www.marchofdimes.com/pregnancy/caffeine-in-pregnancy.aspx. (Accessed April 2014).

17. Centers for Disease Control and Prevention. 2012. Use and binge drinking among women of childbearing age—United States, 2006–2010. *Morbidity and Mortality Weekly Report*. 61(28): 534–538.

18. Martin, T. 2014. Smoking during pregnancy: the risks to our children. Available at http://quitsmoking.about.com/od/tobaccostatistics/a/SGRpregnancy.htm. (Accessed May 2014).

19. American Pregnancy Association. Using illegal drugs during pregnancy. 2013. Available at http://americanpregnancy.org/pregnancyhealth/illegaldrugs.html (Accessed May 2014).

20. Fieril, K. P., M. F. Olsén, A. Glantz, and M. Larsson. 2014. Experiences of exercise during pregnancy among women who perform regular resistance training: a qualitative study. *Physical Therapy*. 94. doi: 10.2522/.

21. Centers for Disease Control and Prevention. Physical Activity: Healthy Pregnant or Postpartum Women. Available at www.cdc.gov/physicalactivity/everyone/guidelines/pregnancy.html. (Accessed May 2014).

22. American Academy of Pediatrics. 2005. Policy Statement: breastfeeding and the use of human milk. *Pediatrics* 115:496–506.

23. Bartick, M., and A. Reinhold. 2010. The burden of suboptimal breastfeeding in the United States: a pediatric cost analysis. *Pediatrics*. 125:e1048–e1056.

24. Clayton, H. B., R. Li, C. G. Perrine, and K. S Scanlon. 2013. Prevalence and reasons for introducing infants early to solid foods: variations by milk feeding type. *Pediatrics*. 131(4):e1108–e1114.

25. Howard, A. J., K. M. Mallan, R. Byrne, A. Magarey, and L. A. Daniels. 2012. Toddlers' food preferences. The impact of novel food exposure, maternal preferences and food neophobia. *Appetite*. 59:818–825.

26. Snow, S. 2013. Most children's meals at large restaurant chains are still unhealthy, a study finds. *The New York Times*. March 28, 2013.

27. The Healthy, Hunger-Free Kids Act of 2010; Public Law No. 111-296.

28. Barnes, M. May 2010. *Solving the Problem of Childhood Obesity. White House Task Force on Childhood Obesity. Report to the President*. Washington, DC: White House Task Force on Childhood Obesity.

29. Adolphus, K., C. L. Lawton, and L. Dye. 2013. The effects of breakfast on behaviour and academic performance in children and adolescents. *Frontiers Human Neurosci*. 7:425. doi:10.3389/fnhum.2013.00425.

30. Rausch, R. 2013. Nutrition and academic performance in school-age children: the relation to obesity and food insufficiency. *J Nutr Food Sci*. 3:190. doi:10.4172/2155-9600.1000190.

31. Hayes, D., M. Spano, J. E. Donnelly, C. H. Hillman, and R. Kleinman. 2014. Proceedings of the Learning Connection Summit: Nutrition, physical activity and student achievement. *Nutrition Today*. 49:18–25.

32. Leidy, H. J., L. C. Ortinau, S. M. Douglas, and H. A. Hoertel. 2013. Beneficial effects of a higher-protein breakfast on the appetitive, hormonal, and neural signals controlling energy intake regulation in overweight/obese "breakfast-skipping", late adolescent girls. *Am J Clin Nutr*. 97:677–688.

33. Fiese, B. H., C. Gundersen, B. Koester, and L. Washington. 2011. Household food insecurity—serious concerns for child development. *Social Policy Report* 25:3–19.

34. Larson, N., R. MacLehose, J. A. Fulkerson, J. M. Berge, M. Story, and D. Neumark-Sztainer. 2013. Eating breakfast and dinner together as a family: associations with sociodemographic characteristics and implications for diet quality and weight status. *J Acad Nutr Diet*. 113:1601–1609.

35. Centers for Disease Control and Prevention. 2013. Physical Activity Facts. Available at www.cdc.gov/healthyyouth/physicalactivity/facts.htm. (Accessed May 2014).

36. Weaver, C. M. 2014. Milk consumption and bone health. *JAMA Pediatr*. 168:12–13.

37. Burris, J., W. Rietkerk, and K. Woolf. 2013. Acne: the role of medical nutrition therapy. *J Acad Nutr Dietet*. 113:416–430.

38. Centers for Disease Control and Prevention. 2013. *The State of Aging and Health in America 2013*. Atlanta, GA: Centers for Disease Control and Prevention, U.S. Department of Health and Human Services.

39. *Huffington Post*. 2013. U.S. Life Expectancy Ranks 26th in the World, OECD Report Shows. Available at www.huffingtonpost.com/2013/11/21/us-life-expectancy-oecd_n_4317367.html. (Accessed May 2014).

40. Rowley, L. 2012. Senior Poverty: Food Insecurity Rising Among Older Americans. *Huffington Post*. Available at www.huffingtonpost.com/2012/08/29/senior-poverty-hunger_n_1834583.html (Accessed May 2014).

41. Food Research and Action Center. 2013. SNAP and public health: the role of the Supplemental Nutrition Assistance Program in improving the health and well-being of Americans. Available at www.frac.org/pdf/snap_and_public_health_2013.pdf. (Accessed May 2013).

Feature Box References

1. The Healthy, Hunger-Free Kids Act of 2010; Public Law No. 111-296.

2. Barnes, M. May 2010. *Solving the Problem of Childhood Obesity. White House Task Force on Childhood Obesity. Report to the President*. Washington, DC: White House Task Force on Childhood Obesity.

3. Adolphus, K., C. L. Lawton, and L. Dye. 2013. The effects of breakfast on behaviour and academic performance in children and adolescents. *Frontiers Human Neurosci* 7:425. doi:10.3389/fnhum.2013.00425.

4. Rausch, R. 2013. Nutrition and academic performance in school-age children: the relation to obesity and food insufficiency. *J Nutr Food Sci* 3:190. doi:10.4172/2155-9600.1000190.

5. Hayes, D., M. Spano, J. E. Donnelly, C. H. Hillman, and R. Kleinman. 2014. Proceedings of the Learning Connection Summit: Nutrition, physical activity ad student achievement. *Nutrition Today* 49:18–25.

6. Leidy, H. J., L. C. Ortinau, S. M. Douglas, and H. A. Hoertel. 2013. Beneficial effects of a higher-protein breakfast on the appetitive, hormonal, and neural signals controlling energy intake regulation in overweight/obese "breakfast-skipping", late adolescent girls. *Am J Clin Nutr*. 97:677–688.

Chapter 12

1. U.S. Centers for Disease Control and Prevention (CDC). 2013. Surveillance for Norovirus Outbreaks. *CDC Features*. Available at http://www.cdc.gov/features/dsNorovirus/. (Accessed October 2013).

2. U.S. Food and Drug Administration. 2014. Recalls, Market Withdrawals, & Safety Alerts. Available at http://www.fda.gov/Safety/Recalls/default.htm#Link_to_Food. (Accessed March 2014).

3. U.S. Centers for Disease Control and Prevention (CDC). Updated 2014, January 8. *Estimates of Foodborne Illness in the United States*. Available at http://www.cdc.gov/foodborneburden/index.html.

4. U.S. Government Accountability Office. 2012. Food Safety: FDA's Advisory and Recall Process Needs Strengthening. Available at http://www.gao.gov/assets/600/593032.pdf. (Accessed July 2012).

5. U.S. Food and Drug Administration. 2013. FDA proposes new food safety standards for foodborne illness prevention and food safety. Available at http://www.fda.gov/newsevents/newsroom/pressannouncements/ucm334156. (Accessed January 2013).

6. U.S. Centers for Disease Control and Prevention (CDC). 2013. Trends in Foodborne Illness in the United States, 2012. Available at http://www.cdc.gov/features/dsfoodnet2012/. (Accessed April 2013).

7. U.S. Centers for Disease Control and Prevention (CDC). 2013. Norovirus. Available at http://www.cdc.gov/norovirus/index.html. (Accessed October 2013).

8. U.S. Centers for Disease Control and Prevention (CDC). 2013. Hepatitis A Information for Health Professionals. Available at http://www.cdc.gov/hepatitis/HAV/HAVfaq.htm#general. (Accessed June 2013).

9. U.S. Centers for Disease Control and Prevention (CDC). 2012. Trichinellosis FAQs. Available at http://www.cdc.gov/parasites/trichinellosis/gen_info/faqs.html. (Accessed August 2012).

10. U.S. Centers for Disease Control and Prevention (CDC). 2013. Parasites: Toxoplasmosis: *Toxoplasma* infection. Available at http://www.cdc.gov/parasites/toxoplasmosis/. (Accessed January 2013).

11. U.S. Centers for Disease Control and Prevention (CDC). 2012. Giardiasis: Frequently Asked Questions (FAQs). Available at http://www.cdc.gov/parasites/giardia/gen_info/faqs.html.

12. U.S. Centers for Disease Control and Prevention (CDC). 2014. A-Z Index for Foodborne Illness. Available at http://www.cdc.gov/foodsafety/diseases/#fungal. (Accessed January 2014).

13. U.S. Department of Agriculture Food Safety and Inspection Service. 2013. Clostridium Botulinum. Available at http://www.fsis.usda.gov/wps/portal/fsis/topics/food-safety-education/get-answers/food-safety-fact-sheets/foodborne-illness-and-disease/clostridium-botulinum. (Accessed August 2013).

14. U.S. Centers for Disease Control and Prevention (CDC). 2010. *Marine Toxins*. Available at www.cdc.gov/nczved/divisions/dfbmd/diseases/marine_toxins/. (Accessed July 2010).

15. Habal, R. 2012. Mushroom Toxicity. *Medscape Reference*. Available at http://emedicine.medscape.com/article/167398-overview. (Accessed December 2012).

16. Woods Hole Oceanographic Institution. 2010. Watch What You Eat. Available at http://www.whoi.edu/page.do?pid=83338&tid=3622&cid=80526. (Accessed August 2010).

17. National Institutes of Health. 2011. Potato plant poisoning: green tubers and sprouts. *MedlinePlus*. www.nlm.nih.gov/medlineplus/ency/article/002875.htm. (Accessed December 2011).

18. U.S. Department of Agriculture Food Safety and Inspection Service. 2013. *Basics for Handling Food Safely*. Available at http://www.fsis.usda.gov/wps/portal/fsis/topics/food-safety-education/get-answers/food-safety-fact-sheets/safe-food-handling/basics-for-handling-food-safely/ct_index. (Accessed August 2013).

19. U.S. Centers for Disease Control and Prevention (CDC). 2012. Multistate Outbreak of Salmonella Bareilly and Salmonella Nchanga Infections Associated with a Raw Scraped Ground Tuna Product. Available at www.cdc.gov/salmonella/bareilly-04-12/index.html. (Accessed May 2012).

20. Center for Science in the Public Interest (CSPI). 2014. Chemical Cuisine. Learn About Food Additives. Available at www.cspinet.org/reports/chemcuisine.htm.

21. U.S. Food and Drug Administration. 2013. FDA Targets Trans Fat in Processed Food. http://www.fda.gov/forconsumers/consumerupdates/ucm372915.htm. (Accessed December 2013).

22. U.S. Department of Agriculture Economic Research Service. 2013. Data Sets: Adoption of Genetically Engineered Crops in the U.S. Available at http://www.ers.usda.gov/data-products/adoption-of-genetically-engineered-crops-in-the-us.aspx#.UxYVOnnIbwI. (Accessed July 2013).

23. U.S. Environmental Protection Agency. 2012. Persistent Organic Pollutants: A Global Issue, A Global Response. Available at www.epa.gov/international/toxics/pop.html. (Accessed July 2012).

24. Food and Drug Administration. 2013. What You Need to Know About Mercury in Fish and Shellfish. Available at www.fda.gov/Food/ResourcesForYou/Consumers/ucm110591.htm. (Accessed June 2013).

25. National Institute of Environmental Health Sciences. 2014. Endocrine Disruptors. Available at http://www.niehs.nih.gov/health/topics/agents/endocrine/#healthstudies. (Accessed March 2014).

26. Buck Louis, G. M., R. Sundaram, A. M. Sweeney, et al. 2014. Urinary bisphenol A, phthalates, and couple fecundity: the Longitudinal Investigation of Fertility and the Environment (LIFE) Study. *Fertil steril.* 2014 Feb 14. pii: S0015-0282(14)00067-3. doi:10.1016/j.fertnstert.2014.01.022.

27. National Institute of Environmental Health Sciences. 2012. Questions and Answers About Bisphenol A. Available at http://www.niehs.nih.gov/health/topics/agents/sya-bpa/index.cfm. (Accessed November 2012).

28. U.S. Environmental Protection Agency. 2012. EPA's Reanalysis of Key Issues Related to Dioxin Toxicity and Response to NAS Comments, Volume 1. EPA 600/R-10/038F. Available at http://www.epa.gov/iris/supdocs/dioxinv1sup.pdf. (Accessed February 2012).

29. U.S. Food and Drug Administration. 2013. *Questions and Answers About Dioxins and Food Safety*. Available at http://www.fda.gov/food/foodborneillnesscontaminants/chemicalcontaminants/ucm077524.htm. (Accessed June 2013).

30. American Academy of Pediatrics. 2012. AAP Makes Recommendations to Reduce Children's Exposure to Pesticides. Available at http://www.aap.org/en-us/about-the-aap/aap-press-room/Pages/AAP-Makes-Recommendations-to-Reduce-Children's-Exposure-to-Pesticides.aspx. (Accessed November 2012).

31. Environmental Protection Agency (EPA). 2012. Pesticides and Food: Healthy, Sensible Food Practices. Available at www.epa.gov/pesticides/food/tips.htm. (Accessed May 2012).

32. American Cancer Society. 2011. Recombinant Bovine Growth Hormone. Available at www.cancer.org/cancer/cancercauses/othercarcinogens/athome/recombinant-bovine-growth-hormone. (Accessed February 2011).

33. Environmental Working Group. 2013. Superbugs invade American supermarkets. Available at http://www.ewg.org/meateatersguide/superbugs/.

34. Smith, T. C., M. J. Male, A. L. Harper, J. S. Kroeger, G. P. Tinkler, et al. 2009. Methicillin-Resistant *Staphylococcus aureus* (MRSA) Strain ST398 Is Present in Midwestern U.S. Swine and Swine Workers. PLoS ONE 4(1): e4258. doi:10.1371/journal.pone.0004258.

35. Pastagia, M., L. C. Kleinman, E. G. Lacerda de la Cruz, and S. G. Jenkins. 2012. Predicting risk for death from MRSA bacteremia. *Emerg Infect Dis.* 2012 Jul;18(7). Available at http://wwwnc.cdc.gov/eid/article/18/7/10-1371_article.

36. United States Department of Agriculture, Agricultural Marketing Service. 2014. National Organic Program. *Welcome to the National Organic Program*. Available at http://www.ams.usda.gov/AMSv1.0/ams.fetchTemplateData.do?template=TemplateA&navID=NOPHomelinkNOPOrganicStandards&rightNav1=NOPHomelinkNOPOrganicStandards&topNav=&leftNav=NationalOrganicProgram&page=NOPNationalOrganicProgramHome&resultType=&acct=nop. (Accessed January 2014).

37. Laux, M. 2013. Organic Foods Trends Profile. Agricultural Marketing Resources Center. Available at http://www.agmrc.org/markets__industries/food/organic-food-trends-profile/. (Accessed November 2013).

38. Brandt, K., C. Leifert, R. Sanderson, and C. J. Seal. 2011. Agro-ecosystem management and nutritional quality of plant foods: the

case of organic fruits and vegetables. *Critical Reviews in Plant Sciences*. 2011 April;30(1–2):177–197.

39. Smith-Spangler C., et al. Are organic foods safer or healthier than conventional alternatives? A systematic review. *Ann Intern Med*. 2012;157(5):348–366. doi:10.7326/0003-4819-157-5-201209040-00007.

40. Baranski, M, et al. 2014. Higher antioxidant and lower cadmium concentrations and lower incidence of pesticide residues in organically grown crops: a systemic literature review and meta-analyses. *British Journal of Nutrition*. 2014 June 26:1–18.

41. Environmental Protection Agency (EPA). n.d. What Is Sustainability? Available at www.epa.gov/sustainability/basicinfo.htm.

42. Louis Bonduelle Foundation. 2012. Biology, varietal improvement & GMOs: summary of the green revolution. Available at http://www.fondation-louisbonduelle.org/france/en/know-your-vegetables/vegetables-benefits/biology-varietal-improvement-omgs-summary-of-the-green-revolution.html#axzz2MIqNojGW. (Accessed March 2012).

43. Imhoff, D., and M. Dimock. 2012. America needs a farm bill that works. *Los Angeles Times*. Available at http://www.latimes.com/news/opinion/commentary/la-oe-imhoff-farm-bill-20120608,0,7923048.story. (Accessed June 2012).

44. Khoury, C. K., et al. 2014. Increasing homogeneity in global food supplies and the implications for food security. *Proc Natl Acad Sci USA*. doi:10.1073/pnas.1313490111.

45. Slow Food USA. 2014. About Us. Accessed March 3, 2014. http://www.slowfoodusa.org/about-us.

46. Edwards-Jones, G. 2010. Does eating local food reduce the environmental impact of food production and enhance consumer health? *Proceedings of the Nutrition Society*. 69, 582–591.

47. United States Department of Agriculture. 2014. Preliminary Report Highlights: U.S. Farms and Farmers. *2012 Census of Agriculture*. Available at http://www.agcensus.usda.gov/Publications/2012/Preliminary_Report/Highlights.pdf. (Accessed February 2014).

48. LocalHarvest. 2014. Community Supported Agriculture. Available at www.localharvest.org/csa/.

49. U.S. Department of Agriculture, Agricultural Marketing Service. 2013. Farmers Markets and Local Food Marketing: 1994–2013. Available at http://www.ams.usda.gov/AMSv1.0/ams.fetchTemplateData.do?template = TemplateS&navID = WholesaleandFarmersMarkets&leftNav = WholesaleandFarmersMarkets&page = WFMFarmersMarketGrowth&description = Farmers%20Market%20Growth&acct = frmrdirmkt. (Accessed August 2013).

50. Eschmeyer, D. 2012. FoodCorps is one of several efforts to give children healthy foods. *Washington Post*. Available at http://www.washingtonpost.com/postlive/foodcorps-is-one-of-several-efforts-to-give-children-healthy-foods/2012/06/18/gJQAepNLoV_story.html. (Accessed June 2012).

51. Wortham, J., and C. Cain Miller. 2013. Venture capitalists are making bigger bets on food start-ups. *The New York Times*. Available at http://www.nytimes.com/2013/04/29/business/venture-capitalists-are-making-bigger-bets-on-food-start-ups.html?pagewanted = 1&_r = 1&ref = global-home. (Accessed April 2013).

52. World Hunger Education Service. 2013. 2013 World hunger and poverty facts and statistics. Available at http://www.worldhunger.org/articles/Learn/world%20hunger%20facts%202002.htm

53. Fanzo, J. C., and P. M. Pronyk. 2011. A review of global progress toward the Millennium Development Goal 1 Hunger Target. *Food Nutr Bull*. 2011 Jun;32(2):144–158.

54. Coleman-Jensen, A., M. Nord, and A. Singh. 2013. *Household Food Security in the United States in 2012*. U.S. Dept. of Agriculture, Economic Research Service. Available at http://www.ers.usda.gov. (Accessed September 2013).

55. U.S. Department of Health & Human Services. 2014 Poverty Guidelines, *Federal Register*, January 24, 2013. Available at http://aspe.hhs.gov/poverty/14poverty.cfm.

56. U.S. Centers for Disease Control and Prevention. 2012. A Look Inside Food Deserts. Available at http://www.cdc.gov/Features/FoodDeserts/. (Accessed September 2012).

57. Healthy Corner Stores Network. 2013. *Food Deserts*. Available at www.healthycornerstores.org/tag/food-deserts. (Accessed July 2013).

58. Moore Lappé, F. 2011. The food movement: its power and possibilities. *The Nation*. Available at www.thenation.com/article/163403/food-movement-its-power-and-possibilities. (Accessed September 2011).

59. Fair Trade USA. 2013. Fair Trade Certified™ Media Kit 2013. Available at http://fairtradeusa.org.

Feature Box References

1. International Society for Infectious Diseases. 2013. *Prion Disease Update 2013*. Available at http://www.promedmail.org. (Accessed October 2013).

2. U.S. Department of Agriculture Animal and Plant Health Inspection Service. 2012. *Update from APHIS Regarding Release of the Final Report on the BSE Epidemiological Investigation*. Available at http://www.aphis.usda.gov/newsroom/2012/08/bse_update.shtml. (Accessed August 2012).

3. U.S. Department of Agriculture. 2013. Press Release: APHIS Finalizes Bovine Import Regulations in Line with International Animal Health Standards. Available at http://www.usda.gov/wps/portal/usda/usdahome?contentid = 2013/11/0207.xml&contentidonly = true. (Accessed November 2013).

4. U.S. Food and Drug Administration. 2013. Food Facts. Eating Outdoors, Handling Food Safely. Available at http://www.fda.gov/food/foodborneillnesscontaminants/buystoreservesafefood/ucm109899.htm. (Accessed May 2013).

5. International Service for the Acquisition of Agri-Biotech Applications. 2012. Global Status of Commercialized Biotech/GM Crops: 2011. ISAAA Brief No. 43-2011: Executive summary. Ithaca, NY: ISAAA. Available at http://www.isaaa.org/resources/publications/briefs/43/executivesummary/default.asp.

6. Benbrook, C. N. 2012. Impacts of genetically engineered crops on pesticide use in the U.S.—The first 16 years. *Environmental Sciences Europe*. 28 September 2012, 24:24.

7. Lincoln P., et al. 2012. Decline of monarch butterflies overwintering in Mexico: is the migratory phenomenon at risk? *Insect Conservation and Diversity*, March. 5(2):95–100.

8. World Health Organization. 20 Questions on Genetically Modified Foods. Accessed 2014. http://www.who.int/foodsafety/publications/biotech/20questions/en/.

9. Union of Concerned Scientists. Genetic Engineering Risks and Impacts. Revised November 7, 2013. Available at http://www.ucsusa.org/food_and_agriculture/our-failing-food-system/genetic-engineering/risks-of-genetic-engineering.html.

10. U.S. Food and Drug Administration. 2013. Questions and Answers on Foods From Genetically Engineered Plants. Available at www.fda.gov/food/foodscienceresearch/biotechnology/ucm346030.htm. (Accessed April 2013).

11. Shiva, V. 2011. Resisting the corporate theft of seeds. *The Nation*. Available at www.thenation.com/article/163401/resisting-corporate-theft-seeds. (Accessed September 2011).

12. Center for Food Safety. 2014. U.S. Polls on GE Food Labeling. Available at http://www.centerforfoodsafety.org/issues/976/ge-food-labeling/us-polls-on-ge-food-labeling#.

answers to Review Questions

Chapter 1
1. d
2. a
3. d
4. b
5. c
6. c
7. b
8. b
9. a
10. b

Chapter 2
1. c
2. d
3. a
4. c
5. a
6. b
7. b
8. b
9. c
10. D

Chapter 3
1. a
2. b
3. c
4. b
5. d
6. d
7. a
8. c
9. b
10. a

Chapter 4
1. c
2. a
3. d
4. d
5. a
6. b
7. c
8. b
9. d
10. c

Chapter 5
1. b
2. b
3. d
4. a
5. c
6. a
7. a
8. d
9. a
10. b

Chapter 6
1. c
2. b
3. d
4. a
5. c
6. d
7. a
8. c
9. d
10. b

Chapter 7
1. c
2. d
3. b
4. a
5. c
6. b
7. b
8. d
9. d
10. a

Chapter 8
1. a
2. b
3. d
4. a
5. c
6. c
7. d
8. b
9. c
10. d

Chapter 9
1. a
2. d
3. a
4. c
5. c
6. b
7. d
8. a
9. d
10. c

Chapter 10
1. d
2. a
3. c
4. d
5. c
6. a
7. b
8. b
9. b
10. c

Chapter 11
1. b
2. a
3. b
4. a
5. c
6. c
7. d
8. d
9. b
10. d

Chapter 12
1. a
2. b
3. c
4. c
5. b
6. d
7. d
8. a
9. d
10. a

glossary

A

absorption   The physiologic process by which molecules of food are taken from the GI tract into the body.

Acceptable Daily Intake (ADI)   An estimate made by the Food and Drug Administration of the amount of a non-nutritive sweetener that someone can consume each day over a lifetime without adverse effects.

Acceptable Macronutrient Distribution Range (AMDR)   A range of intakes for a particular energy source that is associated with reduced risk for chronic disease while providing adequate intake of essential nutrients.

accessory organs   Organs that assist in digestion but are not anatomically part of the GI tract; they include the salivary glands, liver, gallbladder, and pancreas.

added sugars   Sugars and syrups that are added to food during processing or preparation.

adenosine triphosphate (ATP)   The common currency of energy for virtually all cells of the body.

adequate diet   A diet that provides enough energy, nutrients, and fiber to maintain a person's health.

Adequate Intake (AI)   A recommended average daily nutrient intake level based on observed or experimentally determined estimates of nutrient intake by a group of healthy people.

aerobic exercise   Exercise that involves the repetitive movement of large muscle groups, increasing the body's use of oxygen and promoting cardiovascular health.

alcohol poisoning   A potentially fatal condition in which an overdose of alcohol results in cardiac or respiratory failure.

alcohol   A beverage made from fermented fruits, vegetables, or grains.

alpha-linolenic acid   An essential fatty acid found in leafy green vegetables, flaxseed oil, soy oil, fish oil, and fish products; an omega-3 fatty acid.

amenorrhea   The absence of menstruation. In females who had previously been menstruating, the absence of menstrual periods for 3 or more months.

amino acids   Nitrogen-containing molecules that combine to form proteins.

amniotic fluid   The watery fluid contained in the innermost membrane of the sac containing the fetus. It cushions and protects the growing fetus.

anabolic   The term used for a substance that builds muscle and increases strength.

anaerobic   Means "without oxygen"; refers to metabolic reactions that occur in the absence of oxygen.

anencephaly   A fatal neural tube defect in which there is a partial absence of brain tissue, most likely caused by failure of the neural tube to close.

anorexia nervosa   A serious, potentially life-threatening eating disorder that is characterized by self-starvation, which eventually leads to a deficiency in the energy and essential nutrients the body requires to function normally.

antibodies   Defensive proteins of the immune system. Their production is prompted by the presence of bacteria, viruses, toxins, or allergens.

antioxidant   A compound that has the ability to prevent or repair the damage caused by oxidation.

appetite   A psychological desire to consume specific foods.

ariboflavinosis   A condition caused by riboflavin deficiency.

atrophic gastritis   A condition that results in low stomach acid secretion, estimated to occur in about 10% to 30% of adults older than 50 years of age.

B

bacteria   Microorganisms that lack a true nucleus and reproduce by division or by forming spores.

balanced diet   A diet that contains the combinations of foods that provide the proper proportion of nutrients.

basal metabolic rate (BMR)   The energy the body expends to maintain its fundamental physiologic functions.

beriberi   A disease caused by thiamin deficiency.

bile   Fluid produced by the liver and stored in the gallbladder that emulsifies fats in the small intestine.

binge drinking   The consumption of 5 or more alcoholic drinks on one occasion.

binge eating   Consumption of a large amount of food in a short period of time, usually accompanied by a feeling of loss of self-control.

binge-eating disorder   An eating disorder characterized by binge eating an average of twice a week or more, typically without compensatory purging.

bioavailability   The degree to which our body can absorb and use any given nutrient.

biologic age   Physiologic age as determined by health and functional status; often estimated by scored questionnaires.

biomagnification   Process by which persistent organic pollutants become more concentrated in animal tissues as they move from one creature to another through the food chain.

biopesticides   Primarily insecticides, these chemicals use natural methods to reduce damage to crops.

blood volume   The amount of fluid in blood.

body composition   The ratio of a person's body fat to lean body mass.

body image   A person's perception of his or her body's appearance and functioning.

body mass index (BMI)   A measurement representing the ratio of a person's body weight to his or her height.

bone density   The degree of compactness of bone tissue, reflecting the strength of the bones. *Peak bone density* is the point at which a bone is strongest.

brown adipose tissue   A type of adipose tissue that has more mitochondria than white adipose tissue, and which can increase energy expenditure by uncoupling certain steps in the energy production process.

buffers   Proteins that help maintain proper acid–base balance by attaching to, or releasing, hydrogen ions as conditions change in the body.

bulimia nervosa   A serious eating disorder characterized by recurrent episodes of binge eating and compensatory behaviors in order to prevent weight gain, such as self-induced vomiting.

C

cancer   A group of diseases characterized by cells that reproduce spontaneously and independently and may invade other tissues and organs.

carbohydrate   One of the three macronutrients, a compound made up of carbon, hydrogen, and oxygen. It is derived from plants and provides energy.

carbohydrate loading   The practice of altering training and carbohydrate intake so that muscle glycogen storage is maximized; also known as *glycogen loading*.

carbohydrates   The primary fuel source for our body, particularly for the brain and for physical exercise.

carcinogens   Cancer-causing agents, such as certain pesticides, industrial chemicals, and pollutants.

cardiovascular disease   A general term referring to abnormal conditions (dysfunction) of the heart and blood vessels; cardiovascular disease can result in heart attack or stroke.

carotenoid   Fat-soluble plant pigment that the body stores in the liver and adipose tissues. The body is able to convert certain carotenoids to vitamin A.

celiac disease   An immune disease in which consumption of gluten triggers damage to the lining of the small intestine that interferes with the absorption of nutrients.

cell differentiation   The process by which immature, undifferentiated cells develop into highly specialized functional cells of discrete organs and tissues.

cell membrane   The boundary of an animal cell that separates its internal cytoplasm, nucleus, and other structures from the external environment.

cells   The smallest units of matter that exhibit the properties of living things, such as growth, reproduction, and the taking in of nutrients.

chronologic age   Age as defined by calendar years, from date of birth.

chylomicron   A lipoprotein produced in the enterocyte; transports dietary fat out of the intestinal tract.

chyme   Semifluid mass consisting of partially digested food, water, and gastric juice.

cirrhosis   End-stage liver disease characterized by significant abnormalities in liver structure and function; may lead to complete liver failure.

coenzyme   A compound that combines with an inactive enzyme to form an active enzyme.

colic   A condition in infants marked by inconsolable crying for unknown reasons that lasts for hours at a time.

collagen   A protein found in all connective tissues in our body.

colostrum   The first fluid made and secreted by the breasts from late in pregnancy to about a week after birth. It is rich in immune factors and protein.

complementary proteins   Two or more foods that together contain all nine essential amino acids necessary for a complete protein. It is not necessary to eat complementary proteins at the same meal.

complete proteins   Foods that contain all nine essential amino acids.

complex carbohydrate   A nutrient compound consisting of long chains of glucose molecules, such as starch, glycogen, and fiber.

conception   The uniting of an ovum (egg) and sperm to create a fertilized egg.

constipation   A condition characterized by the absence of bowel movements for a period of time that is significantly longer than normal for the individual. When a bowel movement does occur, stools are usually small, hard, and difficult to pass.

cool-down   Activities done after an exercise session is completed; they should be gradual and allow your body to slowly recover from exercise.

cortical bone   A dense bone tissue that makes up the outer surface of all bones as well as the entirety of most small bones of the body; also called compact bone.

creatine phosphate (CP)   A high-energy compound that can be broken down for energy and used to regenerate ATP.

cretinism   A form of mental retardation that occurs in people whose mothers experienced iodine deficiency during pregnancy.

crop rotation   The practice of alternating crops in a particular field to prevent nutrient depletion and erosion of the soil and to help with control of crop-specific pests.

cross-contamination   Contamination of one food by another via the unintended transfer of microorganisms through physical contact.

cytoplasm   The fluid within an animal cell, enclosed by the cell membrane.

D

danger zone   Range of temperature (about 40°F to 140°F [4°C to 60°C]) at which many microorganisms capable of causing human disease thrive.

dehydration   A serious condition of depleted body fluid that results when fluid excretion exceeds fluid intake.

diabetes   A serious, chronic disease in which the body can no longer regulate glucose.

diarrhea   A condition characterized by the frequent passage of loose, watery stools.

dietary fiber   The type of fiber that occurs naturally in foods.

Dietary Guidelines for Americans   A set of principles developed by the U.S. Department of Agriculture and the U.S. Department of Health and Human Services to assist Americans in designing a healthful diet and lifestyle.

Dietary Reference Intakes (DRIs)   A set of nutritional reference values for the United States and Canada that apply to healthy people.

digestion   The process by which foods are broken down into their component molecules, both mechanically and chemically.

disaccharide   A carbohydrate compound consisting of two sugar molecules joined together.

disordered eating   A general term used to describe a variety of abnormal or atypical eating behaviors that are used to keep or maintain a lower body weight.

diuretic   A substance that increases fluid loss via the urine. Common diuretics include alcohol and some prescription medications for high blood pressure and other disorders.

DNA   A molecule present in the nucleus of all body cells that directs the assembly of amino acids into body proteins.

docosahexaenoic acid (DHA)   A type of omega-3 fatty acid that can be made in the body from alpha-linolenic acid and found in our diet primarily in marine plants and animals; together with EPA, it appears to reduce our risk for a heart attack.

drink   The amount of an alcoholic beverage that provides approximately 1/2 fl. oz of pure ethanol.

E

eating disorder   A clinically diagnosed psychiatric disorder characterized by severe disturbances in body image and eating behaviors.

edema   A disorder in which fluids build up in the tissue spaces of the body, causing fluid imbalances and a swollen appearance.

eicosapentaenoic acid (EPA) A type of omega-3 fatty acid that can be made in the body from alpha-linolenic acid and found in our diet primarily in marine plants and animals.

electrolyte A (mineral) substance that dissolves in solution into positively and negatively charged ions and is thus capable of carrying an electrical current.

elimination The process by which the undigested portions of food and waste products are removed from the body.

embryo The human growth and developmental stage lasting from the third week to the end of the eighth week after conception.

empty Calories Calories from solid fats and/or added sugars that provide few or no nutrients.

endocrine disruptors Chemicals that may interfere with the body's endocrine system and produce adverse developmental, reproductive, neurological, and immune effects.

energy cost of physical activity The energy expended on body movement and muscular work above basal levels.

energy expenditure The energy the body expends to maintain its basic functions and to perform all levels of movement and activity.

energy intake The amount of food a person eats; in other words, it is the number of kilocalories consumed.

enzymes Chemicals, usually proteins, that act on other chemicals to speed up body processes.

ergogenic aids Substances used to improve exercise and athletic performance.

esophagus Muscular tube of the GI tract connecting the back of the mouth to the stomach.

essential amino acids Amino acids not produced by the body that must be obtained from food.

essential fatty acids (EFAs) Fatty acids that must be consumed in the diet because they cannot be made by our body. The two essential fatty acids are linoleic acid and alpha-linolenic acid.

Estimated Average Requirement (EAR) The average daily nutrient intake level estimated to meet the requirement of half of the healthy individuals in a particular life stage and gender group.

Estimated Energy Requirement (EER) The average dietary energy intake that is predicted to maintain energy balance in a healthy adult.

evaporative cooling Another term for sweating, which is the primary way in which we dissipate heat.

exercise A subcategory of leisure-time physical activity; any activity that is purposeful, planned, and structured.

F

fair trade A trading partnership promoting equity in international trading relationships and contributing to sustainable development by securing the rights of marginalized producers and workers.

fat-soluble vitamins Vitamins that are not soluble in water but soluble in fat. These include vitamins A, D, E, and K.

fats An important energy source for our body at rest and during low-intensity exercise.

fatty acids Long chains of carbon atoms bound to each other as well as to hydrogen atoms.

female athlete triad A syndrome combining three clinical conditions in some physically active females: low energy availability (with or without eating disorders), menstrual dysfunction, and low bone density.

fetal alcohol spectrum disorders (FASD) An umbrella term describing the range of effects that can occur in the child of a woman who drinks during pregnancy.

fetal alcohol syndrome (FAS) A cluster of birth defects in the children of a mother who consumed alcohol during pregnancy, including facial deformities, impaired growth, and a spectrum of mild to severe cognitive, emotional, and physical problems.

fetus The human growth and developmental stage lasting from the beginning of the ninth week after conception to birth.

fiber-rich carbohydrates A group of foods containing either simple or complex carbohydrates that are rich in dietary fiber. These foods, which include most fruits, vegetables, and whole grains, are typically fresh or only moderately processed.

fiber The nondigestible carbohydrate parts of plants that form the support structures of leaves, stems, and seeds.

fluid A substance composed of molecules that move past one another freely. Fluids are characterized by their ability to conform to the shape of whatever container holds them.

fluorosis A condition marked by staining and pitting of the teeth; caused by an abnormally high intake of fluoride.

food additive A substance or mixture of substances intentionally put into food to enhance its appearance, safety, palatability, and quality.

food allergy An inflammatory reaction caused by an immune system hypersensitivity to a protein component of a food.

food desert Community in which residents lack access to affordable fresh fruits and vegetables and other healthful foods.

food diversity The variety of different species of plant crops or animal sources of food.

food equity Fair distribution of the world's food resources.

food insecurity Condition in which the individual is unable to regularly obtain enough food to provide sufficient energy and nutrients to meet physical needs.

food intolerance A cluster of GI symptoms that occurs following consumption of a particular food but is not caused by an immune system response.

foodborne illness An illness transmitted by food or water contaminated by a pathogenic microorganism, its toxic secretions, or a toxic chemical.

free radical A highly unstable atom with an unpaired electron.

frequency The number of activity sessions per week you perform.

fructose The sweetest natural sugar; a monosaccharide that occurs in fruits and vegetables. Also called *fruit sugar*.

functional fiber The nondigestible forms of carbohydrate that are extracted from plants or manufactured in the laboratory and have known health benefits.

fungi Plantlike, spore-forming organisms that can grow as either single cells or multicellular colonies.

G

galactose A monosaccharide that joins with glucose to create lactose, one of the three most common disaccharides.

gallbladder A sac like accessory organ of digestion that stores bile and secretes it into the small intestine.

gastric juice Acidic liquid secreted within the stomach that contains hydrochloric acid, pepsin, and other chemicals.

gastroesophageal reflux disease (GERD) A chronic disease in which painful episodes of gastroesophageal reflux cause heartburn or other symptoms more than twice per week.

gastrointestinal (GI) tract A long, muscular tube consisting of several organs: the mouth, esophagus, stomach, small intestine, and large intestine.

gene A segment of DNA that carries the instructions for assembling available amino acids into a unique protein.

Generally Recognized as Safe (GRAS) List established by Congress to identify substances used in foods that are generally recognized as safe based on a history of long-term use or on the consensus of qualified research experts.

genetic modification The process of changing an organism by manipulating its genetic material.

gestational diabetes In a pregnant woman, insufficient insulin production or insulin resistance that results in consistently high blood glucose levels; the condition typically resolves after birth occurs.

glucagon A hormone secreted by the alpha cells of the pancreas in response to decreased blood levels of glucose; causes breakdown of liver stores of glycogen into glucose.

gluconeogenesis The generation of glucose from the breakdown of proteins.

glucose The most abundant sugar molecule; a monosaccharide generally found in combination with other sugars. The preferred source of energy for the brain and an important source of energy for all cells.

glycemic index A value that rates the potential of a given food to raise blood glucose and insulin levels.

glycemic load The amount of carbohydrate contained in a given food, multiplied by its glycemic index value.

glycerol An alcohol composed of three carbon atoms; it is the backbone of a triglyceride molecule.

glycogen A polysaccharide stored in animals; the storage form of glucose in animals.

glycolysis The breakdown of glucose; yields two ATP molecules and two pyruvic acid molecules for each molecule of glucose.

goiter A condition marked by enlargement of the thyroid gland, which can be caused by iodine toxicity or deficiency.

grazing The practice of consistently eating small meals throughout the day; done by many athletes to meet their high-energy demands.

green revolution The tremendous increase in global productivity between 1944 and 2000 due to selective cross-breeding or hybridization to produce high-yield grains and industrial farming techniques.

H

healthful diet A diet that provides the proper combination of energy and nutrients and is adequate, moderate, balanced, and varied.

heatstroke A potentially fatal response to high temperature characterized by failure of the body's heat-regulating mechanisms commonly called *sunstroke.*

helminth A multicellular microscopic worm.

heme The iron-containing molecule found in hemoglobin.

heme iron Iron that is part of hemoglobin and myoglobin; found only in animal-based foods, such as meat, fish, and poultry.

hemoglobin The oxygen-carrying protein found in our red blood cells; almost two-thirds of all the iron in our body is found in hemoglobin.

hepatitis Inflammation of the liver; can be caused by a virus or a toxic agent, such as alcohol.

high-density lipoprotein (HDL) A small, dense lipoprotein with a very low cholesterol content and a high protein content.

high-yield varieties Semi-dwarf varieties of plants that are unlikely to fall over in wind and heavy rains and thus can carry larger amounts of seeds, greatly increasing the yield per acre.

homocysteine An amino acid that requires adequate levels of folate, vitamin B_6, and vitamin B_{12} for its metabolism. High levels of homocysteine in the blood are associated with an increased risk for cardiovascular disease.

hormones Chemical messengers secreted into the bloodstream by one of the many glands of the body.

hunger A physical sensation that prompts us to eat.

hydrogenation The process of adding hydrogen to unsaturated fatty acids, making them more saturated and therefore more solid at room temperature.

hypoglycemia A condition marked by blood glucose levels that are below normal fasting levels.

hypothalamus A brain region where sensations such as hunger and thirst are regulated.

hypothesis An educated guess as to why a phenomenon occurs.

I

impaired fasting glucose Fasting blood glucose levels that are higher than normal but not high enough to lead to a diagnosis of type 2 diabetes; also called *pre-diabetes.*

incomplete proteins Foods that do not contain all the essential amino acids in sufficient amounts to support growth and health.

insoluble fibers Fibers that do not dissolve in water.

insulin A hormone secreted by the beta cells of the pancreas in response to increased blood levels of glucose; facilitates uptake of glucose by body cells.

intensity The amount of effort expended during the activity, or how difficult the activity is to perform.

invisible fats Fats that are hidden in foods, such as those found in baked goods, regular-fat dairy products, marbling in meat, and fried foods.

ion An electrically charged particle.

iron-deficiency anemia A disorder in which the production of normal, healthy red blood cells decreases and hemoglobin levels are inadequate to fully oxygenate the body's cells and tissues.

irradiation A sterilization process in which food is exposed to gamma rays or high-energy electron beams to kill microorganisms. Irradiation does not impart any radiation to the food being treated.

irritable bowel syndrome (IBS) A bowel disorder that interferes with normal functions of the colon. IBS causes abdominal cramps, bloating, and diarrhea or constipation.

K

kwashiorkor A form of protein–energy malnutrition that is typically seen in malnourished infants and toddlers and is characterized by wasting, edema, and other signs of protein deficiency.

L

lactic acid A compound that results when pyruvic acid is metabolized.

lactose intolerance A disorder in which the body does not produce sufficient lactase enzyme and therefore cannot digest foods that contain lactose, such as cow's milk.

lactose A disaccharide consisting of one glucose molecule and one galactose molecule; also called *milk sugar.* Found in milk, including human breast milk.

large intestine Final organ of the GI tract consisting of the cecum, colon, rectum, and anal canal and in which most water is absorbed and feces are formed.

leisure-time physical activity   Any activity not related to a person's occupation; includes competitive sports, recreational activities, and planned exercise training.

life expectancy   The expected number of years remaining in one's life, typically stated from the time of birth.

life span   The highest age reached by any member of a species; currently, the human life span is 122 years.

limiting amino acid   The essential amino acid that is missing or in the smallest supply in the amino acid pool and is thus responsible for slowing or halting protein synthesis.

linoleic acid   An essential fatty acid found in vegetable and nut oils; also known as omega-6 fatty acid.

lipids   A diverse group of organic substances that are insoluble in water; lipids include triglycerides, phospholipids, and sterols.

lipoprotein   A spherical (round-shaped) compound in which fat clusters in the center and phospholipids and proteins form the outside of the sphere.

liver   The largest accessory organ of digestion and one of the most important organs of the body. Its functions include production of bile and processing of nutrient-rich blood from the small intestine.

low birth weight   A weight of less than 5.5 lb at birth.

low-density lipoprotein (LDL)   A molecule resulting when a VLDL releases its triglyceride load. Higher cholesterol and protein content makes LDLs somewhat more dense than VLDLs.

low-intensity activities   Activities that cause very mild increases in breathing, sweating, and heart rate.

M

macronutrients   Nutrients that our body needs in relatively large amounts to support normal function and health. Carbohydrates, fats, and proteins are macronutrients.

major minerals   Minerals we need to consume in amounts of at least 100 mg per day, and of which the total amount present in the body is at least 5 grams (5,000 mg).

maltose   A disaccharide consisting of two molecules of glucose. Does not generally occur independently in foods but results as a by-product of digestion. Also called *malt sugar.*

marasmus   A form of protein–energy malnutrition that results from grossly inadequate intake of energy and protein and other nutrients and is characterized by extreme tissue wasting and stunted growth and development.

maximal heart rate   The rate at which your heart beats during maximal-intensity exercise.

megadosing   Taking a dose of a nutrient that is ten or more times greater than the recommended amount.

metabolic water   The water formed as a by-product of our body's metabolic reactions.

metabolism   The chemical reactions occurring in the body in order to maintain life.

metabolism   The sum of all the chemical and physical processes by which the body breaks down and builds up molecules.

micronutrients   Nutrients needed in relatively small amounts to support normal health and body functions. Vitamins and minerals are micronutrients.

minerals   Solid, crystalline substances that do not contain carbon and are not changed by natural processes, including digestion.

moderate-intensity activities   Activities that cause noticeable increases in breathing, sweating, and heart rate.

moderation   Eating the right amounts of foods to maintain a healthy weight and to optimize our body's functioning.

monosaccharide   The simplest of carbohydrates; consists of one sugar molecule, the most common form of which is glucose.

monounsaturated fatty acid (MUFA)   A fatty acid that has two carbons in the chain bound to each other with one double bond; these types of fatty acids are generally liquid at room temperature.

morbid obesity   A condition in which a person's body weight exceeds 100% of normal, putting him or her at very high risk for serious health consequences.

morning sickness   Varying degrees of nausea and vomiting associated with pregnancy, most commonly in the first trimester.

multifactorial disease   Any disease that may be attributable to one or more of a variety of causes.

mutual supplementation   The process of combining two or more incomplete protein sources to make a complete protein.

myoglobin   An iron-containing protein similar to hemoglobin, except that it is found in muscle cells.

MyPlate   The visual representation of the USDA Food Patterns.

N

neural tube   Embryonic tissue that forms a tube, which eventually becomes the brain and spinal cord.

night blindness   A vitamin A–deficiency disorder that results in the loss of the ability to see in dim light.

night-eating syndrome   A disorder characterized by intake of more than 25% of the day's energy late at night. Individuals with this disorder also experience mood and sleep disorders.

non-heme iron   The form of iron that is not a part of hemoglobin or myoglobin; found in animal- and plant-based foods.

non-nutritive sweeteners   Manufactured sweeteners that provide little or no energy; also called *alternative sweeteners.*

nonessential amino acids   Amino acids that can be manufactured by the body in sufficient quantities and therefore do not need to be consumed regularly in our diet.

normal weight   Having an adequate but not excessive level of body fat for health.

nutrient density   The relative amount of nutrients per amount of energy (or number of Calories).

nutrients   Chemicals found in foods that are critical to human growth and function.

Nutrition Facts panel   The label on a food package that contains the nutrition information required by the FDA.

nutrition   The scientific study of food and how food nourishes the body and influences health.

nutritive sweeteners   Sweeteners, such as sucrose, fructose, honey, and brown sugar, that contribute calories (energy).

O

obesity   Having an excess of body fat that adversely affects health, resulting in a person having a weight for a given height that is substantially greater than an accepted standard.

organic   Produced without the use of synthetic fertilizers, toxic and persistent pesticides, genetic engineering, or irradiation.

osteoblasts   Cells that prompt the formation of new bone matrix by laying down the collagen-containing component of bone, which is then mineralized.

osteoclasts   Cells that break down the surface of bones by secreting enzymes and acids that dig grooves into the bone matrix.

osteomalacia   Vitamin D–deficiency disease in adults, in which bones become weak and prone to fractures.

osteoporosis A disease characterized by low bone mass and deterioration of bone tissue, leading to increased bone fragility and fracture risk.

ounce-equivalent (oz-equivalent) A term used to define a serving size that is 1 ounce, or equivalent to an ounce, for the grains section and the protein foods section of MyPlate.

overload principle The principle of placing an extra physical demand on your body to improve your fitness level.

overweight Having a moderate amount of excess body fat, resulting in a person having a weight for a given height that is greater than an accepted standard but is not considered obese.

ovulation The release of an ovum (egg) from a woman's ovary.

P

pancreas Accessory organ of digestion that secretes digestive enzymes into the small intestine via the pancreatic duct; certain pancreatic cells secrete the hormones insulin and glucagon into the bloodstream.

pancreatic amylase An enzyme secreted by the pancreas into the small intestine that digests any remaining starch into maltose.

parasite A microorganism that simultaneously derives benefit from and harms its host.

pasteurization A form of sterilization using high temperatures for short periods of time.

pellagra A disease that results from severe niacin deficiency.

pepsin An enzyme in the stomach that begins the breakdown of proteins into shorter polypeptide chains and single amino acids.

peptic ulcer An area of the GI tract that has been eroded away by the acidic gastric juice of the stomach.

peptide bonds Unique types of chemical bonds in which the amine group of one amino acid binds to the acid group of another to manufacture dipeptides and all larger peptide molecules.

percent daily values (%DV) Information on a Nutrition Facts Panel that tells you how much a serving of food contributes to your overall intake of nutrients listed on the label. The information is based on an energy intake of 2,000 Calories per day.

peristalsis Waves of squeezing and pushing contractions that move food in one direction through the length of the GI tract.

persistent organic pollutants (POPs) Chemicals released into the environment as a result of industry, agriculture, or improper waste disposal; automobile emissions also are considered POPs.

pesticides Chemicals used either in the field or in storage to decrease destruction by predators or disease.

pH Stands for "percentage of hydrogen." It is a measure of the acidity—or level of hydrogen—of any solution, including human blood.

phospholipid A type of lipid in which a fatty acid is combined with another compound that contains phosphate; unlike other lipids, phospholipids are soluble in water.

photosynthesis The process by which plants use sunlight to fuel a chemical reaction that combines carbon and water into glucose, which is then stored in their cells.

physical activity Any movement produced by muscles that increases energy expenditure; includes occupational, household, leisure-time, and transportation activities.

physical fitness The ability to carry out daily tasks with vigor and alertness, without undue fatigue, and with ample energy to enjoy leisure-time pursuits and meet unforeseen emergencies.

phytochemicals Chemicals such as pigments that are present in plants and are believed to have health-promoting effects in humans.

pica An abnormal craving to eat something not fit for food, such as clay, chalk, paint, or other nonfood substances.

placenta A pregnancy-specific organ formed from both maternal and embryonic tissues. It is responsible for oxygen, nutrient, and waste exchange between mother and fetus.

polypharmacy The concurrent use of five or more medications.

polysaccharide A complex carbohydrate consisting of long chains of glucose.

polyunsaturated fatty acids (PUFAs) Fatty acids that have more than one double bond in the chain; these types of fatty acids are generally liquid at room temperature.

prion A protein that misfolds and becomes infectious; prions are not living cellular organisms or viruses.

proof A measure of the alcohol content of a liquid. For example, 100-proof liquor is 50% alcohol by volume, whereas 80-proof liquor is 40% alcohol by volume.

proteases Enzymes that continue the breakdown of polypeptides in the small intestine.

protein–energy malnutrition A disorder caused by inadequate consumption of protein. It is characterized by severe wasting.

proteins Large, complex molecules made up of amino acids and found as essential components of all living cells.

protozoa Single-celled, mobile microorganisms.

provitamin An inactive form of a vitamin that the body can convert to an active form. An example is beta-carotene.

puberty The period of life in which secondary sexual characteristics develop and people are biologically capable of reproducing.

purging An attempt to rid the body of unwanted food by vomiting or other compensatory means, such as excessive exercise, fasting, or laxative abuse.

pyruvic acid The primary end product of glycolysis.

Q

quackery The promotion of an unproven remedy, such as a supplement or other product or service, usually by someone unlicensed and untrained.

R

recombinant bovine growth hormone (rBGH) A genetically engineered hormone injected into dairy cows to enhance their milk output.

recombinant DNA technology A type of genetic modification in which scientists combine DNA from different sources to produce a transgenic organism that expresses a desired trait.

Recommended Dietary Allowance (RDA) The average daily nutrient intake level that meets the nutrient requirements of 97% to 98% of healthy individuals in a particular life stage and gender group.

remodeling The two-step process by which bone tissue is recycled; includes the breakdown of existing bone and the formation of new bone.

residues Chemicals that remain in the foods we eat despite cleaning and processing.

resistance training Exercise in which our muscles act against resistance.

retina The delicate, light-sensitive membrane lining the inner eyeball and connected to the optic nerve. It contains retinal.

rickets A vitamin D–deficiency disease in children. Symptoms include deformities of the skeleton, such as bowed legs and knocked knees.

S

saliva A mixture of water, mucus, enzymes, and other chemicals that moistens the mouth and food, binds food particles together, and begins the digestion of carbohydrates.

salivary amylase An enzyme in saliva that breaks starch into smaller particles and eventually into the disaccharide maltose.

salivary glands A group of glands that together act as an accessory organ of digestion, releasing saliva continually as well as in response to the thought, sight, smell, or presence of food.

saturated fatty acid (SFA) A fatty acid that has no carbons joined together with a double bond; these types of fatty acids are generally solid at room temperature.

set-point theory A theory that suggests that the body raises or lowers energy expenditure in response to increased and decreased food intake and physical activity. This action maintains an individual's body weight within a narrow range.

simple carbohydrate A monosaccharide or disaccharide, such as glucose; commonly called *sugar*.

small intestine The largest portion of the GI tract, in which most digestion and absorption take place.

soluble fibers Fibers that dissolve in water.

solvent A substance that is capable of mixing with and breaking apart a variety of compounds. Water is an excellent solvent.

sphincters Tight rings of muscle separating organs of the GI tract; they open in response to nerve signals, indicating that food is ready to pass into the next section.

spina bifida An embryonic neural tube defect that occurs when the spinal vertebrae fail to completely enclose the spinal cord, allowing it to protrude.

spontaneous abortion The natural termination of a pregnancy and expulsion of the fetus and pregnancy tissues because of a genetic, developmental, or physiologic abnormality that is so severe that the pregnancy cannot be maintained; also known as *miscarriage*.

starch A polysaccharide stored in plants; the storage form of glucose in plants.

sterol A type of lipid found in foods and the body that has a ring structure; cholesterol is the most common sterol that occurs in our diet.

stomach A J-shaped organ in which food is partially digested, churned, and stored until released into the small intestine.

stretching Exercise in which muscles are gently lengthened using slow, controlled movements.

sucrose A disaccharide composed of one glucose molecule and one fructose molecule. It is sweeter than lactose or maltose.

sudden infant death syndrome (SIDS) A condition marked by the sudden death of a previously healthy infant; the most common cause of death in infants more than 1 month of age.

sustainability The ability to meet or satisfy basic economic, social, and security needs now and in the future without undermining the natural resource base and environmental quality on which life depends.

sustainable agriculture Term referring to techniques of food production that preserve the environment indefinitely.

T

teratogen Any substance that can cause a birth defect.

theory A conclusion, or scientific consensus, drawn from repeated experiments.

thermic effect of food The energy expended as a result of processing food consumed.

thirst mechanism A cluster of nerve cells in the hypothalamus that stimulate our conscious desire to drink fluids in response to an increase in the concentration of salt in our blood or a decrease in blood pressure and volume.

thrifty gene theory A theory that suggests that some people possess a gene (or genes) that causes them to be energetically thrifty, resulting in their expending less energy at rest and during physical activity.

time of activity The amount of time that a given exercise session lasts, not including warm-up and cool-down periods.

Tolerable Upper Intake Level (UL) The highest average daily nutrient intake level likely to pose no risk of adverse health effects to almost all individuals in a particular life stage and gender group.

total fiber The sum of dietary fiber and functional fiber.

toxin Any harmful substance; in microbiology, a chemical produced by a microorganism that harms tissues or causes harmful immune responses.

trabecular bone A porous bone tissue found within the ends of the long bones, as well as inside the spinal vertebrae, flat bones (breastbone, ribs, and most bones of the skull), and bones of the pelvis; also called spongy bone.

trace minerals Minerals we need to consume in amounts less than 100 mg per day, and of which the total amount present in the body is less than 5 grams (5,000 mg).

transport proteins Protein molecules that help transport substances throughout the body and across cell membranes.

triglyceride A molecule consisting of three fatty acids attached to a three-carbon glycerol backbone.

trimester Any one of three stages of pregnancy, each lasting 13 to 14 weeks.

tumor Any newly formed mass of undifferentiated cells.

type 1 diabetes The form of diabetes in which the pancreas produces little or no insulin.

type 2 diabetes The form of diabetes in which body cells progressively become less responsive to insulin, or the pancreas does not produce enough insulin.

type of activity The range of physical activities a person can engage in to promote health and physical fitness.

U

umbilical cord The cord containing arteries and veins that connects the baby (from the navel) to the mother via the placenta.

underweight Having too little body fat to maintain health, causing a person to have a weight for a given height that is below an acceptably defined standard.

V

variety Eating different foods each day.

vegetarianism The practice of restricting the diet to food substances of plant origin, including vegetables, fruits, grains, and nuts.

very-low-density lipoprotein (VLDL) A large lipoprotein made up mostly of triglyceride. Functions primarily to transport triglycerides from their source to the body's cells, including to adipose tissues for storage.

vigorous-intensity activities Activities that produce significant increases in breathing, sweating, and heart rate; talking is difficult when exercising at a vigorous intensity.

viruses A group of noncellular infectious agents that are usually smaller than bacteria, lack independent metabolism, and are incapable of growth or reproduction outside living cells.

visible fats Fats that we can see in our foods or see added to foods, such as butter, margarine, cream, shortening, salad dressings, chicken skin, and untrimmed fat on meat.

vitamins Micronutrients that contain carbon and assist us in regulating our body's processes. They are classified as water soluble or fat soluble.

W

warm-up Activities that prepare you for an exercise session, including stretching, calisthenics, and movements specific to the exercise you are about to engage in; also called preliminary exercise.

water intoxication Dilution of body fluid that results when water intake or retention is excessive; it can lead to hyponatremia; also called *overhydration*.

water-soluble vitamins Vitamins that are soluble in water. These include vitamin C and the B-vitamins.

wellness A multidimensional, lifelong process that includes physical, emotional, and spiritual health.

index

credits

Photo Credits

Chapter 1

p. 1: Exactostock/Exactostock; **p. 2:** peangdao/Fotolia; **fig. 1.1:** Yeko Photo Studio/Shutterstock; **p. 7:** Lidante/Shutterstock; **p. 8:** matin/Shutterstock; **p. 10 L:** Photosani/Shutterstock; **p. 10 R:** Forest Badger/Shutterstock; **fig. 1.6:** Samuel Borges Photography/Shutterstock; **fig. 1.7:** Creative Digital Visions; **p. 14:** Alexander Walter/Getty Images; **p. 15:** Andrew Whittuck/Dorling Kindersley Images; **p. 16 T:** Mark Follon/Adams Picture Library t/a apl/lamy; **p. 16 B:** Steve Terrill/Terra/Corbis; **fig. 1-10:** ALEAIMAGE/E+/Getty Images, Kelly Cline/Getty Images, Abbielimages/iStock/Getty Images, Hurst Photo/Shutterstock, Natalia Mylova/Fotolia; **fig. 1.11 a-e:** Pearson Learning Photo Studio; **fig. 1.11 f:** Pearson; **fig. 1.11 g-p:** Pearson Learning Photo Studio; **fig 1.11 q:** Pearson; **fig. 1.11 r-t:** Pearson Learning Photo Studio; **fig. 1.12:** Pearson Education/Pearson Science; **fig. 1.13:** Image Source/Alamy, fotogal/Fotolia, Photodisc/Getty Images, Ragnar Schmuck/Getty Images; **p. 27:** Radius Images/Alamy; **p. 31:** Sandra Baker/Alamy; **p. 32:** Miriam Doerr/Shutterstock

Chapter 2

p. 38: Peathegee Inc/Getty Images; **p. 40:** Howard Kingsnorth/The Image Bank/Getty Images; **p. 41:** Jean Luc Morales/The Image Bank/Getty Images; **fig. 2.2:** Jon Riley/The Image Bank/Getty Images; **p. 42:** Brand X Pictures/Photodisc/Getty Images; **p. 45:** Randy L. Jirtle; **p. 52:** shippee/Shutterstock; **fig. 2.11:** Maridav/Shutterstock, David Musher/Science Source, Steve G. Schmeissner/Science Source, Don W. Fawcett/Science Source; **p. 55:** SPL/Science Source; **p. 56:** Pearson Learning Photo Studio; **fig. 2.15:** MedicalRF.com/Alamy, Dr. E. Walker/Science Photo Library/Photo Researchers, Inc.; **p. 60:** David Murray and Jules Selmes/Dorling Kindersley Images; **p. 62 T:** Cordelia Molloy/Photo Researchers, Inc.; **p. 62 B:** zcw/Shutterstock; **p. 63:** nadi555/Shutterstock; **p. 64:** Susan Van Etten/PhotoEdit

Chapter 3

p. 69: Monkey Business/Fotolia; **p. 73 TL:** Foodcollection/Getty Images; **p. 73 TR:** Danny Smythe/Shutterstock; **p. 73 B:** Monkey Business Images/Shutterstock;

p. 74: Pearson Education/Pearson Science; **fig. 3.6:** Bernd Leitner/Fotolia, Doug Menuez/Photodisc/Getty Images, technotr/Getty Images; **p. 80:** Clive Streeter/Dorling Kindersley Images; **fig. 3.10:** Yuri Arcurs/Shutterstock, Flashon Studio/Shutterstock; **p. 84:** Lawton/SoFood/Corbis; **p. 85:** Ian O'Leary/Dorling Kindersley Images; **p. 87:** Susanna Price/Dorling Kindersley Images; **fig. 3.13:** Alex459/Shutterstock; **p. 89:** Dorling Kindersley Images; **fig. 3.14:** Pearson Education/Pearson Science; **p. 91:** Shoot/AGE Fotostock; **fig. 3.15:** bikeriderlondon/Shutterstock; **p. 96:** sandy young/Alamy

Chapter 4

p. 100: MachineHeadz/Getty Images; **p. 104 T:** Mates/Fotolia; **p. 104 B:** Nikolych/Fotolia; **p. 105:** HLPhoto/Shutterstock; **fig. 4.5:** Myrleen Pearson/PhotoEdit; **p. 107:** Comstock/Thinkstock; **p. 108:** ODD ANDERSEN/AFP/Getty Images; **p. 109:** Kip Peticolas/Fundamental Photographs; **p. 111:** Alex Potemkin/Krakozawr/iStockphoto; **p. 112:** Jeff Greenberg/AGE Fotostock; **p. 113:** James Leynse/Corbis News/Corbis, Pearson Education/Pearson Science, Pearson Education; **fig. 4.8:** Kristin Piljay/Wanderlust Photos/Pearson Education; **p. 115:** Richard Megna/Fundamental Photographs; **p. 118:** Elena Elisseeva/Shutterstock; **p. 120:** Rich Kareckas/AP Images; **fig. 4.11:** Science Photo Library/Science Source, Biophoto Associates/Science Source; **p. 125:** Â© altafulla/Shutterstock.com

Chapter 5

p. 129: ArenaCreative/Fotolia; **p. 132:** Â© Andresr/Shutterstock.com; **fig. 5.3:** Andrew Syred/Science Source; **p. 133:** AlenaKogotkova/Shutterstock; **fig. 5.4:** Pearson Education/Pearson Science; **fig. 5.5:** Mediscan/Medical-on-Line/Alamy; **p. 138:** Ian O'Leary/Dorling Kindersley Images; **p. 139:** Lionel Cironneau/AP Images; **fig. 5.7 (a):** Lucy Deng/FlickrVision/Getty Images; **fig. 5.7 (b):** Christine Osborne Pictures/Alamy; **p. 142:** Ryan McVay/Photodisc/Getty Images; **p. 143:** Ranald MacKechnie/Dorling Kindersley Images; **fig. 5.8:** Kristin Piljay/Wanderlust Photos/Pearson Education; **p. 146:** Pearson Education/Pearson Science; **p. 148:** Rohit Seth/Shutterstock; **fig. 5.9 (a):** Glowimages/Getty Images; **fig. 5.9 (b):** Kevin Schafer/DanitaDelimont; **p. 151:** Ekaterina Nikitina/Shutterstock

Chapter 6

p. 155: Fuse/Getty Images; **fig. 6.1 TL:** pixelman/Shutterstock, J.T. Lewis/Shutterstock; **fig. 6.1 TR:** Jacek Chabraszewski/Shutterstock, Lepas/Shutterstock; **fig. 6.1 BL:** Nikola Bilic/Shutterstock, matka_Wariatka/Shutterstock; **fig. 6.1 BR:** Milos Luzanin/Shutterstock, GoodMood Photo/Shutterstock; **p. 157:** JLP/Sylvia Torres/Flirt/Corbis; **p. 161:** Ian O'Leary/Dorling Kindersley Images; **fig. 6.3:** iStockphoto/Thinkstock; **p. 162:** Susanna Price/Dorling Kindersley Images; **p. 163:** Peter Turnley/Corbis; **fig. 6.4:** Jiri Hera/Shutterstock; **fig. 6.5:** Biophoto Associates/Photo Researchers, Inc.; **fig. 6.8:** Chris Stein/Getty Images; **p. 167:** Philip Dowell/Dorling Kindersley Images; **fig. 6.10:** iStockphoto/Thinkstock; **p. 168:** Valentyn Volkov/Shutterstock; **p. 169:** Pia Tryde/Dorling Kindersley Images; **fig. 6.11:** Mediscan/Alamy; **fig. 6.12:** bluestocking/iStockphoto; **p. 170:** Walter Bibikow/Jon Arnold Images Ltd/Alamy; **p. 171:** David Murray/Dorling Kindersley Images; **fig. 6.13:** Fuat Kose/Getty Images; **fig. 6.14:** Burwell and Burwell Photography/Thinkstock; **fig. 6.15:** Alex Staroseltsev/Shutterstock; **fig. 6.16:** Lester V. Bergman/Encyclopedia/Corbis; **fig. 6.17:** Alasdair Thomson/Getty Images; **p. 174:** Olga Nayashkova/Shutterstock; **fig. 6.18:** istockphoto/Thinkstock; **p. 175:** Steve Moss/Food Features/Alamy; **fig. 6.19:** istockphoto/Thinkstock; **p. 176:** David Murray/Dorling Kindersley Images; **p. 177:** Duncan Smith/Corbis Yellow/Corbis; **fig. 6.21:** Kristin Piljay/Wanderlust Photos/Pearson Education; **p. 180:** Kanusommer/Shutterstock; **p. 183 T:** Quayside/Shutterstock; **p. 183 B:** Courtesy of the USDA; **fig. 6.23:** Southern Illinois University/Science Source, Lew Robertson/Photolibrary/Getty Images, Image Source/Getty Images, Pixtal/AGE Fotostock, Joy Brown /Shutterstock

Chapter 7

p. 192: Mint Images—Tim Robbins/Getty Images; **p. 193:** ZUMA Press, Inc./Alamy; **fig. 7.1 TL:** Eric Gevaert/Shutterstock, Africa Studio/Shutterstock; **fig. 7.1 TR:** Agita Leimane/Shutterstock, amnachphoto/Fotolia; **fig. 7.1 BL:** Lloid/Shutterstock, Jaroslaw Grudzinski/Shutterstock; **fig. 7.1 BR:** Aleksander Skakun/Shutterstock, Loskutnikov/Shutterstock; **p. 194:** Paul prescott/Shutterstock; **p. 197:** Andrea Skjold/Shutterstock;

Text Credits

Chapter 5

p. 146: Source: American Cancer Society. 2013. Soybean. http://www.cancer.org/ treatment/treatmentsandsideeffects/ complementaryandalternativemedicine/ dietandnutrition/soybean; **p. 150:** Source: American Dietetic Association. 2009. Position of the American Dietetic Association: Vegetarian Diet. J. Am. Diet. Assoc. 109:1266–1282.; Albert, C. M., J. M. Gaziano, W. C. Willett, J. E. Mason, and C. H. Hennekens. 2002. Nut consumption and decreased risk of sudden cardiac death in the Physicians' Health Study. Arch. Intern. Med. 162:1382–1387.

Chapter 6

p. 169: Source: National Institute of Allergy and Infectious Diseases. April 13, 2011.

Common Cold. http://www.niaid.nih.gov/ topics/commonCold/Pages/prevention.aspx; **p. 178:** Source: The United States Pharmacopeial Convention. Used with permission.

Chapter 9

p. 267: Source: DONATELLE, REBECCA J., HEALTH: THE BASICS, 11th Ed., ©2015. Reprinted and Electronically reproduced by permission of Pearson Education, Inc., Upper Saddle River, New Jersey.

Chapter 10

p. 294: Source: Based on Heyward, V. and A. Gibson 2014. Advanced Fitness Assessment and Exercise Prescription, 7th edn. Champaign, IL: Human Kinetics.

Chapter 11

p. 330: Source: Data from Rasmussen, K. M., and A. L. Yaktine, eds., Committee to

Reexamine IOM Pregnancy Weight Guidelines; Institute of Medicine; National Research Council. 2009. Weight Gain During Pregnancy: Reexamining the Guidelines. Washington, DC: National Academies Press.

Chapter 12

p. 378: Source: The U.S. Department of Health and Human Services. http:// foodsafety.gov/; **p. 381:** Source: Data from U.S. Food and Drug Administration, Center for Food Safety and Applied Nutrition, 2007. Food Facts. Eating Outdoors. Handling Food Safety; **p. 383:** Source: U.S. Food and Drug Administration; **p. 385:** Source: The Delaney Clause, 1958.